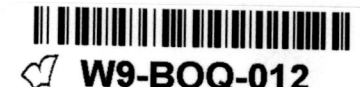

REEDER AND FELSON'S
GAMUTS IN RADIOLOGY

Fourth Edition

Springer
New York
Berlin
Heidelberg
Hong Kong
London
Milan
Paris
Tokyo

Reeder and Felson's

Gamuts in Radiology

Comprehensive Lists of Roentgen Differential Diagnosis

Fourth Edition

MAURICE M. REEDER, MD, FACR

with MRI Gamuts by William G. Bradley, jr., MD, PhD, FACR

and Ultrasound Gamuts by Christopher R. Merritt, MD, FACR

and input from a distinguished 20-member subspecialty

Editorial Board

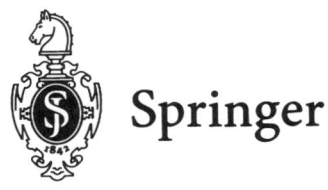 Springer

Maurice M. Reeder, MD, FACR
Adjunct Professor of Radiology
   Uniformed Services University of the Health Sciences
   Bethesda, Maryland
Emeritus Professor and Former Chairman, Section of Radiology
   John A. Burns School of Medicine
   University of Hawaii at Manoa, Honolulu, Hawaii
Colonel, Medical Corps, United States Army, Retired
Formerly Chief, Department of Radiology
   Walter Reed Army Medical Center
Formerly, Radiology Consultant to the Army Surgeon General
Formerly Associate Radiologist
   Registry of Radiologic Pathology
   Armed Forces Institute of Pathology
   Washington, DC

MRI gamuts contributed by:
William G. Bradley, Jr., MD, PhD, FACR
Chairman, Department of Radiology
   University of California, San Diego
   Medical Center
   San Diego, California

Ultrasound gamuts contributed by:
Christopher R. Merritt, MD, FACR
Professor, Department of Radiology
   Division of Ultrasound
   Thomas Jefferson University Hospital
   Philadelphia, Pennsylvania

With 8 illustrations.

Library of Congress Cataloging-in-Publication Data
Reeder, Maurice M. (Maurice Merrick), 1933–
   Reeder and Felson's gamuts in radiology : comprehensive lists of roentgen differential
diagnosis / Maurice M. Reeder.—4th ed.
     p. ; cm.
   Includes bibliographical references and index.
   ISBN 0-387-95588-7 (alk. paper)
   1. Diagnosis, Radioscopic—Outlines, syllabi, etc.   2. Diagnosis, Differential—Outlines,
syllabi, etc.   I. Title: Gamuts in radiology.   II. Felson, Benjamin.   III. Title.
   [DNLM: 1. Radiography—Handbooks.   2. Diagnosis, Differential—Handbooks. WN 39
R325r 2003]
   RC78.17 .R445   2003
   616.07′572—dc21   2002030551

ISBN 0-387-95588-7 Printed on acid-free paper.

Printed in the United States of America.

9 8 7 6 5 4 3 2 1   SPIN 10893188

www.springer-ny.com

Springer-Verlag   New York Berlin Heidelberg
A member of BertelsmannSpringer Science+Business Media GmbH

Editorial Board Members

Section Editors:

Section A: Skull and Brain
Maurice M. Reeder, MD
John B. Campbell, MD

Kelly Koeller, MD, Capt, MC, USN
Chief, Department of Radiologic Pathology
Armed Forces Institute of Pathology
Washington, DC

Christopher Lisanti, MD
Chief, Section of MRI and Brain and Body Imaging
Department of Radiology
Wilford Hall, US Air Force Medical Center
San Antonio, Texas

Section B: Head and Neck
Anton N. Hasso, MD
Professor and Chairman
Department of Radiological Sciences
University of California Irvine Medical Center
Orange, California

Robert Lufkin, MD
Professor, Department of Radiological Sciences
UCLA School of Medicine
Los Angeles, California

Section C: Spine and Its Contents
Mark D. Murphey, MD

Section D: Bone, Joints, and Soft Tissues
Mark D. Murphey, MD

Clyde A. Helms, MD
Professor of Radiology
Duke University Medical Center
Durham, North Carolina

Section E: Cardiovascular
Larry P. Elliott, MD
Clinical Professor of Radiology
University of South Carolina at Charleston Medical
    Center
Formerly, Chairman, Department of Radiology
Georgetown University Medical Center
Washington, DC

Section F: Chest
Nestor L. Müller, MD, PhD

Melissa L. Rosado de Christenson, MD
Professor of Radiology
Ohio State University Medical Center
Columbus, Ohio
Formerly, Chief, Department of Radiologic Pathology
Armed Forces Institute of Pathology
Washington, DC

James C. Reed, MD
Chairman, Department of Diagnostic Radiology
University of Kentucky Medical Center
Lexington, Kentucky

Section G: Gastrointestinal Tract and Abdomen
Ronald L. Eisenberg, MD
Richard M. Gore, MD

Pablo R. Ros, MD
Professor of Radiology and Vice Chairman
Department of Radiology
Harvard University School of Medicine
Brigham & Women's Hospital
Boston, Massachusetts

**Section H: Genitourinary Tract, Retroperitoneum,
    and GYN Ultrasound**
Jeffrey H. Newhouse, MD
Professor of Radiology
Columbia-Presbyterian Medical Center
New York, New York

Christopher R. Merritt, MD

Section I: Mammography: Diseases of the Breast
Ralph L. Smathers, MD
Mammography Specialists, Inc.
Los Gatos, California

Robert McLelland, MD
Clinical Professor of Radiology
University of North Carolina
Chapel Hill, North Carolina
Chairman, American College of Radiology Committee
 on Breast Imaging

Section J: Tropical Medicine and Miscellaneous
Maurice M. Reeder, MD
Adjunct Professor of Radiology and Registrar
International Registry of Tropical Imaging
Uniformed Services University of the Health Sciences
Bethesda, Maryland
Emeritus Professor and Former Chairman of Radiology
University of Hawaii School of Medicine

Section M: MRI of CNS and Body
William G. Bradley, Jr, MD, PhD
Christopher Lisanti, MD

Section O: Obstetrical Ultrasound
Christopher R. Merritt, MD

Consultant for Pediatric Radiology
John B. Campbell, MD

**Consultant for Congenital Syndromes
 and Bone Dysplasias**
Ralph S. Lachman, MD
Professor of Radiology and Pediatrics
UCLA Medical Center
Co-Director, International Skeletal Dysplasia Registry
Los Angeles, California

Consultant for Ultrasound
Christopher R. Merritt, MD

Dedication

This book is dedicated to Colonel William LeRoy Thompson, Medical Corps, U.S. Army (1891-1975)

Colonel Thompson, legendary teacher of morphology in radiology and originator of the Gamut concept, received his M.D. degree from the University of Pennsylvania in 1917, and began his long and illustrious career in the U.S. Army Medical Corps that same year. He had various assignments in general medicine and administration and later became one of the early Army radiologists.

However, it was during his last year before retirement from the Army (1951) that he began his most important work, his major contribution to medicine: the organization of the Registry of Radiologic Pathology at the Armed Forces Institute of Pathology. After retirement, he offered his services, without remuneration, to continue as full-time Registrar and Chief of Radiologic Pathology.

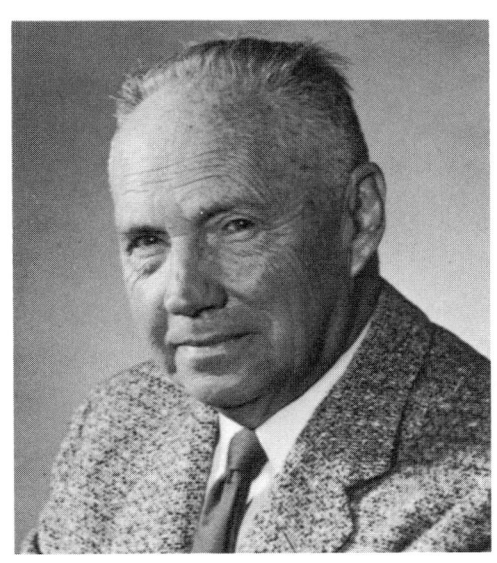

In the ensuing 16 years, Colonel Thompson worked laboriously in accessioning new material and collating the material already in the files of the Institute. He was sustained in this labor by hours of daily contact with his "students." It was here, in seminars at the viewbox, that Colonel Thompson drew upon a lifetime of accumulated knowledge and experience to educate residents, fellows, and practicing physicians from all over the world who came to study under his guidance. In this role, Colonel Thompson was the catalyst, igniting in his students a love of learning and an understanding of the vital role that pathology plays in the discipline of radiology. He was primarily a morphologist, and accepted as such by his colleagues and peers at the AFIP.

Colonel Thompson's down-to-earth nature, his éclat in interpersonal relationships, his obvious deep regard for his students as well as medicine, and his abundant and abiding warmth as a human being made him truly beloved by all who came to know him.

A Tribute to Ben Felson

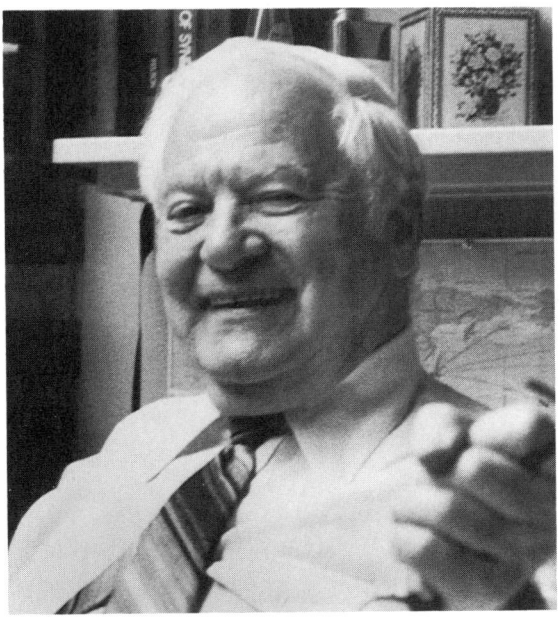

He was certainly the greatest radiologist of his time, and perhaps of all time. He was one of the great men of this century. He was also my very close and dear friend and colleague. He was like a second father to me and his loss to me is monumental, as is his loss to all whose lives he touched in such a profound and positive manner. He lived the fullest life of anyone I ever knew. He was the quintessential student and teacher, the consummate traveler, and the most compassionate, loving, and lovable human most of us have ever known.

He was that rare combination of Will Rogers and William Osler, and wherever he went, from Cincinnati to Colombia to China, he made a lasting impact and lifelong friends. More than anyone else, he enhanced the reputation and knowledge of the fledgling specialty of Radiology through his inquisitiveness and his gift for communication with both the written and spoken word. He nurtured the careers of countless students, residents, and doctors around the world. He will live forever in the hearts and minds of all who knew and loved him.

Godspeed Ben, and continue to smile down on us from above as you did so often during your all-too-brief stay with us on earth.

Maurice M. Reeder, MD

Foreword to the Third Edition

By the late Elias G. Theros, MD

I. Meschan Distinguished Professor of Radiology
Wake Forest University Medical Center
Winston-Salem, North Carolina, USA

Amongst the present generation of radiologists, beguiled by the glamour and excitement of the new high tech imaging and interventional modalities, too few have developed a strong sense of differential diagnosis based on radiologic pattern recognition and its correlation with clinical and laboratory findings. There is no question about the incredible contribution by the new modalities to our diagnostic armamentarium, but, in the evolution of modern-day radiologic practice, the cognitive element has been neglected and our abilities as diagnosticians have suffered.

The advent of this third edition of *Reeder and Felson's Gamuts in Radiology* is timely and welcome. As always, use of the gamut lists will help evoke differential thinking, and this has been enhanced by the addition of more than 250 new gamuts as well as by the updating of more than three-fourths of the existing gamuts. Interestingly, about 130 of the new gamuts are MRI Gamuts developed by Dr. William Bradley, whose enormous experience in clinical MRI has prepared him to think differentially about look-alike patterns and/or locations of lesions displayed by this modality. This is an important step forward in the use of this remarkable new diagnostic tool. It is our fervent hope that some of our very experienced colleagues in CT scanning, sonography, and PET scanning will also organize their findings in terms of gamuts and thus pass their experience to others who can thereby sharpen their diagnostic skills for the benefit of their patients.

Drs. Reeder and Felson, in preparing these gamuts, have made a major contribution to diagnosis in radiology. This they were able to do because of the depth of their own experience and their powers of observation. Those of us who have worked closely with them know that they are radiologists of consummate skills, both in the teaching and practice settings. They are master teachers to whom we all owe much. It is radiology's great fortune that Dr. Reeder has persisted, after Dr. Felson's untimely death, in laboring long hours in gamuts researching and updating. He is providing his professional colleagues with an ever improving powerful diagnostic tool. We are all in his debt.

Table of Contents

A

B

C

D

E

F

G

H

I

J

M

O

Preface to the Fourth Edition

The word *gamut* is defined as the whole range of anything. As used in this book, it indicates a complete list of causes of a particular roentgen finding or pattern.

Most radiologists use the "Gamut approach" without calling it that. You see an epiphyseal lesion of bone and immediately search your memory bank for causes. You recall perhaps six causes, then eliminate two because of rarity or incompatible roentgen pattern. Then with the clinical information at your elbow in the form of an x-ray requisition or a clinician, you weed out two more that don't fit the clinical setting, leaving you with perhaps one or two likely diagnoses.

This process is the basis of the triangulation approach to radiologic diagnosis espoused by the originator of the gamut concept, Colonel William LeRoy Thompson. He taught that roentgen diagnosis begins with accurately interpreting all the nuances and data inherent in the radiograph, then using that information to derive a particular pattern. The second side of the triangle involves reference to a well constructed list of differential diagnoses, which includes not only the common causes, responsible for over 80 percent of the entities, but also the uncommon causes, which are frequently overlooked. The triangle is then completed by reference to the pertinent clinical and laboratory data, age, sex, and other important information concerning the patient.

The purpose of this book is to provide you with complete and accurate lists of differential diagnoses. It is an unobtrusive consultant, quickly available whenever you interpret films or prepare a presentation. In each patient,

the possibilities can be narrowed down to those that fit the roentgen signs and the clinical and laboratory findings. Of course, all the pertinent data on the film must be analyzed to find the appropriate roentgen sign or pattern. Study well—to identify a pattern incorrectly will land you in the wrong gamut, which could lead to an improper diagnosis.

The publication of the fourth edition of *Gamuts in Radiology,* the second prepared without the direct input of

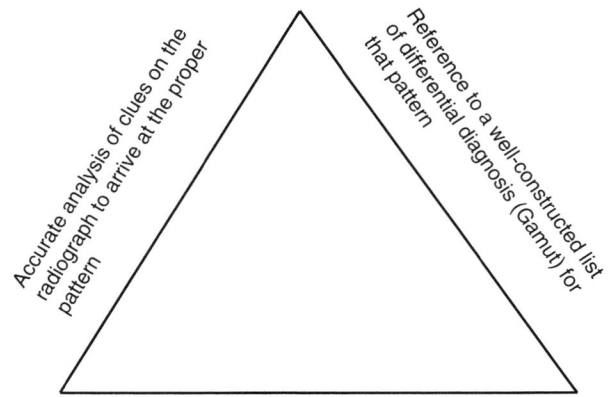

The Triangulation Approach to Radiographic Diagnosis

Accurate analysis of clues on the radiograph to arrive at the proper pattern

Reference to a well-constructed list of differential diagnosis (Gamut) for that pattern

Correlation of radiographic findings and Gamut with patients' clinical and lab findings to arrive at the most likely diagnosis

my widely loved and esteemed colleague, the late Ben Felson, marks many important changes in the book. Most conspicuously, we have added gamuts for over 250 additional patterns, especially in the areas of Ultrasound, Magnetic Resonance Body Imaging, and Head and Neck Imaging, and have updated more than 80 percent of the previously existing gamuts. The end result is a text with approximately 33 percent new material from the third edition, which in turn doubled the information available in the first two editions. Indeed, scarcely a single gamut remains unchanged from the first edition, while the book has tripled in size, reflecting the dramatic advances that have occurred in Radiology over the past three decades, especially in the areas of Ultrasound, CT, and MRI. The three prior editions of the book found wide acceptance—over 50 thousand copies are in circulation throughout North America and Europe, with tens of thousands more present in China, Japan, and most other countries of the world in at least three different languages. However, the information and data banks previously available have been greatly expanded by virtue of this publication.

While the individual gamuts are extensively referenced up to the year 2002, you will note that the majority of current references refer to textbooks rather than journal articles. This is because today's general and subspecialty textbooks are much more likely to refer to the multiple causes for a given pattern than are individual articles, which usually relate to specific entities or procedures. Furthermore, exhaustive lists of references would increase the book's size enormously and undermine its primary goal, which is to provide a quick, efficient reference.

Since the publication of this book's first edition in 1975, it has been flattering to see many of our individual gamuts reproduced in a variety of publications. Many excellent texts have been published that emphasize the gamut or differential diagnosis approach. However, some other authors have in our view lessened the value of the gamuts by culling from our original lists several common causes for a particular pattern and adding a few lines of description (available in most radiology texts) under the guise of providing a brief resume for residents studying for national Board examinations. There are several major disadvantages to this watered-down approach. First, the most common causes for a given pattern should be al-ready known to radiology residents preparing to sit for a Board examination, or else their training program should be suspect. Second, many residents and practitioners who use these abbreviated lists are deprived of the true worth of gamuts, which is to provide a comprehensive listing of the multiple causes, both common and uncommon, for a particular pattern, especially when confronted with difficult or problem cases. The point is to jog your memory to recall all the various possibilities when analyzing an imaging study at the viewbox or monitor. A resident who wants to memorize a few common causes of a particular pattern (for the purpose of passing an examination) need only consult the COMMON heading of the appropriate gamut. Otherwise, this book makes available, in an instant, virtually all possible diagnoses for any given finding.

Dr. Felson and I were always the first to admit that the amount of information and knowledge required to analyze with unerring accuracy and completeness all of the patterns that can present to the radiologist is beyond the comprehension of any two (or perhaps 20) individuals. Nevertheless, our combined experience of over 85 years' practice in major medical centers in the United States, as well as numerous visiting professorships throughout virtually the entire world, gave us sufficient perspective to at least attempt such a prodigious endeavor. Along the way we were greatly aided by our close association with such outstanding radiologists as Colonel William LeRoy Thompson, Elias (Lee) Theros, Harold Jacobson, Richard Marshak, Jerome Wiot, Philip Palmer, and others who broadened our horizons and added invaluable insights in their own specialty areas.

And to each of our 20 Section Editors and Consultants, who have contributed their wisdom and experience in verifying the correctness of the existing gamuts and adding new disease entities to most of them, I extend my profound thanks for a job well done. Along the way they have added several hundred new gamuts to the text. I selected each Section Editor and Consultant because of his or her preeminence in his or her subspecialty area, and they did not disappoint. A personal by-product of their involvement for the first time in the Gamuts projects has been their finding that there were fortunately only a handful of inaccuracies in the original 1500 gamuts compiled by Dr.

Felson and myself, which provides the gratifying bonus of an expert peer review of our prior editions.

Continuing in that collaborative tradition, I am enormously pleased that our Associate Editor, Dr. William Bradley, Jr., has once again lent his incomparable experience in MRI and neuroradiology to the fourth edition of the book. Although there are many experts in MRI today, I can think of no individual better qualified to develop accurate lists of differential diagnosis for the many patterns that have evolved in this exciting and burgeoning modality than Bill Bradley, who has been an innovator and pioneer in the field since its inception. Similarly, I am grateful that Dr. Christopher Merritt has called on his extensive experience in Ultrasound to greatly expand the Sonography gamuts found throughout the various body sections and to create a new Obstetrical Ultrasound section. My longtime friend and former Army Radiology colleague, Dr. Jack Campbell, has provided an enormous contribution by reviewing and updating the hundreds of pediatric and congenital gamuts scattered throughout the various sections of the text.

My first mentor in radiology, the legendary (though not well publicized) Colonel Thompson, is well remembered by his former students and disciples for his insistence on the triangulation approach to radiographic interpretation, a rigorous analytic approach that emphasizes careful study of the film and clinical reasoning. In today's clinical setting, where the proliferation of new technologies is colliding with ever increasing pressures to contain costs and optimize the use of diagnostic tests (as Dr. Theros so eloquently stated in his previous foreword), it is more important than ever that young radiologists learn and apply these principles, which are summarized in these remarks by the Colonel:

The radiograph is to the radiologist what the gross specimen is to the pathologist. It is a window on the disease, monitoring the many changes occurring within the patient during the course of an illness.

The clues to the pattern (and often the diagnosis itself) are almost always on the film if you are observant enough to pay attention to all the data inherent in the radiograph.

Remember that the radiograph is only one-tenth of a second in the history of a disease process. You must always think back to what the findings looked like a day or a week or a year ago (preferably with the help of old films if available, but using intuition or deductive reasoning in their absence) and what the findings are likely to be tomorrow or next week.

A good radiologist must be a good anatomist and morphologist and have a clear understanding of the correlation between what is seen on the radiograph and the underlying gross and microscopic pathology.

Finally, I would like to add a few of my own thoughts that I have passed on to residents over the years:

The radiograph is only one piece of the diagnostic puzzle. It must be evaluated in light of what you know about this patient. The radiologist cannot function as an isolated island unto him- or herself. He or she needs a knowledge of differential diagnosis together with clinical information and interaction with the patient's physician to arrive at the proper solution.

The radiograph is like a single page in a mystery novel. To find out "whodunit" you usually need more detailed information than is available in a single glance or a single moment in time.

Remember that what comes out of the automatic processor so often is not a diagnosis but rather a diagnostic challenge, a pattern for which there may be four or forty possible causes. It is up to us, as the physician's consultant, to interpret this pattern correctly using the triangulation approach.

The ideal radiologist should combine exceptional visual acuity with the intuitiveness of a good detective and the knowledge of odds or probabilities of a smart card player. It is these qualities and attention to detail that set him or her apart from other physicians who "look at" films.

And perhaps the most important advice to young residents: "Work hard and play hard. Enjoy your work and your free time. Life is short."

Indeed, as I sit surrounded by dozens of books and journals spread out over my desk and tables, with my lovely wife, Barbara, and my loyal and lovable West Highland terriers "Kea" and "Pua" nearby, the work is hard but interesting and life is indeed good here in the rolling Potomac countryside outside our nation's capital. Only one thing is missing—my dear friend Ben at my side with his wisdom and counsel and endless tales of the history of radiology and, above all, his great good humor.

Maurice M. Reeder, MD

Acknowledgments

In creating a project of this magnitude, the author inevitably borrows freely from many sources. Specific citations follow most gamuts and a list of more general references appears. For those instances where debts are not acknowledged, the user should understand that lost notes and jaded memories, not ingratitude, are to blame.

The following outstanding radiologists made valuable additions to many of the gamuts found in this and previous editions of the Gamuts book: Drs. Francis A. Burgener, George B. Greenfield, Kenneth R. Kattan, Herbert E. Parks, Andrew K. Poznanski, Leonard E. Swischuk, Hooshang Taybi, and the late John P. Dorst, Harold G. Jacobson, and Elias G. Theros. We are also grateful for the help provided in reviewing specific areas of the text by Dr. Robert McLelland for his review of the Mammography Section I and addition of numerous current references, and by Dr. Hoon Ji for his assistance to Dr. Pablo Ros with the Liver, Spleen, and Pancreas portion of Gastrointestinal Section G.

The production and distribution of this fourth edition of the Gamut book has been greatly aided by Mr. Rob Albano, Ms. Terry Kornak, and others on the Editorial and Production staffs of Springer-Verlag New York, who kept the project on track through its various deadlines to ensure the timely production of a highly refined end product. I am also very grateful to Dr. David Lamel and Mr. Peter Vasilev of Medical Interactive who have used their combined 50 years of experience in producing computerized teaching aids for Radiology and Medicine to aid in the development of a remarkably versatile and user-friendly CD-ROM based on this edition of the Gamuts book, but offering many additional features not possible with the text alone. Finally, my wife, Barbara, and youngest son, Robby, have been towers of strength and support as they guided me through the many landmines of computer quirks and frustrations as I have struggled this past decade to learn the nuances of this brave world of microchips and gigabytes that rightfully belongs to the generations that follow this graying author.

Maurice M. Reeder, MD

An Appreciation

To Barbara Reeder, whose patience, love, and perseverance made possible the timely publication of this present work; and to all the Reeder sons, Dave, Dan, Bill, and Robby, and stepsons, Steve and Eric, in whom previous editions of the book invariably raised a gamut of emotions; and to those colleagues, mentors, and friends, past and present, who have so indelibly defined my own career:

William LeRoy Thompson
Benjamin Felson
Elias G. Theros
Harold G. Jacobson
Philip E.S. Palmer

How to Use This Book

1. SECTIONS

This book is organized into twelve sections, the first eight of which conform to the body systems utilized in the American College of Radiology Index for Roentgen Diagnosis. Each section is denoted by an alphabetical letter. Thus, under D you will find all the gamuts that deal with the skeletal system.

2. TABLE OF CONTENTS

This book has an extensive index. In addition, each section has its own table of contents, the pages of which have been black-edged for quick recognition. You can identify the appropriate table of contents by referring to page xv or by counting down the black index marks along the free edge of the closed book.

It will pay you to take a few minutes to look over the subheadings in the table of contents of each section. Gamuts are grouped in what we consider a logical manner. However, our logic may not be your logic; if you don't find a gamut where you think it belongs, scan the entire table of contents of that section or refer to the index before assuming that it is absent.

3. SUBGAMUTS (eg, A-1-2)

Many times a major gamut will be divided into separate logical components, which are identified by -1, -2, -3, etc. following the number of the parent gamut. These subgamuts amplify or extend the list of diagnoses pertinent to the main gamut to which they belong. For example, a long list of pertinent Congenital Syndromes may be listed as A-1-2 rather than being incorporated into the major heading of Craniosynostosis (A-1-1). Be sure to refer to these associated subgamuts after you have finished with the parent gamut.

4. SUPPLEMENTARY GAMUTS

Most of the gamuts refer to a roentgen sign, pattern, or complex. However, interspersed throughout the book are classifications, tables, drawings, anatomic and physiologic gamuts, and other information useful to the radiologist, which are designated by the letter S following the gamut number. Typical examples are Gamuts D-50-S (Age Range of Highest Incidence of Various Bone Neoplasms) and D-52-S (Sites of Predilection and Eponyms for Avascular Necrosis).

5. INCIDENCE

In most of the gamuts, the entities are subdivided into two groups, COMMON and UNCOMMON. These refer to the relative, rather than absolute, incidence of the disease. Although a bone blister (Gamut D-70) is an uncommon roentgen finding, if you do see one, the diagnosis will generally prove to be giant cell tumor or nonossifying fibroma (two of the conditions listed under COMMON). Conversely, an acute disseminated consolidation (alveolar) pattern (Gamut F-8) is frequently encountered in a busy hospital as a result of the prevalence of pulmonary edema and of pneumonia. Pulmonary hemorrhage is not a rare condition but simply a less common cause of that pattern and consequently is listed under UNCOMMON.

The prevalence of many disorders varies both geographically and from one type of institution to another.

Amebiasis is one of the most common entities in the world, but it is only occasionally seen in most of the United States. A Ewing sarcoma is much more commonly seen at Walter Reed Army Hospital than it is in a county hospital. To avoid such discrepancies, we have based our incidence estimates on our experience at Theoretical General Hospital, Midland, USA.

To attempt to list each cause of a particular pattern in order of its absolute frequency (as some have suggested) would not only be impossible but quite erroneous, since the incidence of various entities varies so remarkably in different countries and continents and even in different communities separated by only a few hundred miles. Thus, in the gamut for *Segmental Narrowing of the Colon*, carcinoma and Crohn's disease, diverticulitis and ulcerative colitis would be common causes in the United States, but quite uncommon or rare in tropical or developing countries where amebiasis, tuberculosis, schistosomiasis and lymphogranuloma venereum would be far more common causes of that pattern.

Admittedly, some of the gamuts deal with seldom seen roentgen signs, but it is in just this type of situation that a gamut is most welcome. It substitutes someone else's experience for your own lack of it.

6. ALPHABETICAL LISTING

The entries in each gamut have been alphabetized for your convenience. Since the entry may not be listed in the form that first comes to your mind, be sure to scan the entire gamut before assuming that a condition is not included.

7. TERMINOLOGY

We have usually selected the most widely used terms for each disease, often furnishing a synonym or eponym as well.

The term *generalized* indicates more or less diffuse involvement (eg, thalassemia of the skeleton); *widespread* means extensive but spotty involvement (eg, Paget's disease of the skeleton); *multiple* means more than one lesion but less than widespread (eg, large metastatic nodules in the lung).

In order to shorten the gamut lists, similar or related conditions are combined, often separated by a comma or semicolon (eg, scleroderma; dermatomyositis). Inclusive group designations, such as primary anemia, lymphoma, and paralytic disorders are often utilized. In these instances you will find the subscript $_g$ which tells you to look in the Glossary (page 949) if you want to know all the entities in that group. Example: Anemia, primary$_g$. If one member of a group is a more likely cause of a particular roentgen finding, it is specifically listed. To illustrate: Anemia, primary$_g$ (e.g., thalassemia). Abbreviations (such as incl., eg, S, ASD, PDA, etc) are listed on p. 947.

8. BRACKETS

Brackets [ ] are used to indicate a condition that does not actually cause the gamuted roentgen finding, but can produce roentgen changes that simulate it. Thus, in Gamut E-45 (Prominence of the Main Pulmonary Artery Segment), *mediastinal or left hilar mass,* which is not a cause, but a mimic, is bracketed.

9. APOSTROPHES

I fully recognize there are many inconsistencies throughout the text with regards to the use of apostrophes when listing diseases or syndromes bearing an individual's name. Recently there has been a growing trend to drop all apostrophes, but the various Medical and Radiology journals and publishers have as yet not adopted a uniform view on the subject. Consequently I have taken the editorial liberty of listing entities according to what appears to be the most commonly accepted terminology and what sounds best to the human ear. I for one cannot readily adapt to the sight or sound of Paget disease or Crohn disease; in ordinary conversation most physicians still refer to Paget's or Crohn's disease, using the apostrophe. On the other hand, many congenital syndromes seem to adapt well to dropping the apostrophe, as in Turner syndrome. My resolve to be nonconformist was heightened by a telephone conversation with my longtime friend and current editor of *AJR,* Dr. Lee Rogers, who agreed with me and said he would expect nothing less from a fellow gray-hair than to buck the current trend by younger authors to drop all apostrophes no matter how badly the resulting terminology offends the human eye or ear.

10. SYNDROMES

S. stands for Syndrome. We must apologize for the great number of congenital syndromes we have included. Since the information is available, we could hardly ignore it. Lump them together? The pediatric roentgenologists have assiduously split them apart. We had a huge tiger by the tail, an animal with variegated stripes and swollen gamuts. Shawl scrotum, Cockayne syndrome, and Prader-Willi syndromes, indeed! They should have their own Gamut book. We can only advise those of you who seldom see dwarfs and other little people to ignore these entries.

11. REFERENCES

References are used to cite only articles, books, and other contributions that have provided a number of the disease entities listed in a gamut. To document each entity would be an impossible task and lengthen the book beyond reason. A listing of general references, updated through 2002, appears in each gamut as appropriate. Some older references for a particular gamut have been retained since they are classical articles or texts with respect to that pattern or several of its causes. Rest assured that, in virtually every case, a listed cause for a particular pattern has been seen or verified by the author or the editorial consultants or documented in the literature.

11. OMISSIONS

We are fully aware that there are omissions on the Gamut lists. Very rare entities or syndromes or single case reports have been deliberately omitted. There are also some inconsistencies in terminology, coverage, and unity. There may even be occasional factual inaccuracies. We hope these flaws are neither too frequent nor too annoying.

Please correct errors if you encounter them; delete entities that you feel do not belong on a gamut; insert additional disorders and add new gamuts as you discover them in the literature or in your practice; create some gamuts yourself. Send us your changes, with documentation, so that they can be incorporated in future editions.

Skull and Brain

BRAIN (See Section "M" for a More Detailed MRI Analysis of the Brain)

A

Gamut A-1-1

PREMATURE CRANIOSYNOSTOSIS (CRANIOSTENOSIS)

COMMON

1. Congenital syndromes and bone dysplasias (See A-1-2)
*2. Decreased intracranial pressure (cerebral atrophy; shunted hydrocephalus "contracting skull") *
3. Primary (idiopathic) craniosynostosis (See A-1-S)

UNCOMMON

*1. Anemia$_g$ (eg, sickle cell disease; thalassemia; iron deficiency)
*2. Cretinism; hypothyroidism (treated)
*3. Hyperthyroidism
*4. Hypervitaminosis D
5. Microcephaly (failure of brain growth)
*6. Polycythemia vera
*7. Rickets (hypophosphatemic, treated; vitamin D resistant)

* Secondary craniosynostosis.

References

1. Cohen MM Jr: Genetic perspective on craniosynostosis and syndromes with craniosynostosis. Neurosurgery 1977;47:886
2. Cohen MM Jr, Maclean RE: Craniosynostosis. Diagnosis, Evaluation, and Management. (ed 2) New York, Oxford Univ Press, 2000
3. David DJ, Poswillo D, Simpson D: The Craniosynostoses. Berlin: Springer Verlag, 1982
4. Duggan CA, Keever EB, Gay BB Jr: Secondary craniosynostosis. AJR 1970;109:277–293
5. Jones KL: Smith's Recognizable Patterns of Human Malformation. (ed 5) Philadelphia: WB Saunders, 1997
6. Newton TH, Potts DG: Radiology of the Skull and Brain. St. Louis: CV Mosby, 1971, vol 1, book 1, pp 222–228
7. Swischuk LE, John SD: Differential Diagnosis in Pediatric Radiology. (ed 2) Baltimore: Williams & Wilkins, 1995
8. Taybi H, Lachman RS: Radiology of Syndromes, Metabolic Disorders, and Skeletal Dysplasias. (ed 4) St. Louis: Mosby-Year Book, Inc., 1996, pp 1000–1002

Gamut A-1-S

CLASSIFICATION OF PRIMARY (IDIOPATHIC) PREMATURE CRANIOSYNOSTOSIS

1. **Brachycephaly** (short, wide, slightly high head with "harlequin" orbits)—bilateral coronal sutures
2. **Microcephaly** (small round head)—all sutures (universal craniosynostosis)
3. **Oxycephaly** (tall, wide, short head) or **turricephaly** (tower-shaped, pointed head with overgrowth of bregma and flat, underdeveloped lower posterior fossa)—bilateral lambdoid and coronal sutures
4. **Plagiocephaly** (oblique asymmetrical head)—unilateral coronal suture (with flattening of ipsilateral frontoparietal region, elevation of ipsilateral sphenoid wing, and unilateral "harlequin" orbit) and/or lambdoid suture
5. **Scaphocephaly** (long, narrow, boat head) or **dolichocephaly** (long, slightly high head)—sagittal suture
6. **Trigonocephaly** (triangular head; narrow in front, broad behind with hypotelorism)—metopic suture
7. **Triphyllocephaly (cloverleaf skull {kleeblattschädel anomaly}**—trilobular skull with frontal and temporal bulges—intrauterine premature closure of sagittal, coronal, and lambdoid sutures with hydrocephalus

References

1. Newton TH, Potts DG: Radiology of the Skull and Brain. St. Louis: CV Mosby, 1971, vol 1, book 1, p 222
2. Silverman FN (ed): Caffey's Pediatric X-ray Diagnosis. (ed 8) Chicago: Year Book Medical Publ, 1985, pp 36–43
3. Swischuk LE, John SD: Differential Diagnosis in Pediatric Radiology. (ed 2) Baltimore: Williams & Wilkins, 1995
4. Swischuk LE: Imaging of the Newborn, Infant, and Young Child. (ed 3) Baltimore: Williams & Wilkins, 1989, pp 906–913

Gamut A-1-2

CONGENITAL SYNDROMES AND BONE DYSPLASIAS WITH PREMATURE CRANIOSYNOSTOSIS

COMMON

1. Achondroplasia (base of skull)
2. Acrocephalopolysyndactyly (Carpenter and other types)
3. Acrocephalosyndactyly (Apert, Pfeiffer, and Saethre-Chotzen types)
4. Asphyxiating thoracic dysplasia (Jeune S.)
5. Chondrodysplasia punctata
6. Cloverleaf skull (kleeblattschädel anomaly)
7. Crouzon S. (craniofacial dysostosis)
8. Fetal rubella S.
9. Hypophosphatasia (late)
10. Mucopolysaccharidoses (eg, Hurler S.; Maroteaux-Lamy S.); mucolipidosis III (pseudo-Hurler polydystrophy); fucosidosis
11. Thanatophoric dysplasia
12. Trisomy 21 S. (Down S.)

UNCOMMON

1. Acro-cranio-facial dysostosis
2. Adrenogenital S.
3. Aminopterin fetopathy
4. Antley-Bixler S.
5. Baller-Gerold S. (craniosynostosis-radial aplasia S.)
6. Bardet-Biedl S.
7. Christian S. (adducted thumbs S.)
8. Chromosomal syndromes (5p-, 7p-, 7q+)
9. Cranio-fronto-nasal dysplasia
10. Craniotelencephalic dysplasia
11. Fetal hydantoin S. (Dilantin embryopathy)
12. Fetal trimethadione S.
13. FG syndrome
14. Hallermann-Streiff S. (oculo-mandibulo-facial S.)
15. Holoprosencephaly (arrhinencephaly)—(results in microcephaly, trigonocephaly, cebocephaly)
16. Meckel S.
17. Metaphyseal chondrodysplasia (Jansen type)
18. Opitz trigonocephaly S. (C syndrome)
19. Pyknodysostosis
20. Seckel S. (bird-headed dwarfism)
21. Trisomy 13 S.
22. Trisomy 18 S.
23. Williams S. (idiopathic hypercalcemia)

References

1. Cohen MM Jr: Genetic perspective on craniosynostosis and syndromes with craniosynostosis. Neurosurgery 1977;47: 886
2. David DJ, Poswillo D, Simpson D: The Craniosynostoses. Berlin: Springer Verlag, 1982
3. Jones KL: Smith's Recognizable Patterns of Human Malformation. (ed 5) Philadelphia: WB Saunders, 1997
4. Newton TH, Potts DG: Radiology of the Skull and Brain. St. Louis: CV Mosby, 1971, vol 1, book 1, pp 222–228
5. Swischuk LE, John SD: Differential Diagnosis in Pediatric Radiology. (ed 2) Baltimore: Williams & Wilkins, 1995
6. Taybi H, Lachman RS: Radiology of Syndromes, Metabolic Disorders, and Skeletal Dysplasias. (ed 4) St. Louis: Mosby-Year Book, Inc., 1996

Gamut A-2

MICROCEPHALY (MICROCRANIA)

COMMON

1. Anencephaly
2. Cerebral atrophy; perinatal brain damage from hypoxia
3. Congenital transplacental infection (eg, toxoplasmosis; rubella; cytomegalovirus; herpes; syphilis)
4. Craniosynostosis, total
5. Encephalocele
6. Micrencephaly (idiopathic small brain)

UNCOMMON

1. Aminopterin fetopathy
2. Aspartylglucosaminuria
3. Beckwith-Wiedemann S.
4. Børjeson-Forssman-Lehman S.

5. Brachmann-de Lange S. (de Lange S.)
6. Cephaloskeletal dysplasia (Taybi-Linder S.)
7. Cerebro-oculo-facio-skeletal S. (Pena–Shokein S. type II)
8. Chondrodysplasia punctata (rhizomelic type)
9. Christian S. (adducted thumbs S.)
10. Chromosome syndromes (eg, 4: del (4p) S.{Wolf-Hirschhorn S.}; 5: del (5p) S. (cat cry S. {cri du chat S.});7: del (7q) S.; 9: dup (9p) S.; 18: del (18q) S.)
11. Cockayne S.
12. Coffin-Siris S.
13. Cohen S.
14. Cutis verticis gyrata
15. Deprivation (pyschosocial) dwarfism
16. Dubowitz S.
17. Dyggve-Melchior-Clausen dysplasia (Smith–McCort S.)
18. Familial
19. Fanconi anemia (pancytopenia-dysmelia S.)
20. Fetal alcohol S.
21. Fetal hydantoin S. (Dilantin embryopathy)
22. Fetal trimethadione S.
23. Fraser S. (cryptophthalmia S.)
24. Freeman-Sheldon S. (whistling face S.)
25. Galloway-Mowat S.
26. Goltz S. (focal dermal hypoplasia)
27. "Happy puppet" S. (Angelman S.)
28. Holoprosencephaly; arrhinencephaly
29. Homocystinuria
30. Incontinentia pigmenti
31. Johanson-Blizzard S.
32. Juberg-Hayward S.
33. Kearns-Sayre S.
34. Krabbe disease (globoid cell leukodystrophy)
35. Lenz microphthalmia S.
36. Lesch-Nyhan S.
37. Lissencephaly syndromes (congenital agyria)
38. Lowry-Wood S.
39. Marden-Walker S.
40. Marinesco-Sjögren S.
41. Maternal phenylketonuria
42. Meckel S.
43. Menkes S. (kinky-hair S.)
44. Microcephalic osteodysplastic dysplasia

45. Microcephaly-lymphedema S.
46. Noonan S.
47. [Normal variant]
48. Oculo-auriculo-vertebral spectrum (Goldenhar-Gorlin S.)
49. Opitz trigonocephaly S. (C syndrome)
50. Prader-Willi S.
51. Prenatal radiation
52. Riley-Day S. (familial dysautonomia)
53. Rubinstein-Taybi S.
54. Seckel S. (bird-headed dwarfism)
55. Smith-Lemli-Opitz S.
56. Trichorhinophalangeal dysplasia, type II (Langer-Giedion) and III (Ruvalcaba S.)
57. Trisomy 9 S.
58. Trisomy 13 S.
59. Trisomy 18 S.
60. Trisomy 21 S. (Down S.)
61. Trisomy 22 S.
62. XXXXX S.

References
1. Felson B (ed): Dwarfs and other little people. Semin Roentgenol 1973:8:133– 263
2. Newton TH, Potts DG: Radiology of the Skull and Brain. St. Louis: CV Mosby, 1971, vol 1, book 1, pp 151–152
3. Jones KL: Smith's Recognizable Patterns of Human Malformation. (ed 5) Philadelphia: WB Saunders, 1997
4. Taybi H, Lachman RS: Radiology of Syndromes, Metabolic Disorders, and Skeletal Dysplasias. (ed 4) St. Louis: Mosby-Year Book, Inc., 1996, pp 1003–1004

Gamut A-3-1

MACROCEPHALY (MACROCRANIA)

COMMON
1. Benign subdural fluid collections of infancy
2. [Calvarial thickening (eg, congenital anemias$_g$)]
*3. Congenital syndromes (See A-3-2)
*4. Craniostenosis
5. Hydrocephalus (See A-114-1)

(continued)

6. Paget's disease
*7. Subdural hematoma

UNCOMMON
1. Aqueduct stenosis
2. Arnold-Chiari malformation
3. Choroid plexus papilloma
*4. Expansion of middle fossa (See A-69)
5. Hydranencephaly
6. Infantile multisystem inflammatory disease (NOMID)
7. Infection causing hydrocephalus (eg, meningitis; toxoplasmosis)
8. Megalencephaly
9. Porencephalic cyst (porencephaly)
10. Posterior fossa cyst (eg, dermoid; teratoma; Dandy-Walker S. (Dandy-Walker malformation))
*11. Tumor or subarachnoid cyst adjacent to calvarium
12. Vein of Galen aneurysm

* May be asymmetrical.

[ ] This condition does not actually cause the gamuted imaging finding, but can produce imaging changes that simulate it.

References
1. Harwood-Nash DC, Fitz CR: Large heads and ventricles in infants. Radiol Clin North Am 1975;13:119–224
2. Kirks DR: Practical Pediatric Imaging. (ed 3) Philadelphia: Lippincott-Raven, 1998, p 151
3. Newton TH, Potts DG: Radiology of the Skull and Brain. St. Louis: CV Mosby, 1971, vol 1, book 1, pp 144–151
4. Scotti LN, Maraviila K, Hardman DR: The enlarging head—angiographic evaluation of megacephaly. American Roentgen Ray Society Scientific Exhibit, Atlanta, 1975
5. Swischuk LE, John SD: Differential Diagnosis in Pediatric Radiology. (ed 2) Baltimore: Williams & Wilkins, 1995, pp 345–347

Gamut A-3-2

CONGENITAL SYNDROMES AND BONE DYSPLASIAS WITH MACROCEPHALY (MEGALENCEPHALY; MACROCRANIA)*

COMMON
1. Achondroplasia; hypochondroplasia
2. Hydrocephalus (See A-114-1)
3. Hyperostosis diseases (eg, osteopetrosis; diaphyseal dysplasia {Camurati-Engelmann disease}; pyknodysostosis; hyperphosphatasia)
4. Mucopolysaccharidoses (incl. Hurler, Hunter, Morquio, Maroteaux-Lamy); mucolipidoses (See J-4-S); GM_1 and GM_2 gangliosidosis
5. Neurofibromatosis
6. Thanatophoric dysplasia

UNCOMMON
1. Achondrogenesis (type II); hypochondrogenesis
2. Acrocollosal S.
3. Aminoacidurias
4. Bannayan-Riley-Ruvalcaba S.
5. Beckwith-Wiedemann S.
6. Campomelic dysplasia
7. Cleidocranial dysplasia
8. Cowden S.
9. Craniodiaphyseal dysplasia
10. Cranioectodermal dysplasia
11. Craniometaphyseal dysplasia
12. Dandy-Walker S. (Dandy-Walker malformation)
13. Endosteal hyperostosis (van Buchem type)
14. FG syndrome
15. Familial megalencephaly; megalencephaly syndromes
16. Fragile X S.
17. Gorlin S. (nevoid basal cell carcinoma S.)
18. Greig cephalopolysyndactyly S.
19. Hydrolethalus
20. Hypomelanosis of Ito
21. Infantile multisystem inflammatory disease (NOMID)

22. Klippel-Trenaunay-Weber S.
23. Kniest dysplasia
24. Lenz-Majewski dysplasia (hyperostolic dwarfism)
25. Lhermitte-Duclos S.
26. Leukodystrophies
27. Marfan S.
28. Marshall-Smith S.
29. Noonan S.
30. Osteogenesis imperfecta
31. Osteopathia striata with cranial sclerosis
32. Pituitary gigantism
33. Proteus S.
34. Riley-Day S. (familial dysautonomia)
35. Robinow S.
36. Schwarz-Lélek S.
37. Sclerosteosis
38. Silver-Russell S.
39. Sotos S. (cerebral gigantism)
40. Tay-Sachs disease
41. Trisomy 8 S.
42. Tuberous sclerosis
43. Weaver S. (Weaver–Smith S.)
44. Zellweger S. (cerebrohepatorenal S.)

* Many dwarfs have relative macrocephaly.

References
1. DeMyer W: Megalencephaly in children: clinical syndromes, genetic patterns, and differential diagnoses from other causes of megalocephaly. Neurology 1972; 22:634–643
2. Holt JF, Kuhns LR: Macrocranium and macrocephaly in neurofibromatosis. Skeletal Radiol 1976;1:25–28
3. Jones KL: Smith's Recognizable Patterns of Human Malformation. (ed 5) Philadelphia: WB Saunders, 1997
4. Swischuk LE, John SD: Differential Diagnosis in Pediatric Radiology. (ed 2) Baltimore: Williams & Wilkins, 1995
5. Taybi H, Lachman RS: Radiology of Syndromes, Metabolic Disorders, and Skeletal Dysplasias. (ed 4) St. Louis: Mosby-Year Book, Inc., 1996, pp 1002–1003

Gamut A-4

ABNORMAL CONTOUR OF THE CALVARIUM (SEE A-1-13)

COMMON
1. Achondroplasia, other congenital syndromes and bone dysplasias (See A-1 to 13)
2. Bone tumor (eg, osteoma; osteosarcoma)
3. Cerebral hemiatrophy (eg, Sturge-Weber S.; Dyke-Davidoff-Masson S.); localized cerebral atrophy
4. Fibrous dysplasia; leontiasis ossea
5. Hydrocephalus
6. Paget's disease (eg, tam-o'-shanter skull) (See A-13)
7. Postoperative deformity
8. Postural flattening, usually occipital (eg, cerebral palsy); postural asymmetry from scoliosis
9. Premature craniosynostosis (See A-1)
10. Trauma (incl. obstetrical); depressed fracture; cephalohematoma

UNCOMMON
1. Acromesomelic dysplasia
2. Arachnoid cyst
3. Craniolacunia
4. Craniopagus twins
5. Crouzon S. (craniofacial dysostosis)
6. Dandy-Walker S. (Dandy-Walker malformation)
7. Encephalocele
8. Hemimegancephaly
9. Hyperphosphatasia
10. Hypertelorism (See B-3); cranium bifidum
11. Hypomelanosis of Ito
12. Microcephaly
13. Neurofibromatosis
14. Osteogenesis imperfecta
15. Porencephalic cyst (porencephaly); cerebral cyst
16. Proteus S.
17. Rickets, healed with bossing
18. Silver-Russell S.
19. Subdural hematoma, chronic; hygroma

Gamut A-5

UNILATERAL SMALL CRANIUM

COMMON

1. Cerebral hemiatrophy (eg, Dyke-Davidoff-Masson S.; Sturge-Weber S.)
2. Head positioning in infancy (postural flattening)
3. Normal (slight)
4. Trauma (depressed skull fracture)
5. Unilateral lambdoid or coronal craniosynostosis (plagiocephaly)

UNCOMMON

1. Radiation therapy
2. Silver-Russell S. (congenital hemiatrophy)

Gamut A-6

FLAT OCCIPUT IN AN INFANT

COMMON

1. Achondroplasia
2. Postural flattening (eg, normal, mental retardation, or immobilized infant)
3. Trisomy 21 S. (Down S.)

UNCOMMON

1. Acrocephalopolysyndactyly (Carpenter type)
2. Acrocephalosyndactyly (Apert, Pfeiffer, Saethre-Chotzen types)
3. Acrodysostosis
4. Brachmann de Lange S. (de Lange S.)
5. Crouzon S. (craniofacial dysostosis)
6. Mucopolysaccharidosis III (Sanfilippo S.)
7. Weaver S. (Weaver–Smith S.)
8. Weill-Marchesani S.
9. XXXXY S.

Reference
1. Jones KL: Smith's Recognizable Patterns of Human Malformation. (ed 5) Philadelphia: WB Saunders, 1997

Gamut A-7

PROMINENT OCCIPUT IN AN INFANT

COMMON

1. Bathrocephaly (idiopathic)
2. Dandy-Walker S. (Dandy-Walker malformation); posterior fossa arachnoid cyst

UNCOMMON

1. Beckwith-Wiedemann S.
2. Campomelic dysplasia
3. Cephalohematoma, occipital
4. Diaphyseal dysplasia (Camurati-Engelmann disease)
5. Hajdu-Cheney S. (idiopathic acro-osteolysis)
6. Meningocele, occipital
7. Mulibrey nanism
8. Otopalatodigital S.
9. Pyknodysostosis
10. Trisomy 9 S.
11. Trisomy 18 S.

Reference
1. Jones KL: Smith's Recognizable Patterns of Human Malformation.(ed 5) Philadelphia: WB Saunders, 1997

Gamut A-8

FRONTAL BOSSING (PROMINENT CENTRAL FOREHEAD)

COMMON

1. Achondroplasia
2. Anemia$_g$ (esp. sickle cell disease; thalassemia)
3. Rickets, healed

UNCOMMON

1. Achondrogenesis
2. Acrocallosal S.
3. Cerebral gigantism (Sotos S.)
4. Cleidocranial dysplasia
5. Coffin-Lowry S.
6. Craniodiaphyseal dysplasia
7. Cranio-fronto-nasal dysplasia
8. Craniometaphyseal dysplasia
9. Craniotelencephalic dysplasia
10. Diaphyseal dysplasia (Camurati-Engelmann disease)
11. Diastrophic dysplasia
12. Frontometaphyseal dysplasia
13. GAPO S.
14. Gorlin S. (nevoid basal cell carcinoma S.)
15. Greig cephalopolysyndactyly S.
16. Hallermann-Streiff S. (oculo-mandibulo-facial S.)
17. Hydrocephalus
18. Hypochondroplasia
19. Infantile multisystem inflammatory disease (NOMID)
20. Larsen S.
21. Lissencephaly syndromes (congenital agyria)
22. Lowe S. (oculocerebrorenal S.)
23. Marshall-Smith S.
24. Megalencephaly
25. Metatropic dysplasia
26. Mucopolysaccharidoses (Hurler S.; Maroteaux-Lamy S.) (See J-4); mucolipidosis II (I-cell disease); GM_1 gangliosidosis; fucosidosis
27. Oculo-auriculo-vertebral spectrum (Goldenhar-Gorlin S.)
28. Oro-facio-digital S. I (Papillon-Leage and Psaume S.)
29. Osteoglophonic dysplasia
30. Osteopetrosis, severe
31. Otopalatodigital S.
32. Progeria
33. Pyknodysostosis
34. Pyle dysplasia (familial metaphyseal dysplasia)
35. Robinow S.
36. Schinzel-Giedion S.
37. Schwarz-Lélek S.
38. Sclerosteosis
39. Silver-Russell S.
40. Sotos S. (cerebral gigantism)
41. Subdural hematoma, chronic
42. Thanatophoric dysplasia
43. 3–M syndrome
44. Trisomy 8 S.

References

1. Jones KL: Smith's Recognizable Patterns of Human Malformation. (ed 5) Philadelphia: WB Saunders, 1997
2. Swischuk LE, John SD: Differential Diagnosis in Pediatric Radiology. (ed 2) Baltimore: Williams & Wilkins, 1995
3. Taybi H, Lachman RS: Radiology of Syndromes, Metabolic Disorders, and Skeletal Dysplasias. (ed 4) St. Louis: Mosby-Year Book, Inc., 1996, p 1002

Gamut A-9

BIPARIETAL BOSSING*

1. Bilateral coronal synostosis, isolated or with Crouzon S. (craniofacial dysostosis)
2. Bilateral subdural hematoma, chronic
3. Cleidocranial dysplasia
4. Cloverleaf skull (kleeblattschädel anomaly)
5. Gorlin S. (nevoid basal cell carcinoma S.)
6. Pyknodysostosis
7. Rickets, healed

* Patients with achondroplasia, hypochondroplasia, and thanatophoric dysplasia have, in addition to frontal bossing, biparietal bossing which can be quite prominent clinically.

Reference

1. Swischuk LE, John SD: Differential Diagnosis in Pediatric Radiology. (ed 2) Baltimore: Williams & Wilkins, 1995, p 352

Gamut A-10

LOCALIZED BULGE OF THE CALVARIUM OR SCALP

COMMON

1. Anemia$_g$, chronic (eg, sickle cell disease; iron deficiency anemia)
2. Cephalohematoma
3. Metastatic carcinoma or neuroblastoma
4. Myeloma
5. Osteoma

UNCOMMON

1. Arachnoid cyst with erosion
2. Dermoid cyst, intradiploic
3. Fibrous dysplasia
4. Intracranial neoplasm (large) with erosion of calvarium
5. Langerhans cell histiocytosis$_g$
6. Leptomeningeal cyst
7. Meningioma
8. Meningocele; encephalocele
9. Neoplasm of skull, other (eg, osteosarcoma; lymphoma$_g$; hemangioma)
10. Paget's disease with secondary malignant neoplasm
11. Porencephalic cyst (porencephaly)
12. Scalp neoplasm or cyst
13. Subdural hematoma

Reference

1. Swischuk LE, John SD: Differential Diagnosis in Pediatric Radiology. (ed 2) Baltimore: Williams & Wilkins, 1995, p 352

Gamut A-11

HYPOPLASIA OF THE BASE OF THE SKULL

COMMON

1. Achondroplasia
2. Cretinism
3. Trisomy 21 S. (Down S.)

UNCOMMON

1. Achondrogenesis; hypochondrogenesis
2. Acrocephalopolysyndactyly (Carpenter type)
3. Acrocephalosyndactyly (Apert and Pfeiffer types)
4. Cranial dysplasia; cleidocranial dysplasia
5. Crouzon S. (craniofacial dysostosis)
6. Diastrophic dysplasia
7. Hallermann-Streiff S. (oculo-mandibulo-facial S.)
8. Hypochondroplasia
9. Metaphyseal chondrodysplasia (Jansen type)
10. Metatropic dysplasia
11. Orbital hypotelorism with arrhinencephaly; trisomy 13 S.
12. Short rib-polydactyly syndromes
13. Spondyloepiphyseal dysplasia congenita
14. Thanatophoric dysplasia

References

1. DuBoulay GH: Principles of X-ray Diagnosis of the Skull. (ed 2) London: Butterworths, 1980, pp 237–243
2. Taybi H, Lachman RS: Radiology of Syndromes, Metabolic Disorders, and Skeletal Dysplasias. (ed 4) St. Louis: Mosby-Year Book, Inc., 1996

Gamut A-12

BASILAR INVAGINATION

COMMON

1. Arnold-Chiari malformation
2. Congenital craniovertebral anomaly (See C-9-1)
   a. Atlantoaxial dislocation with or without congenital separation of odontoid

b. Atlanto-occipital fusion (assimilation)
c. Klippel-Feil S.
d. Stenosis of foramen magnum
e. Unfused posterior arch of atlas
3. Osteogenesis imperfecta
4. Osteomalacia; rickets (See D-44)
5. Paget's disease

UNCOMMON

1. Achondroplasia
2. Ankylosing spondylitis; rheumatoid arthritis; psoriatic arthritis
3. Aqueduct stenosis
4. Cleidocranial dysplasia
5. Crouzon S. (craniofacial dysostosis)
6. Familial
7. Fibrous dysplasia
8. Hajdu-Cheney S. (idiopathic acro-osteolysis)
9. Hydrocephalus, chronic
10. Hyperparathyroidism, primary or secondary (renal osteodystrophy)
11. Hypophosphatasia
12. Langerhans cell histiocytosis$_g$
13. Lowe S. (oculocerebrorenal S.)
14. Metaphyseal chondrodysplasia (Jansen type)
15. Mucopolysaccharidoses (eg, Hurler, Morquio) (See J-4)
16. Occipital craniotomy in a child
17. Osteomyelitis (incl. syphilis; tuberculosis)
18. Osteopetrosis
19. Osteoporosis
20. Pyknodysostosis
21. Sjögren-Larsson S.
22. Trauma, severe
23. Trisomy 21 S. (Down S.)

References

1. Dolan KD: Cervicobasilar relationships. Radiol Clin North Am 1977;15:155–166
2. DuBoulay GH: Principles of X-ray Diagnosis of the Skull. (ed 2) London: Butterworths, 1980, pp 229–235
3. Epstein BS, Epstein JA: The association of cerebellar tonsillar herniation with basilar impression incident to Paget's disease. AJR 1969;107:535–542
4. Taybi H, Lachman RS: Radiology of Syndromes, Metabolic Disorders, and Skeletal Dysplasias. (ed 4) St. Louis: Mosby-Year Book, Inc., 1996, p 1000

Gamut A-13

TAM-O'-SHANTER SKULL (THICKENING OF THE SKULL VAULT WITH BASILAR INVAGINATION)

COMMON

1. Paget's disease

UNCOMMON

1. Fibrous dysplasia
2. Hypophosphatasia
3. Neurofibromatosis
4. Osteogenesis imperfecta
5. Osteomalacia
6. Rickets

Gamut A-14

LOCALIZED INCREASED DENSITY, SCLEROSIS, OR THICKENING OF THE CALVARIUM

COMMON

1. Anatomic variation (eg, sutural sclerosis; external occipital protuberance)
2. Anemia$_g$ (esp. sickle cell disease)
3. [Artifact; hair braid; overlying soft tissue tumor or calcified sebaceous cyst; neurofibroma; neurofibromatosis]
4. Cephalohematoma, calcified; ossified subdural hematoma

(continued)

5. Chronic osteomyelitis or adjacent cellulitis; tuberculosis; syphilis; actinomycosis; mycetoma
6. [Depressed skull fracture]
7. Fibrous dysplasia
8. Hyperostosis frontalis interna (incl. Coffin-Lowry S.; nail-patella S.)
*9. Meningioma
*10. Metastasis, osteoblastic (eg, prostate; breast)
11. Osteoma
12. Paget's disease

UNCOMMON
1. Arteriovenous malformation of dura
2. Cerebral hemiatrophy (Dyke-Davidoff-Masson S.)
3. [Dural calcification]
4. Epidermal nevus S.
5. Frontometaphyseal dysplasia
6. Head-banging, chronic
*7. Hemangioma
8. Hypoparathyroidism
9. Ischemic necrosis (eg, bone flap)
10. Langerhans cell histiocytosis$_g$, healing
11. Lipodystrophy, total (lipoatrophic diabetes)
12. Lymphoma$_g$
13. Mastocytosis
14. Osteoblastoma
15. Osteochondroma
16. Osteosarcoma; infantile fibrosarcoma
17. Radiation osteonecrosis; treated tumor (eg, brown tumor of hyperparathyroidism; lytic metastasis from breast)
18. Tuberous sclerosis

* Sunburst spiculations may be present.

[ ] This condition does not actually cause the gamuted imaging finding, but can produce imaging changes that simulate it.

References
1. DuBoulay GH:,Principles of X-ray Diagnosis of the Skull. (ed 2) London: Butterworths, 1980, pp 113–125
2. Taybi H, Lachman RS: Radiology of Syndromes, Metabolic Disorders, and Skeletal Dysplasias. (ed 4) St. Louis: Mosby-Year Book, Inc., 1996

DIFFUSE OR WIDESPREAD INCREASED DENSITY, SCLEROSIS, OR THICKENING OF THE CALVARIUM

COMMON
1. Acromegaly
*2. Anemia$_g$ (sickle cell disease; thalassemia; iron deficiency anemia; hereditary spherocytosis)
3. Cerebral atrophy in childhood (contracting skull)
4. Congenital syndromes; sclerosing bone dysplasias (eg, osteopetrosis) (See A-15-2)
+5. Fibrous dysplasia; leontiasis ossea
6. Hydrocephalus (postshunting)
7. Hyperostosis interna generalisata; Morgagni-Stewart-Morel S.
8. Normal; idiopathic
*9. Metastases, osteoblastic (eg, prostate; breast)
10. Myelosclerosis
11. Paget's disease ("cotton wool" appearance)
12. Renal osteodystrophy (secondary hyperparathyroidism) (treated, esp. in patients on dialysis)

UNCOMMON
1. Arteriovenous malformation, large
2. Craniosynostosis (See A-1)
3. Cretinism, hypothyroidism (treated)
4. Cyanotic congenital heart disease, longstanding
5. Dilantin (hydantoin) therapy
6. Fluorosis
7. Hemihypertrophy of cranium due to cerebral hemiatrophy (Dyke-Davidoff-Masson S.)
8. Homocystinuria
9. Hyperphosphatasia
10. Hypervitaminosis D
11. Hypoparathyroidism
*12. Leukemia; lymphoma
*13. Meningioma
*14. Metastatic neuroblastoma
15. Microcephaly
16. Myotonic dystrophy

17. Osteomyelitis, chronic; mycetoma; syphilis
*18. Polycythemia (childhood)
19. Rickets, treated ("bossing"); vitamin D-resistant rickets

* May show vertical striations ("hair on end").

+ May develop leontiasis ossea (lion-like facies) due to overgrowth of facial bones.

References

1. Anderson R, et al: Thickening of the skull in surgically treated hydrocephalus. AJR 1970;110:96–101
2. DuBoulay GH: Principles of X-ray Diagnosis of the Skull. (ed 2) London: Butterworths, 1980, pp 98–113
3. Griscom NT, Oh KS: The contracting skull; Inward growth of the inner table as a physiologic response to diminution of intracranial content in children. AJR 1970;110:106–110
4. Kattan KR: Calvarial thickening after Dilantin medication. AJR 1970;110:102–105
5. Swischuk LE, John SD: Differential Diagnosis in Pediatric Radiology. (ed 2) Baltimore: Williams & Wilkins, 1995
6. Taybi H, Lachman RS: Radiology of Syndromes, Metabolic Disorders, and Skeletal Dysplasias. (ed 4) St. Louis: Mosby-Year Book, Inc., 1996, p 1005

Gamut A-15-2

CONGENITAL CONDITIONS WITH INCREASED DENSITY OR THICKENING OF THE SKULL

COMMON

1. Anemia$_g$ (sickle cell disease; thalassemia; pyruvate kinase deficiency; hereditary spherocytosis)
*2. Craniometaphyseal dysplasia; Pyle dysplasia; frontometaphyseal dysplasia
3. Craniosynostosis (See A-1)
4. Cretinism; hypothyroidism
5. Cyanotic congenital heart disease, long standing
6. Diaphyseal dysplasia (Camurati-Engelmann disease)
7. Endosteal hyperostosis (van Buchem and Worth types)
8. Fanconi anemia (pancytopenia-dysmelia S.)
*9. Fibrous dysplasia; leontiasis ossea (incl. polyostotic fibrous dysplasia {McCune-Albright S.})
10. Hemihypertrophy of cranium due to cerebral hemiatrophy (Dyke-Davidoff-Masson S.)
11. Homocystinuria
*12. Hyperphosphatasia
13. Marfan S.
14. Microcephaly
15. Mucopolysaccharidoses (eg, Hurler S.; Hunter S.; Sanfilippo S.; Maroteaux-Lamy S.) (See J-4); GM$_1$ gangliosidosis; mannosidosis; fucosidosis
16. Osteopetrosis
17. Pachydermoperiostosis
18. Pseudohypoparathyroidism; pseudopseudohypoparathyroidism
19. Pyknodysostosis
20. Tuberous sclerosis

UNCOMMON

1. Aase-Smith S.
2. Acrodysostosis (peripheral dysostosis)
3. Cockayne S.
4. Coffin-Lowry S.
5. Craniodiaphyseal dysplasia
6. Distal osteosclerosis
7. Dysosteosclerosis
8. Lenz-Majewski hyperostotic dwarfism
9. Lipodystrophy, total (lipoatrophic diabetes)
10. Marshall S.
11. Melorheostosis
12. Neu-Laxova S.
13. Oculo-dento-osseous dysplasia
14. Osteodysplasty (Melnick-Needles S.)
15. Osteogenesis imperfecta
16. Osteopathia striata with cranial sclerosis
17. Otopalatodigital S., type I
18. Patterson S.
19. POEMS S.
20. Proteus S.
21. Salla disease
22. Schinzel-Giedion S.
23. Schwarz-Lélek S.

(continued)

24. Sclerosteosis
25. Sialidosis (mucolipidosis I); mucolipidosis II (I-cell disease)
26. Trichodentoosseous dysplasia
27. Troell-Junet S.
28. Tubular stenosis (Kenny-Caffey S.)
29. Weill-Marchesani S.
30. Williams S. (idiopathic hypercalcemia)
31. XXXXY S.

* May develop leontiasis ossea (lion-like facies) due to overgrowth of facial bones.

References
1. Kozlowski K, Beighton P: Gamut Index of Skeletal Dysplasias. Berlin: Springer-Verlag, 1984
2. Swischuk LE, John SD: Differential Diagnosis in Pediatric Radiology. (ed 2) Baltimore: Williams & Wilkins, 1995
3. Taybi H, Lachman RS: Radiology of Syndromes, Metabolic Disorders, and Skeletal Dysplasias. (ed 4) St. Louis: Mosby-Year Book, Inc., 1996, p 1005

8. Radiation therapy for invasive carcinoma of ear, sphenoid sinus, or nasopharynx
9. Sarcoma (eg, osteosarcoma; chondrosarcoma; rhabdomyosarcoma)
10. Sphenoid sinusitis; mucocele

References
1. Potter GD: Sclerosis of the base of the skull as a manifestation of nasopharyngeal carcinoma. Radiology 1970;94:35–38
2. Tsai FY, Lisella RS, Lee KF, et al: Osteosclerosis of base of skull as a manifestation of tumor invasion. AJR 1975;124:256–264

Gamut A-17

GENERALIZED INCREASED DENSITY, SCLEROSIS, OR THICKENING OF THE BASE OF THE SKULL (SEE A-16)

COMMON
1. Fibrous dysplasia
2. Paget's disease

UNCOMMON
1. Anemia$_g$, primary (eg, thalassemia; sickle cell disease; pyruvate kinase deficiency; hereditary spherocytosis)
2. Cleidocranial dysplasia
3. Craniodiaphyseal dysplasia
4. Craniometaphyseal dysplasia; frontometaphyseal dysplasia
5. Cretinism; hypothyroidism
6. Diaphyseal dysplasia (Camurati-Engelmann disease)
7. Dysosteosclerosis
8. Endosteal hyperostosis (van Buchem and Worth types)
9. Fluorosis
10. Hyperparathyroidism, primary or secondary (renal osteodystrophy) (treated)

Gamut A-16

LOCALIZED INCREASED DENSITY, SCLEROSIS, OR THICKENING OF THE BASE OF THE SKULL (SEE A-17)

COMMON
1. Fibrous dysplasia
2. Mastoiditis, chronic sclerotic
3. Meningioma

UNCOMMON
1. Chordoma (with calcification)
2. Lymphoepithelioma of nasopharynx or paranasal sinus
3. Lymphoma$_g$
4. Nasopharyngeal infection, chronic (eg, tuberculosis)
5. Osteoblastic metastasis
6. Osteoma; chondroma
7. Petrositis or osteomyelitis, chronic

11. Hyperphosphatasia
12. Hypervitaminosis D
13. Infantile multisystem inflammatory disease (NOMID)
14. Melorheostosis
15. Meningioma (extensive)
16. Metaphyseal chondrodysplasia (Jansen type)
17. Mucopolysaccharidosis (esp. Hurler S.)
18. Neurofibromatosis
19. Osteodysplasty (Melnick-Needles S.)
20. Osteopathia striata with cranial sclerosis
21. Osteopetrosis
22. Otopalatodigital S.
23. Pachydermoperiostosis
24. Pyknodysostosis
25. Pyle dysplasia
26. Ribbing disease (hereditary multiple diaphyseal sclerosis)
27. Sclerosteosis
28. Tricho-dento-osseous S.
29. Vitamin D-resistant rickets (healing)
30. Williams S. (idiopathic hypercalcemia)

References
1. Dornhoffer J, Schwager K. Fibrous dysplasia and ossifying fibroma. Unusual fibro-osseous lesions of the paranasal sinuses. HNO 1995;43:193–196
2. DuBoulay GH: Principles of X-ray Diagnosis of the Skull. (ed 2) London: Butterworths, 1980.
3. Lufkin R, Borges A, Villablanca P: Teaching Atlas of Head and Neck Imaging. New York: Thieme, 2000, pp 13–17
4. Swischuk LE, John SD: Differential Diagnosis in Pediatric Radiology. (ed 2) Baltimore: Williams & Wilkins, 1995, pp 352–355

Gamut A-18

LOCALIZED THINNING OF THE SKULL

COMMON

1. Parietal thinning
2. Subdural hematoma, chronic

UNCOMMON

1. Congenital arachnoid cyst
2. Intracranial tumor, slow growing
3. Leptomeningeal cyst
4. Localized cerebral agenesis or atrophy
5. Localized temporal horn hydrocephalus
6. Necrosis of skull (eg, radiation therapy)
7. Neurofibromatosis
8. Osteoporosis circumscripta (Paget's disease)
9. Porencephalic cyst (porencephaly)

References
1. DuBoulay GH: Principles of X-ray Diagnosis of the Skull. (ed 2) London: Butterworths, 1980
2. Swischuk LE, John SD: Differential Diagnosis in Pediatric Radiology. (ed 2) Baltimore: Williams & Wilkins, 1995

Gamut A-19

GENERALIZED THINNING OF THE SKULL

COMMON

1. Craniolacunia (lacunar skull)
2. Hydrocephalus, long standing (See A-114)
3. Hyperparathyroidism
4. Normal (eg, prominent normal convolutional markings; prematurity)
5. Osteogenesis imperfecta

UNCOMMON

1. Achondrogenesis, type I
2. Aminopterin fetopathy
3. Cleidocranial dysplasia; cranial dysplasia
4. Cushing S.
5. Hypophosphatasia
6. Increased intracranial pressure, other causes (See A-113)
7. Progeria
8. Rickets
9. Trisomy 18 S.

(continued)

References

1. DuBoulay GH: Principles of X-ray Diagnosis of the Skull. (ed 2) London: Butterworths, 1980
2. Osborn AG: Handbook of Neuroradiology. St. Louis: Mosby-Year Book., Inc, 1991, pp 154–155
3. Swischuk LE, John SD: Differential Diagnosis in Pediatric Radiology. (ed 2) Baltimore: Williams & Wilkins, 1995, p 359

Gamut A-20

DIFFUSE OR WIDESPREAD DEMINERALIZATION OR DESTRUCTION OF THE SKULL (INCLUDING "SALT AND PEPPER" SKULL) (SEE A-19)

COMMON
*1. Hyperparathyroidism, primary or secondary (renal osteodystrophy)
*2. Leukemia; lymphoma$_g$
*3. Metastatic carcinoma or neuroblastoma
*4. Multiple myeloma (myelomatosis)
*5. Osteomyelitis, diffuse
6. Osteoporosis (eg, senile; postmenopausal) (See D-43-1)

UNCOMMON
1. Anemia$_g$ (eg, sickle cell disease; thalassemia)
2. Electric burn; thermal burn
3. Idiopathic
4. Meningioma or other meningeal neoplasm
5. Osteomalacia; rickets (See D-44)
6. Osteonecrosis
*7. Paget's disease (osteoporosis circumscripta)
8. Primary malignant neoplasm of skull (eg, Ewing sarcoma)
9. Radiation osteonecrosis; radium poisoning
10. Steroid therapy; Cushing S.
11. Syphilis

* May show mottled or "salt and pepper" destruction of calvarium.

Gamut A-21

EROSION OF THE INNER TABLE OF THE SKULL

COMMON
1. Metastasis
2. Osteomyelitis
3. Pacchionian granulation
4. Subdural hematoma, chronic

UNCOMMON
1. Arteriovenous malformation of brain surface
2. Cisterna magna anomaly
3. Epidermoid
4. Glioma or cyst of superficial brain cortex (eg, oligodendroglioma; leptomeningeal cyst)
5. Hemangioma
6. Langerhans cell histiocytosis$_g$ (esp. eosinophilic granuloma)
7. Meningioma
8. Multiple myeloma
9. Neoplasm of dura, other (eg, sarcoma; melanoma)
10. Porencephalic cyst (porencephaly)
11. Sinus pericranii

Gamut A-22

BUTTON SEQUESTRUM OF THE SKULL*

COMMON
1. Eosinophilic granuloma
2. Metastatic carcinoma (esp. breast)
3. Osteomyelitis (esp. staphylococcal)

UNCOMMON
1. [Burr hole or bone flap]
2. [Calvarial "doughnut," idiopathic]
3. Dermoid cyst

4. Epidermoid (primary cholesteatoma)
5. Fibrosing osteitis
6. [Hemangioma]
7. Meningioma
8. Multiple myeloma
9. Osteonecrosis (eg, radiation therapy; radium poisoning; electric burn; electric shock therapy)
10. Paget's disease
11. Sarcoidosis
12. Syphilis
13. Tuberculosis

* Round radiolucent skull defect with central bony density or sequestrum.

[ ] This condition does not actually cause the gamuted imaging finding, but can produce imaging changes that simulate it.

References

1. Eisenberg RL: Skull and Spine Imaging. An Atlas of Differential Diagnosis. New York: Raven Press, 1994, pp 12–13
2. Newton TH, Potts DG: Radiology of the Skull and Brain. St. Louis: CV Mosby, 1971, p 759
3. Rosen IW, Nadel HI: Button sequestrum of the skull. Radiology 1969;92:969–971
4. Satin R, Usher MS, Goldenberg M: More causes of button sequestrum. J Can Assoc Radiol 1976; 27:288–289
5. Sholkoff SD, Mainzer F: Button sequestrum revisited. Radiology 1971;100:649–652
6. Wells PO: Button sequestrum of eosinophilic granuloma of the skull. Radiology 1956; 67:746–747

Gamut A-23-1

SOLITARY OSTEOLYTIC SKULL LESION (SEE A-23-2)

COMMON

*1. Cholesteatoma (inflammatory)
*2. Epidermoid (primary cholesteatoma)
*3. Fibrous dysplasia
 4. Fracture (esp. depressed)
*5. Hemangioma
*6. Langerhans cell histiocytosis$_g$ (esp. eosinophilic granuloma)

*7. Meningocele; encephalocele; cranium bifidum
 8. Metastasis (esp. from carcinoma of breast, lung, thyroid, or kidney; neuroblastoma)
 9. Myeloma; plasmacytoma
10. Normal variant (eg, venous lake; enlarged emissary channel; inioindineal canal; fontanelle; pacchionian granulation; parietal foramen; parietal thinning) (See A-35-S1)
*11. Osteomyelitis
12. Paget's disease (osteoporosis circumscripta)
*13. Surgical defect (eg, burr hole; craniotomy flap)

UNCOMMON

 1. Aplasia cutis congenita
 2. Arachnoid cyst
 3. Arteriovenous malformation
 4. Bone sarcoma (eg, osteolytic osteosarcoma; Ewing sarcoma; chondrosarcoma)
 5. Brown tumor of hyperparathyroidism
*6. Button sequestrum (See A-22)
*7. Calvarial "doughnut"; idiopathic
 8. Chordoma of clivus
 9. Dermal sinus
10. Dermoid
11. Direct extension from carcinoma of paranasal sinuses or nasopharynx
12. Ectopic intradiploic glial tissue (occipital)
*13. Fungus disease
14. Gaucher's disease; Niemann-Pick disease
15. Glomus jugulare tumor (base)
16. Hydatid disease
17. Leptomeningeal cyst
*18. Lymphoma$_g$
*19. Mucocele or neoplasm of paranasal sinus
*20. Neoplasm of brain or dura with bone erosion (esp. meningioma)
21. Neoplasm or cyst of scalp (eg, carcinoma; rodent ulcer; neurofibroma; sebaceous cyst)
22. Neoplasm of skull, other (eg, chondroid lesion; aneurysmal bone cyst; lymphangioma; giant cell tumor, esp. complicating Paget's disease; malignant fibrous histiocytoma; melanotic progonoma)
23. Neurofibromatosis (eg, asterion or lambdoid suture defect; absent sphenoid wing)

(continued)

*24. Osteonecrosis of skull (eg, radiation therapy; electrical or thermal burn)
*25. Sarcoidosis
 26. Subdural hematoma (intraosseous or chronic)
*27. Syphilis
*28. Tuberculosis

* May have surrounding sclerosis.

References
1. DuBoulay GH; Principles of X-ray Diagnosis of the Skull. (ed 2) London: Butterworths, 1980, pp 57–94
2. Eisenberg RL: Skull and Spine Imaging. An Atlas of Differential Diagnosis. New York: Raven Press, 1994, pp 4–11
3. Lane B: Erosions of the skull. Radiol Clin North Am 1974;12:257–282
4. Taveras JM, Wood EH: Diagnostic Neuroradiology. (ed 2) Baltimore: Williams & Wilkins, vol 1, 1976

Gamut A-23-2

RADIOLUCENT LESION OR BONE DEFECT IN THE SKULL, SOLITARY OR MULTIPLE

CONGENITAL OR DEVELOPMENTAL DEFECT
1. Aplasia cutis congenita
2. Congenital arachnoid cyst
3. Congenital fibromatosis
4. [Craniolacunia (lacunar skull)]
5. Dermal sinus
6. Dermoid
7. Ectopic intradiploic glial tissue
8. Encephalocele; meningoencephalocele; dermal sinus; median cleft face S.; cranium bifidum
9. Epidermoid (primary cholesteatoma)
10. Fibrous dysplasia (incl. cortical)
11. Fontanelle
12. Frontal fenestra
13. Hemangioma or arteriovenous malformation of bone or scalp
14. Inioindineal canal (emissary vein canal)

15. Neurofibromatosis (eg, asterion or lambdoid suture defect; absent sphenoid wing)
16. Pacchionian granulation
17. Parietal foramina
18. Parietal thinning
19. Venous lake or diploic channel
20. Wide sutures (See A-40, 41)

TRAUMATIC
1. Burr hole; surgical defect; craniotomy
2. Fracture, simple or depressed
3. Hematoma (cephalohematoma; intradiploic; subdural); cephalohydrocele
4. Leptomeningeal cyst

INFLAMMATORY OR INFECTIOUS
1. Cholesteatoma
2. Hydatid disease
3. Mucocele of paranasal sinus
4. Osteomyelitis, bacterial or fungal; abscess
5. Sarcoidosis
6. Syphilis; yaws
7. Tuberculosis

NEOPLASTIC
1. Aneurysmal bone cyst
2. Bone sarcoma (eg, Ewing sarcoma; osteosarcoma, chondrosarcoma, fibrosarcoma)
3. Chondroid lesion
4. Chordoma of clivus
5. Giant cell tumor (esp. complicating Paget's)
6. Glomus jugulare tumor
7. Hemangioma; angiomatosis; lymphangioma
8. Intracranial tumor with erosion
9. Lymphoma; leukemia (chloroma)
10. Malignant fibrous histiocytoma
11. Melanotic progonoma
12. Meningioma
13. Metastasis (esp. from neuroblastoma or carcinoma of breast, lung, thyroid, or kidney)
14. Myeloma; plasmacytoma
15. Neoplasm of paranasal sinus or nasopharynx with direct extension

16. Neurofibroma of bone or scalp
17. Skin or scalp tumor with invasion (eg, carcinoma; rodent ulcer)

MISCELLANEOUS

1. Brown tumor of hyperparathyroidism
2. Button sequestrum (See A-22)
3. Calvarial "doughnut"; idiopathic
4. Gaucher disease; Niemann-Pick disease; Weber-Christian disease
5. Hemophilic pseudotumor
6. Langerhans cell histiocytosis$_g$ (eosinophilic granuloma; Hand-Schüller-Christian disease; Letterer-Siwe disease)
7. Infantile cortical hyperostosis (Caffey's disease)
8. Intradiploic neural heterotopia
9. Osteonecrosis (eg, radiation therapy; electrical or thermal burn; postoperative bone flap necrosis)
10. Paget's disease (osteoporosis circumscripta)
11. Parietal thinning, senile

[ ] This condition does not actually cause the gamuted imaging finding, but can produce imaging changes that simulate it.

References

1. DuBoulay GH: Principles of X-ray Diagnosis of the Skull. (ed 2) London: Butterworths, 1980
2. Eisenberg RL: Skull and Spine Imaging. An Atlas of Differential Diagnosis. New York: Raven Press, 1994, pp 4–11
3. Jacobson HG: Personal communication
4. Lane B: Erosions of the skull. Radiol Clin North Am 1974;12:257–282
5. Taveras JM, Wood EH: Diagnostic Neuroradiology. (ed 2) Baltimore: Williams & Wilkins, vol 1, 1976

Gamut A-24

SMALL SELLA TURCICA

COMMON

1. Decreased intracranial pressure (eg, cerebral atrophy; successful shunt for hydrocephalus)
2. Hypopituitarism; growth hormone deficiency
3. Normal variant

UNCOMMON

1. Cockayne S.
2. "Contracting skull" (postinflammatory or post-traumatic cerebral degeneration)
3. Deprivation (pyschosocial) dwarfism
4. Fibrous dysplasia
5. Genetic (primordial) dwarfism
6. Microcephaly (See A-2)
7. Myotonic dystrophy
8. Prader-Willi S.
9. Radiation therapy during childhood
10. Sheehan S. (postpartum pituitary necrosis)
11. Trisomy 21 S. (Down S.)
12. Vestigial or dysplastic sella

References

1. Newton TH, Potts DG: Radiology of the Skull and Brain. St. Louis: CV Mosby, 1971, vol 1, book 1, pp 371–372
2. Oh KS, Ledesma-Medina J, Bender TM: Practical Gamuts and Differential Diagnosis in Pediatric Radiology. Chicago: Year Book Medical Publ, 1982, p 8
3. Taybi H, Lachman RS: Radiology of Syndromes, Metabolic Disorders, and Skeletal Dysplasias. (ed 4) St. Louis: Mosby-Year Book, Inc., 1996, p1004

Gamut A-25-1

ABNORMAL SELLA—J-SHAPED SELLA TURCICA

COMMON

1. Hydrocephalus (mild arrested)
2. Normal variant (5% of normal children)
3. Optic chiasm glioma

UNCOMMON

1. Achondroplasia
2. Cretinism
3. Mucopolysaccharidoses (eg, Hurler S. {gargoylism}; Hunter S.; Maroteaux-Lamy S.); mucolipidoses (See J-4)

(continued)

4. Neurofibromatosis (sphenoid dysplasia)
5. Pituitary tumor extending anteriorly
6. Subarachnoid cyst (intrasellar)
7. Suprasellar tumor

Reference
1. Swischuk LE, John SD: Differential Diagnosis in Pediatric Radiology. (ed 2) Baltimore: Williams & Wilkins, 1995, pp 369–371

Gamut A-25-2

ELONGATED OR STRETCHED SELLA

1. Craniopharyngioma or other juxtasellar or suprasellar neoplasm (eg, meningioma)
2. Enlarging head (eg, storage diseases; chondrodystrophies; hydrocephalus; megalencephaly)
3. Normal variant

Reference
1. Swischuk LE, John SD: Differential Diagnosis in Pediatric Radiology. (ed 2) Baltimore: Williams & Wilkins, 1995, pp 369–371

Gamut A-25-3

OMEGA OR SCOOPED SELLA

COMMON
1. Normal (unilateral)
2. Optic chiasm tumor (glioma; neurofibroma)
3. Pituitary fossa tumor (esp. chromophobe or eosinophilic adenoma)

UNCOMMON
1. Maroteaux-Lamy S.

Reference
1. Swischuk LE, John SD: Differential Diagnosis in Pediatric Radiology. (ed 2) Baltimore: Williams & Wilkins, 1995, pp 369–371

Gamut A-25-4

DYSPLASTIC SELLA

1. Neurofibromatosis

Reference
1. Swischuk LE, John SD: Differential Diagnosis in Pediatric Radiology. (ed 2) Baltimore: Williams & Wilkins, 1995, pp 369–371

Gamut A-26

ENLARGED, ERODED, OR DESTROYED SELLA TURCICA (INCLUDING INTRASELLAR OR PARASELLAR MASS ON CT OR MRI)

COMMON
1. Aneurysm or ectatic internal carotid artery (cavernous or suprasellar segment); carotid-cavernous fistula
2. Craniopharyngioma
3. Cretinism; hypothyroidism
4. Empty sella syndrome; hypopituitarism
5. Increased intracranial pressure, chronic (eg, obstructive hydrocephalus; dilated third ventricle {aqueductal stenosis}; neoplasm; universal craniosynostosis)
6. Juxtasellar or suprasellar neoplasm, other (eg, meningioma; schwannoma of cranial nerves III to VI; optic chiasm glioma; epidermoid; dermoid; teratoma; hamartoma of tuber cinereum; hypothalamic glioma; germinoma; ectopic pinealoma)
7. [Osteoporosis; osteomalacia; hyperparathyroidism]
8. Pituitary adenoma (eg, chromophobe adenoma; eosinophilic adenoma, often with acromegaly or gigantism)

UNCOMMON
1. Abscess (pituitary)

A. Skull and Brain

2. Arachnoid cyst, suprasellar or intrasellar, congenital or acquired (eg, after intracranial bleeding, infection, or with storage disease)
3. Basilar (transsphenoid) encephalocele
4. Benign neoplasm of skull base (eg, ossifying fibroma; osteochondroma; osteoma; chondroma)
5. Chordoma
6. Frontal lobe neoplasm
7. Hypogonadism (incl. Turner S.)
8. Infundibular lesion (eg, metastasis; sarcoidosis)
9. Langerhans cell histiocytosis$_g$ (often leading to diabetes insipidus)
10. Lymphocytic hypophysitis (pituitary enlargement, usually with normal sella, in postpartum woman with thyrotoxicosis)
11. Metastasis (esp. from carcinoma of lung, breast, or kidney; melanoma)
12. Mucocele of sphenoid sinus
13. Mucopolysaccharidoses (esp. Hurler S.); mucolipidosis (See J-4)
14. Neoplasm of sphenoid sinus or nasopharynx with local invasion (eg, carcinoma; juvenile angiofibroma; giant cell tumor; osteosarcoma)
15. Neurofibromatosis
16. Optic nerve neoplasm (eg, glioma; neurofibroma; meningioma)
17. Osteomyelitis, granuloma (eg, syphilis; tuberculosis; sarcoidosis; fungus disease)
18. Oxycephaly
19. Pituitary gland hypertrophy after adrenal ablation (Nelson S.) or with hypothyroidism or primary precocious puberty
20. Pituitary neoplasm, other (eg, adenocarcinoma; carcinosarcoma; lymphoma$_g$; oncocytoma; prolactinoma; choristoma)
21. Postoperative change
22. Rathke cleft cyst

[ ] This condition does not actually cause the gamuted imaging finding, but can produce imaging changes that simulate it.

References

1. Doyle FH: Radiology of the pituitary fossa. In: Lodge T, Steiner RE (eds): Recent Advances in Radiology. New York: Churchill Livingstone, 1979, vol 6, pp 121–143
2. DuBoulay GH: Principles of X-ray Diagnosis of the Skull. (ed 2) London: Butterworths, 1980
3. Kaufman B, Chamberlin WB Jr: The "empty" sella turcica. Acta Radiol 1970; 13:413–425.
4. Lee SH, Rao KC: Cranial Computed Tomography and MRI. (ed 2) New York: McGraw-Hill, 1987, pp 453–477
5. Newton TH, Potts DG: Radiology of the Skull and Brain. St. Louis: CV Mosby, 1971, vol 1, book 1, pp 372–402
6. Sage MR, Chan ESH, Reilly PL: The clinical and radiological features of the empty sella syndrome. Clin Radiol 1980;31:513–519
7. Swischuk LE, John SD: Differential Diagnosis in Pediatric Radiology. (ed 2) Baltimore: Williams & Wilkins, 1995, p 368
8. Taybi H, Lachman RS: Radiology of Syndromes, Metabolic Disorders, and Skeletal Dysplasias. (ed 4) St. Louis: Mosby-Year Book, Inc., 1996, p 1004
9. Taveras JM, Wood EH: Diagnostic Neuroradiology. (ed 2) Baltimore: Williams & Wilkins, 1976, vol 1, pp 65–89
10. Teasdale E, et al: The reliability of radiology in detecting prolactin secreting pituitary microadenomas. Br J Radiol 1981;54:556–571
11. Tindall GT, Hoffman JC Jr: Evaluation of the abnormal sella turcica. Arch Intern Med 1980; 140:1078–1083

Gamut A-27

EROSION OF THE SPHENOID WING

COMMON

1. [Congenital defect, isolated or with neurofibromatosis]
*2. Meningioma

UNCOMMON

1. Benign bone neoplasm (eg, chondroma; giant cell tumor)
2. Chordoma
*3. Craniopharyngioma
4. Expansion of middle fossa (See A-69)
*5. Glioma (eg, optic)
6. Increased intracranial pressure, chronic
7. Langerhans cell histiocytosis$_g$
8. Metastasis

(continued)

9. Parasellar aneurysm of internal carotid artery
10. Pituitary tumor (esp. chromophobe adenoma)
11. Plexiform neurofibroma

* Lesser wing erosion; other lesions listed involve the greater wing.

[ ] This condition does not actually cause the gamuted imaging finding, but can produce imaging changes that simulate it.

References

1. DuBoulay GH: Principles of X-ray Diagnosis of the Skull. (ed 2) London: Butterworths, 1980.
2. Hasso A, Vignaud J, La Masters DL: Pathology of the skull base and vault. In: Newton TH, Hasso AN, Dillon WP (eds): Modern Neuroradiology, vol 3. Computed Tomography of the Head and Neck. New York: Raven Press, 1988, pp 3.1–3.26

Gamut A-28

EROSION OF THE PETROUS RIDGE, PYRAMID, OR APEX

COMMON

1. Acoustic schwannoma
2. Bone neoplasm, benign or malignant (eg, chondroma; hemangioma; osteoblastoma; chordoma)
3. Cholesteatoma, acquired or congenital (epidermoid)
4. Cholesterol granuloma
*5. Metastasis (esp. breast, lung, kidney)

UNCOMMON

*1. Aneurysm of intracavernous or intrapetrous carotid artery
*2. Carcinoma of external auditory meatus
3. Glioma
*4. Glomus jugulare tumor
5. Langerhans cell histiocytosis_g
6. Leptomeningeal cyst
7. Lymphoma_g
8. Malignant neoplasm of nasopharynx (invasive)
9. Meningioma of Meckel's cave

10. Osteomyelitis; apical petrositis (Gradenigo S.)
*11. Rhabdomyosarcoma (child)
12. Schwannoma of V, IX, or X nerve
*13. Tuberculosis

* Middle ear lesion.

References

1. Chapman S, Nakielny R: Aids to Radiological Differential Diagnosis (ed 3) London: WB Saunders, pp 386–387
2. DuBoulay GH: Principles of X-ray Diagnosis of the Skull. (ed 2) London: Butterworths, 1980, pp 193–195
3. Livingstone PA: Differential diagnosis of radiolucent lesions of the temporal bone. Radiol Clin North Am 1974; 12:571–583
4. Newton TH, Potts DG: Radiology of the Skull and Brain. St. Louis: CV Mosby, 1971, vol 1, book 1, pp 424, 447
5. Phelps PD, Lloyd GAS: The radiology of carcinoma of the ear. Br J Radiol 1981;54:103–109
6. Phelps PD, Wright A: Imaging cholesteatoma. Clin Radiol 1990;41:156–162

Gamut A-29

EROSION OR WIDENING OF THE INTERNAL AUDITORY MEATUS

COMMON

1. Acoustic schwannoma
2. [Normal patulous canal]

UNCOMMON

1. Cholesteatoma, inflammatory or congenital (epidermoid)
2. Cyst
3. Glioma of brain stem
4. Increased intracranial pressure; chronic hydrocephalus
5. Meningioma of cerebellopontine angle or petrous apex
6. Metastasis
7. Neurofibromatosis
8. Schwannoma of V or VII nerve

9. Vascular lesion (eg, aneurysm of internal auditory canal artery; arteriovenous malformation; hemangioma)

[ ] This condition does not actually cause the gamuted imaging finding, but can produce imaging changes that simulate it.

References
1. Dubois PJ: Neuro-otology. In: Rosenberg RN (ed): The Clinical Neurosciences. New York: Churchill Livingstone, 1984, vol 4, p 672
2. DuBoulay CH: Principles of X-ray Diagnosis of the Skull (ed 2) London: Butterworths, 1980, pp 186–193
3. Newton TH, Potts DG: Radiology of the Skull and Brain. St. Louis: CV Mosby, 1971, vol 1, book 1, pp 442–446

Gamut A-30

DENSE TEMPORAL BONE LESION

COMMON
1. Fibrous dysplasia
2. Mastoiditis, chronic sclerotic

UNCOMMON
1. Congenital bone dysplasia (eg, osteopetrosis; pyknodysostosis; craniometaphyseal dysplasia)
2. Ossifying fibroma
3. Osteoblastic metastasis
4. Osteosarcoma
5. Otodystrophies (See B-25, B-34)
6. Paget's disease (treated)

Reference
1. Unger JM: Handbook of Head and Neck Imaging. New York: Churchill Livingstone, 1987, pp 160–161

Gamut A-31

NEOPLASM INVOLVING THE TEMPORAL BONE

BENIGN
COMMON
1. Acoustic schwannoma (VIII nerve)
2. [Cholesterol granuloma]
3. Epidermoid (congenital cholesteatoma)
4. [Langerhans cell histiocytosis$_g$ (esp. eosinophilic granuloma)]

UNCOMMON
1. Adenoma (soft tissue); ceruminous gland tumor of external auditory canal
2. Exostosis of external auditory canal
3. Giant cell tumor
4. Glomus jugulare tumor; glomus tympanicum tumor
5. Hemangioma
6. Meningioma
7. Osteoma (cancellous or compact)
8. Schwannoma of V, VII, IX, X, XI, or XII nerve

[ ] This condition does not actually cause the gamuted imaging finding, but can produce imaging changes that simulate it.

MALIGNANT
COMMON
1. Metastasis (esp. from carcinoma of breast, lung, prostate, or kidney; or melanoma) or local extension from parotid carcinoma

UNCOMMON
1. Carcinoma of external auditory canal or rarely the middle ear
2. Lymphoma$_g$; leukemia
3. Myeloma
4. Sarcoma (eg, rhabdomyosarcoma; fibrosarcoma; lymphosarcoma; osteosarcoma; chondrosarcoma; undifferentiated sarcoma)

(continued)

References
1. Unger JM: Handbook of Head and Neck Imaging. New York: Churchill Livingstone, 1987, pp 146–152
2. Valvassori GE, Buckingham RA, Carter BL, Hanafee WN, Mafee MF: Head and Neck Imaging: New York: Thieme Medical Publ, 1988, pp 120–144

Gamut A-32

SMALL OR IRREGULAR FORAMEN MAGNUM

1. Bilateral or unilateral occipitalization (fusion) of C1 to base of skull
2. Chondrodystrophies
   a. Achondroplasia
   b. Achondrogenesis, types I and II
   c. Diastrophic dysplasia
   d. Hypochondroplasia
   e. Metatropic dysplasia
   f. Thanatophoric dysplasia

References
1. Swischuk LE, John SD: Differential Diagnosis in Pediatric Radiology. (ed 2) Baltimore: Williams & Wilkins, 1995, p 371
2. Taybi H, Lachman RS: Radiology of Syndromes, Metabolic Disorders, and Skeletal Dysplasias. (ed 4) St. Louis: Mosby-Year Book, Inc., 1996, p 1002

Gamut A-33

ENLARGED FORAMEN MAGNUM

COMMON

1. Arnold-Chiari malformation
2. Cervical-occipital meningocele or encephalocele
3. Dandy-Walker cyst; other posterior fossa cysts
4. Surgical decompression

UNCOMMON

1. Frontometaphyseal dysplasia
2. Hydrolethalus S.
3. Hypophosphatasia
4. Neoplasm of posterior fossa or upper cervical spine
5. Rubinstein-Taybi S.
6. Syringobulbia

References
1. Swischuk LE, John SD: Differential Diagnosis in Pediatric Radiology. (ed 2) Baltimore: Williams & Wilkins, 1995, p 371
2. Taybi H, Lachman RS: Radiology of Syndromes, Metabolic Disorders, and Skeletal Dysplasias. (ed 4) St. Louis: Mosby-Year Book, Inc., 1996, p 1002

Gamut A-34-S

SKULL AND FACIAL BONES OF MEMBRANOUS ORIGIN

1. Facial bones, including mandible
2. Frontal bone
3. Occipital bone (upper squamosa)
4. Parietal bone
5. Pterygoid (medial plate)
6. Temporal hone (squamosal and tympanic parts)
7. Vomer

Reference
1. Greenfield GB: Radiology of Bone Diseases. (ed 5) Philadelphia: Lippincott, 1990

Gamut A-35-S1

NORMAL SKULL VARIANTS

COMMON

1. Arterial groove (eg, middle meningeal)
2. [Artifact (eg, hair braid; rubber band; skin fold; EEG paste; surgical tape or dressing; skin laceration with air trapping)]
3. Convolutional impressions
4. Crista galli
5. Dural sinus (eg, transverse or sigmoid sinus)
6. Emissary vein; venous lake; diploic channel; sinus groove; other prominent vascular markings
7. Fontanelle
8. Frontal crest
9. Infantile J-shaped sella turcica
10. Metopic suture; mendosal suture
11. Pacchionian granulation
12. Sutural (wormian) bones; interparietal sutures; atypical suture line
13. Torcular Herophili

UNCOMMON

1. Cruciate ridge
2. Inioindineal canal
3. Interparietal bone
4. Kerckring bone (process)
5. Occipital fissure (superior, inferior longitudinal fissure); posterior parietal fissure
6. Parietal foramina
7. Parietal thinning
8. Unfused planum sphenoidale

[ ] This condition does not actually cause the gamuted imaging finding, but can produce imaging changes that simulate it.

References

1. Swischuk LE: The normal pediatric skull: Variations and artifacts. Radiol Clin North Am 1972;10:227–290
2. Tomsick TA: Gamut: Normal skull variant that may simulate a fracture. Semin Roentgenol 1978;13:3

Gamut A-35-S2

NORMAL SKULL VARIANTS THAT MAY SIMULATE A FRACTURE

1. Arterial groove (eg, meningeal vessels; middle temporal branch of superficial temporal artery; deep temporal branches of internal maxillary artery; supraorbital artery)
2. Artifact or soft tissue alteration (eg, skin laceration; skin fold; air trapped beneath skin; matted hair; hair braid; rubber band; tape; dressing; linen)
3. Emissary vein; venous lake; diploic channel; sinus groove
4. Fissure; synchondrosis; suture
    a. Cerebellar synchondrosis
    b. Coronal suture
    c. Innominate synchondrosis
    d. Interparietal suture
    e. Intersphenoid synchondrosis
    f. Lambdoid suture
    g. Lateral fissures of the foramen magnum
    h. Lateral interparietal fissure
    i. Lateral sphenoidal suture
    j. Median occipital fissure
    k. Mendosal suture
    l. Metopic suture
    m. Occipitomastoid suture
    n. Parietal fissure
    o. Parietomastoid suture
    p. Spheno-occipital synchondrosis
    q. Squamosal suture
    r. Transverse occipital suture
    s. Unfused planum sphenoidale
5. Wormian (sutural) bone

References

1. Allen WE, Kier EL, Rothman SLG: Pitfalls in the evaluation of skull trauma. Radiol Clin North Am 1973;11: 479–503
2. Keats TE: Atlas of Normal Roentgen Variants That May Simulate Disease. (ed 4) Chicago: Year Book Medical Publ, 1988

(continued)

3. Swischuk LE: The normal pediatric skull: Variations and ar-tifacts. Radiol Clin North Am 1972;10:277–290
4. Tomsick TA: Gamut: Normal skull variant that may simu-late a fracture. Semin Roentgenol 1978;13:3

Gamut A-36

MULTIPLE WORMIAN (SUTURAL) BONES

COMMON

1. Cleidocranial dysplasia
2. Cretinism; hypothyroidism
3. Hypophosphatasia
4. Normal up to 6 months of age; idiopathic
5. Osteogenesis imperfecta
6. Progeria
7. Pyknodysostosis

UNCOMMON

1. Acrogeria
2. Aminopterin fetopathy
3. Aplasia cutis congenita (Adams-Oliver S.)
4. Chondrodysplasia punctata (Conradi-Hönermann type)
5. Familial idiopathic osteoarthropathy (Currarino S.)
6. Geroderma osteodysplastica
7. Hajdu-Cheney S. (idiopathic acro-osteolysis)
8. Hallermann-Streiff S. (oculo-mandibulo-facial S.)
9. Hydrocephalus (infantile)
10. Infantile multisystem inflammatory disease (NOMID)
11. Mandibuloacral dysplasia
12. Menkes S. (kinky-hair S.); copper deficiency
13. Metaphyseal chondrodysplasia (Jansen type)
14. Osteopetrosis, infantile type; sclerosteosis
15. Otopalatodigital S.
16. Pachydermoperiostosis
17. Prader-Willi S.
18. Schinzel-Giedion S.
19. Trisomy 21 S. (Down S.)
20. Zellweger S. (cerebrohepatorenal S.)

References

1. Cremin B, Goodman H, Spranger J, Beighton P: Wormian bones in osteogenesis imperfecta and other disorders. Skele-tal Radiol 1982; 8:35–38
2. Greenfield GB: Radiology of Bone Diseases. (ed 5) Philadelphia: Lippincott, 1990
3. Kozlowski K, Beighton P: Gamut Index of Skeletal Dys-plasias. Berlin: Springer-Verlag, 1984, pp. 35–36
4. Pryles CV, Khan AJ: Wormian bones. Am J Dis Child 1979;133:380–382
5. Swischuk LE, John SD: Differential Diagnosis in Pediatric Radiology. (ed 2) Baltimore: Williams & Wilkins, 1995, p 374
6. Taybi H, Lachman RS: Radiology of Syndromes, Metabolic Disorders, and Skeletal Dysplasias. (ed 4) St. Louis: Mosby-Year Book, Inc., 1996, p 1006

Gamut A-37

DELAYED OR DEFECTIVE CRANIAL OSSIFICATION

TRANSIENT
(Spontaneous correction before 3 years of age)

1. Aminopterin fetopathy
2. Aplasia cutis congenita (congenital scalp defect— may *not* correct)
3. Craniolacunia (lacunar skull)
4. Cutis laxa; Ehlers-Danlos S.
5. Hypophosphatasia
6. Menkes S. (kinky-hair S.)
7. Metaphyseal chondrodysplasia (Jansen type)
8. Mucopolysaccharidoses (eg, Hunter S.; Hurler S.; Maroteaux-Lamy S.) (See J-4)
9. Osteogenesis imperfecta (does *not* often correct before age 3)
10. Rubinstein-Taybi S.
11. Silver-Russell S.
12. Trisomy 13 S.
13. Trisomy 18 S.
14. Trisomy 21 S. (Down S.)
15. Zellweger S. (cerebrohepatorenal S.)

INTERMEDIATE
(Spontaneous correction between 3 and 10 years)
1. Cretinism; hypothyroidism
2. Osteogenesis imperfecta
3. Otopalatodigital S.
4. Pachydermoperiostosis
5. Progeria
6. Rickets

PROTRACTED
(Persistence beyond 10 years of age)
1. Cleidocranial dysplasia
2. Cranium bifidum occultum
3. Cretinism; hypothyroidism
4. Dermal sinus
5. Encephalocele
6. Frontonasal dysplasia (median cleft face S.)
7. Hallermann-Streiff S. (oculo-mandibulo-facial S.)
8. Hypertelorism with Sprengel's deformity
9. Parietal foramina; occipital foramina
10. Parietal thinning
11. Pyknodysostosis
12. Stanescu dysostosis
13. Tubular stenosis (Kenny-Caffey S.)

LETHAL ENTITIES WITH DEFECTIVE CRANIAL OSSIFICATION
1. Achondrogenesis, type I
2. Fibrochondrogenesis
3. Hypochondrogenesis
4. Hypophosphatasia (prenatal form; severe congenital form)
5. Short rib-polydactyly S., type I (Saldino-Noonan S.)

References
1. Campbell JB: Personal communication.
2. Dorst JP: Personal communication.

SMALL ANTERIOR FONTANELLE

1. Craniosynostosis, primary
2. Craniosynostosis, secondary (eg, chronic anemia$_g$; rickets; hypophosphatasia)
3. Premature closure of sutures (eg, cerebral atrophy; decreased intracranial pressure due to shunted hydrocephalus)
4. Normal variant

Reference
1. Swischuk LE, John SD: Differential Diagnosis in Pediatric Radiology. (ed 2) Baltimore: Williams & Wilkins, 1995, pp 373–374

CONGENITAL SYNDROMES AND BONE DYSPLASIAS WITH LARGE ANTERIOR FONTANELLE OR DELAYED CLOSURE OF FONTANELLES

COMMON
1. Cleidocranial dysplasia
2. Cranium bifidum with lacunar skull
3. Cretinism; hypothyroidism
4. Intrauterine growth retardation (IUGR) or prenatal infection (eg, fetal rubella S.)
5. Normal (esp. in premature)
6. Osteogenesis imperfecta
7. Rickets, severe
8. Trisomy 21 S. (Down S.)

UNCOMMON
1. Aase S.
2. Aminopterin fetopathy
3. Aplasia cutis congenita (congenital scalp defects)
4. Chondrodysplasia punctata

(continued)

5. Coffin-Lowry S.
6. Cutis laxa, type II; occipital horn S.
7. Familial idiopathic osteoarthropathy (Currarino S.)
8. Fetal hydantoin S. (Dilantin embryopathy)
9. Fetal primidone S.
10. Frontonasal dysplasia (median cleft face S.)
11. G syndrome
12. GAPO S.
13. Greig cephalopolysyndactyly S.
14. Hallermann-Streiff S. (oculo-mandibulo-facial S.)
15. Hypochondroplasia
16. Hypophosphatasia
17. Infantile multisystem inflammatory disease (NOMID)
18. Lenz-Majewski dysplasia (hyperostotic dwarfism)
19. Microcephalic osteodysplastic dysplasia
20. Oculo-auriculo-vertebral spectrum (Goldenhar S.)
21. Opitz BBBG syndrome (hypertelorism-hypospadias S.)
22. Opsismodysplasia
23. Osteodysplasty (Melnick-Needles S.)
24. Otopalatodigital S., types I and II
25. Progeria
26. Pyknodysostosis
27. Rubinstein-Taybi S.
28. Schinzel-Giedion S.
29. Silver-Russell S.
30. Trisomy 13 S.
31. Trisomy 18 S.
32. Tubular stenosis dysplasia (Kenny-Caffey S.)
33. Winchester S.
34. Yunis-Varon S.
35. Zellweger S. (cerebrohepatorenal S.)

References
1. Dorst J: Radiological Society of North America Scientific Exhibit, 1972.
2. Felson B (ed): Dwarfs and other little people. Semin Roentgenol 1973;8:133–136
3. Girdany BR, Blank E: Anterior fontanelle bones. AJR 1965;95:148–153
4. Jones KL: Smith's Recognizable Patterns of Human Malformation. (ed 5) Philadelphia: WB Saunders, 1997, pp 778–779
5. Philip AGS: Fontanel size and epiphyseal ossification in neonates with intrauterine growth retardation. J Pediatr 1974;84:204–207
6. Swischuk LE, John SD: Differential Diagnosis in Pediatric Radiology. (ed 2) Baltimore: Williams & Wilkins, 1995, pp 373–374
7. Taybi H, Lachman RS: Radiology of Syndromes, Metabolic Disorders, and Skeletal Dysplasias. (ed 4) St. Louis: Mosby-Year Book, Inc., 1996, p 1002

Gamut A-40

DELAYED CLOSURE, WIDE, AND/OR INCOMPLETE OSSIFICATION OF SUTURES

COMMON
1. Cleidocranial dysplasia
2. Cretinism; hypothyroidism
3. Dandy-Walker S.
4. Hydrocephalus
5. Increased intracranial pressure (esp. brain neoplasm)
6. Infiltration of sutures (eg, metastatic neuroblastoma; leukemia)
7. Intrauterine growth retardation (IUGR) or prenatal infection (eg, fetal rubella S.)
8. Normal; prematurity
9. Osteogenesis imperfecta
10. Osteoporosis, severe
11. Rickets
12. Trisomy 21 S. (Down S.)

UNCOMMON
1. Acrogeria
2. Aminopterin fetopathy
3. Cranium bifidum
4. Diencephalic S.
5. Deprivation (pyschosocial) dwarfism
6. Familial idiopathic osteoarthropathy (Currarino S.)
7. Fetal primidone S.
8. Hajdu-Cheney S. (idiopathic acro-osteolysis)
9. Hallermann-Streiff S. (oculo-mandibulo-facial S.)
10. Hydrolethalus S.

11. Hyperparathyroidism, primary infantile or secondary (renal osteodystrophy)
12. Hypoparathyroidism
13. Hypophosphatasia
14. Laron S. (pituitary dwarfism II); growth hormone deficiency
15. Mandibuloacral dysplasia
16. Neurofibromatosis (bone defect along lambdoid suture)
17. Pachydermoperiostosis
18. Progeria
19. Prolonged parenteral hyperalimentation
20. Pseudotumor cerebri
21. Pyknodysostosis
22. Rubinstein-Taybi S.
23. Schinzel-Giedion S.
24. Silver-Russell S.
25. Trisomy 13 S.
26. Trisomy 18 S.
27. Vitamin A deficiency or intoxication
28. Winchester S.
29. Zellweger S. (cerebrohepatorenal S.)

References
1. Afshani E, Osman M, Girdany BR: Widening of cranial sutures in children with deprivational dwarfism. Radiology 1973;109:141–144
2. Newton TH, Potts DG: Radiology of the Skull and Brain. St. Louis: CV Mosby, 1971, vol 1, book 1, pp 232–236
3. Swischuk LE, John SD: Differential Diagnosis in Pediatric Radiology. (ed 2) Baltimore: Williams & Wilkins, 1995, pp 359–361
4. Taybi H, Lachman RS: Radiology of Syndromes, Metabolic Disorders, and Skeletal Dysplasias. (ed 4) St. Louis: Mosby-Year Book, Inc., 1996, pp 1005–1006

SEPARATION OR INFILTRATION OF SKULL SUTURES IN AN INFANT OR CHILD (See A-40)

COMMON
1. Brain abscess; cerebritis
2. Brain tumor (eg, pinealoma; medulloblastoma)
3. Cerebral edema, hemorrhage, or contusion
4. Hydrocephalus (See A-114); hydranencephaly
5. Incomplete ossification adjacent to sutures (See A-40)
6. Increased intracranial pressure, other causes (See A-113)
7. Lead poisoning; other encephalopathy
8. Leukemia; lymphoma$_g$
9. Meningitis; meningoencephalitis
10. Neuroblastoma, metastatic
11. Normal (esp. prematurity)
12. Subdural hematoma or hygroma
13. Trauma; intracranial injury

UNCOMMON
1. Hydranencephaly
2. Hypervitaminosis A encephalopathy
3. Intracranial cyst, large
4. Megalencephaly
5. Pseudotumor cerebri
6. Rebound growth of brain and body after treatment for hypothyroidism or deprivation (pyschosocial) dwarfism

References
1. Lippe B, Hensen L, Mendoza G, et al: Chronic vitamin A intoxication. Am J Dis Child 1981;135:634–636
2. Swischuk LE, John SD: Differential Diagnosis in Pediatric Radiology. (ed 2) Baltimore: Williams & Wilkins, 1995, pp 359–361
3. Swischuk LE: The growing skull. Semin Roentgenol 1974; 9:115–124
4. Weisberg LA, Chutorian AM: Pseudotumor cerebri of childhood. Am J Dis Child 1977;131:1243–1248

Gamut A-42

DECREASED OR ABSENT CONVOLUTIONAL MARKINGS

COMMON

1. Cerebral atrophy
2. Normal to age 3 years
3. Shunted hydrocephalus

UNCOMMON

1. Cretinism; hypothyroidism
2. Deprivation (pyschosocial) dwarfism
3. Failure to thrive, severe

Reference
1. Swischuk LE, John SD: Differential Diagnosis in Pediatric Radiology. (ed 2) Baltimore: Williams & Wilkins, 1995, p 365

Gamut A-43

INCREASED CONVOLUTIONAL (DIGITAL) MARKINGS

COMMON

1. Craniosynostosis, primary (localized or universal, incl. cloverleaf skull {kleeblattschädel anomaly})
2. Increased intracranial pressure, chronic (eg, brain tumor; cyst; hydrocephalus) (See A-113,114)
3. [Lacunar skull (craniolacunia; luckensch^adel)]
4. Normal

UNCOMMON

1. Craniometaphyseal dysplasia
2. Craniosynostosis, secondary (eg, healing rickets, hypophosphatasia; hypercalcemia; hyperthyroidism; chronic anemia$_g$—esp. thalassemia)

[ ] This condition does not actually cause the gamuted imaging finding, but can produce imaging changes that simulate it.

Reference
1. Swischuk LE, John SD: Differential Diagnosis in Pediatric Radiology. (ed 2) Baltimore: Williams & Wilkins, 1995, pp 363–365

Gamut A-44

INCREASED SIZE OF THE VASCULAR GROOVES OF THE SKULL

COMMON

1. Arteriovenous malformation
2. Hemangioma of skull
3. Meningioma
4. Normal variant

UNCOMMON

1. Collateral circulation (eg, thrombosis of a venous sinus; occlusion of internal carotid artery)
2. Fibrous dysplasia
3. Metastasis (eg, from carcinoma of thyroid or kidney)
4. Pacchionian granulations
5. Paget's disease
6. Sarcoma or other malignant neoplasm of skull

Reference
1. Keats TE: Atlas of Normal Roentgen Variants. (ed 6) St. Louis: Mosby, 1996, pp 8–10

Gamut A-45-1

GENERALIZED "HAIR ON END" PATTERN IN THE SKULL

COMMON

1. Congenital hemolytic anemias$_g$ (thalassemia; sickle cell disease; spherocytosis; elliptocytosis)

UNCOMMON

1. Cyanotic congenital heart disease with secondary polycythemia
2. Hypernephroma with increased erythropoiesis
3. Iron deficiency anemia, severe
4. Leukemia; lymphoma$_g$
5. Multiple myeloma
6. Polycythemia vera
7. Red cell enzyme deficiencies with secondary reticulocytosis (eg, pyruvate kinase, hexokinase, glucose-6–phosphate dehydrogenase)

References

1. Greenfield GB: Radiology of Bone Diseases. (ed 5) Philadelphia: Lippincott, 1990
2. Kohler A, Zimmer EA: Borderlands of the Normal and Early Pathologic in Skeletal Radiology. New York: Grune & Stratton, 1968, p 202
3. Silverman FN, Kuhn JP: Caffey's Pediatric X-ray Diagnosis. (ed 9) St. Louis: Mosby, 1993, pp 57–70
4. Swischuk LE, John SD: Differential Diagnosis in Pediatric Radiology. (ed 2) Baltimore: Williams & Wilkins, 1995
5. Wilson JD, et al: Harrison's Principles of Internal Medicine. (ed 12) New York: McGraw-Hill, 1991

Gamut A-45-2

LOCALIZED "SUNBURST" PATTERN IN THE SKULL

COMMON

1. Hemangioma
2. Meningioma
3. Metastasis (esp. neuroblastoma; carcinoma of prostate or breast)

UNCOMMON

1. Ewing sarcoma
2. Osteosarcoma

References

1. Greenfield GB: Radiology of Bone Diseases. (ed 5) Philadelphia: Lippincott, 1990

2. Silverman FN, Kuhn JP: Caffey's Pediatric X-ray Diagnosis. (ed 9) St. Louis: Mosby, 1993, pp 57–70
3. Swischuk LE, John SD: Differential Diagnosis in Pediatric Radiology. (ed 2) Baltimore: Williams & Wilkins, 1995

Gamut A-46

SOLITARY INTRACRANIAL CALCIFICATION (SEE A-47)

COMMON

1. Arteriosclerosis (esp. carotid siphon)
2. [Artifact; foreign body; calcified sebaceous cyst]
3. Chordoma
4. Choroid plexus
5. Craniopharyngioma
6. Dura (eg, falx; tentorium; superior sagittal sinus)
7. Glioma (eg, low-grade astrocytoma; oligodendroglioma)
8. Habenular commissure
9. Hemangioma; arteriovenous malformation; Sturge-Weber S.
10. Idiopathic
11. Interclinoid ligament (diaphragma sellae)
12. [Skull neoplasm (eg, osteoma; chondroma; osteochondroma; osteosarcoma; chondrosarcoma)]
13. Petroclinoid ligament
14. Pineal gland
15. Tuberculosis (eg, tuberculoma; healed meningitis)

UNCOMMON

1. Aneurysm (incl. vein of Galen "aneurysm")
2. Arachnoid (pacchionian) granulation
3. Basal ganglia; dentate nucleus
4. Choroid plexus papilloma
5. Dermoid; teratoma
6. Encephalitis; meningitis; brain abscess (healed)
7. Ependymoma
8. Epidermoid
9. Fungus disease (esp. cryptococcosis {torulosis}; coccidioidomycosis; zygomycosis {mucormycosis})

(continued)

10. Granuloma (congenital cerebral)
11. Hamartoma
12. Hemangioma
13. Hematoma, chronic (eg, intracerebral; subdural; epidural)
14. Hypophysis
15. [Iatrogenic (eg, contrast medium injection into an abscess or cyst)]
16. Infarct, cerebral
17. Lipoma of corpus callosum
18. Meningioma
19. Metastatic neoplasm (eg, from osteosarcoma; mucinous adenocarcinoma of colon)
20. Parasitic cyst (eg, hydatid; *Cysticercus; Paragonimus*)
21. Pinealoma (eg, germinoma; teratoma)
22. Pituitary adenoma (esp. chromophobe)
23. Pituitary "stone"
24. Porencephalic cyst (porencephaly)
25. Radiation necrosis
26. Scarring; gliosis
27. Schwannoma; neurofibroma
28. Syphilitic gumma
29. Tuberous sclerosis

[ ] This condition does not actually cause the gamuted imaging finding, but can produce imaging changes that simulate it.

References

1. Dähnert W: Radiology Review Manual. (ed 4) Baltimore: Williams & Wilkins, 1999, pp 189–190
2. DuBoulay GH: Principles of X-ray Diagnosis of the Skull (ed 2) London: Butterworths, 1980, pp 244–283
3. Eisenberg RL: Clinical Imaging: An Atlas of Differential Diagnosis. (ed 3) Philadelphia: Lippincott-Raven, 1997, pp 1002–1011
4. Newton TH, Potts DG: Radiology of the Skull and Brain. St. Louis: CV Mosby, 1971, vol 1, book 2, pp 823–873
5. Swischuk LE, John SD: Differential Diagnosis in Pediatric Radiology. (ed 2) Baltimore: Williams & Wilkins, 1995
6. Teplick JG, Haskin ME: Roentgenologic Diagnosis. (ed 3) Philadelphia: WB Saunders, 1976, vol 2

MULTIPLE INTRACRANIAL CALCIFICATIONS (SEE A-46, 49)

COMMON

1. Atherosclerosis (esp. carotid artery siphon)
2. Idiopathic
3. Physiologic (eg, dura {falx, tentorium, superior sagittal sinus}; petroclinoid and interclinoid ligament {diaphragma sellae}; choroid plexi; pineal gland; habenula)

UNCOMMON

1. AIDS with opportunistic infections (eg, toxoplasmosis)
2. Arteriovenous malformation; aneurysms; hemangiomas; Sturge-Weber S.; von Hippel-Lindau disease
3. Basal ganglia (eg, hypoparathyroidism; pseudo-hypoparathyroidism; Fahr disease) (See A-49)
4. Brain abscesses (healed)
5. Calcinosis, metastatic
6. Carbon monoxide intoxication
7. Cockayne S.
8. Encephalitis, viral (eg, congenital transplacental infection*—fetal rubella S.; cytomegalovirus infection; fetal herpes simplex infection); measles; chickenpox; poliomyelitis
9. Folic acid deficiency
10. Fungus disease with basal arachnoiditis (eg, cryptococcosis {torulosis}; coccidioidomycosis; zygomycosis {mucormycosis})
11. Gorlin S. (nevoid basal cell carcinoma S.) (falx; tentorium)
12. Hematomas, old (eg, intracerebral; subdural; epidural)
13. Homocystinuria
14. Hyperparathyroidism, primary or secondary (renal osteodystrophy); renal failure (vascular calcifications)
15. Hypervitaminosis D (dura; pineal gland)

16. [Iatrogenic (eg, Pantopaque or other contrast medium residual)]
17. Lead poisoning
18. Leukemia (treated)
19. Lipoid proteinosis (hyalinosis cutis)
20. Lissencephaly syndromes (congenital agyria) (Miller-Dieker S.)
21. Listeriosis
22. Methotrexate therapy for childhood leukemia
23. Needle-tracks following ventriculography
24. Neoplasms, multiple (eg, meningiomas; gliomas; metastases)
25. Neurofibromatosis (choroid plexi)
26. Parasitic disease (eg, cysticercosis; paragonimiasis; hydatid disease)
27. Pseudoxanthoma elasticum
28. [Scalp (eg, sebaceous cysts; cysticercosis; foreign bodies; EEG paste)]
29. Scarring; gliosis (eg, postradiation therapy; old birth trauma or other injuries)
30. Toxoplasmosis*
31. Tuberculomas; tuberculous meningitis (treated)
32. Tuberous sclerosis
33. Williams S. (idiopathic hypercalcemia) (falx, tentorium)
34. Wilson's disease

* Newborn infantile brain calcifications which can be seen on ultrasound.

[ ] This condition does not actually cause the gamuted imaging finding, but can produce imaging changes that simulate it.

References
1. Babbitt DP, Tang T, Dobbs J, et al: Idiopathic familial cerebrovascular ferrocalcinosis (Fahr's disease) and review of differential diagnosis of intracranial calcification in children. AJR 1969;105:352–358
2. Bentson JR, Wilson GH, Helmer E, et al: Computed tomography in intracranial cysticercosis. J Comput Assist Tomogr 1977;4:464–471
3. DuBoulay CH: Principles of X-ray Diagnosis of the Skull. (ed 2) London: Butterworths, 1980, pp 244–283
4. Eisenberg RL: Clinical Imaging: An Atlas of Differential Diagnosis. (ed 3) Philadelphia: Lippincott-Raven, 1997, pp 1012–1017
5. Kumpe DA, Rao CV, Garcia JH, et al: Intracranial neurosarcoidosis. J Comput Assist Tomogr 1979;3:324–330
6. Newton TH, Potts DG: Radiology of the Skull and Brain. St. Louis: CV Mosby, 1971, vol 1, book 2, pp 823–873
7. Reyes PF, et al: Intracranial calcification in adults with chronic lead exposure. AJR 1986; 146:267–270
8. Schubiger O, Valavanis A, Hayek J: Computed tomography in cerebral aneurysms with special emphasis on giant intracranial aneurysms. J Comput Assist Tomogr 1980;1: 24–32
9. Swischuk LE, John SD: Differential Diagnosis in Pediatric Radiology. (ed 2) Baltimore: Williams & Wilkins, 1995
10. Taybi H, Lachman RS: Radiology of Syndromes, Metabolic Disorders, and Skeletal Dysplasias. (ed 4) St. Louis: Mosby-Year Book, Inc., 1996, pp 1013–1014
11. Teplick JG, Haskin ME: Roentgenologic Diagnosis. (ed 3) Philadelphia: WB Saunders, 1976

SELLAR OR PARASELLAR CALCIFICATION

COMMON
1. Aneurysm of a cerebral artery (eg, giant internal carotid aneurysm; circle of Willis; basilar artery)
2. Atherosclerosis of internal carotid artery siphon in cavernous sinus
3. Craniopharyngioma
4. Normal (petroclinoid or interclinoid ligament-diaphragma sellae)

UNCOMMON
1. Arteriovenous malformation
2. Dermoid
3. Ectopic pinealoma; teratoma
4. Hyperparathyroidism (vascular calcification)
5. Meningioma
6. Optic chiasm glioma (rare)
7. Skull neoplasm (eg, chordoma; osteochondroma; chondroma; osteoma)
8. Pituitary adenoma (esp. chromophobe)
9. Pituitary "stone" in otherwise normal pituitary gland
10. Tuberculous meningitis, healed; granuloma

(continued)

References
1. DuBoulay GH: Principles of X-ray Diagnosis of the Skull. (ed 2) London: Butterworths, 1980
2. Eisenberg RL: Clinical Imaging: An Atlas of Differential Diagnosis. (ed 3) Philadelphia: Lippincott-Raven, 1997, pp 1018–1021

Gamut A-49

BASAL GANGLIA CALCIFICATION

COMMON

1. Hypoparathyroidism; pseudohypoparathyroidism
2. Idiopathic; normal variant; physiologic with aging

UNCOMMON

1. AIDS encephalopathy
2. Atherosclerosis
3. Birth anoxia, hypoxia
4. Carbonic anhydrase II deficiency
5. Carbon monoxide intoxication
6. Cockayne S.
7. Fahr disease (ferrocalcinosis)
8. Familial idiopathic symmetrical basal ganglia calcification and microcephaly
9. Hallervorden-Spatz disease
10. Hemorrhage
11. Hyperparathyroidism
12. Hypothyroidism; cretinism
13. Idiopathic lenticulodentate calcification (Hastings-James S.)
14. Kearns-Sayre S.
15. Lead encephalopathy
16. Lipoid proteinosis (hyalinosis cutis)
17. MELAS syndrome
18. Methotrexate therapy for childhood leukemia
19. Oculo-dento-osseous dysplasia
20. Parasitic disease (eg, toxoplasmosis; cysticercosis)
21. Parkinsonism
22. Phenylketonuria variants
23. Pseudopseudohypoparathyroidism
24. Radiation therapy
25. Trisomy 21 S. (Down S.)
26. Tuberous sclerosis
27. Viral encephalitis, esp. in fetus or newborn (eg, rubella; measles; chickenpox; cytomegalovirus infection); coxsackie B

References
1. Bennett JC, Maffly RH, Steinbach HL: The significance of bilateral basal ganglia calcification. Radiology 1959;72:368–378
2. Cohen CR, Duchesneau PM, Weinstein MA: Calcification of the basal ganglia as visualized by computed tomography. Radiology 1980;134:97–99
3. Dähnert W: Radiology Review Manual. (ed 4) Baltimore: Williams & Wilkins, 1999, p 197
4. Harwood-Nash DCF, Reilly BJ: Calcification of the basal ganglia following radiation therapy. AJR 108:392–395
5. Newton TH, Potts DG: Radiology of the Skull and Brain. St. Louis: CV Mosby, 1971, vol 1, book 2, p 835
6. Numaguchi Y, Hoffman JC Jr, Sones PJ Jr: Basal ganglia calcification as a late radiation effect. AJR 1975;123:27–30
7. Swischuk LE, John SD: Differential Diagnosis in Pediatric Radiology. (ed 2) Baltimore: Williams & Wilkins, 1995, pp 379, 383

Gamut A-50

CURVILINEAR OR RING-LIKE INTRACRANIAL CALCIFICATION

VASCULAR

1. Aneurysm (incl. vein of Galen "aneurysm")
2. Arteriosclerosis (esp. internal carotid artery)
3. Hemangioma; arteriovenous malformation; Sturge-Weber S.
4. Hematoma, chronic (esp. subdural); hygroma

NEOPLASTIC

1. Cystic astrocytoma
2. Cystic craniopharyngioma
3. Lipoma of corpus callosum
4. Pinealoma; teratoma

PARASITIC

1. *Cysticercus* cyst (occasional ring-like calcification)
2. Hydatid cyst
3. *Paragonimus* cyst (often "soap-bubble" calcification)
4. Toxoplasmosis

OTHER

1. Abscess, old
2. Cytomegalovirus infection

Reference
1. Swischuk LE, John SD: Differential Diagnosis in Pediatric Radiology. (ed 2) Baltimore: Williams & Wilkins, 1995, pp 383–385

Gamut A-51-S1

WHO CLASSIFICATION OF TUMORS OF THE NERVOUS SYSTEM

TUMORS OF NEUROEPITHELIAL TISSUE

Astrocytic Tumors	Behavior*
Diffuse astrocytoma	3
Fibrillary astrocytoma	3
Protoplasmic astrocytoma	3
Gemistocytic astrocytoma	3
Anaplastic astrocytoma	3
Glioblastoma	3
Giant cell glioblastoma	3
Gliosarcoma	3
Pilocytic astrocytoma	1
Pleomorphic xanthoastrocytoma	3
Subependymal giant cell astrocytoma	1

Oligodendroglial Tumors	
Oligodendroglioma	3
Anaplastic oligodendroglioma	3

Mixed Gliomas	Behavior*
Oligoastrocytoma	3
Anaplastic oligoastrocytoma	3

Ependymal Tumors	
Ependymoma	3
Cellular	3
Papillary	3
Clear cell	3
Tanycytic	3
Anaplastic ependymoma	3
Myxopapillary ependymoma	1
Subependymoma	1

Choroid Plexus Tumors	
Choroid plexus papilloma	0
Choroid plexus carcinoma	3

Glial Tumors of Uncertain Origin	
Astroblastoma	3
Gliomatosis cerebri	3
Choroid glioma of the 3rd ventricle	1

Neuronal and Mixed Neuronal-Glial Tumors	
Gangliocytoma	0
Dysplastic gangliocytoma of cerebellum (Lhermitte-Duclos)	0
Desmoplastic infantile astrocytoma/ganglioglioma	1
Dysembryoplastic neuroepithelial tumor	0
Ganglioglioma	1
Anaplastic ganglioglioma	3
Central neurocytoma	1
Cerebellar liponeurocytoma	1
Paraganglioma of filum terminale	1

Neuroblastic Tumors	
Olfactory neuroblastoma (Aesthesioneuroblastoma)	3
Olfactory neuroepithelioma	3
Neuroblastomas of the adrenal gland and sympathetic nervous system	3

(continued)

Pineal Parenchymal Tumors	Behavior*
Pineocytoma	1
Pineoblastoma	3
Pineal parenchymal tumor of intermediate differentiation	3

Embryonal Tumors	
Medulloepithelioma	3
Ependymoblastoma	3
Medulloblastoma	3
Desmoplastic medulloblastoma	3
Large cell medulloblastoma	3
Medullomyoblastoma	3
Melanotic medulloblastoma	3
Supratentorial primitive neuroectodermal tumor (PNET)	3
Neuroblastoma	3
Ganglioneuroblastoma	3
Atypical teratoid/rhabdoid tumor	3

TUMORS OF PERIPHERAL NERVES

Schwannoma	
(Neurilemmoma, Neurinoma)	0
Cellular	0
Plexiform	0
Melanotic	0

Neurofibroma	0
Plexiform	0

Perineurinoma	0
Intraneural perineurinoma	0
Soft tissue perineurinoma	0

Malignant Peripheral Nerve Sheath Tumor (MPNST)	3
Epithelioid	3
MPNST with divergent mesnchymal and/or epithelial differentiation	3
Melanotic	3
Melanotic psammomatous	3

TUMORS OF THE MENINGES

Tumors of Meningothelial Cells	Behavior*
Meningioma	0
Meningothelial	0
Fibrous (fibroblastic)	0
Transitional (mixed)	0
Psammomatous	0
Angiomatous	0
Microcystic	0
Secretory	0
Lymphoplasmacyte-rich	0
Metaplastic	0
Clear cell	1
Choroid	1
Atypical	1
Papillary	3
Rhabdoid	3
Anaplastic meningioma	3

Primary Melanocytic Lesions	
Diffuse melanocytosis	0
Melanocytoma	1
Malignant melanoma	3
Meningeal melanomatosis	3

Tumors of Uncertain Histogenesis	
Hemangioblastoma	1

Mesenchymal, Non-meningothelial Tumors	
Lipoma	0
Angiolipoma	0
Hibernoma	0
Liposarcoma (intracranial)	3
Solitary fibrous tumor	0
Fibrosarcoma	3
Malignant fibrous histiocytoma	3
Leiomyoma	0
Leiomyosarcoma	3
Rhabdomyoma	0
Rhabdomyosarcoma	3
Chondroma	0
Chondrosarcoma	3

	Behavior*
Osteoma	0
Osteosarcoma	3
Osteochondroma	0
Hemangioma	0
Epithelioid hemangioendothelioma	1
Hemangiopericytoma	1
Angiosarcoma	3
Kaposi sarcoma	3

LYMPHOMAS AND HEMOPOIETIC NEOPLASMS

Malignant lymphomas	3
Plasmacytoma	3
Granulocytic sarcoma	3

GERM CELL TUMORS

Germinoma	3
Embryonal carcinoma	3
Yolk sac tumor	3
Choriocarcinoma	3
Teratoma	1
Mature	0
Immature	3
Teratoma with malignant transformation	3
Mixed germ cell tumors	3

TUMORS OF THE SELLAR REGION

Craniopharyngioma	1
Adamantinomatous	1
Papillary	1
Granular cell tumor	0

METASTATIC TUMORS

* Tumor behavior is coded 0 for benign tumors, 1 for low or uncertain malignant potential or borderline malignancy, and 3 for malignant tumors.

Gamut A-51-S2

ALTERNATE CLASSIFICATION OF PRIMARY BRAIN TUMORS

GLIOMAS (Glial Neoplasms)
*1. Astrocytoma
    (I and II) Low-grade ("benign") astrocytoma
    (III) Anaplastic ("malignant") astrocytoma
    (IV) Glioblastoma multiforme
2. Oligodendroglioma
*3. Paraglioma
    a. Ependymoma*
    b. Choroid plexus papilloma* or carcinoma

NON-GLIAL NEOPLASMS
Tumors of Primitive Bipotential Precursors and Nerve Cells
  1. Ganglioglioma; gangliocytoma
*2. Medulloblastoma; other $PNET_g$
  3. Neuroblastoma (primary cerebral)

Nerve Sheath Tumors
*1. Neurofibroma
  2. Neurofibrosarcoma
*3. Schwannoma (neurinoma)

Tumors of Mesenchymal Tissue
  1. Hemangioblastoma
*2. Meningioma
  3. Sarcoma (eg, fibrosarcoma and meningeal sarcomatosis; gliosarcoma; hemangiopericytoma)

(continued)

Tumors of the Lymphoreticular System

1. Langerhans cell histiocytosis_g
2. Leukemia
3. Lymphoma (non-Hodgkin's)
4. Myeloma

Tumors of Maldevelopmental Origin
(eg, Arising from Embryonal Remnants)

1. Colloid cyst
*2. Craniopharyngioma
3. Dermoid
4. Epidermoid
5. Germ cell tumors
   a. Germinoma
   b. Teratoid tumor
      i. Choriocarcinoma
      ii. Embryonal carcinoma
      iii. Endodermal sinus (yolk sac) tumor
      iv. Teratoma
      v. Mixed tumor (eg, teratocarcinoma)
6. Hamartoma
7. Lipoma (eg, of corpus callosum)
8. Rathke cleft cyst

Pineal Tumor

1. Germinoma
2. Pineoblastoma
3. Pineocytoma
4. Teratoma
5. Teratocarcinoma

Pituitary Tumor

*1. Adenoma (eosinophilic, basophilic, chromophobe)
2. Carcinoma

Phakomatoses (neurocutaneous syndromes)

*1. Neurofibromatosis (eg, cranial nerve schwanno-
   mas—esp. acoustic; meningiomas; gliomas of optic
   chiasm; cerebral hamartomas)
2. Sturge-Weber S.
*3. Tuberous sclerosis
4. von Hippel-Lindau disease

* Common.

References

1. Dähnert W: Radiology Review Manual. (ed 4) Baltimore: Williams & Wilkins, 1999, pp 190–191
2. Osborn AG: Handbook of Neuroradiology. St. Louis: Mosby-Year Book Inc., 1991, pp 286–318

Gamut A-52-S

INCIDENCE OF BRAIN TUMORS

Percent Incidence in All Age Groups

Classification	Walker	Lane	Dähnert
Glioma			34
Glioblastoma multiforme	23.0	25	
Astrocytoma, low grade	13.0	9	
Ependymoma	1.8	3	
Oligodendroglioma	1.6	2	
Mixed & other gliomas	1.9	3	
Medulloblastoma (PNET)	1.5	3	15+
Meningioma	16.0	14	17
Pituitary adenoma	8.2	11	6
Schwannoma (esp. acoustic)	5.7	7	4
Craniopharyngioma	2.8	3	2
Hemangioblastoma	2.7		2
Sarcoma	2.5		3
Pineal tumor	1.1	1	
Metastases*	13.0		12
Other rare tumors (eg, dermoid, epidermoid, colloid cyst; choroid plexus papilloma)	7.0	3	

Percent Incidence in Pediatric Age Group

Classification	Walker	Lane	Dähnert
Astrocytoma			50
Medulloblastoma			15
Ependymoma			10
Craniopharyngioma			6
Choroid plexus papilloma			2
Others			17

A. Skull and Brain

Percent Incidence in Adult Age Group

Classification	Walker	Lane	Dähnert
Metastases			33
Glioma			25
Meningioma			15
Pituitary adenoma			10
Schwannoma (esp. acoustic)			8
Others			9

* Actual incidence of metastatic tumors is higher since more are being identified with CT and MRI, and many others are not worked up radiologically.
+ In pediatric age group.

References
1. Dähnert W: Radiology Review Manual. (ed 4) Baltimore: Williams & Wilkins, 1999, p 191
2. Lane BA, Moseley IF, Théron J: Intracranial tumors. In: Grainger RG, Allison DJ (eds): Diagnostic Radiology. Edinburgh: Churchill Livingstone, 1992, vol 3, p 1935
3. Walker M: Malignant brain tumors—a synopsis. CA Cancer J for Clinicians 1975;25:114–120

Gamut A-53-1

SUPRATENTORIAL INTRACRANIAL TUMORS IN INFANCY AND CHILDHOOD

CEREBRAL HEMISPHERE TUMORS
*1. Astrocytoma
2. Desmoplastic infantile ganglioglioma
3. Ependymoma
4. Giant cell tumor (in tuberous sclerosis)
5. [Inflammatory pseudotumor (plasma cell granuloma)]
6. Meningioangiomatosis
7. Mixed neuronal-glial tumors (eg, ganglioglioma; gangliocytoma)
8. Oligodendroglioma
9. Primitive neuroectodermal tumor (PNET)$_g$; medulloepithelioma
10. Rhabdoid tumor

SELLAR AND SUPRASELLAR TUMORS
1. Arachnoid cyst
*2. Craniopharyngioma
3. Germ cell tumors (see below)
4. [Granuloma (tuberculosis; sarcoidosis)]
5. Hypothalamic glioma
6. Hypothalamic hamartoma
7. Langerhans cell histiocytosis$_g$
*8. Optic nerve or chiasm glioma
9. Pituitary adenoma (prolactinoma; chromophobe; eosinophilic)
10. Rathke cleft cyst

PINEAL REGION TUMORS
1. Epidermoid; dermoid
*2. Germ cell tumors (germinoma; teratoma; endodermal sinus (yolk sac) tumor; embryonal cell tumor; choriocarcinoma)
3. Pineal and pineal region glioma
4. Pineal cyst; cystic pineal tumor
*5. Pineal parenchymal tumors (pineocytoma; pineoblastoma)

EXTRAPARENCHYMAL TUMORS
1. Calvarial tumors
*2. Choroid plexus papilloma of lateral ventricle
3. Choroid plexus carcinoma
4. Epidermoid; dermoid
5. Langerhans cell histiocytosis$_g$
6. Leukemia; lymphoma$_g$
7. Meningioma; dural sarcoma

* Common.
[ ] This condition does not actually cause the gamuted imaging finding, but can produce imaging changes that simulate it.

References
1. Barkovich AJ: Pediatric Neuroimaging. (ed 3) Philadelphia: Lippincott Williams & Wilkins, 2000, pp 446–543
2. Dähnert W: Radiology Review Manual. (ed 4) Baltimore: Williams & Wilkins, 1999, p 191

Gamut A-53-2

INFRATENTORIAL INTRACRANIAL TUMORS IN INFANCY AND CHILDHOOD

INTRAPARENCHYMAL TUMORS

*1. Brain stem glioma
*2. Cerebellar astrocytoma
*3. Ependymoma of fourth ventricle
 4. Hemangioblastoma
*5. Medulloblastoma; other primitive neuroectodermal tumor (PNET)$_g$
 6. Rhabdoid tumor
 7. Teratoma

EXTRAPARENCHYMAL TUMORS

1. Choroid plexus papilloma of fourth ventricle
2. Enteric cyst
3. Epidermoid; dermoid
4. Schwannoma (neurinoma)
5. Meningioma
6. Skull base tumors
7. Teratoma

* Common.

References
1. Barkovich AJ: Pediatric Neuroimaging. (ed 3) Philadelphia: Lippincott Williams & Wilkins, 2000, pp 446–543
2. Dähnert W: Radiology Review Manual. (ed 4) Baltimore: Williams & Wilkins, 1999, p 191

Gamut A-53-3

BRAIN TUMORS IN CHILDREN UNDER ONE YEAR OF AGE ON CT OR MRI

1. Choroid plexus papilloma or carcinoma
2. Ependymoma
3. Hypothalamic astrocytoma

4. Primitive neuroectodermal tumor (PNET)$_g$ (esp. medulloblastoma)
5. Rhabdoid tumor (eg, rhabdomyosarcoma)
6. Teratoma

Reference
1. Barkovich AJ: Pediatric Neuroimaging. Philadelphia: Lippincott Williams & Wilkins, 2000, pp 543–546

Gamut A-54-S

PRIMARY SITES OF ORIGIN FOR METASTASES TO THE BRAIN, MENINGES, AND SKULL

CEREBRAL PARENCHYMAL METASTASES (seen in approximately 18% of cancer patients) (esp. from carcinoma of lung, breast, GI or GU tract, or paranasal sinus, or melanoma)

HEMORRHAGIC CEREBRAL PARENCHYMAL METASTASES
(esp. from melanoma; choriocarcinoma; thyroid, renal cell, lung or breast carcinoma)

MENINGEAL CARCINOMATOSIS (8% to 10% of all intracranial metastases)
1. Seeding from primary CNS tumors (eg, medulloblastoma, ependymoma, pineoblastoma)
2. Metastatic spread from melanoma, or carcinoma of breast or lung

SKULL METASTASES
1. Adult—from carcinoma of breast or lung; multiple myeloma
2. Child—from neuroblastoma; leukemia

Reference
1. Sze G (New Haven, CT): Lecture at Hawaii Radiological Society Meeting, 1992

Gamut A-55-1

SOLITARY INTRACRANIAL MASS—NEOPLASTIC

PRIMARY (CEREBRAL, CEREBELLAR)

1. Congenital
   a. Chordoma
   b. Craniopharyngioma; Rathke cleft cyst
   c. Dermoid; teratoma
   d. Epidermoid
   e. Hemangioma
   f. Hemangioblastoma
   g. Pineal tumor
2. Cranial nerve origin
   a. Acoustic schwannoma (neurinoma)
   b. Glioma of optic nerve
   c. Trigeminal and other cranial schwannomas (neurinomas)
3. Glioma
   a. Low-grade glioma (grade I and II)
   b. Anaplastic astrocytoma (grade III)
   c. Glioblastoma multiforme (grade IV)
   d. Ependymoma; subependymoma
   e. Mixed glioma
   f. Oligodendroglioma
4. Primitive neuroectodermal tumor (PNET)$_g$
   a. Supratentorial PNET (cerebral neuroblastoma; pineoblastoma)
   b. Medulloblastoma
   c. Medulloepithelioma
   d. Pigmented medulloblastoma (melanotic vermian PNET)
   e. Ependymoblastoma
5. Pineal tumor
   a. Germinoma
   b. Pineoblastoma
   c. Pineocytoma
   d. Teratoma
   e. Teratocarcinoma
6. Intraventricular
   a. Choroid plexus papilloma or carcinoma
   b. Colloid cyst
   c. Meningioma
7. Lymphoma$_g$ (esp. in AIDS)
8. Meningioma
9. Pituitary tumor (esp. eosinophilic or chromophobe adenoma)
10. Sarcoma

METASTATIC CARCINOMA

1. Esp. from carcinoma of lung, breast, kidney or melanoma

Gamut A-55-2

SOLITARY INTRACRANIAL MASS—NONNEOPLASTIC

VASCULAR LESION

1. Aneurysm of internal carotid or vertebral artery or their branches
2. Arteriovenous malformation
3. Cavernous angioma
4. Vein of Galen "aneurysm"

HEMATOMA

1. Epidural
2. Intracerebral (traumatic or spontaneous)
3. Subdural

INFECTION

1. Abscess
   a. Extracerebral
      1. Epidural
      2. Subarachnoid
      3. Subdural
   b. Intracerebral
2. Granulomatous disease
   a. Fungus disease (eg, cryptococcosis {torulosis})
   b. Sarcoidosis

(continued)

   c. Syphilis
   d. Tuberculosis
3. AIDS and its associated conditions
   a. HIV encephalitis
   b. Progressive multifocal leukoencephalopathy (PML)
   c. Toxoplasmosis
   d. [Lymphoma$_g$]
   e. [Kaposi sarcoma]
   f. Cryptococcosis (torulosis)

INFLAMMATORY CONDITION
1. Tumefactive multiple sclerosis
2. Acute disseminated encephalomyelitis (ADEM)

CYST
1. Dandy-Walker syndrome (Dandy-Walker malformation)
2. Leptomeningeal
3. Parasitic (eg, hydatid; *Paragonimus; Cysticercus; Strongyloides*)
4. Porencephalic cyst (porencephaly)

[ ] This condition does not actually cause the gamuted imaging finding, but can produce imaging changes that simulate it.

Gamut A-56-1

MULTIFOCAL INTRACRANIAL LESIONS

COMMON
1. Abscesses (bacterial, fungal; parasitic—toxoplasmosis), intracerebral or extracerebral (subarachnoid; subdural; epidural)
2. AIDS and its associated conditions
   a. HIV encephalitis
   b. Progressive multifocal leukoencephalopathy (PML)
   c. Toxoplasmosis
   d. Cryptococcosis (torulosis)
   e. Lymphoma$_g$

   f. Kaposi sarcoma
3. Aneurysms of internal carotid or vertebral artery or their branches
4. Degenerative and metabolic diseases of brain (esp. Alzheimer's disease)
5. Hematomas (eg, intracerebral ({traumatic or spontaneous}; subdural; epidural)
6. Infarcts
7. Metastases (esp. from carcinoma of lung, breast, kidney, or melanoma)

UNCOMMON
1. Acute disseminated encephalomyelitis (ADEM)
2. Arteriovenous malformations
3. Dysmyelinating or demyelinating diseases (See A-95-1, A-95-2)
4. Granulomatous disease
   a. Fungus disease (eg, cryptococcosis {torulosis})
   b. Sarcoidosis
   c. Syphilis
   d. Tuberculosis
5. Lymphoma (primary multicentric, esp. in AIDS)
6. Meningiomas (multicentric)
7. Metastases from primary CNS tumor (eg, medulloblastoma, other PNET; ependymoma; glioblastoma)
8. Parasitic cysts (neurocysticercosis; paragonimiasis; hydatid disease)
9. Phakomatoses (neurocutaneous syndromes) (See A-56-S)
   a. Neurofibromatosis (meningiomatosis; bilateral acoustic schwannomas; bilateral optic nerve gliomas; cerebral gliomas; choroid plexus papillomas; multiple spine tumors, arteriovenous malformations)
   b. Sturge-Weber S. (intracerebral and cutaneous hemangiomas or arteriovenous malformations)
   c. Tuberous sclerosis (subependymal tubers; intraventricular gliomas {giant cell astrocytoma}; ependymomas)
   d. von Hippel-Lindau disease (retinal angiomatosis; hemangioblastomas)
10. Tumefactive multiple sclerosis

Reference

1. Dähnert W: Radiology Review Manual. (ed 4) Baltimore: Williams & Wilkins, 1999, p 192

Gamut A-56-2

MULTIPLE CNS AND CRANIAL NERVE TUMORS

1. Multiple meningiomas
2. Neurofibromatosis types I and II
3. Neurofibromatosis types I and II mosaicism (segmental NFI or NFII)
4. Schwannomatosis
5. Tuberous sclerosis
6. von Hippel-Lindau S.

Reference

1. Lufkin R, Borges A, Villablanca P: Teaching Atlas of Head and Neck Imaging. New York: Thieme, 2000, pp 395–399

Gamut A-56-S

PHAKOMATOSES (NEUROCUTANEOUS SYNDROMES)

COMMON

1. Neurofibromatosis type 1 (von Recklinghausen's disease) (meningiomatosis; bilateral acoustic schwannomas; bilateral optic nerve gliomas; cerebral gliomas; choroid plexus papillomas; multiple spine tumors, arteriovenous malformations)
2. Sturge-Weber S. (intracerebral and cutaneous hemangiomas or arteriovenous malformations)
3. Tuberous sclerosis (subependymal tubers; intraventricular gliomas {giant cell astrocytoma}; ependymomas)
4. von Hippel-Lindau disease (retinal angiomatosis; hemangioblastomas)

UNCOMMON

1. Ataxia-telangiectasia
2. Epidermal nevus S.
3. Gorlin S. (nevoid basal cell carcinoma S.)
4. Linear nevus sebaceous S.
5. Louis-Bar S.
6. Neurocutaneous melanosis
7. Neurofibromatosis type 2 (bilateral acoustic schwannomas)
8. Proteus S.
9. Wyburn-Mason S.

Reference

1. Osborn AG: Handbook of Neuroradiology. St. Louis: Mosby-Year Book Inc., 1991, pp 187–198

Gamut A-57-1

CT ATTENUATION (DENSITY) OF VARIOUS INTRACRANIAL LESIONS (RELATIVE TO NORMAL BRAIN)—HYPERDENSE

COMMON

1. Acoustic schwannoma (neurinoma)
2. Aneurysm, giant
3. Arteriovenous malformation
4. Craniopharyngioma (solid or calcified)
5. Cysticercosis
6. Hematoma (2 weeks old or less) (eg, acute intracerebral hemorrhage; acute subdural or epidural hematoma)
7. Medulloblastoma; other PNET
8. Meningioma
9. Metastasis, hemorrhagic (esp. melanoma; choriocarcinoma; carcinoma of thyroid, lung, or kidney); calcified metastasis (eg, osteosarcoma; mucinous adenocarcinoma of colon); high density metastasis (eg, carcinoma of colon)
10. Pituitary adenoma (esp. chromophobe)

(continued)

UNCOMMON

1. Choroid plexus papilloma or carcinoma
2. Colloid cyst
3. Ependymoma
4. Glioblastoma multiforme
5. Hamartoma (eg, in tuberous sclerosis)
6. Langerhans cell histiocytosis$_g$
7. Lymphoma$_g$, primary or secondary
8. Oligodendroglioma
9. Paragonimiasis (calcified cysts)
10. Pineoblastoma; pineocytoma; germinoma

References

1. Burgener FA, Kormano M: Differential Diagnosis in Computed Tomography. New York: Thieme Medical Publishers, Inc., 1996, pp 16–31
2. Eisenberg RL: Clinical Imaging: An Atlas of Differential Diagnosis. (ed 3) Philadelphia: Lippincott-Raven, 1997, pp 1062–1064
3. Lee SH, Rao K: Cranial Computed Tomography and MRI. (ed 2) New York: McGraw-Hill, 1987, p 314

5. Glioma of brain stem
6. Granuloma (esp. tuberculoma)
7. Hemangioblastoma (cystic)
8. Langerhans cell histiocytosis$_g$
9. Lymphoma$_g$, primary
10. Pineocytoma; germinoma

References

1. Burgener FA, Kormano M: Differential Diagnosis in Computed Tomography. New York: Thieme Medical Publishers, Inc., 1996, pp 16–31
2. Eisenberg RL: Clinical Imaging: An Atlas of Differential Diagnosis. (ed 3) Philadelphia: Lippincott-Raven, 1997
3. Lee SH, Rao K: Cranial Computed Tomography and MRI. (ed 2) New York: McGraw-Hill, 1987, p 314

Gamut A-57-2

CT ATTENUATION (DENSITY) OF VARIOUS INTRACRANIAL LESIONS—ISODENSE

COMMON

1. Acoustic schwannoma (neurinoma)
2. Astrocytoma, low-grade or high-grade (glioblastoma)
3. Craniopharyngioma (solid or cystic)
4. Hematoma (subacute subdural—2 to 4 weeks old)
5. Metastasis
6. Pituitary adenoma

UNCOMMON

1. Chordoma
2. Colloid cyst
3. Ependymoma
4. Ganglioglioma; ganglioneuroma; neuroblastoma

Gamut A-57-3

CT ATTENUATION (DENSITY) OF VARIOUS SUPRATENTORIAL LESIONS—HYPODENSE

COMMON

1. Abscess (intracerebral or epidural)
2. Astrocytoma (low-grade; cystic; juvenile pilocytic; or high-grade {glioblastoma})
3. Cerebral edema
4. Cerebral infarction
5. Cerebritis (bacterial, tuberculous, fungal, malarial)
6. Cyst
   a. Arachnoid
   b. Leptomeningeal
   c. Parasitic (eg, hydatid, *Paragonimus, Cysticercus, Strongyloides*)
   d. Porencephalic cyst (porencephaly)
7. Cystic neoplasm, other
8. Glioma of brain stem
9. Granuloma (esp. tuberculoma)
10. Hematoma, resolving intracerebral or subdural (3 to 6 weeks old)
11. Metastasis (esp. from squamous cell primary)
12. Multiple sclerosis (periventricular)

UNCOMMON

1. Craniopharyngioma (cystic)
2. Dermoid; teratoma
3. Epidermoid
4. Ganglioglioma; gangliocytoma; ganglioneuroma; neuroblastoma
5. Hemangioblastoma
6. Herpes simplex encephalitis
7. Lipoma
8. Necrosis of globus pallidus (basal ganglia)
9. Oligodendroglioma
10. Progressive multifocal leukoencephalopathy (PML) (periventricular)
11. Prolactinoma
12. Radiation necrosis
13. Subdural empyema

References
1. Burgener FA, Kormano M: Differential Diagnosis in Computed Tomography. New York: Thieme Medical Publishers, Inc., 1996, pp 16–31
2. Eisenberg RL: Clinical Imaging: An Atlas of Differential Diagnosis. (ed 3) Philadelphia: Lippincott-Raven, 1997, pp 1056–1061
3. Lee SH, Rao K: Cranial Computed Tomography and MRI. (ed 2) New York: McGraw-Hill, 1987, p 314

3. Ependymoma
4. Germinoma, teratocarcinoma (pineal)
5. Hemangioblastoma
6. Langerhans cell histiocytosis$_g$
7. Lymphoma$_g$, primary (non-Hodgkins)

References
1. Burgener FA, Kormano M: Differential Diagnosis in Computed Tomography. New York: Thieme Medical Publishers, Inc., 1996, pp 16–31
2. Lange S, Grumme T, Meese W: Computerized Tomography of the Brain. Berlin: Schering Medico-Scientific Book Series, 1980
3. Lee SH, Rao K: Cranial Computed Tomography and MRI. (ed 2) New York: McGraw-Hill, 1987, p 314

Gamut A-58-2

CONTRAST ENHANCEMENT PATTERNS OF INTRACRANIAL MASSES ON CT—MARKED ENHANCEMENT (PATCHY, MIXED, OR RING-LIKE)

COMMON

1. Astrocytoma, anaplastic or high-grade (glioblastoma)
2. Arteriovenous malformation; large aneurysm
3. Metastasis

UNCOMMON

1. Lymphoma$_g$, primary (if necrotic, as in AIDS)
2. Pineoblastoma

References
1. Burgener FA, Kormano M: Differential Diagnosis in Computed Tomography. New York: Thieme Medical Publishers, Inc., 1996, pp 16–31
2. Lange S, Grumme T, Meese W: Computerized Tomography of the Brain. Berlin: Schering Medico-Scientific Book Series, 1980
3. Lee SH, Rao K: Cranial Computed Tomography and MRT. (ed 2) New York: McGraw-Hill, 1987, p 314

Gamut A-58-1

CONTRAST ENHANCEMENT PATTERNS OF INTRACRANIAL MASSES ON CT—MARKED ENHANCEMENT (HOMOGENEOUS)

COMMON

1. Aneurysm, large
2. Meningioma
3. Metastasis
4. Pituitary adenoma

UNCOMMON

1. Acoustic schwannoma (neurinoma)
2. Choroid plexus papilloma or carcinoma

Gamut A-58-3

CONTRAST ENHANCEMENT PATTERNS OF INTRACRANIAL LESIONS ON CT—MODERATE ENHANCEMENT (VARIABLE IN APPEARANCE—HOMOGENEOUS, MIXED, OR RING-LIKE)

COMMON

1. Abscess or cerebritis (ring-like)
2. Astrocytoma (incl. hypothalamic glioma)
3. Cerebral infarction (1–8 weeks—gyral enhancement)
4. Craniopharyngioma (homogeneous, mixed, or ring-like)
5. Cysticercus cyst (ring-like)
6. Ependymoma (homogeneous or patchy)
7. Granuloma (esp. tuberculoma) (ring-like)
8. Hemorrhage (intracerebral or subdural—resolving 3–6 weeks) (ring-like or marginal)
9. Medulloblastoma (homogeneous)

UNCOMMON

1. Chordoma
2. Glomus tumor
3. Hemangioblastoma (homogeneous)
4. Neuroblastoma (mixed)
5. Oligodendroglioma (mixed)
6. Pineocytoma (homogeneous)
7. PNET, other (variable)
8. Radiation necrosis (ring-like)

References

1. Burgener FA, Kormano M: Differential Diagnosis in Computed Tomography. New York: Thieme Medical Publishers, Inc., 1996, pp 16–31
2. Lange S, Grumme T, Meese W: Computerized Tomography of the Brain. Berlin: Schering Medico-Scientific Book Series, 1980
3. Lee SH, Rao K: Cranial Computed Tomography and MRI. (ed 2) New York: McGraw-Hill, 1987, p 314

Gamut A-58-4

CONTRAST ENHANCEMENT PATTERNS OF INTRACRANIAL MASSES ON CT—MINIMAL OR NO ENHANCEMENT

COMMON

1. Astrocytoma, low-grade (mixed) or cystic (homogeneous)
2. Cerebral infarction (12–48 hours)
3. Cyst
   a. Arachnoid
   b. Colloid
   c. Leptomeningeal
   d. Parasitic (eg, hydatid; *Cysticercus; Paragonimus; Strongyloides*)
   e. Pineal
   f. Porencephalic cyst (porencephaly)
4. Hematoma (may show faint ring-like enhancement during resorption—2 to 6 weeks old)

UNCOMMON

1. Craniopharyngioma, cystic
2. Dermoid, teratoma (minimal or no enhancement)
3. Epidermoid (no enhancement)
4. Ganglioglioma; ganglioneuroma (mixed)
5. Lipoma (no enhancement)
6. Oligodendroglioma (minimal or no enhancement)
7. Prolactinoma (no enhancement)

References

1. Burgener FA, Kormano M: Differential Diagnosis in Computed Tomography. New York: Thieme Medical Publishers, Inc., 1996, pp 16–31
2. Lange S, Grumme T, Meese W: Computerized Tomography of the Brain. Berlin: Schering Medico-Scientific Book Series, 1980
3. Lee SH, Rao K: Cranial Computed Tomography and MRI. (ed 2) New York: McGraw-Hill, 1987, p 314

FEATURES USEFUL IN CT IDENTIFICATION
OF VARIOUS TYPES OF INTRACRANIAL TUMORS*

Tumor	Initial density	Frequency calcification	Edema	Enhancement pattern	Age/sex group	Location	Other findings
Meningioma	↑	20%	+1	+3 H	A/F	Dural attachment	Occasional hemorrhage
Pineoblastoma	↑	Rare	0	+3 M	P/M	Pineal region	Irregular margin and hypodense center
Choroid plexus papilloma or carcinoma	↑	Rare	0	+3 H	P	Ventricular system	Occasional hemorrhage, irregular margin
Colloid cyst	↑	0	0	0/+1 H	A	Anterior 3d ventricle	
Germinoma	↑/↔	Rare	0	+3 H	A/M	Pineal region	Meningeal and ependymal seeding
Pituitary adenoma	↔/↑	<5%	0	+3 H	A	Sella	Rare hemorrhage or infarction
Neuroma	↔/↑	0	+1	+3 H	A	Cerebellopontine angle	Occasionally cystic
Pineocytoma	↔/↑	Rare	0	+3 H	P	Pineal region	
Craniopharyngioma	↔/-	30/80%	0	+2 M/R	A/P	Suprasellar	Some cystic
Teratoma	↓	Frequent	+1/0	0	P/A/M	Midline supratentorial	Some cystic, rupture, seeding
Dermoid; epidermoid	↓	Frequent	+1/0	0	P/A/F	Post-fossa base of skull	Some cystic
Lipoma	↓	Rare	+1/0	0	P/A	Supratentorial midline	
Primary lymphoma	↑/↔	0	+2	+2/+3 H	A	Peripheral and deep structures	Irregular margin, multiplicity
Medulloblastoma	↑	10%	+2	+2 H	P	Vermis	Irregular margin
Oligodendroglioma	↑	>90%	+1	+2 M	A	Supratentorial	Irregular margin
Ependymoma	↔/↑	30-40%	+2	+2 H	P	4th ventricle	Irregular margin
Embryonal cell carcinoma	↑/↓	Rare	+1	+3 H	P	Pineal	
Hemangioblastoma	↔	0	+1	+3 H	A	Posterior	Cystic, mural nodule
Ganglioglioma	↓/↔	>30%	0	+1 M	P/A	Temporal lobe	Irregular margin, cystic
Neuroblastoma	↔/↓	Common	+2	+2 M	P	Supratentorial	Hermorrhage
Low-grade astrocytoma	↔/↓	<30%	+1	0/+1 M	A	Supratentorial	Indistinct margin
High-grade astrocytoma (glioblastoma)	↔/↓	Rare	+2	+2-3 M/R	A	Supratentorial	Can be cystic, irregular margin
Brain stem glioma	↓/↔	0	0	+1/M	P	Brain stem	Indistinct margin
Cystic astrocytoma	↓	Rare	+1	+1 H	P	Posterior	Mural tumor nodule

Key: ↑ = Hyperdensity   +1 = Minimal enhancement   H = Homogeneous   A = Adult; P = Pediatric
      ↔ = Isodensity   +2 = Moderate enhancement   M = Mixed   M = Male predominance
      ↓ = Hypodensity   +3 = Intense enhancement   R = Ring pattern   F = Female predominance

* This table was prepared by Russell A. Binder, M.D., and S.H. Lee, M.D. in 1982 and modified by S.H. Lee, M.D. in 1986.

Reference
1. Lee SH, Rao K: Cranial Computed Tomography and MRI. (ed 2), New York: McGraw-Hill, 1987, p 314

Gamut A-60

MULTIPLE ENHANCING LESIONS IN THE CEREBRUM AND CEREBELLUM ON CT OR MRI

COMMON

1. Abscesses (eg, from septicemia; intravenous drug abuse; immunosuppression; cyanotic congenital heart disease; pulmonary AVM)
2. Metastasis (esp. from carcinoma of lung, breast, colon, rectum, or kidney, or melanoma)
3. Multifocal infectious disease (eg, tuberculosis; histoplasmosis)
4. Multiple sclerosis (periventricular demyelinating plaques)
5. Parasitic disease (eg, cysticercosis; toxoplasmosis; paragonimiasis; neurotrichinosis)

UNCOMMON

1. Arteriovenous malformations; aneurysms
2. Cerebral gliomatosis (no enhancement on CT, but some uptake may occur on MRI)
3. Contusions (> 2 weeks old)
4. Infarction, subacute multifocal
   a. Arterial (eg, underperfusion; multiple emboli; cerebral vasculitis due to lupus erythematosus; meningitis)
   b. Venous (superior sagittal sinus thrombosis with parasagittal hemorrhages)
5. Langerhans cell histiocytosis$_g$
6. Lymphoma$_g$, primary (esp. in immunosuppressed or organ transplant patients)
7. Sarcoidosis (usually in meninges)

References
1. Chapman S, Nakielny R: Aids to Radiological Differential Diagnosis. (ed 3) London: WB Saunders, 1995, pp 423–424
2. Eisenberg RL: Clinical Imaging: An Atlas of Differential Diagnosis. (ed 3) Philadelphia: Lippincott-Raven, 1997, pp 1052–1055

Gamut A-61

RING-ENHANCING LESION ON CT OR MRI

COMMON

1. Abscess (bacterial; fungal; parasitic—toxoplasmosis)
2. Cysticercus cyst
*3. Glioblastoma multiforme
4. Hematoma, resolving intracerebral (3–6 weeks old)
*5. Lymphoma$_g$ (eg, if necrotic in transplant recipients or in AIDS)
6. Metastasis
7. Subdural hematoma, resolving (1 to 4 weeks old)

UNCOMMON

1. Aneurysm, large (esp. if thrombosed)
2. Astrocytoma, grade II
3. Craniopharyngioma
4. Demyelinating disease (esp. tumefactive multiple sclerosis; ADEM)
5. Emyema, epidural or subdural
6. Infarction (resolving)
7. Meningioma (atypical)
8. Radiation necrosis

* May cross corpus callosum.

References
1. Eisenberg RL: Clinical Imaging: An Atlas of Differential Diagnosis. (ed 3) Philadelphia: Lippincott-Raven, 1997, pp 1048–1051
2. Lee SH, Rao K: Cranial Computed Tomography and MRI. (ed 2) New York: McGraw-Hill, 1987, p 314

Gamut A-62-1

SIGNAL INTENSITY OF VARIOUS INTRACRANIAL LESIONS ON MRI—HYPERINTENSE T1, HYPERINTENSE T2 SIGNAL

COMMON

1. Aneurysm (with chronic clot or flow phenomenon)
2. Calcification (post-hemorrhagic)
3. Cholesterol cyst or granuloma
4. Chronic or late subacute hematoma
5. Craniopharyngioma
6. Flow (first echo slice entry phenomenon; second echo rephasing)
7. Mucocele of paranasal sinus
8. Normal variant (posterior pituitary bright spot)
9. Rathke cleft cyst

UNCOMMON

1. Dermoid
2. Lipoma (hemorrhagic)
3. Teratoma
4. Xanthogranuloma

Reference
1. Pomeranz SJ: Gamuts and Pearls in MRI. Cincinnati: MRI Education Foundation, Inc., 1990

Gamut A-62-2

HYPERINTENSE T1, HYPOINTENSE T2 SIGNAL ON MRI

COMMON

1. Flow (first echo slice entry phenomenon)
2. Hemorrhagic metastasis (eg, choriocarcinoma; thyroid or renal cell carcinoma; neuroblastoma; embryonal cell carcinoma; malignant melanoma)

3. Lipoma
4. Pantopaque
5. Subacute hematoma

UNCOMMON

1. Colloid cyst
2. Xanthogranuloma (calcified)

Reference
1. Pomeranz SJ: Gamuts and Pearls in MRI. Cincinnati: MRI Education Foundation, Inc., 1990

Gamut A-62-3

HYPO- TO ISOINTENSE T1, HYPOINTENSE T2 SIGNAL ON MRI (1.5 TESLA)

COMMON

1. Acute hematoma
2. Aneurysm with flow phenomenon
3. Calcification (nontraumatic; nonhemorrhagic)
4. Flow (first echo void; second echo rephasing)
5. Iron in brain
6. Meningioma
7. Metastasis (eg, from carcinoma of colon, breast, prostate; osteosarcoma)
8. Neoplasm with acute hemorrhage

UNCOMMON

1. Chloroma
2. Colloid cyst
3. Malignant melanoma

Reference
1. Pomeranz SJ: Gamuts and Pearls in MRI. Cincinnati: MRI Education Foundation, Inc., 1990

Gamut A-62-4

ISOINTENSE T1 AND T2 SIGNAL ON MRI

COMMON

1. Aneurysm with flow phenomenon
2. Flow (combinations of flow void and flow-related hyperintensity)
3. Hamartoma
4. Hematoma, acute (mid field 0.5 Tesla) or subacute (high field)
5. Iron in brain
6. Isointense metastases (from carcinoma of colon, breast, or prostate; osteosarcoma)
7. Meningioma

UNCOMMON

1. Colloid cyst
2. Lymphoma$_g$
3. Medulloblastoma; adult cerebellar sarcoma
4. Tuberculoma

Reference

1. Pomeranz SJ: Gamuts and Pearls in MRI. Cincinnati: MRI Education Foundation, Inc., 1990

Gamut A-62-5

HOMOGENEOUS WATER SIGNAL, VERY HYPOINTENSE T1, VERY HYPERINTENSE T2 ON MRI

COMMON

1. Arachnoid cyst
2. Cystic encephalomalacia
3. Mega cisterna magna (Blake's pouch)
4. Nonependymal-lined cyst
5. Porencephalic cyst

UNCOMMON

1. Dandy-Walker malformation
2. Meningocele
3. Pseudomeningocele (dural leak)
4. Seroma (postsurgical)
5. Trapped fourth ventricle

Reference

1. Pomeranz SJ: Gamuts and Pearls in MRI. Cincinnati: MRI Education Foundation, Inc., 1990

Gamut A-62-6

ISOINTENSE OR HYPOINTENSE T1, HYPERINTENSE T2 SIGNAL ON MRI

COMMON

1. Cerebritis; encephalitis
2. Glial tumors (eg, astrocytoma; glioma; glioblastoma)
3. Infarction (nonhemorrhagic)
4. Lymphoma, primary or secondary
5. Meningioma
6. Metastasis
7. Pituitary adenoma
8. Schwannoma (neurinoma)

UNCOMMON

1. Chordoma
2. Choroid plexus papilloma
3. Craniopharyngioma
4. Ependymoma
5. Gliosis; scar
6. Granuloma (active)
7. Hamartoma
8. Medulloblastoma
9. Pinealoma; pineoblastoma
10. Radiation necrosis
11. Subependymoma
12. Tuberculoma

Reference

1. Pomeranz SJ: Gamuts and Pearls in MRI. Cincinnati: MRI Education Foundation, Inc., 1990

Gamut A-62-7

INHOMOGENEOUS WATER SIGNAL, HYPOINTENSE T1, HYPERINTENSE T2 ON MRI

COMMON

1. Abscess
2. Acute hemorrhage (low field)
3. Arachnoid cyst (complex)
4. Cystic astrocytoma
5. Cystic metastases (from oat cell or squamous cell carcinoma of lung; carcinoma of colon, ovary, or kidney)
6. Hemangioblastoma
7. Hyperacute hemorrhage (high and low field)
8. Mucocele
9. Nonependymal-lined cyst (complex)
10. Porencephalic cyst (complex)

UNCOMMON

1. Amyloidoma
2. Cysticercosis
3. Epidermoid

Reference
1. Pomeranz SJ: Gamuts and Pearls in MRI. Cincinnati: MRI Education Foundation, Inc., 1990

Gamut A-62-8

GYRIFORM CORTICAL/SUBCORTICAL HYPOINTENSE T2 SIGNAL ON HIGH FIELD MRI

COMMON

1. Acute hemorrhagic cortical infarction
2. Luxury flow effect in bland cortical infarct
3. Subacute hemorrhagic cortical infarction (early)

UNCOMMON

1. Acute subarachnoid hemorrhage (high field)
2. Meningitis (flow phenomenon in subcortical U fibers)
3. Superficial siderosis (old subarachnoid hemorrhage)

Reference
1. Pomeranz SJ: Gamuts and Pearls in MRI. Cincinnati: MRI Education Foundation, Inc., 1990

Gamut A-62-9

GYRIFORM CORTICAL/SUBCORTICAL HYPERINTENSE T1 SIGNAL ON MRI

COMMON

1. Chronic or late subacute hemorrhagic cortical infarction
2. Contrast-enhanced subacute cortical infarction
3. Subacute or chronic subarachnoid hemorrhage

UNCOMMON

1. Contrast-enhanced dural/leptomeningeal neoplasm or inflammation
2. Cortical or dural arteriovenous malformation (slice entry or even-echo rephasing)

Reference
1. Pomeranz SJ: Gamuts and Pearls in MRI. Cincinnati: MRI Education Foundation, Inc., 1990

Gamut A-62-10

GYRIFORM CORTICAL HYPERINTENSE T2 SIGNAL WITH PARENCHYMAL LESIONS ON MRI

COMMON

1. Deep white matter and peripheral cortical infarction

UNCOMMON

1. Cryptococcoma with cryptococcal meningitis
2. Granulomatous disease (eg, tuberculosis; sarcoidosis; syphilis)
3. Lymphoma_g
4. Parenchymal metastases with cerebral carcinomatosis
5. Primary brain tumor with subarachnoid or leptomeningeal seeding (eg, ependymoma; ependymoblastoma; medulloblastoma; oligodendroglioma; glioblastoma)
6. Viral meningoencephalitis

Reference
1. Pomeranz SJ: Gamuts and Pearls in MRI. Cincinnati: MRI Education Foundation, Inc., 1990

Gamut A-62-11

BLACK SIGNAL ON MRI

1. Air or gas
2. Bone
3. Calcium
4. Flow
5. Hemosiderin (T2 dependent)
6. Iron, copper, or other metal intracranially
7. Ligaments or tendons
8. Superparamagnetic contrast agents

Reference
1. Pomeranz SJ: Gamuts and Pearls in MRI. Cincinnati: MRI Education Foundation, Inc., 1990

Gamut A-62-12

HYPOINTENSE RINGS ON MRI

1. Abscess (fibrous rim)
2. Chronic hematoma (hemosiderin ring)
3. Glial tumor (eg, astrocytoma; glioma) (susceptibility rim artifact)]
4. Meningioma (pseudocapsule)
5. Parasitic disease (eg, cysticercosis; paragonimiasis; hydatid disease)

Reference
1. Pomeranz SJ: Gamuts and Pearls in MRI. Cincinnati: MRI Education Foundation, Inc., 1990

Gamut A-63

SELLAR AND PARASELLAR MASSES ON CT OR MRI (SEE A-26, 64, 65)

COMMON

1. Aneurysm of internal carotid artery at siphon
2. Craniopharyngioma
3. Glioma of optic chiasm or hypothalamus (often with neurofibromatosis)
4. Pituitary adenoma (macroadenoma or microadenoma) (eg, chromophobe; eosinophilic; basophilic)

UNCOMMON

1. Arachnoid cyst
2. Chordoma
3. Dermoid
4. Ectopic posterior pituitary lobe
5. Epidermoid
6. Germ cell tumor (eg, germinoma; teratoma)
7. Hamartoma of tuber cinereum
8. Infundibular lesion (eg, Langerhans cell histiocytosis_g; sarcoidosis; lipoma)
9. Mandibular nerve (V_3) schwannoma

10. Meningioma (suprasellar)
11. Metastasis (esp. from carcinoma of lung, breast, kidney, or GI tract, or direct spread from carcinoma of nasopharynx or sphenoid sinus)
12. Pituitary hyperplasia (may be normal during puberty or pregnancy)
13. Pituitary neoplasm, other (eg, prolactinoma; choristoma; adenocarcinoma; carcinosarcoma; lymphoma$_g$; oncocytoma)
14. Rathke cleft cyst
15. Sphenoid sinus mass (eg, mucocele; carcinoma)

References
1. Burgener FA, Kormano M: Differential Diagnosis in Computed Tomography. New York: Thieme Medical Publishers, Inc., 1996, pp 34–39
2. Eisenberg RL: Clinical Imaging: An Atlas of Differential Diagnosis. (ed 3) Philadelphia: Lippincott-Raven, 1997, pp 1076–1081

Gamut A-64

ENHANCING SELLAR AND SUPRASELLAR LESIONS ON CT OR MRI

COMMON
1. Aneurysm; arteriovenous malformation
2. Craniopharyngioma
3. Meningioma
4. Pituitary adenoma (eosinophilic; chromophobe)

UNCOMMON
1. Chordoma
2. Choristoma (granular cell tumor of neurohypophysis)
3. Glioma of optic chiasm or hypothalamus
4. Infundibular lesion (eg, Langerhans cell histiocytosis$_g$; sarcoidosis); adenohypophysitis
5. Lymphoma$_g$ (juxtasellar)
6. Meningitis (basal cisterns)
7. Metastasis

8. Pineal tumor (eg, germinoma; pineoblastoma; pineocytoma; teratoma; teratocarcinoma)

References
1. Burgener FA, Kormano M: Differential Diagnosis in Computed Tomography. New York: Thieme Medical Publishers, Inc., 1996, pp 34–39
2. Hatam A, Bergstrøm M, Greitz T: Diagnosis of sellar and parasellar lesions by computed tomography. Neuroradiology 1979;18:249–258
3. Lee SH, Rao K: Cranial Computed Tomography and MRI. (ed 2) New York: McGraw-Hill, 1987, p 314

Gamut A-65-1

SELLAR OR SUPRASELLAR MASS WITH LOW ATTENUATION ON CT

1. Arachnoid cyst
2. Craniopharyngioma (cystic)
3. Dermoid
4. [Empty sella S.]
5. Epidermoid
6. Hypothalamic or optic glioma
7. Lipoma (esp. of infundibulum)
8. Parasitic cyst (eg, *Cysticercus;* hydatid)
9. Pituitary abscess
10. Pituitary cyst (incl. Rathke cleft cyst)
11. Sheehan S. (Simmond's disease) (pituitary apoplexy—necrosis during postpartum period)
12. Teratoma

References
1. Burgener FA, Kormano M: Differential Diagnosis in Computed Tomography. New York: Thieme Medical Publishers, Inc., 1996, pp 34–39
2. Dähnert W: Radiology Review Manual. (ed 4) Baltimore: Williams & Wilkins, 1999, p 199
3. Hatam A, Bergström M, Greitz T: Diagnosis of sellar and parasellar lesions by computed tomography. Neuroradiology 1979;18:249–258
4. Lee SH, Rao K: Cranial Computed Tomography and MRI. (ed 2) New York: McGraw-Hill, 1987, p 314

Gamut A-65-2

SELLAR OR SUPRASELLAR MASS WITH EQUAL (ISODENSE) OR MIXED ATTENUATION ON CT

COMMON

1. Aneurysm of internal carotid artery (thrombosed)
2. Craniopharyngioma
3. Glioma of optic chiasm or hypothalamus (often with neurofibromatosis)
4. Pituitary adenoma (eosinophilic; chromophobe)

UNCOMMON

1. Hamartoma of tuber cinereum
2. Infundibular lesion (metastasis; tuberculosis; sarcoidosis; Langerhans cell histiocytosis$_g$; choristoma); adenohypophysitis
3. Lymphoma$_g$ (juxtasellar)
4. Mucocele or neoplasm of sphenoid sinus (infrasellar)
5. Pineal tumor (eg, germinoma; pineocytoma)
6. [Pituitary hyperplasia]

[ ] This condition does not actually cause the gamuted imaging finding, but can produce imaging changes that simulate it.

References

1. Burgener FA, Kormano M: Differential Diagnosis in Computed Tomography. New York: Thieme Medical Publishers, Inc., 1996, pp 34–39
2. Dähnert W: Radiology Review Manual. (ed 4) Baltimore: Williams & Wilkins, 1999, p 199
3. Hatam A, Bergstrøm M, Greitz T: Diagnosis of sellar and parasellar lesions by computed tomography. Neuroradiology 1979;18:249–258
4. Lee SH, Rao K: Cranial Computed Tomography and MRI. (ed 2) New York: McGraw-Hill, 1987, p 314

Gamut A-65-3

SELLAR OR SUPRASELLAR MASS WITH HIGH ATTENUATION ON CT

1. Aneurysm or ectasia of internal carotid artery
2. Chordoma
3. Craniopharyngioma
4. Germ cell tumor (eg, germinoma; teratoma)
5. Meningioma
6. Metastasis
7. Pineal tumor (eg, pineoblastoma; pineocytoma)
8. Pituitary adenoma (esp. chromophobe)

References

1. Burgener FA, Kormano M: Differential Diagnosis in Computed Tomography. New York: Thieme Medical Publishers, Inc., 1996, pp 34–39
2. Hatam A, Bergstrøm M, Greitz T: Diagnosis of sellar and parasellar lesions by computed tomography. Neuroradiology 1979;18:249–258
3. Lee SH, Rao K: Cranial Computed Tomography and MRI. (ed 2) New York: McGraw-Hill, 1987, p 314

VISUAL ESTIMATION OF CT ATTENUATION* AND ENHANCEMENT IN VARIOUS SELLAR AND PARASELLAR LESIONS

Type of Lesion	No. of Cases	Attenuation relative to that of brain				Enhancement	
		Higher	Lower	Equal	Mixed	Present	Absent
Craniopharyngioma	11	2		4	5	6	1
Chromophobe adenoma	9	4		2	3	7	
Eosinophilic adenoma	4			2	2	2	
Dermoid cyst	2		2				1
Arachnoid cyst	2		2				1
Meningioma	4	4				4	
Optic glioma	2		1		1	2	
Metastasis	1	1				1	
Aneurysm	2	2				2	
Unverified tumor	2				2	1	
Total	39					25	3

* Attenuation relative to that of brain.

Reference

1. Hatam A, Bergstrøm M, Greitz T: Diagnosis of sellar and parasellar lesions by computed tomography. Neuroradiology 1979; 18:249–258

Gamut A-66

HYPOTHALAMIC LESIONS ON MRI

1. Ectopic posterior pituitary gland
2. Germinoma
3. Glioma
4. Hamartoma of tuber cinereum
5. Langerhans cell histiocytosis$_g$
6. Lymphoma$_g$, primary
7. Sarcoidosis; tuberculoisis
8. Wernicke's encephalopathy

Reference

1. Eisenberg RL: Clinical Imaging: An Atlas of Differential Diagnosis. (ed 3) Philadelphia: Lippincott-Raven, 1997, pp 1086–1089

Gamut A-67

MASS INVOLVING THE JUGULAR FORAMEN ON MRI* WITH ENLARGEMENT OF THE JUGULAR CANAL

LESION WITHIN THE CANAL

1. Aneurysm of internal carotid artery
2. Arteriovenous malformation
3. Glomus jugulare tumor
4. [Normal]
5. Schwannoma of cranial nerve IX, X, or XI

LESION ARISING OUTSIDE THE CANAL

1. Carcinoma of nasopharynx
2. Chondroma; chondrosarcoma
3. Chordoma
4. Epidermoid
5. Lymphoma$_g$ (non-Hodgkin's)
6. Meningioma

7. Metastasis
8. Rhabdomyosarcoma

* Usually isointense with brain stem on T_1WI, with high signal intensity on T_2WI, and intense contrast enhancement.
[ ] This condition does not actually cause the gamuted imaging finding, but can produce imaging changes that simulate it.

References

1. Crawford DB, Williams JP, Connaughton PN: Glomus jugulare tumors: The value of lateral tomography. American Roentgen Ray Society Scientific Exhibit, Atlanta, 1975
2. Eisenberg RL: Clinical Imaging: An Atlas of Differential Diagnosis. (ed 3) Philadelphia: Lippincott-Raven, 1997, pp 1112–1115
3. Newton TH, Hasso AN, Dillon WP: Modern Neuroradiology, vol 3. Computed Tomography of the Head and Neck. New York: Raven Press, 1988

Gamut A-68

MASS OR ABNORMAL ENHANCEMENT OF THE TRIGEMINAL NERVE ON CT OR MRI

1. Hemangioma
2. Infection (herpes zoster; Lyme disease; AIDS)
3. Lipoma
4. Meckel's cave lesion (eg, meningioma; metastasis; dermoid; epidermoid)
5. Meningioma (petroclival or cavernous sinus)
6. Metastasis
7. Perineural spread of tumor
8. Sarcoidosis
9. Schwannoma of VII and VIII nerves
10. Trigeminal nerve schwannoma, benign or rarely malignant with neurofibromatosis (plexiform neurofibroma)

References

1. Catalano P, Fang-Hui E, Som PM: Fluid-fluid levels in benign neurogenic tumors. AJNR 1997;l 8:385–387
2. Charabi S, Mantoni M, Tos M, Thomsen J: Cystic vestibular schwannomas: neuroimaging and growth rate. J Laryngol Otol 1994;108:375–379

3. Krishnamurthy S, Holmes B, Powers SK: Schwannomas limited to the infratemporal fossa: report of two cases. J Neuro-Oncol 1998;36:269–277
4. Lufkin R, Borges A, Villablanca P: Teaching Atlas of Head and Neck Imaging. New York: Thieme, 2000, pp 8–12
5. Mautner VF, Lindenau M, Baser MR, et al: The neuroimaging and clinical spectrum of neurofibromatosis II. Neurosurgery 1996;38:880–885
6. Samii M, Migliori MM, Tatagiba M, Babu R: Surgical treatment of trigeminal schwannomas. J Neurosurgery 1995;82:711–718
7. Tegos S, Georgouli G, Gogos C, et al: Primary malignant schwannoma involving simultaneously the right Gasserian ganglion and the distal part of the right mandibular nerve. Case Report. J Neurosurg Sci 1997;41:293–297

MASS IN THE MIDDLE FOSSA ON CT OR MRI WITH EXPANSION OR EROSION OF THE MIDDLE FOSSA FLOOR

COMMON

*1. Aneurysm of internal carotid artery (large); carotid-cavernous fistula; cavernous sinus thrombosis
*2. Arachnoid cyst; temporal lobe agenesis or atrophy with overlying cerebrospinal fluid collection
3. Glomus jugulare or vagale tumor
4. Intra-axial temporal lobe neoplasm (glioma), hematoma, or abscess
*5. Meningioma of sphenoid ridge or middle fossa
6. Nasopharyngeal or paranasal sinus carcinoma or other neoplasm with middle fossa extension
*7. Subdural hematoma, chronic; hygroma

UNCOMMON

1. Benign bone tumor (eg, chondroma; giant cell tumor)
2. [Congenital or postoperative defect]
3. Epidermoid; cholesteatoma

*4. [Increased intracranial pressure, chronic]
5. Langerhans cell histiocytosis$_g$
6. Metastasis
7. Midline neoplasm extending laterally (eg, chordoma; craniopharyngioma; pituitary adenoma)
*8. Neurofibromatosis
*9. [Oxycephaly with partial stenosis of sagittal and metopic sutures]
*10. Porencephalic cyst (porencephaly)
11. Schwannoma (eg, trigeminal; gasserian ganglion)
*12. Temporal horn hydrocephalus, localized
*13. Tolosa-Hunt syndrome (granulomatous invasion of cavernous sinus)

* May cause expansion of middle fossa floor. Other entities usually cause erosion of floor.

[ ] This condition does not actually cause a mass, but can produce expansion or simulate erosion of the middle fossa floor.

References
1. DuBoulay GB: Principles of X-ray Diagnosis of the Skull. (ed 2) London: Butterworths, 1980, pp 180–186
2. Hasso A, Vignaud J, La Masters DL: Pathology of the skull base and vault. In: Newton TH, Hasso AN, Dillon WP (eds): Modern Neuroradiology, vol 3. Computed Tomography of the Head and Neck. New York: Raven Press, 1988, pp 3.1–3.26
3. Newton TH, Potts DG: Radiology of the Skull and Brain. St. Louis: CV Mosby, 1971, vol 1, book 1, pp 311–313

MASS OR DESTRUCTIVE LESION INVOLVING THE CLIVUS, PREPONTINE CISTERN AREA, OR POSTERIOR SKULL BASE ON CT OR MRI

ARISING FROM THE SKULL BASE

1. Bone sarcoma (osteosarcoma; chondrosarcoma)
2. Brown tumor of hyperparathyroidism
3. Chondroid tumor (chondroma; osteochondroma; chondromyxoid fibroma)

(continued)

*4. Chordoma
5. Epidermoid
6. Fibrous dysplasia
7. Giant cell tumor
8. Glomus jugulare tumor
9. Hemangioma
10. Langerhans cell histiocytosis$_g$ (esp. eosinophilic granuloma)
11. Lymphoma$_g$; leukemia; chloroma
12. Metastasis (hematogenous or direct extension with proximal spread from head and neck tumors)
13. Osteomyelitis
14. Plasmacytoma; multiple myeloma
15. Radiation osteonecrosis

ARISING ABOVE THE SKULL BASE OR INTRASELLAR

*1. Aneurysm or ectasia of basilar or vertebral artery
*2. Meningioma (of clivus; petroclival ligament; planum sphenoidale; tuberculum sella)
*3. Parasellar neoplasm with extension (eg, cranio-pharyngioma; optic glioma)
*4. Pituitary macroadenoma (eg, chromophobe; eosinophilic)

ARISING BELOW THE SKULL BASE

*1. Carcinoma of nasopharynx
2. Carcinoma (squamous cell) of sphenoid sinus
3. Mucocele of sphenoid sinus
4. Rhabdomyosarcoma of nasopharynx
5. Schwannoma of trigeminal or lower cranial nerves (See A-68)

* Common.

References

1. Casals MM, Hunter SB, Olson JJ, et al: Metastatic follicular thyroid carcinoma masquerading as a chordoma. Thyroid 1995;5:217–221
2. Doucet V, Peretti-Viton P, Figarella-Branger D, et al: MRI of intracranial chordomas. Extent of tumour and contrast enhancement: criteria for differential diagnosis. Neuroradiology 1997;39:571–576
3. Jansen BP, Pillay M, de Bruin HG, et al: 99mTc-SPECT in the diagnosis of skull base metastasis. Neurology 1997;48:1326–1330
4. Kawase T, Shiobara R, Ohira T, Toya S: Developmental patterns and characteristic symptoms of petroclival meningiomas. Neurologia Medico-Chirurgica 1996;36:1–6
5. Keel S, Bhan AK, Liebsch NJ, Rosenberg AE: Chondromyxoid fibroma of the skull base: a tumor which may be confused with chordoma and chondrosarcoma. A report of three cases and review of the literature. Am J Surg Pathol 1997;21:577–582
6. Lufkin R, Borges A, Villablanca P: Teaching Atlas of Head and Neck Imaging. New York: Thieme, 2000, pp 3–7; 22–26; 27–31
7. Ng SH, Chang TC, Ko SF, et al: Nasopharyngeal carcinoma: MRI and CT assessment. Neuroradiology 1997;39:741–748
8. Pomeranz S, Umansky F, Elidan J, et al: Giant cranial base tumours. Acta Neurochirurgica 1994;129:121–126
9. Tashiro T, Fukuda T, Inoue Y, et al: Intradural chordoma: case report and review of the literature. Neuroradiology 1994;36:313–315
10. Weber AL, Brown EW, Hug EB, Liebsch NJ: Cartilaginous tumors and chordomas of the cranial base. Otolaryngol Clin N Am 1995;28:453–471

Gamut A-71

EXTRA-AXIAL MASSES AND FLUID COLLECTIONS

CONGENITAL AND DEVELOPMENTAL

1. Arachnoid cyst
2. Cerebral atrophy
3. Hydrocephalus (external)
4. Normal variant (eg, mega-cisterna magna)

VASCULAR

1. Aneurysm (esp. giant aneurysm)
2. Arteriovenous malformation; varix
3. Subarachnoid hemorrhage (eg, trauma; ruptured aneurysm or AVM)

TRAUMATIC

1. Epidural hematoma, acute or chronic

2. Subdural hematoma, acute or chronic
3. Subdural shunts or drains

ATROPHIC CONDITIONS WITH DIFFUSE PROMINENCE OF SUBARACHNOID SPACES AND CISTERNS

1. Dehydration
2. Ischemia; hypoxia
3. Infection (eg, meningitis)
4. Malnutrition; deprivational states
5. Neurodegenerative diseases
6. Posttraumatic
7. Steroid therapy
8. Radiation therapy; chemotherapy

INFECTION/INFLAMMATION

1. Idiopathic hypertrophic pachymeningitis
2. Meningitis
3. Sarcoidosis
4. Subdural empyema or effusion
5. Syphilis with hypertrophic pachymeningitis

NEOPLASM

1. Lymphoma; leukemia
2. Metastasis (eg, from carcinoma of lung, breast, prostate, or kidney, or neuroblastoma)
3. Plasmacytoma
4. Primary intracranial extra-axial tumor or cyst
   a. Chordoma
   b. Choroid plexus papilloma or carcinoma
   c. Colloid cyst of third ventricle
   d. Dermoid
   e. Craniopharyngioma
   f. Epidermoid
   g. Lipoma
   h. Meningioma
   i. Pineal tumor (eg, pineoblastoma; pineocytoma; germinoma; teratoma)
   j. Pituitary adenoma (eosinophilic, basophilic, chromophobe)
   k. Schwannoma (neurinoma)—esp. acoustic

References
1. Hasso AN, Smith DS: The cerebellopontine angle. Semin Ultrasound CT MR 1989;10:280–301
2. Osborn AG: Handbook of Neuroradiology. St. Louis: Mosby-Year Book Inc., 1991, pp 234–237

Gamut A-72

MIDLINE SUPRATENTORIAL TUMORS OR CYSTS

TUMORS

COMMON

1. Astrocytoma (giant cell) associated with tuberous sclerosis
2. Craniopharyngioma
3. Optic glioma; hypothalamic glioma
4. Pineal tumor (eg, germinoma; pinealoma; pineoblastoma; teratoma)
5. Pituitary adenoma (esp. chromophobe; eosinophilic)

UNCOMMON

1. Choroid plexus papilloma or carcinoma
2. Lipoma of corpus callosum
3. Meningioma (esp. of tentorium)

CYSTIC STRUCTURES OR LESIONS

1. Arachnoid cyst
2. Cavum septi pellucidi ("fifth ventricle")
3. Cavum veli interpositi
4. Cavum vergae ("sixth ventricle")
5. Colloid cyst of third ventricle
6. Cystic neoplasm (esp. craniopharyngioma)
7. Parasitic cyst (eg, cysticercosis (*Cysticercus* cyst), hydatid disease (echinococcal cyst), paragonimiasis (*Paragonimus* cyst))
8. Pineal cyst

(continued)

VASCULAR LESIONS
1. Aneurysm or ectasia of basilar artery
2. Vein of Galen "aneurysm"

References
1. Chapman S, Nakielny R: Aids to Radiological Differential Diagnosis. (ed 3) London: WB Saunders, 1995, pp 434–435
2. Dähnert W: Radiology Review Manual. (ed 4) Baltimore: Williams & Wilkins, 1999, p 191

Gamut A-73

CYSTIC BRAIN TUMOR WITH A MURAL NODULE

1. Ganglioglioma
2. Glioblastoma multiforme
3. Hemangioblastoma
4. Metastasis (necrotic or hemorrhagic)
5. [Parasitic cyst (*Cysticercus; Paragonimus*)]
6. Pilocytic astrocytoma
7. Pleomorphic xanthoastrocytoma

[ ] This condition does not actually cause the gamuted imaging finding, but can produce imaging changes that simulate it.

Reference
1. Dähnert W: Radiology Review Manual. (ed 4) Baltimore: Williams & Wilkins, 1999, p 188

Gamut A-74

INTRAVENTRICULAR TUMOR OR CYST

COMMON
1. Astrocytoma
   a. Frontal horn most common
   b. Cystic cerebellar astrocytoma in children (4th ventricle mass)
   c. Giant cell astrocytoma in 10% of tuberous sclerosis at foramen of Monro
   d. Pilocytic astrocytoma at foramen of Monro
2. Choroid plexus cyst or papilloma
3. Colloid cyst of third ventricle
4. Cysticercosis
5. Ependymoma
6. Hemangioma in Sturge-Weber S.
7. Meningioma

UNCOMMON
1. Arachnoid cyst
2. Arteriovenous malformation
3. Choroid plexus carcinoma
4. Craniopharyngioma (third ventricle)
5. Dermoid; teratoma
6. Ependymal cyst
7. Epidermoid
8. Germ cell tumor or hypothalamic glioma invading third ventricle
9. Hemangioblastoma
10. Hematoma (congenital hemorrhage in premature; trauma; hypertension)
11. Heterotopic gray matter (subependymal nodules)
12. Lymphoma$_g$
13. Metastasis (esp. from carcinoma of lung or breast; melanoma; medulloblastoma)
14. Neurocytoma (medulloepithelioma); neuroblastoma
15. Oligodendroglioma
16. Primitive neuroectodermal tumor (PNET)$_g$ (medulloblastoma; ependymoblastoma)
17. Sturge-Weber S. (ipsilateral enlargement of choroid plexus in 70% of cases)
18. Subependymoma
19. Trapped ventricle (usually the fourth and usually associated with ventriculitis)
20. Tuberous sclerosis
    a. Paraventricular foci of astrocytes form subependymal nodules
    b. Giant cell astrocytoma adjacent to foramen of Monro in 10% of cases

References
1. Burgener FA, Kormano M: Differential Diagnosis in Computed Tomography. New York: Thieme Medical Publishers, Inc., 1996, pp 49–51

2. Eisenberg RL: Clinical Imaging: An Atlas of Differential Diagnosis. (ed 3) Philadelphia: Lippincott-Raven, 1997, pp 1126–1131
3. Osborn AG: Handbook of Neuroradiology. St. Louis: Mosby-Year Book Inc., 1991, pp 216–222

Gamut A-75

VENTRICULAR WALL NODULE(S)

COMMON
*1. Choroid plexus
 2. Heterotopic gray matter
*3. Neurocysticercosis
 4. Nodular caudate nucleus
*5. Tuberous sclerosis

UNCOMMON
1. Coarctation of lateral ventricles with ependymal adhesions
2. Ependymal seeding from malignant brain tumor (eg, ependymoma; medulloblastoma; glioblastoma)
3. Ependymitis (esp. cryptococcosis {torulosis})
4. Intraventricular neoplasm (eg, ependymoma; subependymoma; epidermoid; meningioma; choroid plexus papilloma or carcinoma)

* May show calcification.

Reference
1. Bergeron RT: Pneumographic demonstration of subependymal heterotopic cortical gray matter in children. AJR 1967; 101:168–177

Gamut A-76

WIDENING OF THE SEPTUM PELLUCIDUM (> 3 MM)

COMMON
1. Cyst or neoplasm of septum pellucidum
2. Noncommunicating cavum septi pellucidi

UNCOMMON
1. Corpus callosum neoplasm infiltrating septum pellucidum
2. Intraventricular astrocytoma extending into septum pellucidum
3. Lipoma of corpus callosum
4. Neoplasm of third ventricle

Gamut A-77-1

MASS INVOLVING THE TRIGONE AND ATRIUM OF THE LATERAL VENTRICLE

CHILD
1. Choroid plexus cyst
2. Choroid plexus papilloma
3. Cysticercosis (*Cysticercus* cyst)
4. Ependymoma
5. Neuroepithelial (noncolloidal) cyst

ADULT
1. Choroid plexus cyst
2. Cysticercosis (*Cysticercus* cyst)
3. Meningioma
4. Neuroepithelial (noncolloidal) cyst

References
1. Burgener FA, Kormano M: Differential Diagnosis in Computed Tomography. New York: Thieme, 1996, p 43
2. Osborn AG: Handbook of Neuroradiology. St. Louis: Mosby-Year Book Inc., 1991, p 220

Gamut A-77-2

MASS INVOLVING THE BODY OF THE LATERAL VENTRICLE

CHILD
1. Choroid plexus papilloma
2. Cysticercosis (*Cysticercus* cyst)
3. Ependymoma
4. Pilocytic astrocytoma
5. Primitive neuroectodermal tumor (PNET)
6. Teratoma

ADULT
1. Cysticercosis (*Cysticercus* cyst)
2. Glioblastoma multiforme
3. Lymphoma$_g$
4. Metastasis
5. Neuroepithelial (noncolloidal) cyst
6. Subependymoma

References
1. Burgener FA, Kormano M: Differential Diagnosis in Computed Tomography. New York: Thieme, 1996, p 43
2. Osborn AG: Handbook of Neuroradiology. St. Louis: Mosby-Year Book Inc., 1991, p 220

Gamut A-78-1

MASS INVOLVING THE FORAMEN OF MONRO AND/OR THE ANTERIOR RECESS AND INFERIOR THIRD VENTRICLE

CHILD
1. Choroid plexus papilloma
2. Craniopharyngioma
3. Germinoma
4. Glioma

5. Langerhans cell histiocytosis$_g$
6. Neurofibromatosis
7. Pilocytic astrocytoma
8. Subependymal giant cell astrocytoma

ADULT
1. Aneurysm
2. Colloid cyst
3. *Cysticercus* cyst
4. Ependymal cyst
5. Glioma
6. Lymphoma$_g$
7. Meningioma
8. Metastasis
9. Pituitary adenoma

References
1. Burgener FA, Kormano M: Differential Diagnosis in Computed Tomography. New York: Thieme, 1996, p 43
2. Osborn AG: Handbook of Neuroradiology. St. Louis: Mosby-Year Book, Inc., 1991, p 221

Gamut A-78-2

MASS INVOLVING THE BODY OR POSTERIOR PORTION OF THE THIRD VENTRICLE

COMMON
1. Choroid plexus papilloma
2. *Cysticercus* cyst
3. Glioma or other neoplasm arising from quadrigeminal body
4. Pinealoma; teratoma
5. Vertebral or basilar artery aneurysm or ectasia

UNCOMMON
1. Cystic pineal gland
2. Ependymal cyst
3. Ependymoma

4. Meningioma (eg, intraventricular or incisural)
5. Quadrigeminal cyst
6. Vascular malformation (incl. vein of Galen "aneurysm")

References
1. Burgener FA, Kormano M: Differential Diagnosis in Computed Tomography. New York: Thieme, 1996, p 43
2. Osborn AG: Handbook of Neuroradiology. St. Louis: Mosby-Year Book, Inc., 1991, p 221

Gamut A-79

PINEAL AREA MASS

COMMON
1. Pineal cyst (cystic pineal gland)
*2. Pineal tumor (eg, germinoma; pineoblastoma; pineocytoma; teratoma; teratocarcinoma; choriocarcinoma)

UNCOMMON
*1. Glioma of nonpineal origin (eg, tumor arising in thalamus, posterior hypothalamus, brain stem, tectal plate of mesencephalon, or splenium with extension into quadrigeminal cistern)
*2. Meningioma (subsplenial)
 3. Metastasis (midline tumor arising from edge of tentorium)
*4. Vein of Galen "aneurysm"
*5. Intensely enhancing lesion on CT or MRI

References
1. Dähnert W: Radiology Review Manual. (ed 4) Baltimore: Williams & Wilkins, 1999, pp 199–200
2. Eisenberg RL: Clinical Imaging: An Atlas of Differential Diagnosis. (ed 3) Philadelphia: Lippincott-Raven, 1997, pp 1082–1085

Gamut A-80-1

INFRATENTORIAL (POSTERIOR FOSSA) LESIONS ON CT OR MRI—FOURTH VENTRICLE (INTRAVENTRICULAR) LESIONS BY LOCATION AND AGE

COMMON
1. Ependymoma

UNCOMMON
1. Arteriovenous malformation; hemangioma
2. Astrocytoma (from brain stem or cerebellum)
3. Choroid plexus papilloma or carcinoma
4. Cysticercosis (*Cysticercus* cyst)
5. Dermoid; teratoma
6. Epidermoid
7. Hemorrhage
8. Medulloblastoma
9. Meningioma
10. Metastasis
11. Subependymoma

BODY OF FOURTH VENTRICLE

CHILD
1. Astrocytoma (from brain stem or cerebellum)
2. Cysticercosis (*Cysticercus* cyst)
3. Ependymoma
4. Medulloblastoma

ADULT
1. Cysticercosis (*Cysticercus* cyst)
2. Dermoid
3. Epidermoid
4. Metastasis

(continued)

LATERAL RECESSES OF FOURTH VENTRICLE

CHILD

1. Ependymoma

ADULT

1. Choroid plexus papilloma

INFERIOR FOURTH VENTRICLE AND OBEX

CHILD

1. Glioma

ADULT

1. Metastasis
2. Subependymoma

References

1. Burgener FA, Kormano M: Differential Diagnosis in Computed Tomography. New York: Thieme, 1996, p 44
2. Bundschuh CV: Posterior fossa abnormalities on 0.3 tesla MRI scanner. Radiological Society of North America Scientific Exhibit, Washington, D.C., 1984
3. Damiano T, Truwit CL: Cerebellar and fourth ventricular tumors in adults. MRI Decisions 1992;6:10–21
4. Eisenberg RL: Clinical Imaging: An Atlas of Differential Diagnosis. (ed 3) Philadelphia: Lippincott-Raven, 1997
5. Hasso AN, et al.: Chapter 27, In: Stark DD, Bradley WG (eds): Magnetic Resonance Imaging. (ed 2) St. Louis: CV Mosby and Co., 1992
6. Osborn AG: Handbook of Neuroradiology. St. Louis: Mosby-Year Book Inc., 1991, p 221

Gamut A-80-2

INFRATENTORIAL LESIONS ON CT OR MRI—CEREBELLAR (PARENCHYMAL) LESIONS

COMMON

1. Astrocytoma
2. Hemangioblastoma (esp. in von Hippel-Lindau syndrome)
3. Hemorrhage
4. Infarction
5. Hypoplasia or aplasia of cerebellum
6. Medulloblastoma, other PNET$_g$ (eg, ependymoblastoma; medulloepithelioma; pigmented medulloblastoma; cerebellar medulloblastoma) (See A-82)
7. Metastasis
8. Neurocysticercosis

UNCOMMON

1. Abscess (pyogenic; tuberculous; fungal)
2. Arteriovenous malformation
3. Dysplastic gangliocytoma of cerebellum—purkingeoma (Lhermitte-Duclos disease)
4. Gliosis (esp. with neurofibromatosis type 1)
5. Lymphoma$_g$
6. Multiple sclerosis
7. Sarcoidosis
8. Sarcoma (lateral medulloblastoma)

References

1. Bundschuh CV: Posterior fossa abnormalities on 0.3 tesla MRI scanner. Radiological Society of North America Scientific Exhibit, Washington, D.C., 1984
2. Damiano T, Truwit CL: Cerebellar and fourth ventricular tumors in adults. MRI Decisions 1992;6:10–21
3. Eisenberg RL: Clinical Imaging: An Atlas of Differential Diagnosis. (ed 3) Philadelphia: Lippincott-Raven, 1997, pp 1090–1099
4. Hasso AN, et al: Chapter 27, In: Stark DD, Bradley WG (eds): Magnetic Resonance Imaging. (ed 2) St. Louis: CV Mosby and Co., 1992

INFRATENTORIAL LESIONS ON CT OR MRI—OTHER POSTERIOR FOSSA LESIONS

COMMON
1. Aneurysm of basilar or vertebral artery
2. Aqueductal stenosis (eg, from midbrain glioma)
3. Arachnoid cyst
4. Cerebellopontine angle neoplasm (eg, acoustic schwannoma; meningioma; epidermoid; glomus jugulare tumor) (See A-81)
5. Chordoma of clivus
6. Glioma (astrocytoma) of brain stem (pons)

UNCOMMON
1. Arteriovenous malformation
2. Other schwannoma (VII, X, XI or XII nerve)
3. Rhabdomyosarcoma

References
1. Bundschuh CV: Posterior fossa abnormalities on 0.3 tesla MRI scanner. Radiological Society of North America Scientific Exhibit, Washington, D.C., 1984
2. Damiano T, Truwit CL: Cerebellar and fourth ventricular tumors in adults. MRI Decisions 1992;6:10–21
3. Eisenberg RL: Clinical Imaging: An Atlas of Differential Diagnosis. (ed 3) Philadelphia: Lippincott-Raven, 1997
4. Hasso AN, et al: Chapter 27, In: Stark DD, Bradley WG (eds): Magnetic Resonance Imaging. (ed 2) St. Louis: CV Mosby and Co., 1992

CEREBELLOPONTINE ANGLE MASS ON CT OR MRI

COMMON
1. Acoustic schwannoma (neurinoma)
2. Aneurysm or ectasia of basilar or vertebral artery

3. Epidermoid (congenital cholesteatoma)
4. Lateral extension of adjacent tumor (eg, pontine glioma; ependymoma or other fourth ventricular tumor; choroid plexus tumor; cerebellar neoplasm {astrocytoma; hemangioblastoma}; chordoma)
5. Meningioma

UNCOMMON
1. Arachnoid cyst
2. Arteriovenous malformation; hemangioma
3. Glomus jugulare tumor (paraganglioma)
4. Langerhans cell histiocytosis$_g$
5. Lipoma
6. [Meningeal enhancement (may rarely appear mass-like—as in bacterial or tuberculous meningitis, syphilis, or sarcoidosis)]
7. Metastasis
8. [Normal variant, pseudotumor (eg, flocculus of cerebellum)]
9. Other schwannoma (trigeminal, VII, X, XI or XII nerve)
10. [Parasellar neoplasm with extension (eg, chromophobe adenoma; optic glioma; craniopharyngioma; nasopharyngeal carcinoma)]
11. Parasitic cyst (eg, *Cysticercus* cyst)
12. Rhabdomyosarcoma

[ ] This condition does not actually cause the gamuted imaging finding, but can produce imaging changes that simulate it.

References
1. Burgener FA, Kormano M: Differential Diagnosis in Computed Tomography. New York: Thieme, 1996, pp 32–34
2. Eisenberg RL: Clinical Imaging: An Atlas of Differential Diagnosis. (ed 3) Philadelphia: Lippincott-Raven, 1997, pp 1100–1107
3. Newton TH, Potts DG: Radiology of the Skull and Brain. St. Louis: CV Mosby, 1971, vol 1, book 1, pp 442–447
4. Smoker WR, Jacoby CG, Mojtahedi S, et al: The CT gamut of cerebellopontine angle lesions. Radiological Society of North America Scientific Exhibit, Washington, D.C., 1984

Gamut A-82

POSTERIOR FOSSA TUMORS
IN CHILDREN (OVER 1 YEAR OF AGE)
ON CT OR MRI

COMMON

1. Brain stem glioma (astrocytoma)
2. Cerebellar astrocytoma (juvenile pilocytic; anaplastic)
3. Ependymoma
4. Primitive neuroectodermal tumor (PNET)$_g$
   a. Cerebellar medulloblastoma
   b. Ependymoblastoma
   c. Medulloepithelioma
   d. Pigmented medulloblastoma (melanotic vermian PNET)

UNCOMMON

1. Acoustic schwannoma (esp. with neurofibromatosis)
2. Dysplastic gangliocytoma of cerebellum–purkingeoma (Lhermitte-Duclos disease)
3. Hemangioblastoma (rare below age 15)
4. Metastasis
5. Other extraparenchymal tumor (eg, dermoid; epidermoid; meningioma; choroid plexus papilloma; skull base tumor)
6. Rhabdoid tumor (eg, rhabdomyosarcoma)
7. Teratoma

References

1. Atlas SW: Magnetic Resonance Imaging of the Brain and Spine. New York: Raven Press, 1991
2. Barkovich AJ: Pediatric Neuroimaging. (ed 3) Philadelphia: Lippincott Williams & Wilkins, 2000, pp 446–487
3. Fitz CR, Rao K: Primary tumors in children. In: Lee SH, Rao K: Cranial Computed Tomography and MRI. (ed 2) New York: McGraw-Hill, 1987, pp 365–381

Gamut A-83

CYSTIC OR NECROTIC MASS
IN THE POSTERIOR FOSSA
(ON CT, MRI, OR ULTRASOUND)

CONGENITAL CRANIOCEREBRAL MASS OR MALFORMATION

1. Arachnoid cyst (extra-axial)
2. Dandy-Walker malformation; Dandy-Walker variant
3. Ependymal cyst
4. Giant cisterna magna
5. [Vein of Galen "aneurysm" (may appear cystic on ultrasound unless Doppler is used)]

INFECTIOUS LESION

1. Abscess (esp. streptococcal; anaerobic)
2. Granulomatous infection (tuberculosis or fungus disease)
3. Parasitic disease (eg, cysticercosis; hydatid disease; paragonimiasis)

BENIGN OR MALIGNANT NEOPLASM

1. Acoustic schwannoma with associated arachnoid cyst (about 5%)
2. Brain stem glioma
3. Cystic astrocytoma (eg, juvenile pilocystic astrocytoma of cerebellum)
4. Dermoid
5. Ependymoma
6. Epidermoid
7. Hemangioblastoma
8. Medulloblastoma (rarely tiny cystic areas, esp. in lateral medulloblastoma {"cerebellar sarcoma"})
9. Metastasis
10. [Tumefactive multiple sclerosis]

TRAPPED FOURTH VENTRICLE (POSTSHUNTING)

Reference
1. Batnitzky S, Price HI, Gilmor RL: Cystic lesions of the posterior fossa. Radiological Society of North America Scientific Exhibit, Washington, D.C., 1984

[ ] This condition does not actually cause the gamuted imaging finding, but can produce imaging changes that simulate it.

Gamut A-84

OBSTRUCTION AT THE FOURTH VENTRICLE OUTLET*

COMMON
1. Atresia of fourth ventricle foramina (eg, Dandy-Walker S. {Dandy-Walker malformation})
2. Basilar arachnoiditis (eg, tuberculous meningitis)
3. Basilar invagination (eg, Paget's disease)
4. Chiari I and Chiari II (Arnold-Chiari) malformations
5. Neoplasm (esp. medulloblastoma; astrocytoma; ependymoma; metastasis)
6. Tonsillar herniation

UNCOMMON
1. Arachnoid cyst
2. *Cysticercus* cyst
3. Fusion deformity at craniovertebral junction
4. Meningocele

* Enlargement of the entire ventricular system with disproportionate dilatation of the fourth ventricle.

Gamut A-85

ENLARGED BRAIN STEM

COMMON
1. Glioma
2. Hemorrhage
3. Metastatic neoplasm

UNCOMMON
1. Abscess
2. Encephalitis
3. Ependymoma
4. Granulomatous disease (eg, tuberculosis; sarcoidosis)
5. Hemangioblastoma
6. Infarction (acute)
7. Medulloblastoma
8. Multiple sclerosis (with mass effect)
9. Other tumors (eg, lipoma; hamartoma; teratoma; epidermoid; lymphoma$_g$)
10. Syringobulbia
11. Vascular anomaly

References
1. Ball JB: Enlarged brain stem. Semin Roentgenol 1984; 19:3–4
2. Eisenberg RL: Clinical Imaging: An Atlas of Differential Diagnosis. (ed 3) Philadelphia: Lippincott-Raven, 1997, pp 1108–1111
3. Harwood-Nash DCF, Fitz CR: Neuroradiology in Infants and Children. St. Louis: CV Mosby, 1976, vol 2, pp 718–724

Gamut A-86

LOW ATTENUATION (HYPODENSE) LESION IN THE BRAIN STEM ON CT (ALSO HYPOINTENSE ON MRI T1-WEIGHTED IMAGES)

COMMON

1. Glioma
2. Infarction
3. Metastasis
4. Multiple sclerosis
5. Normal (decussation of superior cerebellar peduncles at level of inferior colliculi)
6. Syringobulbia (eg, with syringomyelia; Arnold-Chiari malformation; trauma)

UNCOMMON

1. Central pontine myelinolysis
2. Epidermoid
3. Granuloma (eg, tuberculosis or other infection; sarcoidosis)
4. Hamartoma
5. Lipoma
6. Lymphoma$_g$
7. Teratoma

Reference

1. Eisenberg RL: Clinical Imaging: An Atlas of Differential Diagnosis. (ed 3) Philadelphia: Lippincott-Raven, 1997, pp 1108–1111

Gamut A-87

SUBDURAL EMPYEMA ON CT OR MRI

COMMON

1. Sinusitis (frontal or ethmoid) with spread to subdural space
2. Trauma with penetrating injury to skull

UNCOMMON

1. Mastoiditis; middle ear infection
2. Osteomyelitis of skull
3. Purulent meningitis
4. Surgery (craniectomy)

Reference

1. Eisenberg RL: Clinical Imaging: An Atlas of Differential Diagnosis. (ed 3) Philadelphia: Lippincott-Raven, 1997, p 1060

Gamut A-88-1

RIM OR LINEAR ENHANCEMENT OF THE BRAIN SURFACE OR MENINGES ON CT OR MRI
(Indicates abnormal fluid collection over brain surface)

1. Empyema, subdural or epidural
2. Hematoma, subdural or epidural, resolving or chronic (eg, trauma; blood dyscrasia$_g$; anticoagulant therapy)

Gamut A-88-2

DIFFUSE GYRIFORM MENINGEAL ENHANCEMENT ON CT OR MRI
(Indicates disseminated leptomeningeal disease)

1. Benign leptomeningeal fibrosis (eg, scarring from craniotomy, shunt placement, or intrathecal chemotherapy)
2. Langerhans cell histiocytosis$_g$
3. Lymphoma$_g$; leukemia
4. Meningeal carcinomatosis (eg, from carcinoma of breast or lung, or melanoma)
5. Meningitis (eg, bacterial; syphilitic; tuberculous; fungal; viral—esp. herpes simplex; parasitic—neurocysticercosis; chemical)

6. Neoplastic spread or seeding from primary CNS tumor (malignant astroytoma; ependymoma; medulloblastoma; pineoblastoma; germinoma; choroid plexus tumor)
7. Orbital tumor with leptomeningeal spread (eg, retinoblastoma; ocular melanoma)
8. Primary meningeal tumor (eg, meningioma; glioma—primary leptomeningeal glioblastomatosis/gliosarcomatosis; lymphoma; sarcoma)
9. Rheumatoid pachymeningitis
10. Sarcoidosis
11. Subarachnoid hemorrhage, posttraumatic or spontaneous, late with fibroblastic proliferation (in acute or subacute phase, cisternal enhancement can occur)
12. Thrombosis of dural venous sinus (eg, oral contraceptives; infection; dehydration; craniotomy)

References

1. Burrows EH: Surface enhancement of the brain. Clin Radiol 1985;36:233–239
2. Chapman S, Nakielny R: Aids to Radiological Differential Diagnosis. (ed 3) London: WB Saunders, 1995, p 422
3. Dähnert W: Radiology Review Manual. (ed 4) Baltimore: Williams & Wilkins, 1999, pp 181–182
4. Eisenberg RL: Clinical Imaging: An Atlas of Differential Diagnosis. (ed 3) Philadelphia: Lippincott-Raven, 1997, p 1134–1135
5. Osborn AG: Handbook of Neuroradiology. St. Louis: Mosby-Year Book Inc., 1991, pp 227–233
6. Sze G: Diseases of the intracranial meninges: MR imaging features. AJR 1993;160:727–733

Gamut A-88-3

LOCALIZED GYRIFORM MENINGEAL ENHANCEMENT ON CT OR MRI

1. Arteriovenous malformation
*2. Encephalitis
*3. Infarction (esp. subacute)
*4. Glioma
5. Meningioma

6. Meningitis, localized (eg, bacterial, tuberculous, fungal, cysticercosis)

* Parenchymal lesions which infiltrate the cortex and obliterate the sulci.

Gamut A-89

EPENDYMAL AND SUBEPENDYMAL ENHANCEMENT OF VENTRICULAR MARGINS, CISTERNS, AND SUBARACHNOID SPACES ON CT OR MRI

COMMON

1. Meningeal carcinomatosis (esp. metastasis from carcinoma of lung or breast; melanoma of skin or eye; retinoblastoma)
2. Normal (esp, periventricular vascular structures)
3. Subependymal spread or ependymal seeding of primary brain neoplasm (esp. astrocytoma; glioblastoma; ependymoma; medulloblastoma; pineal tumor {germinoma; pineoblastoma}; choroid plexus tumor)
4. Inflammatory (eg, ventriculitis; meningitis)
   a. Abscess or inflammatory cyst rupture
   b. Bacterial, viral, fungal, or parasitic meningitis
   c. Chemical ventriculitis (eg, from shunt placement or intrathecal chemotherapy)
   d. Chronic granulomatous disease (eg, tuberculosis; sarcoidosis; Lyme disease)
   e. Cysticercosis

UNCOMMON

1. Leukemia
2. Lymphoma$_g$, primary or systemic
3. Vascular
   a. Arteriovenous malformation
   b. Collateral venous drainage (dural sinus or cortical vein occlusion; Sturge-Weber S.)
   c. Venous angioma

(continued)

References

1. Burgener FA, Kormano M: Differential Diagnosis in Computed Tomography. New York: Thieme, 1996, pp 52–54
2. Eisenberg RL: Clinical Imaging: An Atlas of Differential Diagnosis. (ed 3) Philadelphia: Lippincott-Raven, 1997, pp 1132–1133
3. Osborn AG: Handbook of Neuroradiology. St. Louis: Mosby-Year Book Inc., 1991, pp 223–226

Gamut A-90-1

INCREASED DENSITY WITHIN THE BASILAR CISTERNS ON NONENHANCED CT

COMMON

1. Iodinated intrathecal contrast media
2. Subarachnoid hemorrhage

UNCOMMON

1. Basilar cistern infection, active (eg, tuberculosis; cryptococcosis {torulosis}; coccidioidomycosis)
2. Bromism
3. En plaque neoplasm (eg, lymphoma$_g$; melanoma; meningioma)
4. Epidermoid
5. Meningeal calcification (eg, prior tuberculous meningitis)
6. Polycythemia
7. Postischemic hypervascularity of the meninges
8. Sarcoidosis

References

1. Enzmann DR: Imaging of Infections and Inflammations of the CNS: CT, Ultrasound and NMR. New York: Raven Press, 1984
2. Lee SH, Rao K: Cranial Computed Tomography and MRI. (ed 2) New York: McGraw-Hill, 1987
3. Masdeau JC, Fine M, Shewmon DA, et al: Post-ischemic hypervascularity of the infant brain: Differential diagnosis on CT. AJNR 1982;3:501–544

4. Osborne DDR, Bohan T, Hudson A: CT demonstration of hyperdense cerebral vasculature due to bromide therapy. J Comput Assist Tomogr 1984;8:982–984
5. Pagani JJ, Libshitz HI, Wallace S: CNS leukemia and lymphoma: CT manifestations. AJNR 1981;2:397–403

Gamut A-90-2

INTENSE ENHANCEMENT OF THE BASILAR CISTERNS ON CT

COMMON

1. Leptomeningeal neoplasm (eg, carcinomatosis; gliomatosis; lymphoma$_g$; leukemia; melanoma; seeding from medulloblastoma or other CNS neoplasm)
2. Meningitis (incl. tuberculous)
3. Subarachnoid hemorrhage, recent

UNCOMMON

1. Cryptococcosis (torulosis)
2. Polycythemia vera
3. Sarcoidosis
4. Siderosis
5. Syphilis

References

1. Enzmann DR: Imaging of Infections and Inflammations of the CNS: CT, Ultrasound and NMR. New York: Raven Press, 1984
2. Holmes S: Personal communication.
3. Kudel TA, Bingham WT, Tubman DE: CT findings of primary malignant leptomeningeal melanoma in neurocutaneous melanosis. AJR 1979;133:950–951
4. Pagani JJ, Libshitz HI, Wallace S: CNS leukemia and lymphoma: CT manifestations. AJNR 1981;2:397–403
5. Pinkston JW, Ballinger WE Jr, Lotz PR, et al: Superficial siderosis: A cause of leptomeningeal enhancement on computed tomography. J Comput Assist Tomogr 1983;7: 1073–1076

Gamut A-91-1

INTRACRANIAL FAT LUCENCY ON CT OR MRI

COMMON
1. Lipoma of corpus callosum

UNCOMMON
1. Dermoid cyst; mature teratoma
2. Epidermoid

Gamut A-91-2

INTRACRANIAL AIR LUCENCY (PNEUMOCEPHALUS) ON PLAIN FILMS, CT, OR MRI

COMMON
1. Trauma (eg, penetrating injury or fracture of a paranasal sinus or mastoid sinus)

UNCOMMON
1. Air embolism in cerebral vessels
2. Iatrogenic (eg, surgery {hypophysectomy; paranasal sinus surgery}; ventriculography)
3. Infection with gas-forming organism (brain abscess; mastoiditis; sinusitis)
4. Neoplasm eroding base of skull arising in a paranasal sinus or nasopharynx (esp. osteoma; carcinoma) or sella (pituitary adenoma); mucocele of paranasal sinus

References
1. Azar-Kia B, Sarwar M, Batnitzky S, et al: Radiology of the intracranial gas. AJR 1975; 124:315–323
2. Kushnet MW, Goldman RL: Lipoma of the corpus callosum associated with a frontal bone defect. AJR 1978;131: 517–518
3. Swischuk LE: Differential Diagnosis in Pediatric Radiology. Baltimore: Williams & Wilkins, 1984, p 378

Gamut A-92

COMMON CONGENITAL MALFORMATIONS OF THE BRAIN SEEN ON CT OR MRI

DISORDERS OF NEURAL TUBE CLOSURE
1. Encephalocele
2. Meningocele

DISORDERS OF NEURONAL MIGRATION
1. Heterotopia
2. Lissencephaly
3. Pachygyria
4. Polymicrogyria
5. Schizencephaly

OTHER DISORDERS OF ORGANOGENESIS
1. Agenesis of corpus callosum
2. Cerebellar aplasia or hypoplasia
3. Chiari malformations (Chiari I, II, and III)
4. Dandy-Walker malformation
5. Holoprosencephaly
6. Lipoma of corpus callosum
7. Septo-optic dysplasia

PHAKOMATOSES (NEUROCUTANEOUS SYNDROMES) (SEE A-56-S)
1. Neurofibromatosis (eg, cranial nerve schwannoma-esp. acoustic; meningioma; glioma of optic chiasm; cerebral hamartomas)
2. Sturge-Weber S.
3. Tuberous sclerosis
4. von Hippel-Lindau S.

Reference
1. Eisenberg RL: Clinical Imaging: An Atlas of Differential Diagnosis. (ed 3) Philadelphia: Lippincott-Raven, 1997, pp 1138–1145

INFECTIONS AND INFLAMMATION OF THE BRAIN AND MENINGES IDENTIFIABLE ON CT OR MRI

FOCAL PARENCHYMAL LESIONS

1. Abscess secondary to emboli
2. Cerebritis
3. Direct extension from sinusitis
4. Trauma with penetrating injury

CYSTIC PARASITIC LESIONS

1. Cysticercosis (parenchymal, intraventricular, subarachnoid)
2. Hydatid disease
3. Paragonimiasis
4. Strongyloidiasis

DIFFUSE PARENCHYMAL INFECTIONS

1. ADEM (slow viruses)
2. AIDS encephalopathy
3. Epstein-Barr encephalitis
4. Herpes simplex encephalitis
5. Malaria
6. Progressive multifocal leukoencephalopathy (PML)

MENINGITIS, EPENDYMITIS

1. Bacterial
2. Tuberculous
3. Viral

EXTRACEREBRAL INFECTIONS— SUBDURAL OR EPIDURAL EMPYEMA

1. Postmeningitis
2. Posttraumatic
3. Secondary to hematogenous or adjacent spread (eg, from sinusitis)

VASCULITIS SECONDARY TO INFECTION

1. Bacterial
2. Granulomatous (eg, tuberculous; fungal)
3. Viral (eg, herpes zoster ophthalmicus)

SARCOIDOSIS (DURAL, LEPTOMENINGEAL, INTRAPARENCHYMAL)

Reference
1. Sze G: Lecture at Hawaii Radiological Society Meeting, 1992

DEGENERATIVE AND METABOLIC DISORDERS OF THE BRAIN ON MRI

DEGENERATIVE DISORDERS

COMMON

1. Alzheimer's disease
2. Parkinson's disease; Parkinsonism-plus syndromes

UNCOMMON

1. Huntington's chorea
2. Jakob-Creutzfeldt disease (spongiform encephalopathy)
3. Olivopontocerebellar atrophy
4. Pick's disease
5. Progressive supranuclear palsy
6. Shy-Drager S.
7. Striatonigral degeneration
8. Wernicke's encephalopathy

METABOLIC DISORDERS

1. Adrenoleukodystrophy
2. Central pontine myelinolysis
3. Hallervorden-Spatz disease
4. Leigh's disease
5. Mucopolysaccharidoses (See J-4)

6. Nonketotic hyperglycemia
7. Phenylketonuria
8. Wilson's disease

Reference
1. Eisenberg RL: Clinical Imaging: An Atlas of Differential Diagnosis. (ed 3) Philadelphia: Lippincott-Raven, 1997, pp 1120–1125

Gamut A-95-1

WHITE MATTER DISEASE OF THE BRAIN ON CT OR MRI— DYSMYELINATING DISEASES
(Abnormal Myelin Formation or Maintenance In Infants and Children)

LYSOSOMAL DISORDERS
1. Krabbe disease (globoid cell leukodystrophy)
2. Metachromatic leukodystrophy

PEROXISOMAL DISORDERS
1. Adrenoleukodystrophy (ALD)—childhood form most common; also neonatal ALD and adult ALD (adrenomyeloneuropathy)
2. Zellweger S. (cerebrohepatorenal S.)

MITOCHONDRIAL DYSFUNCTION
1. Alper's disease (primarily affects grey matter) Kearns-Sayre S.
2. Leigh's disease
3. MELAS (mitochondrial myopathy, encephalopathy, lactic acidosis, and stroke-like episodes)
4. MERRF (myoclonus epilepsy with ragged red fibers)

AMINO ACID AND ORGANIC ACID METABOLIC DISORDERS
1. Canavan's disease (spongiform leukodystrophy)
2. Maple syrup urine disease

UNKNOWN METABOLIC DEFECT
1. Alexander's disease
2. Pelizaeus-Merzbacher disease

References
1. Chapman S, Nakielny R: Aids to Radiological Differential Diagnosis. (ed 3) London: WB Saunders, 1995, pp 448–453
2. Greenberg SB, Faerber EN, Riviello JJ, et al: Subacute necrotizing encephalomyelopathy (Leigh disease): CT and MRI appearances. Pediatr Radiol 1990;21:5–8
3. Hatten HP Jr: Dysmyelinating leukodystrophies: 'LACK Proper Myelin'. Pediatr Radiol 1991;21:477–482
4. Heier L: What importance should be attached to white matter 'dots'? In: Huckman MS (ed): ARRS Neuroradiology Categorical Course Syllabus. Reston: American Roentgen Ray Society, 1992, pp 57–69
5. Lee SH, Rao K: Cranial Computed Tomography and MRI. (ed 2) New York: McGraw-Hill, 1987, pp 717–745
6. Osborn AG: Handbook of Neuroradiology. St. Louis: Mosby-Year Book Inc., 1991, pp 251–262
7. Tien RD, Felsberg GJ, Ferris NJ, Osumi AK: The dementias: correlation of clinical features, pathophysiology, and neuroradiology. AJR 1993;161:245–255

Gamut A-95-2

WHITE MATTER DISEASE OF THE BRAIN ON CT OR MRI—DEMYELINATING (MYELINOCLASTIC) DISEASES*
(Normal Myelin Is Destroyed)

COMMON
1. AIDS encephalitis
2. Multiple sclerosis
3. Progressive multifocal leukoencephalopathy (PML)

UNCOMMON
1. Acute disseminated encephalomyelitis (ADEM)
   a. Allergic (postvaccination)
   b. Fulminating (fatal)
   c. Postinfection (measles; vaccinia; varicella)
   d. Spontaneous or during a respiratory infection

(continued)

2. Acute encephalitis (eg, rubella; measles; chickenpox; mumps; herpes simplex; epidemic encephalopathies
3. Acute hemorrhagic encephalomyelitis
4. Carbon monoxide encephalopathy
5. Central pontine myelinolysis
6. Congenital transplacental infection (eg, rubella; cytomegalovirus; herpes simplex)
7. Disseminated necrotizing leukoencephalopathy (after methotrexate therapy)
8. Hypoxic-ischemic encephalopathy (eg, periventricular leukomalacia in premature infants)
9. Jakob-Creutzfeldt disease
10. Malnutrition; vitamin B_{12} deficiency
11. Marchiafava-Bignami disease (corpus callosum)
12. Radiation therapy (necrosis); chemotherapy
13. Schilder's disease (myelinoclastic diffuse sclerosis)
14. Subacute sclerosing panencephalitis
15. Subcortical arteriosclerotic encephalopathy (SAE; Binswanger's disease)
16. Trauma (white matter shearing injury)
17. Vascular (eg, small vessel disease, lacunar infarcts, migraine, and aging may cause small multifocal white matter lesions)

SECONDARY DEMYELINATING CONDITIONS

1. Anoxia
2. Brain abscess
3. Cerebral infarction
4. Cerebral neoplasm, primary or metastatic
5. Deficiency syndromes
6. Intoxication

* 60% of healthy elderly patients with normal cognitive function may show multiple foci of increased white matter signal on T_2WI.

References

1. Brant-Zawadzki M: Multiple sclerosis and its imitators. In: Huckman MS (ed): ARRS Neuroradiology Categorical Course Syllabus. Reston: American Roentgen Ray Society, 1992, pp 229–232
2. Chapman S, Nakielny R: Aids to Radiological Differential Diagnosis. (ed 3) London: WB Saunders, 1995, pp 448–453
3. Heier L: What importance should be attached to white matter 'dots'? In: Huckman MS (ed): ARRS Neuroradiology Categorical Course Syllabus. Reston: American Roentgen Ray Society, 1992, pp 57–69
4. Lee SH, Rao K: Cranial Computed Tomography and MRI. (ed 2) New York: McGraw-Hill, 1987, pp 717–745
5. Osborn AG: Handbook of Neuroradiology. St. Louis: Mosby-Year Book Inc., 1991, pp 251–262
6. Shaw DWW, Cohen WA: Viral infections of the CNS in children: imaging features. AJR 1993;160:125–133
7. Tien RD, Felsberg GJ, Ferris NJ, Osumi AK: The dementias: correlation of clinical features, pathophysiology, and neuroradiology. AJR 1993;161:245–255

Gamut A-96

PERIVENTRICULAR HYPERINTENSE (BRIGHT) LESION ON T2-WEIGHTED MRI

CHILDREN AND YOUNG ADULTS

1. Acute disseminated encephalomyelitis (ADEM) (postviral leukoencephalopathy)
2. Ependymitis granularis (anterior and lateral to frontal horns in normal individuals)
3. Leukodystrophies
   a. Adrenoleukodystrophy
   b. Alexander's disease
   c. Canavan's disease
   d. Krabbe disease (globoid cell leukodystrophy)
   e. Metachromatic leukodystrophy
   f. Pelizaeus-Merzbacher disease
4. Migraine
5. Mucopolysaccharidoses (See J-4)
6. Multiple sclerosis
7. Vasculitis (lupus erythematosus; sickle cell disease; Behçet S.)
8. Virchow-Robin spaces in putamen

ELDERLY

1. Ischemia of deep white matter (eg, ischemic cardiovascular disease; hypertension; smoking)
2. Lacunar infarction

PATIENTS WITH AIDS

1. Lymphoma
2. Progressive multifocal leukoencephalopathy (PML)
3. Subacute white matter encephalitis (esp. due to HIV or cytomegalovirus infection)
4. Toxoplasmosis

PATIENTS WITH TRAUMA

1. Diffuse axonal/shearing injury
2. Diffuse necrotizing leukoencephalopathy (DNL) (intrathecal methotrexate +/− whole brain radiation
3. Radiation injury to whole brain with demyelination of periventricular white matter

PATIENTS WITH HYDROCEPHALUS

1. Transependymal CSF flow

References

1. Dähnert W: Radiology Review Manual. (ed 4) Baltimore: Williams & Wilkins, 1999, p 187
2. Eisenberg RL: Clinical Imaging: An Atlas of Differential Diagnosis. (ed 3) Philadelphia: Lippincott-Raven, 1997, pp 1116–1119

Gamut A-97

PERIVENTRICULAR HYPODENSE LESION ON CT

1. Cystic neoplasm
2. Encephalomalacia
3. Hematoma (resolving)
4. Parasitic cyst (*Cysticercus; Paragonimus:* hydatid)
5. Porencephalic cyst (porencephaly)

Reference

1. Dähnert W: Radiology Review Manual. (ed 4) Baltimore: Williams & Wilkins, 1999, p 186

Gamut A-98

CEREBRAL INFARCTION (STROKE) ON CT, MRI, OR ANGIOGRAPHY

VASCULAR CAUSES (95% of all strokes)

I. ISCHEMIC STROKE (80%)

A. Arterial Occlusive Disease

1. Arteriolosclerosis (intracerebral arteriolar occlusive disease, esp. with chronic hypertension—lacunar infarct)
2. Atherosclerotic occlusion of a major extracranial or intracranial artery (eg, stenosis; thrombosis; plaque ulceration and embolism)

B. Cardiogenic Emboli

1. Ischemic heart disease with mural thrombus (eg, myocardial infarction; arrhythmia)
2. Left atrial myxoma
3. Nonvalvular atrial fibrillation
4. Valvular heart disease
   a. Infective endocarditis
   b. Nonbacterial thrombotic endocarditis
   c. Prosthetic valve(s)
   d. Rheumatic valvulitis (esp. mitral stenosis)

C. Hypercoaguable State

D. Nonatheromatous Disease

1. Aneurysm (rare)
2. Arteritis; vasculitis
   a. Behçet disease
   b. Collagen vascular disease
   c. Lymphoid granulomatosis
   d. Syphilis
   e. Takayasu arteritis
   f. Temporal arteritis
3. Dissection (spontaneous; traumatic)
4. Elongation, coiling or kinking of artery
5. Fibromuscular dysplasia
6. Moyamoya disease

(continued)

7. Postendartectomy thrombosis, embolism, or restenosis

II. HEMORRHAGIC STROKE (20%)

A. Intracerebral Hemorrhage
1. Amyloid angiopathy
2. Arteriovenous malformation
3. Bleeding diathesis (eg, hemophilia)
4. Drugs (esp. anticoagulants)
5. Hypertensive hemorrhage

B. Vasospasm Due to Nontraumatic Subarachnoid Hemorrhage
1. Arteriovenous malformation
2. Ruptured aneurysm

C. Veno-occlusive Disease, Septic or Aseptic (Involving major venous sinuses, superficial cortical veins, and/or deep venous system)
1. Venous obstruction (eg, thrombosis)

NONVASCULAR CAUSES
(5% of all strokes)

A. Anoxic Ischemic Encephalopathy Due to Acute Respiratory Insufficiency
1. Allergic reaction
2. Carbon monoxide intoxication
3. Drug overdose (eg, central respiratory depressant drugs, esp. alcohol, narcotics, and barbiturates)
4. Heart failure or hypotension (acute)
5. Near-drowning
6. Primary central respiratory failure

B. Brain Tumor

RISK FACTORS FOR STROKE

1. Alcoholism
2. Atrial fibrillation
3. Diabetes
4. Heart failure
5. Heredity
6. Hypercholesterolemia (familial)
7. Hypertension
8. Myocardial infarction
9. Obesity
10. Oral contraceptives
11. Smoking
12. Stress; high anxiety

References
1. Dähnert W: Radiology Review Manual. (ed 4) Baltimore: Williams & Wilkins, 1999, pp 181–182
2. Lee SH, Rao K: Cranial Computed Tomography and MRI. (ed 2) New York: McGraw-Hill, 1987, pp 643–699

Gamut A-99

INTRACEREBRAL HEMORRHAGE OR HEMATOMA ON CT, MRI, OR ANGIOGRAPHY

COMMON
1. Aneurysm (rupture or leakage of berry or infectious aneurysm)
2. Arteriovenous malformation; venous angioma; cavernous angioma
3. Hemorrhagic venous infarction (eg, superior sagittal sinus or other dural sinus thrombosis; cortical vein occlusion)
4. Hypertensive vascular disease (arteriolosclerosis)
5. Neoplasm
   a. Primary—usually in white matter
   b. Metastatic—usually in gray matter (esp. from lung, kidney, melanoma, choriocarcinoma)
6. Stroke (hemorrhagic arterial infarction)
7. Trauma to head

UNCOMMON
1. Amphetamine abuse
2. Amyloid angiopathy
3. Arteritis (See A-102)

4. Bleeding or clotting disorder$_g$ (eg, hemophilia; anti-coagulant therapy)
5. Neonatal germinal matrix hemorrhage (esp. in prematures less than 1500 gm)
6. Surgery; postoperative

References

1. Buonanno FS, Moody DM, Ball MR, et al: Computed cranial tomographic findings in cerebral sinovenous occlusion. J Comput Assist Tomogr 1978;2:281–290
2. Harrington B, Heller A, Dawson D, et al: Intracerebral hemorrhage and oral amphetamine. Arch Neurol 1983;40: 503–507
3. Hickey WF, King RB, Wang AM, et al: Multiple simultaneous intracerebral hematomas: Clinical, radiologic and pathologic findings in two patients. Arch Neurol 1983; 40: 519–522
4. Lee SH, Rao K: Cranial Computed Tomography and MRI. (ed 2) New York: McGraw-Hill, 1987, pp 645, 699–708
5. Osborn AG: Handbook of Neuroradiology. St. Louis: Mosby-Year Book Inc., 1991, pp 271–277
6. Wagle WA, Smith TW, Weiner M: Intracerebral hemorrhage caused by cerebral amyloid angiopathy: Radiographic-pathologic correlation. AJNR 1984;5:171–176

Gamut A-99-S

TIME STAGING OF MRI APPEARANCE OF CEREBRAL HEMATOMA

Stage	Image Type	Appearances	Nature of Hematoma
Acute	T1W	Dark	Intracellular oxyhemoglobin
	T2W	Dark	
1–2 days	T1W	Intermediate	Intracellular deoxyhemoglobin
	T2W	Dark; bright margin	Perifocal edema
3–4 days	T1W	Bright rim appears	Beginning formation of methemoglobin in hematoma
	T2W	Dark with marginal increased signal from edema	
5–7 days	T1W	Bright with dark marginal zone of edema	Methemoglobin with rim of fluid and edema
	T2W	Bright with darker center	
2nd week	T1W	As above	As above
	T2W	Bright with dark rim	Methemoglobin in center with hemosiderin rim
2 months	T1W	Bright with very dark rim	Gliotic or cystic center. Ring of hemosiderin in macrophages

Reference

1. Hackney DB: Location and age of intracranial hemorrhage. ARRS Neuroradiology Categorical Course Syllabus. Reston: American Roentgen Ray Society, 1992, pp 37–45

Gamut A-100

SUBARACHNOID HEMORRHAGE

COMMON
1. Ruptured aneurysm

UNCOMMON
1. Bleeding diathesis$_g$ (eg, anticoagulant therapy)
2. Arteriovenous malformation (brain or spinal canal)
3. Hypertensive intracerebral hemorrhage
4. Idiopathic; no known cause
5. Neoplasm (intracranial or spinal)
6. Trauma (skull or spine fracture or contusion)
7. Vasculopathy

Gamut A-101

PATTERN ANALYSIS OF CEREBRAL VESSELS ON ANGIOGRAPHY (VASCULAR FILLING, SIZE, CONTOUR, AND TRANSIT TIME) (SEE A-102-104)

LACK OF VASCULAR FILLING
1. Compression
2. Dissection
3. Embolization (incl. iatrogenic)
4. Shunt
5. Thrombosis (eg, atherosclerosis; vasculitis)

HYPERVASCULARITY (TOO MANY VESSELS)
1. Arteriovenous malformation; vein of Galen "aneurysm"
2. Collateral circulation
3. Congenital variant
4. Neoplasm (eg, brain tumor; meningioma)

INCREASED SIZE OF VESSELS
1. Aneurysm (incl. vein of Galen "aneurysm")
2. Arteriovenous malformation
3. Carotid-cavernous fistula
4. Ectasia
5. High flow system
6. Neoplasm (eg, brain tumor; meningioma)

DECREASED SIZE OF VESSELS
1. Atherosclerosis
2. Dissection
3. Low flow system
4. Spasm (eg, subarachnoid hemorrhage; migraine)
5. Vasculitis; arteritis

CONTOUR IRREGULARITY OF VESSEL WALLS
1. Atherosclerosis
2. Dissection
3. Fibromuscular hyperplasia
4. Spasm
5. Tumor vascularity or encasement
6. Vasculitis; arteritis

PROLONGED TRANSIT TIME
1. Focal edema
2. Hyperventilation; decreased pCO_2
3. Infarction or occlusion
4. Venous thrombosis

DECREASED TRANSIT TIME AND EARLY VENOUS FILLING
1. Arteriovenous malformation
2. Increased pCO_2
3. Infarction
4. Neoplasm (eg, brain tumor; meningioma)

References
1. Djang WT: Basics of Cerebral Angiography. In: Ravin CE, Cooper C (eds): Review of Radiology. Philadelphia: WB Saunders, 1990, pp 189–191
2. Osborn A: Diagnostic Cerebral Angiography. (ed 2) Philadelphia: Lippincott Williams & Wilkins, 1999

Gamut A-102

ARTERITIS

COMMON

1. Bacterial arteritis; infectious aneurysm (eg, from abscess; meningitis; osteomyelitis; embolism)
2. Connective tissue disease (collagen vascular disease)$_g$ (esp. polyarteritis nodosa; lupus erythematosus)
3. Drug or chemical arteritis (eg, ergot; amphetamine; heroin; arsenic; carbon monoxide)
4. Necrotizing angiitis (eg, rheumatic fever; hypersensitivity angiitis; giant cell {temporal} arteritis; Wegener's granulomatosis; granulomatous angiitis)
5. Takayasu arteritis

UNCOMMON

1. Amyloid angiopathy
2. Behçet syndrome
3. Carotid arteritis (infant or child)
4. Fungal arteritis (esp. cryptococcosis {torulosis}; aspergillosis; phycomycosis); actinomycosis; nocardiosis
5. High-flow angiopathy (associated with arteriovenous malformations or fistulas)
6. Radiation arteritis
7. Rickettsial arteritis
8. Sarcoid arteritis
9. Syphilitic arteritis
10. Tuberculous arteritis
11. Viral arteritis (eg, herpes zoster)

References

1. Ferris EJ, Levine HL: Cerebral arteritis: Classification. Radiology 1973;109:327–341
2. Grainger RG, Allison DJ (eds): Diagnostic Radiology: An Anglo-American Textbook of Imaging, (ed 2) Edinburgh: Churchill Livingstone, 1992, vol 3, pp 1993–1994
3. Hilal SK, Solomon GE, Gold AP, et al: Primary cerebral arterial occlusive disease in children. Radiology 1971; 99: 71–94
4. Leeds NE, Rosenblatt R: Arterial wall irregularities in intracranial neoplasms. Radiology 1972;103:121–124
5. Osborn AG: Handbook of Neuroradiology. St. Louis: Mosby-Year Book, Inc., 1991, pp 112–115

Gamut A-103

CEREBRAL ARTERIAL DISEASE OTHER THAN ARTERITIS ON ANGIOGRAPHY (NARROWING, IRREGULARITY, OCCLUSION, OR ANEURYSM)

1. Arterial spasm (eg, subarachnoid or cerebral hemorrhage; migraine)
2. Arteriosclerosis
3. Arteriovenous malformation
4. Berry aneurysm
5. Cerebral thrombosis (eg, sickle cell disease; oral contraceptives)
6. Embolism (eg, subacute bacterial endocarditis; atrial myxoma)
7. Fibromuscular dysplasia (usually extracranial)
8. Idiopathic
9. [Increased intracranial pressure]
10. Inflammatory disease of brain (eg, abscess; purulent or tuberculous meningitis)
11. Multiple progressive intracranial artery occlusions with telangiectasia (moyamoya)
12. Neoplasm (eg, glioblastoma; lymphoma$_g$; metastasis)
13. Phakomatoses (neurocutaneous syndromes—eg, neurofibromatosis; Sturge-Weber S.; tuberous sclerosis)
14. Trauma

[ ] This condition does not actually cause the gamuted imaging finding, but can produce imaging changes that simulate it.

References

1. Ferris EJ, Levine HL: Cerebral arteritis: Classification. Radiology 1973;109:327–341
2. Grainger RG, Allison DJ (eds): Diagnostic Radiology: An Anglo-American Textbook of Imaging, (ed 2) Edinburgh: Churchill Livingstone, 1992, vol 3, pp 1993–1994
3. Hilal SK, Solomon GE, Gold AP, et al: Primary cerebral arterial occlusive disease in children. Radiology 1971; 99:71–94
4. Leeds NE, Rosenblatt R: Arterial wall irregularities in intracranial neoplasms. Radiology 1972;103:121–124

Gamut A-104

INTRACRANIAL ARTERIOVENOUS SHUNTING AND EARLY VENOUS FILLING ON CEREBRAL ANGIOGRAPHY

COMMON

1. Arteriovenous malformation, congenital or acquired (incl. carotid-cavernous fistula; vein of Galen "aneurysm")
2. Cerebral infarction
3. Occlusive vascular disease
4. Malignant neoplasm of brain, primary or metastatic
5. Meningioma

UNCOMMON

1. Cerebral arteritis
2. Contusion of brain
3. Epilepsy, focal idiopathic
4. Inflammatory lesion (eg, brain abscess)
5. Intracerebral hematoma

References

1. Glickman MG, Mainzer F, Gletne JS: Early venous opacification in cerebral contusion. Radiology 1971;100:615–622
2. Lee SH, Goldberg HI: Hypervascular pattern associated with idiopathic focal status epilepticus. Radiology 1977; 125:159–163

Gamut A-105

AVASCULAR INTRACRANIAL MASS

COMMON

1. Abscess
2. Contusion
3. Edema
4. Epidural hematoma, hygroma, or empyema
5. Hematoma (intracerebral)

6. Neoplasm (low grade glioma {astrocytoma}; oligodendroglioma; metastasis)
7. Subdural hematoma, hygroma, or empyema

UNCOMMON

1. Arachnoid cyst
2. Bone lesion infiltrating dura (eg, metastasis; sarcoma; epidermoid; Langerhans cell histiocytosis$_g$)
3. Colloid cyst of third ventricle
4. Dermoid; teratoma
5. Lipoma of corpus callosum
6. Meningeal neoplasm (eg, avascular meningioma; meningeal involvement by carcinoma, lymphoma$_g$, leukemia, sarcoma, neuroblastoma, or melanoma)
7. Parasitic cyst (eg, *Cysticercus; Paragonimus;* hydatid)
8. Porencephalic cyst (porencephaly)
9. Tuberculoma; other granuloma

Gamut A-106

AVASCULAR ZONE NEAR THE BRAIN SURFACE ON CEREBRAL ANGIOGRAPHY

COMMON

1. Cortical atrophy
2. "Cortical steal" by deep arteriovenous shunt
3. Epidural hematoma, hygroma, or empyema
4. Meningeal neoplasm (eg, avascular meningioma; meningeal involvement by carcinoma, lymphoma$_g$, leukemia, sarcoma, neuroblastoma, or melanoma)
5. Occlusive vascular disease; cerebral infarction
6. Subdural hematoma, hygroma, or empyema

UNCOMMON

1. Arachnoid cyst
2. Bone lesion infiltrating dura (eg, metastasis; sarcoma; epidermoid; Langerhans cell histiocytosis$_g$)
3. Normal large subarachnoid space (infant)

4. Parasitic cyst (eg, *Cysticercus; Paragonimus;* hydatid)
5. Porencephalic cyst (porencephaly)
6. Subdural invasion by glioma
7. Syphilitic pachymeningitis
8. Tuberculoma

Reference
1. Ferris EJ, Lehrer H, Shapiro JH: Pseudo-subdural hematoma. Radiology 1967; 88:75–84

EXTRACRANIAL ISCHEMIC LESION SECONDARILY INVOLVING THE BRAIN

COMMON
1. Occlusion or stenosis of brachiocephalic vessels
2. Steal syndromes (eg, subclavian steal S.) (See A-108)

UNCOMMON
1. Dissecting aneurysm of thoracic aorta
2. Embolization secondary to mitral valve disease or atrial myxoma
3. Takayasu arteritis
4. Trauma to neck
5. Tumor in neck compromising cervical vessels (eg, thyroid adenoma, goiter or carcinoma; neurilemmoma)

Reference
1. Mishkin MM: Extracranial ischemic lesions which secondarily involve the brain. Radiol Clin North Am 1967;5: 395–408

SUBCLAVIAN STEAL SYNDROME

COMMON
1. Atherosclerosis

UNCOMMON
1. Coarctation of aorta with obliteration of subclavian orifice
2. Extravascular obstruction (eg, fibrous band)
3. Hypoplasia, atresia, or isolation of subclavian artery with anomalous aortic arch
4. Ligation for correction of tetralogy of Fallot or coarctation of aorta
5. Obstruction of subclavian artery secondary to cannulation
6. Vascular ring

References
1. Becker AE, Becker MJ, Edwards JE, et al: Congenital anatomic potentials for subclavian steal. Chest 1971; 60:4–13
2. Massumi RA: The congenital variety of the subclavian steal syndrome. Circulation 1963;28:1149–1152
3. Patel A, Toole JF: Subclavian steal syndrome: Reversal of cephalic blood flow. Medicine 1965;44:289–303

LESIONS IDENTIFIABLE ON ULTRASOUND EXAMINATION OF THE INFANT BRAIN

COMMON
1. Hemorrhage involving
   a. Cerebellum
   b. Choroid plexus
   c. Germinal matrix in prematures
   d. Periventricular or intraventricular in full-term infant

(continued)

e. Subdural
f. White matter, in full-term or preterm infant (latter associated with periventricular leukomalacia)
2. Hydrocephalus

UNCOMMON

1. Absent septum pellucidum
2. Agenesis of corpus callosum
3. Arnold-Chiari malformation (Chiari II malformation)
4. Bacterial ventriculitis (occasionally meningitis or encephalitis)
5. Dandy-Walker S.; Dandy-Walker variant
6. Hemimegancephaly
7. Holoprosencephaly
8. Hydranencephaly; anencephaly
9. Hypoxic ischemic injury (diffuse; multifocal; focal; watershed infarcts)
10. Intracranial calcification
11. Lipoma of corpus callosum
12. Lissencephaly
13. Mineralizing vasculopathy
14. Neoplasm (congenital intracranial)
15. Porencephalic cyst (porencephaly) (esp. following periventricular hemorrhage)
16. Schizencephaly
17. Vein of Galen "aneurysm"

References

1. Blomhagen JD, Mack LA: Abnormalities of the neonatal cerebral ventricles. Radiol Clin North Am 1985;23:13–31
2. Chilton SJ, Cremin BJ: Ultrasound diagnosis of CSF cystic lesions in the neonatal brain. Br J Radiol 1983;56:613–620
3. Dewbury K: Ultrasound of the infant brain. In: Grainger RG, Allison DJ (eds): Diagnostic Radiology. Edinburgh: Churchill Livingstone, 1992, vol 3, pp 2089–2095
4. Dewbury KC, Bates RI: Neonatal intracranial hemorrhage: The cause of the ultrasound appearances. Br J Radiol 1983;56:783–789
5. Eisenberg RL: Clinical Imaging: An Atlas of Differential Diagnosis. (ed 3) Philadelphia: Lippincott-Raven, 1997, pp 1146–1149
6. Mack LA, Rumack CM, Johnson ML: Ultrasound evaluation of cystic intracranial lesions in the neonate. Radiology 1980;137:451–455
7. Siegel MJ; Pediatric Sonography (ed 3) Philadelphia: Lippincott Williams & Wilkins, 2002, pp 58–78

Gamut A-110

ECHOGENIC BRAIN LESIONS ON ULTRASOUND

COMMON

1. Calcification
2. Hemorrhage (eg, subependymal)
3. Infarction
4. Normal (choroid plexus; caudothalamic groove)

UNCOMMON

1. Air
2. Arteriovenous malformation
3. Edema
4. Encephalitis
5. Hamartoma
6. Periventricular leukomalacia
7. Tumor

Reference

1. Williamson MR: Chapter 10. Pediatric brain, spine, and hip ultrasonography. In: Essentials of Ultrasound. Philadelphia: WB Saunders, 1996, pp 212, 216

Gamut A-111

CYSTIC BRAIN LESIONS ON ULTRASOUND

COMMON

1. [Aneurysm; arteriovenous malformation]
2. Arachnoid cyst
3. Leptomeningeal cyst
4. Periventricular leukomalacia
5. Porencephalic cyst (porencephaly)

UNCOMMON
1. Agenesis of corpus callosum with midline cyst
2. Choroid plexus cyst
3. Colloid cyst of third ventricle
4. Dandy-Walker cyst
5. Holoprosencephaly (alobar)
6. Parasitic cyst (eg, hydatid; *Cysticercus; Paragonimus*)
7. Schizencephaly
8. Ventricular cyst

[ ] This condition does not actually cause the gamuted imaging finding, but can produce imaging changes that simulate it.

Reference
1. Williamson MR: Chapter 10. Pediatric brain, spine, and hip ultrasonography. In: Essentials of Ultrasound. Philadelphia: WB Saunders, 1996, p 216

Gamut A-112-1

LOW DIASTOLIC FLOW IN INTERNAL CAROTID ARTERY

COMMON
1. Aortic valve insufficiency
2. Distal internal carotid artery stenosis
3. Distal small vessel disease
4. Low cardiac output

UNCOMMON
1. Increased intracranial pressure

Gamut A-112-2

LOW VELOCITY FLOW IN INTERNAL CAROTID ARTERY

COMMON
1. Aortic valve stenosis
2. Distal small vessel disease

3. Low cardiac output
4. Proximal internal carotid artery stenosis
5. Tandem lesions

UNCOMMON
1. Increased intracranial pressure

Gamut A-113

INCREASED INTRACRANIAL PRESSURE

COMMON
1. Brain abscess
2. Cerebral edema, contusion, hemorrhage, or infarction
3. Hematoma (intracerebral, extradural, subdural); hygroma
4. Hydrocephalus, obstructive (See A-114-1)
5. Lead encephalopathy
6. Malignant hypertension
7. Meningitis, meningoencephalitis (eg, tuberculosis; cryptococcosis {torulosis}; toxoplasmosis)
8. Metastatic neoplasm (eg, bronchogenic carcinoma; neuroblastoma)
9. Primary brain tumor

UNCOMMON
1. Aqueductal stenosis
2. Arnold-Chiari malformation
3. Craniostenosis, severe
4. Dandy-Walker S. (Dandy-Walker malformation)
5. Drug therapy (eg, tetracycline)
6. Emphysema, severe with cough
7. Hyperthyroidism
8. Hypervitaminosis A
9. Hypoparathyroidism
10. Increased venous pressure
11. Leukemia; lymphoma$_g$
12. Meningocele

(continued)

13. Parasitic disease (eg, cysticercosis; hydatid disease; paragonimiasis)
14. Pseudotumor cerebri

RADIOLOGIC FEATURES OF INCREASED INTRACRANIAL PRESSURE

1. Increased craniofacial ratio
2. Increased digital markings of calvarium ("hammered silver" appearance)
3. Sellar changes
   a. Decalcification of floor and dorsum of sella
   b. Pointed anterior clinoids
   c. Sellar enlargement
   d. Thinning or loss of posterior clinoids
4. Sutural diastases; unusually deep sutural interdigitations
5. Thinning of calvarium

HYDROCEPHALUS

ATROPHIC HYDROCEPHALUS (CEREBRAL ATROPHY)

1. Arteriovenous malformation; vascular lesion
2. Cerebral maldevelopment (eg, lissencephaly syndromes {congenital agyria}; cerebral hemiatrophy {Dyke-Davidoff-Masson S.})
3. Congenital inflammatory disease (eg, toxoplasmosis; cryptococcosis {torulosis}; fetal cytomegalovirus infection)
4. Demyelinating disease (eg, multiple sclerosis; encephalomyelitis)

5. Drugs (eg, Dilantin; steroids; chemotherapy; marijuana; hard drugs); alcohol
6. Hypertensive cerebral degenerative disease
7. Idiopathic
8. Multi-infarct dementia
9. Normal aging
10. Primary neuronal degeneration (eg, Alzheimer's disease; Pick's disease; Jakob-Creutzfeldt disease; Huntington's chorea)
11. Radiation therapy
12. Trauma

COMMUNICATING (NONABSORPTIVE) HYDROCEPHALUS (SECONDARY TO OBSTRUCTION OF SUBARACHNOID SPACES AT CEREBRAL CONVEXITY, BASAL CISTERNS, OR FORAMEN MAGNUM)

1. Achondroplasia
2. Arnold-Chiari malformation
3. Basilar invagination (See A-12)
4. Dural sinus/cortical venous thrombosis ("Otitic hydrocephalus") (esp. superior sagittal sinus thrombosis)
5. Encephalocele
6. Idiopathic in elderly ("normal pressure hydrocephalus")
7. Leptomeningeal carcinomatosis (metastatic breast carcinoma in adults; medulloblastoma in children; leukemia; lymphoma; ependymoma; pineal germinoma)
8. Meningeal infiltration in storage diseases
9. Meningitis, acute or chronic (esp. tuberculous)
10. Meningomyelocele
11. Neoplasm (eg, brain tumor; meningioma)
12. Subarachnoid or subdural hemorrhage (eg, trauma; bleeding or clotting disorder$_g$; prematurity)

OBSTRUCTIVE (NONCOMMUNICATING) HYDROCEPHALUS (SECONDARY TO INTRAVENTRICULAR, AQUEDUCTAL, FORAMINA OF MONRO, OR FORAMINA OF MAGENDIE AND LUSCHKA OBSTRUCTION)

Intraventricular Mass (See A-74)

1. Choroid plexus papilloma or carcinoma
2. Ependymoma
3. Hematoma; intraventricular hemorrhage or blood clot
   (eg, trauma; arteriovenous malformation)
4. Intraventricular glioma or meningioma
5. Tuberous sclerosis (subependymal nodules)

Foramen of Monro Obstruction (See A-78-1)

1. Aneurysm or ectasia of basilar artery
2. Colloid cyst of third ventricle
3. Craniopharyngioma
4. Glioma of optic chiasm
5. Hypothalamic glioma
6. Pituitary adenoma (chromophobe or eosinophilic)
7. Tuberous sclerosis (giant cell astrocytoma)

Aqueductal Obstruction

1. Congenital aqueductal stenosis or occlusion (usually with Arnold-Chiari malformation)
2. Developmental stenosis
3. Meningioma of tentorium
4. Midbrain neoplasm or hemorrhage
5. Pineal area tumor (eg, pinealoma; teratoma)
6. Vein of Galen "aneurysm"

Fourth Ventricle Obstruction (See A-84)

1. Arachnoid cyst (eg, of suprasellar or quadrigeminal cistern)
2. Brain-stem edema
3. Cerebellopontine angle tumor (eg, large acoustic schwannoma; metastasis)
4. Neoplasm involving fourth ventricle (eg, medulloblastoma {PNET}$_g$; ependymoma; astrocytoma)
5. Outlet obstruction, congenital (eg, Dandy-Walker S. {Dandy-Walker malformation}) or acquired (old hemorrhage or infection)

Other Etiologies Which May Involve One or More of the Above Areas

1. Abscess
2. Basal arachnoiditis (incl. tuberculosis; sarcoidosis; fungus disease)
3. Encephalitis/ventriculitis
4. Parasitic cyst (*Cysticercus; Paragonimus;* hydatid)
5. Tumefactive multiple sclerosis

OVERPRODUCTION OF CEREBROSPINAL FLUID

1. Choroid plexus papilloma

References

1. Bradley WG: Chapter 28, In: Stark DD, Bradley WG (eds): Magnetic Resonance Imaging. (ed 2) St. Louis: CV Mosby, 1992
2. Brucher JA, Salmon JH: Hydrocephalus. Semin Roentgenol 1970;5:186–195
3. Chapman S, Nakielny R: Aids to Radiological Differential Diagnosis. (ed 3) London: WB Saunders, 1995, pp 396–397
4. DuBoulay GH (ed): A Textbook of Radiological Diagnosis. (ed 5) The Head and the Central Nervous System. Philadelphia: WB Saunders, 1984, vol 1, pp 89–94
5. Eisenberg RL: Clinical Imaging: An Atlas of Differential Diagnosis. (ed 3) Philadelphia: Lippincott-Raven, 1997

Gamut A-114-2

CONGENITAL SYNDROMES ASSOCIATED WITH HYDROCEPHALUS

COMMON

1. Achondroplasia
2. Acrocephalosyndactyly (Apert and Pfeiffer types)
3. Arnold-Chiari malformation
4. Crouzon S. (craniofacial dysostosis)
5. Dandy-Walker S. (Dandy-Walker malformation)
6. Fetal alcohol S.
7. Fetal toxoplasmosis infection
8. Huntington's chorea

(continued)

9. Mucopolysaccharidosis I-H (Hurler S.), II (Hunter S.), and VI (Maroteaux-Lamy S.)
10. Osteopetrosis, severe
11. Thanatophoric dysplasia

UNCOMMON

1. Aase-Smith S.
2. Acrocallosal S.
3. Acrodysostosis (peripheral dysostosis)
4. Acromesomelic dysplasia
5. Aicardi S.
6. Aminopterin fetopathy
7. Amniotic band sequence
8. Aplasia cutis congenita (Adams-Oliver S.)
9. Biemond S. II
10. Bobble-head doll S.
11. Caudal dysplasia sequence
12. Cloverleaf skull (kleeblattschädel anomaly)
13. Cockayne S.
14. Craniodiaphyseal dysplasia
15. Craniometaphyseal dysplasia
16. Cystinosis
17. Diencephalic S.
18. Epidermal nevus S.
19. Farber disease (disseminated lipogranulomatosis)
20. Fetal isotretinoin S. (retinoic acid embryopathy)
21. Fetal varicella infection
22. Gorlin S. (nevoid basal cell carcinoma S.)
23. Greig cephalopolysyndactyly S.
24. Hajdu-Cheney S.
25. Hydrolethalus S.
26. Incontinentia pigmenti (Bloch-Sulzberger S.)
27. Infant of the diabetic mother
28. Kasabach-Merritt S.
29. Klüver-Bucy S. (temporal hydrocephalus)
30. Lissencephaly syndromes (congenital agyria); Miller-Dieker S.
31. Mannosidosis
32. Meckel S.
33. MELAS S.
34. Metachromatic leukodystrophies
35. Metatropic dysplasia
36. Mulibrey nanism
37. Neu-Laxova S.
38. Neurocutaneous melanosis
39. Oculo-auriculo-vertebral spectrum (Goldenhar S.)
40. Oro-facio-digital S. I (Papillon-Leage and Psaume S.)
41. Osteogenesis imperfecta
42. Oto-palato-digital S. (type II)
43. Rieger S.
44. Riley-Day S. (familial dysautonomia)
45. Roberts S.
46. Sjögren-Larsson S.
47. Smith-Lemli-Opitz S.
48. Sotos S. (cerebral gigantism)
49. Triploidy (fetal triploidy S.)
50. Trisomy 13 S.; pseudotrisomy 13 S. (holoprosencephaly-polydactyly S.)
51. Tuberous sclerosis
52. VATER association
53. Walker-Warburg S.
54. Warfarin embryopathy (fetal warfarin S.)
55. X-linked hydrocephalus
56. Zellweger S. (cerebrohepatorenal S.)

References

1. Gorlin RJ, Cohen MM Jr, Levin LS: Syndromes of the Head and Neck. (ed 3) New York: Oxford University Press, 1990
2. Jones KL: Smith's Recognizable Patterns of Human Malformation. (ed 5) Philadelphia: WB Saunders, 1997
3. Taybi H, Lachman RS: Radiology of Syndromes, Metabolic Disorders, and Skeletal Dysplasias. (ed 4) St. Louis: Mosby-Year Book, 1996, p 1017

Gamut A-115-1

LARGE HEADS IN INFANTS

WITH LARGE VENTRICLES

1. Hydrocephalus, obstructive communicating or non-communicating (eg, aqueductal stenosis; Arnold-Chiari malformation; Dandy-Walker malformation)
2. Intracranial cyst
3. Neoplasm (posterior fossa or intracranial)

4. Overproduction of CSF (nonobstructive hydro-cephalus)

WITH NORMAL VENTRICLES

1. Calvarial thickening
2. Cerebral edema
3. Macrocephaly; megalencephaly (See A-3)

Reference

1. Harwood-Nash DCF, Fitz CR: Large heads and ventricles in infants. Radiol Clin North Am 1975;13:199–224

Gamut A-115-2

LARGE VENTRICLES IN INFANTS

WITH LARGE HEAD (MACROCEPHALY)

1. Hydrocephalus (See A-114)
2. Intracranial tumor

WITH NORMAL-SIZED OR SMALL HEAD (MICROCEPHALY)

1. Primary failure of brain growth
   a. Dysgenesis (eg, holoprosencephaly; trisomies)
   b. Environmental factors (eg, alcohol or drug abuse; toxins)
   c. Congenital transplacental infection (TORCH—toxoplasmosis; rubella; cytomegalovirus; herpes simplex)
2. Loss of brain substance
   a. Hemorrhage (porencephaly; leukomalacia)
   b. Vascular occlusion (hydranencephaly; poren-cephaly; schizencephaly)
   c. Congenital transplacental infection (TORCH)
3. Natal or postnatal anoxia

References

1. Dähnert W: Radiology Review Manual. (ed 4) Baltimore: Williams & Wilkins, 1999, p 186
2. Harwood-Nash DCF, Fitz CR: Large heads and ventricles in infants. Radiol Clin North Am 1975;13:199–224

Gamut A-116

SMALL VENTRICLES ON CT

1. Increased intracranial pressure
2. Normal variant
3. Postshunting (slitlike ventricles)
6. Pseudotumor cerebri (idiopathic intracranial hyper-tension—ventricles usually normal on CT)

Reference

1. Burgener FA, Kormano M: Differential Diagnosis in Computed Tomography. New York: Thieme, 1996, p 44

Gamut A-117

ABNORMAL CONGENITAL OR DEVELOPMENTAL CONFIGURATION OF THE VENTRICLES

1. Chiari II malformation
2. Corpus callosum agenesis
3. Dandy-Walker syndrome or variant
4. Hamartoma of tuber cinereum
5. Heterotopia
6. Holoprosencephaly (alobar, semilobar, or lobar)
7. Huntington's disease
8. Porencephalic cyst (porencephaly)
9. Schizencephaly
10. Septo-optic dysplasia (absent or hypoplastic septum pelucidum)
11. Ventricular diverticulum

Reference

1. Burgener FA, Kormano M: Differential Diagnosis in Computed Tomography. New York: Thieme, 1996, pp 47–48

(continued)

Gamut A-118

CEREBROSPINAL FLUID RHINORRHEA

COMMON

1. Fracture of frontal or sphenoid sinus, or mastoid sinus
2. Neoplasm of base of skull (esp. osteoma; carcinoma)
3. Postoperative

UNCOMMON

1. Congenital skull defect
2. Hydrocephalus (elevated pressure)
3. Neoplasm of brain or meninges (meningioma) with erosion
4. Osteomyelitis

Reference
1. Lantz EJ, Forbes GS, Brown ML, et al: Radiology of cerebrospinal fluid rhinorrhea. AJR 1980;135:1023–1030

Gamut A-119

CENTRAL NERVOUS SYSTEM COMPLICATIONS OF HIV INFECTION AND AIDS

INFECTIONS

1. Bacterial (meningitis or brain abscess)
   a. Tuberculosis
   b. Atypical mycobacterial infection
   c. Syphilis
   d. Other (*E. coli; Listeria; Nocardia*)
2. Fungal (meningitis or brain abscess)
   a. Aspergillosis
   b. Candidiasis
   c. Coccidioidomycosis
   d. Cryptococcosis (torulosis)
   e. Histoplasmosis
3. Protozoal
   a. Toxoplasmosis (meningoencephalitis)
4. Viral (encephalopathy; encephalitis; diffuse atrophy or white matter disease)
   a. Human immunodeficiency virus (HIV; AIDS)
   b. Cytomegalovirus
   c. Herpes simplex
   d. Papovavirus JC (progressive multifocal leukoencephalopathy—PML)

NEOPLASMS

1. Kaposi sarcoma
2. Lymphoma, primary non-Hodgkin's

CEREBROVASCULAR DISORDERS

1. Cerebral infarction
2. Intracerebral or subarachnoid hemorrhage

CNS SYNDROMES OF UNCERTAIN ETIOLOGY

1. AIDS-related dementia
2. Aseptic meningitis
3. Vacuolar myelopathy

PERIPHERAL NERVOUS SYSTEM DISORDERS

1. Acute polyradiculoneuropathy (eg, Guillain-Barré S.)
2. Chronic inflammatory demyelinating polyneuropathy
3. Distal symmetrical axonal polyneuropathy
4. Mononeuritis multiplex

References
1. Eisenberg RL: Clinical Imaging: An Atlas of Differential Diagnosis. (ed 3) Philadelphia: Lippincott-Raven, 1997, pp 1150–1153
2. Moseley IF, Murray JF, Goodman PC: HIV infection and AIDS: Central nervous system complications. In: Grainger RG, Allison DJ (eds): Diagnostic Radiology. Edinburgh: Churchill Livingstone, 1992, vol 3, pp 1994–1997

B

Head and Neck

B

B

Gamut B-1

MALFORMATION OF THE ORBIT

COMMON

1. Craniosynostosis (See A-1)
2. Enucleation in childhood, traumatic or surgical
3. Fibrous dysplasia; leontiasis ossea
4. Hypertelorism (eg, acrocephalosyndactyly {Apert type}; S.; craniofacial dysostosis (Crouzon S.); Treacher Collins S.) (See B-3)
5. Posttraumatic; postoperative

UNCOMMON

1. Anophthalmos; microphthalmos (eg, Meckel S.)
2. Cerebral atrophy and mental retardation (round orbits)
3. Cyclops
4. Encroachment from adjacent mass (eg, frontal sinus mucocele; frontal encephalocele; antral neoplasm or cyst)
5. Forebrain hypoplasia; holoprosencephaly; arrhinencephaly; cebocephaly (small, round orbits)
6. Hypotelorism (See B-2)
7. Neoplasm (eg, neurofibroma; Burkitt lymphoma)
8. Neurofibromatosis
9. Osteoblastic bone lesion or hyperostosis with encroachment on orbit (eg, meningioma; osteosarcoma; Paget's disease; osteopetrosis; craniometaphyseal dysplasia; hypercalcemia; thalassemia)
10. Radiation therapy

References
1. Swischuk LE, John SD: Differential Diagnosis in Pediatric Radiology. (ed 2) Baltimore: Williams & Wilkins, 1995, pp 397–398
2. Taybi H, Lachman RS: Radiology of Syndromes, Metabolic Disorders, and Skeletal Dysplasias. (ed 4) St. Louis: Mosby-Year Book, 1996, pp 990–992

Gamut B-2

HYPOTELORISM (DECREASED INTERORBITAL DISTANCE)

1. Acrofrontonasal dysostosis
2. CHARGE association
3. Chromosome 20p dup S.
4. Craniotelencephalic dysplasia
5. Forebrain hypoplasia (eg, holoprosencephaly; arrhinencephaly; cebocephaly)
6. Intrauterine growth retardation syndromes (eg, fetal hydantoin S.)
7. Meckel S.
8. Myotonic dystrophy
9. Oculodentoosseous dysplasia
10. Postaxial acrofacial dysostosis (Miller type)
11. Trigonocephaly (craniosynostosis with premature closure of metopic suture)
12. Trichorhinophalangeal dysplasia
13. Trisomy 13 S.
14. Trisomy 21 S. (Down S.)
15. Williams S. (idiopathic hypercalcemia)

References
1. Swischuk LE, John SD: Differential Diagnosis in Pediatric Radiology. (ed 2) Baltimore: Williams & Wilkins, 1995, p 393
2. Taybi H, Lachman RS: Radiology of Syndromes, Metabolic Disorders, and Skeletal Dysplasias. (ed 4) St. Louis: Mosby-Year Book, 1996, p 990

Gamut B-3-1

HYPERTELORISM

1. Anterior meningocele or encephalocele; cranium bifidum
2. Congenital syndromes (See B-3-2)
3. Craniosynostosis of coronal sutures
4. Dermoid (midline)
5. Fibrous dysplasia; leontiasis ossea

(continued)

6. Hydrocephalus in growth period, severe (over-growth of lesser wing of sphenoid)
7. Idiopathic
8. Mucocele
9. Nasal tumor
10. Thalassemia

Gamut B-3-2

CONGENITAL SYNDROMES WITH HYPERTELORISM

COMMON

1. Acrocephalosyndactyly (Apert, Pfeiffer, Saethre-Chotzen types)
2. Cleidocranial dysplasia
3. Crouzon S. (craniofacial dysostosis)
4. Craniosynostosis of coronal sutures
5. Ehlers-Danlos S.
6. Familial hypertelorism; normal variant
7. Fibrous dysplasia; leontiasis ossea
8. Frontonasal dysplasia (median cleft face S.—median cleft nose and palate)
9. Greig cephalopolysyndactyly S.
10. Noonan S.
11. Osteopetrosis
12. Sotos S.
13. Thalassemia
14. Treacher Collins S. (mandibulofacial dysostosis)

UNCOMMON

1. Aarskog S.
2. Acrocallosal S.
3. Acrodysostosis (peripheral dysostosis)
4. Aminopterin fetopathy
5. Beckwith-Wiedemann S.
6. Brachmann-de Lange S. (de Lange S.)
7. Campomelic dysplasia
8. Cardio-facio-cutaneous S.
9. Cat-eye S.

10. Chondrodysplasia punctata
11. Chromosome syndromes (4: del (4p) {Wolf-Hirschhorn S.}; 4: dup (4p); 5: del (5p) {cat cry S. or cri du chat S.}; 18p-)
12. Cloverleaf skull (kleeblattschädel anomaly)
13. Coffin-Lowry S.
14. Craniofrontonasal dysplasia
15. Craniometaphyseal dysplasia
16. Diamond-Blackfan S.
17. DiGeorge S.
18. Dubowitz S.
19. Dyssegmental dysplasia
20. Fetal akinesia sequence (Pena-Shokeir S., type I)
21. FG syndrome
22. Fraser S. (cryptophthalmia S.)
23. Freeman-Sheldon S. (whistling face S.)
24. Frontometaphyseal dysplasia
25. Gorlin S. (nevoid basal cell carcinoma S.)
26. Intrauterine growth retardation syndromes (eg, fetal hydantoin syndrome {Dilantin embryopathy}; fetal isotretinoin S. {retinoic acid embryopathy})
27. Larsen S.
28. Lenz-Majewski dysplasia (hyperostotic dwarfism)
29. LEOPARD S. (multiple lentigenes S.)
30. Marden-Walker S.
31. Metaphyseal chondrodysplasia (Jansen type)
32. Neu-Laxova S.
33. Opitz BBBG syndrome (hypertelorism-hypospadias S.; G S.)
34. Oro-facio-digital S. I and II
35. Oromandibular-limb hypogenesis syndromes
36. Osteoglophonic dysplasia
37. Otopalatodigital S. (types I and II)
38. Pallister-Killian S.
39. Potter sequence
40. Pterygium syndromes
41. Roberts S.
42. Robinow S.
43. Rubinstein-Taybi S.
44. Schinzel-Giedion S.
45. Sclerosteosis
46. Seckel S. (bird-headed dwarfism)
47. Sjögren-Larsson S.
48. Spondyloepiphyseal dysplasia congenita

49. Waardenburg S.
50. Warfarin embryopathy (fetal warfarin S.)
51. Weaver S. (Weaver–Smith S.)
52. XXXXX S.
53. XXXXY S.

References
1. Jones KL: Smith's Recognizable Patterns of Human Malformation. (ed 3) Philadelphia: WB Saunders, 1988
2. MacPherson RI, Wan R, Reed MH: Hypertelorism. American Roentgen Ray Society Scientific Exhibit, San Francisco, 1974
3. Swischuk LE, John SD: Differential Diagnosis in Pediatric Radiology. (ed 2) Baltimore: Williams & Wilkins, 1995, pp 393–397
4. Taybi H, Lachman RS: Radiology of Syndromes, Metabolic Disorders, and Skeletal Dysplasias. (ed 4) St. Louis: Mosby-Year Book, 1996, p 990

5. Forebrain hypoplasia syndromes with hypotelorism (See B-2)
6. Neurofibromatosis (orbital dysplasia)
7. Osteitis (eg, from sphenoid sinusitis)

References
1. Newton TH, Potts DG: Radiology of the Skull and Brain. St. Louis: CV Mosby, vol 1, book 2, 1971, pp 469–470, 502–506
2. Swischuk LE, John SD: Differential Diagnosis in Pediatric Radiology. (ed 2) Baltimore: Williams & Wilkins, 1995, p 393
3. Taybi H, Lachman RS: Radiology of Syndromes, Metabolic Disorders, and Skeletal Dysplasias. (ed 4) St. Louis: Mosby-Year Book, 1996, p 992

Gamut B-4

SMALL ORBIT AND/OR OPTIC CANAL

COMMON

1. Enucleation in childhood
2. Optic nerve atrophy
3. Osteoblastic bone lesion or hyperostosis with encroachment on orbit (eg, meningioma; osteosarcoma; fibrous dysplasia; Paget's disease; osteopetrosis; craniometaphyseal dysplasia; hypercalcemia; thalassemia)
4. Radiation therapy

UNCOMMON

1. Anophthalmos, microphthalmos (eg, Hallermann-Streiff S. (oculo-mandibulo-facial S.); oculovertebral S.-unilateral; trisomy 13 S.; oculo-dento-osseous dysplasia; osteoporosis-pseudoglioma S.)
2. Congenital underdevelopment of globe and face (unilateral)
3. Craniosynostosis of coronal suture
4. Encroachment from adjacent mass (eg, frontal sinus mucocele or neoplasm; antral neoplasm or cyst)

Gamut B-5

LARGE ORBIT

COMMON

1. Coronal craniosynostosis with elevation of orbit
2. Exophthalmos (eg, thyrotoxicosis) (See B-17)
3. Pseudotumor of orbit
4. Tumor, intraconal (eg, hemangioma; optic nerve glioma; neurofibroma; retinoblastoma; metastasis) or extraconal

UNCOMMON

1. Congenital glaucoma (buphthalmos; hydrophthalmos)
2. Congenital serous cyst (often associated with anophthalmos or microphthalmos)
3. Hypoplastic maxilla
4. Langerhans cell histiocytosis$_g$
5. Lymphoma$_g$; Burkitt's lymphoma
6. Neurofibromatosis (orbital dysplasia)
7. [Small contralateral orbit]
8. Varix of orbital vein

[ ] This condition does not actually cause the gamuted imaging finding, but can produce imaging changes that simulate it.

(continued)

References
1. Newton TH, Potts DG: Radiology of the Skull and Brain. St. Louis: CV Mosby, vol 1, book 2, 1971, pp 470–473
2. Taybi H, Lachman RS: Radiology of Syndromes, Metabolic Disorders, and Skeletal Dysplasias. (ed 4) St. Louis: Mosby-Year Book, 1996, p 992

Gamut B-6-1

ORBITAL LESIONS ARISING WITHIN THE ORBIT—INTRAOCULAR OR INTRACONAL MASS

COMMON

1. Cavernous hemangioma
2. Infiltration of retrobulbar fat and intraorbital soft tissues (eg, amyloidosis; Erdheim-Chester disease)
3. Intraocular foreign body
4. Melanoma
5. Meningioma of optic nerve
6. Optic glioma
7. Pseudotumor of orbit

UNCOMMON

1. Benign infantile myxofibromatosis
2. Choroidal osteoma
3. Hamartoma (tuberous sclerosis)
4. Metastasis (esp. from carcinoma of lung or breast)
5. Neurinoma or schwannoma of optic nerve; neurofibroma of cranial nerve III, IV, or V
6. Ophthalmic artery aneurysm
7. Optic neuritis
8. Retinoblastoma
9. Sarcoma (esp. liposarcoma)
10. Vascular lesion, other (eg, capillary hemangioma; hemangiopericytoma; lymphangioma; venous angioma; orbital varices; hematic cyst)

References
1. Arger PH, Mishkin MM, Nenninger RH: An approach to orbital lesions. AJR 1972;115:595–606

2. Bryan RN, Craig JA: The eye: CT of the orbit. In: Bergeron RT, Osborn AG, Som PM: Head and Neck Imaging Excluding the Brain. St. Louis: CV Mosby, 1984, pp 575–616
3. Eisenberg RL: Clinical Imaging: An Atlas of Differential Diagnosis. (ed 3) Philadelphia: Lippincott-Raven, 1997, pp 1158–1163
4. Forbes GS, Sheedy PF II, Waller RR: Orbital tumors evaluated by computed tomography. Radiology 1980;136:101
5. Hershey BL, Roth TC: Orbital infections. Semin Ultrasound CT MR 1997;18:448–459
6. Hesselink JR, Davis KR, Weber AL, et al: Radiological evaluation of orbital metastases, with emphasis on computed tomography. Radiology 1980;137:363
7. Hilal SK, Trokel SL: Computerized tomography of the orbit using thin sections. Semin Roentgenol 1977;12:137–147
8. Levine HL, Ferris EJ, Lessel S, et al: The neuroradiologic evaluation of "optic neuritis." AJR 1975;125:702–716
9. Lufkin R, Borges A, Villablanca P: Teaching Atlas of Head and Neck Imaging. New York: Thieme, 2000, pp 211–213
10. MacPherson P: The radiology of orbital meningioma. Clin Radiol 1979;30:105
11. McKenzie JD, Drayer BP: Computed tomography (CT) and magnetic resonance (MR) imaging of the orbits. Barrow Neurological Institute 1993;9:35–46
12. Peyster RG, Augsburger JJ, Shields JA, Hershey BL, Eagle Jr R, Haskin ME: Intraocular tumors: evaluation with MR imaging. Radiology 1988;168:773–779
13. Rothman M. Orbital trauma. Semin Ultrasound CT MR 1997;18:437–447
14. Weber AL, Jakobiec FA, Sabates NR. Pseudotumor of the orbit. Neuroimaging Clin North Am 1996;6:73–92
15. Weber AL, Sabates NR. Survey of CT and MR imaging of the orbit. Eur J Radiol 1996;22:42–52.

Gamut B-6-2

INTRAOCULAR MASS IN A CHILD (See B-6-1,7-S)

NEOPLASTIC

1. Melanoma (uveal)
2. Metastasis (esp. neuroblastoma)
3. Pseudoglioma (retinal astrocytoma or astrocytic hamartoma, usually with tuberous sclerosis)
4. Retinoblastoma; retinocytoma

NONNEOPLASTIC

1. Chronic retinal detachment
2. Coat's disease
3. Persistent hyperplastic primary vitreous (PHPV)
4. Retinopathy of prematurity or retinal dysplasia (ROP)
5. Toxocariasis or larval granulomatosis
6. Uveitis

References

1. Ainbinder DJ, Haik BG, Frei DF, et al: Gadolinium enhancement: improved MRI detection of retinoblastoma extension into the optic nerve. Neuroradiology 1996;38: 778–781
2. Beets-Tan RG, Hendriks MJ, Ramos LM, Tan KE: Retinoblastoma: CT and MRI. Neuroradiology 1994;36: 59–62
3. Lufkin R, Borges A, Villablanca P: Teaching Atlas of Head and Neck Imaging. New York: Thieme, 2000, pp 223–229
4. Potter PD, Shields CL, Shields JA, Flanders AE: The role of magnetic resonance imaging in children with intraocular tumors and simulating lesions. Ophthalmology 1996:103: 1774–1783
5. Ramji FG, Slovis TL, Baker JD: Orbital sonography in children. Ped Radiology 1996;26:245–258
6. Smirniotopoulos JG, Bargallo N, Mafee MF: Differential diagnosis of leukokoria: radiologic-pathologic correlation. RadioGraphics 1994;14:1059–1082

3. Nevi
4. Retinal cyst
5. Retinal gliosis
6. Retinoblastoma
7. Sarcoidosis

References

1. Gomori JM, et al: Choroidal melanoma: correlation of NMR spectroscopy and MR imaging. Radiology 1986;158: 443–445
2. Lufkin R, Borges A, Villablanca P: Teaching Atlas of Head and Neck Imaging. New York: Thieme, 2000, pp 219–222
3. Mafee MF: Malignant uveal melanoma and simulating lesions. MR imaging evaluation. Radiology 1986;160: 773–780
4. Potter PD, Shields CL, Shields JA, Flanders AE: The role of magnetic resonance imaging in children with intraocular tumors and simulating lesions. Ophthalmology 1996:103: 1774–1783

Gamut B-6-3

ORBITAL LESIONS ARISING WITHIN THE ORBIT—CHOROIDAL MASS

COMMON

1. Hemangioma
2. Hemorrhage
3. Melanoma
4. Metastasis to choroid
5. Retinal/choroidal detachment

UNCOMMON

1. Leiomyoma
2. Neurofibroma; schwannoma

Gamut B-6-4

ORBITAL LESIONS ARISING WITHIN THE ORBIT—EXTRACONAL OR MUSCLE MASS

COMMON

1. Graves' disease, thyrotoxicosis (thyroid ophthalmopathy)
2. Lacrimal gland tumor
3. Lymphoma$_g$; Burkitt's lymphoma
4. Meningioma
5. Metastasis
6. Pseudotumor
7. Trauma
8. Vascular lesion (eg, hemangioma; arteriovenous fistula; lymphangioma; hemangioblastoma; hemangiopericytoma; orbital varices)

UNCOMMON

1. Dacryocystitis
2. Dermoid cyst; epidermoid

(continued)

3. Hematoma
4. Orbital myositis
5. Rhabdomyosarcoma

References
1. See B-6-1 above

Gamut B-6-5

ORBITAL LESIONS ARISING EXTRAORBITALLY OR EXTRACRANIALLY
(eg, From Nasopharynx, Nasal Cavity, Paranasal Sinus, Orbital Bone, or Infratemporal Fossa)

COMMON
1. Bone neoplasm, benign (eg, osteoma)
2. Bone neoplasm, malignant (eg, sarcoma; myeloma; metastasis)
3. Carcinoma of paranasal sinus, nasal cavity, or skin
4. Lymphoma$_g$; Burkitt's lymphoma
5. Orbital abscess or cellulitis (eg, from sinusitis or eyelid infection)
6. Osteomyelitis
7. Paget's disease
8. Trauma (incl. foreign body)

UNCOMMON
1. Bone neoplasm, other benign (eg, osteochondroma; chondroma; aneurysmal bone cyst; ossifying fibroma)
2. Craniofacial malformations
3. Esthesioneuroblastoma (olfactory neuroblastoma)
4. Fibrous dysplasia (leontiasis ossea); other bone dysplasia
5. Granulomatous disease (eg, tuberculosis; sarcoidosis; Wegener's granulomatosis; lethal midline granuloma)

6. Hydatid disease
7. Juvenile angiofibroma (esp. in pterygopalatine fossa)
8. Langerhans cell histiocytosis$_g$
9. Mucocele
10. Neurofibromatosis
11. Osteopetrosis
12. Sinus neoplasm (eg, carcinoma; inverting papilloma)

References
1. See B-6-1 above

Gamut B-6-6

ORBITAL LESIONS ARISING INTRACRANIALLY WITH SECONDARY INVOLVEMENT OF ORBIT

COMMON
1. Meningioma (anterior or middle fossa)

UNCOMMON
1. Aneurysm of internal carotid artery
2. Carotid-cavernous fistula
3. Chiasmatic arachnoiditis
4. Chordoma
5. Craniopharyngioma
6. Encephalomeningocele
7. Hypothalamic tumor
8. Optic glioma
9. Pituitary adenoma

Reference
1. See B-6-1 above

Gamut B-7-S

CT CHARACTERISTICS OF ORBITAL MASSES IN CHILDREN

	Location							Extension		Attenuation		
	Preseptal	Extraconal	Intraconal	Muscle only	Orbital expansion	Bone destruction	Calcification	Intracranial	Facial	High	Low	Enhancement
Optic nerve glioma		+			+			+				+
Rhabdomyosarcoma	+/–	+				+	–		+			+
2° Neuroblastoma	+/–	+				+	+	+	+	+		+
Lymphangioma	+	+	+		+						mixed	+/–
Hemangioma	+	+	+		+						mixed	+ irregular
Histiocytosis X	+/–	+				+	+	+	+			
Infection	+	+							+			+
Leukemia	+	+		+		+						
Lymphoma	+					+			+	+		+
Dermoid	+	+			+					mixed		
Pseudotumor		+	+	+								

References
1. Lallemand DP, Brasch RC, Char DH, Norman D: Orbital tumors in children. Characterisation by computed tomography. Radiology 1984;151:85–88 (slightly modified)
2. Hopper KD, Sherman JL, Boal DK, Eggli KD: CT and MR imaging of the pediatric orbit. RadioGraphics 1992;12:485-503

Gamut B-8

BONY DEFECT, EROSION, OR RADIOLUCENT LESION OF THE ORBIT (See B-11,12)

COMMON

1. Extrinsic tumor invading orbit (eg, meningioma; carcinoma or lymphoma of nasopharynx, nasal cavity, or paranasal sinus; carcinoma of skin or eyelid)
2. Metastasis (eg, from carcinoma of breast or lung; neuroblastoma; Ewing sarcoma)
3. Mucocele
4. Osteomyelitis usually secondary to sinusitis
5. Primary orbital neoplasm (eg, hemangioma; hemangioblastoma; lacrimal gland carcinoma; dermoid; epidermoid; optic glioma; neurofibroma; melanoma; retinoblastoma; rhabdomyosarcoma; lymphoma_g; Burkitt's lymphoma)

(continued)

UNCOMMON

1. Benign infantile myxofibromatosis
2. Encephalomeningocele
3. Juvenile angiofibroma
4. Langerhans cell histiocytosis$_g$
5. Multiple myeloma
6. Neurofibromatosis (orbital dysplasia)—"empty orbit"
7. Primary bone tumor (eg, sarcoma; myeloma; lymphoma$_g$; aneurysmal bone cyst)

References

1. Jacobs L, Weisberg LA, Kinkel WR: Computerized Tomography of the Orbit and Sella Turcica. New York: Raven Press, 1980
2. Newton TH, Potts DG: Radiology of the Skull and Brain. St. Louis: CV Mosby, vol 1, book 2, 1971, pp 476–482
3. Sanchez R, Weber AL, Alexander A, Sweriduk S, Vici G: Paraorbital lesions. Eur J Radiol 1996;22:53–67

Gamut B-9

SCLEROSIS AND THICKENING OF THE ORBITAL ROOF OR WALLS

COMMON

1. Fibrous dysplasia; leontiasis ossea
2. Meningioma
3. Osteitis secondary to chronic sinusitis or mucocele
4. Paget's disease

UNCOMMON

1. Benign infantile myxofibromatosis
2. Craniometaphyseal dysplasia; frontometaphyseal dysplasia
3. Dermoid
4. Langerhans cell histiocytosis$_g$
5. Infantile cortical hyperostosis (Caffey's disease)
6. Lacrimal gland carcinoma
7. Lymphoma$_g$

8. Osteoblastic metastasis (eg, from carcinoma of breast or prostate)
9. Osteoma
10. Osteopetrosis
11. Osteosarcoma
12. Radiation therapy
13. Thalassemia

Reference

1. Newton TH, Potts DG: Radiology of the Skull and Brain. St. Louis: CV Mosby, vol 1, book 2, 1971, pp 482–485

Gamut B-10

NARROWED SUPERIOR ORBITAL (SPHENOIDAL) FISSURE

COMMON

1. Fibrous dysplasia
2. Normal variant; congenital asymmetry or narrowing
3. Paget's disease

UNCOMMON

1. Bone neoplasm (eg, osteoma; osteoblastic metastasis)
2. Meningioma with hyperostosis
3. Osteitis secondary to chronic sinusitis
4. Osteopetrosis
5. Thalassemia

References

1. Newton TH, Potts DG: Radiology of the Skull and Brain. St. Louis: CV Mosby, vol 1, book 2, 1971, pp 521–524
2. Shapiro R, Robinson F: Alterations of the sphenoidal fissure produced by local and systemic processes. AJR 1967; 101:814–827

Gamut B-11

ENLARGED SUPERIOR ORBITAL (SPHENOIDAL) FISSURE (EROSION AND WIDENING)

COMMON

1. Aneurysm of intracavernous portion of internal carotid artery
2. Normal asymmetry
3. Pituitary tumor (esp. chromophobe adenoma)

UNCOMMON

1. Carotid-cavernous fistula
2. Chordoma (parasellar)
3. Craniopharyngioma
4. Extension from orbital or infraorbital mass (eg, hemangioma; arteriovenous malformation; optic glioma; juvenile xanthogranuloma; lymphoma$_g$; Burkitt's lymphoma; neuroblastoma) or from paranasal sinus malignancy
5. Increased intracranial pressure, chronic
6. Langerhans cell histiocytosis$_g$
7. Meningioma, orbital or intracranial
8. Metastatic carcinoma to sphenoid wing
9. Middle fossa mass (eg, infratemporal chronic subdural hematoma or hygroma; arachnoid cyst with temporal lobe agenesis; temporal lobe astrocytoma)
10. Mucocele of sphenoid sinus
11. Neurofibroma
12. Neurofibromatosis (orbital dysplasia)
13. Orbital varix
14. Posterior orbital encephalocele
15. Pseudotumor of orbit
16. Superior orbital fissure syndrome (impairment of cranial nerves III, IV, and VI associated with sphenoid sinusitis)

References
1. DuBoulay GH: Principles of X-ray Diagnosis of the Skull. (ed 2) London: Butterworths, 1980.
2. Newton TH, Potts DG: Radiology of the Skull and Brain. St. Louis: CV Mosby, vol 1, book 2, 1971, pp 508–521

Gamut B-12

LOCALIZED BONY DEFECT OR EROSION ABOUT THE OPTIC CANAL (See B-8,13)

COMMON

1. Aneurysm of internal carotid artery (cavernous portion)
2. Malignant neoplasm arising in orbit, sphenoid sinus, or nasal cavity
3. Pituitary adenoma

UNCOMMON

1. Craniopharyngioma
2. Granuloma (eg, tuberculosis; sarcoidosis)
3. Langerhans cell histiocytosis$_g$
4. Metastasis
5. Mucocele of sphenoid sinus
6. Neoplasm of anterior fossa (eg, meningioma; astrocytoma; glioma)
7. Neurofibroma; neurofibromatosis (orbital dysplasia)
8. Surgical defect

Reference
1. Newton TH, Potts DG: Radiology of the Skull and Brain. St. Louis: CV Mosby, vol 1, book 2, 1971, pp 496–501

Gamut B-13

OPTIC CANAL ENLARGEMENT (OVER 6.5 MM IN DIAMETER) (See B-12,14)

COMMON

1. Glioma of optic nerve
2. Meningioma of optic nerve sheath
3. Metastasis
4. Neurofibromatosis with or without optic neurofibroma or glioma

(continued)

UNCOMMON

1. Aneurysm of ophthalmic artery or cavernous portion of internal carotid artery
2. Arteriovenous malformation with ophthalmic artery involvement
3. Carcinoma of ethmoid or sphenoid sinus
4. Granuloma (eg, tuberculosis; sarcoidosis)
5. Increased intracranial pressure
6. Mucocele of sphenoid sinus
7. Mucopolysaccharidoses (esp. Hurler S.) (See J-4)
8. Pituitary adenoma or craniopharyngioma extending anteriorly
9. Pseudotumor of orbit
10. Retinoblastoma with intracranial extension

References

1. Burgener FA, Kormano M: Differential Diagnosis in Conventional Radiology. (ed 2) New York: Thieme Medical Publ, 1991, pp 156–158
2. Lloyd GAS: Radiology of the Orbit. Philadelphia: WB Saunders, 1975, pp 26–29
3. Newton TH, Potts DG: Radiology of the Skull and Brain. St. Louis: CV Mosby, vol 1, book 2, 1971, pp 492–496

Gamut B-14

OPTIC NERVE ENLARGEMENT (ON CT OR MRI)

NEOPLASTIC

COMMON

1. Meningioma of optic nerve sheath, or of intracranial origin
2. Optic nerve glioma

UNCOMMON

1. Hemangioblastoma; hemangiopericytoma
2. Lymphoma$_g$; leukemia (chloroma)

3. Metastasis or local extension of ocular tumor (eg, retinoblastoma; melanoma); leptomeningeal carcinomatosis
4. Neurofibroma

NONNEOPLASTIC

COMMON

1. Optic neuritis

UNCOMMON

1. Central retinal vein occlusion
2. Connective tissue disease$_g$
3. Cyst of optic nerve sheath
4. Dural ectasia
5. Graves' disease, thyrotoxicosis (thyroid ophthalmopathy) (late)
6. Hematoma, traumatic or other
7. Increased intracranial pressure (with papilledema)
8. Infection (eg, toxoplasmosis; tuberculosis; fungus disease; syphilis; HIV-related optic neuropathies)
9. Multiple sclerosis
10. Pseudotumor of orbit
11. Radiation induced optic neuropathy
12. Sarcoidosis
13. Trauma to optic nerve
14. Vascular lesion (eg, arteriovenous malformation—Wyburn-Mason S.; aneurysm of ophthalmic artery; hemangioma; varix; venous occlusion; ischemia of optic nerve associated with severe hypertension, temporal arteritis, or systemic vasculopathies)

References

1. Azar-Kia B, et al: Optic nerve tumors: Role of magnetic resonance imaging and computed tomography. Radiol Clin North Am 1987;25:561–581
2. Carmody RF, Mafee MF, Goodwin JA, Small K, Haery C: Orbital and optic pathway sarcoidosis: MR findings. Am J Neuroradiol 1994;15:775–783
3. Curtin HD: Pseudotumor. Radiol Clin North Am 1987;25:583–599
4. Eisenberg RL: Clinical Imaging: An Atlas of Differential Diagnosis. (ed 3) Philadelphia: Lippincott-Raven, 1997, pp 1154–1157

5. Flanders AE, et al: Orbital lymphoma: Role of CT and MRI. Radiol Clin North Am 1987;25:601–613
6. Forbes GS: Computed tomography of the orbit. Radiol Clin North Am 1982;20:37–49
7. Johns TT, Citrin CM, Black J: CT evaluation of perineural orbital lesions: Evaluation of the "tram-track" sign. AJNR 1984;5:587–590
8. Lanzieri CF: MRI of the optic nerves and visual pathways. Imag Decisions 1994; May–Jun:21–32
9. Leo JS, Halpern J, Sackler JP: Computed tomography in the evaluation of orbital infections. CT 1980;4:133–138
10. Lufkin R, Borges A, Villablanca P: Teaching Atlas of Head and Neck Imaging. New York: Thieme, 2000, pp 192–202, 214–218
11. Peyster RG, Hoover E: Computed Tomography in Orbital Disease and Neuro-ophthalmology. Chicago: Year Book Medical Publ, 1984
12. Peyster RG, Hoover E, Hershey BL: High resolution CT of lesions of the optic nerve. AJNR 1983;4:169–174
13. Post MJ, Quencer RM, Tabei SZ: CT demonstration of sarcoidosis of the optic nerve, frontal lobes and falx cerebri: Case report and literature review. AJNR 1982;3:523–526
14. Sobel DF, Salvolini U, Newton TH: Ocular and orbital pathology. In: Newton TH, Hasso AN, Dillon WP (eds): Modern Neuroradiology, vol 3. Computed Tomography of the Head and Neck. New York: Raven Press, 1988, pp 9.17–9.24
15. Staubach B: Enlarged optic nerve. Semin Roentgenol 1984;19:83
16. Swenson SA, Forbes GS, Younge BR, et al: Radiologic evaluation of tumors of the optic nerve. AJNR 1982;3:319–326
17. Unsöld R, DeGroot J, Newton TH: Images of the optic nerve: Anatomic-CT correlation. AJNR 1980;1:317–324

3. Hemangioma
4. Lymphoma$_g$; leukemia
5. Metastasis
6. Neurofibroma
7. Normal variant
8. Optic neuritis (esp. in multiple sclerosis)
9. Perioptic hemorrhage
10. Pseudotumor of orbit
11. Retinoblastoma
12. Sarcoidosis

References
1. Johns TT, Citrin CM, Black J: CT evaluation of perineural orbital lesions: Evaluation of the "tram-track" sign. AJNR 1984;5:587–590
2. Lee SH, Rao K: Cranial Computed Tomography and MRI. (ed 2) New York: McGraw-Hill, 1987, p 148
3. Lufkin R, Borges A, Villablanca P: Teaching Atlas of Head and Neck Imaging. New York Thieme, 2000, pp 207–210
4. Peyster RG, Hoover E: Computed Tomography in Orbital Disease and Neuro-ophthalmology. Chicago: Year Book Medical Publ, 1984
5. Post MJ, Quencer RM, Tabei SZ: CT demonstration of sarcoidosis of the optic nerve, frontal lobes and falx cerebri: Case report and literature review. AJNR 1982;3:523–526

Gamut B-16

ENLARGEMENT OF THE RECTUS MUSCLES OF THE EYE (ON CT OR MRI)

COMMON
1. Graves' disease, thyrotoxicosis (thyroid ophthalmopathy)

UNCOMMON
1. Acromegaly
2. Amyloidosis
3. Brown S.
4. Connective tissue disorder$_g$ (eg, rheumatoid arthritis; lupus erythematosus; scleroderma)
5. Granulomatous disease (eg, tuberculosis; sarcoidosis)

Gamut B-15

OPTIC NERVE "TRAM-TRACK" SIGN (DISTINCT OPTIC NERVE WITH PERINEURAL ENHANCEMENT ON CT)

COMMON
1. Optic nerve sheath meningioma

UNCOMMON
1. Carcinomatous infiltration (eg, from lacrimal gland)
2. Erdheim-Chester disease

(continued)

6. Increased venous pressure (eg, extradural arterio-venous fistula; carotid-cavernous fistula; cavernous sinus thrombosis)
7. Lymphoma$_g$; leukemia; Burkitt's lymphoma
8. Metastasis (incl. neuroblastoma)
9. Mikulicz S.
10. Neoplasm, other (eg, hemangioma; hemangiopericytoma; rhabdomyosarcoma; rhabdomyoma; plasmacytoma; neurofibroma of orbit—rarely)
11. Orbital infection, myositis or cellulitis (eg, from adjacent sinusitis)
12. Orbital trauma; foreign body reaction
13. Pseudotumor of orbit
14. Sjögren S.
15. Tolosa-Hunt S. (inflammation of orbital apex)
16. Vasculitis (eg, giant cell arteritis; PAN)
17. Wegener's granulomatosis; lethal midline granuloma

References
1. Bryan RN, Craig JA: The eye: CT of the orbit. In: Bergeron RT, Osborn AG, Som PM: Head and Neck Imaging Excluding the Brain. St. Louis: CV Mosby, 1984, pp 603–606
2. Eisenberg RL: Clinical Imaging: An Atlas of Differential Diagnosis. (ed 3) Philadelphia: Lippincott-Raven, 1997, pp 1164–1165
3. Lufkin R, Borges A, Villablanca P: Teaching Atlas of Head and Neck Imaging. New York: Thieme, 2000, pp 192–202
4. Peyster RG, Hoover E: Computed Tomography in Orbital Disease and Neuro-ophthalmology. Chicago: Year Book Medical Publ, 1984
5. Sobel DF, Salvolini U, Newton TH: Ocular and orbital pathology. In: Newton TH, Hasso AN, Dillon WP (eds): Modern Neuroradiology, vol 3. Computed Tomography of the Head and Neck. New York: Raven Press, 1988, pp 9.25–9.34

Gamut B-17

UNILATERAL EXOPHTHALMOS (PROPTOSIS)

SYSTEMIC DISEASE

COMMON
1. Hyperthyroidism, thyrotoxicosis

BONE DISEASE

COMMON
1. Fracture with retro-orbital hematoma or orbital emphysema
2. Metastasis

UNCOMMON
1. Bone neoplasm, benign or malignant (eg, osteosarcoma)
2. Craniosynostosis, severe (See A-1-1)
3. Fibrous dysplasia; ossifying fibroma
4. Infantile cortical hyperostosis (Caffey's disease)
5. Langerhans cell histiocytosis$_g$
6. Multiple myeloma
7. Neurofibromatosis
8. Osteoma of a paranasal sinus
9. Osteomyelitis
10. Osteopetrosis
11. Paget's disease
12. Thalassemia

PARANASAL SINUS OR NASOPHARYNGEAL DISEASE WITH INTRAORBITAL EXTENSION

COMMON
1. Carcinoma, lymphoepithelioma, or other neoplasm
2. Mucocele

UNCOMMON
1. Sinusitis

PRIMARY ORBITAL SOFT TISSUE DISEASE
(Including Extension From an Intracranial Lesion)

COMMON

1. Abscess, cellulitis, or myositis (retrobulbar or peri-orbital)
2. Granuloma
3. Hemangioma; lymphangioma
4. Lacrimal gland tumor
5. Lymphoma$_g$; leukemia; Burkitt's lymphoma
6. Meningioma (orbital or sphenoid ridge)
7. Metastatic or invasive neoplasm
8. Optic nerve glioma
9. Pseudotumor of orbit
10. Retinoblastoma
11. Spindle cell tumor$_g$, benign or malignant (eg, rhab-domyosarcoma)

UNCOMMON

1. Carotid artery aneurysm; carotid-cavernous fistula; cavernous sinus thrombosis; arteriovenous malformation (congenital or traumatic)
2. Dermoid; teratoma
3. Epidermoid
4. Foreign body
5. Hydatid cyst
6. Liposarcoma
7. Neurofibroma; neurilemmoma
8. Optic neuritis
9. Orbital meningocele or encephalocele (congenital or traumatic)
10. Orbital varices
11. [Pseudoproptosis (eg, large eye; normal asymmetry)]
12. Retrobulbar infarcts in sickle cell disease
13. Sympathicoblastoma; neuroblastoma

[ ] This condition does not actually cause the gamuted imaging finding, but can produce imaging changes that simulate it.

References
1. Bullock LJ, Reeves RJ: Unilateral exophthalmos: Roentgenographic aspects. AJR 1959;82:290–299
2. Lee KF, Hodes PJ, Greenberg L, et al: Three rare causes of unilateral exophthalmos. Radiology 1968;90:1009–1015
3. Lloyd GAS: The radiological investigation of proptosis. Br J Radiol 1970;43:1–18
4. Newton TH, Potts DG: Radiology of the Skull and Brain. St. Louis: CV Mosby, vol 1, book 2, 1971, pp 468–469
5. Price HI, Danziger A: The computerized tomographic findings in pediatric orbital tumors. Clin Radiol 1979;30:435–440
6. Taybi H, Lachman RS: Radiology of Syndromes, Metabolic Disorders, and Skeletal Dysplasias. (ed 4) St. Louis: Mosby-Year Book, 1996, p 989
7. Vade E, Armstrong D: Orbital rhabdomyosarcoma in childhood. Radiol Clin North Am 1987;25:701–714
8. Weber AL, Dallow RL, Momose KJ: Evaluation of orbital and eye lesions by radiographic examination, ultrasound and computerized axial tomography. American Roentgen Ray Society Scientific Exhibit, Atlanta, 1975

Gamut B-18

DEFORMITY AND DIMENSIONAL CHANGES IN THE EYEBALL (ON CT OR MRI)

COMMON

*1. Axial myopia
*2. Coloboma of globe
3. Microphthalmos
*4. Neoplasm (retinal, choroidal, scleral)
5. Phthisis bulbi
6. Surgical scleral banding
7. Trauma

UNCOMMON

1. Aphakia
*2. Congenital glaucoma (buphthalmos)
*3. Macrophthalmos
*4. Posterior staphyloma
5. Pseudotumor of orbit
6. Subchoroidal hemorrhage
7. Wegener's granulomatosis

* May show enlarged eye with increased size of globe.

(continued)

References
1. Bilaniuk LT, Farber M: Imaging of developmental anomalies of the eye and the orbit. Am J Neuroradiol 1992;13: 793–803
2. Osborne DR: CT Analysis of Deformity and Dimensional Changes in the Eyeball. American Roentgen Ray Society Scientific Exhibit, Boston, 1985

Gamut B-19

INTRAORBITAL CALCIFICATION
(See B-20, 21)

COMMON
1. Cataract (lens)
2. [Foreign body; fracture fragment]
3. Phlebolith (eg, orbital varices, venous malformation, cavernous hemangioma, arteriovenous malformation or shunt)
4. Phthisis bulbi (trauma or infection with shrunken globe)
5. Retinoblastoma

UNCOMMON
1. Aneurysm or atherosclerosis of internal carotid or ophthalmic artery; vascular calcification (eg, diabetes)
2. Congenital syndromes
   a. Cryptophthalmia S.
   b. Fetal cytomegalovirus infection
   c. Neurofibromatosis
   d. Oculo-dento-osseous dysplasia
   e. von Hippel-Lindau S.
3. Connective tissue disease (collagen disease)$_g$ (eg, band keratopathy of cornea in rheumatoid arthritis)
4. Drusen
5. Glaucoma
6. Hematoma; myositis ossificans of extraocular muscles
7. Hypercalcemia (conjunctiva or cornea) (eg, in hypervitaminosis D; hyperparathyroidism, primary or secondary {renal osteodystrophy}; metastatic disease; multiple myeloma; milk-alkali S.; Williams S.{idiopathic hypercalcemia})
8. Idiopathic
9. Infection, intraocular (eg, abscess; bacterial ophthalmitis; tuberculosis; syphilis)
10. Intraorbital neoplasm (eg, meningioma; hemangioma; dermoid; teratoma; optic glioma; plexiform neurofibroma; choroidal osteoma; hamartoma; lacrimal gland carcinoma; hemangioendothelioma; metastasis)
11. Mucocele invading orbit
12. [Osteoma; fibrous dysplasia]
13. Parasitic disease (eg, hydatid disease; cysticercosis; toxoplasmosis)
14. Phakoma
15. Radiation therapy
16. Retinal disease (eg, detachment; retinitis; fibrosis; retrolental fibroplasia)

[ ] This condition does not actually cause the gamuted imaging finding, but can produce imaging changes that simulate it.

References
1. Ashton N: Calcareous degeneration and ossification. In: Duke-Elder S (ed): System of Ophthalmology. St. Louis: CV Mosby, 1962
2. Edwards MK, Buncic JR, Harwood-Nash DC: Optic disk drusen: Case report. JCAT 1982;6:383–384
3. Newton TH, Potts DG: Radiology of the Skull and Brain. St. Louis: CV Mosby, vol 1, book 2, 1971, pp 525–540
4. Sundheim JL, Lapayowker MS: Calcification and ossification within the orbit. Radiology 1976;121:391–397

Gamut B-20

GLOBE CALCIFICATION (ON CT) NEOPLASM WITHIN THE GLOBE

COMMON
1. Retinoblastoma

UNCOMMON
1. Choroidal osteoma

NEOPLASM INFILTRATING POSTERIOR GLOBE FROM OPTIC NERVE

COMMON

1. Meningioma of optic nerve sheath

UNCOMMON

1. Hamartoma (tuberous sclerosis)
2. Optic nerve glioma or neurofibroma
3. Sarcoidosis of optic nerve sheath

TRAUMA

COMMON

1. Foreign body in globe
2. Phthisis bulbi (result of chronic post-traumatic degeneration or infection)

UNCOMMON

1. Chronic retinal detachment
2. Postoperative

MISCELLANEOUS

COMMON

1. Drusen
2. Lens (senile cataract)

UNCOMMON

1. Hypercalcemic states
2. Radiation therapy
3. Retrolental fibroplasia
4. Toxoplasmosis
5. Vascular lesion (eg, Sturge-Weber S.; von Hippel-Lindau S.)

References

1. Froula PD, Bartley GB, Garrity JA, Forbes G: The differential diagnosis of orbital calcification as detected on computed tomographic scans. Mayo Clin Proc 1993;68:256–261
2. Johns TT, Citrin CM, Black J: CT evaluation of perineural orbital lesions: Evaluation of the "tram-track" sign. AJNR 1984;5:587–590.

3. Peyster RG, Hoover E: Computed Tomography in Orbital Disease and Neuro-ophthalmology. Chicago: Year Book Medical Publ, 1984.
4. Sobel DF, Salvolini U, Newton TH: Ocular and orbital pathology. In: Newton TH, Hasso AN, Dillon WP (eds): Modern Neuroradiology, vol 3. Computed Tomography of the Head and Neck. New York: Raven Press, 1988.
5. Turner RM, Gutman I, Hilal KS, et al: CT of drusen bodies and other calcific lesions of the optic nerve: Case report and differential diagnosis. AJNR 1983;4:175–178

Gamut B-21

EXTRAGLOBAL CALCIFICATION (ON CT)

COMMON

1. Meningioma of optic nerve sheath
2. Trauma, old
3. Vascular (eg, hemangioma, varices with phleboliths; arteriovenous malformation; atherosclerosis)

UNCOMMON

1. Dermoid
2. Hypercalcemic states
3. Lacrimal gland neoplasm
4. Neuroblastoma
5. Neurofibroma
6. Optic glioma
7. [Orbital wall abnormality (eg, fibrous dysplasia; osteosarcoma; metastasis from prostate or breast carcinoma)]
8. Retinoblastoma (infiltrating)

[This condition does not actually cause the gamuted imaging finding, but can produce imaging changes that simulate it.]

References

1. Froula PD, Bartley GB, Garrity JA, Forbes G: The differential diagnosis of orbital calcification as detected on computed tomographic scans. Mayo Clin Proc 1993;68:256–261

(continued)

2. Johns TT, Citrin CM, Black J: CT evaluation of perineural orbital lesions: Evaluation of the "tram-track" sign. AJNR 1984;5:587–590.
3. Peyster RG, Hoover E: Computed Tomography in Orbital Disease and Neuro-ophthalmology. Chicago: Year Book Medical Publ, 1984.
4. Turner RM, Gutman I, Hilal KS, et al: CT of drusen bodies and other calcific lesions of the optic nerve: Case report and differential diagnosis. AJNR 1983;4:175–178

Gamut B-22

PERIORBITAL SOFT TISSUE SWELLING

1. Orbital infection, cellulitis, or abscess (bacterial, viral, fungal)
2. Orbital inflammation
   a. Connective tissue disorders$_g$
   b. Extension from acute sinusutis or orofacial abscess
   c. Granulomatous diseases (sarcoidosis; Wegener's granulomatosis)
   d. Orbital pseudotumor
   e. Vasculitides

References
1. Davis PC, Newman NJ: Advances in neuroimaging of the visual pathways. Am J Ophthalmol 1996;121:690–705
2. Haugen JR, Ramlo JH: Serious complications of acute sinusitis. Postgrad Med 1993;93:115–118, 122, 125
3. Klapper SR, Patrinely JR, Kaplan SL, Font RL: Atypical mycobacterial infection of the orbit. Ophthalmology, 1995; 102:1536–1541
4. Lufkin R, Borges A, Villablanca P: Teaching Atlas of Head and Neck Imaging. New York: Springer Verlag, 2000, pp 185–188
5. Mauriello Jr JA, Yepez N, Mostafavi R, et al: Invasive rhinosino-orbital aspergillosis with precipitous visual loss. Canad J Ophthalmol 1995;30:124–130
6. Mitchell CS, Nelson Jr MMD: Orofacial abscesses of odontogenic origin in the pediatric patient. Report of two cases. Pediatr Radiol 1993;23:432–434
7. Moll Jr GW, Raila FA, Liu GC, Conerly Sr AW. Rhinocerebral mucormycosis in IDDM. Sequential magnetic resonance imaging of long-term survival with intensive therapy. Diabetes Care 1994;17:1348–1353

8. Sullivan TJ, Patel BC, Aylward GW, Wright JE: Anaerobic orbital abscess secondary to intraorbital wood. Austral N Zeal J Ophthalmol 1993;21:49–52

Gamut B-23

LACRIMAL GLAND ENLARGEMENT

COMMON

1. Benign mixed tumor (pleomorphic adenoma)
3. Carcinoma (esp. adenoid cystic carcinoma; also mucoepidermoid carcinoma; adenocarcinoma)
4. Inflammation (incl. orbital pseudotumor)
   a. Acute dacryoadenitis (usually following a viral infection such as mumps or infectious mononucleosis; also after bacterial or fungus infections)
   b. Chronic dacryoadenitis (eg, sarcoidosis; Sjögren S.; Mikulicz S. [may be associated with tuberculosis, syphilis, or leprosy]; Wegener's granulomatosus)
5. Lymphoma$_g$; leukemia

UNCOMMON

1. Amyloidosis
2. Benign lymphoid hyperplasia
3. Dermoid; epidermoid
4. Metastasis
5. Thyroid ophthalmopathy

References
1. Bilaniuk LT, Farber M: Imaging of developmental anomalies of the eye and the orbit. AJNR 1992;13:793–803
2. Carmody RF, Mafee MF, Goodwin JA, et al: Orbital and optic pathway sarcoidosis: MR findings. AJNR 1994;15: 775–783
3. Krzystolik M, Warner MA: Orbit and adnexal neoplasia. Curr Opin Ophthalmol 1995;6:78–85
4. Lee SH, Rao K: Cranial Computed Tomography in Orbital Disease and Neuro-ophthalmology. Chicago: Year Book Medical Publ, 1984, pp 147–150
5. Lufkin R, Borges A, Villablanca P: Teaching Atlas of Head and Neck Imaging. New York: Springer Verlag, 2000, pp 189–191

6. Poyet C: Orbits. In: Ravin CE, Cooper C (eds): Review of Radiology. Philadelphia: WB Saunders, 1990, p 132
7. Shields CL, Shields JA: Lacrimal gland tumors. Intl Ophthalmol Clin 1993;33:1818
8. Sobel DF, Salvolini U, Newton TH: Ocular and orbital pathology. In: Newton TH, Hasso AN, Dillon WP (eds): Modern Neuroradiology, vol 3. Computed Tomography of the Head and Neck. New York: Raven Press, 1988, pp 9.34–9.37
9. Stewart WB, Krohel GB, Wright JE: Lacrimal gland and fossa lesions: An approach to diagnosis and management. Ophthalmology 1979;86:886

Gamut B-24

CONGENITAL ABNORMALITIES OF THE TEMPORAL BONE

ANOMALIES OF THE SOUND CONDUCTING SYSTEM

1. Stenosis, agenesis, or soft tissue or bony atresia plate of external auditory canal
2. Microtia (deformity of auricle), often with dysplasia of external auditory canal as in:
   a. Mandibular facial dysostosis (eg, Treacher Collins S.; Franceschetti S.)
   b. Hypoplastic mandibular condyle and flat temporomandibular fossa
3. Atresia or hypoplasia of mastoid air cells
4. Hypoplasia or agenesis of middle ear
5. Anomalies of incus and malleus
6. Abnormalities of labyrinthine window and stapes (eg, congenital fixation of stapes footplate; stapedial otosclerosis)

ANOMALIES OF THE FACIAL NERVE

1. Abnormal course, shortening, or ectopia of facial nerve

ANOMALIES OF THE INNER EAR

1. Anomaly or defect in otic capsule
   a. Michel deformity (hypoplasia or aplasia of petrous pyramid and inner ear structures)
   b. Mondini deformity (abnormal cochlea)

VESTIBULAR AQUEDUCT AND SEMICIRCULAR CANAL ANOMALIES

1. Dilated shortened aqueduct
2. Hypoplasia or aplasia of vestibule and semicircular canals (eg, Waardenburg S.)

ANOMALIES OF THE INTERNAL AUDITORY CANAL

1. Hypoplasia of canal
2. Dilated shortened canal (sometimes with chronic hydrocephalus)

DILATED COCHLEAR AQUEDUCT

CONGENITAL OBLITERATIVE LABYRINTHITIS

CONGENITAL CEREBROSPINAL FLUID OTORRHEA (due to defect in internal auditory canal and stapes footplate)

CONGENITAL VASCULAR ANOMALIES

1. High large jugular fossa and bulb
2. Defect in dome of jugular fossa with herniation of bulb into middle ear simulating glomus tumor
3. Ectopic intratemporal course of internal carotid artery (lateral position of artery which may lie in middle ear and be associated with persistent stapedial artery and aberrant middle meningeal artery)

References
1. Unger JM: Handbook of Head and Neck Imaging. New York: Churchill Livingstone, 1987, pp 152–155

(continued)

2. Valvassori GE, Buckingham RA, Carter BL, Hanafee WN, Mafee MF: Head and Neck Imaging. New York: Thieme Medical Publ, 1988, pp 44–64

Gamut B-25

BONE DISORDER ASSOCIATED WITH OTOSCLEROSIS (ON TOMOGRAPHY OR CT)

COMMON
1. Fibrous dysplasia
2. Paget's disease

UNCOMMON
1. Bone tumor, osteogenic (eg, osteoma; osteosarcoma) or chondrogenic (eg, chondrosarcoma)
2. Cleidocranial dysplasia
3. Craniometaphyseal dysplasia
4. Hurler syndrome
5. Osteoblastic metastasis
6. Osteogenesis imperfecta
7. Osteopetrosis

Reference
1. Valvassori GE, Buckingham RA, Carter BL, Hanafee WN, Mafee MF: Head and Neck Imaging. New York: Thieme Medical Publ, 1988, pp 158–172

Gamut B-26

LESION OF THE FACIAL CANAL IN THE TEMPORAL BONE (ON TOMOGRAPHY OR CT)

1. Atresia or hypoplasia of canal
2. Cholesteatoma, congenital or acquired (epidermoid)
3. Extratemporal lesion extending into canal (eg, meningioma; parotid tumor)

4. Hemangioma
5. Infection (eg, herpes zoster; varicella; syphilis)
6. Lymphoma$_g$
7. Malignant external otitis (*Pseudomonas*)
8. Neurinoma of facial nerve
9. Paraganglioma
10. Posttraumatic or postsurgical injury of facial nerve
11. Sarcoidosis

References
1. Petrus LV, Lo WMM: Primary paraganglioma of the facial nerve canal. AJNR 1996;17:171–174
2. Swartz JD, Harnsberger HR, Mukherji SK: The temporal bone. Rad Clin North Am 1998;36:819–853
3. Valvassori GE, Buckingham RA, Carter BL, Hanafee WN, Mafee MF: Head and Neck Imaging. New York: Thieme Medical Publ, 1988

Gamut B-27-1

LESIONS INVOLVING THE FACIAL NERVE OUTSIDE THE TEMPORAL BONE

1. Cholesteatoma
2. Chordoma
3. Hemangioma
4. Idiopathic facial nerve palsy
5. Inflammation/infection (herpes zoster; varicella; sarcoidosis; syphilis)
6. Lymphoma$_g$; leukemic deposits
7. Malignant otitis externa
8. Metastasis
9. Neurinoma; schwannoma

References
1. Lanzieri CF: Head and neck case of the day. AJR 1997;169:275–282
2. Pulec JL: Facial nerve angioma. Ear Nose Throat J 1996;75:225–238
3. Swartz JD, Harnsberger HR, Mukherji SK: The temporal bone. Rad Clin North Am 1998;36:819–853

4. Vogl TJ, Balzer J, Mack M, Steger W: Differential Diagnosis in Head and Neck Imaging. New York: Thieme, 1999, pp 64–67

OSTEOLYSIS OF THE TEMPORAL BONE

FOCAL
1. Langerhans cell histiocytosis$_g$
2. Metastasis
3. Osteomyelitis
4. Retrofenestral/cochlear otosclerosis
5. Syphilis, tertiary (gumma) or osteitis of late congenital syphilis

DIFFUSE
1. Fibrous dysplasia
2. Metastatic disease
3. Multiple myeloma
4. Osteogenesis imperfecta
5. Osteomyelitis (incl. tuberculosis; syphilis)
6. Paget's disease

Gamut B-27-2

FACIAL NERVE PALSY

1. Bell's palsy
2. Benign tumor
   a. Acoustic schwannoma
   b. Choristoma
   c. Epidermoid cyst (congenital cholesteatoma)
   d. Facial nerve tumor (schwannoma; hemangioma; lipoma)
   e. Glomus tympanicum tumor
   f. Meningioma of cerebellopontine angle
3. Herpes zoster oticus
4. Langerhans cell histiocytosis$_g$
5. Malignant tumor
   a. Direct invasion (eg, glomus jugulare tumor; embryonal rhabdomyosarcoma; cystadenocarcinoma of the endolymphatic sac)
   b. Lymphoma$_g$
   c. Metastasis
   d. Perineural spread (parotid or EAC malignancy)
   e. Sarcoma of facial nerve
6. Trauma; temporal bone fracture

Reference
1. Lufkin R, Borges A, Villablanca P: Teaching Atlas of Head and Neck Imaging. New York: Thieme, 2000, pp 417–422

References
1. Arriaga MA, Carrier D: MRI and clinical decisions in cochlear implantation. Am J Otology 1996;17:547–553
2. Lufkin R, Borges A, Villablanca P: Teaching Atlas of Head and Neck Imaging. New York: Thieme, 2000, pp 365–369
3. Mark AS, Seltzer S, Harnsberger HR: Sensorineural hearing loss: more than meets the eye? AJNR 1993;14:37–45
4. Mark AS, Fitzgerald D: MRI of the inner ear. Baillieres Clin Neurology 1994;3:515–535
5. Ross UH, Reinhardt MJ, Berlis A: Localization of active otosclerotic foci by tympano-cochlear scintigraphy (TCS) using correlative imaging. J Laryngol Otol 1995;109:1051–1056
6. Ross UH, Laszig R, Bornemann H, Ulrich C: Osteogenesis imperfecta: clinical symptoms and update findings in computed tomography and tympano-cochlear scintigraphy. Acta Oto-Laryngologica 1993;113:620–624
7. Saunders JE, Derebery MJ, Lo WW: Magnetic resonance imaging of cochlear otosclerosis. Ann Otol Rhinol Laryngol 1995;104:826–829
8. Valvassori GE: Imaging of otosclerosis. Otolaryngol Clin N Am 1993;26:359–371
9. Weissman JL. Hearing loss. Radiology 1996;199:593–611

(continued)

10. Woollford TJ, Roberts GR, Hartley C, Ramsden RT: Etiology of hearing loss and cochlear computed tomography: findings in preimplant assessment. Ann Otol Rhinol Laryngol 1995(Suppl);166:201–206

Gamut B-29

DESTRUCTIVE LESIONS IN THE PETROUS APEX

INFECTIOUS/INFLAMMATORY LESIONS
1. Abscess of petrous apex
2. Malignant otitis externa (osteomyelitis of skull base)
3. Petrous apicitis; petrous apex syndrome (Gradenigo S.)

BENIGN TUMORS
1. Cholesteatoma
2. Cholesterol granuloma
3. Meningioma
4. Paraganglioma

MALIGNANT TUMORS
1. Carcinoma of nasopharynx
2. Chondrosarcoma of skull base
3. Chordoma
4. Lymphoma$_g$
5. Metastasis
6. Plasmacytoma; multiple myeloma

References
1. Bourne RR, Maclaren RE: lntracranial plasmacytoma masquerading as Gradenigo's syndrome (letter). Brit J Ophthalmol 1998;82:458–459
2. Frates MC, Oates E: Partous apicitis: evaluation by bone SPECT and magnetic resonance imaging. Clin Nucl Med 1990;15:293–294
3. Gadre AK, Brodie HA, Fayad JN, O'Leary MJ: Venous channels of the petrous apex: their presence and clinical importance. Otolaryngol Head Neck Surg 1997;ll6:168–174

4. Hardjasudarma M, Edwards RL, Ganley JP, Aarstad RF: Magnetic resonance imaging features of Gradenigo's syndrome. Am J Otolaryngol 1995;116:247–250
5. Horn KL, Erasmus MD, Akiya FI: Suppurative petrous apicitis: osteitis or osteomyelitis? An imaging case report. Am J Otolaryngol 1996;17:54–57
6. Jackler RK, Parker DA: Radiographic differential diagnosis of petrous apex lesions. Am J Otology 1992;13:561–574
7. Lufkin R, Borges A, Villablanca P: Teaching Atlas of Head and Neck Imaging. New York: Thieme, 2000, pp 370–374
8. Murakami T, Tsubaki J, Tahara Y, Nagashima T: Gradenigo's syndrome: CT and MRI findings. Pediatr Radiol 1996;26:684–685

Gamut B-30

VASCULAR MIDDLE EAR MASS (INTRA- or RETROTYMPANIC)

1. Aberrant or exposed internal carotid artery
2. Aneurysm of carotid artery
3. Chronic inflammation (eg, cholesterol granuloma; inflammatory debris with hemorrhage)
4. Exposed, high riding jugular bulb
5. Glomus jugulare or glomus tympanicum tumor
6. Hemangioma
7. Persistent stapedial artery

References
1. Ashikaga R, Araki Y, Ishida O: Bilateral aberrant internal carotid arteries. Neuroradiology 1995;37:655–657
2. Dietz RR, Davis WL, Harnsberger HR, et al: MR imaging and MR angiography in the evaluation of pulsatile tinnitus. AJNR 1994;15:879–889
3. Guinto Jr FC, Garrabrant EC, Radcliffe WB: Radiology of the persistent stapedial artery. Radiology 1972;105: 365–369
4. Lufkin R, Borges A, Villablanca P: Teaching Atlas of Head and Neck Imaging. New York: Thieme, 2000, pp 339-343,400–403
5. Pirodda A, Sorrenti G, Marliani AF, Capello I: Arterial anomalies of the middle ear associated with stapes ankylosis. J Laryngol Otol 1994;108:237–239
6. Rodgers GK, Applegate L, de La Cruz A, Lo W: Magnetic resonance angiography: analysis of vascular lesions of the temporal bone and skull base. Am J Otology 1993;14:56–62

7. Shankar L, Metha AL, Hawke M, Rutka J: High resolution CT of an aberrant internal carotid artery. J Otolaryngol 1992;21:373–375
8. Takahashi S, Higano S, Kuriara N, Shirane R, et al: Congenital absence and aberrant course of the internal carotid artery. Europ Radiol 1996;6:571–573

Gamut B-31

SOFT TISSUE IN THE MIDDLE EAR

1. Cholesteatoma, acquired (pars flaccida or pars tensa) (See B-31-S)
2. Cholesterol granuloma
3. Chronic otitis media
4. Glomus tympanicum tumor
5. Granulation tissue
6. Malignant otitis externa
7. Neoplasm (squamous cell carcinoma in adults; rhabdomyosarcoma in children)

Reference
1. Lufkin R, Borges A, Villablanca P: Teaching Atlas of Head and Neck Imaging. New York: Thieme, 2000, pp 381–387

Gamut B-31-S

COMPLICATIONS ASSOCIATED WITH CHOLESTEATOMA

1. Abscess
2. Encephalitis
3. Facial nerve paralysis
4. Labyrinthine fistula
5. Meningitis
6. Petrous apex syndrome (Gradenigo S.)
7. Sinus thrombosis

Reference
1. Lufkin R, Borges A, Villablanca P: Teaching Atlas of Head and Neck Imaging. New York: Thieme, 2000, pp 381–387

Gamut B-32

EROSION OR DESTRUCTION OF TYMPANIC PORTION OF PETROUS BONE, MIDDLE EAR, OR MASTOID

COMMON
1. Cholesteatoma, acquired or congenital (epidermoid—rare in mastoid)
2. Cholesterol granuloma
3. Chronic otitis media (incus and rarely malleus)
4. Fracture of the temporal bone
5. Mastoiditis, acute or chronic
6. [Postoperative defect; simple or radical mastoidectomy]

UNCOMMON
1. Bone neoplasm, benign or malignant (eg, hemangioma; embryonal rhabdomyosarcoma)
2. Carcinoma of mastoid, external auditory meatus, or middle ear
3. Ceruminous gland tumor
4. Dermoid cyst
5. Epidural mastoid cyst or pneumatocele
6. Glomus jugulare tumor; glomus tympanicum tumor (nonchromaffin paraganglioma)
7. Granuloma (esp. tuberculosis)
8. Keratosis obturans
9. Langerhans cell histiocytosis$_g$
10. [Large mastoid air cell]
11. Lymphoma$_g$
12. Malignant necrotizing external otitis (acute osteomyelitis of temporal bone in aged diabetic due to *Pseudomonas aeruginosa*)
13. Meningioma
14. Metastasis
15. Nasopharyngeal neoplasm (invasive)
16. Neurinoma
17. Postmastoidectomy meningocele or meningoencephalocele

(continued)

18. Sarcoidosis
19. Syphilis
20. Venous malformation

[ ] This condition does not actually cause the gamuted imaging finding, but can produce imaging changes that simulate it.

References
1. DuBoulay GH: Principles of X-ray Diagnosis of the Skull. (ed 2) London: Butterworths, 1980, p 195
2. Duggan CA, Hoffman JC, Brylski JR: The efficacy of angiography in the evaluation of glomus tympanicum tumors. Radiology 1970;97:45–49
3. Healy JF, Wong W: Unsuspected and unrelated pathology noted on limited computed tomographic scans of the paranasal sinuses and temporal bone. Clin Imag 1997;21: 155–162
4. Livingstone PA: Differential diagnosis of radiolucent lesions of the temporal bone. Radiol Clin North Am 1974; 12:571–583
5. Mendez G Jr, Quencer RM, Post JD, et al: Malignant external otitis: A radiographic-clinical correlation. AJR 1979; 132:957–961
6. Newton TH, Potts DG: Radiology of the Skull and Brain. St. Louis: CV Mosby, vol 1, book 1, 1971, pp 424–442
7. Phelps PD, Lloyd GAS: The radiology of cholesteatoma. Clin Radiol 1980;31:501–512
8. Phelps PD, Lloyd GAS: The radiology of carcinoma of the ear. Br J Radiol 1981;54:103–109
9. Valvassori GE, Buckingham RA, Carter BL, Hanafee WN, Mafee MF: Head and Neck Imaging. New York: Thieme Medical Publ, 1988, pp 74–114

Gamut B-33-1

SYNDROMES WITH MASTOID ABNORMALITIES—MASTOIDITIS

1. Achondroplasia
2. Chronic granulomatous disease of childhood (petrositis)
3. Gradenigo S. (apical petrositis)
4. Hyperimmunoglobulinemia E S. (Buckley S. or Job S.)
5. Immotile cilia S.

6. Langerhans cell histiocytosis$_g$
7. Wiskott-Aldrich S.

References
1. Taybi H, Lachman RS: Radiology of Syndromes, Metabolic Disorders, and Skeletal Dysplasias. (ed 4) St. Louis: Mosby-Year Book, 1996, p 986

Gamut B-33-2

SYNDROMES WITH MASTOID ABNORMALITIES— UNDERDEVELOPMENT OF MASTOIDS

1. Cleidocranial dysplasia
2. Cockayne S.
3. Craniodiaphyseal dysplasia
4. Craniometaphyseal dysplasia
5. Diaphyseal dysplasia (Camurati-Engelmann disease)
6. Endosteal hyperostosis (van Buchem type)
7. Frontometaphyseal dysplasia
8. Hypothyroidism, infantile (cretinism)
9. Mucopolysaccharidoses (See J-4)
10. Osteopathia striata (Voorhoeve disease)
11. Osteopetrosis
12. Otopalatodigital S. (type I)
13. Polyostotic fibrous dysplasia (McCune-Albright S.)
14. Pyknodysostosis
15. Treacher Collins S.

Reference
1. Taybi H, Lachman RS: Radiology of Syndromes, Metabolic Disorders, and Skeletal Dysplasias. (ed 4) St. Louis: Mosby-Year Book, 1996, p 986

Gamut B-33-3

SYNDROMES WITH MASTOID ABNORMALITIES—INCREASED PNEUMATIZATION OF MASTOIDS

1. Acromegaly
2. Adrenogenital S.
3. Cerebral hemiatrophy (Dyke-Davidoff-Masson S.)
4. Lipodystrophy (lipoatrophic diabetes)

Reference
1. Taybi H, Lachman RS: Radiology of Syndromes, Metabolic Disorders, and Skeletal Dysplasias. (ed 4) St. Louis: Mosby-Year Book, 1996, p 986

Gamut B-34

ABSENCE OR STENOSIS (BONY NARROWING) OF THE EXTERNAL AUDITORY CANAL

CONGENITAL
1. Bony or membranous atresia or stenosis of the EAC
2. Cleidocranial dysplasia
3. Congenital rubeola
4. Crouzon S. (craniofacial dysostosis)
5. Goldenhar S.
6. Klippel-Feil S.
7. Osteopetrosis
8. Thalidomide embryopathy
9. Treacher Collins S.

ACQUIRED
1. Exostosis of the EAC (swimmer's ear)
2. Fibrous dysplasia
3. Neoplasm (eg, osteoma; chondroid tumors); other benign and malignant bone tumors (rare)
4. Paget's disease

5. Postsurgical changes
6. Recurrent external otitis

References
1. Chandrasekhar SS, De La Cruz A, Garrido E: Surgery of congenital aural atresia. Am J Otology 1995;16:713–717
2. Cremers WR, Smeets JH: Acquired atresia of the external auditory canal. Surgical treatment and results. Arch Otolaryngol Head Neck Surg 1993;119:162–164; Laryngoscope 1987;97(suppl 45):15–17.
3. Deleyiannis FW, Cockcroft BD, Pinczower EF: Exostoses of the external auditory canal in Oregon surfers. Am J Otolaryngol 1996;17:303–307
4. Fisher EW, McManus TC: Surgery for external auditory canal exostoses and osteomata. J Laryngol Otol 1994; 108:106–110
5. Jahrsdoerfer RA, Jacobson JT: Treacher Collins syndrome: otologic and auditory management. J Amer Acad Audiol 1995;6:93–102
6. Lambert PR, Dodson EE: Congenital malformations of the external auditory canal. Otolaryngol Clin North Am 1996; 29:741–760.
7. Lufkin R, Borges A, Villablanca P: Teaching Atlas of Head and Neck Imaging. New York: Thieme, 2000, pp 344–348
8. Lumbroso C, Sebag G, Argyropoulou M, et al: Preoperative x-ray computed tomographic evaluation of major aplasia of the ear in children. Journal de Radiologie 1995;76:185–189
9. Mayer TE, Brueckmann H, Siegert R, et al: High-resolution CT of the temporal bone in dysplasia of the auricle and external auditory canal. Am J Neuroradiology 1997;18:53–65
10. Murphy TP, Burstein F, Cohen S: Management of congenital atresia of the external auditory canal. Otolaryngol Head Neck Surg 1997;116:580–584
11. Vallino-Napoli LD: Audiologic and otologic characteristics of Pfeiffer syndrome. Cleft Palate-Craniofacial J 1996; 33:524–529

Gamut B-35

EXTERNAL AUDITORY CANAL TUMOR

COMMON
1. Carcinoma (esp. squamous cell; also basal cell carcinoma; melanoma; metastasis)
2. Exostosis

(continued)

UNCOMMON

1. Adenomatous tumor (adenoma; pleomorphic adenoma; adenoid cystic carcinoma; adenocarcinoma)
2. Ceruminoma (benign ceruminous adenoma)
3. Cholesteatoma
4. Keratosis obturans; invasive keratitis
5. Osteoma (ivory or cancellous)
6. Retroauricular proliferating hemangioma
7. Skin lesion, benign (eg, lipoma; fibroma; sebaceous cyst)

References
1. Bergeron RT, Osborn AG, Som PM: Head and Neck Imaging Excluding the Brain. St. Louis: CV Mosby, 1984, pp 813–817
2. Powell T, Jenkins JPR: Ear, nose and throat: In: Grainger RG, Allison DJ: Diagnostic Radiology. (ed 2) Edinburgh: Churchill Livingstone, 1992, vol 3, p 2141

Gamut B-36

CALCIFICATION IN EAR CARTILAGE (PINNA)

COMMON

1. Boxing or other trauma
2. Frostbite
3. Gout

UNCOMMON

1. Acromegaly
2. Addison's disease
3. Connective tissue disease (collagen disease)$_g$
4. CPPD crystal deposition disease
5. Diabetes mellitus
6. Diastrophic dysplasia
7. Familial cold hypersensitivity
8. Hypercalcemia
9. Hypercorticism (Cushing S.)
10. Hyperparathyroidism, primary or secondary (renal osteodystrophy)
11. Hyperthyroidism
12. Hypoparathyroidism
13. Hypopituitarism (anterior lobe)
14. Idiopathic
15. Inflammation; infection
16. Keutel S.
17. Ochronosis (alkaptonuria)
18. Relapsing polychondritis
19. Sarcoidosis
20. Senility; aging
21. Syphilitic perichondritis
22. von Meyenberg disease (systemic chondromalacia)

References
1. Gordon DL: Calcification of auricular cartilage. Arch Intern Med 1964;113:23–27
2. Greenfield GB: Radiology of Bone Diseases. (ed 5) Philadelphia: Lippincott, 1990
3. Rubin AB, Chan KF: Case report 109. Pinnal calcification associated with acromegaly. Skeletal Radiol 1980;5:51–52
4. Taybi H, Lachman RS: Radiology of Syndromes, Metabolic Disorders, and Skeletal Dysplasias. (ed 4) St. Louis: Mosby-Year Book, 1996, p 983

Gamut B-37

DEFORMITY, ASYMMETRY, OR OPACIFICATION OF THE NASAL CAVITY

COMMON

1. Congenital deformity of nasal septum
2. Fracture of nasal plates or septum
3. Mucosal swelling (inflammatory, allergic, traumatic)
4. Pseudopolyp or polyp (incl. allergic polyposis; polypoid rhinosinusitis; cystic fibrosis {mucoviscidosis})
5. Rhinolith; foreign body
6. Turbinate abnormality (eg, enlargement; congenital absence)

UNCOMMON

1. Antrochoanal polyp
2. Benign neoplasm (eg, fibroma; neurofibroma; ossifying fibroma; osteoma)
3. Carcinoma of nose or antrum
4. Choanal atresia or stenosis
5. Dermoid cyst; mature nasopharyngeal teratoma
6. Encephalomeningocele, transsphenoid
7. Esthesioneuroblastoma (olfactory neuroblastoma)
8. Fibrosarcoma
9. Hypoplasia of nasal bones in various congenital syndromes
10. Inverting papilloma
11. Lymphoma$_g$
12. Mucocele
13. Rhinoscleroma with granulomatous mass
14. Wegener's granulomatosis

References
1. Castillo M, Mukherji SK: Imaging of facial anomalies. Curr Prob Diagn Radiol 1996;25:169–188
2. DuBoulay GH: Principles of X-ray Diagnosis of the Skull. (ed 2) London: Butterworths, 1980
3. Hall RE, Delbalso AM, Carter LC: Radiography of the sinonasal tract. In: Delbalso AM: Maxillofacial Imaging. Philadelphia: WB Saunders, 1990, pp 139–207
4. Hasso AN: MRI Atlas of the Head and Neck. Pratt Street, London: Martin Dunitz, Ltd., 1993, pp 58–59
5. Rao VM, El-Noueam KI: Sinonasal imaging: anatomy and pathology. Rad Clin North Am 1998;36:921–939

Gamut B-38

UNILATERAL NASAL CAVITY MASS

1. Carcinoma (squamous cell) of maxillary sinus
2. Granulomatous disease (eg, fungus disease; tuberculosis; syphilis; rhinoscleroma; Wegener's granulomatosis; lethal midline granuloma)
3. Inverted papilloma
4. Mucocele
5. Nasopharyngeal angiofibroma
6. Polyp (angiomatous polyp; nasoantral polyp)

References
1. Hug EB, Wang CC, Montgomery WW, Goodman ML: Management of inverted papilloma of the nasal cavity and paranasal sinuses: importance of radiation therapy. Intl J Rad Oncol Biol Physics 1993;26:67–72
2. Lawson W, Ho BT, Shaari CM, Biller HF: Inverted papilloma: a report of 112 cases. Laryngoscope 1995;105(3 Pt 1):282–288
3. Lufkin R, Borges A, Villablanca P: Teaching Atlas of Head and Neck Imaging. New York: Thieme, 2000, pp 319–323
4. Michaels L. Benign mucosal tumors of the nose and paranasal sinuses. Semin Diagn Pathol 1996;13:113–117
5. Roobottom CA, Jewell FM, Kabala J: Primary and recurrent inverting papilloma: appearances with magnetic resonance imaging. Clin Radiol 1995;50:472–475
6. Vrabec DP: The inverted Schneiderian papilloma: a 25-year study. Laryngoscope 1994;104(5 Pt 1):582–605
7. Woodruff WW, Vrabec DP: Inverted papilloma of the nasal vault and paranasal sinuses: spectrum of CT findings. AJR 1994;162:419–423

Gamut B-39

NASAL SEPTUM PERFORATION

1. Carcinoma (squamous cell)
2. Cocaine abuse
3. Fungus disease
4. Lymphoma$_g$ (esp. nasal T-cell lymphoma; Burkitt lymphoma)
5. Rhinoscleroma
6. Sarcoidosis
7. Syphilis
8. Trauma
9. Wegener's granulomatosis; lethal midline granuloma

References
1. Borisch B, Hennig I, Laeng RH, et al: Association of the subtype 2 of the Epstein-Barr virus with T-cell non-Hodgkin's lymphoma of the midline granuloma type. Blood 1993;82:858–864
2. Chen HH, Fong L, Su IJ, Ting LL, et al: Experience of radiotherapy in lethal midline granuloma with special emphasis on centrofacial T-cell lymphoma: a retrospective analysis covering a 34-year period. Radiotherapy & Oncol 1996;38:1–6

(continued)

3. Hartig G, Montone K, Wasik M, et al: Nasal T-cell lymphoma and the lethal midline granuloma syndrome. Otolaryngol Head Neck Surg 1996;114:653–656
4. Lufkin R, Borges A, Villablanca P: Teaching Atlas of Head and Neck Imaging. New York: Thieme, 2000, pp 324–327
5. Ramsay AD, Rooney N: Lymphomas of the head and neck. I: Nasofacial T-cell lymphoma. Europ J Cancer. Part B, Oral Oncology 1993;29B:99–102
6. Sevinsky LD, Woscoff A, Jaimovich L, Terzian A: Nasal cocaine abuse mimicking midline granuloma. J Am Acad Dermatol 1995;32:286–287

Gamut B-40

NASAL RIDGE MASS IN A CHILD

Congenital/Developmental Lesions

1. Dermal sinus
2. Fibrous dysplasia involving the nasal bones and forehead (cherubism)
3. Nasal dermoid/epidermoid
4. Nasal encephalocele
5. Nasal glioma

Inflammatory/Infectious Lesions

1. Cellulitis/phlegmon or abscess
2. Congenital syphilis
3. Inflammatory polyp
4. Pott's puffy tumor (tuberculosis)

Benign and Malignant Neoplasms

1. Angioma
2. Langerhans cell histiocytosis$_g$ (esp. eosinophilic granuloma)
3. Lymphoma$_g$; Burkitt lymphoma
4. Metastasis
5. Neurofibroma
6. Olfactory neuroblastoma
7. Rhabdomyosarcoma
8. Teratoma

Trauma to the Nasal Bones

References

1. Albery SM, Chaljub G, Cho NL, et al: MR imaging of nasal masses. RadioGraphics 1995;15:1311–1327
2. Cauchois R, Laccourreye O, Bremond D, et al: Nasal dermal sinus cyst. Ann Otol Rhinol Laryngol 1994;103(8 pt 1):615–618
3. Fitzpatrick E, Miller RH: Congenital midline masses: dermoids, gliomas and encephaloceles. J Louisiana State Med Soc 1996;148:93–96
4. Hladky JP, Le Jeune JP, Pertuson B, et al: Nasofrontal dermoid fistulae and cysts: 19 cases. Neuro-Chirurgie 1995; 41:337–342
5. Lufkin R, Borges A, Villablanca P: Teaching Atlas of Head and Neck Imaging. New York: Thieme, 2000, pp 295–298
6. Nocini PF, Barbaglio A, Dolci M, Salgarelli A: Dermoid cyst of the nose: a case report and review of the literature. J Oral Maxillofac Surg 1996;54:357–362
7. Posnick JC, Bortoluzzi P, Amstrong DC, Drake JM: Intracranial nasal dermoid sinus cysts: computed tomographic scan findings and surgical results. Plastic Reconstructive Surg 1994;93:745–754, discussion 755–756
8. Reilly JR, Koopman CF, Cotton R: Nasal mass in a pediatric patient (clinical conference). Head and Neck 1992;14: 415–418
9. Sweet RM: Lesions of the nasal radix in pediatric patients: diagnosis and management. South Med J 1992;85:164–169.

Gamut B-41-1

BENIGN AND MALIGNANT LESIONS OF THE NASOPHARYNX, NASAL CAVITY, AND PARANASAL SINUSES

BENIGN

COMMON

1. Inflammatory polyp; polypoid rhinosinusitis
2. Juvenile angiofibroma
3. [Lymphoid tissue; adenoids]
4. Mucocele
5. Mucous retention cyst
6. Osteoma

UNCOMMON

1. Adenoma
2. Ameloblastoma
3. Amyloidosis
4. Antrochoanal polyp
5. Arteriovenous malformation or fistula
6. Branchial cleft cyst
7. Chondroma
8. Dentigerous (follicular) cyst
9. Dermoid; teratoma
10. Encephalocele; meningocele
11. Epithelial papilloma (inverting and squamous)
12. Fibroma; desmoid tumor
13. Giant cell reparative granuloma
14. Giant cell tumor
15. Granuloma (eg, tuberculosis; sarcoidosis)
16. Hamartoma
17. Hemangioma
18. Histiocytosis$_g$
19. Inclusion cyst
20. Lipoma
21. Lymphangioma
22. Mucormycosis
23. Nasoalveolar cyst
24. Neurogenic tumor$_g$ (eg, neurinoma of IX, X, or XI nerve)
25. [Rhinolith, foreign body]
26. Rhinoscleroma
27. Salivary gland tumor (eg, Warthin tumor)
28. Tornwaldt cyst (notochord remnant)

MALIGNANT

COMMON

1. Carcinoma (esp. squamous cell; also adenocarcinoma; adenoid cystic carcinoma);
2. Lymphoepithelioma (incl. Schmincke tumor)
3. Lymphoma$_g$; Burkitt lymphoma
4. Metastasis (incl. retropharyngeal lymphadenopathy)

UNCOMMON

1. Chordoma
2. Esthesioneuroblastoma (olfactory neuroblastoma)
3. Hemangiopericytoma

4. Malignant histiocytoma
5. Melanoma
6. Plasmacytoma (extramedullary); myeloma
7. Salivary gland neoplasm (eg, carcinoma; mixed tumor)
8. Sarcoma (eg, neurosarcoma; rhabdomyosarcoma; spindle cell sarcoma; fibrosarcoma)
9. Wegener's granulomatosis; lethal midline granuloma

[ ] This condition does not actually cause the gamuted imaging finding, but can produce imaging changes that simulate it.

References

1. Braun IF: MRI of the nasopharynx. Rad Clin North Am 1989;27:327
2. Hall RE, Delbalso AM, Carter LC: Radiography of the sinonasal tract. In: Delbalso AM: Maxillofacial Imaging. Philadelphia: WB Saunders, 1990, pp 139–207
3. Kieserman SP, Stern J: Malignant transformation of nasopharyngeal lymphoid hyperplasia. Otolaryngol Head Neck Surg 1995;113:474–476
4. Lufkin R, Borges A, Villablanca P: Teaching Atlas of Head and Neck Imaging. New York: Thieme, 2000, pp 89–91, 101–104
5. Rao VM, El-Noueam KI: Sinonasal imaging: anatomy and pathology. Rad Clin North Am 1998;36:921–939
6. Teresi LM, Lufkin RB, Hanafee W: MRI of the nasopharynx and floor of the middle cranial fossa. Part II. Malignant tumors, etc. Radiology 1987;164:817
7. Teresi LM, et al: Chapter 37. In: Stark DD, Bradley WG (eds): Magnetic Resonance Imaging. (ed 2) St. Louis: CV Mosby and Co., 1992
8. Unger JM: Handbook of Head and Neck Imaging. New York: Churchill Livingstone, 1987, pp 85–91
9. Valvassori GE, Buckingham RA, Carter BL, Hanafee WN, Mafee MF: Head and Neck Imaging. New York: Thieme Medical Publ, 1988, pp 219–234
10. Woodruff WW, Vrabec DP: Inverted papilloma of the nasal vault and paranasal sinuses: spectrum of CT findings. AJR 1994;162:419–423

Gamut B-41-2

CYSTIC NASOPHARYNGEAL MASS

1. Atypical lymph node
2. Encephalomeningocele
3. Pharyngeal cyst
4. Tornwaldt cyst

References
1. Lufkin R, Borges A, Villablanca P: Teaching Atlas of Head and Neck Imaging. New York: Thieme, 2000, pp 75–77
2. Miyahara H, Matsunaga T: Tornwaldt's disease. Acta Oto-Laryngol (Suppl) 1994;517:36–39

Gamut B-42

AGGRESSIVE NASOPHARYNGEAL MASS IN A CHILD

1. Carcinoma of nasopharynx
2. Chloroma
3. Esthesioneuroblastoma
4. Hemangiopericytoma
5. Infection, aggressive (fungal, tuberculous, bacterial cocci)
6. Langerhans cell histiocytosis$_g$
7. Lymphoma$_g$, incl. Burkitt's lymphoma
8. Metastatic neuroblastoma
9. Minor salivary gland malignancy
10. Rhabdomyosarcoma; other soft tissue sarcomas (incl. fibrosarcoma; angiosarcoma; mesenchymal chondrosarcoma; malignant mesenchymoma)

References
1. Gilles R, Couanet D, Sigal R, et al: Head and neck rhabdomyosarcomas in children: value of clinical and CT findings in the detection of loco-regional relapses. Clin Radiol 1994;49:412–415
2. Kraus DH, Saenz NC, Gollamudi S, et al: Pediatric rhabdomyosarcoma of the head and neck. Am J Surg 1997;174:556–560
3. Kowalski LP, San CI: Prognostic factors in head and neck soft tissue sarcomas: analysis of 128 cases. J Surg Oncol 1994;56:83–88
4. Lee JH, Lee MS, Lee BH, et al: Rhabdomyosarcoma of the head and neck in adults: MR and CT findings. AJNR 1996;17:1923–1928
5. Lufkin R, Borges A, Villablanca P: Teaching Atlas of Head and Neck Imaging. New York: Thieme, 2000, pp 96–100
6. Lyos AT, Goepfert H, Luna MA, et al: Soft tissue sarcoma of the head and neck in children and adolescents. Cancer 1996;77:193–200
7. Odell PF: Head and neck sarcomas: a review. J Otolaryngol 1996;25:7–13
8. Park YW: Evaluation of neck masses in children. Amer Fam Phys 1995;51:1904–1912
9. Yang WT, Kwan WH, Li CK, Metreweli C: Imaging of pediatric head and neck rhabdomyosarcomas with emphasis on magnetic resonance imaging and a review of the literature. Pediatr Hematol Oncol 1997;14:243–257

Gamut B-43

EXTENSION OF NEOPLASM FROM INTRACRANIAL CAVITY TO NASOPHARYNX

COMMON

1. Chromophobe adenoma

UNCOMMON

1. Craniopharyngioma
2. Malignant otitis externa extending medially
3. Meningioma
4. Neurinoma; neurofibroma
5. Paraganglioma (glomus jugulare, glomus vagale, or carotid body tumor)

References
1. Hall RE, Delbalso AM, Carter LC: Radiography of the sinonasal tract. In: Delbalso AM: Maxillofacial Imaging. Philadelphia: WB Saunders, 1990, pp 139–207
2. Rao VM, El-Noueam KI: Sinonasal imaging: anatomy and pathology. Rad Clin North Am 1998;36:921–939

3. Teresi LM, et al: Chapter 37. In: Stark DD, Bradley WG (eds): Magnetic Resonance Imaging. (ed 2) St. Louis: CV Mosby and Co., 1992
4. Unger JM: Handbook of Head and Neck Imaging. New York: Churchill Livingstone, 1987, pp 85–91
5. Valvassori GE, Buckingham RA, Carter BL, Hanafee WN, Mafee MF: Head and Neck Imaging. New York: Thieme Medical Publ, 1988, pp 219–234

Gamut B-44

NASOPHARYNGEAL (AND/OR INFRATEMPORAL FOSSA) LESION

COMMON

1. Abscess (retropharyngeal) or cellulitis
2. Cervical spine lesion, including fracture
3. Enlarged adenoids, tonsils
4. Hematoma
5. Juvenile angiofibroma
6. Malignant nasopharyngeal neoplasm (esp. carcinoma; lymphoepithelioma; lymphoma$_g$; rhabdomyosarcoma; plasmacytoma) (See B-41-1)

UNCOMMON

1. Amyloidosis
2. Aneurysm of internal carotid artery
3. Antrochoanal polyp
4. Arteriovenous malformation
5. Benign nasopharyngeal neoplasm, other (See B-41-1)
6. Bone sarcoma (eg, chondrosarcoma; osteosarcoma)
7. Chordoma of clivus
8. Encephalocele, transsphenoid
9. Foreign body
10. Inflammatory polyp; polypoid rhinosinusitis
11. Lymphadenopathy, other (eg, infectious mononucleosis; sinus histiocytosis)

12. Meningioma of skull base
13. Metastasis
14. Mucocele
15. Nasal polyp; enlarged turbinate
16. Neoplasm extending from sphenoid, ethmoid, or maxillary sinus, nasal fossa, or parotid gland
17. Papillomas (Schneiderian)
18. Rhinoscleroma
19. Sarcoidosis
20. Tornwaldt cyst (notochord remnant)
21. Tuberculosis of nasopharynx or cervical spine

References
1. Jing B: Tumors of the nasopharynx. Radiol Clin North Am 1970;8:323–342
2. Newton TH, Potts DG: Radiology of the Skull and Brain. St. Louis: CV Mosby, vol 1, book 1, 1971, pp 251–258
3. Swischuk LE: Imaging of the Newborn, Infant, and Young Child. (ed 3) Baltimore: Williams & Wilkins, 1989
4. Unger JM: Handbook of Head and Neck Imaging. New York: Churchill Livingstone, 1987
5. Valvassori GE, Buckingham RA, Carter BL, Hanafee WN, Mafee MF: Head and Neck Imaging. New York: Thieme Medical Publ, 1988

Gamut B-45

LESIONS OF THE PTERYGOPALATINE (SPHENOMAXILLARY) FOSSA

COMMON

1. Juvenile angiofibroma
2. Malignant neoplasm, invasive (eg, carcinoma; melanoma; rhabdomyosarcoma; esthesioneuroblastoma {olfactory neuroblastoma})
3. Meningioma of sphenoid wing or nasal fossa
4. Metastasis
5. Trauma with fracture of pterygoid plates (eg, zygomatico-maxillary and Le Fort fractures)

(continued)

UNCOMMON

1. Aneurysm (carotid-cavernous sinus; paraclinoid)
2. Hyperostotic bone disease (eg, fibrous dysplasia; Paget's disease; meningioma; chronic osteomyelitis)
3. Inflammatory disease (eg, necrotizing granuloma; fungus infection; chronic hypertrophic polypoid rhinosinusitis)
4. Inverting papilloma
5. Mucocele (sphenoethmoid)
6. Pituitary adenoma or trigeminal neurinoma extending into base of pterygoid plates
7. Soft tissue tumor extension from parotid gland, nasopharynx, or cervical nodes

References

1. Osborn AG: The pterygopalatine (sphenomaxillary) fossa. In: Bergeron RT, Osborn AG, Som PM: Head and Neck Imaging Excluding the Brain. St. Louis: CV Mosby, 1984, pp 172–185
2. Woodruff WW, Vrabec DP: Inverted papilloma of the nasal vault and paranasal sinuses: spectrum of CT findings. AJR 1994;162:419–423

3. Curtin H: Separation of the masticator space from the parapharyngeal space. Radiology 1987;163:195–204
4. Jansen JC, Baatenburg de Jong RJ, Schipper J, et al: Color Doppler imaging of paragangliomas in the neck. J Clin Ultras 1997;25:481–485
5. Kramer LA, Mafee MF: Chapter 27. In: Stark DD, Bradley WG (eds): Magnetic Resonance Imaging. (ed 2) St. Louis: Mosby, 1992
6. Lasjaunias P, Berenstein A: Surgical Neuroangiography, vol. 2. Endovascular Treatment of Craniofacial Lesions. New York: Springer-Verlag, 1987
7. Leverstein H, Castelijns JA, Snow GB: The value of magnetic resonance imaging in the differential diagnosis of parapharyngeal space tumours. Clin Otolaryngol 1995;20:428–433
8. Lufkin R, Borges A, Villablanca P: Teaching Atlas of Head and Neck Imaging. New York: Thieme, 2000, pp 82–88
9. Pensak ML, Gluckman JL, Shumrick KA: Parapharyngeal space tumors: an algorithm for evaluation and management. Laryngoscope 1994:104:1170–1173
10. Som PM, Sacher M, Stollman AL: Common tumors of the parapharyngeal space: refined imaging diagnosis. Radiology 1988;169:81–85
11. Som PM, Curtin HD: Lesions of the parapharyngeal space. Role of MR imaging. Otolaryngol Clin North Am 1995; 28:515–542
12. Zak FG, Lawson W: The Paraganglionic Chemoreceptor System. Physiology, Pathology, and Clinical Medicine. New York: Springer-Verlag, 1982

Gamut B-46

POST-STYLOID PARAPHARYNGEAL (CAROTID) SPACE MASS

1. Enlarged lateral retropharyngeal lymph node
2. Glomus jugulare or vagale tumor (paraganglioma)
3. Meningioma
4. Metastasis
5. Pleomorphic adenoma (benign mixed tumor from accessory salivary tissue)
4. Schwannoma

References

1. Batsakis JG: Tumors of the Head and Neck: Clinical and Pathological Considerations. (ed 2) Baltimore: Williams & Wilkins, 1979
2. Cole JM, Beiler D: Long-term results of treatment for glomus jugulare and glomus vagale tumors with radiotherapy. Laryngoscope 1994;104:1461–1465

GAMUT B-47-1

LESIONS OF THE PARAPHARYNGEAL SPACE

1. Abscess
2. Branchial cleft cyst
3. Carcinoma (adenocarcinoma; adenoid cystic carcinoma; mucoepidermoid carcinoma)
4. Epidermoid inclusion cyst
5. Fibromatosis
6. Jugular vein thrombosis (chronic)
7. Lipoma; other fatty lesions (See B-47-2)
8. Lymphadenopathy
9. Meningioma
10. Minor salivary gland tumor
11. Neurinoma; schwannoma

12. Paraganglioma
13. Pleomorphic adenoma
14. Sarcoma
15. Thrombosed aneurysm of the internal carotid artery
16. Vascular malformation (rarely pure venous)

References

1. Elango S: Parapharyngeal space lipoma. Ear Nose Throat J 1995;74:52–53
2. Hamza A, Fagan JJ, Weissman JL, Myers EN: Neurilemmomas of the parapharyngeal space. Arch Otolaryngol 1997;123:622–626
3. Helmberger RC, Stringer SP, Mancuso AA: Rhabdomyosarcoma of the pharyngeal musculature extending into the prestyloid parapharyngeal space. AJNR 1996;17:1115–1118
4. Miller FR, Wanamaker JR, Lavertu P, Wood BG: Magnetic resonance imaging and the management of parapharyngeal space tumors. Head & Neck 1996;18:67–77
5. Mukherji SK, Castillo M: A simplified approach to the spaces of the suprahyoid neck. Rad Clin North Am 1998; 36:761–780
6. Porter MJ, Suen WM, John DG, Van Hasselt CA: Fibromatosis of the parapharyngeal space. J Laryngol Otol 1994; 108:1102–1104
7. Sigal R: Infrahyoid neck. Rad Clin North Am 1998;36: 781–799
8. Tillich M, Ranner G, Humer-Fuchs U, Lang-Loidolt D: Synovial sarcoma of the parapharyngeal space: CT and MRI. Neuroradiology 1998;40:261–263
9. Vogl TJ, Balzer J, Mack M, Steger W: Differential Diagnosis in Head and Neck Imaging. New York: Thieme, 1999, pp 217–228
10. Weissman JL: Imaging of the salivary glands. Semin Ultrasound CT MR 1995;16:546–568

References

1. Abdullah BJ, Liam CK, Kaur H, Mathew KM: Parapharyngeal space lipoma causing sleep-apnoea. Brit J Radiol 1997;70:1063–1065
2. Collins MH, Chatten J: Lipoblastoma/lipoblastomatosis: a clinicopathologic study of 25 tumors. Am J Surg Pathol 1997;21:1131–1137
3. Kraus MD, Guillou L, Fletcher CD: Well-differentiated inflammatory liposarcoma: an uncommon and easily overlooked variant of a common sarcoma. Am J Surg Pathol 1997;21:518–527
4. Lufkin R, Borges A, Villablanca P: Teaching Atlas of Head and Neck Imaging. New York: Thieme, 2000, pp 92–95
5. Saddik M, Oldring DJ, Mourad WA: Liposarcoma of the base of tongue and tonsillar fossa: A possibly underdiagnosed neoplasm. Arch Path Lab Med 1996;120:292–295
6. Stewart MG, Schwartz MR, Alford BR: Atypical and malignant lipomatous lesions of the head and neck. Arch Otolaryngol Head Neck Surg 1994;120:1151–1155

Gamut B-48

LESIONS OF THE MASTICATOR SPACE

1. Abscess (odontogenic)
2. Accessory parotid gland
3. Benign masseteric hypertrophy
4. Carcinoma (squamous cell)
5. Hemangioma
6. Hemangiopericytoma
7. Leiomyoma
8. Lymphangioma
9. Lymphoma (non-Hodgkins)
10. Metastasis
11. Minor salivary gland tumor
12. Neurofibroma; schwannoma
13. Osteoblastoma
14. Osteomyelitis of mandible
15. Sarcoma (chondrosarcoma; osteosarcoma; rhabdomyosarcoma; leiomyosarcoma)
16. Trigeminal (V_3) denervation atrophy

Gamut B-47-2

FATTY LESIONS IN THE PRESTYLOID PARAPHARYNGEAL SPACE (PPS)

1. Angiolipoma
2. Benign symmetric lipomatosis (Madelung disease)
3. Dermoid cyst; teratoma
4. Hibernoma
5. Lipoblastoma; lipoblastomatosis (pediatric patient)
6. Lipoma
7. Liposarcoma

(continued)

References
1. Daniels RL, Haller JR, Harnsberger HR: Hemangiopericytoma of the masticator space. Ann Otol Rhinol Laryngol 1996;105:162–165
2. Hasso AN: MRI Atlas of the Head and Neck. Pratt Street, London: Martin Dunitz, Ltd., 1993, pp 159–160
3. Mukherji SK, Castillo M: A simplified approach to the spaces of the suprahyoid neck. Rad Clin North Am 1998; 36:761–780
4. Som PM, Curtin HD, Silvers AR: A reevaluation of imaging criteria to access aggressive masticator space tumors. Head & Neck 1997;19:335–342
5. Vogl TJ, Balzer J, Mack M, Steger W: Differential Diagnosis in Head and Neck Imaging. New York: Thieme, 1999, pp 216–218

Gamut B-49-1

ABNORMALITIES OF THE PHARYNX—CONGENITAL

1. Choanal atresia
2. Cleft palate
3. Cyst (Tornwaldt cyst {notochord remnant}; para-pharyngeal cyst)
4. Encephalocele; meningocele

Reference
1. Valvassori GE, Buckingham RA, Carter BL, Hanafee WN, Mafee MF: Head and Neck Imaging. New York: Thieme Medical Publ, 1988

Gamut B-49-2

ABNORMALITIES OF THE PHARYNX— FUNCTIONAL DISORDER

1. Functional nasopharyngeal obstruction by enlarged adenoids or uvula (eg, pickwickian S. {marked obesity}; hypersomnolence states)
2. Swallowing disorder (eg, myasthenia gravis, scleroderma, dysautonomia) (See G-1, G-2)

Gamut B-49-3

ABNORMALITIES OF THE PHARYNX—TRAUMA

1. Fracture (eg, pterygoid plates; angle of mandible)
2. Puncture wound of nasophyarynx or pharynx (air in soft tissues; abscess; airway distortion)
3. Thorotrast injury to pharyngeal soft tissues and carotid arteries

Gamut B-49-4

ABNORMALITIES OF THE PHARYNX—INFECTION

1. Abscess
2. Adenoid hypertrophy; tonsillitis
3. Fungus disease$_g$ (eg, mucormycosis; actinomycosis; candidiasis)
4. Granulomatous disease (eg, tuberculosis; sarcoidosis; rhinoscleroma)

Reference
1. Valvassori GE, Buckingham RA, Carter BL, Hanafee WN, Mafee MF: Head and Neck Imaging. New York: Thieme Medical Publ, 1988

Gamut B-49-5

NEOPLASMS OF THE PHARYNX

1. Neoplasms of nasopharynx (See B-41-1)
2. Neoplasms of oropharynx (See B-106)
3. Neoplasms of hypopharynx (See B-111)

HYPOPLASTIC OR ABSENT PARANASAL SINUSES (USUALLY FRONTAL)

COMMON
1. Anemia$_g$, primary (esp. thalassemia; also sickle cell disease)
2. Congenital absence or hypoplasia
3. Cretinism; hypothyroidism
4. Fibrous dysplasia; leontiasis ossea
5. Kartagener S.
6. Paget's disease
7. Trisomy 21 S. (Down S.)

UNCOMMON
1. Binder S. (maxillonasal dysplasia)
2. Cleidocranial dysplasia
3. Cockayne S.
4. Craniometaphyseal dysplasia
5. Diaphyseal dysplasia (Camurati-Engelmann disease); craniodiaphyseal dysplasia
6. Frontometaphyseal dysplasia
7. Frontonasal dysplasia (median cleft face S.)
8. Hyperphosphatasia
9. Hypopituitarism
10. Metaphyseal chondrodysplasia (Jansen type)
11. Osteodysplasty (Melnick-Needles S.)
12. Osteopathia striata with cranial sclerosis
13. Osteopetrosis
14. Otopalatodigital S.
15. Prader-Willi S.
16. Pyknodysostosis
17. Schwarz-Lélek S.
18. Treacher Collins S.

References
1. Rao VM, El-Noueam KI: Sinonasal imaging: anatomy and pathology. Rad Clin North Am 1998;36:921–939
2. Taybi H, Lachman RS: Radiology of Syndromes, Metabolic Disorders, and Skeletal Dysplasias. (ed 4) St. Louis: Mosby-Year Book, 1996, p 1000

OPACIFICATION OF ONE OR MORE PARANASAL SINUSES

COMMON
*1. Hemorrhage or edema from trauma or surgery; epistaxis; barotrauma
2. [Hypoplasia or aplasia of a sinus]
3. Inflammatory mass (eg, nonsecretory cyst; mucous retention cyst; polyp; mucocele; pyocele)
4. Sinusitis
5. [Spurious opacification (eg, swelling of soft tissues of cheek; technical factors—poor positioning; increased thickness of adjacent bone—eg, fibrous dysplasia; Paget's disease; thalassemia; craniometaphyseal dysplasia)]

UNCOMMON
1. Cystic fibrosis (mucoviscidosis)
*2. Granulomatous or other infectious disease
   a. Fungus disease (eg, mucormycosis; aspergillosis; actinomycosis; blastomycosis; rhinosporidiosis)
   b. Leprosy
   c. Rhinoscleroma
   d. Sarcoidosis
   e. Syphilis
   f. Tuberculosis
3. Kartagener S.; immotile cilia S. (sinusitis)
*4. Neoplasm, benign or malignant (eg, carcinoma; lymphoma$_g$, incl. Burkitt lymphoma)
*5. Polypoid rhinosinusitis
*6. Wegener's granulomatosis; lethal midline granuloma

* Often with bone destruction.

[ ] This condition does not actually cause the gamuted imaging finding, but can produce imaging changes that simulate it.

References
1. Smoker WRK: The paranasal sinuses and temporomandibular joint. Categorical Course on Body Magnetic Resonance Imaging, pp 153–164

(continued)

2. Yousem D: Imaging of sinonasal inflammatory disease. Radiology 1993;188:303–314

Gamut B-52

FLUID LEVEL IN A PARANASAL SINUS

COMMON

1. Fracture of sinus wall with hemorrhage
2. Sinusitis, acute

UNCOMMON

1. Iatrogenic (eg, maxillary antral lavage; nasal packing for epistaxis; indwelling nasogastric tube)
2. Neoplasm (eg, osteoma or carcinoma of sinus)
3. Normal (infant)

Reference
1. Ogawa TK, Bergeron RT, Whitaker CW, et al: Air-fluid levels in the sphenoid sinus in epistaxis and nasal packing. Radiology 1976;118:351–354

Gamut B-53

MASS IN A PARANASAL SINUS

COMMON

*1. Carcinoma (esp. squamous cell; also adenocarcinoma; adenoid cystic; cylindroma)
 2. Encapsulated exudate, pus, or blood
*3. Extrinsic neoplasm invading sinus (eg, pituitary, orbital, oral, or nasopharyngeal; chordoma; juvenile angiofibroma; lymphoepithelioma; Burkitt lymphoma)
*4. Fracture with hematoma (eg, blow-out fracture of orbit)
 5. Impacted tooth (maxillary sinus)

 6. Mucocele (esp. frontal or ethmoid)
 7. Mucosal edema or inflammation (eg, from sinusitis due to allergy or infection)
 8. Mucous retention cyst; serous or nonsecretory cyst
*9. Osteoma (esp. frontal or ethmoid)
10. Polyp or pseudopolyp (incl. cystic fibrosis {mucoviscidosis})
*11. [Spurious opacification (eg, swelling of soft tissues of cheek; technical factors—poor positioning; increased thickness of adjacent bone—fibrous dysplasia, Paget's disease, thalassemia, craniometaphyseal dysplasia)]

UNCOMMON

 1. Antrochoanal polyp (maxillary sinus)
 2. Barotrauma
*3. Benign neoplasm, other (eg, osteochondroma; hemangioma; hemangiopericytoma; dermoid; lipoma; ossifying fibroma; osteoid osteoma; osteoblastoma; giant cell tumor; aneurysmal bone cyst)
*4. Bone sarcoma (eg, osteosarcoma; chondrosarcoma).
*5. Encephalocele
 6. Epithelial papilloma (squamous and inverting)
 7. Foreign body
*8. Granulomatous disease (eg, tuberculosis; syphilis; leprosy; glanders; fungus disease$_g$; sarcoidosis; rhinoscleroma; giant cell granuloma)
*9. Langerhans cell histocytosis$_g$
*10. Metastasis (esp. from carcinoma of kidney, lung, or breast)
*11. Myeloma, plasmacytoma (extramedullary)
*12. Neurogenic tumor$_g$ (eg, schwannoma; neurofibroma; neurocele; meningioma)
*13. Odontogenic cyst or tumor (eg, dentigerous cyst; globulomaxillary cyst; odontoma) at base of maxillary antrum
*14. Polypoid rhinosinusitis
15. Sinolith (calcified secretions)
*16. Surgical ciliated cyst (post Caldwell-Luc operation)

*17. Wegener's granulomatosis; lethal midline granuloma

* Usually with bone involvement.

[ ] This condition does not actually cause the gamuted imaging finding, but can produce imaging changes that simulate it.

References
1. Atallah N, Jay MM: Osteomas of the paranasal sinuses. J Laryngol Otol 1981;95:291–304
2. Chalijub G, Cho NL, Rassekh CH, John SD, Guinto FC: MR imaging of nasal masses. RadioGraphics 1995;15:1311–1327
3. Han MH, Chang KH, Lee CH, et al: Cystic expansile masses of the maxilla: differential diagnosis with CT and MR. AJNR 1995;16:333–338
4. Healy JF, Wong W: Unsuspected and unrelated pathology noted on limited computed tomographic scans of the paranasal sinuses and temporal bone. Clin Imag 1997;21:155–162
5. Holness RO, Attia E: Osteoma of the frontoethmoid sinus with secondary brain abscess and intracranial mucocele: case report (letter). Neurosurgery 1994;35:796–797
6. Koivunen P, Löppönen H, Fors AP, Jokinen K: The growth rate of osteomas of the paranasal sinuses. Clin Otolaryngol 1997;22:111–114
7. Lufkin R, Borges A, Villablanca P: Teaching Atlas of Head and Neck Imaging. New York: Thieme, 2000, pp 303–307
8. Mosesson RE, Som PM: The radiographic evaluation of sinonasal tumors: an overview. Otolaryngol Clin North Am 1995;28:1097–1115
9. Rao VM, El-Noueam KI: Sinonasal imaging: anatomy and pathology. Rad Clin North Am 1998;36:921–939
10. Rappaport JM, Attia EL: Pneumocephalus in frontal sinus osteoma: a case report. J Otolaryngol 1994;23:430–436
11. Unger JM: Handbook of Head and Neck Imaging. New York: Churchill Livingstone, 1987
12. Woodruff WW, Vrabec DP: Inverted papilloma of the nasal vault and paranasal sinuses: spectrum of CT findings. AJR 1994;162:419–423

Gamut B-54

LIQUID SINUS MASS (ON CT OR MRI)

1. Acute sinusitis
2. Cyst (odontogenic; keratocyst)

3. Iatrogenic (previous tooth extraction; sinus surgery)
4. Meningoencephalocele
5. Mucocele
6. Necrotic malignant tumor
7. Trauma

References
1. Som PM, Curtin HD: Head and Neck Imaging. (ed 3) St. Louis: Mosby-Year Book, 1996, pp 140–160
2. Vogl TJ, Balzer J, Mack M, Steger W: Differential Diagnosis in Head and Neck Imaging. New York: Thieme, 1999, pp 171–172

Gamut B-55

SINUS DISEASE WITH BONE DESTRUCTION

AGGRESSIVE INFECTION
1. Actinomycosis
2. Aspergillosis
3. Bacterial osteomyelitis
4. Candidiasis
5. Cryptococcosis
6. Histoplasmosis
7. Nocardiosis
8. Mucormycosis
9. Rhinoscleroma
10. Syphilis
11. Tuberculosis

NONINFECTIOUS GRANULOMATOUS PROCESSES
1. Idiopathic midline granuloma
2. Sarcoidosis
3. Wegener's granulomatosis

(continued)

NEOPLASM

1. Bone sarcoma (osteosarcoma; chondrosarcoma; Ewing sarcoma; fibrosarcoma)
2. Carcinoma (adenocarcinoma; squamous cell carcinoma)
3. Esthesioneuroblastoma
4. Lymphoma$_g$; Burkitt lymphoma
5. Malignant fibrous histiocytoma
6. Melanoma
7. Metastasis
8. Minor salivary gland neoplasm
9. Plasmacytoma; multiple myeloma
10. Rhabdomyosarcoma

MISCELLANEOUS

1. Langerhans cell histiocytosis$_g$ (esp. eosinophilic granuloma)
2. Nasal abuse from cocaine or chromate salts
3. Radiation injury
4. Trauma with fracture

Note: In an HIV-positive patient, aggressive infections either bacterial (nocardiosis) or fungal (aspergillosis, mucormycosis, candidiasis, cryptococcosis) are likely, as is an aggressive lymphoma.

References

1. Blitzer A, Lawson W: Fungal infections of the nose and paranasal sinuses, Part 1. Otolaryngol Clin North Am 1993; 26:1007–1035
2. Carinci F, Curioni C, Padula E, Calearo C: Cancer of the nasal cavity and paranasal sinuses: a new staging system. Internat J Oral Maxillofacial Surgery 1996;25:34–39
3. De Shazo RD, Sweain RE: Diagnostic criteria for allergic fungal sinusitis. J Allergy Clin Immunol 1995;96:24–35
4. Harbo G, Grau C, Bundgaard T, et al: Cancer of the nasal cavity and paranasal sinuses. A clinico-pathological study of 277 patients. Acta Oncologica 1997;36:45–50
5. Jakobsen MH, Larsen SK, Kirkegaard J, Hansen HS: Cancer of the nasal cavity and paranasal sinuses. Prognosis and outcome of treatment. Acta Oncologica 1997;36:27–31
6. Johnson CD, Brandes W: Invasive aspergillosis of the sphenoethmoid sinuses in an immunocompetent host. J Amer Osteopath Assoc 1992;92:1047–1051
7. Lawson W, Blitzer A: Fungal infections of the nose and paranasal sinuses, Part II. Otolaryngol Clin North Am 1993;26:1037–1068
8. Lufkin R, Borges A, Villablanca P: Teaching Atlas of Head and Neck Imaging. New York: Thieme, 2000, pp 314–318, 328–332
9. Parsons JT, Kimsey FC, Mendenhall Wm, et al: Radiation therapy for sinus malignancies. Otolaryngologic Clin North Am 1995;28:1259–1268
10. Som PM, Curtin HD: Chronic inflammatory sinonasal diseases including fungal infections—the role of imaging. Radiol Clin North Am 1993;31:33–34
11. Som PM, Silvers AR, Catalano PJ, et al: Adenosquamous carcinoma of the facial bones, skull base, and calvaria: CT and MR manifestations. Am J Neuroradiol 1997;18:173–175
12. Terk MR, Underwood DZ, Zee CS, Colletti PM: MR imaging in rhinocerebral and intracranial mucormycosis with CT and pathologic correlation. Magn Reson Imag 1992;10:81–87

Gamut B-56

TEMPOROMANDIBULAR JOINT DISEASE

COMMON

1. Condylar morphological abnormality (congenital or acquired); abnormal condylar excursion
2. Degenerative arthritis
3. Rheumatoid arthritis
4. Temporomandibular joint syndrome (limited excursion of mandibular condyle with displacement of the meniscus, usually anteriorly, occasionally posteriorly, best seen on MRI)
   a. Anterior dislocation with or without reduction
   b. Combined dislocations (both in frontal and sagittal planes)
   c. Disc perforation
5. Postsurgical changes
6. Posttraumatic changes

UNCOMMON

1. Adjacent bony disease (eg, Paget's disease; fibrous dysplasia)
2. Ankylosing spondylitis

3. Erosive (inflammatory) arthritis
4. Gout (rare)
5. Iatrogenic (eg, multiple steroid injections)
6. Infectious arthritis
7. Juvenile rheumatoid arthritis
8. Loose body
9. Neoplasm (eg, osteochondroma)
10. Osteochondritis dissecans (avascular necrosis)
11. Pigmented villonodular synovitis
12. Psoriatic arthritis

References
1. Barthelemy CR: The temporomandibular joint. In: Unger JM: Handbook of Head and Neck Imaging. New York: Churchill Livingstone, 1987, pp 189–205
2. Brady AP, McDevitt L, Stack JP, Downey D: A technique for magnetic resonance imaging of the temporomandibular joint. Clin Radiol 1993;47:127–133
3. DelBalso AM: An approach to the diagnostic imaging of jaw lesions, dental implants, and the temporomandibular joint. Rad Clin North Am 1998;36:855–890
4. Dorsay TA, Youngberg RA, Orr FE, Mulrean J: Cine MRI in the evaluation of the Proplast-Teflon TMJ interpositional implant. J Comput Assist Tomogr 1995;19:800–803
5. Dorsay TA, Youngberg RA: Cine MRI of the TMJ: need for initial closed mouth images without the Burnett device. J Comput Assist Tomogr 1995;19:163–164
6. Katzberg RW, Westesson PL, Tallents RH, Drake CM: Anatomic disorders of the temporomandibular joint disc in asymptomatic subjects. J Oral Maxillofac Surg 1996; 54:147–153
7. Lufkin R, Borges A, Villablanca P: Teaching Atlas of Head and Neck Imaging. New York: Thieme, 2000, pp 431–436
8. Muller-Leisse C, Augthun M, Bauer W, et al: Anterior disc displacement without reduction in the temporomandibular joint: MRI and associated clinical findings. J Magn Reson Imag 1996;6:769–774
9. Ramamelsberg P, Pospiech PR, Jager L, et al: Variability of disc position in asymptomatic volunteers and patients with internal derangements of the TMJ. Oral Surg Oral Med Oral Path Oral Radiol Endodontics 1997;83:393–399
10. Rao VM: Imaging of the temporomandibular joint. Semin Ultrasound CT MR 1995;l6:513–526
11. Simmons HC, Gibbs SJ: Recapture of temporomandibular joint discs using anterior repositioning appliances: an MRI study. Cranio 1995;13:227–237
12. Smoker WRK: The paranasal sinuses and temporomandibular joint. Categorical Course on Body Magnetic Resonance Imaging, pp 153–164
13. Takebayashi S, Takama T, Okada S, Masuda G, Matsubara S. MRI of the TMJ disc with intravenous administration of gadopentetate dimeglumine. J Comput Assist Tomogr 1997;21:209–215

Gamut B-57-1

PROGNATHISM

COMMON
1. Acromegaly
2. Normal variant; idiopathic

UNCOMMON
1. Cherubism (fibrous dysplasia)
2. Congenital syndromes (See B-57-2)
3. Edentulous mandible
4. Epidermolysis bullosa dystrophica
5. Hypothyroidism (juvenile)
6. Lymphangioma of tongue; other congenital tongue enlargements
7. Paget's disease

Gamut B-57-2

CONGENITAL SYNDROMES AND BONE DYSPLASIAS WITH PROGNATHISM

COMMON
1. Cherubism (fibrous dysplasia)
2. Cleidocranial dysplasia
3. Crouzon S. (craniofacial dysostosis)

UNCOMMON
1. Acrocephalosyndactyly (Apert type)
2. Acrodysostosis (peripheral dysostosis)
3. Beckwith-Wiedemann S.
4. Binder S. (maxillonasal dysplasia)

(continued)

5. Cloverleaf skull (kleeblattschädel anomaly)
6. Cockayne S.
7. Craniodiaphyseal dysplasia
8. Craniometaphyseal dysplasia
9. Endosteal hyperostosis (van Buchem and Worth types)
10. Facial hemihypertrophy (unilateral prognathism)
11. Gorlin S. (nevoid basal cell carcinoma S.)
12. Hajdu-Cheney S. (idiopathic acro-osteolysis)
13. "Happy puppet" S.
14. Hypothyroidism (juvenile)
15. LEOPARD S.
16. Mucolipidosis III (pseudo-Hurler polydystrophy)
17. Myotonic dystrophy
18. Normal variant
19. Oculo-dento-osseous dysplasia
20. Opitz BBBG S. (G syndrome)
21. Osteoglophonic dwarfism
22. Pyle dysplasia (familial metaphyseal dysplasia)
23. Rieger S.
24. Sclerosteosis
25. Sotos S. (cerebral gigantism)
26. Williams S. (idiopathic hypercalcemia)
27. XXXXY S.

Reference
1. Taybi H, Lachman RS: Radiology of Syndromes, Metabolic Disorders, and Skeletal Dysplasias. (ed 4) St. Louis: Mosby-Year Book, 1996, p 996

Gamut B-58

BILATERAL ENLARGEMENT OF THE MANDIBLE IN A CHILD

1. Fibrous dysplasia; cherubism
2. Multiple dentigerous cysts, esp. Gorlin S. (nevoid basal cell carcinoma S.)

References
1. Ayoub AF, el-Mofty SS: Cherubism: report of an aggressive case and review of the literature. J Oral Maxillofac Surg 1993;51:702–705

2. Banjar AA, Gangopadhyay K: Imaging quiz case 2. Cherubism. Arch Otolaryngol Head Neck Surg 1997;123:111–113
3. Hitomi G, Nishide N, Mitsui K: Cherubism: diagnostic imaging and review of the literature in Japan. Oral Surg Oral Med Oral Pathol Oral Radiol Endodontics 1996; 81:623–628
4. Katz JO, Underhill TE: Multilocular radiolucencies. Dental Clin North Am 1994;38:63–81
5. Penfold CN, McCullagh P, Eveson JW, Ramsay A: Giant cell lesions complicating fibro-osseous conditions of the jaws. Intl J Oral Maxillofac Surg 1993;22:158–162
6. Pierce AM, Sampson WJ, Wilson DF, Goss AN: Fifteen-year follow-up of a family with inherited craniofacial fibrous dysplasia. J Oral Maxillofac Surg 1996;54:780–788

Gamut B-59

MICROGNATHIA

COMMON

1. Pierre Robin S. (Robin sequence)
2. Primary or secondary absence (severe hypoplasia) of the tongue
3. Treacher Collins S. (mandibulofacial dysostosis)

UNCOMMON

1. Acrofacial dysostosis (Nager, Miller, or Weyers types)
2. Acrogeria
3. Aminopterin fetopathy
4. Arthrogryposis
5. Atelosteogenesis
6. Brachmann-de Lange S. (de Lange S.)
7. Campomelic dysplasia
8. Cat cry S. (cri du chat S.)
9. Catel-Manzke S.
10. Cerebro-costo-mandibular S.
11. Cerebro-oculo-facio-skeletal S. (Pena-Shakein S. type II)
12. Chondrodysplasia punctata
13. Chromosome 4p- S. (Wolf S.)
14. Chromosome 18: del (18p) S.
15. Cockayne S.

16. Cohen S.
17. Contractural arachnodactyly
18. Cowden S. (multiple hamartoma S.)
19. DiGeorge sequence
20. Diastrophic dysplasia
21. Dubowitz S.
22. Dyssegmental dysplasia
23. Ehlers-Danlos S.
24. Femoral hypoplasia-unusual facies S.
25. Fetal akinesia sequence (Pena-Shokeir S., type I)
26. Fetal alcohol S.
27. Fetal valproate S.
28. FG S.
29. Freeman-Sheldon S. (whistling face S.)
30. Frontometaphyseal dysplasia
31. Fryns S.
32. GAPO S.
33. Hajdu-Cheney S.
34. Hallermann-Streiff S. (oculo-mandibulo-facial S.)
35. Hypoglossia-hypodactylia S. (aglossia-adactylia S.)
36. Infantile cortical hyperostosis (Caffey's disease) (late sequela)
37. Johanson-Blizzard S.
38. Klippel-Feil S.
39. Larsen S.
40. Lissencephaly syndromes (congenital agyria) (Miller-Dieker S.)
41. Mandibuloacral dysplasia
42. Marden-Walker S.
43. Marshall-Smith S.
44. Meckel S.
45. Mesomelic dysplasia (Langer type)
46. Metaphyseal chondrodysplasia (Jansen type)
47. Möbius S.
48. Neu-Laxova S.
49. Noonan S.
50. Oculo-auriculo-vertebral spectrum (Goldenhar S.)
51. Opitz BBBG S. (G syndrome)
52. Opitz trigonocephaly S. (C syndrome)
53. Oro-facio-digital S. I (Papillon-Leage and Psaume S.) and II (Mohr S.)
54. Oromandibular-limb hypogenesis S. (incl. Hanhart S.)

55. Osteodysplasty (Melnick-Needles S.)
56. Osteolysis with nephropathy
57. Otopalatodigital S., type II
58. Oto-spondylo-megaepiphyseal dysplasia (OSMED)
59. Pallister-Hall S.
60. Pallister-Killian S. (only in infancy)
61. Potter sequence
62. Progeria
63. Pterygium syndromes
64. Pyknodysostosis
65. Roberts S.
66. Robinow S.
67. Rubinstein-Taybi S.
68. Schwartz-Jampel S. (osteochondromuscular dystrophy)
69. Seckel S. (bird-headed dwarfism)
70. Short rib-polydactyly syndromes (Saldino-Noonan and Majewski types)
71. Silver-Russell S.
72. Smith-Lemli-Opitz S.
73. Stickler S. (arthro-ophthalmopathy)
74. TAR S. (thrombocytopenia-absent radius S.)
75. Tricho-rhino-phalangeal dysplasia, types I and II
76. Trisomy syndromes (13, 18, 22)
77. Turner S.
78. Weissenbacher-Zweymüller phenotype
79. Williams S. (idiopathic hypercalcemia)
80. Yunis-Varón S.
81. Zellweger S. (cerebrohepatorenal syndrome)

References
1. Felson B (ed): Dwarfs and other little people. Semin Roentgenol 1973:8:258.
2. Jones KL: Smith's Recognizable Patterns of Human Malformation. Philadelphia: WB Saunders, 1988.
3. Swischuk LE: Differential Diagnosis in Pediatric Radiology. Baltimore: Williams & Wilkins, 1984, p. 122.
4. Taybi H, Lachman RS: Radiology of Syndromes, Metabolic Disorders, and Skeletal Dysplasias. (ed 4) St. Louis: Mosby-Year Book, 1996, pp 995–996

Gamut B-60

CONGENITAL SYNDROMES AND BONE DYSPLASIAS WITH MIDFACE (MAXILLARY AND/OR MALAR -ZYGOMATIC) HYPOPLASIA

COMMON
1. Achondroplasia
2. Chondrodysplasia punctata
3. Cleidocranial dysplasia
4. Crouzon S. (craniofacial dysostosis)
5. Treacher Collins S. (mandibulofacial dysostosis)
6. Trisomy 21 S. (Down S.)

UNCOMMON
1. Aarskog S.
2. Acrocephalosyndactyly (Apert type)
3. Acrodysostosis (peripheral dysostosis)
4. Acrofacial dysostosis (Nager and Miller types)
5. Acromesomelic dysplasia
6. Antley-Bixler S.
7. Atelosteogenesis
8. Binder S. (maxillonasal dysplasia)
9. Bloom S.
10. Campomelic dysplasia
11. Chromosome 18q- S.
12. Cowden S. (multiple hamartoma-neoplasia S.)
13. Craniofrontonasal dysplasia
14. Dysosteosclerosis
15. Dyssegmental dysplasia
16. Fetal alcohol S.
17. Fetal valproate S.
18. Freeman-Sheldon S. (whistling face S.)
19. Frontonasal dysplasia (median cleft face S.)
20. GAPO S.
21. Geroderma osteodysplastica
22. Hajdu-Cheney S.
23. Hallermann-Streiff S. (oculo-mandibulo-facial S.)
24. Hypochondroplasia
25. Keutel S.
26. Kyphomelic dysplasia
27. Larsen S.
28. Mandibuloacral dysplasia
29. Oculo-auriculo-vertebral spectrum (Goldenhar S.)
30. Osteoglophonic dysplasia
31. Otopalatodigital dysplasia, type II
32. Progeria
33. Pyknodysostosis
34. Rieger S.
35. Schinzel-Giedion S.
36. Schneckenbecken dysplasia
37. Seckel S. (bird-headed dwarfism)
38. Silver-Russell S.
39. Sponastrime dysplasia
40. Stanescu dysostosis
41. Stickler S. (arthro-ophthalmopathy)
42. Thanatophoric dysplasia
43. 3-M S.
44. Trichorhinophalangeal dysplasia
45. Trisomy 18 S.
46. Weill-Marchesani S.
47. Weissenbacher-Zweymüller phenotype
48. Wildervanck S.
49. Yunis-Varón S.

Reference

1. Taybi H, Lachman RS: Radiology of Syndromes, Metabolic Disorders, and Skeletal Dysplasias. (ed 4) St. Louis: Mosby-Year Book, 1996, pp 994–995

Gamut B-61-1

DELAYED ERUPTION OR NON-ERUPTION OF TEETH

CONGENITAL SYNDROMES (See B-61-2)

ENDOCRINOPATHIES
1. Hypoparathyroidism
2. Hypopituitarism (anterior lobe)
3. Hypothyroidism; cretinism

FAMILIAL TENDENCY

IDIOPATHIC

LOCAL FACTORS
1. Developmental
   a. Cleft lip and/or cleft palate
   b. Disorientation of tooth germ
   c. Ectopic eruption
   d. Lack of space
   e. Prolonged retention of deciduous teeth
   f. Submersion and ankylosis
   g. Supernumerary teeth
2. Hereditary (eg, amelogenesis imperfecta)
3. Iatrogenic
   a. Improperly contoured restoration (eg, stainless steel crowns)
   b. Lack of space (eg, premature extraction of deciduous teeth and loss of space for permanent successor)
   c. Over-retained roots of deciduous teeth
4. Inflammatory (eg, Garré's sclerosing osteomyelitis)
5. Mechanical (eg, fibrosis of alveolar mucosa; dilaceration of tooth; impacted tooth)
6. Nonodontogenic jaw lesion
   a. Fibrous dysplasia; cherubism
   b. Giant cell reparative granuloma
   c. Ossifying fibroma
7. Obstruction by dentigerous or radicular cyst
8. Odontogenic tumor
   a. Adenoameloblastoma
   b. Ameloblastic fibroma and myxoma
   c. Ameloblastic fibro-odontoma
   d. Neuroectodermal tumor of infancy (melanotic progonoma)
   e. Odontogenic myxoma and fibroma
   f. Odontoma (compound or complex)
9. Traumatic (eg, injury to deciduous teeth early in life; jaw fracture)

References
1. Berkman MD: Pedodontic radiographic interpretation. Dental Radiogr Photogr 1971;44:27–39
2. Taybi H, Lachman RS: Radiology of Syndromes, Metabolic Disorders, and Skeletal Dysplasias. (ed 4) St. Louis: Mosby-Year Book, 1996, p 1008

Gamut B-61-2

CONGENITAL SYNDROMES AND BONE DYSPLASIAS WITH DELAYED ERUPTION OR NONERUPTION OF TEETH (See B-62)

COMMON
1. Chondroectodermal dysplasia (Ellis-van Creveld S.)
2. Cleidocranial dysplasia
3. Fetal rubella S.
4. Gardner S.
5. Hypoparathyroidism; pseudohypoparathyroidism
6. [Hypophosphatemic rickets]
7. Hypopituitarism (anterior lobe)
8. Hypothyroidism; cretinism
9. Mucopolysaccharidoses (See J-4-S)
10. Osteogenesis imperfecta
11. Osteopetrosis
12. Progeria
13. Pyknodysostosis
14. Trisomy 21 S. (Down S.)
15. Williams S. (idiopathic hypercalcemia)

UNCOMMON
1. Aarskog S.
2. Acrodysostosis (peripheral dysostosis)

(continued)

3. Acrocephalosyndactyly (Apert type)
4. Brachmann-de Lange S. (de Lange S.)
5. Dubowitz S.
6. Ectodermal dysplasia (hypohidrotic)
7. GAPO S.
8. Goltz S. (focal dermal hypoplasia)
9. Hallermann-Streiff S. (oculo-mandibulo-facial S.)
10. Hanhart S.
11. Incontinentia pigmenti
12. Kocher-Debré-Sémélaigne S.
13. Lacrimo-auriculo-dento-digital S. (LADD S.)
14. Osteoglophonic dysplasia
15. Robinow S.
16. Romberg S.
17. Tricho-dento-osseous S.
18. Trichorhinopharyngeal dysplasia (type I)
19. Winchester S.

[ ] This condition does not actually cause the gamuted imaging finding, but can produce imaging changes that simulate it.

References

1. Berkman MD: Pedodontic radiographic interpretation. Dental Radiogr Photogr 1971;44:27–39
2. Taybi H, Lachman RS: Radiology of Syndromes, Metabolic Disorders, and Skeletal Dysplasias. (ed 4) St. Louis: Mosby-Year Book, 1996, p 1008

Gamut B-62

CONGENITAL SYNDROMES AND BONE DYSPLASIAS WITH DEFECTIVE AND/OR DELAYED DENTITION
(See B-61-2)

COMMON

1. Cherubism; polyostotic fibrous dysplasia (McCune-Albright S.) (delayed eruption or agenesis; displaced teeth)
2. Chondroectodermal dysplasia (Ellis-van Creveld S.) (neonatal teeth; conical peg-shaped teeth; partial anodontia; delayed eruption)
3. Cleidocranial dysplasia (delayed eruption; supernumerary teeth; partial anodontia; malformed roots; enamel hypoplasia; early loss)
4. Cretinism; hypothyroidism (delayed eruption)
5. Ehlers-Danlos S. (small, irregular teeth; partial anodontia)
6. [Fluorosis]
7. Gorlin S. (nevoid basal cell carcinoma S.) (odontogenic cyst; irregular placement; caries)
8. Homocystinuria (irregular, crowded teeth)
9. Hypoparathyroidism; pseudohypoparathyroidism (hypodontia; delayed eruption; enamel hypoplasia; caries)
10. Hypophosphatasia (early loss; poor dentin; caries)
11. [Hypophosphatemic rickets (delayed eruption; enamel hypoplasia; gingival and periapical infection)]
12. Hypopituitarism (anterior lobe) (delayed eruption)
13. Mucopolysaccharidoses (eg, Hurler S.; Hunter S.; Morquio S.) (small malaligned teeth; thin enamel) (See J-4)
14. Osteogenesis imperfecta I, III, and IV (hypodontia; delayed eruption; poor dentin; short roots; opalescent teeth)
15. Osteopetrosis (delayed eruption)
16. Progeria (delayed eruption; crowded teeth)
17. Pyknodysostosis (delayed eruption; partial anodontia; irregular placement; persistent deciduous teeth)
18. Pyle dysplasia (poor teeth)
19. [Syphilis, congenital (Hutchinson's teeth)]
20. Trisomy 21 S. (Down S.) (hypodontia; microdontia; delayed eruption)

UNCOMMON

1. Aarskog S. (delayed eruption; hypodontia; malocclusion; enamel hypoplasia)
2. Acrocephalosyndactyly (Apert type) (delayed eruption)
3. Aglossia-adactylia S. (missing incisors)
4. Aminopterin fetopathy
5. Bardet-Biedl S.
6. Brachmann-de Lange S. (de Lange S.) (delayed eruption)

7. Cerebro-costo-mandibular S.
8. Cockayne S. (caries)
9. Coffin-Lowry S.
10. Cohen S.
11. Congenital insensitivity to pain (early loss)
12. Cranioectodermal dysplasia (microdontia; hypodontia, fusion; enamel dysplasia)
13. Craniometaphyseal dysplasia
14. Crouzon S. (craniofacial dysostosis) (partial anodontia; wide spacing)
15. DOOR S.
16. Dyskeratosis congenita S. (caries; malalignment)
17. Dysosteosclerosis
18. Ectodermal dysplasias (eg, hereditary, anhidrotic, hypohidrotic, or Robinson type) (partial anodontia; conical teeth)
19. Endosteal hyperostosis (Worth type)
20. Epidermal nevus S. (odontodysplasia)
21. Frontometaphyseal dysplasia (hypodontia)
22. Gardner S. (delayed eruption)
23. Goltz S. (focal dermal hypoplasia) (hypodontia; enamel hypoplasia; delayed eruption; malformed teeth; irregular placement)
24. Hajdu-Cheney S. (idiopathic acro-osteolysis) (early loss)
25. Hallermann-Streiff S. (oculo-mandibulo-facial S.) (hypodontia; supernumerary teeth; neonatal teeth; delayed eruption)
26. Hanhart S. (hypodontia; delayed eruption)
27. Hyperphosphatasia (early loss)
28. Hypoglossia-hypodactylia S. (neonatal teeth)
29. Hypomelanosis of Ito (irregular spacing; peglike incisors)
30. Incontinentia pigmenti (hypodontia; delayed eruption; conical teeth)
31. Johanson-Blizzard S. (oligodontia; small teeth)
32. KBG S. (macrodontia; oligodontia; malposition; enamel hypoplasia)
33. Kocher-Debré-Sémélaigne S. (delayed eruption)
34. Lacrimo-auriculo-dento-digital S. (LADD S.) (delayed eruption; anodontia; enamel dysplasia)
35. Lenz microphthalmia S.
36. Lenz-Majewski dysplasia
37. Lowe S. (oculo-cerebro-renal S.) (cysts)
38. Marinesco-Sjögren S. (irregular teeth)
39. Marshall S. (prominent upper incisors)
40. Mesomelic dysplasias
41. Oculo-auriculo-vertebral spectrum (Goldenhar S.) (delayed eruption; missing teeth)
42. Oculo-dento-osseous dysplasia (hypodontia; microdontia; enamel hypoplasia)
43. Oro-facio-digital S. I (Papillon-Leage and Psaume S.) (missing lower central and lateral incisors; supernumerary cuspids and bicuspids; enamel hypoplasia; malocclusion)
44. Oro-facio-digital S. II (Mohr S.) (missing central incisors)
45. Osteodysplasty (Melnick-Needles S.) (malaligned teeth)
46. Osteoglophonic dysplasia (delayed eruption)
47. Osteolysis (familial expansile) (progressive tooth mobility and fracture; pulpitis)
48. Otopalatodigital S. (types I and II) (hypodontia)
49. Pachyonychia congenita (caries; early loss)
50. Papillon-Lefèvre S. (early loss)
51. Prader-Willi S. (dental caries; enamel hypoplasia)
52. Rieger S. (hypodontia; microdontia)
53. Robinow S. (delayed eruption)
54. Romberg S. (delayed eruption)
55. Rothmund-Thomson S. (microdontia; hypodontia; delayed eruption; supernumerary teeth)
56. Rubinstein-Taybi S.
57. Sclerosteosis
58. Seckel S. (bird-headed dwarfism) (missing teeth)
59. Short rib-polydactyly S. (type I)
60. Singleton-Merten S.
61. Sjögren-Larsson S. (dental dysplasia)
62. Stanescu dysostosis (small, crowded teeth; enamel hypoplasia)
63. Stickler S. (arthro-ophthalmopathy) (malocclusion; dental maleruption)
64. Thalidomide embryopathy
65. Treacher Collins S. (mandibulofacial dysostosis)
66. Tricho-dento-osseous S. (delayed eruption; early loss)
67. Weill-Marchesani S. (malformed teeth)
68. Werner S.
69. Weyers acrodental dysostosis

(continued)

70. Wildervanck S. (defective teeth)
71. Williams S. (idiopathic hypercalcemia) (delayed eruption; microdontia)
72. Winchester S. (delayed eruption)
73. XXXXY S. (hypodontia)
74. Yunis-Varón S. (hypodontia; impacted teeth)

[ ] This condition does not actually cause the gamuted imaging finding, but can produce imaging changes that simulate it.

References

1. Berkman MD: Pedodontic radiographic interpretation. Dental Radiogr Photogr 1971;44:27–39
2. Greenfield GB: Radiology of Bone Diseases. (ed 5) Philadelphia: Lippincott, 1990
3. Jones KL: Smith's Recognizable Patterns of Human Malformation. (ed 3) Philadelphia: WB Saunders, 1988
4. Taybi H, Lachman RS: Radiology of Syndromes, Metabolic Disorders, and Skeletal Dysplasias. (ed 4) St. Louis: Mosby-Year Book, 1996, pp 1006–1008

13. Metastatic disease (esp. neuroblastoma; rhabdomyosarcoma)
14. Papillon-Lefèvre S.
15. Pyknodysostosis
16. Rickets, severe
17. Sheehan S. (Simmonds disease) (postpartum pituitary necrosis)
18. Trichodento-osseous S.
19. Werner S.

References

1. Farman AG, Nortje CJ, Wood RE: Oral and Maxillofacial Diagnostic Imaging. St. Louis: Mosby-Year Book, 1993, p 21
2. Taybi H, Lachman RS: Radiology of Syndromes, Metabolic Disorders, and Skeletal Dysplasias. (ed 4) St. Louis: Mosby-Year Book, 1996, p 1008

Gamut B-63

EARLY LOSS OF TEETH

COMMON

1. Dental caries, advanced
2. Juvenile periodontitis
3. Trauma

UNCOMMON

1. Acroosteolysis
2. Chédiak-Higashi S.
3. Cleidocranial dysplasia
4. Congenital insensitivity to pain
5. Cyclic neutropenia
6. Hajdu-Cheney S.
7. Heavy metal poisoning
8. Hyperparathyroidism
9. Hyperphosphatasia
10. Langerhans cell histiocytosis$_g$
11. Leukemia
12. Mandibuloacral dysplasia

Gamut B-64

CONGENITAL SYNDROMES WITH MULTIPLE MISSING TEETH (ANODONTIA OR HYPODONTIA) (See B-61-2)

COMMON

1. Cherubism (fibrous dysplasia)
2. Chondroectodermal dysplasia (Ellis-van Creveld S.)
3. Cleidocranial dysplasia
4. Crouzon S. (craniofacial dysostosis)
5. Ehlers-Danlos S.
6. Idiopathic
7. Osteogenesis imperfecta
8. Pseudohypoparathyroidism
9. Trisomy 21 S. (Down S.)

UNCOMMON

1. Aarskog S.
2. Acrofacial dysostosis (peripheral dysostosis)
3. Böök S.
4. Coffin-Lowry S.

5. Ectodermal dysplasia (hypohidrotic)
6. EEC S.
7. Frontometaphyseal dysplasia
8. Goltz S. (focal dermal hypoplasia)
9. Hallermann-Streiff S. (oculo-mandibulo-facial S.)
10. Hanhart S.
11. [Hereditary]
12. Hypoglossia-hypodactylia S.; aglossia-adactylia S.
13. Hypophosphatasia
14. [Idiopathic; nonfamilial]
15. Incontinentia pigmenti
16. Johanson-Blizzard S.
17. Lacrimo-auriculo-dento-digital S. (LADD S.)
18. Oculo-dento-osseous dysplasia
19. Oro-facio-digital S. I (Papillon-Leage and Psaume S.)
20. Oro-facio-digital S. II (Mohr S.)
21. Otopalatodigital S.
22. Progeria
23. Pyknodysostosis
24. Rieger S.
25. Rothmund-Thomson S.
26. Seckel S. (bird-headed dwarfism)
27. XXXXY S.

[ ] This condition does not actually cause the gamuted imaging finding, but can produce imaging changes that simulate it.

References

1. Berkman MD: Pedodontic radiographic interpretation. Dental Radiogr Photogr 1971;44:27–39
2. Farman AG, Nortje CJ, Wood RE: Oral and Maxillofacial Diagnostic Imaging. St. Louis: Mosby-Year Book, 1993, p 20
3. Taybi H, Lachman RS: Radiology of Syndromes, Metabolic Disorders, and Skeletal Dysplasias. (ed 4) St. Louis: Mosby-Year Book, 1996, p 1006

Gamut B-65

HYPERDONTIA

COMMON

1. Cleft palate
2. Cleidocranial dysplasia
3. Compound odontoma
4. Idiopathic

UNCOMMON

1. Achondroplasia
2. Ehlers-Danlos S.
3. Gardner S.
4. Hallermann-Streiff S. (oculo-mandibulo-facial S.)
5. Orofaciodigital S.

Reference

1. Farman AG, Nortjé CJ, Wood RE: Oral and Maxillofacial Diagnostic Imaging. St. Louis: Mosby-Year Book, 1993, p 20

Gamut B-66

LOSS OF LAMINA DURA OF THE TEETH

COMMON

1. Hyperparathyroidism, primary or secondary (renal osteodystrophy)
2. Local inflammatory disease; periodontitis (eg, gingivitis; pyorrhea; dental caries; periodontal abscess; periapical granuloma or abscess; radicular cyst; sclerosing osteomyelitis)
3. Osteoporosis (esp. postmenopausal)
4. Periodontosis (noninflammatory, degenerative)

UNCOMMON

1. Anemia$_g$ (eg, thalassemia; sickle cell)
2. Burkitt's lymphoma

(continued)

3. Cushing S.; steroid therapy
4. Fibrous dysplasia
5. Hyperphosphatasia
6. Hypertvitaminosis D
7. Hypoparathyroidism
8. Hypothyroidism
9. Langerhans cell histiocytosis$_g$ (esp. eosinophilic granuloma)
10. Leukemia
11. Metastasis (esp. from carcinoma of breast)
12. Multiple myeloma
13. Neoplasm, primary (eg, malignant tumor; fibrous histiocytoma)
14. Osteomalacia; rickets (severe)
15. Paget's disease
16. Periapical cemental dysplasia
17. Removal of opposing tooth
18. Renal acidosis; oxalosis
19. Scleroderma (widened periodontal membrane)
20. Scurvy
21. Traumatic (hemorrhagic) bone cyst

References
1. Berry HM Jr: The lore and the lure o' the lamina dura. Radiology 1973;109:525–528
2. Farman AG, Nortje CJ, Wood RE: Oral and Maxillofacial Diagnostic Imaging. St. Louis: Mosby-Year Book, 1993, pp 24–25
3. Ferris RA, Hakkal HG, Cigtay OS: Radiologic manifestations of North American Burkitt's lymphoma. AJR 1975; 123:614–620
4. Greenfield GB: Radiology of Bone Diseases. (ed 5) Philadelphia: Lippincott, 1990

Gamut B-67

FLOATING TEETH

COMMON

1. Langerhans cell histiocytosis$_g$ (esp. eosinophilic granuloma)
2. Periodontitis, severe; periapical abscess

UNCOMMON

1. Agranulocytosis and cyclic neutropenia
2. Ameloblastoma
3. Calcifying odontogenic cyst (Gorlin cyst)
4. Carcinoma of mouth
5. Desmoplastic fibroma
6. Fibrous dysplasia
7. Giant cell reparative granuloma
8. Hemangioma or lymphangioma of mandible
9. Hyperparathyroidism, primary or secondary (renal osteodystrophy)
10. Hypophosphatasia
11. Lymphoma$_g$; leukemia, Burkitt's lymphoma
12. Melanotic progonoma
13. Mercury poisoning
14. Metastatic neoplasm (esp. neuroblastoma)
15. Myeloma; plasmacytoma
16. Odontogenic myxoma; odontogenic fibroma
17. Papillon-Lefèvre syndrome (juvenile periodontosis)
18. Sarcoma (esp. osteosarcoma; Ewing sarcoma)
19. Traumatic (hemorrhagic) bone cyst

References
1. Keusch KD, Poole CA, King DR: The significance of "floating teeth" in children. Radiology 1966;86:215–219
2. Prein J, Remagen W, Spiessl B, et al: Atlas of Tumors of the Facial Skeleton. Berlin: Springer-Verlag, 1986
3. Shafer WG, Hine MK, Levy BM: A Textbook of Oral Pathology. (ed 3) Philadelphia: WB Saunders, 1974

Gamut B-68

MANDIBULAR PERIOSTITIS

LAMINAR PERIOSTEAL NEW BONE

COMMON

1. Bone sarcoma (esp. osteosarcoma; Ewing sarcoma)
2. Langerhans cell histiocytosis$_g$ (esp. eosinophilic granuloma)
3. Malignant neoplasm, primary (eg, carcinoma of mouth) or metastatic

4. Osteomyelitis (pyogenic; Garré's sclerosing osteomyelitis)
5. Reactive periostitis to adjacent soft tissue infection

UNCOMMON
1. Actinomycosis
2. Hypervitaminosis A
3. Idiopathic (eg, with dysproteinemia)
4. Infantile cortical hyperostosis (Caffey's disease)
5. Leukemia; lymphoma
6. Necrosis (thermal, chemical, radiation)
7. Scurvy
8. Syphilis
9. Tuberculosis

SPICULATED PERIOSTEAL NEW BONE PERPENDICULAR TO CORTEX
COMMON
1. Bone sarcoma (osteosarcoma; Ewing sarcoma)
2. Metastatic disease (eg, osteoblastic metastases; neuroblastoma)

UNCOMMON
1. Anemia, primary$_g$ (eg, thalassemia; sickle cell disease)
2. Burkitt lymphoma
3. Hemangioma
4. Syphilis

References
1. Farman AG, Nortje CJ, Wood RE: Oral and Maxillofacial Diagnostic Imaging. St. Louis: Mosby-Year Book, 1993, pp 24–25
2. Jayne HE, Hays RA, O'Brien FW: Cysts and tumors of the mandible: Their differential diagnosis. AJR 1961;86: 292–309
3. Kilcoyne RF, Krolls SO, Allman RM: Luetic osteomyelitis of the mandible. RPC of the month from the AFIP. Radiology 1970;94:687–691
4. Stafne EC, Gibilisco JA: Oral Roentgenographic Diagnosis. (ed 4) Philadelphia: WB Saunders, 1975
5. Thoma KH: Oral Surgery. (ed 5) St. Louis: CV Mosby, 1969
6. Wood NK, Goaz PW: Differential Diagnosis of Oral Lesions. (ed 4) St. Louis: Mosby-Year Book, 1991

Gamut B-69

GENERALIZED OSTEOPENIA OR OSTEOLYSIS OF THE JAW

COMMON
1. Anemia$_g$ (esp. thalassemia; sickle cell disease; spherocytosis)
2. Cachectic diseases (eg, malignancy); malnutrition; protein-deficient states
3. Connective tissue diseases$_g$ (esp. rheumatoid arthritis)
4. Diabetes
5. Hyperparathyroidism, primary or secondary (renal osteodystrophy)
6. Immobilization, prolonged
7. Langerhans cell histiocytosis$_g$
8. Leukemia; lymphoma$_g$; Burkitt's lymphoma; lymphosarcoma
9. Metastases (carcinomatosis)
10. Multiple myeloma
11. [Normal anatomic variations in radiodensity of bone]
12. Osteomalacia; rickets (eg, calcium or Vitamin D deficiency; long term anticonvulsant therapy) (See D-44)
13. Osteoporosis (eg, senile; postmenopausal; drug or steroid-induced; Cushing S.; thyrotoxicosis) (See D-43-1)
14. Paget's disease (lytic phase)

UNCOMMON
1. Acromegaly (pseudo-osteoporosis)
2. Cyclic neutropenia; agranulocytosis
3. Gaucher's disease
4. Hemangioma (central cavernous)
5. Hypogonadism, incl. Turner S. (XO S.); Klinefelter S. (XXY S.)
6. Hypoparathyroidism
7. Hypophosphatasia
8. Hypovitaminosis C
9. Massive osteolysis (Gorham's disease)

(continued)

10. Myelofibrosis
11. Osteogenesis imperfecta
12. Oxalosis
13. Progeria
14. Radiation therapy
15. Sarcoidosis
16. Squamous cell carcinoma of mandible; other diffuse local malignancy

[ ] This condition does not actually cause the gamuted imaging finding, but can produce imaging changes that simulate it.

References
1. Farman AG, Nortjé CJ, Wood RE: Oral and Maxillofacial Diagnostic Imaging. St. Louis: Mosby-Year Book, 1993, p 30
2. Wood NK, Goaz PW: Differential Diagnosis of Oral Lesions. (ed 5) St. Louis: Mosby-Year Book, 1997, pp 392–413

Gamut B-70-S

NORMAL ANATOMIC RADIOLUCENCIES IN THE JAW (MAXILLA AND MANDIBLE)

MAXILLA
1. Greater palatine foramen
2. Incisive foramen, incisive canal; superior foramina of incisive canal
3. Intermaxillary suture
4. Maxillary sinus
5. Nasolacrimal duct or canal

MANDIBLE
1. Anterior buccal mandibular depression
2. Cortical plate mandibular defects
3. Lingual foramen
4. Mandibular canal (inferior dental canal)
5. Mandibular foramen
6. Medial sigmoid depression of ramus
7. Mental foramen
8. Mental fossa
9. Midline symphysis
10. Pseudocyst of the condyle
11. Submandibular fossa

MANDIBLE AND MAXILLA
1. Marrow space
2. Nutrient canal
3. Periodontal ligament space
4. Pulp chamber and root canal
5. Tooth crypt (developing)

Reference
1. Wood NK, Goaz PW: Differential Diagnosis of Oral Lesions. (ed 5) St. Louis: Mosby-Year Book, 1997, pp 238–251

Gamut B-71

NONODONTOGENIC RADIOLUCENT LESIONS OF THE JAWS

COMMON
1. Fibrous dysplasia (cherubism)
2. Giant cell granuloma
3. Multiple myeloma
4. Metastatic or invasive neoplasm (esp. from carcinoma of mouth, lung, breast, or kidney)
5. Osteomyelitis

UNCOMMON
1. Aneurysmal bone cyst
2. Bone cyst (solitary; traumatic; hemorrhagic)
3. Brown tumor of hyperparathyroidism
4. Desmoplastic fibroma
5. Giant cell tumor (rare)
6. Incisive canal cyst (nasopalatine canal cyst); mid-palatal cyst
7. Langerhans cell histiocytosis$_g$ (esp. eosinophilic granuloma)
8. Lingual mandibular bone defect (Stafne cyst)
9. Malignant neoplasm, primary
   a. Chondrosarcoma
   b. Ewing sarcoma
   c. Fibrosarcoma

d. Lymphoma$_g$; Burkitt lymphoma
e. Osteolytic osteosarcoma
10. Neurogenic tumor
11. Ossifying fibroma, early
12. Radiation necrosis
13. Surgical defect
14. Vascular lesion (eg, arteriovenous malformation; angioma)

References

1. Blaschke DP, Osborn AG: The mandible and teeth. In: Bergeron RT, Osborn AG, Som PM: Head and Neck Imaging Excluding the Brain. St. Louis: CV Mosby, 1984, pp 299–343
3. Kumar R, et al: Lytic lesions of the mandible. RSNA Scientific Exhibit, Washington, DC, 1984
3. Prein J, Remagen W, Spiessl B, et al: Atlas of Tumors of the Facial Skeleton. Berlin: Springer-Verlag, 1986

Gamut B-72

WELL-DEFINED LYTIC (CYST-LIKE) LESIONS OF THE JAW
(See B-73 to B-81)

COMMON

*1. Ameloblastoma
*2. Dentigerous (follicular) cyst
*3. Giant cell reparative granuloma
 4. Normal anatomic variation (eg, marrow space; follicle nutrient canal; foramen)
 5. Periapical granuloma or abscess
 6. Periodontal cyst (radicular, dental, periapical, or residual cyst)
 7. Postsurgical or postextraction defect

UNCOMMON

 1. Adenomatoid odontogenic tumor (adenoameloblastoma), early
 2. Ameloblastic fibroma and myxoma
*3. Ameloblastic fibrosarcoma
*4. Aneurysmal bone cyst
*5. Bone cyst (solitary; traumatic; hemorrhagic)
*6. Bone sarcoma (eg, chondrosarcoma; fibrosarcoma)
*7. Brown tumor of hyperparathyroidism
*8. Calcifying epithelial odontogenic tumor (Pindborg tumor)
*9. Calcifying odontogenic cyst (Gorlin cyst)
 10. Cementifying fibroma, early
 11. Cementoma, early; periapical cemental dysplasia
*12. Desmoplastic fibroma
 13. Developmental lingual mandibular salivary gland defect (Stafne cyst)
*14. Fibrous dysplasia (cherubism)
 15. Fissural developmental cyst (eg, globulomaxillary; median palatal; median mandibular; median alveolar; incisive canal; nasopalatine)
*16. Giant cell tumor (rare)
*17. Hemangioma (central); arteriovenous malformation
*18. Hydatid cyst
 19. Langerhans cell histiocytosis$_g$ (esp. eosinophilic granuloma)
 20. Lingual mandibular bone defect (Stafne cyst)
 21. Melanotic neuroectodermal tumor of infancy
*22. Metastasis
*23. Multiple myeloma; plasmacytoma
 24. Neurogenic tumor (esp. neurofibroma arising from mandibular nerve); neurofibromatosis
 25. Odontogenic fibroma
 26. Odontogenic keratocyst (primordial cyst)
*27. Odontogenic myxoma
 28. Odontoma, compound
 29. Ossifying fibroma, immature
 30. Tuberculosis (cystic)

* May be expansile.

References

1. Blaschke DP, Osborn AG: The mandible and teeth. In: Bergeron RT, Osborn AG, Som PM: Head and Neck Imaging Excluding the Brain. St. Louis: CV Mosby, 1984, pp 299–343
2. Burgener FA, Kormano M: Differential Diagnosis in Conventional Radiology. (ed 2) New York: Thieme Medical Publ, 1991, pp 171–175
3. Eversole LR, Rovin S: Differential radiographic diagnosis of lesions of the jawbones. Radiology 1972;105:277–284

(continued)

4. Farman AG, Nortjé CJ, Wood RE: Oral and Maxillofacial Diagnostic Imaging. St. Louis: Mosby-Year Book, 1993, p 28
5. Kumar R, et al: Lytic lesions of the mandible. RSNA Scientific Exhibit, Washington, DC, 1984
6. McIvor J: Maxillofacial radiology. In: Grainger RG, Allison DJ (eds): Diagnostic Radiology. Edinburgh: Churchill Livingstone, 1986, vol 3, pp 1914–1915
7. Prein J, Remagen W, Spiessl B, et al: Atlas of Tumors of the Facial Skeleton. Berlin: Springer-Verlag, 1986

Gamut B-73

UNILOCULAR CYSTIC LESIONS OF THE MANDIBLE

ODONTOGENIC CYSTS

1. Ameloblastoma
2. Dentigerous (follicular) cyst
3. Odontogenic keratocyst
4. Primordial cyst
5. Radicular cyst
6. Residual cyst

NONODONTOGENIC CYSTS

1. Developmental cortical bone defect (Stafne cyst)
2. Traumatic cyst

References

1. Lufkin R, Borges A, Villablanca P: Teaching Atlas of Head and Neck Imaging. New York: Thieme, 2000, pp 437–442
2. Mass E, Kaplan I, Hirshberg A: A clinical and histopathological study of radicular cysts associated with primary molars. J Oral Path Med 1995;24:458–461
3. Minami M, Kaneda T, Ozawa K, et al: Cystic lesions of the maxillomandibular region: MR imaging distinction of odontogenic keratocysts and ameloblastomas from other cysts. AJR 1996;66:943–949
4. Shrout MK, Hall JM , Hildebolt CE: Differentiation of periapical granulomas and radicular cysts by digital radiometric analysis. Oral Surg Oral Med Oral Path 1993;76:356–361
5. White SC, Sapp JP, Seto BG, Mankovich NJ: Absence of radiometric differentiation between periapical cysts and granulomas. Oral Surg Oral Med Oral Path 1994;78:650–654

Gamut B-74

MULTILOCULAR LESIONS OF THE JAW

COMMON

1. Ameloblastoma
2. Giant cell granuloma
3. Multilocular radicular or residual cyst
4. Odontogenic keratocyst (incl. Gorlin-Goltz S.)
5. Odontogenic myxoma

UNCOMMON

1. Ameloblastic fibroma
2. Aneurysmal bone cyst
3. Arteriovenous malformation; hemangioma
4. Brown tumor of hyperparathyroidism
5. Calcifying odontogenic cyst (Gorlin cyst)
6. Fibrous dysplasia; cherubism
7. Giant cell tumor
8. Langerhans cell histiocytosis$_g$ (esp. eosinophilic granuloma)
9. Metastasis
10. Mucoepidermoid tumor
11. Multiple myeloma
12. Odontoma (developing)
13. Traumatic bone cyst

References

1. Absi EG, Sim RL: Odontogenic keratocyst involving the maxillary sinus: report of two cases. Dento-Maxillofac Radiol 1994;23:226–229
2. Anand VK, Arrowood Jr JP, Krolls SO: Odontogenic keratocysts: a study of 50 patients. Laryngoscope 1995;105:14–16
3. Farman AG, Nortjé CJ, Wood RE: Oral and Maxillofacial Diagnostic Imaging. St. Louis: Mosby-Year Book, 1993, p 31
4. Lufkin R, Borges A, Villablanca P: Teaching Atlas of Head and Neck Imaging. New York: Thieme, 2000, pp 448–450
5. Marker P, Brondum N, Clausen PP, Bastian HL: Treatment of large odontogenic keratocysts by decompression and later cystectomy: a long-term follow-up and a histologic study of 23 cases. Oral Surg Oral Med Oral Pathol Oral Radiol Endodontics 1996;82:122–131

6. Meara JG, Li KK, Shah SS, Cunningham MJ: Odontogenic keratocysts in the pediatric population. Arch Otolaryngol Head Neck Surg 1996;122:725–728
7. Nohl FS, Gulabivala K: Odontogenic keratocyst as periradicular radiolucency in the anterior mandible: two case reports. Oral Surg Oral Med Oral Pathol Oral Radiol Endodontics 1996;81:103–109

References

1. Daley TED, Wysocki GP: New developments in selected cysts of the jaws. J Canad Dental Assoc. J de L Association Dentaire Canadienne 1997;63:526–527, 530–532
2. Han MH, Chang KH, Lee CH, et al: Cystic expansile masses of the maxilla: differential diagnosis with CT and MR. AJNR 1995;6:333–338
3. Harris IR, Brown JE: Application of cross-sectional imaging in the differential diagnosis of apical radiolucency. Intl Endodontic J 1997;30:288–290
4. Krolls SO: Personal communication
5. Lufkin R, Borges A, Villablanca P: Teaching Atlas of Head and Neck Imaging. New York: Thieme, 2000, pp 299–302
6. Prein J, Remagen W, Spiessl B, et al: Atlas of Tumors of the Facial Skeleton. Berlin: Springer-Verlag, 1986
7. Wood NK, Goaz PW: Differential Diagnosis of Oral Lesions. (ed 5) St. Louis: Mosby-Year Book, 1997

Gamut B-75

CYSTIC LESIONS IN THE MAXILLA

ODONTOGENIC CYSTS

1. Cystic ameloblastoma
2. Dentigerous (follicular) cyst
3. Odontogenic keratocyst
4. Primordial cyst
5. Radicular cyst
6. Residual cyst

FISSURAL CYSTS

A. Midline:
   1. Cyst of papilla palatina
   2. Incisive canal cyst (nasopalatine duct cyst)
   3. Median alveolar cyst
   4. Median palatal cyst
B. Lateral:
   1. Globulomaxillary cyst
   2. Nasolabial or nasoalveolar cyst (soft tissue)
   3. Surgical ciliated cyst of maxillary sinus

BONE CYSTS

1. Aneurysmal bone cyst
2. Hemorrhagic cyst
3. Simple unicameral bone cyst

ANTRAL LESION EXTENDING INTO THE MAXILLARY ALVEOLAR RIDGE

1. Mucocele

Gamut B-76

PERIAPICAL RADIOLUCENCY IN THE JAWS

COMMON

*1. [Anatomic (false) periapical lucency (eg, dental papilla; greater palatine foramen; incisive foramen and canal; mandibular canal; marrow spaces; maxillary sinus; mental foramen; naris; nasolacrimal duct; submandibular and sublingual fossae)]
*2. Dentigerous (follicular) cyst
3. Malignant neoplasm (eg, metastasis; multiple myeloma; leukemia; lymphoma$_g$; Burkitt lymphoma; squamous cell carcinoma; malignant salivary gland tumor; osteolytic osteosarcoma; chondrosarcoma; Ewing sarcoma; fibrosarcoma)
4. [Other nonodontogenic radiolucent lesions of the jaws] (See B-71)
*5. Periapical cementoosseous dysplasia, early
*6. Periodontal cyst, other (eg, residual, paradental, incisive canal, median mandibular, midpalatal, or primordial)
*7. Pulpoperiapical disease
   a. Periapical granuloma

(continued)

b. Radicular cyst
c. Scar; fibrous healing defect
d. Chronic and acute dentoalveolar abscess
e. Osteomyelitis
f. Hyperplasia of maxillary sinus lining
8. Surgical defect
9. Traumatic bone cyst

UNCOMMON

*1. Ameloblastic variants
*2. Ameloblastoma
3. Aneurysmal bone cyst
4. Brown tumor of hyperparathyroidism
*5. Buccal cyst
*6. Cementoossifying fibroma (early)
*7. Cementoblastoma (early)
*8. Central odontogenic fibroma—WHO type
*9. Dentin dysplasia
10. Fibrous dysplasia; cherubism
11. Gaucher's disease
*12. Giant cell granuloma
13. Juvenile ossifying fibroma
14. Langerhans cell histiocytosis$_g$ (esp. eosinophilic granuloma)
*15. Odontoma (early)
16. Pseudotumor of hemophilia

* Odontogenic periapical radiolucency.
[ ] This condition does not actually cause the gamuted imaging finding, but can produce imaging changes that simulate it.

References
1. Farman AG, Nortjé CJ, Wood RE: Oral and Maxillofacial Diagnostic Imaging. St. Louis: Mosby-Year Book, 1993, p 27
2. Wood NK, Goaz PW: Differential Diagnosis of Oral Lesions. (ed 5) St. Louis: Mosby-Year Book, 1997, pp 252–278

Gamut B-77

PERICORONAL RADIOLUCENCY IN THE JAWS (AROUND AN IMPACTED OR UNERUPTED TOOTH)

COMMON
*1. Adenomatoid odontogenic tumor (adenoameloblastoma)
*2. Ameloblastic fibroma
*3. Ameloblastoma (multilocular or unicystic mural)
*4. Calcifying odontogenic cyst (Gorlin cyst), early
*5. [Dental follicle (pericoronal space); follicular hyperplasia]
*6. Dentigerous (follicular) cyst
7. Malignant neoplasm (eg, metastasis; multiple myeloma; leukemia; lymphoma$_g$; Burkitt lymphoma; squamous cell or odontogenic carcinoma; malignant salivary gland tumor; osteolytic osteosarcoma; chondrosarcoma; Ewing sarcoma; teratoma)
8. [Other nonodontogenic radiolucent lesions of the jaws] (See B-71)

UNCOMMON
*1. Ameloblastic fibrosarcoma
*2. Calcifying epithelial odontogenic tumor (Pindborg tumor)
3. Gardner S.
*4. Gorlin-Goltz S. (odontogenic keratocyst-basal cell nevus S.)
5. Juvenile ossifying fibroma
6. Langerhans cell histiocytosis$_g$ (esp. eosinophilic granuloma)
*7. Odontogenic fibroma, myxoma, or fibromyxoma
*8. Odontogenic keratocyst; other primordial cysts
*9. Odontoma or ameloblastic fibroodontoma (premineralized stage)
*10. Paradental cyst
11. [Postextraction socket]

12. Pseudotumor of hemophilia
*13. Squamous odontogenic tumor

* Odontogenic pericoronal lesion.

[ ] This condition does not actually cause the gamuted imaging finding, but can produce imaging changes that simulate it.

References

1. Benn A, Altini M: Dentigerous cysts of inflammatory origin. A clinicopathologic study. Oral Surg Oral Med Oral Pathol Oral Radiol Endodontics 1996;81:203–209
2. Blaschke DP, Osborn AG: The mandible and teeth. In: Bergeron RT, Osborn AG, Som PM: Head and Neck Imaging Excluding the Brain. St. Louis: CV Mosby, 1984, pp 299–343
3. Carr MM, Anderson RD, Clarke KD: Multiple dentigerous cysts in childhood. J Otolaryngol 1996;25:267–270
4. Daley TD, Wysocki P: The small dentigerous cyst. A diagnostic dilemma. Oral Surg Oral Med Oral Pathol Oral Radiol Endodontics 1995;79:77–81
5. Farman AG, Nortjé CJ, Wood RE: Oral and Maxillofacial Diagnostic Imaging. St. Louis: Mosby-Year Book, 1993, p 27
6. Johnson LM, Sapp JP, McIntire DN: Squamous cell carcinoma arising in a dentigerous cyst. J Oral Maxillofac Surg 1994;52:987–990
7. Kumar R, et al: Lytic lesions of the mandible. RSNA Scientific Exhibit, Washington, DC, 1984
8. Prein J, Remagen W, Spiessl B, et al: Atlas of Tumors of the Facial Skeleton. Berlin: Springer-Verlag, 1986
9. Sadeghi EM, Sewall SR, Dohse A, Novak TS: Odontogenic tumors that mimic a dentigerous cyst. Compend Continuing Educ Dentistry 1995;16:500, 502–504
10. Toller MO, Sipahier M, Acikgoz A: CT display of multiple dentigerous cysts of the mandible: a case report. J Clin Pediatr Dentistry 1995;l9:135–137
11. Wood NK, Goaz PW: Differential Diagnosis of Oral Lesions. (ed 5) St. Louis: Mosby-Year Book, 1997, pp 279–295

INTERRADICULAR RADIOLUCENCY IN THE JAW (BETWEEN THE ROOTS OF TEETH OR AT THE SIDE OF A TOOTH ROOT)

COMMON

1. Anatomic radiolucency (eg, primary tooth crypt; mental foramen and canal; maxillary sinus; incisive foramen; lateral fossa between lateral incisor and canine teeth; bone marrow pattern; nutrient canal)
2. Benign nonodontogenic tumor or tumor-like condition (See B-71)
3. Extension of disease from adjacent tooth
4. Furcation involvement (eg, advanced periodontal disease)
5. Globulomaxillary radiolucencies (esp. cyst)
6. Incisive canal cyst (nasopalatine canal cyst)
7. Lateral periodontal cyst (inflammatory or developmental)
8. Lateral canal periapical (radicular) cyst
9. Malignant neoplasm (eg, metastasis; multiple myeloma; leukemia; lymphoma$_g$; squamous cell or odontogenic carcinoma; bone sarcoma)
10. Median mandibular cyst
11. Odontogenic cyst, other (eg, dentigerous cyst; paradental cyst; odontogenic keratocyst {primordial cyst}; buccal cyst)
12. Odontogenic tumors (See B-76, 77)
13. Perforation of root during endodontic therapy
14. Periodontal abscess
15. Periodontal bony pocket
16. Traumatic bone cyst

UNCOMMON

1. Adenomatoid odontogenic tumor (adenoameloblastoma)
2. Giant cell granuloma
3. Langerhans cell histiocytosis$_g$ (eosinophilic granuloma)

(continued)

4. Melanotic neuroectodermal tumor of infancy (usually in anterior maxilla)
5. Radiation osteonecrosis

References

1. Farman AG, Nortjé CJ, Wood RE: Oral and Maxillofacial Diagnostic Imaging. St. Louis: Mosby-Year Book, 1993, p 28
2. Wood NK, Goaz PW: Differential Diagnosis of Oral Lesions. (ed 5) St. Louis: Mosby-Year Book, 1997, pp 296–308

Gamut B-79

WELL-DEFINED (CYST-LIKE) LESIONS OF THE JAW (NOT NECESSARILY CONTACTING TEETH)

COMMON

1. Ameloblastoma (multilocular or unicystic)
2. [Anatomic patterns (eg, marrow spaces; maxillary sinus; early stage of tooth crypts; median sigmoid depression)]
3. Brown tumor of hyperparathyroidism
4. Cementoosseous dysplasia (focal)
5. Cementoossifying fibroma (early)
6. Dentigerous (follicular) cyst
7. Giant cell granuloma
8. Focal osteoporotic bone marrow (hematopoietic) defect of the jaw
9. Incisive canal cyst (nasopalatine canal cyst); mid-palatine cyst
10. Lingual mandibular bone defect (Stafne cyst)
11. Metastasis
12. Odontogenic keratocyst; other primordial cysts
13. [Periapical granuloma or abscess; radicular cyst]
14. Residual cyst
15. Surgical defect; postextraction socket
16. Traumatic (hemorrhagic, simple) bone cyst

UNCOMMON

1. Adenomatoid odontogenic tumor (adenoameloblastoma), early
2. Ameloblastic fibroma and myxoma
3. Ameloblastic fibrosarcoma
4. Aneurysmal bone cyst
5. [Artifact]
6. Benign nonodontogenic tumor (eg, lipoma; myxoma; fibroma; giant cell tumor; osteoblastoma–early)
7. Bone sarcoma (eg, chondrosarcoma; fibrosarcoma)
8. Calcifying epithelial odontogenic tumor (Pindborg tumor)
9. Calcifying odontogenic cyst (Gorlin cyst)
10. Central squamous cell carcinoma in cyst lining
11. Dentinoma (immature)
12. Desmoplastic fibroma
13. Fibrous dysplasia; cherubism
14. Hemangioma (central); arteriovenous malformation; aneurysm in bone
15. Hydatid cyst
16. Langerhans cell histiocytosis$_g$ (esp. eosinophilic granuloma)
17. Minor salivary gland tumor in bone
18. Myeloma; plasmacytoma
19. Neurofibroma arising from mandibular nerve; schwannoma; neurofibromatosis; amputation neuroma
20. Odontogenic fibroma or myxoma
21. Odontoma, early
22. Ossifying fibroma, immature
23. Postoperative maxillary cyst
24. Pseudotumor of hemophilia
25. Squamous odontogenic tumor
26. Tuberculosis, cystic

[ ] This condition does not actually cause the gamuted imaging finding, but can produce imaging changes that simulate it.

References

1. DelBalso AM: Lesions of the jaws. Semin Ultrasound CT MR 1995;16:487–512
2. DelBalso AM: An approach to the diagnostic imaging of jaw lesions, dental implants, and the temporomandibular joint. Rad Clin North Am 1998;36:855–890

3. Farman AG, Nortjé CJ, Wood RE: Oral and Maxillofacial Diagnostic Imaging. St. Louis: Mosby-Year Book, 1993, p 28
4. Stafne EC, Gibilisco JA: Oral Roentgenographic Diagnosis. (ed 4) Philadelphia: WB Saunders, 1975
5. Wood NK, Goaz PW: Differential Diagnosis of Oral Lesions. (ed 5) St. Louis: Mosby-Year Book, 1997, pp 309–332

Gamut B-80

MULTIPLE SEPARATE WELL-DEFINED LUCENT LESIONS OF THE JAW

COMMON

1. Anatomic variations (eg, focal osteoporotic marrow defects; postextraction sockets)
2. Cysts (eg, dentigerous, radicular, primordial)
3. Gorlin S. (nevoid basal cell carcinoma S.)
*4. Langerhans cell histiocytosis$_g$
*5. Metastases
*6. Multiple myeloma
7. Periapical granulomas

UNCOMMON

1. Ameloblastomas
2. Brown tumors of hyperparathyroidism
3. Cementoosseous dysplasia (early)
4. Cherubism (fibrous dysplasia)
5. Gaucher disease; Niemann-Pick disease
6. Giant cell reparative granulomas
*7. Hemangiomas
*8. Leukemia; lymphoma$_g$; Burkitt lymphoma
9. Mucopolysaccharidoses (esp. Hurler S.; Hunter S.; Maroteaux-Lamy S.; Sanfilippo S.; Scheie S.)
10. Multiple dental cysts with arachnodactyly (Marfan S.)
11. Neurofibromatosis
12. Nodular cemental masses; periapical cemental dysplasia (early)
13. Noonan S. (odontogenic keratocysts)

14. Oxalosis
15. Papillon-Lefèvre S.
16. Squamous odontogenic tumors
17. Traumatic bone cysts

* Multiple osteolytic lesions with punched-out margins.

References
1. Farman AG, Nortjé CJ, Wood RE: Oral and Maxillofacial Diagnostic Imaging. St. Louis: Mosby-Year Book, 1993, p 35
2. Wood NK, Goaz PW: Differential Diagnosis of Oral Lesions. (ed 5) St. Louis: Mosby-Year Book, 1997, pp 380–391

Gamut B-81

EXPANSILE RADIOLUCENT LESIONS OF THE JAWS (INCLUDING MULTILOCULAR LESIONS) WITH DISCRETE MARGINS

COMMON

*1. Ameloblastoma
*2. Aneurysmal bone cyst
*3. Cherubism (fibrous dysplasia)
4. Dentigerous (follicular) cyst
*5. Giant cell granuloma
6. Metastasis (esp. from carcinoma of lung, breast, GI tract, or kidney)
7. [Normal anatomic pattern (eg, maxillary sinus compartments; marrow spaces)]
*8. Odontogenic keratocyst (other primordial cysts)
*9. Odontogenic myxoma

UNCOMMON

1. Ameloblastic fibrosarcoma
2. Ameloblastic odontoma
*3. Arteriovenous malformation; central hemangioma
4. Bone cyst
*5. Brown tumor of hyperparathyroidism

(continued)

---

*6. Calcifying epithelial odontogenic tumor (Pindborg tumor)
*7. Calcifying odontogenic cyst (Gorlin cyst)
8. Carcinoma (central mucoepidermoid or adenoid cystic)
*9. Cementoossifying fibroma
10. Central mucoepidermoid carcinoma of mandible
11. Chondroma
12. Desmoplastic fibroma
13. Giant cell tumor (rare)
14. Hemangiopericytoma
*15. Hydatid cyst
16. Langerhans cell histiocytosis$_g$ (esp. eosinophilic granuloma)
17. Lymphoma$_g$; Burkitt lymphoma
18. Myeloma; plasmacytoma
19. Neuroectodermal tumor of infancy
20. Neurofibromatosis; neurofibroma of mandibular nerve
*21. Odontogenic fibroma
22. Odontoma (immature)
23. Osteosarcoma (eg, telangiectatic)
*24. Pseudotumor of hemophilia
25. Residual cyst
26. Squamous odontogenic tumor

* May be multilocular.

[ ] This condition does not actually cause the gamuted imaging finding, but can produce imaging changes that simulate it.

References
1. Eversole LR, Rovin S: Differential radiographic diagnosis of lesions of the jawbones. Radiology 1972;105:277–284
2. Farman AG, Nortjé CJ, Wood RE: Oral and Maxillofacial Diagnostic Imaging. St. Louis: Mosby-Year Book, 1993, p 32
3. Langlais RP: Radiology of the jaws. In: Delbalso AM: Maxillofacial Imaging. Philadelphia: WB Saunders, 1990, pp 313–373
4. Prein J, Remagen W, Spiessl B, et al: Atlas of Tumors of the Facial Skeleton. Berlin: Springer-Verlag, 1986
5. Wood NK, Goaz PW: Differential Diagnosis of Oral Lesions. (ed 5) St. Louis: Mosby-Year Book, 1997, pp 333–355

Gamut B-82

EXPANSILE RADIOLUCENT LESIONS OF THE JAWS WITH ILL-DEFINED MARGINS

COMMON
1. Metastasis
2. Myeloma; plasmacytoma

UNCOMMON
*1. Ameloblastoma
*2. Aneurysmal bone cyst (rapid growth)
3. Bone sarcoma (eg, chondrosarcoma; fibrosarcoma)
4. Brown tumor of hyperparathyroidism
5. Burkitt's lymphoma
6. Langerhans cell histiocytosis$_g$ (esp. eosinophilic granuloma)

* May be multilocular.

References
1. Eversole LR, Rovin S: Differential radiographic diagnosis of lesions of the jawbones. Radiology 1972;105:277–284
2. Langlais RP: Radiology of the jaws. In: Delbalso AM: Maxillofacial Imaging. Philadelphia: WB Saunders, 1990, pp 313–373
3. Prein J, Remagen W, Spiessl B, et al: Atlas of Tumors of the Facial Skeleton. Berlin: Springer-Verlag, 1986
4. Wood NK, Goaz PW: Differential Diagnosis of Oral Lesions. (ed 5) St. Louis: Mosby-Year Book, 1997, 333–355

Gamut B-83

ILL-DEFINED LYTIC LESIONS OF THE JAWS

COMMON
1. Bone sarcoma (eg, osteolytic osteosarcoma; Ewing sarcoma; chondrosarcoma; fibrosarcoma; hemangioendothelioma {angiosarcoma}; liposarcoma; neurosarcoma)

2. Carcinoma of oral cavity (esp. squamous cell)
3. Chronic osteitis (chronic alveolar abscess)
4. Langerhans cell histiocytosis$_g$ (esp. eosinophilic granuloma)
5. Metastasis (esp. from carcinoma of breast, lung, GI tract, or kidney; melanoma; neuroblastoma)
6. Multiple myeloma; plasmacytoma
7. Osteomyelitis; actinomycosis

UNCOMMON

1. Ameloblastoma (esp. malignant)
2. Aneurysmal bone cyst (rapid growth)
3. Desmoplastic fibroma
4. Fibrous dysplasia (early)
5. Arteriovenous malformation; hemangioma
6. Hematopoietic bone marrow defect
7. Lymphoma$_g$ (incl. leukemia; Burkitt lymphoma; lymphosarcoma)
8. Malignant fibrous histiocytoma
9. Malignant minor salivary gland tumor
10. Massive osteolysis (Gorham's disease)
11. Neuroectodermal tumor of infancy
12. Odontogenic myxoma or fibroma
13. Odontogenic sarcoma
14. Osteoblastoma
15. Paget's disease (early)
16. Primary intraosseous carcinoma; spindle cell carcinoma
17. Radiation necrosis
18. Sarcoidosis
19. Surgical defect
20. Tuberculosis

References
1. DelBalso AM: Lesions of the jaws. Semin Ultrasound CT MR 1995;16:487–512
2. DelBalso AM: An approach to the diagnostic imaging of jaw lesions, dental implants, and the temporomandibular joint. Rad Clin North Am 1998;36:855–890
3. Eversole LR, Rovin S: Differential radiographic diagnosis of lesions of the jawbones. Radiology 1972;105:277–284
4. Farman AG, Nortjé CJ, Wood RE: Oral and Maxillofacial Diagnostic Imaging. St. Louis: Mosby-Year Book, 1993, p 28

5. Kumar R: Lytic lesions of the mandible. RSNA Scientific Exhibit, Washington, D.C.,1984
6. Wood NK, Goaz PW: Differential Diagnosis of Oral Lesions. (ed 5) St. Louis: Mosby-Year Book, 1997, pp 356–379

Gamut B-84

LYTIC LESIONS OF THE JAW WITH INTERNAL RESIDUAL BONE

COMMON

1. Ameloblastoma
2. Hemangioma
3. Invasive squamous cell carcinoma
4. Odontogenic myxoma

UNCOMMON

1. Bone sarcoma (esp. Ewing sarcoma; osteosarcoma)
2. Fibrous dysplasia
3. Lymphoma$_g$
4. Ossifying fibroma

Reference
1. Farman AG, Nortjé CJ, Wood RE: Oral and Maxillofacial Diagnostic Imaging. St. Louis: Mosby-Year Book, 1993, p 43

Gamut B-85-1

MIXED RADIOLUCENT AND RADIOPAQUE PERIAPICAL LESIONS OF THE JAWS

COMMON

1. Calcifying crown of developing tooth
2. Cementoossifying fibroma
3. Periapical cementoosseous dysplasia (intermediate stage of cementoma)

(continued)

4. Rarefying and condensing osteitis
5. Tooth root with rarefying osteitis

UNCOMMON

1. Calcifying odontogenic cyst
2. Cementoblastoma (intermediate stage)
3. Complex and compound odontoma (intermediate stage)
4. Foreign body (eg, root canal cement)
5. Nodular cemental masses
6. Osteomyelitis (chronic)
7. Paget's disease

References
1. Farman AG, Nortjé CJ, Wood RE: Oral and Maxillofacial Diagnostic Imaging. St. Louis: Mosby-Year Book, 1993, p 36
2. Wood NK, Goaz PW: Differential Diagnosis of Oral Lesions. (ed 5) St. Louis: Mosby-Year Book, 1997, pp 415–432

References
1. Farman AG, Nortjé CJ, Wood RE: Oral and Maxillofacial Diagnostic Imaging. St. Louis: Mosby-Year Book, 1993, p 36
2. Wood NK, Goaz PW: Differential Diagnosis of Oral Lesions. (ed 5) St. Louis: Mosby-Year Book, 1997, pp 415–432

Gamut B-85-3

MIXED RADIOLUCENT AND RADIOPAQUE LESIONS OF THE JAWS NOT NECESSARILY CONTACTING TEETH (INCLUDING TARGET LESION)

COMMON

1. Bone island
*2. Cementoosseous dysplasia (focal or florid)
*3. Cementoossifying fibroma
4. Desmoplastic ameloblastoma
5. Fibrous dysplasia; cherubism
6. Ossifying postsurgical bone defect
7. Ossifying subperiosteal hematoma
8. Osteoblastic metastasis (esp. from breast or prostate)
9. Osteomyelitis, chronic (pyogenic with sequestrum*; Brodie abscess; Garré's sclerosing osteomyelitis; complicating a malignant tumor)
10. Paget's disease
*11. Periapical cemental dysplasia; sclerosing cemental masses
*12. Retained deciduous tooth root; infected residual permanent root tip

UNCOMMON

*1. Adenomatoid odontogenic tumor (adenoameloblastoma)
2. Ameloblastic fibro-odontoma or fibrodentinoma

Gamut B-85-2

MIXED PADIOLUCENT AND RADIOPAQUE PERICORONAL LESIONS OF THE JAWS

COMMON

1. Adenomatoid odontogenic tumor (adenoameloblastoma)
2. Ameloblastic fibroodontoma
3. Calcifying epithelial odontogenic tumor (Pindborg tumor)
4. Calcifying odontogenic cyst
5. Complex or compound odontoma (intermediate stage)

UNCOMMON

1. Ameloblastic fibrodentinoma
2. Calcifying hyperplastic dental follicle
3. Cystic odontoma

*3. Bone sarcoma (eg, osteosarcoma; chondrosarcoma; Ewing sarcoma)

*4. Calcifying epithelial odontogenic tumor (Pindborg tumor)

5. Calcifying odontogenic cyst (Gorlin cyst)

*6. Cementoblastoma

*7. Chondroma

*8. Complex and compound odontoma (intermediate stage)

*9. Hemangioma

10. Langerhans cell histiocytosis$_g$, healing

11. Lymphoma$_g$

12. Odontodysplasia

*13. Ossifying fibroma

*14. Osteoblastoma (intermediate)

15. Osteoid osteoma

16. Osteonecrosis (eg, radiation)

17. [Superimposed soft tissue calcification (eg, sialolith)]

* Radiopaque lesion of the jaw, which may have a peripheral lucent shadow (target lesion).

[ ] This condition does not actually cause the gamuted imaging finding, but can produce imaging changes that simulate it.

References

1. DelBalso AM: Lesions of the jaws. Semin Ultrasound CT MR 1995;16:487–512
2. DelBalso AM: An approach to the diagnostic imaging of jaw lesions, dental implants, and the temporomandibular joint. Rad Clin North Am 1998;36:855–890
3. Eversole LR, Rovin S: Differential radiographic diagnosis of lesions of the jawbones. Radiology 1972;105:277–284
4. Farman AG, Nortjé CJ, Wood RE: Oral and Maxillofacial Diagnostic Imaging. St. Louis: Mosby-Year Book, 1993, pp 37, 40
5. Prein J, Remagen W, Spiessl B, et al: Atlas of Tumors of the Facial Skeleton. Berlin: Springer-Verlag, 1986
6. Wood NK, Goaz PW: Differential Diagnosis of Oral Lesions. (ed 5) St. Louis: Mosby-Year Book, 1997, pp 433–448

Gamut B-85-4

SOLITARY OPACITY IN THE JAW NOT NECESSARILY CONTACTING TEETH

COMMON

1. Bone island; osteoma

*2. Cemento-osseous dysplasia (focal)

3. Complex odontoma

4. Condensing or sclerosing osteitis

5. Idiopathic osteosclerosis

6. Ossifying subperiosteal hematoma

7. Osteomyelitis, chronic (pyogenic with sequestrum; Garré's sclerosing osteomyelitis)

8. [Periapical cemental dysplasia; sclerosing cemental masses]

9. Retained tooth root

10. Tori; exostosis

11. Unerupted, impacted, or supernumerary tooth

UNCOMMON

*1. Bone sarcoma (eg, osteosarcoma; chondrosarcoma)

*2. Cementoossifying fibroma

3. Chondroma

4. Fibrous dysplasia

5. Foreign body

*6. Hemangioma

7. Langerhans cell histiocytosis$_g$ (healed)

8. Lymphoma$_g$

* 9. Ossifying fibroma

10. Ossifying postsurgical bone defect

11. Osteoblastic metastasis (esp. from breast or prostate)

*12. Osteoblastoma; osteoid osteoma

13. Osteonecrosis (eg, radiation)

14. Paget's disease

15. [Superimposed soft tissue calcification (eg, sialolith; antrolith; calcified lymph nodes)]

* Radiolucent lesion of the jaw, which may have a central opacity (target lesion).

(continued)

[ ] This condition does not actually cause the gamuted imaging finding, but can produce imaging changes that simulate it.

References

1. DelBalso AM: Lesions of the jaws. Semin Ultrasound CT MR 1995;16:487–512
2. DelBalso AM: An approach to the diagnostic imaging of jaw lesions, dental implants, and the temporomandibular joint. Rad Clin North Am 1998;36:855–890
3. Eversole LR, Rovin S: Differential radiographic diagnosis of lesions of the jawbones. Radiology 1972;105:277–284
4. Farman AG, Nortjé CJ, Wood RE: Oral and Maxillofacial Diagnostic Imaging. St. Louis: Mosby-Year Book, 1993, p 37
5. Prein J, Remagen W, Spiessl B, et al: Atlas of Tumors of the Facial Skeleton. Berlin: Springer-Verlag, 1986
6. Wood NK, Goaz PW: Differential Diagnosis of Oral Lesions. (ed 5) St. Louis: Mosby-Year Book, 1997, pp 477–499

Gamut B-86

PERIAPICAL RADIOPACITIES

COMMON

1. Bone island; periapical idiopathic osteosclerosis; osteoma (incl. Gardner S.)
2. Condensing or sclerosing osteitis
3. Foreign body
4. Hypercementosis
5. [Odontoma, compound or complex]
6. Periapical or focal cementoosseous dysplasia
7. [Unerupted succedaneous tooth; impacted tooth; retained root]

UNCOMMON

1. Calcifying odontogenic cyst
2. Cementoossifying fibroma
3. Cementoblastoma
4. Chondroma; chondrosarcoma
5. Focal or diffuse sclerosing osteomyelitis
6. Hamartoma
7. Osteoblastic metastasis

8. Osteoblastoma
9. Osteosarcoma
10. Paget's disease
11. [Superimposed sialolith, antrolith, phlebolith, calcified lymph node]
12. Torus mandibularis or palatinus; exostosis

[ ] This condition does not actually cause the gamuted imaging finding, but can produce imaging changes that simulate it.

References

1. DelBalso AM: Lesions of the jaws. Semin Ultrasound CT MR 1995;16:487–512
2. DelBalso AM: An approach to the diagnostic imaging of jaw lesions, dental implants, and the temporomandibular joint. Rad Clin North Am 1998;36:855–890
3. Eversole LR, Rovin S: Differential radiographic diagnosis of lesions of the jawbones. Radiology 1972;105:277–284
4. Farman AG, Nortjé CJ, Wood RE: Oral and Maxillofacial Diagnostic Imaging. St. Louis: Mosby-Year Book, 1993, pp 36–37
5. Langlais RP: Radiology of the jaws. In: Delbalso AM: Maxillofacial Imaging. Philadelphia: WB Saunders, 1990, pp 313–373
6. McIvor J: Maxillofacial radiology. In: Grainger RG, Allison DJ: Diagnostic Radiology. Edinburgh: Churchill Livingstone, 1986, vol 3, pp 1914–1915
7. Prein J, Remagen W, Spiessl B, et al: Atlas of Tumors of the Facial Skeleton. Berlin: Springer-Verlag, 1986
8. Wood NK, Goaz PW: Differential Diagnosis of Oral Lesions. (ed 5) St. Louis: Mosby-Year Book, 1997, pp 457–476

Gamut B-87

MULTIPLE OR GENERALIZED OPAQUE LESIONS OF THE JAW

COMMON

1. Cementoosseous dysplasia (florid)
2. Fibrous dysplasia (eg, McCune-Albright S.)
3. Multiple hypercementoses
4. Multiple periapical condensing osteitis
5. Multiple periapical or focal cementoosseous dysplasia

6. Multiple socket sclerosis
7. Paget's disease
8. Sclerosing osteomyelitis (eg, Garré's sclerosing osteomyeiitis; chronic diffuse sclerosing osteomyelitis; actinomycosis)
9. Unerupted or impacted teeth; retained roots

UNCOMMON

1. Cleidocranial dysplasia
2. Cretinism (unerupted teeth)
3. Enchondromatosis (Ollier's disease)
4. Familial gigantiform cementomas
5. Generalized hyperostosis diseases (eg, fluorosis; endosteal hyperostosis {van Buchem type}; osteopetrosis; hyperphosphatasia; dysosteosclerosis; craniometaphyseal dysplasia; diaphyseal dysplasia; craniodiaphyseal dysplasia; pyknodysostosis)
6. Hypercementosis
7. Infantile cortical hyperostosis (Caffey's disease)
8. Multiple odontomas
9. Multiple osteomas (eg, Gardner S.)
10. Muliple tori, exostoses, or osteochondromas
11. Osteoblastic metastases
12. [Superimposed sialoliths, phleboliths, calcified lymph nodes]

[ ] This condition does not actually cause the gamuted imaging finding, but can produce imaging changes that simulate it.

References
1. DelBalso AM: Lesions of the jaws. Semin Ultrasound CT MR 1995;16:487–512
2. DelBalso AM: An approach to the diagnostic imaging of jaw lesions, dental implants, and the temporomandibular joint. Rad Clin North Am 1998;36:855–890
3. Eversole LR, Rovin S: Differential radiographic diagnosis of lesions of the jawbones. Radiology 1972;105:277–284
4. Farman AG, Nortjé CJ, Wood RE: Oral and Maxillofacial Diagnostic Imaging. St. Louis: Mosby-Year Book, 1993, pp 36–37
5. Langlais RP: Radiology of the jaws. In: Delbalso AM: Maxillofacial Imaging. Philadelphia: WB Saunders, 1990, pp 313–373
6. McIvor J: Maxillofacial radiology. In: Grainger RG, Allison DJ: Diagnostic Radiology. Edinburgh: Churchill Livingstone, 1986, vol 3, pp 1914–1915

7. Prein J, Remagen W, Spiessl B, et al: Atlas of Tumors of the Facial Skeleton. Berlin: Springer-Verlag, 1986
8. Wood NK, Goaz PW: Differential Diagnosis of Oral Lesions. (ed 5) St. Louis: Mosby-Year Book, 1997, pp 500–518

Gamut B-88

SYNDROMES WITH SALIVARY GLAND ABNORMALITY

1. Cystic fibrosis (mucoviscidosis)
2. Hyperparathyroidism, primary
3. Hypoglossia-hypodactylia S. (aplasia-adactylia S.)
4. Lacrimo-auriculo-dento-digital S. (LADD S. or Levy-Hollister S.)
*5. Mikulicz S.
6. Oculo-auriculo-vertebral spectrum (Goldenhar S.)
*7. Sjögren S.
8. Treacher Collins S.

* Salivary duct ectasia.

References
1. Silvers AR, Som PM: Salivary glands. Rad Clin North Am 1998;36:941–966
2. Som PM, Brandwein MS, Silvers A: Nodel inclusion cysts of the parotid gland and parapharyngeal space: a discussion of lymphoepithelial, AIDS-related parotid, and branchial cysts, cystic Warthin's tumors, and cysts in Sjögren's syndrome. Laryngoscope 1995;105:1122–1128
3. Taybi H, Lachman RS: Radiology of Syndromes, Metabolic Disorders, and Skeletal Dysplasias. (ed 4) St. Louis: Mosby-Year Book, 1996, p 998

Gamut B-89

SALIVARY DUCT STRICTURE ON SIALOGRAPHY

1. Carcinoma
2. Congenital
3. Infection; inflammation; scarring

(continued)

4. Radiation therapy
5. Stone
6. Trauma, including surgical

References
1. Kreel L: Outline of Radiology. New York: Appleton-Century-Crofts, 1971, p 92
2. Valvassori GE, Buckingham RA, Carter BL, Hanafee WN, Mafee MR: Head and Neck Imaging. New York: Thieme Medical Publ, 1988, p 301

Gamut B-90

PAROTID OR OTHER SALIVARY GLAND ENLARGEMENT

COMMON

1. Mumps
2. Neoplasm, benign (esp. pleomorphic adenoma [mixed tumor]; monomorphic adenoma-Warthin tumor; oncocytoma; hemangioma; lymphangioma; lipoma) (See B-91)
3. Neoplasm, malignant (esp. adenoid cystic {cylindroma} and mucoepidermoid carcinoma; also acinic cell tumor and adenocarcinoma)
4. Stone in duct (esp. in submandibular gland)
5. Suppurative sialadenitis, acute; abscess
6. Trauma with hemorrhage, edema, fistula, or sialocele

UNCOMMON

1. Alcoholism; cirrhosis
2. Allergic or drug reaction (eg, sulfa; iodides)
3. Chronic punctate sialadenitis (benign lymphoepithelial disease, sicca S.)
4. Cyst (eg, lymphoepithelial {esp. in AIDS patients}; dermoid; branchial cleft; mucous retention; ranula)
5. Cystic fibrosis (mucoviscidosis)
6. Granulomatous disease involving parotid gland and lymph nodes (eg, sarcoidosis; tuberculosis; atypical mycobacterial infection; actinomycosis; Wegener's granulomatosis; cat-scratch fever)
7. Hormonal disturbance (eg, diabetes; hypothyroidism; pregnancy)
8. Idiopathic; lipomatous pseudohypertrophy of parotid
9. Infection, other (eg, acute parotitis; recurrent pyogenic parotitis; sialodochitis)
10. Lymph node (esp. intraparotid)
11. Malnutrition; kwashiorkor
12. [Masseter muscle hypertrophy]
13. Metastasis (eg, melanoma; squamous cell carcinoma)
14. Mikulicz S. (bilateral salivary enlargement due to lymphoma$_g$, sarcoidosis, or other disease)
15. Mucocele
16. Radiation therapy
17. Sialodochitis fibrinosa
18. Sjögren S. (primary or associated with rheumatoid arthritis, lupus, scleroderma, or lymphoproliferative disorders)
19. Stricture of duct (See B-89)

[ ] This condition does not actually cause the gamuted imaging finding, but can produce imaging changes that simulate it.

References
1. Kreel L: Outline of Radiology. New York: Appleton-Century-Crofts, 1971, p 91
2. Krolls SO: Salivary gland diseases. J Oral Med 1972;27: 96–99
3. Silvers AR, Som PM: Salivary glands. Rad Clin North Am 1998;36:941–966
4. Slone RM, Fisher AJ: Pocket Guide to Body CT Differential Diagnosis. New York: McGraw-Hill, 1999, pp 20–21
5. Som PM, Sanders DE: The salivary glands. In: Bergeron RJ, Osborn AG, Som PM: Head and Neck Imaging Excluding the Brain. St. Louis: CV Mosby, 1984, pp 186–234
6. Valvassori GE, Buckingham RA, Carter BL, Hanafee WN, Mafee MF: Head and Neck Imaging. New York: Thieme Medical Publ, 1988
7. Weissman JL: Imaging of the salivary glands. Rad Clin North Am 1998;36:941–966

Gamut B-91

SALIVARY GLAND NEOPLASM

BENIGN

COMMON

1. Hemangioma; lymphangioma
2. Monomorphic adenoma, esp. Warthin's tumor (papillary adenocystoma lymphomatosum; cystadenolymphoma)
3. Pleomorphic adenoma (mixed tumor)

UNCOMMON

1. Lipoma
2. Neurinoma; neurofibroma
3. Oncocytoma (oxyphilic adenoma)

MALIGNANT

COMMON

1. Carcinoma
   a. Adenoid cystic (cylindroma)
   b. Carcinoma in pleomorphic adenoma (malignant mixed tumor)
   c. Mucoepidermoid

UNCOMMON

1. Acinic cell tumor
2. Carcinoma, other types
   a. Adenocarcinoma
   b. Epidermoid (squamous cell)
   c. Undifferentiated
3. Lymphoma_g
4. Metastasis (esp. melanoma; carcinoma of skin)
5. Sarcoma

References

1. Batsakis JG: Tumors of the Head and Neck: Clinical and Pathological Considerations. (ed 2) Baltimore: Williams & Wilkins, 1979, pp 21–26
2. Curtin HD: Assessment of salivary gland pathology. Otolaryngol Clin North Am 1988;21:547–573
3. Lufkin R, Borges A, Villablanca P: Teaching Atlas of Head and Neck Imaging. New York: Thieme, 2000; pp 275–278, 289–291
4. Seifert G, Miehlke A, Haubrich J, Chilla R: Diseases of the Salivary Glands. New York: Thieme, 1986, pp 171–318.
5. Silvers AR, Som PM: Salivary glands. Rad Clin North Am 1998;36:941–966
6. Som PM, Sanders DE: The salivary glands. In: Bergeron RT, Osborn AG, Som PM: Head and Neck Imaging Excluding the Brain. St. Louis: CV Mosby, 1984, pp 216–231
7. Som PM, Shugar JM, Sacher M, et al: Benign and malignant parotid pleomorphic adenomas: CT and MR studies. J Comput Assist Tomogr 1988;25:65–69
8. Som PM, Biller HF: High grade malignancies of the parotid gland: identification with MR imaging. Radiology 1989; 173:823–826
9. Som PM, Braun IF, Shapiro MD, Reede DL, et al: Tumors of the parapharyngeal space and upper neck. MR imaging characteristics. Radiology 1987;164:823–829
10. Swartz JD, Rothman MI, Marlowe FI, Berger AS: MR imaging of parotid mass lesions: attempts at histopathologic differentiation. J Comput Assist Tomogr 1989;13:789–796
11. Tabor EK, Curtin HD: MR of the salivary glands. Rad Clin North Am 1989;27:379–392
12. Teresi LM, Lufkin RB, Wortham DG, et al: Parotid masses. MR imaging. Radiology 1987;163:405–409
13. Weissman JL: Imaging of the salivary glands. Rad Clin North Am 1998;36:941-966

Gamut B-92

CYSTIC MASS OF THE PAROTID AND OTHER SALIVARY GLANDS

1. Abscess
*2. Branchial cleft cyst
3. Cystic lymphoma_g
4. Dermoid cyst
5. Hematoma
6. Lymphangioma
*7. Lymphoepithelial cysts (esp. in AIDS)
*8. Necrotic tumor or lymph node metastasis (esp. intraparotid)
*9. Pleomorphic adenoma (mixed tumor), cystic
*10. Primary cyst formation
11. Retention cyst (mucocele)

(continued)

12. Sialocele
*13. Sjögren S.
*14. Warthin tumor

* May be bilateral.

References

1. Beitler JJ, Vikram B, Silver CE, Rubin JS, et al: Low-dose radiotherapy for multicystic benign lymphoepithelial lesions of the parotid gland in HIV-positive patients: long-term results. Head & Neck 1995;17:31–35
2. Bruneton JN, Mourou MY: Ultrasound in salivary gland disease. J Oto-Rhino-Laryngol Related Specialties 1993; 55:284–289
3. Cohen MN, Rao U, Shedd DP: Benign cysts of the parotid gland. J Surg Oncol 1984;27:1156–1179
4. Finfer MD, Schinella RA, Rothstein SG, et al: Cystic parotid lesions in patients at risk for the acquired immunodeficiency syndrome. Arch Otolaryngol Head Neck Surg 1988;114:1290–1294
5. Holliday RA, Cohen WA, Schinella RA, et al: Benign lymphoepithelial parotid cysts and hyperplastic cervical adenopathy in AIDS-risk patients: a new CT appearance. Radiology 1988;168:439–441
6. Joe VQ, Westesson PL: Tumors of the parotid gland: MR imaging characteristics of various histologic types. AJR 1994;163:433–438
7. Lufkin R, Borges A, Villablanca P: Teaching Atlas of Head and Neck Imaging. New York: Thieme, 2000, pp 233–236, 279–281
8. Martinoli C, Pretolesi F, Del Bono V, et al: Benign lymphoepithelial parotid lesions in HIV-positive patients: spectrum of findings at gray-scale and Doppler sonography. AJR 1995;165:975–979
9. Minami M, Tanioka H, Oyama K, Itai Y, et al: Warthin tumor of the parotid gland: MR-pathologic correlation. Am J Neuroradiol 1993;14:209–214
10. Schrot RJ, Adelman HM, Linden CN, Wallach PM: Cystic parotid gland enlargement in HIV disease. The diffuse infiltrative lymphocytosis syndrome. JAMA 1997;278: 166–167
11. Seddon BM, Padley SP, Gazzard BG: Differential diagnosis of parotid masses in HIV positive men: report of five cases and review. Intl J Stds AIDS 1996;7:224–227
12. Som PM, Brandwein MS, Silvers A: Nodal inclusion cysts of the parotid gland and parapharyngeal space: a discussion of lymphoepithelial, AIDS-related parotid, and branchial cysts, Warthin's tumors, and cysts in Sjögren's syndrome. Laryngoscope 1995;105:1122–1128
13. Teresi LM, Lufkin RB, Warthan DG, et al: Parotid masses: MR imaging. Radiology 1987;163:405–409
14. Vogl TJ, Balzer J, Mack M, Steger W: Differential Diagnosis in Head and Neck Imaging. New York: Thieme, 1999, p 251
15. Weissman JL: Imaging of the salivary glands. Semin Ultrasound CT MR 1995;16:546–568

MULTIPLE DISCRETE INTRAPAROTID LESIONS

1. Lymphadenopathy, inflammatory (eg, local or regional infection; sarcoidosis; Kimura's disease) or metastatic (lymphoma$_g$; melanoma; squamous cell carcinoma of the external auditory canal, midface, or scalp)
2. Multicentric oncocytomas
3. Multicentric Warthin tumors
4. Multiple benign lymphoepithelial cysts (esp. in AIDS)
5. Multiple branchial cleft cysts
6. Multiple intraparotid cysts
7. Multiple pleomorphic adenomas
8. Sjögren S.

Reference

1. Lufkin R, Borges A, Villablanca P: Teaching Atlas of Head and Neck Imaging. New York: Thieme, 2000; pp 282–285

BILATERAL PAROTID ENLARGEMENT WITH PARENCHYMAL HETEROGENEITY (US, CT, MRI)

SIALOADENOSIS

1. Chronic alcoholism
2. Diabetes
3. Drug reaction
4. Hyperlipidemia

5. Malnutrition (nutritional mumps)
6. Postradiation therapy

SIALADENITIS
1. Infectious (viral parotitis; lymphoepithelial cysts {esp. in AIDS})
2. Inflammatory (eg, sarcoidosis; graft vs. host disease; Mikulicz S.)

BILATERAL PAROTID NEOPLASMS
1. Oncocytoma
2. Pleomorphic adenoma
3. Warthin's tumor

MULTIPLE INTRAPAROTID LYMPHADENOPATHY
1. Lymphoma$_g$
2. Metastatic disease
3. Reactive

OTHERS
1. Amyloidosis
2. Clear cell oncocytosis
3. Polycystic (dysgenetic) disease

References
1. Bohuslavizki KH, Brenner W, Wolf H, et al: Value of quantitative salivary gland scintigraphy in the early stage of Sjögren's syndrome. Nucl Med Commun 1995;16:917–922
2. Izumi M, Eguchi K, Uetani M, et al: MR features of the lacrimal gland in Sjögren's syndrome. AJR 1998;170:1661–1666
3. Izumi M, Eguchi K, Nakamura H, et al: Premature fat deposition in the salivary glands associated with Sjögren syndrome: MR and CT evidence. AJR 1997;168:951–958
4. Izumi M, Eguchi K, Ohki M, et al: MR imaging of the parotid gland in Sjögren's syndrome: a proposal for new diagnostic criteria. AJR 1996;l66:1483–1487
5. Lufkin R, Borges A, Villablanca P: Teaching Atlas of Head and Neck Imaging. New York: Thieme, 2000, pp 270–274
6. Makula E, Pokorny G, Rajtar M, et al: Parotid gland ultrasonography as a diagnostic tool in primary Sjögren's syndrome. Brit J Rheumatol 1996;35:972–977
7. Saito T, Fukuda H, Horikawa M, et al: Salivary gland scintigraphy with 99m Tc-pertechnetate in Sjögren's syndrome: relationship to clinicopathologic features of salivary and lacrimal glands. J Oral Path Med 1997;26:46–50
8. Som PM, Brandwein MS, Silvers A: Nodal inclusion cysts of the parotid gland and parapharyngeal space: a discussion of lymphoepithelial, AIDS-related parotid and branchial cysts, cystic Warthin's tumors, and cysts in Sjögren's syndrome. Laryngoscope 1995;l05:1122–1128
9. Yoshiura K, Yuasa K, Tabata O, et al: Reliability of ultrasonography and sialography in the diagnosis of Sjögren's syndrome. Oral Surg Oral Med Oral Path Oral Radiol Endodontics 1997;83:400–407

Gamut B-95
SMALL PAROTID GLAND

1. Chronic postobstructive atrophy
2. Normal variant
3. Postoperative superficial or total parotidectomy
4. Postradiation therapy

References
1. Lufkin R, Borges A, Villablanca P: Teaching Atlas of Head and Neck Imaging. New York: Thieme, 2000, pp 267–269
2. Yamashita T, Tomoda K, Kumazawa T: The usefulness of partial parotidectomy for benign parotid gland tumors. A retrospective study of 306 cases. Acta Oto-Laryngolica (Suppl) 1993;500:113–116

Gamut B-96
BILATERAL CHEEK MASSES

PSEUDOMASSES
1. Benign masseteric hypertrophy
2. Bilateral accessory parotid gland tissue
3. Bilateral facial processes of the parotid glands

INFECTION/INFLAMMATION
1. Bilateral lymphoepithelial cysts (HIV-associated)
2. Mikulicz S.

(continued)

3. Sarcoidosis
4. Sjögren S. (early inflammatory stage)
5. Viral parotitis

NEOPLASM

1. Bilateral intraparotid lymphadenopathy
   (eg, lymphoma$_g$)
2. Bilateral parotid gland tumors (eg, pleomorphic adenoma, Warthin's tumor, oncocytoma)

OTHER

1. Bilateral parotid gland hypertrophy secondary to alcoholism

References

1. Honda T, Sasaki K, Takeuchi M, Nozaki M: Endoscope-assisted intraoral approach for masseteric hypertrophy. Ann Plastic Surg 1997;38:9–14
2. Mandel L, Kaynar A: Masseteric hypertrophy. NY State Dental J 1994;60:44–47
3. Morse MH: Enlargement of the pterygo-masseteric muscle complex. Clin Radiol 1994;49:71
4. Nishida M, Iizuka T: Intraoral removal of the enlarged mandibular angle associated with masseteric hypertrophy. J Oral Maxillofac Surg 1995;53:1476–1479
5. Rosa RA, Kotkin HC: That acquired masseteric look. ASDC J Dentistry Child 1996;63:105–107
6. Smyth AG: Botulinum toxin treatment of bilateral masseteric hypertrophy. Brit J Oral Maxillofac Surg 1994;32:29–33
7. Tart RP, Kotzur IM, Mancuso AA, et al: CT and MR imaging of the buccal space and buccal space masses. RadioGraphics 1995;15: 531–550

Gamut B-97

LESIONS OF THE SUBMANDIBULAR SPACE

1. Benign tumor of submandibular gland
2. Branchial cleft cyst
3. Calculus in a salivary gland
4. Carcinoma (adenoid cystic; mucoepidermoid; acinar cell)
5. Cystic hygroma (lymphangioma)
6. Epidermoid; dermoid
7. Hemangioma
8. Lipoma
9. Ludwig angina secondary to abscess or cellulitis
10. Lymphadenopathy (reactive or metastatic)
11. Pseudotumor secondary to motor atrophy of cranial nerve
12. Ranula
13. Thyroglossal duct cyst

References

1. Fine MJ, Holliday RA, Roland JT: Clinically unsuspected venous malformations limited to the submandibular triangle: CT findings. AJNR 1995;16:491–494
2. Mukherji SK, Castillo M: A simplified approach to the spaces of the suprahyoid neck. Rad Clin North Am 1998; 36:761–780
3. Weissman JL: Imaging of the salivary glands. Semin Ultrasound CT MR 1995;16:546–568
4. Weissman JL, Carrau RL: Anterior facial vein and submandibular gland together: predicting the histology of submandibular masses with CT or MR imaging. Radiology 1998;208:441–446

Gamut B-98

LESIONS OF THE SUBLINGUAL SPACE

1. Abscess
2. Benign mixed tumor of salivary glands
3. Carcinoma (squamous cell; adenoid cystic; mucoepidermoid)
4. Cystic hygroma (lymphangioma)
5. Dilated excretory duct of submandibular gland
6. Epidermoid; dermoid
7. Hemangioma
8. Hypoglossal nerve atrophy
9. Lingual thyroid tissue
10. Ludwig angina; cellulitis
11. Ranula

References

1. Mukherji SK, Castillo M: A simplified approach to the spaces of the suprahyoid neck. Rad Clin North Am 1998; 36:761–780
2. Weissman JL: Imaging of the salivary glands. Semin Ultrasound CT MR 1995;16:546–568

Gamut B-99

SOFT TISSUE MASS IN THE NECK

CYSTIC MASS

1. Abscess (eg, from tonsillitis, pharyngitis, parotid infection, dental procedure, or trauma)
2. Aneurysm of the carotid artery or jugular vein
3. Branchial cleft cyst (first or second)
4. Cervical thymic cyst
5. Dermoid cyst; teratoma; epidermoid
6. Diverticulum, air-filled (eg, lateral pharyngeal, tracheal, Zenker's)
7. Laryngocele (external)
8. Lymphangioma (cystic hygroma)
9. Necrotic lymph node (esp. from tonsillar or nasopharyngeal malignancy)
10. Neurogenic tumor (eg, cystic schwannoma or neurofibroma)
11. Parathyroid cyst
12. [Subcutaneous emphysema]
13. Thyroglossal duct cyst
14. Thyroid cyst

SOLID MASS

1. Abscess
2. Actinomycosis
3. Carotid body tumor (paraganglioma; chemodectoma)
4. Cervical thymus gland
5. Epidermoid
6. Lipoma; liposarcoma
7. Lymphadenopathy, esp. metastatic from squamous cell carcinoma, melanoma, or thyroid carcinoma

(See B-101-S); tuberculous (scrofula); sarcoidosis; also benign lymphoid hyperplasia; acute lymphadenitis; systemic lymph node enlargement (eg, infectious mononucleosis; cat-scratch disease)

8. Lymphoma$_g$; Burkitt lymphoma
9. Mesenchymal tumor
10. Neurogenic tumor$_g$ (schwannoma; neurofibroma; plexiform neurofibroma; neuroblastoma)
11. Parathyroid adenoma
12. Sebaceous cyst
13. Salivary gland enlargement (eg, mumps; stone in duct; neoplasm-pleomorphic adenoma) (See B-90); ectopic salivary gland tissue
14. Thyroid tumor (eg, adenoma; goiter; carcinoma); thyroiditis; ectopic thyroid

VASCULAR MASS

1. Aneurysm of the carotid artery or jugular vein
2. Arteriovenous fistula
3. Carotid body tumor (paraganglioma; chemodectoma)
4. Cervical aortic arch
5. Dilated jugular lymph sac
6. Hemangioma
7. Hemangiopericytoma
8. Hematoma
9. Jugular vein ectasia or asymmetry
10. Jugular vein thrombosis (bland, septic or metastatic clot) (See B-100)
    a. Septic—Lemierre S. (necrobacilioisis), a suppurative thrombophlebitis of the IJV secondary to an oropharyngeal infection
    b. Placement of central venous lines and indwelling catheters
    c. Puncture of IJV by intravenous drug abusers
11. Lymphangioma (cystic hygroma)
12. Posttraumatic pseudoaneurysm

PSEUDOMASS

1. Hypertrophy of the sternocleidomastoid muscle
2. Status post-unilateral radical neck dissection

[ ] This condition does not actually cause the gamuted imaging finding, but can produce imaging changes that simulate it.

(continued)

References

1. Chong VFH, Fan YF: Pictorial review: radiology of the carotid space. Clin Radiol 1996;51:762–768
2. Finn JP, Zisk JH, Edelman RR, et al: Central venous occlusion. MR angiography. Radiology 1993;l 87:245–251
3. Ginsberg LE: Inflammatory and infectious lesions of the neck. Semin Ultrasound, CT, MR 1997;18:205–219
4. Gudinchet F, Maeder P, Neveceral P, Schnyder P: Lemierre's syndrome in children: high-resolution CT and color Doppler sonography patterns. Chest 1997;112:271–273
5. Harnsberger HR, Dillon WP: Cystic masses of the head and neck: rare lesions with characteristic radiologic features. Taken in part from Head and Neck Imaging (ed. 2) St. Louis: Mosby-Year Book, 1994, pp 617–629
6. Harnsberger HR, Osborn AG: Differential diagnosis of head and neck lesions based on their space of origin. 1. The suprahyoid part of the neck. AJR 1991;157:147–154
7. Johnson IJ, Smith I, Akintunde MO, et al: Assessment of preoperative investigations of thyroglossal cysts. J Royal Coll Surg Edinburgh 1996;41:48–49
8. Kawanaka M, Sugimoto Y, Suehiro M, Fukuchi M: Thyroid imaging in a typical case of acute suppurative thyroiditis with abscess formation due to infection from a persistent thyroglossal duct. Ann Nucl Med 1994;8:159–162
9. Lim-Dunham JE, Feinstein KA, Yousefzadeh DK, Ben-Ami T: Sonographic demonstration of a normal thyroid gland excludes ectopic thyroid in patients with thyroglossal duct cyst. AJR 1995;164:1489–1491
10. Lufkin R, Borges A, Villablanca P: Teaching Atlas of Head and Neck Imaging. New York: Thieme, 2000, pp 122-126, 521–539
11. Reede DL, Bergeron RT, Osborn AG: CT of the soft tissues of the neck. In: Bergeron RT, Osborn AG, Som PM: Head and Neck Imaging Excluding the Brain. St. Louis: CV Mosby, 1984, pp 491–530
12. Sakai O, Nakashima N, Shibayama C, et al: Asymmetrical or heterogeneous enhancement of the internal jugular veins in contrast-enhanced CT of the head and neck. Neuroradiology 1997;39:292–295
13. Slone RM, Fisher AJ: Pocket Guide to Body CT Differential Diagnosis.New York: McGraw-Hill, 1999, pp 12–16
14. Stocks RM, Milburn M, Thompson J: Unusual neck masses secondary to jugular venous abnormalities: case report and discussion. Amer Surg 1997;63:305–309
15. Warpeha RL: Masses in the neck. In: Wood NK, Goaz PW: Differential Diagnosis of Oral Lesions. (ed 4) St. Louis: Mosby-Year Book, 1991, pp 616–637

Gamut B-100-S

PATHOGENESIS OF INTERNAL JUGULAR VEIN THROMBOSIS

1. Hypercoaguable states (eg, malignancies; paraproteinemias; connective tissue disorders$_g$ {esp. lupus erythematosus}; pregnancy; coagulation defects {eg, deficiency of protein C and S, antithrombin III}
2. Placement of central venous lines and indwelling catheters
3. Puncture of IJV by intravenous drug abusers
4. Radiation therapy
5. Sepsis, infection—Lemierre S. (necrobacilioisis), a suppurative thrombophlebitis of the IJV secondary to tonsillitis or other oropharyngeal infection, otitis, mastoiditis, or dental infection
6. Stasis of blood (eg, hypotension; dehydration; immobilization)
7. Surgical trauma during head and neck procedures
8. Thrombus extension from an intracrania venous sinus (esp. sigmoid and transverse sinuses)
9. Trauma to neck (open or blunt)

References

1. Duffey DC, Billings KR, Eichel BS, Sercarz JA: Internal jugular vein thrombosis. Ann Otol Rhinol Laryngol 1995; 104:899–904
2. Leontsinis TG, Currie AR, Mannell A: Internal jugular vein thrombosis following functional neck dissection, Laryngoscope 1995;105:169–174
3. Lufkin R, Borges A, Villablanca P: Teaching Atlas of Head and Neck Imaging. New York: Thieme, 2000, pp 122–126
4. Poe LB, Manzione JV, Wasenko JJ, Kellman RM: Acute internal jugular vein thrombosis associated with pseudoabscess of the retropharyngeal space. AJNR 1995;16(Suppl): 892–896
5. Terada Y, Mitsui T, Jikuya T, et al: Infected thrombophlebitis of the right internal jugular vein. J Vasc Surg 1996;24: 1066–1067

Gamut B-101-S

METASTATIC CERVICAL LYMPHADENOPATHY ON CT OR MRI (LOCATION OF LYMPH NODES AND SUSPECTED PRIMARY SITE OF MALIGNANCY)

UPPER CERVICAL NODES
1. Base of tongue
2. Maxillary or ethmoid sinus
3. Nasopharynx
4. Tonsil

MIDDLE AND LOWER JUGULAR NODES
1. Esophagus
2. Larynx
3. Pharynx
4. Thyroid

MIDLINE OR PARATRACHEAL NODES
1. Larynx
2. Lung
3. Thyroid

SUBMAXILLARY NODES
1. Floor of mouth
2. Tongue

SUPRACLAVICULAR NODES
1. Breast
2. Esophagus
3. Lung
4. Stomach

Reference
1. Reede DL, Bergeron RT, Osborn AG: CT of the soft tissues of the neck. In: Bergeron RT, Osborn AG, Som PM: Head and Neck Imaging Excluding the Brain. St. Louis: CV Mosby, 1984, p 529

Gamut B-102

SOLID MASS IN THE CAROTID SHEATH

1. Lymphadenopathy, inflammatory or infectious
2. Traumatic neuroma
3. Tumor
4. Benign
   a. Granular cell tumor (rhabdomyoblastoma)
   b. Hemangiolymphangioma
   c. Lipoma
   d. Nerve sheath tumor (schwannoma; neurofibroma; ganglioneuroma; ganglioblastoma; ganglioneuroblastoma)
   e. Paraganglioma (glomus jugulare or glomus vagale tumor; carotid body tumor)
   f. Thyroid and parathyroid tumors (eg, adenoma)
5. Malignant
   a. Lymphoma$_g$
   b. Metastatic lymphadenopathy

References
1. Catalano P, Fang-Hui E, Som PM: Fluid-fluid levels in benign neurogenic tumors. AJNR 1997;18:385–387
2. Furukawa M, Furukawa MK, Katoh K, Tsukuda M: Differentiation between schwannoma of the vagus nerve and schwannoma of the cervical sympathetic chain by imaging diagnosis. Laryngoscope 1996;106:1548–1552
3. Ganesan S, Harar RP, Owen RA, et al: Horner's syndrome: a rare presentation of cervical sympathetic chain schwannoma. J Laryngol Otol 1997;111:493–495
4. George B, Lot G: Neurinomas of the first two cervical nerve roots: a series of 42 cases. J Neurosurgery 1995;82:917–923
5. Kumchev Y, Kalnev B: A neurofibroma affecting the first right cervical sympathetic ganglion and entering the jugular foramen of the skull base. Folia Medica 1997;39:15–19
6. Lufkin R, Borges A, Villablanca P: Teaching Atlas of Head and Neck Imaging. New York: Thieme, 2000, pp 147–151
7. Sairyo K, Henmi T, Endo H: Foramen magnum schwannoma with an unusual clinical presentation, case report. Spinal Cord 1997;35:554–556
8. Sheridan MF, Yim DW: Cervical sympathetic schwannoma: a case report and review of the English literature. Otolaryngol Head Neck Surg 1997;117:S206–210
9. Silver AJ, Mawad ME, Hilal SK, et al: Computed tomography of the carotid space and related cervical spaces. Radiology 1984;150:723–728

Gamut B-103-1

THYROID LESIONS (See also B-103-2)

COMMON

1. Adenoma (eg, adenomatous hyperplasia; follicular adenoma; parathyroid adenoma)
2. Carcinoma (eg, papillary; follicular; anaplastic; medullary; Hürthle cell)
3. Cystic lesion (eg, cystic thyroid nodule; colloid cyst; colloid-filled macrofollicle in a goiter; simple cyst; necrotic papillary carcinoma, adenoma, or goiter; cystic parathyroid adenoma)
4. Goiter
5. Thyroiditis (incl. acute suppurative; Riedel's)

UNCOMMON

1. Abscess
2. Hemorrhage within an adenoma or colloid nodule
3. Lymphoma_g
4. Metastasis (esp. carcinoma of lung, breast, or kidney; melanoma)

References
1. See B-103-2
2. Slone RM, Fisher AJ: Pocket Guide to Body CT Differential Diagnosis. New York: McGraw-Hill, 1999, pp 18–19

Gamut B-103-2

ILL-DEFINED ENLARGEMENT OF THE THYROID GLAND WITH EXTRATHYROID EXTENSION

INFECTIOUS/INFLAMMATORY

1. Acute suppurative thyroiditis (bacterial or fungal)
2. Riedel's thyroiditis (invasive fibrous thyroiditis)

NEOPLASTIC

1. Carcinoma of thyroid (eg, anaplastic; squamous cell)
2. Lymphoma_g of thyroid
3. Metastasis (esp. carcinoma of breast, lung, or kidney; melanoma)
4. Sarcoma (rare)

IATROGENIC

1. Postradiation therapy (radiation-induced thyroiditis)
2. Postsurgical changes

References
1. Bagnasco M, Passalacqua G, Pronzato C, et al: Fibrous invasive (Riedel's) thyroiditis with critical response to steroid treatment. J Endocrinol Invest 1995;18:305–307
2. Brady OH, Hehir DJ, Heffernan SJ: Riedel's thyroiditis—case report and literature review. Irish J Med Sci 1994;163:176–177
3. Elewaut D, Rubens R, Elewaut A, Kunnen M: Lusoria dysphagia in a patient with retroperitoneal fibrosis and Riedel's thyroiditis. J Int Med 1996;239:75–78
4. Intenzo CM, Park CH, Kim SM, et al: Clinical, laboratory and scintigraphic manifestations of subacute and chronic thyroiditis. Clin Nucl Med 1993;18:302–306
5. Julie C, Vieillefond A, Desligneres S, et al: Hashimoto's thyroiditis associated with Riedel's thyroiditis and retroperitoneal fibrosis. Pathol Res Pract 1997;193:573–578
6. Lufkin R, Borges A, Villablanca P: Teaching Atlas of Head and Neck Imaging. New York: Thieme, 2000, pp 157–162, 169–173
7. Nakahara H, Noguchi S, Murakami N, et al: Gadolinium enhanced MR imaging of thyroid and parathyroid masses. Radiology 1997;202:765–772
8. Russell P, Lean CL, Delbridge L, et al: Proton magnetic resonance and human thyroid neoplasia. I: Discrimination between benign and malignant neoplasms. Am J Med 1994;96:383–388
9. Wan SK, Chan JK, Tang SK: Paucicellular variant of anaplastic thyroid carcinoma. A mimic of Riedel's thyroiditis. Am J Clin Pathol 1996;105:388–393
10. Zimmerman-Belsing T, Feldt-Rasmussen U: Riedel's thyroiditis: an autoimmune or primary fibrotic disease? (see comments). J Int Med 1994;235:271–274

Gamut B-104-1

FATTY TUMORS OF THE NECK

SOLITARY
WITH NO CONTRAST ENHANCEMENT
1. Dermoid cyst
2. Lipoma

WITH CONTRAST ENHANCEMENT
1. Angiolipoma
2. Hibernoma
3. Lipoblastoma; lipoblastomatosis
4. Liposarcoma

MULTIPLE
1. Benign symmetric lipomatosis (Madelung disease)
2. Cushing syndrome

References
1. Abdullah BJ, Liam CK, Kaur H, Matthew KM: Parapharyngeal space lipoma causing sleep apnoea. Brit J Radiol 1997;70:1063–1065
2. Eckel HE, Jungehülsing M: Lipoma of the hypopharynx: preoperative diagnosis and transoral resection. J Laryngol Otol 1994;108:174–177
3. Elango S: Parapharyngeal space lipoma. Ear Nose Throat J 1995;74:52–53
4. Kransdorf MJ: Benign soft-tissue tumors in a large referral population: distribution of specific diagnoses by age, sex and location. AJR 1995;164:395–402
5. Lufkin R, Borges A, Villablanca P: Teaching Atlas of Head and Neck Imaging. New York: Thieme, 2000, pp 127–131
6. Tsunoda A: Lipoma in the peri-tonsillar space. J Laryngol Otol 1994;108:693–695
7. Worsey J, McGuirt W, Carrau RL, Peitzman AB: Hibernoma of the neck: a rare cause of neck mass. Am J Otolaryngol 1994;15:152–154
8. Zelger BW, Zelger BG, Plörer A, et al: Dermal spindle cell lipoma: plexiform and nodular variants. Histopathology 1995;27:533–540

Gamut B-104-2

DIFFUSE LIPOMATOSIS OF THE NECK

WITHOUT INFLAMMATORY SIGNS
1. Benign or multiple symmetric lipomatosis
2. Cushing syndrome
3. Lipoblastomatosis (children)
4. Liposarcoma
5. Morbid obesity
6. Multiple familial lipomatosis

WITH INFLAMMATORY SIGNS
1. Dercum's disease (acute panniculitis)
2. Progressive nodular lipomatosis
3. Weber-Christian disease (painful adiposis)

References
1. Borges A, Torrinha F, Lufkin RB, Abemayor E: Laryngeal involvement in multiple symmetric lipomatosis: the role of computed tomography in diagnosis. Am J Otolaryngol 1997;18:127–130
2. Chung JY, Ramos-Caro FA, Beers B, et al: Multiple lipomas, angiolipomas, and parathyroid adenomas in a patient with Birt-Hogg-Dube syndrome. Intl J Dermatol 1996;35:365–367
3. Feldman DR, Schabel Si: Multiple symmetrical lipomatosis: computed tomographic appearance. South Med J 1995;88:681–682
4. Kitano H, Nakanishi Y, Takeuchi E, Nagahara K: Multiple symmetrical lipomatosis: no longer just a Mediterranean disease? J Oto Rhino Laryngol Related Specialties 1994;56:177–180
5. Lufkin R, Borges A, Villablanca P: Teaching Atlas of Head and Neck Imaging. New York: Thieme, 2000, pp 132–136
6. Martin DS, Sharafuddin M, Boozan J, et al Multiple symmetric lipomatosis (Madelung's disease). Skeletal Radiol 1995;24:72–73
7. Murty KD, Murty PS, George S, et al: Lipoma of the larynx. Am J Otolaryngol 1994;15:149–151
8. Parmar C, Blackburn C: Madelung's disease: an uncommon disorder of unknown aetiology? Brit J Oral Maxillofac Surg 1996;34:467–470

Gamut B-105-1

INCREASED RETROPHARYNGEAL (PREVERTEBRAL) SPACE IN AN INFANT OR CHILD

COMMON

1. Enlarged adenoids and lymphoid tissue
2. Hematoma or edema from cervical spine injury or fracture
3. Retropharyngeal abscess or cellulitis (eg, from pyogenic adenitis; perforation of pharynx by foreign body or intubation)
4. Retropharyngeal inflammatory lymphadenopathy (bacterial, viral, tuberculous, histoplasmic)
5. [Technical factors (eg, buckling of airway; crying; expiratory film; improper positioning with flexion or obliquity of neck; superimposed ear lobe)]

UNCOMMON

1. Branchial cleft cyst (third)
2. Dilated jugular veins and carotid arteries from vein of Galen aneurysm or other large intracranial arteriovenous malformation
3. Enteric or duplication cyst
4. Lymph fluid
5. Lymphadenopathy, noninflammatory (eg, metastatic disease; Langerhans cell histiocytosis$_g$; leukemia; lymphoma$_g$; sinus histiocytosis)
6. Myxedema (hypothyroidism)
7. Neoplasm (eg, hemangioma; lymphangioma {cystic hygroma}; angiofibroma; plexiform neurofibroma; ganglioneuroma; neuroblastoma; lipoma; teratoma; rhabdomyosarcoma)
8. Retropharyngeal goiter
9. Spinal disease (eg, osteomyelitis; tuberculosis; metastasis; primary neoplasm; fracture)
10. Superior vena cava obstruction with edema
11. Traumatic pseudodiverticulum of pharynx (from finger in infant's mouth during delivery)

[ ] This condition does not actually cause the gamuted imaging finding, but can produce imaging changes that simulate it.

References

1. Babl FE, Pascucci R: Images in clinical medicine. Retropharyngeal abscess. NEJM 1997;337:472
2. Daniello NJ, Goldstein SI: Retropharyngeal hematoma secondary to minor blunt head and neck trauma. ENT 1994; 73:41–43
3. Davis WL, Harnsberger HR, Smoker WRK, Watanabe AS: Retropharyngeal space: evaluation of normal anatomy and diseases with CT and MR imaging. Radiology 1990; 174:59–64
4. el-Sayed Y, al Dousary S: Deep neck space abscesses. J Otolaryngol 1996;25:227–233
5. Gianoli GJ, Espinola TE, Guarisco JL, Miller RH: Retropharyngeal space infection: changing trends. Otolaryngol Head Neck Surg 1991;105:92–100
6. Goldenberg D, Golz A, Joachims HZ: Retropharyngeal abscess: a clinical review. J Laryngol Otol 1997;111:546–550
7. Grünebaum M, Moskowitz G: The retropharyngeal soft tissues in young infants with hypothyroidism. AJR 1970; 108:543–545
8. Hayden CK Jr, Swischuk LE: Retropharyngeal edema, airway obstruction, and caval thrombosis. AJR 1982;138: 757–758
9. Hewel K, Kioumehr F, So G, Wang M: Infected third bronchial cleft cyst: retropharyngeal extension to the superior mediastinum. Canad Assoc Radiologists J 1996;47: 111–113
10. Lazor B, Cunningham MJ, Eavey RD, Weber AL: Comparison of computed tomography and surgical findings in deep neck infections. Otolaryngol Head Neck Surg 1994;111: 746–750
11. Lufkin R, Borges A, Villablanca P: Teaching Atlas of Head and Neck Imaging. New York: Thieme, 2000, pp 137–142
12. Marra S, Hotaling AJ: Deep neck infections. Am J Otolaryngol 1996;17:287–298
13. McCook TA, Felman AH: Retropharyngeal masses in infants and young children. Am J Dis Child 1979;133:41–43
14. Swischuk LE, John SD: Differential Diagnosis in Pediatric Radiology. (ed 2) Baltimore: Williams & Wilkins, 1995, pp 118–122
15. Wong YK, Novotny GM: Retropharyngeal space—a review of anatomy, pathology, and clinical presentation. J Otolaryngol 1978;7:528–535

Gamut B-105-2

INCREASED RETROPHARYNGEAL (PREVERTEBRAL) SPACE IN AN ADULT

COMMON

1. Abscess or cellulitis
2. Direct invasion from nasopharyngeal or oropharyngeal squamous cell carcinoma
3. Lymphadenopathy (eg, metastatic disease; lymphoma$_g$; tuberculosis)
4. Postcricoid carcinoma
5. Spinal disease (eg, osteophytes; primary or metastatic neoplasm; inflammation or osteomyelitis)
6. Tortuous carotid artery
7. Trauma (prevertebral edema or hematoma; spine fracture)

UNCOMMON

1. Chordoma
2. Lymphangioma; hemangioma; lipoma
3. Myxedema (hypothyroidism)
4. Retropharyngeal goiter
5. Zenker's diverticulum

References
1. Babl FE, Pascucci R: Images in clinical medicine. Retropharyngeal abscess. NEJM 1997;337:472
2. Cheung YK, Sham JST, Chan FL, et al: Computed tomography of the paranasopharyngeal spaces: normal variations and criteria for tumor extension. Clin Radiol 1992;45: 109–113
3. Daniello NJ, Goldstein SI: Retropharyngeal hematoma secondary to minor blunt head and neck trauma. ENT 1994; 73:41–43
4. Davis WL, Harnsberger HR, Smoker WRK, Watanabe AS: Retropharyngeal space: evaluation of normal anatomy and diseases with CT and MR imaging. Radiology 1990;174: 59 64
5. el-Sayed Y, al Dousary S: Deep neck space abscesses. J Otolaryngol 1996;25:227–233
6. Gianoli GJ, Espinola TE, Guarisco JL, Miller RH: Retropharyngeal space infection: changing trends. Otolaryngol Head Neck Surg 1991;105:92–100
7. Goldenberg D, Golz A, Joachims HZ: Retropharyngeal abscess: a clinical review. J Laryngol Otol 1997;111:546–550
8. Lazor B, Cunningham MJ, Eavey RD, Weber AL: Comparison of computed tomography and surgical findings in deep neck infections. Otolaryngol Head Neck Surg 1994;111: 746 750
9. Lufkin R, Borges A, Villablanca P: Teaching Atlas of Head and Neck Imaging. New York: Thieme, 2000, pp 137–142
10. Marra S, Hotaling AJ: Deep neck infections. Am J Otolaryngol 1996;17:287–298
11. Nokes SR, Adametz J, Gardner G, Beaton JN: Radiological case of the month. Blastomycosis osteomyelitis with epidural and retropharyngeal abscess. J Arkansas Med Soc 1995;92:253–254
12. Poe LB, Manzione JV, Wasenko JJ, Kellman RM: Acute internal jugular vein thrombosis associated with pseudo-abscess of the retropharyngeal space. AJNR 1995;116: 892–896
13. Som PM, Biller HF, Lawson W, et al: Parapharyngeal space masses: an updated protocol based upon 104 cases. Radiology 1984;153:149–156
14. Wong YK, Novotny GM: Retropharyngeal space—a review of anatomy, pathology, and clinical presentation. J Otolaryngol 1978;7:528–535

Gamut B-106

LESIONS OF THE OROPHARYNX

COMMON

1. Carcinoma of tonsil, soft palate, or base of tongue (esp. squamous cell; rarely lymphoepithelioma or transitional cell)
2. Extension of nasopharyngeal or hypopharyngeal tumor to oropharynx
3. Macroglossia (eg, neoplasm of tongue—esp. carcinoma or granular cell myoblastoma; ranula; sialocyst; amyloidosis; congenital—Down S.; cretinism) (See B-108)
4. [Normal variant (eg, lingual tonsil hypertrophy; prolapse of mucosa through thyrohyoid membrane mimicking oropharyngeal diverticulum)]
5. Thyroglossal duct cyst
6. Tonsillitis; peritonsillar abscess

(continued)

UNCOMMON

1. Abscess/bacterial cellulitis (Vincent's angina)
2. Branchial cleft cyst
3. Dermoid
4. Lipoma
5. Lymphangioma (cystic hygroma)
6. Metastasis
7. Minor salivary gland malignancy (adenoid cystic carcinoma; mucoepidermoid carcinoma; adeno-carcinoma)
8. Schwannoma; neurofibroma
9. Venous malformation

[ ] This condition does not actually cause the gamuted imaging finding, but can produce imaging changes that simulate it.

Reference

1. Unger JM: Handbook of Head and Neck Imaging. New York: Churchill Livingstone, 1987, pp 91–99

Gamut B-107

LESIONS OF THE HARD AND SOFT PALATE

1. Carcinoma (squamous cell)
2. Fistula
3. Lymphoma$_g$; Burkitt lymphoma
4. Minor salivary gland tumor
5. Sarcoma (eg, osteosarcoma)

References

1. Eustace S, Suojanen J, Marianacci E, et al: Osteosarcoma of the hard palate. Skeletal Radiol 1995;24:392–394
2. Som PM, Curtin HD: Head and Neck Imaging. (ed 3) St. Louis: Mosby-Year Book, 1996, pp 449–452

Gamut B-108

LARGE TONGUE (MACROGLOSSIA)

COMMON

1. Amyloidosis

2. Cretinism; hypothyroidism
3. Trisomy 21 S. (Down S.)

UNCOMMON

1. Acromegaly
2. Beckwith-Wiedeman S.
3. Chromosome 4:dup (4p) S.
4. Cyst (eg, duplication; lingual; thyroglossal duct; dermoid)
5. Glycogen storage disease, type II (Pompe's disease)
6. Infant of diabetic mother
7. Jaw or dental deformity with increased mouth size
8. Kocher-Debré-Sémélaigne S.
9. Lingual thyroid
10. Mucopolysaccharidoses (esp. Hurler S.) (See J-4-S); GM$_1$ gangliosidosis
11. Multiple endocrine neoplasia, type IIB (MEN IIB; mucosal neuroma S.)
12. Muscular dystrophy; myotonia congenita
13. Neoplasm of tongue (eg, hemangioma; lymphan-gioma; granular cell myoblastoma; rhabdomyoma; rhabdomyosarcoma; carcinoma)
14. Ranula; sialocyst
15. Robinow S.
16. Trauma

References

1. Jones KL: Smith's Recognizable Patterns of Human Mal-formation. (ed 3) Philadelphia: WB Saunders, 1988
2. Morfit HM: Lymphangioma of the tongue. Arch Surg 1960;81:761–767
3. Taybi H, Lachman RS: Radiology of Syndromes, Metabolic Disorders, and Skeletal Dysplasias. (ed 4) St. Louis: Mosby-Year Book, 1996

Gamut B-109

MASS IN THE MIDLINE OR AT BASE OF TONGUE

1. Carcinoma (squamous cell) of tongue
2. Dermoid
3. Hemangioma
4. Lingual thyroid

5. Lingual tonsil (esp. with lymphoid hyperplasia)
6. Lymphoma$_g$
7. Metastasis
8. Ranula, atypical
9. Schwannoma
10. Thyroglossal duct cyst

References

1. Douglas PS, Baker AW: Lingual thyroid. Brit J Oral Maxillofac Surg 1994;32:123–124
2. Giovagnorio F, Cordier A, Romeo R: Lingual thyroid: value of integrated imaging. Europ Radiol 1996;6:105–107
3. Hsu CY, Wang SJ: Thyroid hemiagenesis accompanying an ectopic sublingual thyroid. Clin Nucl Med 1994;19:546
4. Jayaram G, Kakar A, Prakash R: Papillary carcinoma arising in sublingual ectopic thyroid concentrating both Tc-99m pertechnetate and I-131. Diagnosis by fine needle aspiration cytology. Clin Nucl Med 1995;20:381–383
5. Lufkin R, Borges A, Villablanca P: Teaching Atlas of Head and Neck Imaging. New York: Thieme, 2000, pp 233–236, 247–251
6. Teresi LM, et al: Chapter 36. In: Stark DD, Bradley WG (eds): Magnetic Resonance Imaging. (ed 2) St. Louis: Mosby, 1992
7. Vogl T, Mees K, Muhling M, Lissner J: Magnetic resonance imaging in diagnosing diseases of the neck. Hospimedica 1987;Jan–Feb:17–23
8. Vogl T, Brüning R, Grevers G, et al: MR imaging of the oropharynx and tongue: comparison of plain and Gd-DTPA studies. J Comput Assist Tomogr 1988;12:427–433

Gamut B-110

CYSTIC FLOOR OF THE MOUTH MASS

1. Abscess/bacterial cellulitis (Vincent's angina)
2. Branchial cleft cyst, atypical
3. Dermoid cyst; epidermoid
4. Lymphangioma (cystic hygroma)
5. Necrotic neoplasm
6. Ranula (simple or plunging)
7. Salivary gland neoplasm, cystic
8. Thyroglossal duct cyst

References

1. Batsakis JG: Tumors of the Head and Neck. Clinical and Pathological Considerations. (ed 2) Baltimore: Williams & Wilkins, 1979, pp 226–228

2. Coit WE, et al: Ranulas and their mimics: CT evaluation. Radiology 1987;163:211–216
3. Davidson HD, Ouchi T, Steiner RE: NMR imaging of congenital intracranial germinal layer neoplasms. Neuroradiology 1985;27:301–303
4. Davison MJ, Morton RP, McIvor NP: Plunging ranula: clinical observations. Head and Neck 1998;20:63–68
5. Dillon WP, Miller EM: Cervical soft tissues. In: Newton TH, Hasso AN, Dillon WP (eds), Modern Neuroradiology, vol. 3: Computed Tomography of the Head and Neck. New York: Raven Press, 1988,11.31–11.33
6. Garcia CJ, Flores PA, Arce JD, Chuaqui B, Schwartz DS: Ultrasonography in the study of salivary gland lesions in children. Pediatr Radiol 1998;28:418–425
7. Hunter TB, Palplanus SH, Chernin MM, Coulthara SW: Dermoid cyst of the floor of the mouth: CT appearance. AJR 1983;141:1239–1240
8. Lufkin R, Borges A, Villablanca P: Teaching Atlas of Head and Neck Imaging. New York: Thieme, 2000, pp 237–240, 241–243

Gamut B-111

LESIONS OF THE HYPOPHARYNX, LARYNX, AND UPPER TRACHEA

COMMON

1. Carcinoma of hypopharynx (esp. in pyriform sinus, posterolateral wall, or postcricoid)
2. Carcinoma of larynx (See B-119)
3. Congenital (eg, tracheoesophageal fistula; atresia; hypoplasia; web; stenosis; laryngomalacia)
4. Epiglottic enlargement (esp. epiglottitis) (See B-114)
5. Foreign body
6. Hemangioma, esp. subglottic in children
7. Infection (eg, *Clostridium tetani;* tuberculosis; fungus disease—esp. candidiasis)
8. Juvenile papillomatosis
9. Laryngocele (esp. in glassblowers or musicians, or with chronic coughing)
10. Papilloma, squamous cell (solitary)
11. Polyp
12. Retropharyngeal abscess
13. Tracheal tumor

(continued)

14. Trauma (incl. intubation)
15. Vocal cord paralysis (eg, involvement of recurrent laryngeal nerve by malignancy; trauma; congenital)
16. Zenker's diverticulum

UNCOMMON

1. Adenoma
2. Amyloidosis
3. Benign neoplasm of larynx (eg, chondroma; angiofibroma; fibroma; myoma; lipoma; paraganglioma; neurofibroma) (See B-119)
4. Cyst
5. Kaposi sarcoma
6. Lymphoma$_g$
7. Metastasis
8. Midline granuloma
9. Plasmacytoma
10. Rhinoscleroma
11. Sarcoidosis
12. Sarcoma
13. Wegener's granulomatosis

References
1. Unger JM: Handbook of Head and Neck Imaging. New York: Churchill Livingstone, 1987, pp 100–135
2. Vogl TJ: Chapter 38. In: Stark DD, Bradley WG (eds): Magnetic Resonance Imaging. (ed 2) St. Louis: CV Mosby, 1992

Gamut B-112

VALLECULAR MASS

CYSTIC

1. Dermoid; teratoma
2. Laryngocele
3. Lymphangioma (cystic hygroma)
4. Thyroglossal duct cyst
5. Tongue base cyst
6. Vallecular cyst

SOLID

1. Carcinoma (squamous cell)
2. Ectopic thyroid
3. Hemangioma

References
1. Lufkin R, Borges A, Villablanca P: Teaching Atlas of Head and Neck Imaging. New York: Thieme, 2000; pp 50–53.
2. Wang CR, Lim KE: Vallecular cysts: report of two cases. Pediatr Radiol 1995;25(Suppl 1):S218–S219
3. Wong KS, Li HY, Huang TS: Vallecular cyst synchronous with laryngomalacia, presentation of two cases. Otolaryngol Head Neck Surg 1995;13:621–624

Gamut B-113

PYRIFORM SINUS MASS

1. Carcinoma of pyriform sinus
2. Lymphoma$_g$
3. Mesenchymal tumor
4. Metastasis
5. Postoperative scarring
6. Postradiation edema

References
1. Allal AS: Cancer of the pyriform sinus: trends towards conservative treatment. Bull Cancer 1997;84:757–762
2. Elias MM, Hilgers FJ, Keus RB, et al: Carcinoma of the pyriform sinus: a retrospective analysis of treatment results over a 20-year period. Clin Otolaryngol 1995;20:249–253
3. Larsson SV, Mancuso A, Hoover L, Hanafee W: Differentiation of pyriform sinus cancer from supraglottic laryngeal cancer by computed tomography. Radiology 1981;141:427–432
4. Lufkin R, Borges A, Villablanca P: Teaching Atlas of Head and Neck Imaging. New York: Thieme, 2000; pp 66–68

Gamut B-114

EPIGLOTTIC ENLARGEMENT

COMMON

1. Epiglottitis (esp. Haemophilus influenzae, type B)

UNCOMMON

1. Allergy (esp. angioneurotic edema; drug reaction)
2. Amyloidosis
3. Bleeding disorder (esp. hemophilia)
4. Carcinoma (squamous cell)
5. Congenital aryepiglottic enlargement
6. Congenital "omega" epiglottis
7. Edematous reaction to foreign body, hot air, or smoke
8. Hypothyroidism
9. Infection, other (eg, tuberculosis; sarcoidosis; candidiasis {moniliasis}; leishmaniasis; syphilis)
10. Laryngocele, atypical
11. Lye ingestion
12. Neoplasm, other (eg, hemangioma; lymphangioma; lymphoma$_g$)
13. [Pseudothickening of aryepiglottic folds due to buckling caused by poor inspiration or laryngomalacia]
14. Radiation therapy (edema)
15. Retention cyst
16. Trauma (incl. intubation)

[ ] This condition does not actually cause the gamuted imaging finding, but can produce imaging changes that simulate it.

References

1. Barrow HN, Vastola AP, Wang RC: Adult supraglottitis. Otolaryngol Head Neck Surg 1993;109:474–477
2. Dawson KP, Steinberg A, Capaldi N: The lateral radiograph of neck in laryngotracheo-bronchitis (croup). J Quality in Clin Pract 1994;14:39–43
3. Frantz TD, Rasgon BM: Acute epiglottitis, changing epidemiologic pattern. Otolaryngol Head Neck Surg 1993;109: 457–460
4. John SD, Swischuk LE, Kayden Jr CK, Freeman Jr DH: Aryepiglottic fold width in patients with epiglottitis: where should measurements be obtained? Radiology 1994;190: 123–125
5. Kass EG, McFadden EA, Jacobson S, Toohill RJ: Acute epiglottitis in the adult: experience with a seasonal presentation. Laryngoscope 1993;103:841–844
6. Lufkin R, Borges A, Villablanca P: Teaching Atlas of Head and Neck Imaging. New York: Thieme, 2000; pp 35–37
7. Nemzek WR, Katzberg RW, Van Slyke MA, Bickley LS: A reappraisal of the radiologic findings of acute inflammation of the epiglottis and supraglottic structures in adults. AJNR 1995;16:495–502
8. Smith MM, Mukherji SK, Thompson JE, Castillo M: CT in adult supraglottitis. AJNR 1996;17:1355–1358

Gamut B-115

SUPRAGLOTTIC MASS

1. Amyloidosis
2. Carcinoma of larynx (supraglottic)
   a. Anterior carcinoma arising on epiglottis and anterior false cords
   b. Posterolateral carcinoma arising from medial surface of the aryepiglottic folds and the paralaryngeal spaces (marginal tumors)
3. Chondroma
4. Hemangioma
5. Laryngocele
6. Lymphoma$_g$
7. Metastasis
8. Papilloma
9. Posttraumatic deformity (pseudomass)

References

1. Katsounaakis J, Remy H, Vuong T, et al: Impact of magnetic resonance imaging and computed tomography on the staging of laryngeal cancer. Europ Arch Oto-Rhino-Laryngol 1995;252:206–208
2. Larsson SV, Mancuso A, Hoover L, Hanafee W: Differentiation of pyriform sinus cancer from supraglottic laryngeal cancer by computed tomography. Radiology,1981;141: 427–432
3. Lufkin R, Borges A, Villablanca P: Teaching Atlas of Head and Neck Imaging. New York: Thieme, 2000; pp 62–65

(continued)

4. Myers EN, Alvi A: Management of carcinoma of the supra-glottic larynx: evolution, current concepts, and future trends. Laryngoscope 1996;106(Pt 1):559–567
5. Thabet HM, Sessions DG, Gado MH, et al: Comparison of clinical evaluation and computed tomographic diagnostic accuracy for tumors of the larynx and hypopharynx. Laryngoscope 1996;106(Pt 1):589–594

Gamut B-116

PARALARYNGEAL CYSTIC MASS

1. Branchial cleft cyst
2. Congenital laryngeal cyst
3. Cyst of the epiglottis
4. Dermoid; teratoma
5. Laryngocele
6. Lymphangioma (cystic hygroma)
7. Neoplasm with necrosis simulating cyst
8. Thyroglossal duct cyst
9. Vallecular cyst

References
1. Curtin HD: Imaging of the larynx: current concepts. Radiology 1989;173:1–11
2. Lufkin R, Borges A, Villablanca P: Teaching Atlas of Head and Neck Imaging. New York: Thieme, 2000; pp 38–41
3. Teresi LM, Lufkin RB, Hanafee WN: Magnetic resonance imaging of the larynx. Radiol Clin North Am 1989;27:393–406

Gamut B-117

LARYNGEAL ASYMMETRY

1. Arytenoid dislocation
2. Carcinoma of larynx
3. Laryngocele
4. Recurrent laryngeal nerve paralysis
5. Superior laryngeal nerve paralysis
6. Traumatic deformity

References
1. Decker GAG, du Plessis DJ: Lee McGregor's Synopsis of Surgical Anatomy. (ed 12) Bristol: John Wright & Sons, Ltd., 1986, p 372
2. Gacek M, Gacek RR: Cricoarytenoid joint mobility after chronic vocal cord paralysis. Laryngoscope 1996;106(12 Pt 1):1528–1530
3. Jacobs CJ, Harnsberger HR, Lufkin RB, et al: Vagal neuropathy: evaluation with CT and MR imaging. Radiology 1987;164:97–102
4. Tanaka S, Hirano M, Umeno H: Laryngeal behavior in unilateral superior laryngeal nerve paralysis. Ann Otol Rhinol Laryngol 1994;103:93–97

Gamut B-118

ABNORMAL SHAPE OF THE LARYNGEAL CARTILAGE (INCLUDING EXPANSILE OR DESTRUCTIVE LESIONS)

1. Carcinoma of larynx (esp. squamous cell)
*2. Chondroma
*3. Chondrosarcoma
4. Congenital deformity
*5. Metastasis to cartilage (esp.from melanoma; carcinoma of kidney, breast, lung or prostate)
6. Postsurgical changes
*7. Posttraumatic deformity (chronic)
8. Trauma to larynx, acute

* May cause an expansile lesion of laryngeal cartilage.

References
1. Batsakis JF, Luna MA, Byers RM: Metastases to the larynx. Head Neck Surg 1948;5:458–460
2. Bent III JP, Porubsky ES: The management of blunt fractures of the thyroid cartilage. Otolaryngol Head Neck Surg 1994;110:195–202
3. Bogdan CJ, Maniglia AJ, Eliachar I, Katz RL: Chondrosarcoma of the larynx: challenges in diagnosis and management. Head Neck 1994;16:127–134
4. Bough Jr ID, Chiles PJ, Fratalli MA, Vernose G: Laryngeal chondrosarcoma: two unusual cases. Am J Otolaryngol 1995;16:126–131

5. Browne JD: Management of nonepidermoid cancer of the larynx. Otolaryngol Clin North Am 1997;30:215–229
6. Cavicchi O, Farneti G, Occhiuzzi L, Sorrenti G: Laryngeal metastasis from colonic adenocarcinoma. J Laryngol Otol 1990;104:730–732
7. Chui L, Lufkin R, Hanafee W: The use of MRI in the identification of posttraumatic laryngeal deformities. Clin Imag 1990;14:127–130
8. Chui LD, Rasgon BM: Laryngeal chondroma, a benign process with long-term clinical implications. Ear Nose Throat J 1996;75:540–542, 544–549
9. Cullen JR: Ovarian carcinoma metastatic to the larynx. J Laryngol Otol 1990;104:48–49
10. Ferlito A, Caruso G, Recher G: Secondary laryngeal tumors. Arch Otolaryngol Head Neck Surg 1988;114:635–639
11. Fields JA: Renal carcinoma metastasis to larynx. Laryngoscope 1966;76:99–101
12. Grignon DJ, Ro JY, Ayala AG, et al: Carcinoma of the prostate metastasizing to vocal cord. Urology 1990;36:85–88
13. Hanson DG, Mancuso AA, Hanafee WN: Pseudomass lesions due to occult trauma of the larynx. Laryngoscope 1982;92:1249–1253
14. Lewis JE, Olsen KD, Inwards CY: Cartilaginous tumors of the larynx: clinicopathologic review of 47 cases. Ann Otol Rhinol Laryngol 1997;106:94–100
15. Lufkin R, Borges A, Villablanca P: Teaching Atlas of Head and Neck Imaging. New York: Thieme, 2000; pp 46–49, 54–57, 69–71
16. Whicker JH, Carder GA, Devine KD: Metastasis to the larynx: report of a case and review of the literature. Arch Otolaryngol 1972;96:182–184

Gamut B-119

LARYNGEAL TUMOR

COMMON

1. Carcinoma, supraglottic, glottic, or subglottic (esp. squamous cell; occasionally adenocarcinoma or carcinosarcoma)
2. Juvenile papillomatosis

UNCOMMON

1. [Amyloidosis]
2. Benign neoplasm (eg, chondroma; granular cell myoblastoma; plasma cell granuloma; chemodectoma; neurofibroma; angiofibroma; fibroma; myoma; lipoma)
3. Cyst (congenital retention)
4. [Laryngocele]
5. Lymphoma$_g$
6. Metastasis
7. Papilloma, squamous cell (solitary)
8. Polyp
9. Sarcoma (eg, rhabdomyosarcoma; fibrosarcoma)
10. [Subglottic hemangioma or other tumor]
   (See B-122)

[ ] This condition does not actually cause the gamuted imaging finding, but can produce imaging changes that simulate it.

References

1. Hayden CK Jr, Swischuk LE: Head and neck lesions in children. In: Bergeron RT, Osborn AG, Som PM: Head and Neck Imaging Excluding the Brain. St. Louis: CV Mosby, 1984, pp 708–715
2. Unger JM: Handbook of Head and Neck Imaging. New York: Churchill Livingstone, 1987, pp 112–129

Gamut B-120

VOCAL CORD ASYMMETRY

1. Carcinoma of glottis (90% squamous cell)
2. Papilloma of vocal cord
3. Recurrent laryngeal nerve paralysis
4. Teflon injection of vocal cord

References

1. Katsounakis J, Remy H, Vuong T, et al: Impact of magnetic resonance imaging and computed tomography on the staging of laryngeal cancer. Europ Arch Oto-Rhino-Laryngol 1995;252:206–208
2. Lufkin R, Borges A, Villablanca P: Teaching Atlas of Head and Neck Imaging. New York: Thieme, 2000; pp 58–61
3. Mukherji SK, Castillo M, Huda W, et al: Comparison of dynamic and spiral CT for imaging the glottic larynx. J Comput Assist Tomogr 1995;19:899–904
4. Teresi LM, Lufkin RB, Hanafee WN: Magnetic resonance imaging of the larynx. Radiol Clin North Am 1989;27:393–406

(continued)

5. Weinstein GS, Laccourreye O, Brasnu D, Yousem DM: The role of computed tomography and magnetic resonance imaging in planning for conservation laryngeal surgery. Neuroimag Clin North Am 1996;6:497–504

Gamut B-121

PARALYZED OR PARETIC VOCAL CORD

COMMON

1. Aortic aneurysm
2. Carcinoma, metastatic or invasive (esp. thyroid, esophagus, lung, breast)
3. Laryngeal disease (carcinoma; infection)
4. Mediastinal neoplasm (esp. thyroid tumor; lymphoma$_g$)
5. Postoperative (eg, thyroidectomy, radical neck dissection, mediastinal surgery)
6. Recurrent laryngeal nerve pathology (insult to brain stem, skull base, neck, or mediastinum)
7. Superior sulcus tumor
8. Trauma (eg, gunshot wound)

UNCOMMON

1. Arytenoid dislocation
2. Cerebral lesion; Chiari malformation; intracranial tumor; birth injury
3. Diabetic neuropathy
4. Idiopathic
5. Inflammatory lesion within thorax (eg, tuberculosis)
6. Jugular foramen neoplasm
7. Laryngocele
8. Vascular ring

References

1. Glazer HS, Aronberg DJ, Lee JKT, et al: Extralaryngeal causes of vocal cord paraylsis: CT evaluation. AJR 1983;141:527–530
2. Lufkin R, Borges A, Villablanca P: Teaching Atlas of Head and Neck Imaging. New York: Thieme, 2000, pp 42–45

Gamut B-122

SUBGLOTTIC TRACHEAL NARROWING

COMMON

1. Acquired subglottic stenosis (eg, external trauma; hematoma; post-intubation; posttracheostomy fibrosis; postoperative repair of esophageal atresia)
2. Carcinoma
3. Croup (laryngotracheobronchitis)
4. Extrinsic mass, other (eg, paratracheal cyst; goiter; lymphadenopathy; lymphoma$_g$; lymphangioma; localized retropharyngeal abscess)
5. Normal (eg, expiratory collapse {"floppy trachea"}; anterior tracheal indentation in infants)
6. Subglottic hemangioma (esp. infants)
7. Tracheomalacia
8. Vascular compression (eg, right aortic arch; double aortic arch; aberrant left subclavian artery; innominate artery compression S.)

UNCOMMON

1. Amyloidosis
2. Congenital subglottic stenosis (primary tracheal stenosis)
3. Ectopic intratracheal thyroid or thymus tissue; ectopic goiter
4. Epidermolysis bullosa
5. Foreign body aspiration into trachea or esophagus, impacted food
6. Injury to larynx or upper trachea, other (eg, intense heat; smoke; lye; acid)
7. Juvenile papillomatosis
8. Laryngeal web
9. Lipoid proteinosis
10. Radiation therapy
11. Scleroma (rhinoscleroma)
12. Subglottic mass, other (eg, mucocele, inflammatory histiocytoma; lipoma; fibroma; adenoma; polyp; papilloma; polypoid hemangioendothelioma; cyst)
13. Tuberculosis

References
1. Ebel K-D, Blickman H, Willich E, Richter E: Differential Diagnosis in Pediatric Radiology. Stuttgart: Thieme, 1999, pp 9–12
2. Hayden CK Jr, Swischuk LE: Head and neck lesions in children. In: Bergeron RT, Osborn AG, Som PM: Head and Neck Imaging Excluding the Brain. St. Louis: CV Mosby, 1984
3. Swischuk LE, John SD: Differential Diagnosis in Pediatric Radiology. (ed 2) Baltimore: Williams & Wilkins, 1995, pp 126–129

Gamut B-123

UPPER AIRWAY OBSTRUCTION IN A CHILD—ACUTE OR CHRONIC (See B-105-1, 106, 111, 114, 122)

ACUTE

COMMON

1. Abscess (peritonsillar, retropharyngeal, mediastinal)
2. Choanal atresia
3. Croup (laryngotracheobronchitis)
4. Epiglottitis, other epiglottic enlargement (See B-114)
5. Foreign body
6. Laryngeal edema (eg, allergic, anaphylactic, or hereditary angioneurotic edema; inhalation of noxious gases; posttraumatic)
7. Retropharyngeal hemorrhage (eg, bleeding or clotting disorder$_g$; hematoma from trauma or neck surgery)

UNCOMMON

1. Diphtheria
2. Laryngeal spasm (eg, tetany)
3. Ludwig's angina

CHRONIC

COMMON

1. Esophageal atresia; tracheoesophageal fistula
2. Extrinsic mass (eg, neoplasm; thyroid mass; cervical lymphadenopathy; cystic hygroma; thyroglossal duct cyst)
3. Tonsil and adenoid hypertrophy
4. Tracheal mass, intrinsic (eg, subglottic hemangioma; cyst; polyp; hamartochondroma; lipoma; chloroma; scleroma; ectopic thyroid tissue; web) (See F-81-1, F-81-2)
5. Tracheal stricture or stenosis (traumatic; prolonged intubation; postoperative; inflammatory; burn; congenital)
6. Vascular ring (esp. double aortic arch) (See E-21-S); innominate artery compression

UNCOMMON

1. Antrochoanal polyp
2. Cyst of epiglottis or aryepiglottic folds
3. Esophageal neoplasm
4. Laryngeal web
5. Macroglossia (eg, myxedema {hypothyroidism})
6. Micrognathia with glossoptosis (eg, Pierre Robin S. (Robin sequence), Möbius S.; isolated micrognathia)
7. Nasal angiofibroma
8. Papillomatosis
9. Tracheomalacia; laryngomalacia
10. Vocal cord lesion (eg, laryngeal polyp, papilloma, or cyst)

References
1. Dunbar JS: Upper respiratory tract obstruction in infants and children. Caldwell Lecture, 1969. AJR 1970;109:227–246
2. Kushner DC, Clifton Harris GB: Obstructive lesions of the larynx and trachea in infants and children. Radiol Clin North Am 1978;16:181–194
3. Schapiro RL, Evans ET: Surgical disorders causing neonatal respiratory distress. AJR 1972;114:305–321
4. Strife JL: Upper airway and tracheal obstruction in infants and children. Radiol Clin North Am 1988;26:309–322
5. Swischuk LE, John SD: Differential Diagnosis in Pediatric Radiology. (ed 2) Baltimore: Williams & Wilkins, 1995

Spine and Its Contents

C

CONGENITAL SYNDROMES AND BONE DYSPLASIAS WITH VERTEBRAL ABNORMALITY
(See also C-11–17 and C-21–25)

COMMON

1. Achondroplasia (narrow lumbar spinal canal; lower thoracic kyphosis; lumbar lordosis)
2. Acrocephalosyndactyly (Apert, Pfeiffer, and Saethre-Chotzen types) (cervical and lumbar vertebral fusion)
3. Cleidocranial dysplasia (spina bifida; kyphoscoliosis)
4. Cretinism; hypothyroidism (kyphosis; beaked, flat vertebrae)
5. Diastrophic dysplasia (kyphoscoliosis; platyspondyly; narrow lumbar spinal canal)
6. Fanconi anemia (scoliosis; kyphosis; Klippel-Feil S.; spina bifida; sacral agenesis)
7. Fetal alcohol S. (scoliosis; hemivertebrae; Klippel-Feil S.)
8. Holt-Oram S. (scoliosis; fusion; hemivertebrae)
9. Homocystinuria (kyphoscoliosis; osteoporosis; "codfish vertebrae")
10. Hypophosphatasia (osteoporosis with collapsed vertebrae)
11. Klippel-Feil S. (cervical block vertebrae; hemivertebrae; atlantooccipital fusion; atlantoaxial instability; spinal stenosis)
12. Marfan S. (scoliosis; spondylolisthesis)
13. Mucopolysaccharidoses, esp. Morquio S. (See J-4) (atlantoaxial subluxation; narrow spinal canal; kyphoscoliosis)
14. Multiple epiphyseal dysplasia (Fairbank) (hemivertebrae; platyspondyly)
15. Neurofibromatosis (kyphoscoliosis)
16. Noonan S. (scoliosis; kyphosis; Klippel-Feil S.)
17. Osteogenesis imperfecta (scoliosis; fractured vertebrae)
18. Osteopetrosis (dense vertebrae; fractures)
19. Pseudoachondroplasia (kyphoscoliosis)
20. Spondyloepiphyseal dysplasia, all forms (kyphoscoliosis; platyspondyly)
21. Spondylometaphyseal dysplasia (kyphoscoliosis)
22. Thanatophoric dysplasia (platyspondyly; narrow spinal canal)
23. Trisomy 21 S. (Down S.) (atlantoaxial subluxation)

UNCOMMON

1. Achondrogenesis, types I and II (lumbar vertebrae et al. appear absent)
2. Acrodysostosis (peripheral dysostosis) (narrow spinal canal)
3. Aicardi S. (block vertebrae; hemivertebrae; spina bifida; scoliosis; Arnold-Chiari malformation)
4. Alagille S. (arteriohepatic S.) (butterfly vertebrae; narrow spinal canal)
5. Atelosteogenesis (coronal and sagittal clefts; thoracic vertebral hypoplasia; platyspondyly; scoliosis)
6. Binder S. (cervical spine anomalies with kyphosis or scoliosis; spina bifida; block vertebrae)
7. Brachyolmia (scoliosis; platyspondyly with square or round edges; narrow disk spaces)
8. Campomelic dysplasia (hypoplastic cervical spine; kyphosis)
9. Caudal dysplasia sequence (variable vertebral agenesis in lumbosacral spine; tethered cord; diastematomyelia; lipoma; syringomyelia)
10. CHILD S. (scoliosis; hemivertebrae; fused vertebrae)
11. Chondrodysplasia punctata (kyphoscoliosis; atlantoaxial subluxation)
12. Cockayne S. (ovoid, biconcave or scalloped vertebrae; kyphosis; intervertebral calcification)
13. Crouzon S. (craniofacial dysostosis) (craniocervical junction abnormalities)
14. Currarino triad (sacral hypoplasia with anterior meningocele or teratoma; tethered cord)
15. de la Chapelle dysplasia (small vertebrae; platyspondyly)
16. Dysosteosclerosis (platyspondyly)
17. Dyssegmental dysplasia (short spine; ovoid or misshapen vertebrae)
18. Dysspondylochondromaosis (kyphoscoliosis; hemivertebrae; anisospondyly)

(continued)

19. Ehlers-Danlos S. (scoliosis; spondylolisthesis)
20. Enchondromatosis (Ollier's disease) (kyphoscoliosis)
21. Femoral hypoplasia—unusual facies S. (missing or hemivertebrae; scoliosis; sacral dysplasia)
22. Freeman-Sheldon S. (whistling face S.)
23. Geroderma osteodysplastica (platyspondyly)
24. GM$_1$ gangliosidosis; fucosidosis (platyspondyly)
25. Goltz S. (focal dermal hypoplasia) (scoliosis; vertebral malsegmentation)
26. Gorlin S. (nevoid basal cell carcinoma S.) (kyphoscoliosis; multiple anomalies)
27. Hajdu-Cheney S. (idiopathic acro-osteolysis) (kyphoscoliosis; osteoporosis)
28. Hallermann-Streiff S. (oculo-mandibulo-facial S.) (spina bifida)
29. Hyperphosphatasia (scoliosis, biconcave vertebrae)
30. Hypochondroplasia (narrow spinal canal; lordosis; platyspondyly)
31. Incontinentia pigmenti (scoliosis; vertebral anomalies)
32. Kniest dysplasia (platyspondyly; lordosis; kyphoscoliosis; narrow spinal canal)
33. Larsen S. (cervical kyphosis)
34. LEOPARD S. (kyphoscoliosis with cervical and posterior spinal fusion)
35. Marshall S. (platyspondyly)
36. Metaphyseal chondrodysplasia (Jansen and McKusick types) (atlantoaxial instability)
37. Metatropic dysplasia (kyphoscoliosis; platyspondyly; atlantoaxial subluxation)
38. Multiple pterygium S. (scoliosis; multiple vertebral anomalies)
39. Nail-patella S. (osteo-onychodysplasia) (spina bifida)
40. Narrow lumbar spinal canal S.
41. Oculo-auriculo-vertebral spectrum (Goldenhar S.) (hemivertebrae; block vertebrae; Klippel-Feil S.; spina bifida)
42. Oculovertebral S. (hemivertebrae; block vertebrae)
43. Osteodysplasty (Melnick-Needles S.) (tall vertebrae with anterior concavity)
44. Osteoglophonic dwarfism (platyspondyly; narrow spinal canal)
45. Otopalatodigital S. (posterior spinal defects)
46. Parastremmatic dysplasia (kyphoscoliosis; platyspondyly)
47. Patterson S. (cervical platyspondyly; ovoid thoracic and lumbar vertebrae)
48. Poland sequence (scoliosis; vertebral anomalies)
49. Popliteal pterygium S. (spina bifida)
50. Prader-Willi S. (scoliosis; kyphosis; osteoporosis)
51. Progeria (osteoporosis; infantile, ovoid vertebrae)
52. Pyle dysplasia (familial metaphyseal dysplasia) (platyspondyly)
53. Robin sequence (Pierre Robin S.) (occipito-atlanto-axial hypermobility with arch defects of atlas)
54. Robinow S. (hemivertebrae; vertebral fusions)
55. Rothmund-Thomson S. (flat, elongated vertebrae)
56. Rubinstein-Taybi S. (odontoid hypoplasia; C1-C2 instability; vertebral anomalies)
57. Schwartz-Jampel S. (osteochondromuscular dystrophy) (kyphoscoliosis; platyspondyly)
58. Seckel S. (bird-headed dwarfism) (kyphoscoliosis)
59. Shawl scrotum S. (hypoplastic C1; subluxation C1-C2)
60. Short rib-polydactyly syndromes (misshapen, poorly ossified vertebrae; coronal clefts)
61. Smith-McCort S. (platyspondyly)
62. Split notochord S. (spina bifida anterior and posterior; split cord; spinal cord and nerve defects; neuroenteric cyst)
63. Sponastrine dysplasia
64. Spondylocarpotarsal fusion S. (scoliosis; vertebral fusion; narrow disks)
65. Spondylocostal dysostosis (Jarcho-Levine S.) (fused, absent, butterfly, or hemivertebrae; kyphoscoliosis)
66. Spondyloepimetaphyseal dysplasia (kyphoscoliosis)
67. Spondyloperipheral dysplasia (platyspondyly)
68. Stickler S. (arthro-ophthalmopathy) (kyphoscoliosis; irregular end plates with anterior wedging of vertebrae; cervical spine stenosis and myelopathy)
69. Tethered cord S. (numerous anomalies in lower spine)
70. Trisomy 13 S. (spina bifida)
71. Trisomy 18 S. (kyphoscoliosis; meningomyelocele)

72. VATER association (cervical kyphosis; Klippel-Feil S.)
73. Wildervanck S. (cervico-oculo-acoustic S.) (cervical segmentation malformation)
74. Williams S. (idiopathic hypercalcemia) (dense vertebrae; kyphoscoliosis)

References

1. Felson B, (ed): Dwarfs and other little people. Semin Roentgenol 1973;8:258–259
2. Jones KL: Smith's Recognizable Patterns of Human Malformation. Philadelphia: WB Saunders, 1988
3. Kozlowski K, Beighton P: Gamut Index of Skeletal Dysplasias. Berlin: Springer-Verlag, 1984, p 41
4. Taybi H, Lachman RS: Radiology of Syndromes, Metabolic Disorders, and Skeletal Dysplasias. (ed 4) St. Louis: Mosby-Year Book Inc., 1996, pp 1045–1048

Gamut C-2-S

NONSPINAL CONDITIONS ASSOCIATED WITH VERTEBRAL ANOMALIES

COMMON

1. Cloacal abnormality
2. Congenital heart disease
3. Genitourinary abnormality
4. Imperforate anus (sacral)
5. Maternal diabetes
6. Neurofibromatosis
7. Sprengel's deformity

UNCOMMON

1. Aplasia or hypoplasia of lung
2. Neurenteric cyst; duplication cyst
3. Venolobar S. (eg, scimitar S.; lobar agenesis)

Gamut C-3-1

KYPHOSIS

COMMON

1. Congenital spinal anomaly (eg, fused vertebrae; hemivertebra; spina bifida with meningocele; bony bar)
2. Congenital syndromes (esp. achondroplasia; other osteochondrodysplasias; storage diseases; neurofibromatosis) (See C-1)
3. Fracture, traumatic or pathologic; dislocation
4. Idiopathic
5. Infection (eg, spinal osteomyelitis or tuberculosis (Pott's disease))
6. Neoplasm of spine, primary or metastatic; multiple myeloma
7. Neuromuscular disorder$_g$ with hypotonia (eg, cerebral palsy; muscular dystrophy; myasthenia gravis)
8. [Normal in infants (thoracolumbar; C2-3 angulation)]
9. Osteoporosis (esp. juvenile, senile or post-menopausal) (See D-43-1)
10. Paget's disease
11. Paralysis (eg, poliomyelitis; paraplegia)
12. Posture, faulty or occupational (upper thoracic; changes with position)
13. Rheumatoid or ankylosing spondylitis
14. Scheuermann disease (juvenile kyphosis)

UNCOMMON

1. Acromegaly; excessive endocrine growth
2. Charcot spine; neuropathic osteoarthropathy
3. Cretinism; hypothyroidism
4. Generalized weakness
5. Hyperparathyroidism (primary)
6. Osteomalacia; rickets
7. Radiation therapy atrophy
8. Syringomyelia
9. Tuberous sclerosis

[ ] This condition does not actually cause the gamuted imaging finding, but can produce imaging changes that simulate it.

(continued)

References
1. Resnick D: Diagnosis of Bone and Joint Disorders. (ed 3) Philadelphia: WB Saunders, 1995, pp 3413–3442, 4245–4268
2. Schmorl G, Junghanns H: The Human Spine in Health and Disease. (ed 2) New York: Grune and Stratton, 1971, pp 344–362

Gamut C-3-2

CERVICAL KYPHOSIS

1. Binder S.
2. Burton S.
3. Campomelic dysplasia
4. Compression fracture
5. Desbuquois dysplasia
6. Diastrophic dysplasia
7. Larsen S.
8. Metnick-Needles S. (lethal variety)
9. Neurofibromatosis type 1
10. Pseudodiastrophic dysplasia
11. Retropharyngeal abscess

References
1. Gorlin RJ, Cohen MM, Jr, Levin LS: Syndromes of the Head and Neck. (ed 3) New York: Oxford University Press, 1990, pp 181, 813
2. Taybi H, Lachman RS: Radiology of Syndromes, Metabolic Disorders, and Skeletal Dysplasias. (ed 4) St. Louis: Mosby-Year Book, Inc, 1996, p 1046

Gamut C-3-3

THORACOLUMBAR GIBBUS

ACQUIRED

1. Compression fracture
2. Infantile multisystem inflammatory disease (NOMID)
3. Langerhans cell histiocytosis$_g$ (esp. eosinophilic granuloma)

4. Neoplasm of spine, primary or metastatic
5. Pyogenic osteomyelitis
6. Scheuermann disease, severe
7. Tuberculous spondylitis (Pott's disease)

CONGENITAL

1. Achondroplasia
2. Coffin-Lowry S.
3. GM$_1$ gangliosidosis; fucosidosis
4. Hypothyroidism (cretinism)
5. Mucolipidosis II (Leroy's I-cell disease)
6. Mucopolysaccharidoses (Hurler S.; Hunter S.; Maroteaux-Lamy S.)

References
1. Taybi H, Lachman RS: Radiology of Syndromes, Metabolic Disorders, and Skeletal Dysplasias. (ed 4) St. Louis: Mosby-Year Book, Inc, 1996

Gamut C-4

SCOLIOSIS

COMMON

1. Chest wall abnormality (eg, asymmetric chest; congenital rib anomalies; Sprengel deformity)
2. Congenital spinal anomaly (eg, fusion of posterior elements; unilateral bar; meningomyelocele; segmentation anomaly; wedge vertebra; hemivertebra; Klippel-Feil S.)
3. Congenital syndromes (esp. Ehlers-Danlos S.; fetal alcohol S.; Marfan S.; homocystinuria; osteogenesis imperfecta; campomelic dysplasia; storage diseases; neurofibromatosis; Proteus S.) (See C-1)
4. Degenerative spondylosis
5. Degenerative disc disease
6. Idiopathic
7. Infection (eg, spinal tuberculosis, osteomyelitis)
8. Leg shortening or amputation; pelvic tilt; foot deformity

9. Neoplasm, intraspinal or extraspinal, primary or metastatic; multiple myeloma
10. Neuromuscular disorder$_g$ with hypotonia (eg, cerebral palsy; muscular dystrophy; Friedreich's ataxia; myotonic dystrophy)
11. Osteoporosis (See D-43-1)
12. Paralysis (eg, poliomyelitis; paraplegia; hemiparesis; hemiplegia)
13. Postoperative (eg, thoracoplasty; pneumonectomy)
14. [Postural; changes with position]
15. Pulmonary or pleural disease, unilateral (eg, fibrosis; fibrothorax; empyema; hypoplastic lung)
16. Spasm (eg, retroperitoneal, psoas, or abdominal abscess, inflammation, or hemorrhage; ureteral or renal calculus)
17. Trauma (fracture; subluxation)

UNCOMMON

1. Congenital heart disease (eg, ASD; tetralogy)
2. Hyperparathyroidism (primary)
3. Neurenteric cyst; duplication cyst
4. Osteoid osteoma
5. Radiation therapy atrophy
6. Rickets
7. Syringomyelia

[ ] This condition does not actually cause the gamuted imaging finding, but can produce imaging changes that simulate it.

References

1. Resnick D: Diagnosis of Bone and Joint Disorders. (ed 3) Philadelphia: WB Saunders, 1995, pp 4245–4268
2. Schmorl G, Junghanns H: The Human Spine in Health and Disease. (ed 2) New York: Grune and Stratton, 1971, pp 364–374

PARASPINAL SOFT TISSUE MASS
(See F-90, F-99)

COMMON

1. Abscess
2. Aortic aneurysm; tortuous aorta
3. Esophageal dilatation; achalasia
4. Hematoma, traumatic or spontaneous
5. [Hiatal hernia]
6. Idiopathic; anatomic variant
7. Lymphadenopathy, any cause
8. Lymphoma$_g$; leukemia
9. Metastatic neoplasm
10. Multiple myeloma
11. Neurogenic tumor (neurofibroma; neurilemmoma; ganglioneuroma; neuroblastoma; malignant peripheral nerve sheath tumor; neurofibromatosis with neurofibroma or dural estasia); intraspinal tumor of hourglass type
12. Osteoarthritis (spondylosis deformans); other arthritis with spur formation; DISH; extruded disk
13. Osteomyelitis of spine with abscess (eg, tuberculous, sarcoid, fungal, brucellar, *Salmonella,* other bacterial); nonspecific spondylitis
14. Pleural effusion; empyema
15. [Pneumonia; atelectasis]

UNCOMMON

1. Amyloidosis
2. Bochdalek hernia
3. Bronchogenic cyst
4. Chemodectoma
5. Dilated azygos system (eg, superior or inferior vena cava obstruction); mediastinal varices
6. Langerhans cell histiocytosis$_g$ (esp. eosinophilic granuloma of vertebra)
7. Extramedullary hematopoiesis (esp. in thalassemia)
8. Fibromatosis
9. Hydatid disease
10. Hydroureter; retrocaval ureter
11. Meningocele (all types)

(continued)

12. Mesothelioma
13. Mustard operation for transposition of great vessels
14. Neoplasm of spine, primary (eg, giant cell tumor; chordoma; sarcoma)
15. Neurenteric cyst; duplication cyst
16. Other posterior mediastinal or retroperitoneal neoplasm (See F-90)
17. Paget's disease
18. Pancreatic pseudocyst or neoplasm
19. Pheochromocytoma; other adrenal neoplasm
20. Retroperitoneal fibrosis
21. Rhabdomyosarcoma; other soft tissue sarcoma
22. Sequestration, extrapulmonary
23. Splenosis
24. Thoracic kidney

[ ] This condition does not actually cause the gamuted imaging finding, but can produce imaging changes that simulate it.

References

1. Gupta SK, Mohan V: The thoracic paraspinal line: Further significance. Clin Radiol 1979;30:329–335
2. Greenfield GB: Radiology of Bone Diseases. (ed 5) Philadelphia: Lippincott, 1990
3. Kransdorf MJ, Murphey MD: Imaging of Soft Tissue Tumors. Philadelphia: WB Saunders, 1997
4. Polansky SM, Culham JAG: Paraspinal densities developing after repair of transposition of the great arteries. AJR 1980;134:394–396

Gamut C-6-S1

CERVICAL SPINE INJURIES: MECHANISM OF INJURY

FLEXION

1. Anterior subluxation (hyperflexion sprain)
2. Bilateral interfacetal dislocation
3. Clay-shoveler's fracture
4. Flexion teardrop fracture
5. Simple wedge fracture

FLEXION—ROTATION

1. Rotatory dislocation with interlocking
2. Unilateral interfacetal dislocation or fracture-dislocation

EXTENSION—ROTATION

1. Pillar fracture
2. Pedicolaminar fracture separation

VERTICAL COMPRESSION

1. Burst fracture
   a. Burst fracture of lower cervical vertebrae
   b. Fracture of occipital condyle
   c. Jefferson fracture of atlas

EXTENSION

1. Avulsion fracture anterior arch of atlas
2. Extension teardrop fracture
3. Hyperextension dislocation or fracture-dislocation
4. Laminar fracture
5. Posterior dislocation of atlas with fractured odontoid
6. Posterior neural arch fracture of atlas
7. Spinous process fracture
8. Traumatic spondylolisthesis; hangman's fracture (deceleration; hyperextension)

LATERAL FLEXION

1. Jefferson fracture, asymmetric (Jefferson variant)
2. Lateral compression fracture
3. Occipital condyle fracture
4. Transverse process fracture
5. Uncinate process fracture

COMPLEX OR POORLY UNDERSTOOD MECHANISM

1. Acute traumatic transverse atlantal ligament rupture
2. Occipitoatlantal dissociation
3. Odontoid fracture
4. Rotary subluxation/fixation C1-2 (torticollis)
5. Acute traumatic rotary atlantoaxial dissociation

References
1. Bonakdarpour A: Cervical Spine Trauma. American Roentgen Ray Society Refresher Course, Washington, 1986
2. Daffner D: Imaging of Vertebral Trauma. (ed 2) Philadelphia: Lippincott Williams & Wilkins, 1998
3. Harris JH Jr, Mirvis SE: The Radiology of Acute Cervical Spine Trauma. (ed 3) Baltimore: Williams & Wilkins, 1996
4. Kattan KR: Trauma and No-trauma of the Cervical Spine. Springfield, IL: CC Thomas, 1975
5. Murphey MD, Batnitsky S, Bramble JM: Diagnostic imaging of spinal trauma. Radiol Clin North Am 1989;27: 855–872

References
1. Bonakdarpour A: Cervical Spine Trauma. American Roentgen Ray Society Refresher Course, Washington, 1986
2. Daffner D: Imaging of Vertebral Trauma. (ed 2) Philadelphia: Lippincott Williams & Wilkins, 1998
3. Harris JH Jr, Mirvis SE: The Radiology of Acute Cervical Spine Trauma. (ed 3) Baltimore: Williams & Wilkins, 1996
4. Kattan KR: Trauma and No-trauma of the Cervical Spine. Springfield, IL: CC Thomas, 1975
5. Murphey MD, Batnitsky S, Bramble JM: Diagnostic imaging of spinal trauma. Radiol Clin North Am 1989;27: 855–872

Gamut C-6-S2

CERVICAL SPINE INJURIES: STABILITY

STABLE

1. Anterior subluxation
2. Avulsion of anterior arch of C1
3. Burst fracture (lower cervical vertebrae)
4. Clay-shoveler's fracture
5. Laminar fracture
6. Pillar fracture
7. Posterior neural arch fracture of atlas
8. Simple wedge fracture
9. Spinous process fracture
10. Torticollis
11. Unilateral interfacetal dislocation

UNSTABLE

1. Bilateral interfacetal dislocation
2. Extension teardrop fracture (stable in flexion, unstable in extension)
3. Flexion teardrop fracture
4. Hyperextension dislocation and fracture-dislocation
5. Jefferson fracture of atlas
6. Occipitoatlantal dissociation
7. Odontoid fracture (all types)
8. Pedicolaminar fracture separation
9. Traumatic spondylolisthesis (hangman's fracture)

Gamut C-6-S3

RADIOLOGIC SIGNS OF SPINE INSTABILITY

1. Loss of vertebral height (<25% cervical spine; >50% dorsolumbar spine)
2. Vertebral displacement > 2mm
3. Widened interlaminar space (>2mm than levels above or below)
4. Widened interspinous space (>2mm than levels above or below)
5. Widened facet joints (>2mm than levels above or below)
6. Widened interpedicular distance (>2mm than levels above or below)
7. Disruption of posterior vertebral body line
8. Focal narrowing or widening of intervertebral disc space
9. Focal angulation >11N (cervical spine)

Reference
1. Daffner R: Imaging of Vertebral Trauma. Philadelphia: Lippincott-Raven, 1996

Gamut C-7-1

ATLANTOAXIAL SUBLUXATION OR INSTABILITY

COMMON

1. Incompetence of transverse atlantoaxial ligament (congenital, traumatic, or hyperemic condition)
2. [Normal widening of C1-dens distance in children (up to 4–5 mm)]
3. Rheumatoid arthritis; juvenile chronic arthritis
4. Occipitalization of atlas
5. Trauma (with fracture of odontoid or torn transverse ligaments)

UNCOMMON

1. Absent anterior arch of atlas
2. Absent, hypoplastic, or separate odontoid process (os odontoideum)
3. Arthritis, other—with laxity of transverse ligament or erosion of odontoid (eg, ankylosing spondylitis; psoriatic arthritis; Reiter S.; gout)
4. Atlantooccipital fusion
5. Behçet S.
6. Block vertebra C2-C3
7. Calcium pyrophosphate dihydrate deposition disease (CPPD)
8. Collagen vascular disease$_g$ (lupus erythematosus; scleroderma; CREST S.)
9. Congenital syndromes (esp. trisomy 21 S. {Down S.}; Morquio S.; other storage diseases; Marfan S.) (See C-7-2)
10. Infection, esp. in children (eg, retropharyngeal or nasopharyngeal infection or abscess; mastoiditis; parotitis; cervical adenitis; tooth abscess)
11. Tuberculosis

[ ] This condition does not actually cause the gamuted imaging finding, but can produce imaging changes that simulate it.

References

1. Dähnert W: Radiology Review Manual. (ed 4) Baltimore: Williams & Wilkins, 1999, p 148
2. Elliott S: The odontoid process in children—is it hypoplastic? Clin Radiol 1988;39:391–393
3. Kattan KR: Trauma and No-trauma of the Cervical Spine. Springfield, IL: CC Thomas, 1975
4. Koss JC, Dalinka MK: Atlantoaxial subluxation in Behçet's syndrome. AJR 1980;134:392–393
5. Martel W: The occipito-atlanto-axial joints in rheumatoid arthritis and ankylosing spondylitis. AJR 1961;86:223–240
6. Resnick D: Diagnosis of Bone and Joint Disorders. (ed 3) Philadelphia: WB Saunders, 1995
7. Swischuk LE, John SD: Differential Diagnosis in Pediatric Radiology. (ed 2) Baltimore: Williams & Wilkins, 1995, pp 442–443
8. Wortzman G, Dewar FP: Rotary fixation of the atlantoaxial joint: rotational atlantoaxial subluxation. Radiology 1968; 90:479–487

Gamut C-7-2

CONGENITAL SYNDROMES AND BONE DYSPLASIAS WITH ATLANTOAXIAL SUBLUXATION OR INSTABILITY*

COMMON

1. Chondrodysplasia punctata (Conradi-Hönermann type)
2. [Congenital anomalies (eg, absent anterior arch of atlas; incompetence of transverse atlantoaxial ligament; odontoid anomalies)]
3. Marfan S.
4. Mucopolysaccharidosis (eg, Morquio S.) (See J-4)
5. Trisomy 21 S. (Down S.)

UNCOMMON

1. Aarskog S.
2. Campomelic dysplasia
3. Diastrophic dysplasia
4. Dyggve-Melchior-Clausen dysplasia (Smith-McCort S.)
5. Grisel S.
6. Hypochondrogenesis
7. Klippel-Feil S.
8. Metaphyseal chondrodysplasia (McKusick type)

9. Metatropic dysplasia
10. Mucolipidosis III (pseudo-Hurler polydystrophy)
11. Neurofibromatosis I
12. Opsismodysplasia
13. Patterson S.
14. Pseudoachondroplasia
15. Spondyloepimetaphyseal dysplasia (Strudwick and short limb-hand types)
16. Spondyloepiphyseal dysplasia congenita and tarda
17. Spondylometaphyseal dysplasia
18. Winchester S.

* Congenital laxity of ligaments and associated hypoplasia of dens and C1.
[ ] This condition does not actually cause the gamuted imaging finding, but can produce imaging changes that simulate it.

References

1. Rosenbaum DM, Blumhagen JD, King HA: Atlanto-occipital instability in Down syndrome. AJR 1986;146:1269–1272
2. Swischuk LE, John SD: Differential Diagnosis in Pediatric Radiology. (ed 2) Baltimore: Williams & Wilkins, 1995, pp 442–443
3. Taybi H, Lachman RS: Radiology of Syndromes, Metabolic Disorders, and Skeletal Dysplasias. (ed 4) St. Louis: Mosby-Year Book Inc., 1996, pp 1045–1046

Gamut C-8

ODONTOID (DENS) ABSENCE, HYPOPLASIA, FRAGMENTATION OR EROSION

COMMON

1. Arthritis (eg, rheumatoid; gout; psoriasis; ankylosing spondylitis; lupus erythematosus)
2. Craniovertebral junction anomaly (eg, occipitalization of atlas; atlantoaxial fusion; os odontoideum)
3. Klippel-Feil S.
4. Morquio S.
5. Trauma (eg, resorption after cervical spine trauma in infancy)
6. Trisomy 21 S. (Down S.)

UNCOMMON

1. Aarskog S.
2. Campomelic dysplasia
3. Chondrodysplasia punctata (Conradi-Hönermann type and others)
4. CREST S.
5. Diastrophic dysplasia
6. Dyggve-Melchior-Clausen dysplasia
7. Gorlin S. (nevoid basal cell carcinoma S.)
8. Kniest dysplasia
9. Marshall-Smith S.
10. Metaphyseal chondrodysplasia (McKusick type)
11. Metastasis
12. Metatropic dysplasia
13. Microcephalic osteodysplastic dysplasia
14. Mucopolysaccharidoses, other (esp. Hurler S.; Maroteaux-Lamy S.); mucolipidosis II (I-cell disease) and III (pseudo-Hurler polydystrophy); fucosidosis (See J-4)
15. Multiple epiphyseal dysplasia (Fairbank)
16. Patterson S.
17. Rubenstein-Taybi S.
18. Smith-McCort S.
19. Spondyloepimetaphyseal dysplasias
20. Spondyloepiphyseal dysplasia congenita and tarda
21. Tuberculous spondylitis

References

1. Elliott S: The odontoid process in children—is it hypoplastic? Clin Radiol 1988;39:391–393
2. Epstein BS: The Spine. Philadelphia: Lea & Febiger, 1976
3. Garber JN: Abnormalities of the atlas and axis vertebrae—congenital and traumatic. J Bone Joint Surg 1964;46A:1782–1791
4. Gwinn JL, Smith JL: Acquired and congenital absence of the odontoid process. AJR 1962;88:424–431
5. Kozlowski K, Beighton P: Gamut Index of Skeletal Dysplasias. Berlin: Springer-Verlag, 1984, p 47
6. Resnick D: Diagnosis of Bone and Joint Disorders. (ed 3) Philadelphia: WB Saunders, 1995, pp 866–870
7. Schlesinger S: Small or hypoplastic dens. Semin Roentgenol 1986;21:241–242
8. Swischuk LE, John SD: Differential Diagnosis in Pediatric Radiology. (ed 2) Baltimore: Williams & Wilkins, 1995, pp 441–442

(continued)

9. Taybi H, Lachman RS: Radiology of Syndromes, Metabolic Disorders, and Skeletal Dysplasias. (ed 4) St. Louis: Mosby-Year Book Inc., 1996, p 1046
10. Wackenheim A: Roentgen Diagnosis of the Craniovertebral Region. Berlin: Springer-Verlag, 1974, pp 363–366

2. Resnick D: Diagnosis of Bone and Joint Disorders. (ed 3) Philadelphia: WB Saunders, 1995, pp 4245–4268
3. Shapiro R, Robinson F: Anomalies of the craniovertebral border. AJR 1976;127:281–287

Gamut C-9-1

CRANIOVERTEBRAL JUNCTION ABNORMALTTY—CONGENITAL

BONE ABNORMALITY, ASYMPTOMATIC

1. Asymmetric atlantoaxial joint
2. Asymmetric atlanto-occipital joint
3. Posterior arch of atlas defect
4. Rachischisis of C-1
5. Third occipital (tertiary) condyle

BONE ABNORMALITY, SYMPTOM-PRODUCING

1. Atlantoaxial fusion or malsegmentation
2. Atlantooccipital fusion (occipitalization of atlas); hypoplasia of occipital condyle
3. Basilar invagination (See A-12)
4. Crouzon S. (craniofacial dysostosis)
5. Odontoid dysplasia with atlantoaxial dislocation; os odontoideum (separate odontoid); hypoplasia or aplasia of dens
6. Stenosis of foramen magnum
7. Stenosis of cervical spinal canal

CERVICOMEDULLARY ANOMALY

1. Arteriovenous malformation
2. Chiari malformations
3. Hydromyelia

References

1. Guinto FC Jr, Kumar R, Mirfakhree M: Radiological Society of North America Scientific Exhibit, Washington, DC, 1984

Gamut C-9-2

CRANIOVERTEBRAL JUNCTION ABNORMALITY—ACQUIRED

BONE LESION

1. Fibrous dysplasia
2. Inflammatory disease
3. Neoplasm of skull base (primary or metastatic)
4. Paget's disease
5. Posttraumatic or degenerative lesion

EXTRAMEDULLARY LESION

1. Aneurysm
2. Cystic lesion (eg, arachnoid cyst; epidermoid cyst)
3. Neoplasm (eg, meningioma; neurofibroma; lipoma)

INTRAMEDULLARY LESION

1. Glioma
2. Hemangioblastoma
3. Syringomyelia

References

1. Guinto FC Jr, Kumar R, Mirfakhree M: Radiological Society of North America Scientific Exhibit, Washington, DC, 1984
2. Resnick D: Diagnosis of Bone and Joint Disorders. (ed 3) Philadelphia: WB Saunders, 1995, pp 4245–4268

Gamut C-10

FUSION OF THE CERVICAL SPINE

COMMON
1. Ankylosing spondylitis
2. Block vertebrae, congenital or acquired (eg, post-traumatic; surgical fusion; tuberculosis or other infection)
3. Diffuse idiopathic skeletal hyperostsosis (DISH)
4. Juvenile chronic arthritis (Still's disease)
5. Rheumatoid arthritis (incl. juvenile)

UNCOMMON
1. Acrocephalosyndactyly (Apert, Pfeiffer, and Saethre-Chotzen types)
2. Fibrodysplasia (myositis) ossificans progressiva
3. Fluorosis
4. Hypervitaminosis A
5. Hypoparathyroidism
6. Klippel-Feil S.
7. Psoriatic arthritis
8. Reiter S.
9. SAPHO S.
10. Vertebral malsegmentation (See C-11)

References
1. Boutin RD, Resnick D: The SAPHO syndrome: An evolving concept for unifying several idiopathic disorders of bone and skin. AJR 1998;170:585–591
2. Connor JM, Smith R: The cervical spine in fibrodysplasia ossificans progressiva. Br J Radiol 1982;55:492–496
3. Dihlmann VW, Friedmann G: Die röntgenkriterien der juvenilrheumatischen zervikalsynostose im erwachsenenalter. Fortschr Røntgenstr 1977;126:536–541
4. Resnick D: Diagnosis of Bone and Joint Disorders. (ed 3) Philadelphia: WB Saunders, 1995
5. Taybi H, Lachman RS: Radiology of Syndromes, Metabolic Disorders, and Skeletal Dysplasias. (ed 4) St. Louis: Mosby-Year Book, Inc., 1996, p 1048

Gamut C-11

CONGENITAL VERTEBRAL MALSEGMENTATION (SUPERNUMERARY, PARTIALLY FORMED OR HEMIVERTEBRAE, FUSED OR BLOCK VERTEBRAE)

COMMON
1. Chondrodysplasia punctata
2. Diastematomyelia
3. Isolated anomaly
4. Klippel-Feil S.
5. Meningomyelocele

UNCOMMON
1. Acrocephalosyndactyly (Apert, Pfeiffer, and Saethre-Chotzen types)
2. Aicardi S.
3. Alagille S. (arteriohepatic S.)
4. Binder S.
5. Cat cry S. (cri du chat S.)
6. Caudal dysplasia sequence
7. CHILD S.
8. Dysspondylochondromatosis
9. Dyssegmental dysplasia
10. Fanconi anemia
11. Femoral hypoplasia-unusual facies S.
12. Fetal alcohol S.
13. Goltz S. (focal dermal hypoplasia)
14. Gorlin S. (nevoid basal cell carcinoma S.)
15. Holt-Oram S.
16. Hypophosphatasia (perinatal lethal)
17. Incontinentia pigmenti
18. Larsen S.
19. LEOPARD S. (multiple lentigenes S.)
20. Multiple pterygium S.
21. MURCS association
22. Noonan S.
23. Oculo-auriculo-vertebral spectrum (Goldenhar S.)
24. Poland S. (pectoral muscle aplasia-syndactyly)

(continued)

25. Robinow S.
26. Split notochord S.
27. Spondylocarpotarsal fusion S.
28. Spondylocostal dysostosis (Jarcho-Levin S.)
29. Tethered cord S.
30. Trisomy 8 S.
31. Trisomy 18 S.
32. VATER association
33. Wildervanck S. (cervico-oculo-acoustic S.)

References

1. Kozlowski K, Beighton P: Gamut Index of Skeletal Dysplasias. Berlin: Springer-Verlag, 1984, p 45
2. Taybi H, Lachman RS: Radiology of Syndromes, Metabolic Disorders, and Skeletal Dysplasias. (ed 4) St. Louis: Mosby-Year Book, Inc., 1996, p1048

Gamut C-12

ABSENT OR MINIMALLY OSSIFIED VERTEBRAE

1. Achondrogenesis
2. Atelosteogenesis
3. Boomerang dysplasia
4. Caudal dysplasia sequence (caudal regression S.)
5. Dyssegmental dysplasia
6. Hypochondrogenesis
7. Opsismodysplasia
8. Schneckenbecken dysplasia
9. Spondylomegaepiphyseal-metaphyseal dysplasia

Reference

1. Taybi H, Lachman RS: Radiology of Syndromes, Metabolic Disorders, and Skeletal Dysplasias. (ed 4) St. Louis: Mosby-Year Book, Inc., 1996, p1047

Gamut C-13

CORONAL CLEFT VERTEBRAE

COMMON

1. Chondrodysplasia punctata (all types)
2. Kniest dysplasia
3. Mesomelic dysplasias
4. Metatropic dysplasia
5. Normal variant (esp. in lower thoracic-upper lumbar spine of premature male infant)

UNCOMMON

1. Atelosteogenesis
2. Desbuquois dysplasia
3. Dyssegmental dysplasia
4. Fibrochondrogenesis
5. Humerospinal dysostosis
6. Malsegmentation of spine
7. Otospondylomegaepiphyseal dysplasia (OSMED)
8. Short rib-polydactyly S., type I (Saldino-Noonan S.)
9. Spondyloepimetaphyseal dysplasia (Iraqi type)
10. Trisomy 13 S.
11. Weissenbacher-Zweymüller S. (incl. micrognathic dwarfism)

References

1. Fielden P, Russell JGB: Coronally cleft vertebra. Clin Radiol 1970;21:327–328
2. Kozlowski K, Beighton P: Gamut Index of Skeletal Dysplasias. Berlin: Springer-Verlag, 1984, p 46
3. Rowley KA: Coronal cleft vertebra. J Fac Radiol 1955; 6:267–274
4. Swischuk LE, John SD: Differential Diagnosis in Pediatric Radiology. (ed 2) Baltimore: Williams & Wilkins, 1995, p 408
5. Taybi H, Lachman RS: Radiology of Syndromes, Metabolic Disorders, and Skeletal Dysplasias. (ed 4) St. Louis: Mosby-Year Book Inc., 1996, p 1047–1048
6. Wollin DG, Elliott GB: Coronal cleft vertebrae and persistent notochordal derivatives of infancy. J Can Assoc Radiol 1961;12:78–81

Gamut C-14

PROMINENT ANTERIOR CANAL (CENTRAL VEIN GROOVE) OF A VERTEBRAL BODY

COMMON

1. Hypothyroidism; infantile (cretinism)
2. Normal (up to age 7)
3. Sickle cell disease

UNCOMMON

1. Cockayne S.
2. Gaucher's disease
3. Leukemia, lymphoma$_g$
4. Metastatic neuroblastoma
5. Osteopetrosis
6. Progeria
7. Thalassemia major

References

1. Greenfield GB: Radiology of Bone Diseases. (ed 5) Philadelphia: Lippincott, 1990
2. Mandell A, Kricum ME: Exaggerated anterior vertebral notching. Radiology 1979;131:367–369
3. Swischuk LE, John SD: Differential Diagnosis in Pediatric Radiology. (ed 2) Baltimore: Williams & Wilkins, 1995, p 409

Gamut C-15

CONGENITAL PLATYSPONDYLY

COMMON

1. Anemia$_g$ (eg, sickle cell disease; thalassemia)
2. Hypothyroidism, juvenile; cretinism
3. Metatropic dysplasia
4. Morquio S.
5. [Osteogenesis imperfecta congenita with numerous compression fractures]

6. Spondyloepiphyseal dysplasia, all forms
7. Thanatophoric dysplasia and variants

UNCOMMON

1. Achondrogenesis
2. Achondroplasia (homozygous)
3. Atelosteogenesis (type I)
4. Brachyolmia
5. Cephaloskeletal dysplasia (Taybi-Linder S.)
6. de la Chapelle S.
7. Diastrophic dysplasia
8. Dyggve-Melchior-Clausen dysplasia
9. Dysosteosclerosis
10. Ehlers-Danlos S.
11. Fibrochondrogenesis
12. Freeman-Sheldon S. (whistling face S.)
13. Gaucher disease
14. Geroderma osteodysplastica
15. GM$_1$ gangliosidosis; fucosidosis
16. Hallermann-Streiff S. (oculo-mandibulo-facial S.)
17. Homocystinuria
18. Hyperphosphatasia
19. Hypochondrogenesis
20. Hypophosphatasia, severe
21. Hypopituitarism (anterior lobe)
22. [Idiopathic juvenile osteoporosis]
23. Kniest dysplasia
24. Larsen S.
25. Lethal osteosclerotic skeletal dysplasias
26. Marshall S.
27. Opsismodysplasia
28. Osteoglophonic dwarfism
29. Otospondylomegaepiphyseal dysplasia
30. Parastremmatic dwarfism
31. Patterson S. (cervical spine)
32. Pseudoachondroplasia
33. Pseudodiastrophic dysplasia
34. Rothmund-Thomson S.
35. Schwartz-Jampel S. (osteochondromuscular dystrophy)
36. Short rib-polydactyly S., type I (Saldino-Noonan S.)
37. Smith-McCort S.
38. Spondyloenchondromatosis

(continued)

39. Spondyloepimetaphyseal dysplasia
40. Spondylometaphyseal dysplasia (Kozlowski and other types)
41. Spondyloperipheral dysplasia
42. Wolcott-Rallison dysplasia

[ ] This condition does not actually cause the gamuted imaging finding, but can produce imaging changes that simulate it.

References

1. Kozlowski K: Platyspondyly in childhood. Pediatr Radiol 1974;2:81–88
2. Kozlowski K, Beighton P: Gamut Index of Skeletal Dysplasias. Berlin: Springer-Verlag, 1984, p 43
3. Schorr S, Legum C: Radiological aspects of the vertebral components of osteochondrodysplasias. Br J Radiol 1977; 50:302–311
4. Swischuk LE, John SD: Differential Diagnosis in Pediatric Radiology. (ed 2) Baltimore: Williams & Wilkins, 1995, pp 411–414
5. Taybi H, Lachman RS: Radiology of Syndromes, Metabolic Disorders, and Skeletal Dysplasias. (ed 4) St. Louis: Mosby-Year Book Inc., 1996, pp 1046–1047

Gamut C-16

ANISOSPONDYLY*

1. Campomelic dysplasia
2. Dyssegmental dysplasia
3. Homocystinuria
4. Kniest dysplasia
5. Osteogenesis imperfecta
6. Spondyloepimetaphyseal dysplasia
7. Spondyloepiphyseal dysplasia
8. Spondylometaphyseal dysplasia
9. Stickler S. (arthro-ophthalmopathy)

* Congenital irregular flattening of two or more vertebral bodies in the presence of other normal vertebrae.

Reference

1. Kozlowski K, Beighton P: Gamut Index of Skeletal Dysplasias. (ed 2) London: Springer-Verlag, 1995, p 44

Gamut C-17

SOLITARY COLLAPSED VERTEBRA (INCLUDING VERTEBRA PLANA) (See C-18)

COMMON

1. Brown tumor of hyperparathyroidism
*2. Eosinophilic granuloma (Langerhans cell histiocytosis$_g$)
*3. Fracture, traumatic or pathologic
*4. Hemangioma
*5. Lymphoma$_g$; leukemia
*6. Metastasis (incl. neuroblastoma)
7. Myeloma; plasmacytoma
8. [Normal developmental variant (eg, C5 or C6 or a thoracic vertebra reduced in height)]
9. Osteomyelitis (eg, tuberculous, fungal, pyogenic, brucellar, typhoid, syphilitic)
10. Osteoporosis (eg, senile, postmenopausal) (See D-43-1)
*11. Paget's disease
12. Steroid therapy; Cushing S.

UNCOMMON

1. Amyloidosis
2. Benign bone tumor, other (eg, giant cell tumor; aneurysmal bone cyst)
3. Chordoma
4. Hydatid disease
5. Neuropathy (eg, diabetes; syphilis; congenital insensitivity to pain)
6. Osteomalacia
7. Sarcoidosis
8. Sarcoma (eg, Ewing sarcoma; osteosarcoma; chondrosarcoma)
9. Scheuermann's disease
*10. Traumatic ischemic necrosis (eg, Kömmell's disease)

* May produce vertebra plana.
[ ] This condition does not actually cause the gamuted imaging finding, but can produce imaging changes that simulate it.

Gamut C-18

MULTIPLE COLLAPSED VERTEBRAE
(See C-17)

COMMON

1. Fractures, traumatic or pathologic
2. Hyperparathyroidism, primary or secondary (renal osteodystrophy)
3. Metastases
4. Multiple myeloma
5. Neuropathy (eg, diabetes; syphilis; congenital insensitivity to pain)
6. Osteomalacia (See D-44)
7. Osteomyelitis (eg, tuberculous, fungal, pyogenic, brucellar, syphilitic)
8. Osteoporosis (eg, senile, postmenopausal, or idiopathic juvenile osteoporosis; hypogonadism; prolonged immobilization) (See D-43-1)
9. Scheuermann's disease
10. Sickle cell disease; other anemias
11. Steroid therapy; Cushing S.

UNCOMMON

1. Amyloidosis
2. Congenital fibromatosis
3. Convulsions (eg, tetanus; tetany; hypoglycemia; electroshock therapy)
4. Gaucher's disease
5. Hajdu-Cheney S. (idiopathic acro-osteolysis)
6. Hemangiomatosis (Gorham's vanishing bone disease)
7. Hydatid disease
8. Hyperphosphatasia
9. Hypophosphatasia
10. Langerhans cell histiocytosis$_g$
11. Lymphoma$_g$; leukemia
12. Osteogenesis imperfecta
13. Paget's disease
14. [Platyspondyly, esp. dwarf syndromes (eg, Morquio S.; spondyloepiphyseal dysplasia; pseudoachondroplasia; thanatophoric dysplasia)] (See C-15)

15. Radiation therapy
16. Rheumatoid arthritis

[ ] This condition does not actually cause the gamuted imaging finding, but can produce imaging changes that simulate it.

Gamut C-19

BICONCAVE ("FISH") VERTEBRAE
(INCLUDING STEP-LIKE VERTEBRAE*)

COMMON

1. Hyperparathyroidism, primary or secondary (renal osteodystrophy)*
2. Metastatic disease
3. Osteomalacia; rickets (See D-44)
4. Osteoporosis (eg, senile or postmenopausal; malnutrition; steroid therapy) (See D-43-1)
5. Paget's disease
*6. Schmorl's nodes
*7. Sickle cell disease

UNCOMMON

*1. Anemias, other (eg, thalassemia; hereditary spherocytosis; iron deficiency)
*2. Gaucher's disease
*3. Homocystinuria
4. Lymphoma$_g$
5. Osteogenesis imperfecta
6. Sponastrine dysplasia

* "Step-like" vertebra with H-shaped or Lincoln log configuration may occur.

References

1. Greenfield GB: Radiology of Bone Diseases. (ed 5) Philadelphia: Lippincott, 1990
2. Rohlfing BM: Vertebral end-plate depression: Report of two patients without hemoglobinopathy. AJR 1977;128:599–600
3. Schwartz AM, Homer MJ, McCauley RGK: Step-off vertebral body: Gaucher's disease versus sickle cell hemoglobinopathy. AJR 1979, 132:81–85

(continued)

4. Swischuk LE, John SD: Differential Diagnosis in Pediatric Radiology. (ed 2) Baltimore: Williams & Wilkins, 1995, pp 414–416
5. Westerman MP, Greenfield GB, Wong PWK: "Fish vertebrae," homocystinuria, and sickle cell anemia. JAMA 1974; 230:261–262
6. Ziter FMH Jr: Central vertebral end-plate depression in chronic renal disease: Report of two cases. AJR 1979; 132:809–811

Gamut C-20

WEDGED VERTEBRA*

1. Chronic hyperflexion of spine; muscular hypotonia
2. Congenital syndromes and bone dysplasias with thoracolumbar wedging (eg, achondroplasia; hypothyroidism; mucopolysaccharidoses—See J-4)
3. Hemivertebra (gibbus or lateral wedging)
4. Kyphosis (See C-3)
5. Normal variant (minimal wedging in thoracic spine or at C3 or C4 in infant or young child)
6. Pathologic fracture in weakened vertebra (eg, osteoporosis; infection; metastasis; multiple myeloma; primary neoplasm)
7. Rotoscoliosis (lateral wedging)
8. Scheuermann's disease
9. Trauma (compression fracture)
10. Tuberculosis (gibbus); other chronic infection of spine (spondylitis)

* Primarily anterior wedging unless otherwise indicated.

References

1. Swischuk LE, John SD: Differential Diagnosis in Pediatric Radiology. (ed 2) Baltimore: Williams & Wilkins, 1995, pp 417–419
2. Swischuk LE, Swischuk PN, John SD: Wedging of C3 in infants and children: usually a normal finding and not a fracture. Radiology 1993;188:523–526

Gamut C-21

ANTERIOR BEAKED VERTEBRAE IN A CHILD

COMMON

1. Achondroplasia (central anterior wedging)
2. Cretinism; hypothyroidism (inferior beak)
3. Mucopolysaccharidoses (esp. Morquio S.—central beak; Hunter S., Hurler S., Maroteaux-Lamy S.—inferior beak) (See J-4)
4. Neuromuscular disease with generalized hypotonia (eg, Werdnig-Hoffmann disease; Niemann-Pick disease; phenylketonuria; mental retardation)
5. Normal variant in infants (thoracolumbar junction; C2-3 angulation)
6. Scheuermann's disease
7. Trauma, acute or chronic; battered child S. (hyperflexion-decompression spinal injury)

UNCOMMON

1. Adenosine deaminase deficiency with severe combined immunodeficiency and chondro-osseous dysplasia
2. Aspartylglucosaminuria
3. Diastrophic dysplasia
4. Dyggve-Melchior-Clausen dysplasia (Smith-McCort S.)
5. Marshall S.
6. Mucolipidoses; GM_1 gangliosidosis; fucosidosis; mannosidosis; sialidosis (See J-4)
7. Neurofibromatosis (dysplastic vertebrae)
8. Pseudoachondroplasia
9. Spondyloepimetaphyseal dysplasia (short limb-hand type)
10. Spondyloepiphyseal dysplasia congenita
11. Trisomy 21 S. (Down S.)

References

1. Swischuk LE: The beaked, notched, or hooked vertebra; its significance in infants and young children. Radiology 1970; 95:661–664.

2. Swischuk LE, John SD: Differential Diagnosis in Pediatric Radiology. (ed 2) Baltimore: Williams & Wilkins, 1995, pp 418–421
3. Taybi H, Lachman RS: Radiology of Syndromes, Metabolic Disorders, and Skeletal Dysplasias. (ed 4) St. Louis: Mosby-Year Book Inc., 1996, p 1047

Gamut C-22

CUBOID VERTEBRAE

COMMON

1. Achondroplasia
2. Normal variant (cervical spine and thoracolumbar junction)

UNCOMMON

1. Diastrophic dysplasia
2. Gorlin S. (nevoid basal cell carcinoma S.)
3. Hypochondroplasia
4. Mucopolysaccharidoses (See J-4)
5. Pseudodiastrophic dysplasia
6. Short rib-polydactyly syndromes (eg, Saldino-Noonan S.; Majewski S.)
7. Thanatophoric dysplasia

References

1. Swischuk LE, John SD: Differential Diagnosis in Pediatric Radiology. (ed 2) Baltimore: Williams & Wilkins, 1995, p 414

Gamut C-23

ROUND VERTEBRAE

COMMON

1. Cretinism; hypothyroidism (untreated)
2. Normal in neonate (esp. thoracolumbar junction) or child with delayed appearance of ring epiphyses

3. Vertebral body underdevelopment (eg, meningomyelocele)

UNCOMMON

1. Bone dysplasias with "pear shaped" vertebrae (eg, Morquio S.;
   a. Acromesomelic dysplasia
   b. Chondroectodermal dysplasia
   c. Cranioectodermal dysplasia
   d. Dyggve-Melchior-Clausen dysplasia (Smith-McCort S.)
   e. Hypochondrogenesis
   f. Schneckenbecken dysplasia
   g. Spondyloepiphyseal dysplasia congenita
   h. Spondyloepimetaphyseal dysplasia
   i. Spondylometaphyseal dysplasia)
2. Patterson S. (ovoid thoracic and lumbar bodies)
3. Pseudoachondroplasia
4. Short rib-polydactyly syndromes (eg, Saldino-Noonan S.; Majewski S.)
5. Smith-Lemli-Opitz S. (type II) (high ovoid lumbar bodies)
6. Weill-Marchesani S.

References

1. Kramer PPG, Scheers IM: Round anterior margin of lumbar vertebral bodies in children with a meningocele. Pediatr Radiol 1987;17:263
2. Swischuk LE, John SD: Differential Diagnosis in Pediatric Radiology. (ed 2) Baltimore: Williams & Wilkins, 1995, pp 418–421

Gamut C-24

TALL VERTEBRAE

COMMON

1. Block or fused vertebra (See C-25)
2. Hypotonia (eg, neuromuscular disorders$_g$; mental retardation); nonweight bearing
3. Trisomy 21 S. (Down S.)

(continued)

UNCOMMON
1. Antley-Bixler S.
2. Chromosome 4:del (4p) S. (Wolf-Hirschhorn S.)
3. Dolichospondylic dysplasia
4. Dyssegmental dysplasia
5. Freeman-Sheldon S. (whistling face S.)
6. Hadju-Cheney S.
7. Infantile multisystem inflammatory disease
8. Marfan S.; arachnodactyly
9. Osteodysplasty (Melnick-Needles S.)
10. Proteus S.
11. Spondylocostal dysplasia

References
1. Gooding CA, Neuhauser EBD: Growth and development of the vertebral bodies in the presence and absence of normal stress. AJR 1965;93:388–393
2. Kozlowski K, Beighton P: Gamut Index of Skeletal Dysplasias. (ed 2) London: Springer-Verlag, 1995, p 44
3. Swischuk LE, John SD: Differential Diagnosis in Pediatric Radiology. (ed 2) Baltimore: Williams & Wilkins, 1995, pp 416–417
4. Taybi H, Lachman RS: Radiology of Syndromes, Metabolic Disorders, and Skeletal Dysplasias. (ed 4) St. Louis: Mosby-Year Book, Inc., 1996, p 1048

Gamut C-25

FUSED OR BLOCK VERTEBRAE
(Congenital and Acquired)

CONGENITAL

COMMON
1. Acrocephalosyndactyly (Apert and Pfeiffer types)
2. Crouzon S. (craniofacial dysostosis)
3. Fetal alcohol S.
4. Fibrodysplasia (myositis) ossificans progressiva
5. Goltz S. (focal dermal hypoplasia) (anterior fusion)
6. Holt-Oram S.
7. Isolated anomaly (esp. C2-3)
8. Klippel-Feil S.
9. With spinal dysraphism

UNCOMMON
1. Aicardi S.
2. Binder S.
3. CHILD S.
4. Diamond-Blackfan S. (cervical spine)
5. Hypomelanosis of Ito
6. LEOPARD S.
7. Multiple synostosis S.
8. Mayer-Rokitansky-Kuster S.
9. Noonan S.
10. Oculo-auriculo-vertebral spectrum (Goldenhar S.)
11. Proteus S.
12. Robinow S.
13. Spondylocostal dysostoses (esp. Jarcho-Levin S.)
14. Wildervanck S.

ACQUIRED

COMMON
1. Ankylosing spondylitis
2. Infection (esp. tuberculosis); juvenile discitis (healed)
3. Rheumatoid arthritis (esp. juvenile)
4. Scheuermann's disease
5. Surgical fusion
6. Trauma (severe)

References
1. Swischuk LE, John SD: Differential Diagnosis in Pediatric Radiology. (ed 2) Baltimore: Williams & Wilkins, 1995, pp 421–423
2. Taybi H, Lachman RS: Radiology of Syndromes, Metabolic Disorders, and Skeletal Dysplasias. (ed 4) St. Louis: Mosby-Year Book, Inc., 1996, p 1048

Gamut C-26

ENLARGEMENT OF ONE OR MORE VERTEBRAE

COMMON
1. Acromegaly; gigantism
2. Congenital (eg, block vertebra—See C-25)
3. Paget's disease

UNCOMMON

1. Benign bone tumor (eg, giant cell tumor; hemangioma; aneurysmal bone cyst; osteoblastoma)
2. Compensatory enlargement from nonweight bearing (eg, paralysis$_g$)
3. Fibrous dysplasia
4. Hydatid disease
5. Hyperphosphatasia

References
1. Epstein BS: The Spine. (ed 4) Philadelphia: Lea & Febiger, 1976
2. Greenfield GB: Radiology of Bone Diseases. (ed 5) Philadelphia: Lippincott, 1990
3. Murphey MD, Andrews CL, Flemming DJ, et al: Primary tumors of the spine: Radiologic-pathologic correlation. RadioGraphics 1996; 16:1131–1158

Gamut C-27

"SQUARING" OF ONE OR MORE VERTEBRAL BODIES*

COMMON

1. Ankylosing spondylitis
2. Normal variant
3. Paget's disease

UNCOMMON

1. Hypervitaminosis A
2. Psoriatic arthritis
3. Reiter S.
4. Rheumatoid arthritis
5. SAPHO S.
6. Wilson disease

* Acquired diseases causing squared vertebrae. For congenital cuboid or occasionally squared vertebrae, see Gamut C-22.

References
1. Jacobson HG: Personal communication.
2. Resnick D: Diagnosis of Bone and Joint Disorders. (ed 3) Philadelphia: WB Saunders, 1995

Gamut C-28

SPOOL-SHAPED VERTEBRAE (ANTERIOR AND POSTERIOR SCALLOPING)

COMMON

1. Hypotonia
2. Neurofibromatosis
3. Normal (occasionally mild in lumbar spine)

UNCOMMON

1. Cockayne S.
2. Mucopolysaccharidoses (See J-4)
3. Osteodysplasty (Melnick-Needles S.)
4. Trisomy 21 S. (Down S.); other trisomies

Reference
1. Swischuk LE, John SD: Differential Diagnosis in Pediatric Radiology. (ed 2) Baltimore: Williams & Wilkins, 1995, p 420

Gamut C-29

ANTERIOR GOUGE DEFECT (SCALLOPING) OF ONE OR MORE VERTEBRAL BODIES

COMMON

1. Aneurysm of aorta
2. Lymphoma$_g$; chronic leukemia
3. Lymphadenopathy from metastases or inflammation
*4. Neurofibromatosis (dysplastic vertebra)
5. Normal variant (lower thoracic, upper lumbar)
6. Tuberculosis (spondylitis)

UNCOMMON

1. Adjacent intraabdominal neoplasm or cyst
*2. Chondrodystrophies and storage diseases

(continued)

3. Cockayne S.
*4. Glycogen storage disease
5. Multiple myeloma (paravertebral soft tissue mass)
*6. Osteodysplasty (Melnick-Needles S.)
*7. Trisomy 21 S. (Down S.)

* Often have spindle- or spool-shaped vertebrae with both anterior and posterior scalloping.

References

1. Resnick D: Diagnosis of Bone and Joint Disorders. (ed 3) Philadelphia: WB Saunders, 1995
2. Swischuk LE, John SD: Differential Diagnosis in Pediatric Radiology. (ed 2) Baltimore: Williams & Wilkins, 1995, pp 409–411

Gamut C-30

EXAGGERATED CONCAVITY (SCALLOPING) OF THE POSTERIOR SURFACE OF ONE OR MORE VERTEBRAL BODIES

COMMON

1. Achondroplasia; other chondrodystrophies with a narrow spinal canal (See Uncommon #4)
2. Increased intraspinal pressure (eg, severe communicating hydrocephalus; neoplasm)
3. Neoplasm of spinal canal (eg, ependymoma; dermoid; lipoma; neurofibroma; meningioma)
4. Neurofibromatosis with or without neurofibroma ("dural ectasia"); congenital expansion of the subarachnoid space ("intraspinal meningocele")
5. Normal variant (physiologic scalloping—esp. L4, L5)

UNCOMMON

1. Acromegaly
2. Cyst of spinal canal
3. Hydatid disease

4. Other congenital syndromes and bone dysplasias
   a. Cockayne S.
   b. Diastrophic dysplasia
   c. Dyggve-Melchior-Clausen dysplasia
   d. Ehlers-Danlos S. (dural ectasia)
   e. Marfan S. (dural ectasia)
   f. Metatropic dysplasia
   g. Mucopolysaccharidoses (eg, Hurler S; Hunter S.; Morquio S.; Sanfilippo S.); mucolipidosis II (I-cell disease) (See J-4)
   h. Osteogenesis imperfecta
   i. Smith-McCort S.
   j. Thanatophoric dysplasia
5. Spinal dysraphism; meningomyelocele
6. Syringomyelia; hydromyelia

References

1. Greenfield GB: Radiology of Bone Diseases. (ed 5) Philadelphia: Lippincott, 1990
2. Heard G, Payne EE: Scalloping of the vertebral bodies in von Recklinghausen's disease of the nervous system (neurofibromatosis). J Neurol Neurosurg Psychiatry 1962; 25:345–351
3. Howieson J, Norrell HA, Wilson CB: Expansion of the subarachnoid space in the lumbosacral region. Radiology 1968; 90:488–492
4. Kozlowski K, Beighton P: Gamut Index of Skeletal Dysplasias. Berlin: Springer-Verlag, 1984, p 46
5. Leeds NE, Jacobson HG: Plain film examination of the spinal canal. Semin Roentgenol 1972;7:179–196
6. Mitchell GE, Lourie H, Berne AS: The various causes of scalloped vertebrae with notes on their pathogenesis. Radiology 1967;89:67–74
7. Salerno NR, Edeiken J: Vertebral scalloping in neurofibromatosis. Radiology 1970;97:509–510
8. Swischuk LE, John SD: Differential Diagnosis in Pediatric Radiology. (ed 2) Baltimore: Williams & Wilkins, 1995, pp 409–411

Gamut C-31

INCREASED BAND(S) OF DENSITY IN THE SUBCHONDRAL ZONES OF VERTEBRAE (INCLUDING RUGGER JERSEY SPINE)

COMMON

1. Compression fracture
2. Hypercorticism; Cushing S.; steroid therapy
*3. Hyperparathyroidism, primary or secondary (renal osteodystrophy)
*4. Osteopetrosis
5. Paget's disease
6. Sclerosing spondylosis in the elderly

UNCOMMON

1. Growth arrest lines
2. Heavy metals (eg, Thorotrast; lead)
3. Hypoparathyroidism; pseudohypoparathyroidism
*4. Lead poisoning, chronic
5. Leukemia, treated
*6. Lipid granulomatosis (Erdheim-Chester disease)
*7. Myeloid metaplasia (myelosclerosis)
*8. Osteomesopyknosis
9. Radiation therapy
*10. Williams S. (idiopathic hypercalcemia)

* May have the appearance of a "rugger jersey."

References
1. Proshek R, Labelle H, Bard C, Morton D: Osteomesopyknosis: A benign familial disorder of bone. J Bone Joint Surg (Am) 1985;67:652–653
2. Swischuk LE, John SD: Differential Diagnosis in Pediatric Radiology. (ed 2) Baltimore: Williams & Wilkins, 1995, p 401

Gamut C-32

BONE-IN-BONE OR SANDWICH VERTEBRA

COMMON

*1. Osteopetrosis
2. Paget's disease
3. Physiologic in newborn (often premature) infant
*4. Renal osteodystrophy (secondary hyperparathyroidism), healing

UNCOMMON

1. Chronic illness (growth arrest lines)
*2. Hypercalcemia; hypervitaminosis D
*3. Lead poisoning, chronic
4. Radiation therapy
5. Thorotrast

* May have a "rugger jersey spine" or "sandwich vertebra" appearance.

Reference
1. Swischuk LE, John SD: Differential Diagnosis in Pediatric Radiology. (ed 2) Baltimore: Williams & Wilkins, 1995, p 401

Gamut C-33

INCREASED VERTICAL (PIN-STRIPE OR CORDUROY) TRABECULATION OF ONE OR MORE VERTEBRAL BODIES

COMMON

1. Anemia, primary$_g$
2. Hemangioma
3. Osteoporosis
4. Paget's disease

UNCOMMON

1. Axial osteomalacia
2. Fibrogenesis imperfecta ossium

(continued)

3. Lymphoma$_g$; leukemia
4. Metastatic disease (incl. carcinomatosis)
5. Multiple myeloma (incl. myelomatosis)

* Due to loss of the minor bone trabeculae, with the remaining major trabeculae aligned vertically for support.

Reference

1. Wang CSF, Steinbach LS, Campbell JB, et al: Fibrogenesis imperfecta ossium: imaging correlation in three new patients. Skeletal Radiol 1999;28:390–395

13. Sarcoidosis
14. Sclerotic pedicle (See C-42)
15. Tuberous sclerosis

References

1. Murphey MD, Andrews CL, Flemming DJ, et al: Primary tumors of the spine. Radiologic-pathologic correlation. RadioGraphics 1996;16:1131–1158
2. Swischuk LE, John SD: Differential Diagnosis in Pediatric Radiology. (ed 2) Baltimore: Williams & Wilkins, 1995, pp 401–402

Gamut C-34

FOCAL AREA OF SCLEROSIS IN A VERTEBRA

COMMON

1. Enostosis (bone island)
2. Fracture (compression or healing or healed)
3. Idiopathic
4. Osteoblastic metastasis
5. Sclerosis of apophyseal joints due to arthritis or malalignment
6. Spondylosis (discogenic sclerosis)

UNCOMMON

1. Bone sarcoma (esp. osteosarcoma; chondrosarcoma; Ewing sarcoma)
2. Chordoma
3. Hemangioma
4. Langerhans cell histiocytosis$_g$ (healed)
5. Lymphoma$_g$
6. Mastocytosis
7. Melorheostosis
8. Myeloma (eg, POEMS S.)
9. Osteoblastoma
10. Osteoid osteoma
11. Osteoma
12. Osteomyelitis (esp. chronic from tuberculosis, brucellosis, fungus disease, or typhoid fever)

Gamut C-35

DENSE SCLEROTIC VERTEBRA, SOLITARY OR MULTIPLE (INCLUDING IVORY VERTEBRA)

COMMON

1. Fracture (compression or healing)
2. Hemangioma
*3. Lymphoma$_g$
*4. Myelosclerosis (myeloid metaplasia)
*5. Osteoblastic metastasis
*6. Osteomyelitis, chronic sclerosing (eg, tuberculosis; syphilis; brucellosis; typhoid)
*7. Paget's disease
8. Renal osteodystrophy (secondary hyperparathyroidism)

UNCOMMON

1. Bone sarcoma (eg, osteosarcoma*; chondrosarcoma; Ewing sarcoma)
*2. Chordoma
*3. Fluorosis
4. Hypervitaminosis D
5. Idiopathic (eg, nondiscogenic sclerosis)
6. Lenz-Majewski dysplasia (hyperostolic dwarfism)
7. Mastocytosis
8. Multiple myeloma (rarely—<3%); POEMS S.
9. Osteoblastoma

10. Osteoma; enostosis (bone island)
*11. Osteopetrosis
12. Radiation therapy; radium poisoning
13. Rickets (healing)
14. Sarcoidosis
15. Sickle cell disease
16. Spondylosis (discogenic sclerosis)
17. Tuberous sclerosis
18. Williams S. (idiopathic hypercalcemia)

* Can cause "ivory" vertebra(e).

References
1. Murphey MD, Andrews CL, Flemming DJ, et al: Primary tumors of the spine. Radiologic-pathologic correlation. RadioGraphics 1996;16:1131–1158
2. Resnick D: Diagnosis of Bone and Joint Disorders. (ed 3) Philadelphia: WB Saunders, 1995

Gamut C-36

SPINAL OSTEOPENIA (LOSS OF DENSITY)

COMMON
1. Anemia$_g$ (esp. sickle cell disease; thalassemia)
2. Arthritis (esp. rheumatoid, incl. juvenile rheumatoid)
3. Carcinomatosis
4. Hyperparathyroidism, primary or secondary (renal osteodystrophy)
5. Multiple myeloma
6. Osteomalacia (See D-44)
7. Osteoporosis (esp. juvenile, senile, or post-menopausal; prolonged immobilization) (See D-43-1)
8. Steroid therapy; Cushing S.

UNCOMMON
1. Acromegaly
2. Amyloidosis
3. Fibrogenesis imperfecta ossium
4. Gaucher's disease; Niemann-Pick disease
5. Homocystinuria
6. Hyperthyroidism
7. Hypogonadism (eg, Fröhlich S.; Turner S.)

8. Leukemia; lymphoma$_g$
9. Osteogenesis imperfecta
10. Sponastrine dysplasia

Reference
1. Greenfield GB: Radiology of Bone Diseases. (ed 5) Philadelphia: Lippincott, 1990

Gamut C-37

LYTIC LESION OF THE SPINE

COMMON
1. Chordoma; notochordal remnant
2. Fracture (esp. insufficiency fracture of sacrum)
3. Hemangioma
4. Langerhans cell histiocytosis$_g$ (esp. eosinophilic granuloma)
5. Metastasis
6. Myeloma; plasmacytoma
7. Spondylodiskitis (osteomyelitis/diskitis) (eg, tuberculous, sarcoid, fungal, brucellar, other bacterial)
8. Paget's disease
9. Rheumatoid arthritis
10. Schmorl's nodes

UNCOMMON
1. Aneurysmal bone cyst
2. Bone sarcoma (eg, Ewing sarcoma; osteolytic osteosarcoma; chondrosarcoma; fibrosarcoma malignant fibrous histiocytoma; rhabdomyosarcoma)
3. Brown tumor of hyperparathyroidism
4. Chondroid lesion
5. Fibrous dysplasia
6. Giant cell tumor
7. Gout
8. Hemangioendothelioma; hemangiopericytoma
9. Hydatid disease
10. Intraspinal neoplasm with erosion of vertebra (eg, neurofibroma; meningioma)
11. Lymphoma$_g$

(continued)

12. Meningocele; diastematomyelia
13. Nonossifying fibroma
14. Osteoblastoma
15. Osteoid osteoma
16. Traumatic ischemic necrosis (Kòmmell's disease)

Gamut C-38-S

VERTEBRAL NEOPLASMS AND LOOK-ALIKES

BENIGN

COMMON

1. Aneurysmal bone cyst
2. Hemangioma
3. Osteoblastoma

UNCOMMON

1. Enostosis (bone island); osteoma
2. Giant cell tumor
3. Osteochondroma
4. Osteoid osteoma

MALIGNANT

COMMON

1. Chordoma
2. Ewing sarcoma
3. Lymphoma$_g$; leukemia
4. Metastasis
5. Multiple myeloma; plasmacytoma

UNCOMMON

1. Angiosarcoma
2. Chondrosarcoma
3. Fibrosarcoma
4. Malignant giant cell tumor
5. Malignant fibrous histiocytoma

6. Malignant hemangioendothelioma and hemangiopericytoma
7. Osteosarcoma
8. PNET
9. Rhabdomyosarcoma

LOOK-ALIKES

1. Arthritic spondylitis (eg, rheumatoid; gout; psoriatic)
2. Eosinophilic granuloma (Langerhans cell histiocytosis$_g$)
3. Fibrous dysplasia
4. Hydatid disease
5. Paget's disease
6. Spondylodiskitis (osteomyelitis/diskitis) (eg, tuberculous, sarcoid, fungal, brucellar, other bacterial)

Reference

1. Dähnert W: Radiology Teaching Manual. (ed 4) Baltimore: Williams & Wilkins, 1999, pp 151–152

Gamut C-39

LESIONS OF THE VERTEBRAL BODY AND/OR APPENDAGES WITH PROMINENT EXPANSILE REMODELING

COMMON

1. Aneurysmal bone cyst
2. Hemangioma
3. Osteoblastoma

UNCOMMON

1. Chondroid lesion
2. Fibrous dysplasia
3. Giant cell tumor
4. Gout
5. Hydatid cyst
6. Metastasis
7. Multiple myeloma; plasmacytoma

Gamut C-40-1

ABNORMAL SIZE OR SHAPE OF A VERTEBRAL PEDICLE—ABSENT OR HYPOPLASTIC PEDICLE

1. Congenital absence or hypoplasia
2. Destroyed pedicle (See C-41)
3. Mucopolysaccharidoses (esp. Hunter S.)
4. Neurofibromatosis
5. [Poorly visualized pedicles C2-C5]
6. Radiation therapy

[ ] This condition does not actually cause the gamuted imaging finding, but can produce imaging changes that simulate it.

References
1. Mandell GA: The pedicle in neurofibromatosis. AJR 1978;130:675–678
2. Morin ME, Palacios E: The aplastic hypoplastic lumbar pedicle. AJR 1974;122:639–642
3. Swischuk LE, John SD: Differential Diagnosis in Pediatric Radiology. (ed 2) Baltimore: Williams & Wilkins, 1995, pp 403–405
4. Wiener MD, Martinez S, Forsberg DA: Congenital absence of a cervical spine pedicle: clinical and radiographic findings. AJR 1990;155:1037–1041

Gamut C-40-2

ENLARGED PEDICLE

1. Compensatory hypertrophy with contralateral deficiency of neural arch
2. Neoplasm (eg, osteoid osteoma; osteoblastoma; hemangioma)

Reference
1. Swischuk LE, John SD: Differential Diagnosis in Pediatric Radiology. (ed 2) Baltimore: Williams & Wilkins, 1995, pp 403–404

Gamut C-40-3

DYSPLASTIC PEDICLE

COMMON
1. Neurofibromatosis
2. Part of other congenital anomaly

UNCOMMON
1. Diastematomyelia
2. Klippel-Feil S.
3. Meningomyelocele

Reference
1. Swischuk LE, John SD: Differential Diagnosis in Pediatric Radiology. (ed 2) Baltimore: Williams & Wilkins, 1995, p 403

Gamut C-40-4

FLATTENED PEDICLE

1. Intraspinal expanding neoplasm or cyst; arteriovenous malformation
2. Normal (eg, upper lumbar spine)
3. Syringomyelia; hydromyelia

Reference
1. Swischuk LE, John SD: Differential Diagnosis in Pediatric Radiology. (ed 2) Baltimore: Williams & Wilkins, 1995, p 403

Gamut C-41

VERTEBRAL PEDICLE EROSION OR DESTRUCTION

COMMON

1. Intraspinal neoplasm or cyst (esp. neurofibroma; meningioma)
2. Metastasis
3. Tuberculosis, fungus or other infectious disease

UNCOMMON

1. Benign bone tumor (eg, aneurysmal bone cyst; giant cell tumor; hemangiopericytoma)
2. [Congenital absence of pedicle]
3. Eosinophilic granuloma (Langerhans cell histiocytosis$_g$)
4. Hydatid disease
5. Lymphoma$_g$
6. Multiple myeloma
7. Syringomyelia; hydromyelia
8. Vertebral artery aneurysm or tortuosity (cervical spine); arteriovenous malformation

[ ] This condition does not actually cause the gamuted imaging finding, but can produce imaging changes that simulate it.

Gamut C-42

VERTEBRAL PEDICLE SCLEROSIS

COMMON

1. Metastasis (osteoblastic)
2. Osteoblastoma
3. Osteoid osteoma
4. Stress-induced
   a. Congenital absence or hypoplasia of contralateral posterior elements
   b. Malalignment of apophyseal joints
   c. Spondylolisthesis

UNCOMMON

1. Idiopathic
2. Lymphoma$_g$
3. Osteosarcoma; Ewing sarcoma
4. Paget's disease
5. Posttraumatic (healed fracture)

References

1. Pettine K, Klassen R: Osteoid osteoma and osteoblastoma of the spine. J Bone Joint Surg 1986;68A:354–361
2. Swischuk LE, John SD: Differential Diagnosis in Pediatric Radiology. (ed 2) Baltimore: Williams & Wilkins, 1995, p 403
3. Wilkinson RH, Hall JE: The sclerotic pedicle: Tumor or pseudotumor? Radiology 1974;111:683–688

Gamut C-43

SMALL OR NARROW INTERVERTEBRAL FORAMEN

COMMON

1. Degenerative or posttraumatic arthritis with hypertrophic bony ridging and spurring

UNCOMMON

1. Diastematomyelia
2. Fused vertebra
3. Klippel-Feil S.
4. Meningomyelocele
5. Posterior subluxation of cervical spine
6. Unilateral bar resulting in scoliosis

Reference

1. Swischuk LE, John SD: Differential Diagnosis in Pediatric Radiology. (ed 2) Baltimore: Williams & Wilkins, 1995, pp 425–427

Gamut C-44

ENLARGED INTERVERTEBRAL FORAMEN

COMMON
1. Congenital with other anomalies
2. Neurofibroma

UNCOMMON
1. Congenital absence or hypoplasia of pedicle or neural arch
2. Dermoid; teratoma
3. Dejerine-Sottas S. (hypertrophic interstitial polyneuritis)
4. Dural ectasia (eg, idiopathic; neurofibromatosis; Marfan S.; Ehlers-Danlos S.)
5. Fibroma of spinal ligaments
6. Hydatid disease
7. Lateral thoracic meningocele
8. Lymphoma$_g$
9. Metastasis to spine or nerve
10. Neuroblastoma, ganglioneuroma (dumbbell tumors)
11. Neurofibromatosis (bony dysplasia; dural ectasia)
12. Postsurgical
13. Posttraumatic (eg, fracture; avulsed nerve root "diverticulum")
14. Primary neoplasm of spine or spinal cord (eg, chordoma; meningioma; lipoma)
15. Spondylolysis
16. Vertebral artery aneurysm or tortuosity (eg, coarctation of aorta)

References
1. Anderson RE, Shealy CN: Cervical pedicle erosion and rootlet compression caused by a tortuous vertebral artery. Radiology 1970;96:537–538
2. Danziger J, Bloch S: The widened cervical intervertebral foramen. Radiology 1975; 116:671–674
3. Patel DV, Ferguson RJL, Schey WL: Enlargement of the intervertebral foramen, an unusual cause. AJR 1978;131:911–913
4. Swischuk LE, John SD: Differential Diagnosis in Pediatric Radiology. (ed 2) Baltimore: Williams & Wilkins, 1995, pp 425–427

Gamut C-45-1

DEFECTIVE OR DESTROYED POSTERIOR NEURAL ARCHES—CONGENITAL DEFECTS

1. Defect in posterior arch of C1 (rarely C2 or other vertebrae)
2. Diastematomyelia
3. Meningocele; meningomyelocele; sacral dimple
*4. [Normal synchondroses between body and arches seen on oblique views]
5. Spina bifida occulta (usually L5 or S1)
+6. Spondylolysis

* Note: Must differentiate the normal synchondrosis occurring between the dens and arch of C2 from a hangman's fracture.
+ Believed to be due to stress fractures but may have a tendency to occur with some frequency in hypoplastic neural arches)
[ ] This condition does not actually cause the gamuted imaging finding, but can produce imaging changes that simulate it.

References
1. Charlton OP, Gehweiler JA Jr, Morgan CL, et al: Spondylolysis and spondylolisthesis of the cervical spine. Skeletal Radiol 1978;3:79–84
2. Swischuk LE, Hayden CK Jr, Sarwar M: The dens-arch synchondrosis versus the hangman's fracture. Pediatr Radiol 1979;8:100–112
3. Swischuk LE, John SD: Differential Diagnosis in Pediatric Radiology. (ed 2) Baltimore: Williams & Wilkins, 1995, pp 405–408

Gamut C-45-2

DEFECTIVE OR DESTROYED POSTERIOR NEURAL ARCHES—ACQUIRED DEFECTS OR DESTRUCTION

1. Fracture with hyperextension injury (eg, hangman's fracture of C2)
2. Hydatid disease

(continued)

3. Langerhans cell histiocytosis$_g$
4. Metastasis
5. Multiple myeloma
6. Osteomyelitis
7. Primary neoplasm of spine (eg, hemangioma; aneurysmal bone cyst; osteoblastoma; osteoid osteoma; giant cell tumor; Ewing sarcoma; other bone sarcoma)
8. Spondylolysis, spondylolisthesis (pars interarticularis defects or stress fractures)

References

1. Beeler JW: Further evidence on the acquired nature of spondylolysis and spondylolisthesis. AJR 1970:108:796–798
2. Swischuk LE, John SD: Differential Diagnosis in Pediatric Radiology. (ed 2) Baltimore: Williams & Wilkins, 1995, pp 405–408

Gamut C-46-1

SPINA BIFIDA OCCULTA*

COMMON

1. Isolated anomaly

UNCOMMON

1. Aarskog S.
2. Aicardi S.
3. Bardet-Biedl S.
4. Dermoid (intraspinal)
5. Diastematomyelia
6. Dorsal dermal sinus
7. Epidermoid cyst
8. Fanconi anemia
9. Filum terminate lipoma
10. Freeman-Sheldon S. (whistling face S.)
11. Gorlin S. (nevoid basal cell carcinoma S.)
12. Hallermann-Streiff S. (oculo-mandibulo-facial S.)
13. Klinefelter S. (XXY S.)
14. Klippel-Feil S.
15. LEOPARD S.

16. Lipomeningocele
17. Meningocele
18. Otopalatodigital S. (type I)
19. Split notochord S.
20. Tethered cord S.
21. Wildervanck S.

* Skin-covered defect in posterior neural arch, commonly seen in the lower lumbar spine or upper sacrum and rarely associated with neurologic defect by itself.

References

1. Dähnert W: Radiology Review Manual. (ed 4) Baltimore: Williams & Wilkins, 1999, p 149
2. Taybi H, Lachman RS: Radiology of Syndromes, Metabolic Disorders, and Skeletal Dysplasias. (ed 4) St. Louis: Mosby-Year Book Inc., 1996

Gamut C-46-2

SPINA BIFIDA APERTA*

1. Meningocele
2. Meningomyelocele
3. Myelocele
4. Myeloschisis

* Incomplete fusion of posterior elements of vertebrae and overlying soft tissues; posterior protrusion of all or parts of the contents of the spinal canal through a bony spina bifida; almost always associated with neurologic defect.

Reference

1. Dähnert W: Radiology Review Manual. (ed 4) Baltimore: Williams & Wilkins, 1999, p 149

Gamut C-47

SACRAL AGENESIS OR HYPOPLASIA

1. Caudal regression S. or mermaid S. (sirenomelia) (usually in infants of diabetic mothers)
2. Fanconi anemia
3. Femoral-facies S.

4. Oculo-auriculo-vertebral spectrum (Goldenhar S.)
5. Roberts S.
6. Silver-Russell S.
7. Teratoma (presacral)

References
1. Kenefick JS: Hereditary sacral agenesis associated with presacral tumors. Br J Surg 1973;60: 271–274
2. Passarge E, Lenz W: Syndrome of caudal regression in infants of diabetic mothers: observations of further cases. Pediatrics 1966;37:672–675
3. Swischuk LE, John SD: Differential Diagnosis in Pediatric Radiology. (ed 2) Baltimore: Williams & Wilkins, 1995, pp 444–445
4. Taybi H, Lachman RS: Radiology of Syndromes, Metabolic Disorders, and Skeletal Dysplasias. (ed 4) St. Louis: Mosby-Year Book Inc., 1996
5. Tsuchida Y, Watanasupt W, Nakajo T: Anorectal malformations associated with a presacral tumor and sacral defect. Pediatr Surg Int 1989;4:398–402

Gamut C-48-2
SACROCOCCYGEAL "TAIL" OR APPENDAGE

1. Association with other anomalies (eg, spinal dysraphism; omphalocele)
2. Crouzon S. (craniofacial dysostosis)
3. Goltz S. (focal dermal hypoplasia)
4. Isolated anomaly; idiopathic
5. Metatropic dysplasia
6. Pallister-Killian S.
7. Simpson-Golabi-Behmel S.

Reference
1. Taybi H, Lachman RS: Radiology of Syndromes, Metabolic Disorders, and Skeletal Dysplasias. (ed 4) St. Louis: Mosby-Year Book Inc., 1996, p 1047

Gamut C-48-1
SACRAL DEFORMITY (Curved or Sickle-Shaped Sacrum)

1. Currarino triad
2. Imperforate anus
3. Meningocele (anterior, lateral, or intrasacral)
4. Teratoma (presacral)
5. Tethered cord S. (often with spinal lipoma)

References
1. Swischuk LE, John SD: Differential Diagnosis in Pediatric Radiology. (ed 2) Baltimore: Williams & Wilkins, 1995, pp 444–445
2. Taybi H, Lachman RS: Radiology of Syndromes, Metabolic Disorders, and Skeletal Dysplasias. (ed 4) St. Louis: Mosby-Year Book Inc., 1996

Gamut C-49-1
SACROILIAC JOINT DISEASE (EROSION, WIDENING, SCLEROSIS AND/OR FUSION)

COMMON
+*1. Ankylosing spondylitis
 *2. Infectious arthritis or osteomyelitis (eg, pyogenic; tuberculous)
+3. Osteitis condensans ilii
 4. Osteoarthritis, degenerative or posttraumatic
*5. Psoriatic arthritis
*6. Reiter S. (reactive arthritis)
 7. Rheumatoid arthritis (incl. juvenile)

UNCOMMON
1. Agenesis (caudal dysplasia)
2. Behçet S.
3. Bone neoplasm of sacrum, primary (eg, giant cell tumor; chordoma; sarcoma) or metastatic

(continued)

4. Calcium pyrophosphate crystal deposition disease
5. Enteropathic arthritis due to inflammatory bowel disease (eg, ulcerative colitis; Crohn's disease; Whipple's disease)
6. Familial Mediterranean fever (familial recurrent polyserositis)
*7. Gaucher's disease
8. Gout
+9. Hyperparathyroidism, primary or secondary (renal osteodystrophy)
+10. Leukemia; lymphomag
+11. Multicentric reticulohistiocytosis (lipoid derma-toarthritis)
*12. Occupational acro-osteolysis (eg, polyvinylchloride osteolysis)
*13. Paraplegia, paralysis$_g$
14. Pseudohypoparathyroidism
*15. Relapsing polychondritis
16. SAPHO S.
17. Sacroiliitis circumscripta

* Fusion of sacroiliac joint(s) may occur.
\+ Usually bilateral symmetrical.

References

1. Boutin RD, Resnick D: The SAPHO Syndrome: An evolving concept for unifying several idiopathic disorders of bone and skin. AJR 1998;170:585–591
2. Brower AC: Arthritis in Black and White. (ed 2) Philadelphia: WB Saunders Co., 1997
3. Burgener FA, Kormano M: Differential Diagnosis in Conventional Radiology. (ed 2) New York: Thieme Medical Publ, 1991, p 183
4. Resnik CS, Resnick D: Radiology of disorders of the sacroiliac joints. JAMA 1985;253:2863–2866

Gamut C-49-2

SACROILIAC JOINT ABNORMALITIES— SYMMETRICAL VS. ASYMMETRICAL AND UNILATERAL VS. BILATERAL

SYMMETRICAL INVOLVEMENT

COMMON

1. Ankylosing spondylitis
2. Inflammatory bowel disease (Crohn disease; ulcerative colitis; Whipple S.)
3. Osteitis condensans ilii
4. Osteoarthritis
5. Reiter/reactive disease
6. Rheumatoid arthritis (adult)

UNCOMMON

1. Behçet S.
2. Familial Mediterranean fever
3. Gout
4. Hyperparathyroidism
5. Juvenile rheumatoid arthritis
6. Mixed connective tissue disease (overlap S.)
7. Psoriatic arthritis
8. Relapsing polychondritis
9. SAPHO S.

ASYMMETRICAL INVOLVEMENT

COMMON

1. Osteoarthritis
2. Psoriatic arthritis
3. Reiter/reactive disease

UNCOMMON

1. Behçet S.
2. Familial Mediterranean fever
3. Gout
4. Infection
5. Juvenile rheumatoid arthritis
6. Mixed connective tissue disease (overlap S.)

7. Relapsing polychondritis
8. Rheumatoid arthritis (adult)
9. SAPHO S.

UNILATERAL INVOLVEMENT

COMMON

1. Infection
2. Osteoarthritis
3. Psoriatic arthritis
4. Reiter/reactive disease

UNCOMMON

1. Behçet S.
2. Familial Mediterranean fever
3. Gout
4. Juvenile rheumatoid arthritis
5. Mixed connective tissue disease (overlap S.)
6. Relapsing polychondritis
7. Rheumatoid arthritis (adult)
8. SAPHO S.

Gamut C-50

SACROCOCCYGEAL OR PRESACRAL MASS (See C-51)

COMMON

1. Abscess (eg, rectal perforation from trauma or surgery; sinus tract from Crohn's disease, ulcerative colitis, amebiasis, schistosomiasis, tuberculosis, or lymphogranuloma venereum)
2. Bone cyst or neoplasm, benign (eg, aneurysmal bone cyst; giant cell tumor)
3. Carcinoma of prostate
4. Hematoma; fracture
5. Malignant neoplasm of sacrum (eg, chordoma; sarcoma; metastasis; myeloma)
6. Normal variant or after pelvic surgery
7. Teratoma; dermoid cyst

UNCOMMON

1. Arachnoid, extradural, or perineural cyst
2. Ectopic kidney
3. Hamartoma
4. Hydatid cyst
5. Hydroureter; urinoma
6. Intraspinal neoplasm, other (eg, ependymoma; lipoma)
7. Lymphocele
8. Lymphoma$_g$
9. Meningocele (anterior sacral)
10. Neurenteric cyst
11. Neurofibromatosis I
12. Neurogenic tumor
13. Osteomyelitis of sacrum
14. Ovarian cyst or neoplasm; tubo-ovarian abscess
15. Rectal duplication

References

1. Epstein BS: The Spine. (ed 4) Philadelphia: Lea & Febiger, 1976
2. Keslar PJ, Buck JL, Suarez ES: Germ cell tumors of the sacrococcygeal region: Radiologic-pathologic correlation. RadioGraphics 1994;14:607–622
3. Kransdorf MJ, Murphey MD: Imaging of Soft Tissue Tumors. Philadelphia: WB Saunders Co., 1997
4. Lombardi G, Passerini A: Spinal Cord Diseases: A Radiologic and Myelographic Analysis. Baltimore: Williams & Wilkins, 1964
5. Murphey MD, Andrews CL, Flemming DJ, et al: Primary tumors of the spine: Radiologic-pathologic correlation. RadioGraphics 1996;16:1131–1158
6. Silverman FN (ed): Caffey's Pediatric X-ray Diagnosis. (ed 8) Chicago: Year Book Medical Publ, 1985
7. Taybi H, Lachman RS: Radiology of Syndromes, Metabolic Disorders, and Skeletal Dysplasias. (ed 4) St. Louis: Mosby-Year Book Inc., 1996, p 1047
8. Werner JL, Taybi H: Presacral masses in childhood. AJR 1970;109:403–410
9. Wetzel L, Levine E: Pictorial Essay. MR imaging of sacral and presacral lesions. AJR 1990;154:771–775

Gamut C-51

SACRAL NEOPLASM (See C-50)

BENIGN

COMMON

1. Aneurysmal bone cyst
2. Benign neurogenic tumor (neurofibroma; neurilemmoma); notochordal rest
3. Giant cell tumor
4. Teratoma (sacrococcygeal)

UNCOMMON

1. Osteoblastoma
2. Osteochondroma
3. Osteoma

MALIGNANT

COMMON

1. Chondrosarcoma
2. Chordoma
3. Ewing sarcoma
4. Lymphoma$_g$
5. Metastasis (esp. from carcinoma of breast, prostate, kidney, colon, or cervix)
6. Multiple myeloma; plasmacytoma

UNCOMMON

1. Fibrosarcoma; malignant fibrous histiocytoma
2. Malignant giant cell tumor
3. Malignant peripheral nerve sheath tumor (MPNST); neuroblastoma
4. Osteosarcoma
5. Paget's sarcoma
6. Radiation-induced sarcoma

References

1. Murphey MD, Andrews CL, Flemming DJ, et al: Primary tumors of the spine: Radiologic-pathologic correlation. RadioGraphics 1996;16:1131–1158
2. Smith J: International Skeletal Society Lecture. Philadelphia, 1984

Gamut C-52

NARROW DISK SPACES

COMMON

1. Ankylosing spondylitis
2. Block vertebra, congenital or acquired (See C-25)
*3. Degenerative disk disease (usually associated with osteoarthritis)
*4. Discitis; spondyloarthritis (juvenile)
*5. Herniated disk
*6. Kyphosis; scoliosis (severe)
*7. Neuropathic arthropathy (eg, diabetes; syringomyelia; tabes dorsalis)
*8. Osteomyelitis (eg, pyogenic; tuberculous; sarcoid; brucellar; typhoid)
*9. Rheumatoid arthritis; other inflammatory arthritis
10. Scheuermann's disease
*11. Trauma (flexion-rotation injury)

UNCOMMON

*1. Calcium pyrophosphate crystal deposition disease
2. Cockayne S.
3. Kniest dysplasia
4. Morquio S.
5. Neoplasm (rarely)
*6. Ochronosis (alkaptonuria)
7. Ruvalcaba S.
8. Spondyloepiphyseal dysplasia tarda

* Often with adjacent sclerosis of the vertebral margins.

References

1. Alexander CJ: The aetiology of juvenile spondyloarthritis (discitis). Clin Radiol 1970;21:178–187
2. Forster A, Pothmann R, Winter K, Bauman-Rath CA: Magnetic resonance imaging in non-specific discitis. Pediatr Radiol 1987;17:162–163
3. Frank P, Gleeson J: Destructive vertebral lesions in ankylosing spondylitis. Br J Radiol 1975;48:755–758
4. Martel W: Pathogenesis of cervical discovertebral destruction in rheumatoid arthritis. Arthritis Rheum 1977;20:1217–1225
5. Swischuk LE, John SD: Differential Diagnosis in Pediatric Radiology. (ed 2) Baltimore: Williams & Wilkins, 1995, pp 432–434

6. Szalay EA, Green NE, Heller RM, et al: Magnetic resonance imaging in the childhood diagnosis of discitis. J Pediatr Orthop 1987;7:164–167
7. Wenger DR, Bobechko WP, Gilday DL: The spectrum of intervertebral disc-space infection in children. J Bone Joint Surg 1978;60A:100–108

3. Metastasis
4. Myeloma

Reference
1. Murphey, MD Andrews CL, Flemming DJ, et al: Primary tumors of the spine: Radiologic-pathologic correlation. RadioGraphics 1996;16:1131–1158

Gamut C-53

WIDE DISK SPACES

1. Acromegaly
2. Biconcave vertebrae (See C-19)
3. Calcific discitis
4. Endplate infarction (eg, sickle cell disease; Gaucher's disease)
5. Osteomalacia (See D-44)
6. Osteoporosis (See D-43-1)
7. Platyspondyly (esp. Morquio S.; osteogenesis imperfecta; cretinism; metatropic dysplasia) (See C-15)
8. Trauma (hyperextension injury to spine)

Reference
1. Swischuk LE, John SD: Differential Diagnosis in Pediatric Radiology. (ed 2) Baltimore: Williams & Wilkins, 1995, pp 433–435

Gamut C-54

TUMORS THAT CAN CROSS THE INTERVERTEBRAL DISK

COMMON
1. Chondroma
2. Chondrosarcoma
3. Lymphoma$_g$

UNCOMMON
1. Ewing sarcoma
2. Giant cell tumor

Gamut C-55

CALCIFICATION OF ONE OR MORE INTERVERTEBRAL DISKS

COMMON
*1. Degenerative spondylosis
2. Idiopathic (eg, transient calcification in children, esp. in cervical spine; persistent type in adults)
*3. Ochronosis (alkaptonuria)
*4. Posttraumatic
5. Spinal fusion (eg, congenital block vertebra; Klippel-Feil S.; fibrodysplasia {myositis} ossificans progressiva; surgical fusion)

UNCOMMON
1. Aarskog S.
2. Acromegaly
3. Amyloidosis
*4. Ankylosing spondylitis
5. Calcium pyrophosphate dihydrate deposition disease
6. Chondrocalcinosis; other causes (See D-242)
7. Cockayne S.
8. Diffuse idiopathic skeletal hyperostosis (DISH)
9. Gout
10. Hemochromatosis
11. Homocystinuria
12. Hypercalcemia
13. Hyperparathyroidism
14. Hypervitaminosis D
15. Hypophosphatasia
*16. Infection (eg, brucellosis)

(continued)

17. Mucolipidosis II (I-cell disease)
18. Paraplegia; poliomyelitis
19. Rheumatoid spondylitis (incl. juvenile chronic arthritis)
20. Spondyloepiphyseal dysplasia tarda
21. Wilson disease

* Can cause disk ossification.

References

1. Dähnert W: Radiology Review Manual. (ed 4) Baltimore: Williams & Wilkins,1999, p 153
2. Dussault RG, Kaye JJ: Intervertebral disk calcification associated with spine fusion. Radiology 1977;125:57–61
3. Edeiken J, Dalinka M, Karasick D: Edeiken's Roentgen Diagnosis of Diseases of Bone. (ed 4) Baltimore: Williams & Wilkins, 1989
4. Greenfield GB: Radiology of Bone Diseases. (ed 5) Philadelphia: Lippincott, 1990
5. Kozlowski K, Beighton P: Gamut Index of Skeletal Dysplasias. Berlin: Springer-Verlag, 1984, pp 48–49
6. Mainzer F: Herniation of the nucleus pulposus. A rare complication of intervertebral-disk calcification in children. Radiology 1973;107:167–170
7. Murray RO, Jacobson HG, Stoker D: The Radiology of Skeletal Disorders. (ed 3) Edinburgh: Churchill Livingstone, 1990
8. Swischuk LE, John SD: Differential Diagnosis in Pediatric Radiology. (ed 2) Baltimore: Williams & Wilkins, 1995, pp 433–437
9. Taybi H, Lachman RS: Radiology of Syndromes, Metabolic Disorders, and Skeletal Dysplasias. (ed 4) St. Louis: Mosby-Year Book Inc., 1996, p 1046
10. Weinberger A, Myers AR: Intervertebral disc calcification in adults: a review. Semin Arthritis Rheum 1978;18:69–75

GAS IN AN INTERVERTEBRAL DISK (VACUUM DISK)*

COMMON

1. Degeneration of nucleus pulposus
2. Schmorl's nodes (intraosseous herniation of disk) (on CT)
3. Spondylosis deformans

UNCOMMON

1. Fractured vertebra
2. Metastatic disease to adjacent vertebra with vertebral collapse
3. Osteomyelitis of vertebra (rare)
4. Osteonecrosis with vertebral collapse (Kömmell's disease)

* Nitrogen gas from surrounding tissues enters into clefts of a disk with an abnormal nucleus pulposus or annulus attachment.

References

1. Dähnert W: Radiology Review Manual. (ed 4) Baltimore: Williams & Wilkins, 1999, pp 152–153
2. Greenfield GB: Radiology of Bone Diseases. (ed 5) Philadelphia: Lippincott, 1990

CONGENITAL SYNDROMES AND BONE DYSPLASIAS WITH A NARROW SPINAL CANAL (NARROW INTERPEDICULAR DISTANCE): SPINAL STENOSIS

COMMON

1. Achondroplasia; hypochondroplasia
2. Acromegaly
3. Diastrophic dysplasia
4. Klippel-Feil S.

UNCOMMON

1. Acrodysostosis (peripheral dysostosis)
2. Acromesomelic dysplasia
3. Alagille S. (arteriohepatic S.)
4. Brachyolmia
5. Calcium pyrophosphate crystal deposition disease
6. Cauda equina S. (narrow lumbar spinal canal S.)
7. Cerebrocostomandibular S.
8. Chondroectodermal dysplasia (Ellis-van Creveld S.)
9. Dyggve-Melchior-Clausen dysplasia (Smith-Mc-Cort S.)

10. Dyschondrosteosis
11. Gordon S.
12. Kniest dysplasia
13. Metatropic dysplasia
14. Mucolipidosis II (early infancy)
15. Osteoglophonic dysplasia
16. Pseudohypoparathyroidism; pseudopseudohypoparathyroidism
17. Robinow S.
18. Schneckenbecken dysplasia
19. Spondylometaphyseal dysplasia
20. Stickler S.
21. Thanatophoric dysplasia
22. Trisomy 8 S.
23. Turner S.
24. Weill-Marchesani S.

References
1. Kozlowski K, Beighton P: Gamut Index of Skeletal Dysplasias. Berlin: Springer-Verlag, 1984, pp 47–48
2. Taybi H, Lachman RS: Radiology of Syndromes, Metabolic Disorders, and Skeletal Dysplasias. (ed 4) St. Louis: Mosby-Year Book Inc., 1996, p 1047

4. Idiopathic
5. Marfan S.
6. Mucopolysaccharidoses (esp. Hurler S.; Hunter S.; Morquio S.)
7. Neurofibromatosis I; dural ectasia
8. Otopalatodigital S. (type I)
9. Syringomyelia; hydromyelia
10. Tethered cord S.

[ ] This condition does not actually cause the gamuted imaging finding, but can produce imaging changes that simulate it.

Reference
1. Taybi H, Lachman RS: Radiology of Syndromes, Metabolic Disorders, and Skeletal Dysplasias. (ed 4) St. Louis: Mosby-Year Book Inc., 1996, p 1047

Gamut C-58

WIDE SPINAL CANAL (INCREASED INTERPEDICULAR DISTANCE) (See C-59, 61)

COMMON
1. Intraspinal neoplasm (eg, ependymoma; astrocytoma; neurofibroma; lipoma) or cyst
2. Meningocele; meningomyelocele
3. [Rotation of vertebra due to scoliosis or poor radiographic positioning]

UNCOMMON
1. Arteriovenous malformation
2. Diastematomyelia
3. Frontometaphyseal dysplasia

Gamut C-59

INTRAMEDULLARY LESION (WIDENING OF SPINAL CORD ON MYELOGRAPHY, CT, OR MR)

COMMON
1. [Extrinsic compression (eg, by cervical ridge; herniated disk; large extramedullary or extradural tumor)]
2. Infection (eg, abscess; myelitis—viral or bacterial; HIV; Lyme disease; cytomegalovirus; progressive multifocal leukoencephalopathy {PML})
3. Inflammation (eg, multiple sclerosis; acute transverse myelitis; acute disseminated encephalomyelitis {ADEM}; Devic S.)
4. Intramedullary tumor (esp. ependymoma and astrocytoma; also rarely oligodendroglioma; ganglioglioma; hemangioblastoma; primary melanoma; lipoma; lymphoma$_g$)
5. Syringomyelia; hydromyelia

UNCOMMON
1. Arteriovenous malformation; angioma
2. Dermoid; teratoma; epidermoid

(continued)

3. Diastematomyelia
4. Granuloma (eg, sarcoidosis; tuberculosis)
5. Hematoma, contusion, or edema of cord (post-traumatic or anticoagulant therapy)
6. Infarct of spinal cord (eg, anterior spinal artery infarct; venous infarct/ischemia)
7. Meningomyelocele
8. Metastasis (eg, breast, lung, melanoma); drop metastasis through the central canal (eg, medullo-blastoma)
9. Postradiation myelopathy
10. [Spinal cord atrophy] (See C-60)
11. Transection of cord

[ ] This condition does not actually cause the gamuted imaging finding, but can produce imaging changes that simulate it.

References

1. Dähnert W: Radiology Review Manual. (ed 4) Baltimore: Williams & Wilkins,1999, pp 153–155
2. Epstein BS: Spinal canal mass lesions. Radiol Clin North Am 1966;4:185–202
3. Epstein BS: The Spine: A Radiological Text and Atlas. (ed 4) Philadelphia: Lea & Febiger, 1976
4. Lewtas N: The Spine and Myelography. In: Sutton D (ed): Textbook of Radiology and Imaging. (ed 4) Edinburgh: Churchill Livingstone, 1987
5. Moseley IF: Myelography. In: DuBoulay GH (ed): A Textbook of Radiological Diagnosis. (ed 5) London: HK Lewis, 1984, p 530
6. Stevens JM: The Spine and Spinal Cord. In: Sutton D, Young JWR (eds): A Short Textbook of Clinical Imaging. London: Springer-Verlag, 1990, pp. 806–811

Gamut C-60

SPINAL CORD ATROPHY

COMMON

1. Amyotrophic lateral sclerosis
2. Multiple sclerosis
3. Posttraumatic
4. Spondylosis; disk hernation (esp. cervical)
5. Syringomyelia, hydromyelia (after collapse)

UNCOMMON

1. Arteriovenous malformation of cord
2. Friedreich's ataxia
3. Ischemia with cord infarction
4. Other motor neuron disease or motor and sensory neuropathies
5. Postradiation myelopathy
6. Subacute combined degeneration
7. Tabes dorsalis

Reference

1. Stevens JM: The Spine and Spinal Cord. In: Sutton D, Young JWR (eds): A Short Textbook of Clinical Imaging. London: Springer-Verlag, 1990, p 811

Gamut C-61

INTRADURAL, EXTRAMEDULLARY LESION (ON MYELOGRAPHY, CT, OR MR)

COMMON

1. Arachnoiditis (See C-62)
2. Meningioma
3. Metastasis, esp. leptomeningeal "drop" seeding from CNS tumor (eg, medulloblastoma; glioblas-toma; pinealoma; ependymoma; PNET) or hematogenous (eg, from carcinoma of lung or breast; melanoma; lymphoma$_g$)
4. Neurofibroma

UNCOMMON

1. Arachnoid cyst
2. Cysticercosis (cysts)
3. Dermoid; teratoma; epidermoid
4. Ependymoma of filum terminale
5. Granuloma (eg, tuberculoma; fungal—aspergilloma; sarcoid)
6. Hemangioblastoma; hemangiopericytoma
7. Lipoma (lipomyeloschisis)
8. Meningocele

9. Neurenteric cyst
10. Tortuosity of nerve roots
11. Vascular malformation; angioma; varices

Reference
1. Stevens JM: The Spine and Spinal Cord. In: Sutton D, Young JWR (eds): A Short Textbook of Clinical Imaging. London: Springer-Verlag, 1990, pp 802–806

Gamut C-62

ARACHNOIDITIS

1. Cysticercosis
2. Pantopaque myelography
3. Postoperative
4. Posttraumatic
5. Spinal meningitis
   a. Bacterial
   b. Fungal
   c. HIV 1
   d. Sarcoid
   e. Tuberculous

Gamut C-63

EXTRADURAL LESION (ON MYELOGRAPHY, CT, OR MR)

COMMON
1. Dermoid; teratoma; epidermoid
2. Disk disease (bulging disk; herniated or sequestered nucleus pulposus)
3. Epidural metastasis (eg, lymphoma$_g$)
4. Epidural scar (eg, after disk surgery)
5. Fracture fragment or dislocation from vertebral trauma
6. Hematoma (traumatic, spontaneous, or bleeding hemangioma)

7. [Iatrogenic (needle point defect; extradural injection of Pantopaque)]
8. Ligamentum flavum thickening; intraspinal ligament ossification (eg, DISH; primary—esp. in Japanese)
9. Lipomatosis (obesity; steroid therapy; Cushing S.)
10. Meningioma (with intradural component)
11. Metastasis (esp. from carcinoma of lung, breast, prostate, or colon)
12. Neurogenic tumor (esp. neurofibroma with intradural component; also ganglioneuroma; ganglioneuroblastoma; neuroblastoma)
13. Osteomyelitis; epidural abscess (esp. tuberculous; pyogenic)
14. Spinal stenosis; spondylosis; osteophyte
15. Vertebral neoplasm with intraspinal extension (eg, sarcoma; myeloma; chordoma; hemangioma; giant cell tumor; aneurysmal bone cyst; osteoblastoma; osteochondroma)

UNCOMMON
1. Amyloidosis
2. Arachnoid cyst
3. Arachnoiditis (See C-62)
4. Epidural granuloma (eg, tuberculous; fungal; sarcoid)
5. Extramedullary hematopoiesis
6. Lipoma; fibroma
7. Paget's disease
8. Parasitic infection (eg, cysticercosis; hydatid disease; schistosomiasis)
9. Retroperitoneal neoplasm extending through intervertebral foramen (eg, neuroblastoma; lymphoma$_g$)

[ ] This condition does not actually cause the gamuted imaging finding, but can produce imaging changes that simulate it.

References
1. DuBoulay GH (ed): A Textbook of X-Ray Diagnosis by British Authors. Neuroradiology. London: AK Lewis, 1984
2. Epstein BS: Spinal canal mass lesions. Radiol Clin North Am 1966;4:185–202
3. Stevens JM: The Spine and Spinal Cord. In: Sutton D, Young JWR (eds): A Short Textbook of Clinical Imaging. London: Springer-Verlag, 1990, pp 791–802

(continued)

4. Taveras JM, Wood EH: Diagnostic Neuroradiology. (ed 2) Baltimore: Williams & Wilkins, 1976

12. Meningioma
13. Osteomyelitis of spine
14. Paget's disease

References
1. Greenfield GB: Radiology of Bone Diseases. (ed 5) Philadelphia: Lippincott, 1990
2. O'Carroll MP, Witcombe JB: Primary disorders of bone with "spinal block." Clin Radiol 1979;30:299–306

Gamut C-64

SPINAL BLOCK (ON MYELOGRAPHY, CT, OR MR)

COMMON

1. Fracture, traumatic or pathologic
2. Hemorrhage (traumatic; spontaneous; anticoagulant therapy)
3. Herniated disk
4. Intervertebral joint disorder
5. Metastasis or contiguous spread of malignancy
6. Neoplasm of spine, primary (eg, sarcoma; myeloma; chordoma; giant cell tumor)
7. Neurogenic tumor (esp. neurofibroma)
8. Spinal stenosis

UNCOMMON

1. Abscess, epidural
2. Achondroplasia
3. Arachnoiditis (See C-62)
4. Cyst of spinal canal (eg, congenital; arachnoid; dermoid; *Cysticercus;* hydatid)
5. Fibrous dysplasia
6. Granuloma (eg, tuberculosis; schistosomiasis)
7. Hemangioma of vertebra
8. Intramedullary lesion, large (eg, syringomyelia; ependymoma; lipoma)
9. Klippel-Feil S.
10. Lipoma of canal
11. Lymphoma$_g$

Gamut C-65

TORTUOUS FILLING DEFECT ON LUMBAR MYELOGRAPHY

COMMON

1. Nerve root elongation, redundancy, or displacement (eg, spinal stenosis or arthrosis; disk herniation; achondroplasia)

UNCOMMON

1. Arachnoiditis (See C-62)
2. Extradural or intradural neoplasm
3. Multiple lesions at same or adjacent levels
4. Vascular abnormality (eg, arteriovenous malformation; venous angioma; varices)

Reference
1. Cronquist S, Thulin C-A: Significance of tortuous filling defects at lumbar myelography. Acta Radiologica Diag 1979; 20:561–568

D

Bone, Joints, and Soft Tissues

I. BONE—GENERALIZED

D

D

D

II. BONE—ANATOMIC

D

D

D. Bone, Joints, and Soft Tissues

D

D

IV. SOFT TISSUES

D

D

GAMUT D-1-S

INTERNATIONAL NOMENCLATURE AND CLASSIFICATION OF THE OSTEOCHONDRODYSPLASIAS (1997)

1. Achondroplasia group

Osteochondrodysplasia	Mode of Inheritance*
Thanatophoric dysplasia, Type I (includes San Diego Type)	AD
Thanatophoric dysplasia, Type II	AD
Achondroplasia	AD
Hypochondroplasia	AD
Hypochondroplasia	AD
SADDAN (severe achondroplasia, developmental delay, acanthosis nigricans)	AD

2. Severe Spondylodyplastic dysplasias

Lethal platyspondylic skeletal dysplasias (Torrance Type, Luton Type)	SP
Achondrogenesis Type 1A	AR
Opsismodysplasia	AR
SMD Sedaghatian Type	AR

3. Metatropic dysplasia group

Fibrochondrogenesis	AR
Schneckenbecken dysplasia	AR
Metatropic dysplasia (various forms)	AD

4. Short-rib dysplasia (SRP) (with or without polydactyly) group

SRP type I/III (Saldino-Noonan/ Verma-Naumoff)	AR
SRP type II (Majewski)	AR
SRP type IV (Beemer)	AR
Asphyxiating thoracic dysplasia (Jeune)	AR
Chondroectodermal Dysplasia (Ellis-van Creveld dysplasia)	AR
Thoracolaryngopelvic dysplasia (Barnes)	AD

5. Atelosteogenesis-Omodysplasia group

Osteochondrodysplasia	Mode of Inheritance*
Atelosteogenesis type I (includes "Bommerang dysplasia")	SP
Omodysplasia I (Maroteaux)	AD
Omodysplasia II (Borochowitz)	AR
Atelosteogenesis Type III	AD
de la Chapelle dysplasia	AR

6. Diastrophic dysplasia group

Achondrogenesis 1B	AR
Diastrophic dysplasia	AR
MED Autosomal Recessive Type	AR

7. Dyssegmental dysplasia group

Dyssegmental dysplasia, Silverman-Handmaker Type	AR
Dyssegmental dysplasia, Rolland-Desbuquois Type	AR

8. Type II collagenopathies

Achondrogenesis II (Langer-Saldino)	AD
Hypochondrogenesis	AD
Spondyloepiphyseal dysplasia (SED) congenita	AD
Spondyloepimetaphyseal dysplasia (SEMD) Strudwick Type	AD
Kniest dysplasia	AD
SED Namaqualand Type	AD
Spondyloperipheral dysplasia	AD
Mild SED with premature onset arthrosis	AD
Stickler dysplasia Type I	AD

9. Type XI collagenopathies

Stickler dysplasia Type II	AD
Stickler dysplasia Type III	AD
Marshall syndrome	AD
Otospondylomegaepiphyseal dysplasia (OSMED)	AR
Otospondylomegaepiphyseal dysplasia (OSMED	AD

(continued)

10. Other spondyloepi-(meta)-physeal [SE(M)D] dysplasias

Osteochondrodysplasia	Mode of Inheritance*
X-linked SED tarda	XLD
SEMD Handigodu Type	AD?
Progressive pseudorheumatoid dysplasia	AR
Dyggve-Melchior-Clausen dysplasia	AR
Wolcott-Rallison dysplasia	AR
Immuno-osseous dysplasia (Schimke)	AR
Schwartz-Jampel syndrome	AR
SEMD with joint laxity (SEMDJL)	AR
SEMD with multiple dislocations (Hall) (leptodactylic Type)	
SPONASTRIME dysplasia	AR
SEMD short limb - abnormal calcification type	AR
SEMD Pakistani Type	AR
Anauxetic dysplasia	AR

11. Multiple epiphyseal dysplasia & pseudoachondroplasia

Pseudoachondroplasia	AD
Multiple epiphyseal dysplasia (MED)	AD
(Fairbanks and Ribbing Types)	AD
	AD
Familial hip dysplasia (Beukes)	AD

12. Chondrodysplasia punctata (CDP) (stippled epiphyses group)

Rhizomelic CDP Type 1	AR
Rhizomelic CDP Type 2	AR
Rhizomelic CDP Type 3	AR
CDP Conradi-Hünermann Type	XLD
CDP X-linked recessive Type (brachytelephalangic)	XLR
CDP Tibia-metacarpal Type	AD
CHILD (limb-reduction-icthyosis)	XLD
CHILD (limb-reduction-icthyosis)	XLD
Hydrops-ectopic calcification-moth-eaten appearance HEM (Greenberg dysplasia)	AR
Dappled diaphyseal dysplasia	AR

13. Metaphyseal dysplasias

Osteochondrodysplasia	Mode of Inheritance*
Jansen Type	AD
Schmid Type	AD
Cartilage-Hair-Hypoplasia (McKusick)	AR
Metaphyseal anadysplasia (various types)	AD/XLD
Metaphyseal dysplasia with pancreatic insufficiency and cyclic neutropenia (Shwachmann Diamond)	AR
Adenosine deaminase (ADA) deficiency	AR
Metaphyseal chondrodysplasia Spahr Type	AR
Acroscyphodysplasia (various types)	AR

14. Spondylometaphyseal dysplasias (SMD)

Spondylometaphyseal dysplasia Kozlowski Type	AD
Spondylometaphyseal dysplasia (Sutcliffe/corner fracture Type)	AD
SMD with severe genu valgum (includes Schmidt and Algerian Types)	AD

15. Brachyolmia spondylodysplasias

Hobaek (includes Toledo Type)	AR
Maroteaux Type	AR
Autosomal dominant Type	AD

16. Mesomelic dysplasias

Dyschondrosteosis (Leri-Weill)	AD
Langer type (homozygous dyschondrosteosis)	AR
Nievergelt Type	AD
Kozlowski-Reardon Type	AR
Reinhardt-Pfeiffer Type	AD
Werner Type	AD
Robinow Type, dominant	AD
Robinow Type, recessive	AR
Mesomelic dysplasia with synostoses	AD
Mesomelic dysplasia Kantaputra Type	AD
Mesomelic dysplasia Verloes Type	AD
Mesomelic dysplasia Savarirayan Type	

17. Acromelic dysplasias

Osteochondrodysplasia	Mode of Inheritance*
Acromicric dysplasia	AD
Geleophysic dysplasia	AR
Myhre dysplasia	
Weill-Marchesani dysplasia	AR
Trichorhinophalangeal dysplasia Types I/III	AD
Trichorhinophalangeal dysplasia Type II (Langer-Giedion)	AD
Brachydactyly Type A1	AD
Brachydactyly Type A2	AD
Brachydactyly Type A3	
Brachydactyly Type B	AD
Brachydactyly Type C	AD
Brachydactyly Type D	AD
Brachydactyly Type E	AD
Pseudohypoparathyroidism (Albright Hereditary Osteodystrophy)	AD
Acrodysostosis	SP(AD)
Saldino-Mainzer dysplasia	AR
Brachydactyly-hypertension dysplasia (Bilginturan)	AD
Craniofacial conodysplasia	AD
Angel-shaped phalango-epiphyseal dysplasia (ASPED)	AD
Camptodactyly arthropathy coxa vara pericarditis (CACP)	AR
Christian Brachydactyly	AD

18. Acromesomelic dysplasias

Acromesomelic dysplasia Type Maroteaux	AR
Acromesomelic dysplasia Type Campailla-Martinelli	AR
Acromesomelic dysplasia Type Ferraz/Ohba	AD
Acromesomelic dysplasia Type Osebold Remondini	AD
Grebe dysplasia	AR
Cranioectodermal dysplasia	AR

19. Dysplasias with predominant membranous bone involvement

Osteochondrodysplasia	Mode of Inheritance*
Cleidocranial dysplasia	AD
Yunis-Varon dysplasia	AR
Parietal foramina (isolated)	AD
Parietal foramina (isolated)	AD

20. Bent-bone dysplasia group

Campomelic dysplasia	AD
Cumming syndrome	AR
Stüve-Wiedemann dysplasia (neonatal Schwartz-Jampel)	AR

21. Multiple dislocations with dysplasias

Larsen syndrome	AD
Larsen-like syndromes (including La Reunion Island)	AR
Desbuquois dysplasia	AR
Pseudodiastrophic dysplasia	AR

22. Dysostosis multiplex group

Mucopolysaccharidosis IH	AR
Mucopolysaccharidosis IS	AR
Mucopolysaccharidosis II	XLR
Mucopolysaccharidosis IIIA	AR
Mucopolysaccharidosis IIIB	AR
Mucopolysaccharidosis IIIC	AR
Mucopolysaccharidosis IIID	AR
Mucopolysaccharidosis IVA	AR
Mucopolysaccharidosis IVB	AR
Mucopolysaccharidosis VI	AR
Mucopolysaccharidosis VII	AR
Fucosidosis	AR
a-Mannosidosis	AR
b-Mannosidosis	AR
Aspartylglucosaminuria	AR
GM1 Gangliosidosis, several forms	AR
Sialidosis, several forms	AR
Sialic acid storage disease	AR
Galactosialidosis, several forms	AR
Multiple sulfatase deficiency	AR
Mucolipidosis II	AR
Mucolipidosis III	AR

(continued)

23. Low birthweight slender bone group

Osteochondrodysplasia	Mode of Inheritance*
Type I microcephalic osteodysplastic dysplasia	AR
Type II microcephalic osteodysplastic dysplasia	AR
Microcephalic osteodysplastic dysplasia (Saul Wilson)	AR
3M syndrome	AR

24. Dysplasias with decreased bone density

Osteogenesis imperfecta I (normal teeth)	AD
Osteogenesis imperfecta I (normal teeth)	AD
Osteogenesis imperfecta I (opalescent teeth)	AD
Osteogenesis imperfecta II	AD
Osteogenesis imperfecta III	AD
	AD
	AR
	AR
Osteogenesis imperfecta IV (normal teeth)	AD
Osteogenesis imperfecta IV (opalescent teeth)	AD
Osteogenesis imperfecta V	
Osteogenesis imperfecta VI	
Cole-Carpenter dysplasia	SP
Bruck dysplasia I	AR
Bruck dysplasia II	
Singleton-Merton dysplasia	AR
Osteopenia with radiolucent lesions of the mandible	AD
Osteoporosis-pseudoglioma dysplasia	AR
Geroderma osteodysplasticum	AR
Idiopathic juvenile osteoporosis	SP

25. Dysplasias with defective mineralization

Hypophosphatasia- perinatal lethal and infantile forms	AR
Hypophosphatasia dult form	AD
Hypophosphatemic rickets	XLD
	AD
Neonatal hyperparathyroidism	AR
Transient neonatal hyperparathyroidism	AD
with hypocalciuric hypercalcemia	AD

26. Increased bone density without modification of bone shape

Osteochondrodysplasia	Mode of Inheritance*
Osteopetrosis	
Infantile form (OPB)	AR
With infantile neuroaxonal dysplasia	AR?
Delayed form Type I (OPA1)	AD
Delayed form Type II (OPA2)	AD
Intermediate form (possibly heterogeneous)	AR
With ectodermal dysplasia and immune defect (OLEDAID)	XL
Dysosteosclerosis	AR
Osteomesopyknosis	AD
Cranial osteosclerosis with bamboo hair (Netherton)	
Pyknodysostosis	AR
Osteosclerosis Stanescu Type	AD
Osteopathia striata (isolated)	SP
Osteopathia striata with cranial sclerosis	AD/XLD?
Melorheostosis	SP
Osteopoikilosis	SP
Mixed sclerosing bone dysplasia	SP

27. Increased bone density with diaphyseal involvement

Osteochondrodysplasia	Mode of Inheritance*
Diaphyseal dysplasia	AD
Camurati Engelmann	
Diaphyseal dysplasia with anemia (Ghosal)	AR
Craniodiaphyseal dysplasia	AR
Lenz Majewski dysplasia	
Endosteal hyperostosis	
van Buchem Type	AR
Sclerosteosis	AR
Worth Type	AD
Sclero-osteo-cerebellar dysplasia	AR
Kenny Caffey dysplasia Type I	AR
Kenny Caffey dysplasia Type II	AD
Osteoectasia with hyperphosphatasia (Juvenile Paget disease)	AR

Osteochondrodysplasia	Mode of Inheritance*
Diaphyseal medullary stenosis with bone malignancy	AD
Oculodentoosseous dysplasia	AR
Trichodentoosseous dysplasia	AD

28. Increased bone density with metaphyseal involvement

Pyle dysplasia	AR
Craniometaphyseal dysplasia	
Severe Type	AR
Mild Type	AD

29. Craniotubular digital dysplasias

Frontometaphyseal dysplasia	XLR
Osteodysplasty, Melnick-Needles	XLD
Precocious osteodysplasty (terHaar dysplasia)	AR
Otopalatodigital syndrome Type I	XLD
Otopalatodigital syndrome Type II	XLR

30. Neonatal severe osteosclerotic dysplasias

Blomstrand dysplasia	AR
Raine dysplasia	AR
Caffey disease with prenatal onset	AD
Astley-Kendall dysplasia	AR

31. Disorganized development of cartilaginous and fibrous components of the skeleton

Dysplasia epiphysealis hemimelica	SP
Multiple cartilaginous with hemangiomata (Maffucci)	SP
Spondyloenchondromatosis	AR
Spondyloenchondromatosis with basal ganglia calcification	AR
Dysspondyloenchondromatosis	
Metachondromatosis	AD
Osteoglophonic dysplasia	AD
Genochondromatosis	AD
Carpotarsal osteochondromatosis	AD
Fibrous dysplasia (McCune-Albright and others) mosaic	SP

Osteochondrodysplasia	Mode of Inheritance*
Jaffe Campanacci Type	SP
Fibrodysplasia ossificans progressiva	AD
Cherubism	AD
Cherubism with gingival fibromatosis	AR

32. Osteolyses
Multicentric -hands and feet

Multicentric carpal-tarsal osteolysis with and without nephropathy	AD
Winchester syndrome	AR
Torg syndrome	AR

Distal phalanges

Hadju-Cheney syndrome	AD
Mandibuloacral syndrome	AR

Diaphyses and metaphyses

Familial expansile osteolysis	AD
Juvenile hyaline fibromatosis (includes systemic juvenile hyalinosis)	AR

33. Patella dysplasias

Nail patella dysplasia	AD
Patella hypoplasia/aplasia	AD
Ischiopubic patellar dysplasia	AD
Genitopatellar syndrome	AR?
Ear patella short stature syndrome (Meier Gorlin)	AR

LOCALIZED SKELETAL MALFORMATIONS (DYSOSTOSES)

A. Localized disorders with predominant cranial and facial involvement

Apert syndrome	AD
Pfeiffer syndrome	AD
Pfeiffer syndrome	AD
Crouzon syndrome	AD
Craniosynostosis (Crouzon-like) with Acanthosis Nigricans	AD
Jackson-Weiss syndrome	AD
Jackson-Weiss syndrome	AD

(continued)

Osteochondrodysplasia	Mode of Inheritance*
Saethre-Chotzen syndrome	AD
Craniosynostosis Muenke Type	AD
Craniosynostosis Boston Type	AD
Craniosynostosis Adelaide Type	AD
Craniosynostosis with polydactyly (Carpenter)	AR
Antley-Bixler syndrome	AD
Craniosynostosis with cutis gyrata (Beare-Stevenson)	AD
Oral-facial-digital syndrome Type I	XLR
Cephalo-polysyndactyly (Greig)	AD
Craniofrontonasal dysplasia	XLD
Mandibulo-facial dysostosis (Treacher-Collins)	AD

B. Localized disorders with predominant axial involvement

Spondylocostal dysplasia	AD
Spondylocostal dysplasia	AR
COVESDEM (COsto VErtebral Segmentation DEfect with Mesomelial and peculiar face)	AR
Oculo-vertebral syndrome (Weyer)	AD

C. Localized disorders with predominant involvement of the extremitites

Isolated SHFM3	AD
Isolated SHFM4	AD
Syndromic SHFM1 with deafness and MR	AD
Isolated SHFM2	XL
Ectrodactyly-ectodermal dysplasia clfet-palate syndrome	AD
Symphalangism - proximal	AD
Rubinstein-Taybi syndrome	?AD
Coffin-Siris syndrome	AR
Coffin-Siris syndrome	AR
Fanconi syndrome Group A	AR
Fanconi syndrome Group C	AR
Fanconi syndrome Group D	AR
Fanconi syndrome Group E	AR
Fanconi syndrome Group F	AR

Osteochondrodysplasia	Mode of Inheritance*
Fanconi syndrome Group G	AR
Multiple synostoses	AD
Hand foot genital syndrome	AD

*AD autosomal dominant. AR autosomal recessive. SP sporadic. XLD X-liked dominant. XLR X-linked recessive

Gamut D-2

SCLEROSING BONE DYSPLASIAS

COMMON

1. Craniometaphyseal dysplasia
2. Diaphyseal dysplasia (Camurati-Engelmann disease)
3. Endosteal hyperostosis (van Buchem and Worth types); sclerosteosis
4. Hyperphosphatasia
5. Melorheostosis
6. Oculodentoosseous dysplasia
7. Osteopathia striata (Voorhoeve disease); osteopathia striata with cranial sclerosis
8. Osteopetrosis
9. Osteopoikilosis
10. Pachydermoperiostosis
11. Pyknodysostosis
12. Pyle dysplasia

UNCOMMON

1. Craniodiaphyseal dysplasia
2. Dysosteosclerosis
3. Frontometaphyseal dysplasia
4. Lenz-Majewski dysplasia (hyperostotic dwarfism)
5. Ribbing disease (hereditary multiple diaphyseal sclerosis)

References

1. Beighton P, et al: International Classification of Osteochondrodysplasias, 1992 (modified)

2. Rimoin DL: International Nomenclature and Classification of the Osteochondrodysplasias (1997). Am J Med Genetics 1998;79:376–382
3. Taybi H, Lachman RS: Radiology of Syndromes, Metabolic Disorders, and Skeletal Dysplasias. (ed 4) St. Louis: Mosby-Year Book Inc, 1996, p 1103

Gamut D-2-S

CLASSIFICATION OF SCLEROSING BONE DYSPLASIAS

DYSPLASIAS OF ENDOCHONDRAL BONE FORMATION

Affecting primary spongiosa (immature bone)
1. Osteopetrosis (Albers-Schönberg disease)
   a. Autosomal-recessive type (lethal)
   b. Autosomal-dominant type
   c. Intermediate-recessive type
   d. Autosomal-recessive type with tubular acidosis (Sly disease)
2. Pyknodysostosis

Affecting spongiosa (mature bone)
1. Bone island (enostosis)
2. Osteopathia striata (Voorhoeve disease)
3. Osteopoikilosis

DYSPLASIAS OF INTRAMEMBRANOUS BONE FORMATION
1. Diaphyseal dysplasia (Camurati-Engelmann disease)
2. Endosteal hyperostosis (hyperostosis corticalis generalisata)
   a. Autosomal-recessive form
      i. Van Buchem type
      ii. Sclerosteosis
   b. Autosomal-dominant form
      i. Worth type
      ii. Nakamura disease

3. Ribbing disease (hereditary multiple diaphyseal sclerosis)

MIXED SCLEROSING DYSPLASIAS (affecting both endochondral and intramembranous ossification)

Affecting predominantly endochondral ossification
1. Craniometaphyseal dysplasia
2. Dysosteosclerosis
3. Pyle dysplasia

Affecting predominantly intramembranous ossification
1. Craniodiaphyseal dysplasia
2. Melorheostosis
3. Progressive diaphyseal dysplasia with skull base involvement (Neuhauser variant)

COEXISTENCE OF TWO OR MORE SCLEROSING BONE DYSPLASIAS
1. Melorheostosis with osteopoikilosis and osteopathia striata
2. Osteopathia striata with cranial sclerosis (Horan-Beighton S.)
3. Osteopathia striata with osteopoikilosis and cranial sclerosis
4. Osteopathia striata with osteopoikilosis
5. Osteopathia striata with generalized cortical hyperostosis
6. Osteopathia striata with osteopetrosis
7. Osteopoikilosis with progressive diaphyseal dysplasia

Reference
1. Greenspan A: Sclerosing bone dysplasias—a target-site approach. Skeletal Radiol 1991; 20:561-583

Gamut D-3

LETHAL FORMS OF DWARFISM AND SKELETAL DYSPLASIAS*

COMMON

1. Achondrogenesis (types I & II)
2. Achondroplasia (homozygous form)
+3. Campomelic dysplasia
4. Chondrodysplasia punctata (rhizomelic type)
+5. [Congenital transplacental infection (eg, cytomegalovirus infection; herpes simplex; rarely rubella)]
6. Hypochondrogenesis
7. Hypophosphatasia, severe
8. Osteogenesis imperfecta (type II)
9. Short rib syndromes (with or without polydactyly)
   a. Type I (Saldino-Noonan)
   b. Type II (Majewski)
   c. Type III (lethal thoracic dysplasia)
10. Thanatophoric dysplasia (with or without cloverleaf skull deformity (kleeblattschädel anomaly)

UNCOMMON

+1. Arthrogryposis
+2. Asphyxiating thoracic dysplasia (Jeune S.)
3. Atelosteogenesis
4. Cephaloskeletal dysplasia (Taybi-Linder S.)
5. Diastrophic dysplasia (rare lethal form)
6. Dyssegmental dysplasia
7. Fibrochondrogenesis
8. Metatropic dysplasia (rare lethal form)
9. Neu-Laxova S.
10. Opsismodysplasia
11. Osteodysplasty (Melnick-Needles S.) (lethal male)
12. Osteopetrosis with precocious manifestations (rarely lethal)
13. Potter S.
14. Pseudodiastrophic dysplasia
15. Schneckenbecken dysplasia
16. Spondylocostal dysostosis (Jarcho-Levin S.)
+17. Spondyloepiphyseal dysplasia congenita

18. Spondylometaphyseal dysplasia (Sedaghatian type)
19. Warfarin embryopathy

* Death usually occurs in perinatal period or within first month of life; however, some of these entities are not invariably fatal, especially those preceded by the plus sign (+).

References
1. Kozlowski K, Beighton P: Gamut Index of Skeletal Dysplasias. (ed 2) Berlin: Springer-Verlag, 2000
2. Kozlowski K, et al: Neonatal death dwarfism. Fortschr Röntgenstr 1978; 129:626–633
3. Taybi H, Lachman RS: Radiology of Syndromes, Metabolic Disorders, and Skeletal Dysplasias. (ed 4) St. Louis: Mosby-Year Book Inc, 1996, pp 1054–1055

Gamut D-4

LATE-ONSET DWARFISM (IDENTIFIABLE BEYOND INFANCY)

COMMON

1. Dyschondrosteosis
2. Hypochondroplasia
3. Multiple epiphyseal dysplasia (Fairbank and other forms)
4. Pseudoachondroplasia (pseudoachondroplastic spondyloepiphyseal dysplasia)
5. Spondyloepimetaphyseal dysplasia (several forms)
6. Spondyloepiphyseal dysplasia tarda and other forms
7. Spondylometaphyseal dysplasia (Kozlowski and other types)
8. Stickler S. (arthro-ophthalmopathy)

UNCOMMON

1. Acrodysplasia with retinitis pigmentosa and nephropathy (Saldino-Mainzer S.)
2. Brachyolmia
3. Dyggve-Melchior-Clausen dysplasia (Smith-McCort S.)
4. Metaphyseal chondrodysplasia (Jansen, Schmid, McKusick, Shwachman types)

5. Otospondylomegaepiphyseal dysplasia (OSMED)
6. Parastremmatic dysplasia
7. Progressive pseudorheumatoid chondrodysplasia
8. Schwartz-Jampel S. (chondrodystrophic myotonia)
9. Spondyloperipheral dysplasia
10. Trichorhinophalangeal dysplasia

Reference
1. Lachman RS: International Nomenclature and Classification of the Osteochondrodysplasias (1997). Pediatr Radiol 1998:28:737–744

Gamut D-5-1

MAJOR SYNDROMES OF SHORT LIMB DWARFISM—RHIZOMELIC DWARFISM (PROXIMAL LIMB SHORTENING—HUMERUS, FEMUR)

COMMON
1. Achondrogenesis
2. Achondroplasia
3. Hypochondroplasia
4. Pseudoachondroplasia (pseudoachondroplastic spondyloepiphyseal dysplasia)
5. Spondyloepimetaphyseal dysplasias
6. Thanatophoric dysplasia

UNCOMMON
1. Atelosteogenesis
2. Chondrodysplasia punctata (rhizomelic type)
3. Femoral hypoplasia-unusual facies S.
4. Kyphomelic dysplasia
5. Metatropic dysplasia
6. Omodysplasia
7. Opsismodysplasia
8. Oto-spondylo-megaepiphyseal dysplasia (OSMED)
9. Pseudodiastrophic dysplasia
10. Spondyloenchondrodysplasia
11. Spondylometaphyseal dysplasia
12. Stanescu dysostosis
13. Weissenbacher-Zweymüller phenotype

References
1. Kozlowski K, Beighton P: Gamut Index of Skeletal Dysplasias. (ed 2) Berlin: Springer-Verlag, 2000
2. Lachman RS: International Nomenclature and Classification of the Osteochondrodysplasias (1997). Pediatr Radiol 1998:28:737–744
3. Taybi H, Lachman RS: Radiology of Syndromes, Metabolic Disorders, and Skeletal Dysplasias. (ed 4) St. Louis: Mosby-Year Book Inc, 1996, p 1040

Gamut D-5-2

MAJOR SYNDROMES OF SHORT LIMB DWARFISM—MESOMELIC DWARFISM (Middle segment limb shortening—radius, ulna or tibia, fibula)

Mesomelia with Normal Hands and Feet
1. Dyschondrosteosis
2. Mesomelic dysplasia (eg, Langer and Reinhardt-Pfeiffer types)

Acromesomelia with Hand and Foot Abnormalities
1. Acromesomelic dysplasia (Maroteaux and Campailla-Martinelli types)
2. Campomelic dysplasia
3. Chondroectodermal dysplasia (Ellis-van Creveld S.)
4. Grebe chondrodysplasia
5. Kyphomelic dysplasia
6. Mesomelic dysplasia (Nievergelt, Robinow, and Werner types)
7. Schinzel-Giedion S.
8. Short rib-polydactyly S. type II (Majewski)

References
1. Kozlowski K, Beighton P: Gamut Index of Skeletal Dysplasias. (ed 2) Berlin: Springer-Verlag, 2000
2. Taybi H, Lachman RS: Radiology of Syndromes, Metabolic Disorders, and Skeletal Dysplasias. (ed 4) St. Louis: Mosby-Year Book Inc, 1996, p 1036

Gamut D-5-3

MAJOR SYNDROMES OF SHORT LIMB DWARFISM—ACROMELIC DWARFISM
(Distal segment shortening— hands, feet)

COMMON

1. Achondroplasia
2. Acrodysostosis (peripheral dysostosis)
3. Asphyxiating thoracic dysplasia (Jeune S.)
4. Chondroectodermal dysplasia (Ellis-van Creveld S.)
5. Diastrophic dysplasia
6. Otopalatodigital S. (types I and II)
7. Pseudoachondroplasia (pseudoachondroplastic spondyloepiphyseal dysplasia)
8. Thanatophoric dysplasia

UNCOMMON

1. Acrodysplasia with retinitis pigmentosa and nephropathy (Saldino-Mainzer S.)
2. Acromesomelic dysplasia
3. Acromicric dysplasia
4. Brachydactyly syndromes (esp. type E)
5. Chondrodysplasia punctata (brachytelephalangic type)
6. Grebe chondrodysplasia (achondrogenesis, Brazilian type)
7. Spondylometaphyseal dysplasia (Sedaghatian type)
8. Spondyloperipheral dysplasia

References
1. Kozlowski K, Beighton P: Gamut Index of Skeletal Dysplasias. (ed 2) Berlin: Springer-Verlag, 2000
2. Taybi H, Lachman RS: Radiology of Syndromes, Metabolic Disorders, and Skeletal Dysplasias. (ed 4) St. Louis: Mosby-Year Book Inc, 1996

Gamut D-6

CONGENITAL SYNDROMES AND SKELETAL DYSPLASIAS WITH SHORT LIMBS

COMMON

1. Achondroplasia
2. Chondrodysplasia punctata (all types)
3. Dyschondrosteosis; Madelung deformity
4. Enchondromatosis (Ollier disease); Maffucci S.
5. Hereditary multiple exostoses (multiple cartilaginous exostoses; osteochondromatosis)
6. Hypophosphatasia
7. Mucopolysaccharidoses (eg, Hurler S.) (See J-4)
8. Multiple epiphyseal dysplasia (Fairbank)
9. Osteogenesis imperfecta (type II)
10. Phocomelia (incl. thalidomide embryopathy; infant of diabetic mother)
11. Pseudoachondroplasia (pseudoachondroplastic spondyloepiphyseal dysplasia)
12. Thanatophoric dysplasia
13. Turner S.

UNCOMMON

1. Acrodysostosis (peripheral dysostosis)
2. Acromesomelic dysplasia
3. Aminopterin fetopathy
4. Asphyxiating thoracic dysplasia (Jeune S.)
5. Atelosteogenesis
6. Bloom S.
7. Brachmann-de Lange S. (de Lange S.)
8. Campomelic dysplasia
9. Cephaloskeletal dysplasia (Taybi-Linder S.)
10. CHILD S. (ichthyosis-limb reduction S.)
11. Chondroectodermal dysplasia (Ellis-van Creveld S.)
12. Diastrophic dysplasia
13. Dyggve-Melchior-Clausen dysplasia
14. Dyssegmental dysplasia
15. Fibrochondrogenesis
16. GM_1 gangliosidosis

17. Grebe chondrodysplasia (achondrogenesis, Brazilian type)
18. Holt-Oram S.
19. Hyperphosphatasia
20. Hypochondroplasia
21. Kniest dysplasia
22. Larsen S.
23. Mesomelic dysplasia (Langer, Nievergelt, Robinow types)
24. Metaphyseal chondrodysplasia (Jansen, McKusick, Schmid types)
25. Metatropic dysplasia
26. Mietens-Weber S.
27. Orofaciodigital syndrome I (Papillon-Leage and Psaume S.)
28. Oto-spondylo-megaepiphyseal dysplasia (OSMED)
29. Patterson S.
30. Roberts S. (pseudothalidomide S.)
31. Seckel S. (bird-headed dwarfism)
32. Short rib-polydactyly syndromes
33. Spondyloepiphyseal dysplasias
34. Spondylometaphyseal dysplasia
35. TAR S. (thrombocytopenia-absent radius S.)
36. Warfarin embryopathy
37. Weill-Marchesani S.

References

1. Felson B (ed): Dwarfs and other little people. Semin Roentgenol 1973; 8:255
2. Swischuk LE, John SD: Differential Diagnosis in Pediatric Radiology. (ed 2) Baltimore: Williams & Wilkins, 1995
3. Taybi H, Lachman RS: Radiology of Syndromes, Metabolic Disorders, and Skeletal Dysplasias. (ed 4) St. Louis: Mosby-Year Book Inc, 1996, p 1035

Gamut D-7

SHORT SQUAT BONES

COMMON

1. Achondroplasia

2. Epiphyseal-metaphyseal injury (trauma; infection; radiation; hypervitaminosis A)
3. Mucopolysaccharidoses (esp. Hunter; Hurler; Maroteaux-Lamy); mucolipidosis II (I-cell disease); GM_1 gangliosidosis (See J-4)

UNCOMMON

1. Achondrogenesis
2. Asphyxiating thoracic dysplasia (Jeune S.)
3. Brachmann-de Lange S. (de Lange S.)
4. Campomelic dysplasia
5. Chondroectodermal dysplasia (Ellis-van Creveld S.)
6. Diastrophic dysplasia
7. Dyggve-Melchior-Clausen dysplasia
8. Dyschondrosteosis; Madelung deformity
9. Hyperphosphatasia
10. Hypochondroplasia
11. Hypophosphatasia
12. Hypothyroidism
13. Kniest dysplasia
14. Larsen S.
15. Metaphyseal chondrodysplasia (Jansen type)
16. Metatropic dysplasia
17. Neonatal dwarfs, other
18. Osteogenesis imperfecta (type II)
19. Phocomelia (eg, thalidomide embryopathy; infant of diabetic mother)
20. Pseudoachondroplasia (pseudoachondroplastic spondyloepiphyseal dysplasia)
21. Rickets (vitamin D-deficient, type B)
22. Short rib-polydactyly syndromes type I (Saldino-Noonan) and type II (Majewski)
23. Thanatophoric dysplasia
24. Turner S.
25. Weissenbacher-Zweymüller phenotype
26. Chondrodysplasia punctata, rhizomelic type

Reference

1. Swischuk LE, John SD: Differential Diagnosis in Pediatric Radiology. (ed 2) Baltimore: Williams & Wilkins, 1995, pp 192–195

Gamut D-8

BOWED BONES, SINGLE OR MULTIPLE

COMMON

*1. Achondroplasia
*2. Bow legs, physiologic (See D-185)
3. Enchondromatosis (Ollier disease); Maffucci S.
4. Fibrous dysplasia (incl. polyostotic fibrous dyspla-sia (McCune-Albright S.)
5. Fracture, traumatic or pathologic (esp. greenstick fracture; plastic bowing; healed fracture)
6. Hydatid disease
7. Hyperparathyroidism (osteitis fibrosa cystica)
*8. Neurofibromatosis (esp. tibia, fibula)
*9. Osteogenesis imperfecta
10. Osteomalacia (See D-44)
11. Osteomyelitis, severe (eg, bacterial; tuberculous; smallpox residual)
12. Paget's disease
13. Paralysis or restricted movement during growth (eg, neuromuscular disorder_g; poliomyelitis; mus-cular dystrophy; juvenile rheumatoid arthritis)
*14. Prenatal bowing of long bones
15. Renal osteodystrophy (secondary hyperparathy-roidism)
16. Rickets (all types)
17. Syphilis (saber shin); yaws (boomerang tibia)
18. Tibia vara (Blount disease)

UNCOMMON

*1. Achondrogenesis (types I and II)
*2. Acromesomelic dysplasia
*3. Antley-Bixler S.
*4. Asphyxiating thoracic dysplasia (Jeune S.)
*5. Atelosteogenesis
*6. Brachmann-de Lange S. (de Lange S.)
*7. Campomelic dysplasia
*8. Chondroectodermal dysplasia (Ellis-van Creveld S.)
*9. Cloverleaf skull deformity (kleeblattschädel anomaly) with thanatophoric dysplasia
*10. Congenital pseudoarthrosis
*11. Contractural arachnodactyly
*12. Diastrophic dysplasia
13. Dyschondrosteosis (radius and tibia); Madelung deformity
*14. Dyssegmental dysplasia
*15. Epidermal nevus S.
*16. Fibrochondrogenesis
*17. Frontometaphyseal dysplasia
18. Hajdu-Cheney S.
19. Homocystinuria
*20. Hydrolethalus S.
*21. Hyperphosphatasia
*22. Hypochondroplasia
*23. Hypophosphatasia
*24. Infantile cortical hyperostosis (Caffey disease) (late)
*25. Intrauterine positional deformity
*26. Isolated anomaly
*27. Kyphomelic dysplasia
*28. Larsen S.
*29. Mesomelic dysplasia
*30. Metaphyseal chondrodysplasia (Jansen and other types)
*31. Mucopolysaccharidosis (Morquio; Maroteaux-Lamy); mucolipidosis; GM_1 gangliosidosis
*32. Schwartz-Jampel S. (chondrodystrophic myotonia)
*33. Occipital horn S.
*34. Opsismodysplasia
*35. Osteodysplasty (Melnick-Needles S.)
*36. Osteopetrosis
*37. Otopalatodigital S. (types I and II)
*38. Pallister-Hall S.
*39. Parastremmatic dysplasia
*40. Pseudoachondroplasia (pseudoachondroplastic spondyloepiphyseal dysplasia)
*41. Pseudohypoparathyroidism
*42. Roberts S.
*43. Short rib-polydactyly syndromes
*44. Spondyloepimetaphyseal dysplasia
*45. Spondylometaphyseal dysplasia (Kozlowski and Sedaghatian types)
*46. Thanatophoric dysplasia
*47. Tibial bowing with or without absent fibula
48. Weismann-Netter S. (saber shin)

* Bowed limbs in infancy.

References

1. Swischuk LE, John SD: Differential Diagnosis in Pediatric Radiology. (ed 2) Baltimore: Williams & Wilkins, 1995, pp 200–205
2. Taybi H, Lachman RS: Radiology of Syndromes, Metabolic Disorders, and Skeletal Dysplasias. (ed 4) St. Louis: Mosby-Year Book Inc, 1996, pp 1021–1022

Gamut D-9

TWISTED BONES

COMMON

1. Fibrous dysplasia
2. Hyperparathyroidism (osteitis fibrosa cystica)
3. Neurofibromatosis
4. Osteodysplasty (Melnick-Needles S.)
5. Osteogenesis imperfecta
6. Osteomyelitis (late sequela)
7. Posttraumatic; postoperative (esp. regenerated rib)

UNCOMMON

1. Frontometaphyseal dysplasia
2. Gorlin S. (nevoid basal cell carcinoma S.)
3. Idiopathic
4. Otopalatodigital S. (types I and II)
5. Pyle dysplasia

Reference

1. Swischuk LE, John SD: Differential Diagnosis in Pediatric Radiology. (ed 2) Baltimore: Williams & Wilkins, 1995, p 206

Gamut D-10

OVERCONSTRICTION OR OVERTUBULATION (NARROW DIAMETAPHYSIS, LONG THIN BONES)

COMMON

1. Chronic illness with hypotonia or immobilization
2. Disuse atrophy
3. Marfan S.
4. Muscular disorders$_g$ (eg, arthrogryposis; amyotonia congenita {Oppenheim disease}; progressive muscular dystrophy; Werdnig-Hoffmann disease; myotubular myopathy; myotonic dystrophy)
5. Paralytic disorders$_g$ (eg, poliomyelitis; cerebral palsy; congenital malformation of brain or spinal cord)

UNCOMMON

1. Acromegaly (phalanges)
2. Antley-Bixler S.
3. Atelosteogenesis
4. Brachmann-de Lange S. (de Lange S.)
5. Caudal dysplasia sequence (caudal regression S.)
6. Chromosome 4: del(4p) S. (Wolf-Hirschhorn S.)
7. Cockayne S.
8. Congenital pseudoarthrosis
9. Contractural arachnodactyly
10. Dermatomyositis
11. Epidermolysis bullosa
12. Fetal akinesia deformation sequence (Pena-Shokeir S. type I)
13. Fetal hydantoin S. (Dilantin embryopathy)
14. Glycogen storage disease type I (von Gierke disease)
15. Hallermann-Streiff S. (oculomandibulofacial S.)
16. Homocystinuria
17. Hypopituitarism (eg, primordial dwarfism)
18. Juvenile rheumatoid arthritis
19. Marden-Walker S.
20. Marshall-Smith S
21. Mulibrey nanism

(continued)

22. Multiple pterygium S.
23. Neurofibromatosis
24. Osteogenesis imperfecta (type III)
25. Prader-Willi S.
26. Progeria
27. Restrictive dermopathy (stiff skin S.)
28. Schwartz-Jampel S. (chondrodystrophic myotonia)
29. Silver-Russell S.
30. Spondylocostal dysostosis (Jarcho-Levin S.)
31. Stickler S. (arthro-ophthalmopathy)
32. 3-M syndrome
33. Trisomy 8 S.
34. Trisomy 18 S.
35. Tubular stenosis dysplasia (Kenny-Caffey S.)
36. Werner S.
37. Winchester S.

References

1. Greenfield GB: Radiology of Bone Diseases. (ed 5) Philadelphia: Lippincott, 1990
2. Kozlowski K, Beighton P: Gamut Index of Skeletal Dysplasias. Berlin: Springer-Verlag, 1984, p 902
3. Swischuk LE, John SD: Differential Diagnosis in Pediatric Radiology. (ed 2) Baltimore: Williams & Wilkins, 1995, pp 197–198
4. Taybi H, Lachman RS: Radiology of Syndromes, Metabolic Disorders, and Skeletal Dysplasias. (ed 4) St. Louis: Mosby-Year Book, Inc, 1996, p 1040

Gamut D-11

UNDERCONSTRICTION OR UNDERTUBULATION (WIDE DIAMETAPHYSIS), LOCALIZED OR GENERALIZED (See D-34)

COMMON

1. Achondroplasia; other chondrodysplasias (See D-1)
2. Anemia$_g$ (eg, thalassemia; sickle cell disease)
3. Bone cyst or benign expansile neoplasm
4. Fibrous dysplasia
5. Gaucher disease; Niemann-Pick disease
6. Healing or healed fracture; metaphyseal injury
7. Osteomyelitis, chronic productive (eg, Garré sclerosing osteomyelitis; congenital syphilis)
8. Paget's disease

UNCOMMON

1. Achondrogenesis (types I and II)
2. Acrodysostosis (peripheral dysostosis)
3. Cleidocranial dysplasia
4. Craniometaphyseal dysplasia; Craniodiaphyseal dysplasia
5. Diaphyseal dysplasia (Camurati-Engelmann disease)
6. Dysosteosclerosis
7. Dyssegmental dysplasia
8. Enchondromatosis (Ollier disease)
9. Endosteal hyperostosis (van Buchem and Worth types)
10. Fibrogenesis imperfecta ossium
11. Hereditary multiple exostoses (multiple cartilaginous exostoses; osteochondromatosis)
12. Hyperphosphatasia
13. Hypervitaminosis A or D
14. Hypochondrogenesis
15. Hypochondroplasia
16. Hypophosphatasia
17. Infantile cortical hyperostosis (Caffey disease)
18. Kyphomelic dysplasia
19. Lead poisoning (late)
20. Lenz-Majewski dysplasia
21. Léri S. (pleonosteosis)
22. Mastocytosis
23. Mesomelic dysplasia (Langer type)
24. Metaphyseal chondrodysplasia (Jansen type)
25. Mucopolysaccharidoses (esp. Morquio S., Hurler S.); mucolipidoses; GM$_1$ gangliosidosis (See J-4)
26. Neu-Laxova S.
27. Oculodentoosseous dysplasia
28. Omodysplasia
29. Opsismodysplasia
30. Osteogenesis imperfecta (type II)
31. Osteopetrosis
32. Pyle dysplasia
33. Rickets (healing)

34. Schinzel-Giedion S.
35. Scurvy (healing)
36. Trisomy 8 S.
37. Weill-Marchesani S.

References
1. Greenfield GB: Radiology of Bone Diseases. (ed 5) Phila-delphia: Lippincott, 1990
2. Silverman FN (ed): Caffey's Pediatric X-ray Diagnosis. (ed 9) Chicago: Year Book Medical Publ, 1995, p 1924
3. Swischuk LE, John SD: Differential Diagnosis in Pediatric Radiology. (ed 2) Baltimore: Williams & Wilkins, 1995, pp 198–199
4. Taybi H, Lachman RS: Radiology of Syndromes, Metabolic Disorders, and Skeletal Dysplasias. (ed 4) St. Louis: Mosby-Year Book, Inc, 1996, p 1024

Gamut D-12

BALLOONED BONES (WIDE DIAPHYSES, OFTEN THIN CORTICES): LOCALIZED OR GENERALIZED BROAD TUBULAR BONES

COMMON

*1. Anemia$_g$, severe (esp. thalassemia; sickle cell disease)
*2. Bone cyst or benign expansile neoplasm (eg, enchondroma)
*3. Fibrous dysplasia
4. Osteomyelitis, esp. spina ventosa* (tuberculosis); also chronic productive (eg, Garré sclerosing osteomyelitis; syphilis; yaws; tropical ulcer)
5. Paget's disease
6. Subperiosteal hemorrhage (eg, trauma; fracture; battered child S.; leukemia; hemophilia; scurvy)

UNCOMMON

*1. Craniodiaphyseal dysplasia
*2. Diaphyseal dysplasia (Camurati-Engelmann disease)

*3. Dysosteosclerosis
4. Endosteal hyperostosis (van Buchem and Worth types)
*5. Gaucher disease; Niemann-Pick disease
*6. Hyperparathyroidism, severe (eg, brown tumor)
7. Hyperphosphatasia
*8. Hypophosphatasia
9. Infantile cortical hyperostosis (Caffey disease)
10. Infantile multisystem inflammatory disease (NOMID)
11. Léri S. (pleonosteosis)
*12. Mastocytosis
13. Mesomelic dysplasia (Langer, Nievergelt types)
14. Metaphyseal chondrodysplasia (Jansen type)
15. Mucopolysaccharidoses; mucolipidosis II (I-cell disease); GM$_1$ gangliosidosis (See J-4)
16. Neu-Laxova S.
17. Oculodentoosseous dysplasia
18. Osteopetrosis
*19. Otopalatodigital S. (types I and II)
20. Pachydermoperiostosis
*21. Pyle dysplasia
22. Schwarz-Lélek S.
23. Singleton-Merten S.
24. Thanatophoric dysplasia

* Thin cortices.

References
1. Kozlowski K, Beighton P: Gamut Index of Skeletal Dysplasias. (ed 2) Berlin: Springer-Verlag, 2000
2. Swischuk LE, John SD: Differential Diagnosis in Pediatric Radiology. (ed 2) Baltimore: Williams & Wilkins, 1995, pp 198–200
3. Taybi H, Lachman RS: Radiology of Syndromes, Metabolic Disorders, and Skeletal Dysplasias. (ed 4) St. Louis: Mosby-Year Book, Inc, 1996, p 1024

ASYMMETRY IN SIZE OF A BONE OR LIMB (HEMIHYPERTROPHY OR HEMIATROPHY), LOCALIZED OR GENERALIZED (See D-14, D-29)

WITH BONE DYSPLASIA, DYSOSTOSIS, OR SYNDROME

1. Beckwith-Wiedemann S.
2. Chondrodysplasia punctata (Conradi-Hünermann type)
3. Coffin-Lowry S.
4. Dysplasia epiphysealis hemimelica (Trevor disease)
5. Enchondromatosis (Ollier disease); Maffucci S.
6. Femoral hypoplasia-unusual facies S.
7. Fibrous dysplasia (incl. McCune-Albright S.)
8. Goltz S. (focal dermal hypoplasia)
9. Hereditary multiple exostoses (multiple cartilaginous exostoses; osteochondromatosis)
10. Idiopathic; congenital hemihypertrophy
11. Melorheostosis
12. Oculoauriculovertebral spectrum (Goldenhar S.)
13. Osteogenesis imperfecta
14. Phocomelia (eg, thalidomide embryopathy); other congenital limb hypoplasias
15. Prader-Willi S.
16. Proteus S.
17. Seckel S. (bird-headed dwarfism)
18. Silver-Russell S.

WITH VASCULAR MALFORMATIONS

1. Hemangioma; arteriovenous malformation; Klippel-Trenaunay S.; Parkes Weber S.; Maffucci S.
2. Lymphangioma
3. Lymphatic abnormality

WITH NEUROCUTANEOUS OR CUTANEOUS SYNDROMES OR SOFT TISSUE ABNORMALITY

1. CHILD S. (ichthyosis-limb reduction S.)
2. Hypomelanosis of Ito
3. Incontinentia pigmenti
4. Macrodystrophia lipomatosa
5. Neurofibromatosis
6. Poland S. (pectoral muscle aplasia-syndactyly)
7. Romberg S. (esp. mandible)
8. Sturge-Weber S.
9. Tuberous sclerosis
10. von Hippel-Lindau S.

WITH NEOPLASM ASSOCIATION

1. Adrenal gland neoplasm (adrenocortical carcinoma, adenoma)
2. Gonadal neoplasm (gonadoblastoma)
3. Hepatic neoplasm (hepatoblastoma)
4. Renal neoplasm (Wilms' tumor)

WITH ACQUIRED (SECONDARY) ASYMMETRY

1. Endocrine disorder (eg, adrenogenital S.)
2. Hyperemia, any cause (eg, from chronic infection; juvenile chronic arthritis; juvenile rheumatoid arthritis; hemophilia); also conditions leading to decreased blood supply to a limb
3. Hypospadias; cryptorchidism
4. Infantile cortical hyperostosis (Caffey disease)
5. Lymphangiectasia (extremity)
6. Neuromuscular disorder$_g$ (eg, cerebral palsy; poliomyelitis)
7. Osteomyelitis (eg, bacterial; yaws; smallpox residual)
8. Radiation injury
9. Scurvy (with epiphyseal trauma)
10. Trauma (eg, burn; epiphyseal injury; impacted or distracted fracture; surgical procedure)

References

1. Kozlowski K, Beighton P: Gamut Index of Skeletal Dysplasias. Berlin: Springer-Verlag, 1984, pp 22–23

2. Taybi H, Lachman RS: Radiology of Syndromes, Metabolic Disorders, and Skeletal Dysplasias. (ed 4) St. Louis: Mosby-Year Book, Inc, 1996, pp 1066–1067

Gamut D-14

LOCALIZED ACCELERATED MATURATION, ELONGATION, OR OVERGROWTH OF A BONE, DIGIT, OR LIMB

COMMON

1. Arteriovenous fistula; hemangioma; lymphangioma
2. Chronic arthritis (eg, tuberculous; juvenile rheumatoid)
3. Chronic osteomyelitis (eg, Garré sclerosing osteomyelitis; tuberculosis; tropical ulcer)
4. Hemihypertrophy (See D-13)
5. Hyperemia, any cause
6. Idiopathic
7. Neurofibromatosis
8. Trauma; injury (eg, healing fracture)

UNCOMMON

1. Congenital macrodactyly
2. Dysplasia epiphysealis hemimelica (Trevor disease)
3. Epidermal nevus S.
4. Fibrous dysplasia
5. Hemophilia (hemarthrosis)
6. Infantile cortical hyperostosis (Caffey disease)
7. Klippel-Trenaunay S.; Parkes Weber S.
8. Lymphatic obstruction, chronic (eg, lymphangiectasia; congenital hypoplasia of lymphatics; filariasis; elephantiasis; neoplasm)
9. Macrodystrophia lipomatosa
10. Maffucci S. (enchondromatosis with hemangiomas)
11. Melorheostosis
12. Neoplasm (eg, infiltrating angiolipoma)
13. Proteus S.

Reference
1. Greenfield GB: Radiology of Bone Diseases. (ed 5) Philadelphia: Lippincott, 1990

Gamut D-15

GENERALIZED OR WIDESPREAD OVERGROWTH OR ELONGATION OF THE SKELETON (GIGANTISM)

COMMON

1. Adrenogenital S. (prior to premature closure of epiphyses)
2. Beckwith-Wiedemann S.
3. Congenital total lipodystrophy (lipoatrophic diabetes)
4. Constitutional or familial tall stature
5. Hemihypertrophy (See D-13)
6. Homocystinuria
7. Hyperpituitarism; pituitary gigantism; acromegaly
8. Hyperthyroidism (in early childhood)
9. Klinefelter S. (XXY S.)
10. Marfan S.
11. Neurofibromatosis
12. Polyostotic fibrous dysplasia (McCune-Albright S.)
13. Sotos S. (cerebral gigantism)

UNCOMMON

1. Bannayan-Riley-Ruvalcaba S.
2. Fragile X S.
3. Infant of diabetic mother
4. Marshall-Smith S.
5. Perlman S.
6. Sclerosteosis
7. Simpson-Golabi-Behmel S. (gigantism-dysplasia S.)
8. Weaver-Smith S.
9. XXX S.; XYY S.

References
1. Green M: Pediatric Diagnosis. (ed 6) Philadelphia: Saunders, 1998, p 285
2. Greenfield GB: Radiology of Bone Diseases. (ed 5) Philadelphia: Lippincott, 1990
3. Silverman FN (ed): Caffey's Pediatric X-ray Diagnosis. (ed 9) Chicago: Year Book Medical Publ, 1993, p 1528
4. Taybi H, Lachman RS: Radiology of Syndromes, Metabolic Disorders, and Skeletal Dysplasias. (ed 4) St. Louis: Mosby-Year Book, Inc, 1996, p 1068

Gamut D-16

GENERALIZED ACCELERATED SKELETAL MATURATION (INCREASED BONE AGE)

COMMON

1. Adrenogenital S. (adrenocortical tumor or hyperplasia)
2. Constitutional or familial tall stature
3. Excessive androgen, estrogen or steroid administration or production (eg, virilizing adrenal or gonadal neoplasm or hyperplasia; Cushing S.)
4. Hypothalamic or parathalamic lesion with sexual precocity (eg, craniopharyngioma; astrocytoma; hamartoma; optic chiasm glioma; tuberculosis)
5. Idiopathic isosexual precocious puberty
6. Pituitary gigantism; hyperpituitarism
7. Polyostotic fibrous dysplasia (McCune-Albright S.)
8. Sotos S. (cerebral gigantism)

UNCOMMON

1. Congenital syndromes and skeletal dysplasias, other
   a. Acrodysostosis (peripheral dysostosis)
   *b. Asphyxiating thoracic dysplasia (Jeune S.) (hips)
   *c. Bannayan-Riley-Ruvalcaba S.
   *d. Beckwith-Wiedemann S.
   e. Chondroectodermal dysplasia (Ellis-van Creveld S.)
   f. Congenital total lipodystrophy (lipoatrophic diabetes)
   g. Contractural arachnodactyly
   h. Diastrophic dysplasia (hands)
   *i. Greig cephalopolysyndactyly S.
   *j. Marshall-Smith S.
   k. Otopalatodigital S. (type II)
   l. Otospondylomegaepiphyseal dysplasia (OSMED)
   m. Pseudohypoparathyroidism (hands)
   *n. Schneckenbecken dysplasia (carpals, tarsals)
   o. Trisomy 8 S.
   p. Tuberous sclerosis (with sexual precosity)
   *q. Weaver S.
2. Ectopic gonadotropin production (hepatoma; choriocarcinoma; teratoma)
3. Encephalitis
4. Exogenous obesity with overgrowth and tall stature
5. Homocystinuria
*6. Hyperthyroidism (maternal or acquired)
7. Pinealoma, primary or ectopic
8. Primary hyperaldosteronism (Conn S.)

* Advanced bone age in the newborn.

References

1. Greenfield GB: Radiology of Bone Diseases. (ed 5) Philadelphia: Lippincott, 1990
2. Poznanski AK: The Hand in Radiologic Diagnosis. (ed 2) Philadelphia: WB Saunders, 1984, pp 67–96
3. Rieth KG, et al: CT of cerebral abnormalities in precocious puberty. AJR 1987; 148:1231–1238
4. Taybi H, Lachman RS: Radiology of Syndromes, Metabolic Disorders, and Skeletal Dysplasias. (ed 4) St. Louis: Mosby-Year Book, Inc, 1996, p 1052

Gamut D-17-1

GENERALIZED RETARDED SKELETAL MATURATION (DELAYED BONE AGE)

COMMON

1. Congenital heart disease (esp. cyanotic)
2. Congenital syndromes of dwarfism or mental retardation (See D-17-2)
3. Constitutional delay of growth and adolescence; nonspecific or idiopathic retardation
4. Cretinism; hypothyroidism
5. Deprivation (psychosocial) dwarfism
6. Diabetes, juvenile
7. Hypogonadism (eg, Turner S.)
8. Hypopituitarism with growth hormone deficiency (eg, idiopathic; craniopharyngioma)
9. Idiopathic; familial short stature

10. Intrauterine growth retardation (IUGR); infant of toxemic mother
11. Malnutrition; failure to thrive
12. Neurologic disorders$_g$; cerebral hypoplasia
13. Renal disease (eg, nephrosis; chronic renal failure; cystinosis; renal tubular acidosis)
14. Severe constitutional disease or chronic illness (eg, celiac disease; cystic fibrosis {mucoviscidosis}; ulcerative colitis)
15. Small for gestational age neonate

UNCOMMON

1. Addison disease (adrenal insufficiency)
2. Aminopterin fetopathy
3. Anemia$_g$, chronic (eg, sickle cell disease; thalassemia)
4. Copper deficiency, nutritional; Menkes S. (kinky-hair S.)
5. Hypoparathyroidism
6. Idiopathic juvenile osteoporosis
7. Langerhans cell histiocytosis$_g$
8. Lesch-Nyhan S. (congenital hyperuricosuria)
9. Phenylketonuria
10. Rickets (all types)
11. Steroid therapy; Cushing S.

References

1. Green M: Pediatric Diagnosis. (ed 6) Philadelphia: WB Saunders, 1998, p 276
2. Greenfield GB: Radiology of Bone Diseases. (ed 5) Philadelphia: Lippincott, 1990
3. Poznanski AK: The Hand in Radiologic Diagnosis. (ed 2) Philadelphia: WB Saunders, 1984
4. Taybi H, Lachman RS: Radiology of Syndromes, Metabolic Disorders, and Skeletal Dysplasias. (ed 4) St. Louis: Mosby-Year Book, Inc, 1996, p 1053
5. Teplick JG, Haskin ME: Roentgenologic Diagnosis. (ed 3) Philadelphia: WB Saunders, 1976

Gamut D-17-2

CONGENITAL SYNDROMES AND SKELETAL DYSPLASIAS WITH RETARDED OR DYSHARMONIC SKELETAL MATURATION*

COMMON

1. Achondroplasia
2. Hypothyroidism; cretinism
3. Mucopolysaccharidoses (esp. Morquio S.); mucolipidosis II (I-cell disease) and III (pseudo-Hurler polydystrophy); fucosidosis (See J-4)
4. Trisomy 21 S. (Down S.)
5. Turner S.

UNCOMMON

1. Achondrogenesis
2. Aminopterin fetopathy
3. Brachmann-de Lange S. (de Lange S.)
4. Campomelic dysplasia
5. Celiac disease (gluten-induced enteropathy)
6. Cephaloskeletal dysplasia (Taybi-Linder S.)
7. Chondroectodermal dysplasia (Ellis-van Creveld S.)
8. Cleidocranial dysplasia
9. Cloverleaf skull deformity (kleeblattschädel anomaly)
10. Cockayne S.
11. Coffin-Lowry S.
12. Coffin-Siris S.
13. Cystinosis
14. de Morsier S.
15. Diastrophic dysplasia
16. Dubowitz S.
17. Fanconi anemia (pancytopenia-dysmelia S.)
18. Fetal rubella infection
19. Floating-harbor S.
20. Freeman-Sheldon S. (whistling face S.)
21. GAPO S.
22. Glycogen storage disease type I (von Gierke disease)
23. Incontinentia pigmenti
24. Infant of toxemic mother

(continued)

25. Johanson-Blizzard S.
26. Kocher-Debré-Sémélaigne S.
27. Laron S. (pituitary dwarfism II)
28. Larsen S.
29. Lenz-Majewski dysplasia
30. LEOPARD syndrome (multiple lentigenes S.)
31. Leprechaunism; Patterson S.
32. Léri S. (pleonosteosis)
33. Lesch-Nyhan S. (congenital hyperuricosuria)
34. Lowe S. (oculocerebrorenal S.)
35. Mauriac S.
36. Metatropic dysplasia
37. Multiple epiphyseal dysplasia (Fairbank)
38. Noonan S.
39. Opitz trigonocephaly S. (C syndrome)
40. Osteodysplasty (Melnick-Needles S.)
41. Papillon-Lefèvre S.
42. Phenylketonuria
43. Pituitary dwarfism (Levi-Lorain S.); hypopituitarism
44. Prader-Willi S.
45. Prasad S. (geophagia S.)
46. Riley-Day S. (familial dysautonomia)
47. Rubinstein-Taybi S.
48. Silver-Russell S.
49. Spondyloepimetaphyseal dysplasia
50. Spondyloepiphyseal dysplasia
51. Spondylometaphyseal dysplasia (esp. Kozlowski type)
52. Thanatophoric dysplasia
53. 3-M syndrome
54. Trichorhinophalangeal dysplasia, type I (Giedion S.)
55. Trisomy 18 S.
56. Tubular stenosis dysplasia (Kenny-Caffey S.)
57. Weill-Marchesani S.
58. Wilson disease (hepatolenticular degeneration)
59. XXXXY S.
60. Zellweger S. (cerebrohepatorenal S.)

* Most skeletal dysplasias, especially those with epiphyseal abnormalities, have delayed or dysharmonic skeletal maturation. The same is true for many dysmorphology syndromes.

References
1. Felson B (ed): Dwarfs and other little people. Semin Roentgenol 1973; 8:255
2. Kozlowski K, Beighton P: Gamut Index of Skeletal Dysplasias. Berlin: Springer-Verlag, 1984, pp 18–19
3. Poznanski AK: The Hand in Radiologic Diagnosis. (ed 2) Philadelphia: WB Saunders, 1984, pp 67–96
4. Swischuk LE, John SD: Differential Diagnosis in Pediatric Radiology. (ed 2) Baltimore: Williams & Wilkins, 1995
5. Taybi H, Lachman RS: Radiology of Syndromes, Metabolic Disorders, and Skeletal Dysplasias. (ed 4) St. Louis: Mosby-Year Book, Inc, 1996, p 1053

Gamut D-18

PSEUDOEPIPHYSES AND ACCESSORY EPIPHYSES

COMMON
1. Cleidocranial dysplasia
2. Idiopathic; normal variant
*3. Otopalatodigital S. (types I and II)
*4. Trisomy 21 S. (Down S.)

UNCOMMON
1. Acrodysostosis (peripheral dysostosis)
2. Acromicric dysplasia
3. Brachydactyly C
4. Catel-Manzke S.
5. Chromosome 4: del (4p) S. (Wolf-Hirschhorn S.)
6. Chromosome 9: dup(9p) S.
*7. Cockayne S.
8. Diastrophic dysplasia
9. Dyggve-Melchior-Clausen dysplasia
10. Fanconi anemia (pancytopenia-dysmelia S.) (thumb)
11. Fetal hydantoin S. (Dilantin embryopathy)
12. Fibrodysplasia (myositis) ossificans progressiva
*13. Gordon S. (distal arthrogryposis)
14. Hand-foot-genital S.
15. Hypoglossia-hypodactylia S. (aglossia-adactylia S.)
16. Hypothyroidism; cretinism
17. Kniest dysplasia
18. Larsen S.
19. Pseudoachondroplasia

20. Pseudohypoparathyroidism
21. Silver-Russell S.
22. Spondyloepiphyseal dysplasia
*23. 3-M syndrome
24. Townes-Brocks S.
*25. XXXXY S.; XXXXX S.

* Affecting primarily the second metacarpal.

References

1. Gorlin RJ, Cohen MM, Levin LS: Syndromes of the Head and Neck. (ed 3) New York: Oxford University Press, 1990
2. Greenfield GB: Radiology of Bone Diseases. (ed 5) Philadelphia: Lippincott, 1990
3. Kozlowski K, Beighton P: Gamut Index of Skeletal Dysplasias. Berlin: Springer-Verlag, 1984, pp 73–74
4. Poznanski AK: The Hand in Radiologic Diagnosis. (ed 2) Philadelphia: WB Saunders, 1984, p 154
5. Resnick D: Diagnosis of Bone and Joint Disorders. (ed 3) Philadelphia: WB Saunders, 1995, p 2065

5. Juvenile chronic arthritis (eg, juvenile rheumatoid arthritis)
6. Osteomyelitis (eg, Listeria monocytogenes*); congenital transplacental infections
7. Pituitary gigantism
8. Rickets
9. Thiemann disease (hand)
10. Trauma
*11. Vitamin K reductase deficiency

*Stippled epiphyses.

Reference

1. Greenfield GB: Radiology of Bone Diseases. (ed 5) Philadelphia: Lippincott, 1990

Gamut D-19-1

IRREGULARITY, FRAGMENTATION, OR STIPPLING OF MULTIPLE EPIPHYSEAL OSSIFICATION CENTERS

COMMON

1. Avascular necrosis (eg, Legg-Perthes disease; steroid therapy; sickle cell disease) (See D-48)
*2. Congenital syndromes (See D-19-2)
3. Cretinism; hypothyroidism
*4. Normal, age related (eg, distal femur, capitellum)
5. Osteochondroses

UNCOMMON

1. Dysplasia epiphysealis hemimelica (Trevor disease)
2. Frostbite
3. Hypo-hyperparathyroidism
*4. Hypopituitarism (anterior lobe) with growth hormone deficiency

Gamut D-19-2

CONGENITAL SYNDROMES AND BONE DYSPLASIAS WITH IRREGULARITY, FRAGMENTATION, OR STIPPLING OF MULTIPLE EPIPHYSEAL OSSIFICATION CENTERS

COMMON

*1. Chondrodysplasia punctata (all types)
  a. Conradi-Hünermann (CP-CH)
  b. Brachytelephalangic type (CP-BT)
  c. Rhizomelic type
  d. Sheffield type
  e. Tibial-metacarpal type (CP-MT)
  f. X-linked dominant (Happle) type
  g. X-linked recessive (Curry) type
2. Cretinism; hypothyroidism
3. Dysplasia epiphysealis hemimelica (Trevor disease)
4. Mucopolysaccharidoses (eg, Morquio S.) (See J-4)
*5. Multiple epiphyseal dysplasia (Fairbank)
*6. Osteopoikilosis
*7. Pseudoachondroplasia (pseudoachondroplastic spondyloepiphyseal dysplasia)

(continued)

*8. Spondyloepiphyseal dysplasia (congenita or tarda)

*9. Trisomy 21 S. (Down S.)

UNCOMMON

1. Acrodysostosis (peripheral dysostosis)
*2. Brachmann-de Lange S. (de Lange S.)
*3. CHILD S.
*4. Chromosome disorders, many
*5. Congenital transplacental infections (TORCH)
6. Cutis laxa (hips)
7. Diastrophic dysplasia
8. Dyggve-Melchior-Clausen dysplasia (Smith-McCort S.)
9. Enchondromatosis (Ollier disease); Maffucci S.
*10. Fetal alcohol S. (esp. lower extremities, calcaneus)
*11. Fetal hydantoin S.
12. Homocystinuria
13. Infantile multisystem inflammatory disease (NOMID)
14. Kniest dysplasia
15. Metatropic dysplasia
16. Meyer dysplasia of femoral head
*17. Mucolipidosis II (I-cell disease); GM_1 gangliosidosis
18. Nail-patella S. (osteo-onychodysplasia)
19. Osteopathia striata (Voorhoeve disease)
*20. Pacman dysplasia
21. Parastremmatic dysplasia
*22. Smith-Lemli-Opitz S.
23. Spondyloepimetaphyseal dysplasia (short limb-hand type)
24. Stickler S. (arthro-ophthalmopathy)
25. Trichorhinophalangeal dysplasia (hips)
*26. Trisomy 18 S.
*27. Warfarin embryopathy
28. Winchester S.
*29. Zellweger S. (cerebrohepatorenal S.)

* Stippled epiphyses.

References

1. Felson B (ed): Dwarfs and other little people. Semin Roentgenol 1973; 8:255
2. Kozlowski K. Beighton P: Gamut Index of Skeletal Dysplasias. Berlin: Springer-Verlag, 1984, pp. 68–69
3. Poznanski AK: Punctate epiphyses: a radiologic sign, not a disease. Pediatr Radiol 1994;24:418–424
4. Taybi H, Lachman RS: Radiology of Syndromes, Metabolic Disorders, and Skeletal Dysplasias. (ed 4) St. Louis: Mosby-Year Book, Inc, 1996, pp 1029, 1057

Gamut D-19-3

STIPPLED OR PUNCTATE EPIPHYSES

COMMON

1. Chondrodysplasia punctata (all types)
    a. Conradi-Hünermann (CP-CH)
    b. Brachytelephalangic type (CP-BT)
    c. Rhizomelic type
    d. Sheffield type
    e. Tibial-metacarpal type (CP-MT)
    f. X-linked dominant (Happle) type
    g. X-linked recessive (Curry) type
2. Normal, age related (eg, distal femur, capitellum)
3. Osteopoikilosis
4. Pseudoachondroplasia (pseudoachondroplastic spondyloepiphyseal dysplasia)
5. Spondyloepiphyseal dysplasia (congenita or tarda)
6. Trisomy 21 S. (Down S.)

UNCOMMON

1. Brachmann-de Lange S. (de Lange S.)
2. CHILD S.
3. Chromosome disorders, many
4. Congenital transplacental infections (TORCH)
5. Fetal alcohol S. (esp. lower extremities, calcaneus)
6. Fetal hydantoin S.
7. Hypopituitarism (anterior lobe) with growth hormone deficiency
8. *Listeria monocytogenes* osteomyelitis
9. Mucolipidosis II (I-cell disease); GM_1 gangliosidosis
10. Pacman dysplasia
11. Smith-Lemli-Opitz S.
12. Trisomy 18 S.

13. Vitamin K reductase deficiency
14. Warfarin embryopathy
15. Zellweger S. (cerebrohepatorenal S.)

References
1. Felson B (ed): Dwarfs and other little people. Semin Roentgenol 1973; 8:255
2. Greenfield GB: Radiology of Bone Diseases. (ed 5) Philadelphia: Lippincott, 1990
3. Kozlowski K. Beighton P: Gamut Index of Skeletal Dysplasias. Berlin: Springer-Verlag, 1984, pp. 68–69
4. Poznanski AK: Punctate epiphyses: a radiologic sign, not a disease. Pediatr Radiol 1994;24:418–424
5. Taybi H, Lachman RS: Radiology of Syndromes, Metabolic Disorders, and Skeletal Dysplasias. (ed 4) St. Louis: Mosby-Year Book, Inc, 1996, pp 1029, 1057

Gamut D-20

ALTERATION IN SIZE OR APPEARANCE OF MULTIPLE EPIPHYSES (See D-19, D-21 to D-27)

COMMON

1. Arthritis (eg, juvenile chronic; juvenile rheumatoid; rheumatoid; psoriatic)
2. Avascular necrosis (eg, sickle cell disease; steroid therapy; Cushing S.); osteochondroses (See D-48, D-48-S)
3. Cone-shaped epiphyses (See D-27)
4. Congenital syndromes with irregular, fragmented, or stippled epiphyses (See D-19)
5. Cretinism; hypothyroidism
6. Delayed or increased skeletal maturation (See D-16, 17)
7. Dense (ivory) epiphyses (See D-26)
8. Diabetes, juvenile
9. Hemophilia
10. Hyperparathyroidism, primary or secondary (renal osteodystrophy)
11. Malnutrition; malabsorption
12. Mucopolysaccharidoses (eg, Hurler; Hunter; Morquio) (See J-4)
13. Multiple epiphyseal dysplasia (Fairbank)

14. Neurologic disorders$_g$
15. Normal variant
16. Osteomyelitis (eg, tuberculosis; smallpox residual; *Listeria monocytogenes*); congenital transplacental infections (TORCH)
17. Osteoporosis
18. Radiation injury
19. Rickets; osteomalacia
20. Scurvy
21. Thermal injury (eg, frostbite; burn; electrical injury)
22. Trauma (incl. battered child S.)

UNCOMMON

1. Achondroplasia
2. Acrodysostosis (peripheral dysostosis)
3. Adrenogenital S.
4. Beckwith-Wiedemann S.
5. Chondrodysplasia punctata (all forms)
6. Chondroectodermal dysplasia (Ellis-van Creveld S.)
7. Chromosome disorders, many
8. Congenital heart disease, cyanotic
9. Cutis laxa (hips)
10. Deprivation (psychosocial) dwarfism
11. Diastrophic dysplasia
12. Dyggve-Melchior-Clausen dysplasia (Smith-McCort S.)
13. Dysplasia epiphysealis hemimelica (Trevor disease)
14. Enchondromatosis (Ollier disease); Maffucci S.
15. Homocystinuria
16. Hormone-secreting neoplasm leading to precocious puberty (eg, gonadal tumor; teratoma; pinealoma; hepatoblastoma)
17. Hyperthyroidism
18. Hypochondroplasia
19. Hypo-hyperparathyroidism
20. Hypophosphatasia
21. Hypopituitarism (anterior lobe) with growth hormone deficiency
22. Idiopathic isosexual precocious puberty
23. Infantile multisystem inflammatory disease (NOMID)
24. Kniest dysplasia

(continued)

---

25. Metaphyseal chondrodysplasia (Jansen and other types)
26. Metatropic dysplasia
27. Meyer dysplasia of femoral head
28. Mucolipidosis II (I-cell disease) and III (pseudo-Hurler polydystrophy); GM_1 gangliosidosis
29. Nail-patella S. (osteo-onychodysplasia)
30. Osteogenesis imperfecta
31. Osteopathia striata (Voorhoeve disease); osteopathia striata with cranial sclerosis
32. Osteopoikilosis
33. Otospondylomegaepiphyseal dysplasia (OSMED)
34. Parastremmatic dysplasia
35. Pituitary gigantism
36. Pseudoachondroplasia (pseudoachondroplastic spondyloepiphyseal dysplasia)
37. Schwartz-Jampel S. (chondrodystrophic myotonia)
38. Smith-Lemli-Opitz S.
39. Sotos S. (cerebral gigantism)
40. Spondyloepimetaphyseal dysplasia (short limb-hand type)
41. Spondyloepiphyseal dysplasia (congenita or tarda)
42. Spondylo-megaepiphyseal-metaphyseal dysplasia
43. Stickler S. (arthro-ophthalmopathy)
44. Thiemann disease (hand)
45. Trichorhinophalangeal dysplasia
46. Trisomy 18 S.
47. Trisomy 21 S. (Down S.)
48. Warfarin embryopathy
49. Winchester S.
50. Zellweger S. (cerebrohepatorenal S.)

References

1. Felson B (ed): Dwarfs and other little people. Semin Roentgenol 1973; 8:255
2. Kozlowski K. Beighton P: Gamut Index of Skeletal Dysplasias. Berlin: Springer-Verlag, 1984, pp. 68–69
3. Oh KS, Ledesma-Medina J, Bender TM: Practical Gamuts and Differential Diagnosis in Pediatric Radiology. Chicago: Year Book Medical Publ, 1982, p 146
4. Swischuk LE, John SD: Differential Diagnosis in Pediatric Radiology. (ed 2) Baltimore: Williams & Wilkins, 1995
5. Taybi H, Lachman RS: Radiology of Syndromes, Metabolic Disorders, and Skeletal Dysplasias. (ed 4) St. Louis: Mosby-Year Book, Inc, 1996, pp 1029, 1057

Gamut D-21-1

SMALL EPIPHYSES—GENERALIZED

COMMON
1. Cretinism; hypothyroidism
2. Delayed skeletal maturation, any cause (See D-17)
3. Normal variant

UNCOMMON
1. Acromesomelic dysplasia
2. Congenital heart disease, cyanotic
3. Deprivation (psychosocial) dwarfism
4. Diabetes, juvenile
5. Diastrophic dysplasia
6. Hypopituitarism (eg, idiopathic; cranio-pharyngioma)
7. Juvenile chronic arthritis (eg, juvenile rheumatoid arthritis)
8. Malnutrition; malabsorption
9. Microepiphyseal dysplasia (proximal femur)
10. Mucolipidosis III (pseudo-Hurler polydystrophy)
11. Mucopolysaccharidoses (esp. Morquio S.)
12. Multiple epiphyseal dysplasia (Fairbank)
13. Progressive pseudorheumatoid chondrodysplasia
14. Pseudoachondroplasia (pseudoachondroplastic spondyloepiphyseal dysplasia)
15. Rickets
16. Spondyloepimetaphyseal dysplasias
17. Spondyloepiphyseal dysplasia (congenita or tarda)
18. Steroid therapy, prolonged; Cushing S.
19. Stickler S. (arthro-ophthalmopathy)
20. Winchester S.

References

1. Oh KS, Ledesma-Medina J, Bender TM: Practical Gamuts and Differential Diagnosis in Pediatric Radiology. Chicago: Year Book Medical Publ, 1982, p 146
2. Swischuk LE, John SD: Differential Diagnosis in Pediatric Radiology. (ed 2) Baltimore: Williams & Wilkins, 1995, pp 242–244
3. Taybi H, Lachman RS: Radiology of Syndromes, Metabolic Disorders, and Skeletal Dysplasias. (ed 4) St. Louis: Mosby-Year Book Inc, 1996, p 1030

Gamut D-21-2

SMALL EPIPHYSES—LOCALIZED

COMMON
1. Developmental dysplasia of the hip—DDH (congenital hip dysplasia or dislocation)
2. Disuse of an extremity (eg, neuromuscular disorder$_g$; arthritis)
3. Infection
4. Legg-Perthes disease, early; other avascular necrosis (See D-48)
5. Trauma

UNCOMMON
1. Metaphyseal chondrodysplasia (McKusick type) (proximal femur)
2. Meyer dysplasia of femoral head
3. Nail-patella S. (osteo-onychodysplasia)
4. Osteopathia striata with cranial sclerosis (proximal femur)
5. Otospondylomegaepiphyseal dysplasia (OSMED) (proximal femur)
6. Small patella S.
7. Trichorhinophalangeal dysplasia, type I (Giedion S.) and II (Giedion-Langer S.) (proximal femur)

References
1. Oh KS, Ledesma-Medina J, Bender TM: Practical Gamuts and Differential Diagnosis in Pediatric Radiology. Chicago: Year Book Medical Publ, 1982, p 146
2. Swischuk LE, John SD: Differential Diagnosis in Pediatric Radiology. (ed 2) Baltimore: Williams & Wilkins, 1995, pp 242–244
3. Taybi H, Lachman RS: Radiology of Syndromes, Metabolic Disorders, and Skeletal Dysplasias. (ed 4) St. Louis: Mosby-Year Book Inc, 1996, p 1030

Gamut D-22-1

LARGE EPIPHYSES—GENERALIZED

COMMON
1. [Diseases leading to thin diaphyses (eg, neurologic disorders$_g$; osteogenesis imperfecta)] (See D-10)
2. Juvenile chronic arthritis (eg, juvenile rheumatoid arthritis)

UNCOMMON
1. Adrenogenital S.
2. Beckwith-Wiedemann S.
3. Chromosome 4: del (4p) S. (Wolf-Hirschhorn S.)
4. Cockayne S.
5. Congenital total lipodystrophy (lipoatrophic diabetes)
6. Hemophilia
7. Hormone-secreting neoplasm leading to precocious puberty (eg, gonadal tumor; teratoma; pinealoma; hepatoblastoma)
8. Hyperthyroidism
9. Idiopathic isosexual precocious puberty
10. Infantile multisystem inflammatory disease (NOMID)
11. Kniest dysplasia (hands)
12. Mesomelic dysplasia (Langer type)
13. Metaphyseal chondrodysplasia (Jansen type)
14. Otospondylomegaepiphyseal dysplasia (OSMED)
15. Progressive pseudorheumatoid chondrodysplasia
16. Sotos S. (cerebral gigantism)
17. Spondyloepiphyseal dysplasia with macroepiphyses (Kozlowski type)
18. Spondylomegaepiphyseal-metaphyseal dysplasia

[ ] This condition does not actually cause the gamuted imaging finding, but can produce imaging changes that simulate it.

References
1. Oh KS, Ledesma-Medina J, Bender TM: Practical Gamuts and Differential Diagnosis in Pediatric Radiology. Chicago: Year Book Medical Publ, 1982, pp 142–144

(continued)

2. Swischuk LE, John SD: Differential Diagnosis in Pediatric Radiology. (ed 2) Baltimore: Williams & Wilkins, 1995, pp 242–244
3. Taybi H, Lachman RS: Radiology of Syndromes, Metabolic Disorders, and Skeletal Dysplasias. (ed 4) St. Louis: Mosby-Year Book Inc, 1996, pp 1029–1030

Gamut D-22-2

LARGE EPIPHYSES—LOCALIZED

COMMON

1. Arthritis (chronic sequelae from septic, tuberculous, or fungal)
2. Coxa magna and plana (eg, healed Legg-Perthes disease)
3. Hemophilic hemarthrosis
4. Juvenile chronic arthritis (eg, juvenile rheumatoid arthritis)
5. Posttraumatic; healing fracture

UNCOMMON

1. Angiomatous lesion (esp. hemangioma); arteriovenous malformation
2. Dysplasia epiphysealis hemimelica (Trevor disease)
3. Idiopathic localized gigantism
4. Localized hyperemia; other causes
5. Metaphyseal chondrodysplasia (Schmid type) (proximal femur)
6. Neurofibromatosis
7. Postsurgical (eg, open reduction with internal fixation)
8. Proteus S. (Perthes-like femoral heads)

References
1. Oh KS, Ledesma-Medina J, Bender TM: Practical Gamuts and Differential Diagnosis in Pediatric Radiology. Chicago: Year Book Medical Publ, 1982, pp 142–144
2. Swischuk LE, John SD: Differential Diagnosis in Pediatric Radiology. (ed 2) Baltimore: Williams & Wilkins, 1995, pp 242–244

Gamut D-23

THIN EPIPHYSES

COMMON

1. Hypothyroidism; cretinism
2. Renal osteodystrophy (secondary hyperparathyroidism)
3. Rickets

UNCOMMON

1. Acromesomelic dysplasia
2. Diastrophic dysplasia
3. Dyggve-Melchior-Clausen dysplasia
4. Kniest dysplasia
5. Microepiphyseal dysplasia (Elsbach)
6. Multiple epiphyseal dysplasia (Fairbank)
7. Schwartz-Jampel S. (chondrodystrophic myotonia)
8. Stickler S. (arthro-ophthalmopathy)
9. Thiemann disease

References
1. Poznanski AK: The Hand in Radiologic Diagnosis. (ed 2) Philadelphia: WB Saunders, 1984, p 900
2. Taybi H, Lachman RS: Radiology of Syndromes, Metabolic Disorders, and Skeletal Dysplasias. (ed 4) St. Louis: Mosby-Year Book Inc, 1996

Gamut D-24

INDISTINCT OR FUZZY EPIPHYSES

COMMON

1. Hyperparathyroidism, primary or secondary (renal osteodystrophy)
2. Hypothyroidism; cretinism
3. Osteomalacia
4. Rickets

UNCOMMON

1. Hypophosphatasia
2. Metaphyseal chondrodysplasia (Jansen type)
3. Mucolipidosis II (I-cell disease); GM$_1$ gangliosidosis

Reference

1. Swischuk LE, John SD: Differential Diagnosis in Pediatric Radiology. (ed 2) Baltimore: Williams & Wilkins, 1995, pp 245–246

Gamut D-25

RING EPIPHYSES (DENSE CORTEX WITH LUCENT CENTER)

COMMON

1. Osteoporosis, severe (esp. disuse atrophy)
2. Scurvy (Wimberger ring)

UNCOMMON

1. Hemophilia
2. Hyperparathyroidism, primary or secondary (renal osteodystrophy), healing
3. Hypothyroidism, healing
4. Juvenile osteoporosis
5. Lead poisoning
6. Osteogenesis imperfecta
7. Rickets, healing
8. Williams S. (idiopathic hypercalcemia)

References

1. Swischuk LE, John SD: Differential Diagnosis in Pediatric Radiology. (ed 2) Baltimore: Williams & Wilkins, 1995, pp 245–246
2. Taybi H, Lachman RS: Radiology of Syndromes, Metabolic Disorders, and Skeletal Dysplasias. (ed 4) St. Louis: Mosby-Year Book Inc, 1996, p 1029

Gamut D-26

DENSE (IVORY) EPIPHYSES OF HANDS AND FEET

ACQUIRED

COMMON

1. Hypopituitarism
2. Normal variant (esp. distal phalanges)
3. Retarded skeletal maturation (See D-17)

UNCOMMON

1. Connective tissue disease (collagen disease)$_g$ (eg, lupus erythematosus; scleroderma)
2. Deprivation (psychosocial) dwarfism
3. Hypothyroidism
4. Renal osteodystrophy (secondary hyperparathyroidism)

CONGENITAL

COMMON

1. Multiple epiphyseal dysplasia (Fairbank)
2. Thiemann disease
3. Trichorhinophalangeal dysplasia, type I (Giedion S.) and II (Giedion-Langer S.)

UNCOMMON

1. Cockayne S.
2. Coffin-Lowry S.
3. Coffin-Siris S.
4. Dyggve-Melchior-Clausen dysplasia
5. Homocystinuria
6. Lesch-Nyhan S. (congenital hyperuricosuria)
7. Morquio S.
8. Mucolipidosis III (pseudo-Hurler polydystrophy)
9. Osteopetrosis
10. Robinow S.
11. Seckel S. (bird-headed dwarfism)
12. Silver-Russell S.
13. Spondyloepiphyseal dysplasia congenita

(continued)

14. Stickler S. (arthro-ophthalmopathy)
15. Trisomy 21 S. (Down S.)
16. Turner S.
17. Williams S. (idiopathic hypercalcemia)

References

1. Kuhns LR, Poznanski AK, Shaw HAS, et al: Ivory epiphyses. Radiology 1973; 109:643–648
2. Poznanski AK: The Hand in Radiologic Diagnosis. (ed 2) Philadelphia: WB Saunders, 1984, pp 147–152
3. Swischuk LE, John SD: Differential Diagnosis in Pediatric Radiology. (ed 2) Baltimore: Williams & Wilkins, 1995, p 240
4. Taybi H, Lachman RS: Radiology of Syndromes, Metabolic Disorders, and Skeletal Dysplasias. (ed 4) St. Louis: Mosby-Year Book Inc, 1996, p 1029

Gamut D-27

CONE-SHAPED EPIPHYSES

COMMON

1. Dactylitis (esp. bone infarction—sickle cell disease, vasculitis; osteomyelitis-postmeningococcemia; smallpox residual; frostbite; burn)
2. Idiopathic or normal
3. Trauma; epiphyseal-metaphyseal fracture; battered child S.

UNCOMMON

1. Achondroplasia
2. Acrocephalosyndactyly (Apert type)
3. Acrodysostosis (peripheral dysostosis)
4. Acrodysplasia with retinitis pigmentosa and nephropathy (Saldino-Mainzer S.); other conorenal syndromes
5. Acromesomelic dysplasia
6. Acromicric dysplasia
7. Asphyxiating thoracic dysplasia (Jeune S.)
8. Brachydactyly syndromes (esp. type E)
9. Chondroectodermal dysplasia (Ellis-van Creveld S.)
10. Cleidocranial dysplasia
11. Cockayne S.
12. Coffin-Siris S.
13. Diastrophic dysplasia
14. DOOR S.
15. Dyggve-Melchior-Clausen dysplasia
16. Hereditary multiple exostoses (multiple cartilaginous exostoses; osteochondromatosis) (lateral cone)
17. Hyperthyroidism, neonatal
18. Hypervitaminosis A, chronic
19. Hypochondroplasia
20. Hypophosphatasia (knees)
21. Infantile multisystem inflammatory disease (NOMID)
22. Kashin-Beck disease
23. Metaphyseal chondrodysplasia (Jansen, McKusick and Schmid types)
24. Multiple epiphyseal dysplasia (Fairbank)
25. Orofaciodigital syndrome I (Papillon-Leage and Psaume S.)
26. Osteogenesis imperfecta
27. Osteoglophonic dysplasia
28. Osteopetrosis
29. Otopalatodigital S. (type I)
30. Pseudoachondroplasia (pseudoachondroplastic spondyloepiphyseal dysplasia)
31. Pseudohypoparathyroidism; pseudopseudohypoparathyroidism
32. Radiation injury
33. Ruvalcaba S. (trichorhinophalangeal S., type III)
34. Scurvy
35. Seckel S. (bird-headed dwarfism)
36. Spondyloepimetaphyseal dysplasia (cone-shaped epiphyses type)
37. Trichorhinophalangeal dysplasia, type I (Giedion S.) and II (Giedion-Langer S.)
38. Weill-Marchesani S.

References

1. Giedion A: Cone-shaped epiphyses of the hands and their diagnostic value. The tricho-rhino-phalangeal syndrome. Ann Radiol 1967; 10:322–329
2. Poznanski AK: The Hand in Radiologic Diagnosis. (ed 2) Philadelphia: WB Saunders, 1984, pp 155–161
3. Silverman FN (ed): Caffey's Pediatric X-ray Diagnosis. (ed 9) Chicago: Year Book Medical Publ, 1993

4. Swischuk LE, John SD: Differential Diagnosis in Pediatric Radiology. (ed 2) Baltimore: Williams & Wilkins, 1995
5. Taybi H, Lachman RS: Radiology of Syndromes, Metabolic Disorders, and Skeletal Dysplasias. (ed 4) St. Louis: Mosby-Year Book Inc, 1996, p 1029

References
1. Greenfield GB: Radiology of Bone Diseases. (ed 5) Philadelphia: Lippincott, 1990
2. Silverman FN (ed): Caffey's Pediatric X-ray Diagnosis. (ed 9) Chicago: Year Book Medical Publ, 1993, pp 1754–1759
3. Spranger JW, Langer LO Jr., Wiedemann H-R: Bone Dysplasias. Philadelphia: WB Saunders, 1974, pp 269–273
4. Swischuk LE, John SD: Differential Diagnosis in Pediatric Radiology. (ed 2) Baltimore: Williams & Wilkins, 1995, p 264

Gamut D-28-1

WIDE EPIPHYSEAL PLATE (PHYSIS)— GENERALIZED

COMMON

1. Growth hormone excess (eg, pituitary tumor; gigantism; treatment with growth hormone)
2. Hyperparathyroidism, primary or esp. secondary (renal osteodystrophy)
3. Maturation delay (endocrine, constitutional, other causes) (wide for age)
4. Rickets (all types) (See D-44)

UNCOMMON

1. Aminoaciduria (eg, phenylketonuria; homocystinuria)
2. Copper deficiency, nutritional; Menkes S. (kinky-hair S.) (neonate and young infant)
3. Dyggve-Melchior-Clausen dysplasia
4. Hypophosphatasia
5. Hypothyroidism; cretinism
6. Infection (eg, congenital transplacental infection—syphilis, rubella)
7. Metaphyseal chondrodysplasia (Jansen, McKusick, Schmid types)
8. Mucolipidosis II (I-cell disease); GM_1 gangliosidosis
9. Mucopolysaccharidosis VI (Maroteaux-Lamy S.)
10. Osteogenesis imperfecta (types II and III)
11. Scurvy, advanced
12. Spondylometaphyseal dysplasia (esp. Kozlowski type)
13. Total parenteral nutrition (neonate and young infant)

Gamut D-28-2

WIDE EPIPHYSEAL PLATE (PHYSIS)— LOCALIZED

COMMON

1. Pathologic fracture (eg, scurvy; rickets; leukemia; metastasis)
2. Slipped capital femoral epiphysis
3. Trauma, esp. epiphyseal-metaphyseal fracture (Salter-Harris)

UNCOMMON

1. Congenital insensitivity to pain (fracture)
2. Infection (incl. congenital transplacental infection—syphilis, rubella)
3. Kirner deformity
4. Metaphyseal dysplasia (Shwachman type) (proximal femur)
5. Myelodysplasia (with absent or diminished pain sensitivity) (fracture)
6. Radiation injury
7. Riley-Day S. (familial dysautonomia) (fracture)
8. Spondylometaphyseal dysplasias

References
1. Greenfield GB: Radiology of Bone Diseases. (ed 5) Philadelphia: Lippincott, 1990
2. Silverman FN (ed): Caffey's Pediatric X-ray Diagnosis. (ed 9) Chicago: Year Book Medical Publ, 1993, pp 1754–1759
3. Swischuk LE, John SD: Differential Diagnosis in Pediatric Radiology. (ed 2) Baltimore: Williams & Wilkins, 1995, p 264

LOCALIZED EPIPHYSEAL OR METAPHYSEAL LESION RESULTING IN PREMATURE CLOSURE OF GROWTH PLATE AND A SHORTENED BONE

COMMON

1. Local hyperemia (eg, infection; juvenile chronic arthritis; juvenile rheumatoid arthritis; hemophilia; arteriovenous malformation)
2. Osteomyelitis (eg, bacterial; tuberculous; meningococcal; yaws; smallpox residual)
3. Trauma; battered child S.; surgical trauma

UNCOMMON

1. Bone infarction (eg, sickle cell disease)
2. Disuse (eg, immobilization; postfracture)
3. Enchondromatosis (Ollier disease); Maffucci S.
4. Hypervitaminosis A
5. Infantile multisystem inflammatory disease (NOMID)
6. Hereditary multiple exostoses (multiple cartilaginous exostoses; osteochondromatosis)
7. Neoplasm invading growth plate
8. Pseudohypoparathyroidism; pseudopseudo-hypoparathyroidism
9. Radiation injury
10. Rickets
11. Scurvy
12. Thermal injury (burn; frostbite)

References
1. Greenfield GB: Radiology of Bone Diseases. (ed 5) Philadelphia: Lippincott, 1990
2. Silverman FN (ed): Caffey's Pediatric X-ray Diagnosis. (ed 9) Chicago: Year Book Medical Publ, 1995, pp 1759, 1761

GROSS DISRUPTION OF EPIPHYSEAL-METAPHYSEAL REGION

COMMON

1. Battered child S.; other severe trauma with epiphyseal-metaphyseal fracture
2. Fracture in neurologic or neuromuscular disorder$_g$
3. Fracture in weakened bone
   a. Bone infarction (esp. sickle cell disease)
   b. Congenital transplacental infection (eg, syphilis; rubella; cytomegalovirus infection)
   c. Hyperparathyroidism
   d. Metastatic disease
   e. Osteomyelitis (eg, bacterial; smallpox residual)
   f. Rickets (all types)

UNCOMMON

1. Bone sarcoma
2. Langerhans cell histiocytosis$_g$ (esp. eosinophilic granuloma)
3. Metaphyseal chondrodysplasia (Jansen type)
4. Osteogenesis imperfecta
5. Pseudoachondroplasia (pseudoachondroplastic spondyloepiphyseal dysplasia)
6. Scurvy
7. Sensory neuropathy
   a. Amyotrophic lateral sclerosis
   b. Congenital insensitivity to pain
   c. Diabetes
   d. Leprosy
   e. Myelodysplasia
   f. Peripheral nerve injury
   g. Syphilis (tabes dorsalis)
   h. Syringomyelia; hydromyelia
8. Spondyloepimetaphyseal dysplasia (Strudwick type)

Reference
1. Swischuk LE, John SD: Differential Diagnosis in Pediatric Radiology. (ed 2) Baltimore: Williams & Wilkins, 1995, pp 262–264

Gamut D-31

RADIOLUCENT METAPHYSEAL BANDS

COMMON

*1. Congenital transplacental infection (eg, toxoplas-
mosis; rubella; cytomegalovirus infection; herpes;
syphilis)
2. Leukemia
3. Metastatic disease (esp. neuroblastoma)
4. Normal variant (esp. in neonate); prematurity
*5. Systemic illness or stress in childhood, infancy,
or in utero (eg, asthma; diabetes; cystic fibrosis
{mucoviscidosis}; juvenile chronic arthritis;
juvenile rheumatoid arthritis; malnutrition)
*6. Trauma; fractures; battered child S.; deprivation
(psychosocial) dwarfism

UNCOMMON

*1. Chemotherapy; radiation injury
2. Erythroblastosis fetalis
3. Fetal hydantoin S. (Dilantin embryopathy)
4. Heavy metal or chemical poisoning, esp. lead
(alternating with dense lines)
5. Hypervitaminosis D
6. Hypophosphatasia
7. Infection, postnatal (eg, brucellosis)
8. Intrauterine gut perforation with meconium
peritonitis
*9. Osteopetrosis
10. Oxalosis
11. Prolonged parenteral hyperalimentation; total
parenteral nutrition
*12. Rickets, healing
13. Scurvy
*14. Williams S. (idiopathic hypercalcemia)

* May have alternating radiolucent and radiopaque transverse metaphyseal bands.

References

1. Greenfield GB: Radiology of Bone Diseases. (ed 5) Philadelphia: Lippincott, 1990
2. Oh KS, Ledesma-Medina J, Bender TM: Practical Gamuts
and Differential Diagnosis in Pediatric Radiology. Chicago:
Year Book Medical Publ, 1982, pp 148–149
3. Poznanski AK: Annual oration—diagnostic clues in the
growing ends of bone. J Can Assoc Radiol 1978; 29:7–21
4. Swischuk LE, John SD: Differential Diagnosis in Pediatric
Radiology. (ed 2) Baltimore: Williams & Wilkins, 1995,
p 251
5. Wolfson JJ, Engel RR: Anticipating meconium peritonitis
from metaphyseal bands. Radiology 1969; 92:1055–1060

Gamut D-32

TRANSVERSE LINES OR ZONES
OF INCREASED DENSITY
IN THE METAPHYSES

COMMON

1. Anemia$_g$, chronic (eg, sickle cell disease; thalassemia)
2. Chemotherapy (eg, methotrexate)
3. Growth acceleration lines following growth arrest
due to systemic illness or stress in infancy or childhood (eg, asthma; diabetes; cystic fibrosis {muco-
viscidosis}; juvenile chronic arthritis; juvenile
rheumatoid arthritis; malnutrition)
4. Lead poisoning
5. Leukemia, treated
6. Normal variant (esp. in neonate—dense zone of
provisional calcification)
7. Renal osteodystrophy (secondary hyperparathyroidism), healing
8. Rickets, healing
9. Trauma; battered child S.; stress fracture

UNCOMMON

1. Aminopterin fetopathy
2. Biphosphonate therapy
3. Chronic recurrent multifocal osteomyelitis

(continued)

4. Congenital transplacental infection, healing (eg, toxo-plasmosis; rubella; cytomegalovirus infection; herpes; syphilis)
5. Deprivation (psychosocial) dwarfism with trauma
6. Drug or hormone therapy in high dosage (eg, steroids; parathormone; methotrexate; estrogen or heavy metal therapy to mother during pregnancy)
7. Dysosteosclerosis
8. Heavy metal or chemical poisoning, other (eg, bismuth; arsenic; phosphorus; fluoride; mercury; lithium; radium; thorotrast)
9. Hypervitaminosis D
10. Hypoparathyroidism; pseudohypoparathyroidism
11. Hypothyroidism; cretinism (treated)
12. Meconium peritonitis (neonatal dense bands)
13. Metaphyseal chondrodysplasias
14. Osteopetrosis
15. Oxalosis
16. Parathormone therapy
17. Patterson S.
18. Radiation injury from bone-seeking isotopes (Sr^{90}, Y^{90}, P^{32})
19. Sclerosteosis (esp. knees)
20. Scurvy, healing
21. Spondyloepimetaphyseal dysplasias
22. Spondylometaphyseal dysplasias
23. Vascular injury
24. Williams S. (idiopathic hypercalcemia)

References
1. Follis RH Jr, Park EA: Some observations on bone growth, with particular respect to zones and transverse lines of increased density in the metaphysis. AJR 1952; 68:709–724
2. Poznanski AK: The Hand in Radiologic Diagnosis. (ed 2) Philadelphia: WB Saunders, 1984, pp 143–144
3. Silverman FN (ed): Caffey's Pediatric X-ray Diagnosis. (ed 9) Chicago: Year Book Medical Publ, 1993, pp 1762–1763
4. Taybi H, Lachman RS: Radiology of Syndromes, Metabolic Disorders, and Skeletal Dysplasias. (ed 4) St. Louis: Mosby-Year Book Inc, 1996, p 1037

Gamut D-33

DENSE VERTICAL METAPHYSEAL LINES

COMMON
1. Congenital transplacental infections ("celery stalk" metaphyses) (eg, rubella; cytomegalovirus infection; syphilis)
2. Metaphyseal injury (localized)
3. Osteopathia striata (Voorhoeve disease)

UNCOMMON
1. Enchondromatosis, early (Ollier disease); Maffucci S.
2. Goltz S. (focal dermal hypoplasia)
3. Hypophosphatasia
4. Metaphyseal chondrodysplasias
5. Mixed sclerosing bone dysplasia
6. Normal variant
7. Osteopathia striata with cranial sclerosis
8. Phenylketonuria
9. Sponastrime dysplasia

References
1. Chapman S, Nakielny R: Aids to Radiological Differential Diagnosis. (ed 3) London: WB Saunders, 1995, p 52
2. Swischuk LE, John SD: Differential Diagnosis in Pediatric Radiology. (ed 2) Baltimore: Williams & Wilkins, 1995, pp 252–254

Gamut D-34-1

SPLAYING, FLARING, OR WIDENING OF THE METAPHYSES (INCLUDING ERLENMEYER FLASK DEFORMITY) (See D-34-2 and -3)

COMMON
*1. Anemia$_g$, primary (eg, thalassemia; sickle cell disease)

2. Bone cyst or benign expansile bone neoplasm
3. Fibrous dysplasia (incl. McCune-Albright S.)
4. Fracture; epiphyseal-metaphyseal injury
*5. Gaucher disease; Niemann-Pick disease
6. Normal variant
7. Rickets, incl. biliary rickets

UNCOMMON

*1. Congenital syndromes and bone dysplasias (esp. osteopetrosis; achondroplasia; Pyle dysplasia) (See D-34-2)
2. Fetal hydantoin S. (Dilantin embryopathy)
3. Hypervitaminosis A
4. Hypophosphatasia
5. Immunologic disorders$_g$
6. Langerhans cell histiocytosis$_g$
*7. Lead poisoning, chronic
*8. Mastocytosis
9. Phenylketonuria
10. Renal osteodystrophy (secondary hyperparathyroidism)
11. Scurvy

* May have Erlenmeyer flask-like deformity.

References

1. Kozlowski K, Beighton P: Gamut Index of Skeletal Dysplasias. Berlin: Springer-Verlag, 1984, p 63
2. Swischuk LE, John SD: Differential Diagnosis in Pediatric Radiology. (ed 2) Baltimore: Williams & Wilkins, 1995, pp 257–259

Gamut D-34-2

CONGENITAL SYNDROMES AND SKELETAL DYSPLASIAS WITH SPLAYING, FLARING, OR WIDENING OF THE METAPHYSES

COMMON

1. Achondroplasia
2. Enchondromatosis (Ollier disease); Maffucci S.

3. Chondrodysplasia punctata (multiple types, esp. rhizomelic)
4. Chondroectodermal dysplasia (Ellis-van Creveld S.)
*5. Gaucher disease; Niemann-Pick disease
*6. Hereditary multiple exostoses (multiple cartilaginous exostoses; osteochondromatosis)
*7. Osteopetrosis
*8. Pyle dysplasia

UNCOMMON

1. Achondrogenesis
2. Acromesomelic dysplasia
3. Cephaloskeletal dysplasia (Taybi-Linder S.)
4. Cockayne S.
*5. Craniometaphyseal dysplasia; craniodiaphyseal dysplasia
6. de la Chapelle dysplasia
7. Diastrophic dysplasia
*8. Dysosteosclerosis
9. Dyssegmental dysplasia
10. Fibrochondrogenesis
*11. Frontometaphyseal dysplasia
12. Hypochondroplasia
*13. Hypophosphatasia (adult)
14. Infantile multisystem inflammatory disease (NOMID)
*15. Kniest dysplasia
*16. Membranous lipodystrophy
17. Mesomelic dysplasia (Langer type)
18. Metaphyseal chondrodysplasia (Jansen, McKusick, Schmid types)
19. Metatropic dysplasia
20. Morquio S.
21. Mucolipidosis II (I-cell disease)
22. Oculodento-osseous dysplasia
*23. Osteodysplasty (Melnick-Needles S.)
24. Osteogenesis imperfecta (rare "cystic" form)
*25. Otopalatodigital S. (type I)
26. Phenylketonuria
27. Progressive pseudorheumatoid chondrodysplasia
28. Pseudoachondroplasia (pseudoachondroplastic spondyloepiphyseal dysplasia)
*29. Schwarz-Lélek S.

(continued)

---

30. Short rib-polydactyly syndromes
31. Spondyloepiphyseal dysplasia congenita
32. Spondylomegaepiphyseal-metaphyseal dysplasia
33. Spondylometaphyseal dysplasia (Sedaghatian and corner fracture types)
34. Stickler S. (arthro-ophthalmopathy) (infants)
35. Thanatophoric dysplasia
*36. Weaver S.
37. Weissenbacher-Zweymüller phenotype
38. Williams S. (idiopathic hypercalcemia) (distal femurs)

* May have Erlenmeyer flask-like deformity.

References
1. Kozlowski K, Beighton P: Gamut Index of Skeletal Dysplasias. Berlin: Springer-Verlag, 1984, p 63
2. Swischuk LE, John SD: Differential Diagnosis in Pediatric Radiology. (ed 2) Baltimore: Williams & Wilkins, 1995, pp 257–259
3. Taybi H, Lachman RS: Radiology of Syndromes, Metabolic Disorders, and Skeletal Dysplasias. (ed 4) St. Louis: Mosby-Year Book Inc, 1996, pp 1030, 1037–1038

4. Hypophosphatasia (adult)
5. Kniest dysplasia
6. Lead poisoning, chronic
7. Mastocytosis
8. Membranous lipodystrophy
9. Osteodysplasty (Melnick-Needles S.)
10. Otopalatodigital S. (type I)
11. Rickets, healing
12. Schwarz-Lélek S.
13. Weaver S.

References
1. Greenfield GB: Radiology of Bone Diseases. (ed 5) Philadelphia: Lippincott, 1990
2. Swischuk LE, John SD: Differential Diagnosis in Pediatric Radiology. (ed 2) Baltimore: Williams & Wilkins, 1995, pp 257–259
3. Taybi H, Lachman RS: Radiology of Syndromes, Metabolic Disorders, and Skeletal Dysplasias. (ed 4) St. Louis: Mosby-Year Book Inc, 1996, pp 1030, 1037–1038

Gamut D-34-3

ERLENMEYER FLASK DEFORMITY OF METAPHYSIS (See D-34-1 and -2)

COMMON

1. Anemia$_g$, primary (eg, thalassemia; sickle cell disease)
2. Gaucher disease; Niemann-Pick disease
3. Hereditary multiple exostoses (multiple cartilaginous exostoses; osteochondromatosis)
4. Osteopetrosis
5. Pyle dysplasia (familial metaphyseal dysplasia)

UNCOMMON

1. Craniometaphyseal dysplasia
2. Dysosteosclerosis
3. Frontometaphyseal dysplasia

Gamut D-35

DUMBBELL BONES (SHORT LONG BONES WITH PRONOUNCED METAPHYSEAL FLARING)

COMMON

1. Achondroplasia
2. Kniest dysplasia
3. Metatropic dysplasia
4. Pseudoachondroplasia (pseudoachondroplastic spondyloepiphyseal dysplasia), severe

UNCOMMON

1. Chondrodysplasia punctata, rhizomelic type
2. Chondroectodermal dysplasia (Ellis-van Creveld S.)
3. Diastrophic dysplasia
4. Dyssegmental dysplasia
5. Fibrochondrogenesis
6. Omodysplasia

7. Osteogenesis imperfecta (type III)
8. Otospondylomegaepiphyseal dysplasia (OSMED)
9. Weissenbacher-Zweymüller phenotype

References
1. Swischuk LE: Differential Diagnosis in Pediatric Radiology. Baltimore: Williams & Wilkins, 1984, p 166
2. Taybi H, Lachman RS: Radiology of Syndromes, Metabolic Disorders, and Skeletal Dysplasias. (ed 4) St. Louis: Mosby-Year Book Inc, 1996, p 1028

Gamut D-36-1

METAPHYSEAL CUPPING

COMMON

1. Cone-shaped epiphyses (See D-27)
2. Congenital syndromes and bone dysplasias (See D-36-2)
3. Normal variant (eg, distal ulna and fibula; triangular-shaped finger and toe phalanges)
4. Prolonged immobilization of joints causing distal metaphyseal cupping (eg, poliomyelitis; tuberculosis or pyarthrosis of hip; slipped capital femoral epiphysis; developmental dysplasia of the hip—DDH {congenital hip dysplasia or dislocation})
5. Rickets (all types) (See D-44)
6. Trauma (to cartilage); epiphyseal-metaphyseal injury

UNCOMMON

1. Bone infarction; hypovascularity
2. Hypervitaminosis A
3. Leukemia
4. Osteomyelitis (eg, bacterial-esp. meningococcemia; syphilis; yaws; smallpox-prior to eradication)
5. Radiation injury
6. Scurvy (after a compression fracture)
7. Sickle cell disease
8. Thermal injury (frostbite; burn)

References
1. Caffey J: Traumatic cupping of the metaphyses of growing bones. AJR 1970; 108:451–460

2. Greenfield GB: Radiology of Bone Diseases. (ed 5) Philadelphia: Lippincott, 1990
3. Poznanski AK: The Hand in Radiologic Diagnosis. (ed 2) Philadelphia: WB Saunders, 1984, p 900
4. Swischuk LE, John SD: Differential Diagnosis in Pediatric Radiology. (ed 2) Baltimore: Williams & Wilkins, 1995, pp 257–258

Gamut D-36-2

CONGENITAL SYNDROMES AND SKELETAL DYSPLASIAS WITH METAPHYSEAL CUPPING

COMMON

1. Achondroplasia
2. Chondroectodermal dysplasia (Ellis-van Creveld S.)
3. Congenital insensitivity to pain
4. Hypophosphatasia
5. Sickle cell disease

UNCOMMON

1. Achondrogenesis (type II)
2. Acrodysostosis (peripheral dysostosis)
3. Cephaloskeletal dysplasia (Taybi-Linder S.)
4. Chondrodysplasia punctata (rhizomelic and X-linked recessive types)
5. Copper deficiency, nutritional; Menkes S. (kinky-hair S.) (spurs)
6. Diastrophic dysplasia
7. Dyssegmental dysplasia
8. Hyperparathyroidism, neonatal
9. Hypochondroplasia
10. Immune deficiency syndromes (eg, metaphyseal dysplasia with thymolymphopenia; Shwachman S.; adenosine deaminase deficiency)
11. Infantile multisystem inflammatory disease (NOMID)
12. Metaphyseal chondrodysplasia (all types)
13. Metatropic dysplasia
14. Mucolipidosis II (I-cell disease) (in infants); GM_1 gangliosidosis

(continued)

15. Mucopolysaccharidoses (See J-4)
16. Opsismodysplasia
17. Osteodysplasty (Melnick-Needles S.)
18. Phenylketonuria
19. Pseudoachondroplasia (pseudoachondroplastic spondyloepiphyseal dysplasia)
20. Schneckenbecken dysplasia
21. Short rib-polydactyly S. type III
22. Spondylomegaepiphyseal-metaphyseal dysplasia
23. Spondylometaphyseal dysplasia (Kozlowski and Sedaghatian types)
24. Thanatophoric dysplasia
25. Trichorhinophalangeal dysplasia, type I (Giedion S.) and type II (Langer-Giedion S.)
26. Vitamin K deficiency embryopathy

References
1. Poznanski AK: The Hand in Radiologic Diagnosis. (ed 2) Philadelphia: WB Saunders, 1984, p 900
2. Swischuk LE, John SD: Differential Diagnosis in Pediatric Radiology. (ed 2) Baltimore: Williams & Wilkins, 1995, pp 257–258
3. Taybi H, Lachman RS: Radiology of Syndromes, Metabolic Disorders, and Skeletal Dysplasias. (ed 4) St. Louis: Mosby-Year Book Inc, 1996, p 1037

Gamut D-37

METAPHYSEAL BEAKS, SPURS, OR FRAGMENTATION

COMMON

1. Bow legs, other causes (See D-185)
2. Fracture, epiphyseal-metaphyseal (eg, normal bones; battered child S.; breech delivery)
3. Normal, esp. knees with physiologic bow legs
4. Osteomyelitis; congenital transplacental infections (eg, rubella; cytomegalovirus infection; syphilis)
5. Rickets (all types)
6. Tibia vara (Blount's disease)

UNCOMMON

1. Adenosine deaminase deficiency
2. Copper deficiency, nutritional; Menkes S. (kinky-hair S.)
3. Deferoxamine-induced bone dysplasia
4. Dyschondrosteosis (medial tibial metaphysis)
5. Hyperparathyroidism
6. Hypophosphatasia
7. Leukemia
8. Maroteaux-Lamy S.
9. Metaphyseal dysplasia (Jansen and anadysplasia types)
10. Metastatic disease (esp. neuroblastoma)
11. Neurologic disease$_g$ with bone atrophy
12. Opsismodysplasia
13. Patterson S.
14. Scurvy (Pelkan spurs)
15. Short rib-polydactyly S. type II (Majewski) and III
16. Spondyloepimetaphyseal dysplasia (Strudwick type)
17. Spondylometaphyseal dysplasia (corner fracture type)

References
1. Kleinman PK, Belanger PL, Karellas A, Spevak MR: Pictorial essay: normal metaphyseal radiologic variants not to be confused with findings of infant abuse. AJR 1991; 156: 781–783
2. Oh KS, Ledesma-Medina J, Bender TM: Practical Gamuts and Differential Diagnosis in Pediatric Radiology. Chicago: Year Book Medical Publ, 1982, p 154
3. Spranger JW, Langer LO, Wiedemann H-R: Bone Dysplasias. Philadelphia: WB Saunders, 1974
4. Swischuk LE, John SD: Differential Diagnosis in Pediatric Radiology. (ed 2) Baltimore: Williams & Wilkins, 1995, pp 256–257
5. Taybi H, Lachman RS: Radiology of Syndromes, Metabolic Disorders, and Skeletal Dysplasias. (ed 4) St. Louis: Mosby-Year Book, Inc, 1996, p 1037

Gamut D-38

INDISTINCT FRAYED METAPHYSES

COMMON

1. Osteomalacia
2. Rickets (all types) (See D-44)

UNCOMMON

1. Chronic stress (eg, in wrists of adolescent gymnasts)
2. Congenital transplacental infections (rubella; syphilis)
3. Copper deficiency, nutritional; Menkes S. (kinky-hair S.)
4. Dyggve-Melchior-Clausen dysplasia
5. Hyperparathyroidism, severe
6. Hypophosphatasia
7. Metaphyseal chondrodysplasia (Jansen and other types)
8. Morquio S.
9. Oxalosis
10. Patterson S.
11. Scurvy

References

1. Carter SR, et al: Stress changes of the wrist in adolescent gymnasts. Br J Radiol 1988; 61:109–112
2. Greenfield GB: Radiology of Bone Disease. (ed 5) Philadelphia: Lippincott, 1990
3. Grünebaum M, Horodniceanu C, Steinherz R: The radiographic manifestations of bone changes in copper deficiency. Pediatr Radiol 1980; 9:101–104
4. Swischuk LE, John SD: Differential Diagnosis in Pediatric Radiology. (ed 2) Baltimore: Williams & Wilkins, 1995, p 255

Gamut D-39

EROSION OF THE MEDIAL ASPECT OF THE PROXIMAL METAPHYSES OF LONG BONES (ESPECIALLY THE HUMERUS, FEMUR, AND TIBIA)

COMMON

1. Hyperparathyroidism, primary or secondary (renal osteodystrophy)
2. Leukemia
3. Metastatic neuroblastoma
4. Rheumatoid arthritis (humeral notch)

UNCOMMON

1. Gaucher disease; Niemann-Pick disease (esp. humerus)
2. Hurler S.
3. Juxtacortical chondroma
4. Normal variant
5. Rickets
6. Syphilis, congenital

Reference

1. Li JKW, Birch PD, Davies AM: Proximal humerus defects in Gaucher's disease. Br J Radiol 1988; 61:579–583

Gamut D-40-S

DIFFERENTIAL DIAGNOSIS OF VARIOUS METAPHYSEAL DISTURBANCES

Disturbance	Epiphysis	Physis	Zone of Provisional Calcification	Fraying	Cupping	Radiolucent Metaphyseal Band	Metaphyseal Fracture	Periosteal Reaction	Age of Onset (May be present at)
Rickets	Ill-defined	Widened	Early stage —ill-defined	+					6 months— rarely at birth (osteomalacic mothers)
			Healing stage —widened		+	–	–	+	
Scurvy	Ringed	Narrow, normal	Widened	–	From infarction	+	+	+	3 months
Hypophosphatasia	Ill-defined	Widened	Ill-defined	+	+	–	–	+	Birth
Metaphyseal dysplasia	Normal	Widened	Ill-defined	+	+	–	–	–	Birth
Phenylketonuria	May be retarded	Spicules of calcium protrude	Normal	–	+	–	–	–	1 month
Infantile trauma	May be displaced	May be widened	Normal	–	–	–	+	+	Birth injury
Rubella	Ill-defined	Normal	Absent	+	–	+	–	–	Birth
Syphilis	Normal	Widened	Widened	+	+	+	+	+	Birth
Leukemia	Ill-defined, destructive foci	Normal	Normal	–	–	+	–	+	Birth

Reference
1. Greenfield GB: Radiology of Bone Diseases. (ed 4) Philadelphia: Lippincott, 1986, p 254

Gamut D-41

SUBPERIOSTEAL BONE RESORPTION
(See D-39, D-105)

COMMON

*1. Chronic avulsive injury of cortex (eg, cortical/ periosteal desmoid)
2. Hyperparathyroidism, primary or secondary (renal osteodystrophy)

UNCOMMON

1. Erdheim-Chester disease
+2. Farber disease (disseminated lipogranulomatosis)
+3. Metaphyseal chondrodysplasia (Jansen type)
+4. Mucolipidoses; GM$_1$ gangliosidosis
5. Pseudohypohyperparathyroidism
6. Rickets, severe
*7. Subperiosteal hematoma
*8. Subperiosteal osteomyelitis

* Focal.
+ In infants.

References
1. Resnick D: Diagnosis of Bone and Joint Disorders (ed 3). Philadelphia: Saunders, 1995
2. Swischuk LE, John SD: Differential Diagnosis in Pediatric Radiology (ed 2). Baltimore: Williams & Wilkins,1995, pp 218–220

Gamut D-41-S

SITES OF OSSEOUS RESORPTION IN PRIMARY AND SECONDARY HYPERPARATHYROIDISM

A. Subperiosteal

1. Hands (middle phalanges of 2nd and 3rd fingers, radial aspect; also terminal phalangeal tufts; sesamoid bones)
2. Femur, tibia, humerus (predominantly proximal medial aspect)
3. Other long bones (proximal or distal)
4. Lamina dura of teeth
5. Ribs (upper or lower border)

B. Subchondral

1. Clavicle (acromioclavicular and sternoclavicular joints)
2. Pubic symphysis
3. Hands and feet (interphalangeal joints, MCP and MTP joints)
4. Sacroiliac joint (greater on iliac side)
5. Discovertebral junction
6. Patellofemoral joint
7. Tibiofemoral joint
8. Glenohumeral joint
9. Sella turcica (endosteal resorption)
10. Calvarium, inner and outer table (endosteal resorption)

C. Subligamentous or Subtendinous

1. Clavicle (distal undersurface—coracoclavicular ligament)

2. Humerus (proximal—rotator cuff)
3. Olecranon process of ulna (anconeus attachment)
4. Anterior superior iliac spine (sartorius attachment)
5. Anterior inferior iliac spine (rectus femoris attachment)
6. Ischial tuberosities (hamstring attachment)
7. Calcaneus (posterior superior and inferior surfaces—achilles and aponeurosis attachments)

References
1. Murphey MD, Sartoris DJ, Quale JL, Pathria MN, Martin NL: Musculoskeletal manifestations of chronic renal insufficiency.
2. Murray RO, Jacobson HG, Stoker DJ: The Radiology of Skeletal Disorders. (ed 3) Edinburgh: Churchill Livingstone, 1990

Gamut D-42

LOCALIZED OR REGIONAL OSTEOPOROSIS; BONE ATROPHY (INCLUDING SUDECK'S ATROPHY)

COMMON

1. Acro-osteolysis (See D-127)
2. Arthritis (esp. rheumatoid; juvenile chronic; juvenile rheumatoid; Reiter S.; septic; tuberculous; fungal—mycetoma) (See D-228); synovitis
3. Disuse atrophy; immobilization (eg, fracture; cast); neural or muscular paralysis
4. Hemorrhage (eg, trauma; hemophilia)
5. Neoplasm, benign or malignant (esp. myeloma; osteolytic metastasis)
6. Osteomyelitis (eg, bacterial; tuberculous; fungal)
7. Osteonecrosis (incl. radiation); bone infarct or avascular necrosis, early
8. Soft tissue infection adjacent to bone; human or animal bite
9. Sudeck's atrophy (reflex sympathetic dystrophy)
10. Thermal injury (eg, burn; frostbite); electroshock

(continued)

11. Trauma with or without fracture; fracture complications (eg, nonunion; malunion; infection)
12. Vascular insufficiency, arterial or venous (eg, arteriosclerosis obliterans; Buerger disease (thromboangiitis obliterans); Raynaud disease)

UNCOMMON

1. Arteriovenous malformation; hemangioma
2. Bone marrow edema S. (transient osteoporosis of hip)
3. Congenital pseudarthrosis
4. Denervation or tendon transection
5. Diabetes (diabetic osteopathy)
6. Idiopathic
7. Paget's disease (eg, osteoporosis circumscripta of skull)
8. Regional migratory osteoporosis of legs
9. Sarcoidosis
10. Shoulder-hand S. (eg, myocardial infarction; scalenus anticus S.)

Gamut D-43-1

GENERALIZED OSTEOPOROSIS

I. CONGENITAL SYNDROMES (See D-43-2)
II. DEFICIENCY DUE TO MALASSIMILATION

COMMON

1. Alcoholism
2. Calcium, phosphorus deficiency
3. Malabsorption (eg, sprue; celiac disease; cystic fibrosis {mucoviscidosis}; inflammatory small bowel disease; postgastrectomy; blind loop S.)
4. Malnutrition; kwashiorkor; starvation; anorexia nervosa
5. Protein deficiency
6. Vitamin C deficiency (scurvy)
7. [Vitamin D deficiency (rickets)]

UNCOMMON

1. Copper deficiency, nutritional; Menkes S. (kinky-hair S.) (in infants)

III. DISUSE ATROPHY (MUSCLE WEAKNESS; LACK OF STRESS STIMULUS OR WEIGHT BEARING)

COMMON

1. Cerebral palsy
2. Immobilization (eg, chronic disease; major fracture; cast)
3. Muscular dystrophy; neuromuscular disorder$_g$
4. Spinal cord disease

UNCOMMON

1. Arthrogryposis
2. Space flight osteoporosis

IV. ENDOCRINE

COMMON

1. Adrenocortical abnormality (eg, adrenal atrophy—adrenopause; Addison disease; Cushing S.)
2. Hypogonadism
   a. Ovarian—estrogen deficiency (eg, menopause; oophorectomy; Turner S.)
   b. Testicular (eg, eunuchoidism; prepubertal castration S.; Klinefelter S. (XXY S.)
3. Pancreatic abnormality (eg, poorly controlled diabetes; pancreatic insufficiency; cystic fibrosis {mucoviscidosis}; pancreatitis)
4. Parathyroid abnormality (eg, hyperparathyroidism, primary or secondary {renal osteodystrophy}; hypoparathyroidism with steatorrhea)
5. Thyroid abnormality (eg, hyperthyroidism; thyrotoxicosis; hypothyroidism; cretinism)

UNCOMMON

1. Pituitary abnormality (eg, acromegaly; Cushing S. due to basophilic adenoma; hypopituitarism; craniopharyngioma)

2. Steroid-producing nonendocrine neoplasm (eg, oat cell carcinoma of lung)

V. MISCELLANEOUS

COMMON

1. Anemia$_g$ (eg, sickle cell disease; thalassemia; spherocytosis; pyruvate kinase deficiency; severe iron deficiency)
2. Connective tissue disease (collagen disease)$_g$ (eg, lupus erythematosus; scleroderma; dermatomyositis; CREST syndrome; MCTD)
3. Iatrogenic; drug therapy (eg, excessive steroids, heparin); hypervitaminosis A and D; biphosphonate therapy; chemotherapy; aluminum-induced bone disease; experimental hyperoxia
4. Idiopathic (eg, idiopathic juvenile osteoporosis)
5. Liver disease (eg, jaundice; biliary atresia; Wilson disease {hepatolenticular degeneration}; large or multiple liver tumors or cysts with protein disturbance)
6. Metastatic disease (eg, carcinomatosis)
7. Multiple myeloma
8. [Osteomalacia]
9. Pregnancy
10. Renal disease (eg, nephrosis; renal tubular acidosis; oxalosis; renal osteodystrophy—secondary hyperparathyroidism)
11. Rheumatoid arthritis
12. Senile or postmenopausal osteoporosis

UNCOMMON

1. Amyloidosis
2. Deprivation (psychosocial) dwarfism
3. Epidermolysis bullosa (dystrophica and acquired)
4. Gaucher disease; Niemann-Pick disease
5. Hemochromatosis
6. Hemophilia
7. Histiocytic medullary reticulocytosis
8. Hydroxyapatite deposition disease (HADD)
9. Hypoxemia (eg, chronic pulmonary disease; congenital heart disease)
10. Kawasaki S.
11. Leukemia, acute

12. Mastocytosis
13. Ochronosis (alkaptonuria)
14. Reflex sympathetic dystrophy, widespread
15. Seronegative spondyloarthropathy (esp. ankylosing spondylitis)
16. Tylosis
17. Vascular tumors of bone, widespread (eg, angiomatosis; massive osteolysis {Gorham vanishing bone disease})
18. Waldenström macroglobulinemia
19. Wegener granulomatosis

[ ] This condition does not actually cause the gamuted imaging finding, but can produce imaging changes that simulate it.

References

1. Greenfield GB: Radiology of Bone Diseases. (ed 5) Philadelphia: Lippincott, 1990
2. Taybi H, Lachman RS: Radiology of Syndromes, Metabolic Disorders, and Skeletal Dysplasias. (ed 4) St. Louis: Mosby-Year Book, Inc, 1996, pp 1055–1056
3. Teplick JG, Haskin ME: Roentgenologic Diagnosis. (ed 3) Philadelphia: WB Saunders, 1976

Gamut D-43-2

CONGENITAL SYNDROMES AND SKELETAL DYSPLASIAS WITH GENERALIZED OSTEOPOROSIS

COMMON

1. Anemia$_g$ (eg, sickle cell disease; thalassemia; spherocytosis; pyruvate kinase deficiency)
2. Cystic fibrosis (mucoviscidosis)
3. Metabolic error (eg, homocystinuria; hypophosphatasia; phenylketonuria)
4. Neuromuscular disorders and dystrophies$_g$ (eg, arthrogryposis; myotonica congenita; Duchenne muscular dystrophy)
5. Osteogenesis imperfecta (all types)

(continued)

UNCOMMON

1. Aspartylglucosaminuria
2. Cerebro-oculo-facial-skeletal S. (Pena-Shokeir S. type II)
3. Cockayne S.
4. Contractural arachnodactyly
5. Cranioectodermal dysplasia
6. Ehlers-Danlos S.
7. Familial Mediterranean fever (familial recurrent polyserositis)
8. Fanconi anemia (pancytopenia-dysmelia S.)
9. Farber disease (disseminated lipogranulomatosis)
10. Fibrodysplasia (myositis) ossificans progressiva
11. Fibrogenesis imperfecta ossium
12. Gaucher disease; Niemann-Pick disease
13. Geroderma osteodysplastica
14. Glycogen storage disease type I (von Gierke disease)
15. Goltz S. (focal dermal hypoplasia)
16. Hallermann-Streiff S. (oculomandibulofacial S.)
17. Infantile multisystem inflammatory disease (NOMID)
18. Infantile Refsum disease
19. Klinefelter S. (XXY S.)
20. Laron S. (pituitary dwarfism II)
21. Lowe S. (oculocerebrorenal S.)
22. Mauriac S.
23. Membranous lipodystrophy
24. Menkes S. (kinky-hair S.)
25. Metachromatic leukodystrophies
26. Mucopolysaccharidoses; mucolipidoses; GM_1 gangliosidosis; mannosidosis (See J-4)
27. Osteochondrodysplasias (eg, Pyle dysplasia; diaphyseal dysplasia; metaphyseal dysplasia {Jansen type}; achondrogenesis)
28. Osteolysis syndromes (incl. Hajdu-Cheney S.; osteolysis with nephropathy)
29. Osteoporosis-pseudoglioma S.
30. Otopalatodigital S.
31. Papillon-Lefèvre S.
32. Parastremmatic dysplasia
33. Prader-Willi S.
34. Progeria; Werner S.

35. Pseudohypoparathyroidism; pseudopseudo-hypoparathyroidism
36. Rothmund-Thomson S.
37. Singleton-Merten S.
38. Thevenard S. (acrodystrophic neuropathy)
39. Trisomy 13 S.
40. Trisomy 18 S.
41. Turner S.
42. Williams S. (idiopathic hypercalcemia), late
43. Wilson disease (hepatolenticular degeneration)
44. Winchester S.
45. Wolman disease (familial xanthomatosis)

References

1. Greenfield GB: Radiology of Bone Diseases. (ed 5) Philadelphia: Lippincott, 1990
2. Kozlowski K, Beighton P: Gamut Index of Skeletal Dysplasias. Berlin: Springer-Verlag, 1984, pp 3–4
3. Poznanski AK: The Hand in Radiologic Diagnosis. (ed 2) Philadelphia: WB Saunders, 1984, p 922
4. Taybi H, Lachman RS: Radiology of Syndromes, Metabolic Disorders, and Skeletal Dysplasias. (ed 4) St. Louis: Mosby-Year Book, Inc, 1996, pp 1055–1056

Gamut D-44

OSTEOMALACIA AND RICKETS

I. DEFICIENT ABSORPTION OF CALCIUM OR PHOSPHORUS

A. Malabsorption states

1. Cathartic abuse (esp. oily cathartics; phenolphthalein; magnesium sulfate)
2. Mesenteric disease
3. Pancreatic insufficiency (exocrine); pancreatitis
4. Postoperative gastric or small bowel resection; small bowel bypass
5. Primary small bowel disease (eg, celiac disease; sprue; amyloidosis; scleroderma; Crohn's disease; lymphoma; small bowel fistula; blind loop S.)
6. Steatorrhea, idiopathic

B. Obstructive jaundice or liver failure

1. Acquired chronic biliary obstruction
2. Biliary atresia

II. EXCESSIVE RENAL EXCRETION OF CALCIUM OR PHOSPHORUS

A. Glomerular (hyperphosphatemic)

1. Renal osteodystrophy (secondary hyperparathyroidism)
2. Renal osteomalacia

B. Tubular (hypophosphatemic)

1. Fanconi syndromes (de Toni-Debré-Fanconi S.) (osteomalacia or rickets, growth retardation, renal tubular acidosis, phosphaturia, glycosuria, aminoaciduria, and proteinuria)
   a. Primary (idiopathic)
       i. Childhood type, with cystinosis
       ii. Adult type, without cystinosis
   b. Secondary (acquired)
       i. Beryllium poisoning
       ii. Drugs (eg, amphoteracin B; lithium salts; outdated tetracycline)
       iii. Heavy metal poisoning (eg, lead; cadmium; fluoride)
       iv. Hypervitaminosis D in adults
       v. Multiple myeloma
       vi. Nephrotic syndrome
       vii. Neurofibromatosis
       viii. Renal transplantation
1. Inborn metabolic disturbances (eg, galactosemia; oxalosis; tyrosinosis; Wilson disease {hepatolenticular degeneration}; GM_1 gangliosidosis; hereditary fructose intolerance)
3. Vitamin D-resistant rickets (hypophosphatemic familial rickets)

III. EXCESSIVE UTILIZATION OF CALCIUM AS FIXED BASE

1. Chronic obstructive renal disease
2. Idiopathic hypercalciuria
3. Polycystic kidney disease
4. Renal tubular acidosis
5. Ureterosigmoidostomy (hyperchloremia)

IV. MISCELLANEOUS

1. Aluminum-induced bone disease (eg, phosphate deficiency from aluminum hydroxide hemodialysis; antacid-induced osteomalacia and nephrolithiasis)
2. Anticonvulsant drug therapy (eg, Dilantin; tranquilizers) (accelerated hepatic degradation of vitamin D3 and 25-HCC)
3. Congenital rickets (maternal magnesium sulfate therapy; mother with osteomalacia)
4. Decreased deposition of calcium in bone (eg, diphosphonate treatment for Paget's disease)
5. Dietary calcium deficiency (rare)
6. Enzyme abnormality (eg, hypophosphatasia)
7. Excessive excretion of calcium or phosphorus via breast or placenta (puerperal osteomalacia)
8. Fibrogenesis imperfecta ossium; axial osteomalacia (with acquired vitamin D resistance)
9. Immunologic disorders$_g$
10. Paraneoplastic syndromes (humoral syndromes) (See D-44-S)
11. Pernicious anemia
12. Pseudovitamin D-deficiency rickets or osteomalacia
13. Vitamin D deficient rickets (dietary or lack of sunshine)

NOTE: In infants less than 6 months of age, consider chiefly:

1. Biliary atresia
2. Hypophosphatasia
3. Maternal magnesium sulfate therapy
4. Neonatal rickets (premature infants with combined dietary deficiency and impaired hepatic hydroxylation of vitamin D)
5. Vitamin D-dependent rickets (associated with severe myopathy; dietary intake of vitamin D is adequate)

References
1. Greenfield GB: Radiology of Bone Diseases. (ed 5) Philadelphia: Lippincott, 1990

(continued)

2. Murray RO, Jacobson HG, Stoker DJ: The Radiology of Skeletal Disorders. (ed 3) Edinburgh: Churchill Livingstone, 1990
3. Taybi H, Lachman RS: Radiology of Syndromes, Metabolic Disorders, and Skeletal Dysplasias. (ed 4) St. Louis: Mosby-Year Book, Inc, 1996, p 713
4. Turner ML, Dalinka MK: Osteomalacia: Uncommon causes. AJR 1979; 133:539–540

3. Resnick D: Diagnosis of Bone and Joint Disorders. (ed 3) Philadelphia: Saunders, 1995
4. Weidner N: Review and update: Oncogenic osteomalacia-rickets. Ultrastruct Pathol 1991; 15:317–333

Gamut D-44-S

ONCOGENIC (TUMOR-INDUCED) OSTEOMALACIA: BONE AND SOFT TISSUE NEOPLASM ASSOCIATIONS*

COMMON

1. Hemangiopericytoma
2. Hemangioma, cavernous or sclerosing
3. Mesenchymal tumor (prominent fibrous and vascular components)

UNCOMMON

1. Angiosarcoma
2. Fibrous dysplasia
3. Giant cell granuloma (reparative)
4. Giant cell tumor (benign and malignant)
5. Gorlin S. (nevoid basal cell carcinoma S.)
6. Malignant fibrous histiocytoma
7. Malignant peripheral nerve sheath tumor (MPNST)
8. Metastatic disease (esp. blastic-prostate; also neuroblastoma)
9. Nasopharyngeal angiofibroma
10. Nonossifying fibroma (fibroxanthoma); fibrous cortical defect
11. Osteoblastoma

* All related to production of ectopic humoral substance.

References

1. Greenfield GB: Radiology of Bone Disease. (ed 5) Philadelphia: Lippincott, 1990
2. McAllister WH, Siegel MJ: Oncogenic rickets (Feuerstein and Mims Syndrome with resistant rickets). AJR 1989; 152:1330–1331

Gamut D-45-S

CAUSES OF ALTERED CALCIUM AND PHOSPHORUS CONCENTRATIONS

HYPERCALCEMIA

1. Adrenal insufficiency
2. Hyperparathyroidism
3. Hyperthyroidism
4. Hypervitaminosis D
5. Hypophosphatasia
6. Hypothyroidism
7. Leukemia; lymphoma
8. Metaphyseal chondrodysplasia (Jansen type)
9. Milk-alkali S.
10. Multiple myeloma (myelomatosis)
11. Reticuloses
12. Sarcoidosis
13. Secretion of parathormone-like substance from malignant neoplasms
14. Skeletal metastases (carcinomatosis)
15. Werner S. (familial multiple endocrine neoplasms-MEN S., type I)
16. Widespread bone destruction; rapid deossification
17. Williams S. (idiopathic hypercalcemia)

HYPERPHOSPHATEMIA

1. Acromegaly
2. Glomerular failure
3. Hypervitaminosis D
4. Hypoparathyroidism; pseudohypoparathyroidism
5. Skeletal metastases (carcinomatosis)

HYPOCALCEMIA

1. Acidosis
2. Hypoalbuminemia

3. Hypoparathyroidism; pseudohypoparathyroidism
4. Malabsorption with reduced calcium absorption from intestine
5. Normal neonate
6. Pancreatitis
7. Uremia; renal osteodystrophy (secondary hyperparathyroidism)
8. Vitamin D deficiency (hypovitaminosis D)

HYPOPHOSPHATEMIA

1. Dietary deficiency
2. Hyperparathyroidism
3. Hypovitaminosis D (eg, Vitamin D-deficiency rickets; osteomalacia)
4. Increased carbohydrate metabolism
5. Malabsorption
6. Pregnancy
7. Renal tubular dysfunction (eg, Fanconi S.; Vitamin D-resistant rickets)
8. Skeletal metastases (carcinomatosis)

HYPERCALCIURIA

1. Acidosis
2. Hypercalcemia
3. Hypervitaminosis D
4. Hyperparathyroidism, primary
5. Osteoporosis, active
6. Renal tubular dysfunction
7. Sarcoidosis
8. Widespread bone destruction; rapid deossification

HYPOCALCIURIA

1. Active reconstruction of bone
2. Alkalosis
3. Decreased glomerular filtration rate
4. Hypocalcemia
5. Malabsorption with reduced calcium absorption from intestine
6. Vitamin D deficiency (hypovitaminosis D)

Reference

1. Greenfield GB: Radiology of Bone Diseases. (ed 5) Philadelphia: Lippincott, 1990

WIDESPREAD OR GENERALIZED DEMINERALIZATION WITH COARSE TRABECULATION

COMMON

1. Anemia$_g$, primary (esp. sickle cell disease, thalassemia)
2. Carcinomatosis
3. Hyperparathyroidism, primary or secondary (renal osteodystrophy)
4. Multiple myeloma (myelomatosis)
5. Osteomalacia, rickets (eg, biliary atresia; alimentary tract disorder) (See D-44)
6. Osteoporosis (See D-43)
7. Paget's disease
8. Paralysis

UNCOMMON

1. Acromegaly
2. Fibrogenesis imperfecta ossium
3. Gaucher disease
4. Hemophilia
5. Idiopathic axial osteomalacia
6. Leukemia
7. Osteogenesis imperfecta
8. Recalcification after disuse osteoporosis

SCATTERED AREAS OF DECREASED AND INCREASED BONE DENSITY IN THE SKELETON

COMMON

1. Lymphoma$_g$; leukemia
2. Metastases (esp. breast)
3. Osteomyelitis (esp. unusual infection—eg, tuberculosis; syphilis)

(continued)

---

4. Paget's disease
5. Renal osteodystrophy (secondary hyperparathyroidism)

UNCOMMON
1. Fibrous dysplasia
2. Hyperparathyroidism, primary
3. Hyperphosphatasia
4. Langerhans cell histiocytosis$_g$
5. Mastocytosis
6. Tuberous sclerosis

Gamut D-48

AVASCULAR NECROSIS (EPIPHYSEAL ISCHEMIA)

COMMON
1. Anemia$_g$, primary (esp. sickle cell disease)
2. Idiopathic; Legg-Perthes disease
3. Occlusive vascular disease (eg, arteriosclerosis; Leriche S.; thromboembolic disease; giant cell arteritis)
4. Osteochondritis dissecans (localized form of avascular necrosis)
5. Steroid therapy; Cushing S.
6. Trauma (eg, fracture—esp. of femoral neck or proximal scaphoid; dislocation; surgical correction of congenital hip; slipped capital femoral epiphysis; hip nailing; microfracture; battered child S.; congenital insensitivity to pain)

UNCOMMON
1. Burn; frostbite; electrical injury
2. Caisson disease (dysbaric osteonecrosis)
3. Connective tissue disease (collagen disease)$_g$ (eg, lupus erythematosus; polyarteritis nodosa; scleroderma)
4. Diabetes
5. Drug therapy (eg, anti-inflammatory agents—Butazolidin, Indocin; immunosuppressives; cytotoxic therapy; methotrexate)
6. Fabry disease
7. Fat embolism (eg, alcoholism; liver disease; pancreatitis; trauma)
8. Gaucher disease
9. Gout
10. Hemophilia
11. Hyperlipoproteinemia
12. Hypothyroidism
13. Infection (eg, pyogenic arthritis; osteomyelitis; subacute bacterial endocarditis)
14. Langerhans cell histiocytosis$_g$
15. Lymphoma$_g$; leukemia
16. Meyer dysplasia of femoral head
17. Multiple epiphyseal dysplasia (Fairbank) (femoral heads)
18. Neuropathic arthropathy (Charcot joint)
19. Osteoporosis, generalized
20. Polycythemia vera
21. Pregnancy
22. Radiation injury; radium poisoning
23. Rheumatoid arthritis
24. Spontaneous osteonecrosis of the knee
25. Thiemann disease (phalanges)
26. Trichorhinophalangeal dysplasia, type I (Giedion S.)
27. Winchester S.

References

1. Beltran J, Herman LJ, Burk JM, et al: Femoral head avascular necrosis: MR imaging with clinical-pathologic and radionuclide correlation. Radiology 1988; 166: 215–220
2. Bjorkergren AG, Al Rowaih A, Lindstrand A, Wingstrand H, Thorngren K-G, Pettersson H: Spontaneous osteonocrosis of the knee: Value of MR imaging in determining prognosis. AJR 1990; 154:331–336
3. Edeiken J, Hodes PJ, Libshitz HI, et al: Bone ischemia. Radiol Clin North Am 1967; 5:515–529
4. Edeiken J, Dalinka M, Karasick D: Edeiken's Roentgen Diagnosis of Diseases of Bone. Baltimore: Williams & Wilkins,1990
5. Griffiths HJ: Etiology, pathogenesis, and early diagnosis of ischemic necrosis of the hip. JAMA 1981; 246:2615–2617
6. Hunder GG, Worthington JW, Bickel WH: Avascular necrosis of the femoral head in a patient with gout. JAMA 1968; 203:47–49

7. Jacobson HG, Siegelman SS: Some miscellaneous solitary bone lesions. Semin Roentgenol 1966; 1:314–335
8. Jaffe HL: Ischemic necrosis of bone. Med Radiogr Photogr 1969; 45:58–86
9. Lecouvet FE, Vandeberg BC, Maldague BE, et al: Early irreversible osteonecrosis versus transient lesions of the femoral condyles: Prognostic value of subchondral bone and marrow changes on MR imaging. AJR 1998; 170:71–77
10. Mallory TH: Avascular necrosis of the femoral head in the adult. Ohio State Med J 1975; 71:548-550
11. Martel W, Sitterley BH: Roentgenologic manifestations of osteonecrosis. AJR 1969; 106:509-522
12. Mitchell DG, Rao VM, Dalinka MK, et al: Femoral head avascular necrosis: correlation of MR imaging, radiographic staging, radionuclide imaging and clinical findings. Radiology 1987; 162:709-715
13. Murray RO, Jacobson HG, Stoker DJ: The Radiology of Skeletal Disorders. (ed 3) Edinburgh: Churchill Livingstone, 1990
14. Resnick D. Diagnosis of Bone and Joint Disorders. (ed 3) Philadelphia, Saunders, 1995
15. Salimi, Wezel Vas, Sundaram M: Avascular necrosis: in an untreated case of chronic myelogenous leukemia. Skeletal Radiol 1988; 17:353–355
16. Swischuk LE, John SD: Differential Diagnosis in Pediatric Radiology. (ed 2) Baltimore: Williams & Wilkins, 1995
17. Vandeberg BC, Malghem J, Labaisse MA, Noel H, Maldague B: Avascular necrosis of the hip: Comparison of contrast enhanced and nonenhanced MR imaging with histologic correlation. Radiology 1992; 182:445–450

Gamut D-48-S

SITES OF PREDILECTION AND EPONYMS FOR AVASCULAR NECROSIS

COMMON

1. Carpal lunate	Kienböck 1910
2. Femoral capital epiphysis	Legg-Calvé-Perthes 1910
3. Medial femoral condyle (occasionally lateral femoral condyle)	
4. Medial tibial condyle	Blount 1937
5. [Osteochondritis dissecans]	König 1887
6. Second metatarsal head (occasionally third or fourth)	Freiberg 1914
7. Secondary patellar center	Sinding-Larsen 1921
8. Talus (trochlea)	Diaz 1928
9. Tarsal navicular	Köhler 1908
10. Tibial tubercle	Osgood-Schlatter 1903
11. Vertebral body	Calvé and Kümmell 1925
12. Vertebral epiphysis	Scheuermann 1921

UNCOMMON

1. Bases of phalanges	Thiemann 1909
*2. Calcaneal apophysis	Sever 1912
3. Capitulum of humerus	Panner 1927
4. Carpal scaphoid	Preiser 1911
5. Distal tibial epiphysis	Liffert and Arkin 1950
6. Distal ulna	Burns 1921
7. Entire carpus bilaterally	Caffey 1945
8. Fifth metatarsal base	Iselin 1912
9. Greater trochanter of femur	Mandl 1922
10. Head of humerus	Hass 1921
11. Head of radius	Brailsford
12. Heads of metacarpals	Mauclaire 1927; Dietrich 1932
*13. Iliac crest	Buchman 1927
14. Intercondylar spines of tibia	Caffey 1956
15. Ischial apophysis	Milch 1953
*16. Ischiopubic synchondrosis	Van Neck 1924
17. Os tibiale externum	Haglund 1908
18. Primary patellar center	Köhler 1908
19. Symphysis pubis	Pierson 1929

* Now considered a normal variant.
[ ] This condition does not actually cause the gamuted imaging finding, but can produce imaging changes that simulate it.

Reference

1. Greenfield GB: Radiology of Bone Diseases. (ed 5) Philadelphia: Lippincott, 1990

Gamut D-49

BONE INFARCT (DIAMETAPHYSEAL ISCHEMIA)

COMMON

1. Anemia$_g$, primary (esp. sickle cell disease)
2. Idiopathic
3. Occlusive vascular disease (arteriosclerosis; Buerger disease {thromboangiitis obliterans}; thromboembolic disease)

UNCOMMON

1. Caisson disease (dysbaric osteonecrosis)
2. Connective tissue disease (collagen disease)$_g$ (eg, lupus erythematosus, scleroderma)
3. Fat embolism (eg, alcoholism)
4. Gaucher disease
5. Infection; osteomyelitis
6. Pancreatitis with fat necrosis
7. Pheochromocytoma
8. Polyarteritis nodosa (vasculitis)
9. Radiation injury; radium poisoning

References

1. Edeiken J, Hodes PJ, Libshitz HI, et al: Bone ischemia. Radiol Clin North Am 1967; 5:515–529
2. Edeiken J, Dalinka M, Karasick D: Edeiken's Roentgen Diagnosis of Diseases of Bone. Baltimore: Williams & Wilkins, 1990

Gamut D-50

"BONE WITHIN A BONE" APPEARANCE

COMMON

1. Bone infarct (eg, sickle cell disease)
2. [Growth arrest and recovery, "growth lines" (eg, due to severe childhood disease; infection; scurvy; rickets; stress; immobilization; leukemia chemotherapy)]
3. Idiopathic
4. Normal neonate (esp. spine)
5. Osteopetrosis
6. Paget's disease

UNCOMMON

1. Acromegaly
2. Bone diseases with a split or double layer cortex (See D-103)
3. Chronic osteomyelitis with sequestrum and involucrum (eg, pyogenic; syphilis)
4. Erdheim-Chester disease
5. Heavy metal poisoning (eg, lead; phosphorus; bismuth; cadmium; fluoride)
6. Hypervitaminosis D
7. Oxalosis
8. Prostaglandin E$_1$ therapy
9. Subcortical osteoporosis (eg, Sudeck's atrophy {reflex sympathetic dystrophy} involving carpals or tarsals; leukemia; metastatic disease)
10. Subperiosteal hemorrhage
11. Thorotrast; radiation osteitis

References

1. Brill PW, Baker DH, Ewing ML: Bone-within-bone in the neonatal spine. Radiology 1973; 108:363–366
2. Frager DH, Subbarao K: The bone within a bone. JAMA 1983; 249:77–79
3. Greenfield GB: Radiology of Bone Diseases. (ed 5) Philadelphia: Lippincott, 1990
4. Matzinger MA, Briggs VA, Dunlap HJ, et al: Plain film and CT observations in prostaglandin-induced bone changes. Pediatr Radiol 1992;22:264–266
5. Murray RO, Jacobson HG: The Radiology of Skeletal Disorders. (ed 3) Edinburgh: Churchill Livingstone, 1990
6. O'Brien JP: The manifestations of arrested bone growth: The appearance of a vertebra within a vertebra. J Bone Joint Surg 1969; 51A:1376–1378
7. Sutton D: A Textbook of Radiology and Imaging. (ed 4) Edinburgh: Churchill Livingstone, 1987

Gamut D-51

BONE LESION WITH SEQUESTRUM OR SEQUESTRUM-LIKE REGION

COMMON

*1. Brodie abscess; osteomyelitis
*2. Button sequestrum in skull (See A-22)
 3. Osteoid osteoma
*4. Osteonecrosis; bone infarct

UNCOMMON

1. Langerhans cell histiocytosis$_g$ (esp. eosinophilic granuloma)
2. Lymphoma$_g$
3. Malignant fibrous histiocytoma; fibrosarcoma
4. Metastasis (esp. breast or other carcinoma with button sequestrum in skull)
5. Osteoblastoma
*6. Syphilis; yaws
*7. Tropical ulcer
*8. Tuberculosis

* Lesions which contain true sequestra (devitalized bone surrounded by granulation tissue) are the result of infection or infarction.

Gamut D-52

MULTIPLE SCLEROTIC FOCI OR CALCIFIC STREAKING IN INFANTS AND CHILDREN (See D-33)

NEONATES AND INFANTS

1. Chondrodysplasia punctata (all types)
2. Chromosomal disorders (esp. trisomy 18 and 21)
3. Congenital transplacental infections ("celery stalk" metaphyses) (eg, rubella; cytomegalovirus infection; syphilis)
4. Healed fractures (eg, stress fracture; battered child S.; osteogenesis imperfecta)

5. Mucolipidosis II (I-cell disease); GM$_1$ gangliosidosis
6. Phenylketonuria
7. Smith-Lemli-Opitz S.
8. Sponastrime dysplasia
9. Warfarin embryopathy
10. Zellweger S. (cerebrohepatorenal S.)

OLDER CHILDREN

1. Angiomatosis (rarely)
2. Bone infarcts; avascular necroses (eg, sickle cell disease; acute pancreatitis)
3. Bone islands (enostoses)
4. Enchondromatosis (Ollier disease); Maffucci S.
5. Gardner S.
6. Goltz S. (focal dermal hypoplasia)
7. Gorlin S. (nevoid basal cell carcinoma S.) (osteopoikilosis-like changes)
8. Healed fractures (incl. osteogenesis imperfecta)
9. Langerhans cell histiocytosis$_g$, healed or healing
10. Lymphoma$_g$
11. Mastocytosis
12. Melorheostosis
13. Metaphyseal chondrodysplasia (Jansen type)
14. Mixed sclerosing bone dysplasia
15. Osteomyelitis, multiple sites, healed or healing; yaws; fungal-mycetoma
16. Osteopathia striata (Voorhoeve disease); osteopathia striata with cranial sclerosis
17. Osteopetrosis
18. Osteopoikilosis
19. Osteosarcomatosis; osteoblastic metastases
20. Parastremmatic dysplasia
21. Patterson S.
22. Pyle dysplasia, in infancy; craniometaphyseal dysplasia; frontometaphyseal dysplasia; craniodiaphyseal dysplasia
23. Tuberous sclerosis

References

1. Kozlowski K, Beighton P: Gamut Index of Skeletal Dysplasias. Berlin: Springer-Verlag, 1984, pp 9, 61
2. Silverman FN (ed): Caffey's Pediatric X-ray Diagnosis. (ed 9) Chicago: Year Book Medical Publ, 1995, p 170

Gamut D-53

SOLITARY OSTEOSCLEROTIC BONE LESION (See D-54)

COMMON

1. Avascular necrosis (See D-48)
2. Bone infarct (See D-49)
3. Bone island or enostosis; idiopathic sclerosis
4. Callus (healed or healing fracture); stress fracture
5. Chondroid lesion (eg, enchondroma; osteochondroma)
6. Healed or healing benign bone lesion (eg, bone cyst; nonossifying fibroma {fibroxanthoma}; fibrous cortical defect; brown tumor of hyperparathyroidism; Langerhans cell histiocytosis$_g$, esp. eosinophilic granuloma)
7. Hyperostosis frontalis interna (skull)
8. Osteoblastic metastasis (esp. breast; prostate) (See D-85)
9. Osteochondritis dissecans
10. Osteoid osteoma
11. Osteoma
12. Osteomyelitis, chronic or healed (eg, Garré sclerosing osteomyelitis; Brodie abscess; granuloma; mycetoma; tropical ulcer)
13. Osteonecrosis (eg, radiation)
14. Paget's disease

UNCOMMON

1. Bone sarcoma (eg, osteosarcoma; chondrosarcoma; Ewing sarcoma; parosteal sarcoma)
2. Condensing osteitis of clavicle
3. Fibrous dysplasia
4. Lymphoma$_g$; leukemia
5. Lytic metastasis following radiation or chemotherapy
6. Medullary calcification in a long bone following removal of an intramedullary rod
7. Mastocytosis
8. Melorheostosis
9. Meningioma (skull)
10. Ossifying fibroma (face, jaws)
11. Osteitis condensans ilii (unilateral)
12. Osteoblastoma
13. Plasma cell granuloma
14. Sternocostoclavicular hyperostosis (SAPHO S.)
15. Syphilis; yaws

References

1. Burgener FA, Kormano M: Differential Diagnosis in Conventional Radiology. (ed 2) New York: Thieme Medical Publ, 1991
2. Swee RG, McLeod RA, Beabout JW: Osteoid osteoma: Detection, diagnosis, and localization. Radiology 1979; 130:117–123
3. Swischuk LE, John SD: Differential Diagnosis in Pediatric Radiology. (ed 2) Baltimore: Williams & Wilkins, 1995, p 228

Gamut D-54

MULTIPLE OSTEOSCLEROTIC BONE LESIONS

COMMON

1. Bone infarcts
2. Bone islands (enostoses)
3. Callus (eg, healed rib fractures; battered child S.)
4. Osteitis condensans ilii
5. Osteoblastic metastases (esp. breast; prostate) (See D-85)
6. Osteomyelitis, chronic or healed (eg, tuberculous; fungal)
7. Paget's disease

UNCOMMON

1. Avascular necroses
2. Chondrodysplasia punctata
3. Congenital total lipodystrophy (lipoatrophic diabetes)
4. Enchondromatosis (Ollier disease); Maffucci S.
5. Erdheim-Chester disease
6. Fibrous dysplasia
7. Heavy metal poisoning (eg, lead; phosphorus; bismuth; cadmium; fluoride)

8. Hereditary multiple exostoses (multiple cartilaginous exostoses; osteochondromatosis)
9. Infantile cortical hyperostosis (Caffey disease)
10. Lymphoma$_g$; leukemia
11. Lytic metastases or multiple myeloma following radiation or chemotherapy
12. Mastocytosis
13. Melorheostosis
14. Mixed sclerosing bone dysplasia
15. Multiple enchondromas; osteochondromas
16. Multiple healed or healing benign bone lesions (eg, nonossifying fibromas {fibroxanthomas}; fibrous cortical defects; brown tumors of hyperparathyroidism; Gaucher disease; Langerhans cell histiocytosis$_g$; angiomatosis)
17. Multiple myeloma (rarely); POEMS S.
18. Osteomas (eg, Gardner S.)
19. Osteomesopyknosis
20. Osteopathia striata (Voorhoeve disease); osteopathia striata with cranial sclerosis
21. Osteopoikilosis
22. Osteosarcomatosis
23. Pyknodysostosis
24. Sarcoidosis
25. Sternocostoclavicular hyperostosis (SAPHO S.)
26. Syphilis; yaws
27. Tuberous sclerosis

References

1. Boutin RD, Resnick D: The SAPHO Syndrome: an evolving concept for unifying several idiopathic disorders of bone and skin. AJR 1998:170;585–591
2. Burgener FA, Kormano M: Differential Diagnosis in Conventional Radiology. (ed 2) New York: Thieme Medical Publ, 1991
3. Resnick D, Greenway GD, Bardwick PA, et al: Plasma-cell dyscrasia with polyneuropathy, organomegaly, endocrinopathy, M-protein, and skin changes. The POEMS syndrome. Radiology 1981; 140:17–22
4. Resnick D: Diagnosis of Bone and Joint Disorders. (ed 3) Philadelphia: Saunders, 1995

Gamut D-55-1

GENERALIZED OR WIDESPREAD OSTEOSCLEROSIS

COMMON

1. Myelofibrosis; myelosclerosis; myeloid metaplasia
2. Osteoblastic metastases (esp. breast; prostate)
3. Paget's disease
*4. Physiologic osteosclerosis of newborn (normal variant, esp. in prematures)
5. Renal osteodystrophy (secondary hypoparathyroidism) (esp. healing phase)
6. Sickle cell disease (rarely other anemias)

UNCOMMON

*1. Congenital cyanotic heart disease
2. Congenital syndromes; other (See D-55-2)
3. Congenital transplacental infection (eg, congenital syphilis; rubella; toxoplasmosis; cytomegalovirus infection)
*4. Diaphyseal dysplasia (Camurati-Engelmann disease)
*5. Diffuse idiopathic skeletal hyperostosis (DISH)
*6. Endosteal hyperostosis (van Buchem and Worth types)
7. Erdheim-Chester disease
8. Erythroblastosis fetalis
9. Fluorosis
10. Gaucher disease
11. Heavy metal poisoning (eg, lead; phosphorus; bismuth; cadmium, fluoride); thorotrast injection
12. Hyperparathyroidism (almost exclusively secondary {renal osteodystrophy}, esp. treated or in the young)
13. Hyperphosphatasia
*14. Hypertrophic osteoarthropathy (See D-98)
15. Hypervitaminosis A and D, chronic
16. Hypoparathyroidism; pseudohypoparathyroidism; pseudopseudohypoparathyroidism
17. Hypothyroidism; cretinism
18. Idiopathic osteosclerosis (familial)

(continued)

*19. Infantile cortical hyperostosis (Caffey disease)
20. Lymphoma$_g$; leukemia (treated)
21. Mastocytosis
*22. Melorheostosis
23. Multiple myeloma (rare); POEMS S.
*24. Neurofibromatosis
25. Osteodysplasty (Melnick-Needles S.)
26. Osteomalacia, rickets (healing)
27. Osteopathia striata (Voorhoeve disease); osteopathia striata with cranial sclerosis
28. Osteopetrosis
29. Osteopoikilosis
30. Osteosarcomatosis
31. Oxalosis
*32. Pachydermoperiostosis
33. Polyostotic fibrous dysplasia (McCune-Albright S.)
34. Pyknodysostosis
35. Pyle dysplasia, in infancy; craniometaphyseal dysplasia
36. Sarcoidosis
37. Syphilis; yaws
38. Tuberous sclerosis
39. Tubular stenosis dysplasia (Kenny-Caffey S.)
40. Williams S. (idiopathic hypercalcemia)

* Changes predominantly on bone surface.

References

1. Brancaccio D, Poggi A, Ciccarelli C, et al: Bone changes in end-stage oxalosis. AJR 1981; 136:935–939
2. Burgener FA, Kormano M: Differential Diagnosis in Conventional Radiology. (ed 2) New York: Thieme Medical Publ, 1991
3. Greenfield GB: Radiology of Bone Diseases. (ed 5) Philadelphia: Lippincott, 1990
4. Kozlowski K, Beighton P: Gamut Index of Skeletal Dysplasias. Berlin: Springer-Verlag, 1984, pp 7–9
5. Resnick D: Diagnosis of Bone and Joint Disorders. (ed 3) Philadelphia: Saunders, 1995
6. Taybi H, Lachman S: Radiology of Syndromes, Metabolic Disorders, and Skeletal Dysplasias. (ed 4) St. Louis: Mosby-Year Book, 1996, p 1056
7. Teplick JG, Haskin ME: Roentgenologic Diagnosis. (ed 3) Philadelphia: Saunders, 1976

Gamut D-55-2

CONGENITAL SYNDROMES AND SKELETAL DYSPLASIAS WITH GENERALIZED OR WIDESPREAD OSTEOSCLEROSIS

COMMON

1. Diaphyseal dysplasia (Camurati-Engelmann disease)
2. Endosteal hyperostosis (van Buchem and Worth types)
3. Gaucher disease
4. Hyperphosphatasia
5. Hypothyroidism; cretinism
6. Infantile cortical hyperostosis (Caffey disease)
7. Melorheostosis
8. Neurofibromatosis
9. Osteodysplasty (Melnick-Needles S.)
10. Osteopathia striata (Voorhoeve disease); osteopathia striata with cranial sclerosis
11. Osteopetrosis
12. Osteopoikilosis
13. Pachydermoperiostosis
14. [Physiologic osteosclerosis of newborn]
15. Polyostotic fibrous dysplasia (McCune-Albright S.)
16. Pseudohypoparathyroidism
17. Pyknodysostosis
18. Pyle dysplasia, in infancy; craniometaphyseal dysplasia; frontometaphyseal dysplasia; craniodiaphyseal dysplasia
19. Tuberous sclerosis
20. Williams S. (idiopathic hypercalcemia)

UNCOMMON

1. Congenital total lipodystrophy (lipoatrophic diabetes)
2. Dysosteosclerosis
3. Epidermal nevus S.
4. Erdheim-Chester disease
5. Gardner S.

6. Idiopathic osteosclerosis (familial)
7. Lenz-Majewski dysplasia
8. Lethal osteosclerotic skeletal dysplasias
9. Mixed sclerosing bone dysplasia
10. Oculodentoosseous dysplasia
11. Osteomesopyknosis
12. Otopalatodigital S.
13. Oxalosis
14. Patterson S.
15. POEMS S.
16. Robinow S.
17. Rothmund-Thomson S.
18. Schwarz-Lélek S.
19. Sclerosteosis
20. Stanescu dysostosis
21. Trichodentoosseous S.
22. Tubular stenosis dysplasia (Kenny-Caffey S.)
23. Weismann-Netter S.

[ ] This condition does not actually cause the gamuted imaging finding, but can produce imaging changes that simulate it.

References
1. Beighton P, Cremin BJ: Sclerosing Bone Dysplasias. Berlin: Springer-Verlag, 1980
2. Kozlowski K, Beighton P: Gamut Index of Skeletal Dysplasias. Berlin: Springer-Verlag, 1984, pp 7-9
3. Taybi H, Lachman RS: Radiology of Syndromes, Metabolic Disorders, and Skeletal Dysplasias. (ed 4) St. Louis: Mosby-Year Book Inc, 1996, pp 1056–1057

Gamut D-56-S

GENERALIZED OR WIDESPREAD OSTEOSCLEROSIS: A CLASSIFICATION BASED ON ITS LOCATION WITHIN BONE

PREDOMINANTLY INVOLVING MEDULLARY BONE

1. Erdheim-Chester disease
2. Fluorosis
3. Gaucher disease; Niemann-Pick disease
4. Hyperparathyroidism, primary (esp. in children)

5. Hypervitaminosis D
6. Lymphoma$_g$; leukemia
7. Mastocytosis
8. Multiple myeloma
9. Myelofibrosis; myelosclerosis
10. Osteoblastic metastases (See D-85)
11. Osteopathia striata (Voorhoeve disease); osteopathia striata with cranial sclerosis
12. Osteopoikilosis
13. Osteosarcomatosis
14. Oxalosis
15. Polycythemia vera
16. Polyostotic fibrous dysplasia (McCune-Albright S.)
17. Renal osteodystrophy (secondary hyperparathyroidism)
18. Rickets (hypophosphatemic vitamin D-resistant rickets in adults)
19. Sarcoidosis
20. Sickle cell disease and variants$_g$

PREDOMINANTLY INVOLVING CORTICAL BONE

1. Congenital cyanotic heart disease
2. Diaphyseal dysplasia (Camurati-Engelmann disease)
3. Diffuse idiopathic skeletal hyperostosis (DISH)
4. Endosteal hyperostosis (van Buchem and Worth types)
5. Hypertrophic osteoarthropathy (See D-98)
6. Hypervitaminosis A
7. Hypothyroidism; cretinism
8. Infantile cortical hyperostosis (Caffey disease)
9. Melorheostosis
10. Pyle dysplasia; craniometaphyseal dysplasia; craniodiaphyseal dysplasia
11. Osteosclerosis, autosomal dominant
12. Pachydermoperiostosis
13. Ribbing disease (hereditary multiple diaphyseal sclerosis)

(continued)

INVOLVING MEDULLARY AND CORTICAL BONE

1. Dysosteosclerosis
2. Hypoparathyroidism; pseudohypoparathyroidism; pseudopseudohypoparathyroidism
3. Neurofibromatosis
4. Osteomalacia, rickets (healing)
5. Osteopetrosis
6. Osteosclerosis with dentine dysplasia
7. Paget's disease
8. Physiologic osteosclerosis of newborn
9. Pyknodysostosis
10. Sclerosteosis
11. Syphilis; yaws
12. Tuberous sclerosis
13. Tubular stenosis dysplasia (Kenny-Caffey S.)
14. Williams S. (idiopathic hypercalcemia)

References
1. Genant HK: Review of the osteoscleroses. In: Diagnostic Radiology Proceedings of the Annual Postgraduate Course in Diagnostic Radiology. San Francisco: Univ. of California School of Medicine, 1981, pp 109–122
2. Resnick D: Diagnosis of Bone and Joint Disorders. (ed 3) Philadelphia, Saunders, 1995

Gamut D-57-1

PREFERENTIAL SITE WITHIN BONE OF VARIOUS OSSEOUS LESIONS— EPIPHYSIS/APOPHYSIS/SESAMOID (See D-58)

1. Chondroblastoma (Codman tumor)
2. Clear cell chondrosarcoma
3. Giant cell tumor (after fusion of epiphyseal plate; originates in metaphysis)
4. Intraosseous ganglion
5. Langerhans cell histiocytosis$_g$ (esp. eosinophilic granuloma)

6. Osteoid osteoma
7. Osteomyelitis (esp. infants and adults)
8. Subchondral cyst (related to osteoarthritis, inflammatory arthritis, or osteochondral injury)

Gamut D-57-2

PREFERENTIAL SITE OF VARIOUS OSSEOUS LESIONS—METAPHYSIS (See D-59)

1. Aneurysmal bone cyst
2. Bone cyst (active)
3. Chondromyxoid fibroma
4. Chondrosarcoma
5. Cortical/periosteal desmoid
6. Desmoplastic fibroma
7. Enchondroma
8. Giant cell tumor (rare in skeletally immature patient)
9. Lipoma
10. Malignant fibrous histiocytoma; fibrosarcoma
11. Metastasis
12. Nonossifying fibroma (fibroxanthoma); fibrous cortical defect
13. Osteoblastoma
14. Osteochondroma; exostosis
15. Osteomyelitis (child)
16. Osteosarcoma (90% in metaphysis)
17. Parosteal sarcoma
18. Periosteal chondroma or fibroma

Gamut D-57-3

PREFERENTIAL SITE OF VARIOUS OSSEOUS LESIONS—DIAMETAPHYSIS
(See D-59)

1. Bone cyst (late-latent)
2. Bone infarct
3. Chondromyxoid fibroma
4. Chondrosarcoma
5. Enchondroma
6. Ewing sarcoma
7. Fibrous dysplasia
8. Hemangioma; lymphangioma
9. Lipoma
10. Lymphoma$_g$
11. Malignant fibrous histiocytoma; fibrosarcoma
12. Metastasis
13. Multiple myeloma; plasmacytoma
14. Nonossifying fibroma (fibroxanthoma); fibrous cortical defect
15. Osteomyelitis
16. Periosteal chondroma or fibroma

Gamut D-57-4

PREFERENTIAL SITE OF VARIOUS OSSEOUS LESIONS—DIAPHYSIS
(See D-60)

1. Adamantinoma (esp. tibia)
2. Bone cyst (late-latent)
3. Chondrosarcoma (esp. arising from previous benign chondroid lesion)
4. Enchondroma
5. Ewing sarcoma
6. Fibrous dysplasia
7. Hemangioma (esp. tibia)
8. Langerhans cell histiocytosis$_g$
9. Lymphoma$_g$
10. Malignant fibrous histiocytoma; fibrosarcoma (esp. arising in fibrous lesion or bone infarct)
11. Metastasis
12. Multiple myeloma; plasmacytoma
13. Osteofibrous dysplasia (esp. tibia)
14. Osteoid osteoma
15. Osteosarcoma (10% in diaphysis)

Gamut D-57-S

FAVORED SITES OF ORIGIN OF VARIOUS BONE LESIONS (THE "FIELD THEORY" OF THE ORIGIN OF BONE TUMORS)

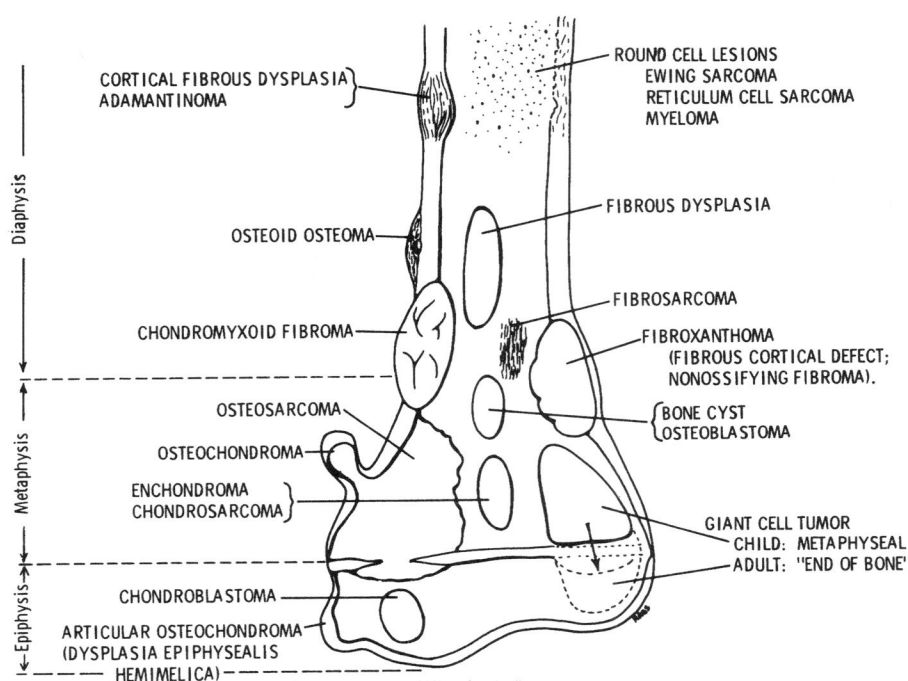

Composite diagram illustrating frequent sites of bone tumors. The diagram depicts the end of a long bone that has been divided into the epiphysis, metaphysis, and diaphysis. The typical sites of common primary bone tumors are labeled. Bone tumors tend to predominate in those ends of long bone that undergo the greatest growth and remodeling, and hence have the greatest number of cells and amount of cell activity (shoulder and knee regions). When small tumors, presumably detected early, are analyzed, preferential sites of tumor origin become apparent within each bone, as shown in this illustration. This suggests a relationship between the type of tumor and the anatomic site affected. In general, a tumor of a given cell type arises in the field where the homologous normal cells are most active. These regional variations suggest that the composition of the tumor is affected or may be determined by the metabolic field in which it arises.

References
1. Johnson LC: A general theory of bone tumors. Bull NY Acad Med 1953;29:164–171
2. Madewell JE, Ragsdale BD, Sweet DE: Radiologic and pathologic analysis of solitary bone lesions. Part I: Internal margins. Radiol Clin North Am 1981;19:715–748

Gamut D-58

SOLITARY LYTIC EPIPHYSEAL OR EPIPHYSEAL-METAPHYSEAL LESION OF BONE

COMMON

1. Arthritic lesion (eg, gout; rheumatoid arthritis; tuberculosis; hemophilic pseudotumor; osteoarthritis with degenerative cyst or geode)
2. Avascular necrosis (See D-48)
3. Chondroblastoma (Codman tumor)
*4. Giant cell tumor
5. [Normal femoral condylar or femoral head defect (eg, fovea centralis)]
6. Osteochondritis dissecans (See D-48-S)
*7. Osteomyelitis (infant or adult-epiphysis; child-metaphysis—esp. tuberculous or poorly treated bacterial); Brodie abscess
8. Synovial lesion (eg, pigmented villonodular synovitis); synovial herniation pit or erosion in metaphysis of femoral neck

UNCOMMON

1. Amyloidosis
*2. Aneurysmal bone cyst
*3. Angiomatous lesion$_g$
*4. Bone cyst
*5. Bone sarcoma (eg, arising in benign fibrous or chondroid lesion; clear cell chondrosarcoma)
6. Defect from avulsion fracture (esp. knee)
*7. Enchondroma
*8. Hydatid cyst
9. Intraosseous ganglion
10. Langerhans cell histiocytosis$_g$ (eosinophilic granuloma)
*11. Lipoma
*12. Metastasis
*13. Osteoid osteoma
*14. Plasmacytoma (myeloma)

*Epiphyseal-metaphyseal location.

[ ] This condition does not actually cause the gamuted imaging finding, but can produce imaging changes that simulate it.

Reference
1. Bullough PG, Bansal M: The differential diagnosis of geodes. Radiol Clin North Am 1988; 26:1165–1184

Gamut D-59-1

SOLITARY LYTIC METAPHYSEAL OR DIAMETAPHYSEAL LESION— WELL-DEFINED GEOGRAPHIC LESION

1. Adamantinoma (esp. tibia)
2. Angiomatous lesion (eg, hemangioma; lymphangioma, cystic type)
3. Bone cyst
4. Bone infarct
5. Brown tumor of hyperparathyroidism
6. Chondromyxoid fibroma
7. Cortical/periosteal desmoid
8. Enchondroma
9. Fibrous dysplasia
10. Giant cell tumor (rare in skeletally immature patient)
11. Langerhans cell histiocytosis$_g$
12. Lipoma
13. Metastasis
14. Multiple myeloma (punched out lesion)
15. Nonossifying fibroma (fibroxanthoma); fibrous cortical defect
16. Osteoblastoma
17. Osteoid osteoma
18. Osteomyelitis, subacute to chronic (Brodie abscess) or due to unusual/low virulent organism
19. Periosteal chondroma or fibroma
20. Tropical ulcer, benign

Gamut D-59-2

SOLITARY LYTIC METAPHYSEAL OR DIAMETAPHYSEAL LESION— ILL-DEFINED GEOGRAPHIC LESION

1. Adamantinoma (esp. tibia)
2. Bone infarct (eg, in sickle cell disease—usually well-defined)
3. Bone sarcoma (eg, osteosarcoma; chondrosarcoma; fibrosarcoma)
4. Chondromyxoid fibroma (usually well-defined)
5. Cortical/periosteal desmoid
6. Desmoplastic fibroma
7. Giant cell granuloma
8. Giant cell tumor (rare in skeletally immature patient)
9. Hydatid cyst
10. Langerhans cell histiocytosis$_g$
11. Lymphoma$_g$
12. Malignant fibrous histiocytoma
13. Metastasis
14. Multiple myeloma; plasmacytoma
15. Osteomyelitis
16. Syphilis (eg, Wimberger sign); yaws
17. Tropical ulcer, malignant

Gamut D-59-3

SOLITARY LYTIC METAPHYSEAL OR DIAMETAPHYSEAL LESION— MOTHEATEN OR PERMEATIVE LESION

1. Bone sarcoma (esp. Ewing sarcoma; osteosarcoma; chondrosarcoma; fibrosarcoma)
2. Langerhans cell histiocytosis$_g$ (esp. eosinophilic granuloma in patients less than 10 years of age)
3. Lymphoma$_g$

4. Malignant fibrous histiocytoma
5. Metastasis
6. Multiple myeloma
7. Osteomyelitis (usually acute bacterial)

Gamut D-60

SOLITARY LYTIC DIAPHYSEAL LESION

COMMON

1. Bone cyst (late-latent)
2. Bone infarct
*3. Bone sarcoma (esp. round cell neoplasm such as Ewing sarcoma)
4. Diametaphyseal lesion extending into diaphysis (eg, nonossifying fibroma) (See D-59)
5. Enchondroma
6. Fibrous dysplasia
*7. Langerhans cell histiocytosis$_g$ (esp. eosinophilic granuloma)
*8. Metastasis
*9. Myeloma; plasmacytoma
10. Osteoid osteoma
*11. Osteomyelitis

UNCOMMON

*1. Adamantinoma (esp. tibia)
2. Brown tumor of hyperparathyroidism
3. Osteofibrous dysplasia (esp. tibia)
4. Hemophilic pseudotumor
*5. Hydatid cyst
*6. Lymphoma$_g$
*7. Malignant fibrous histiocytoma; fibrosarcoma
*8. Osteosarcoma
9. Paget's disease
*10. Syphilis; yaws
*11. Tropical ulcer

*May be motheaten or permeative pattern.

Gamut D-61-S

DIAGRAM OF PATTERNS OF BONE DESTRUCTION

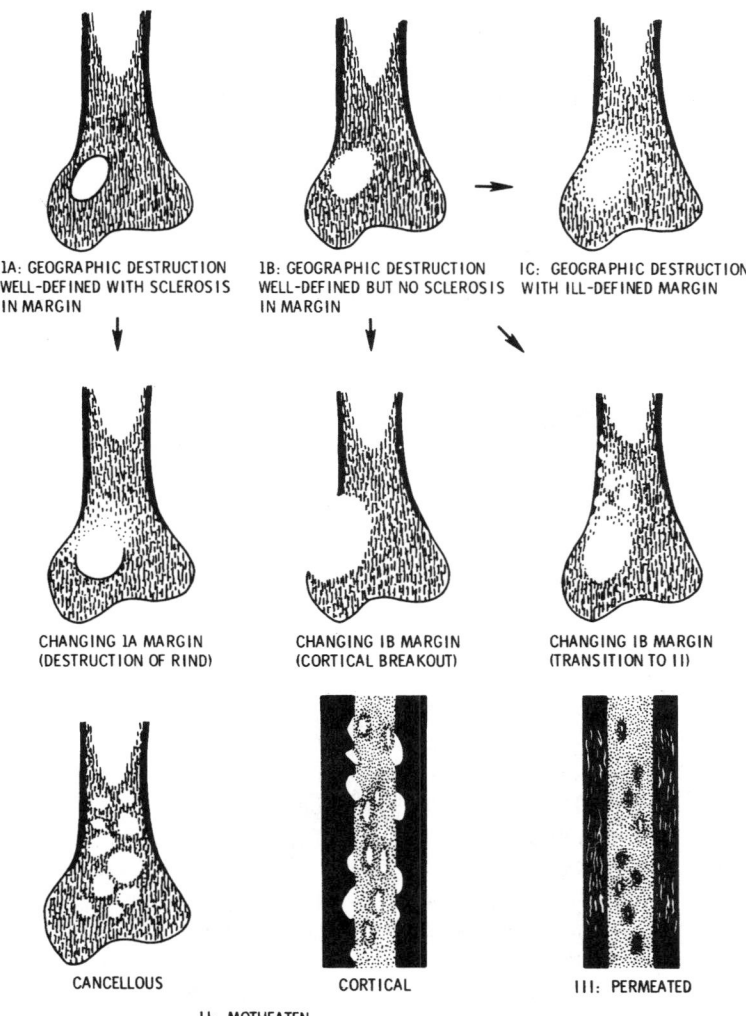

1A: GEOGRAPHIC DESTRUCTION WELL-DEFINED WITH SCLEROSIS IN MARGIN

1B: GEOGRAPHIC DESTRUCTION WELL-DEFINED BUT NO SCLEROSIS IN MARGIN

1C: GEOGRAPHIC DESTRUCTION WITH ILL-DEFINED MARGIN

CHANGING 1A MARGIN (DESTRUCTION OF RIND)

CHANGING 1B MARGIN (CORTICAL BREAKOUT)

CHANGING 1B MARGIN (TRANSITION TO II)

CANCELLOUS

CORTICAL

III: PERMEATED

II: MOTHEATEN

Schematic diagram of patterns of bone destruction (types IA, IB, IC, II, III) and their margins. Arrows indicate the most frequent transitions or combinations of these margins. Transitions imply increased activity and a greater probability of malignancy.

Reference
1. Madewell JE, Ragsdale BD, Sweet DE: Radiologic and pathologic analysis of solitary bone lesions. Part I: Internal margins. Radiol Clin North Am 1981;19:715–748

COMMON BONE LESIONS AND THEIR TYPICAL PATTERNS OF BONE DESTRUCTION

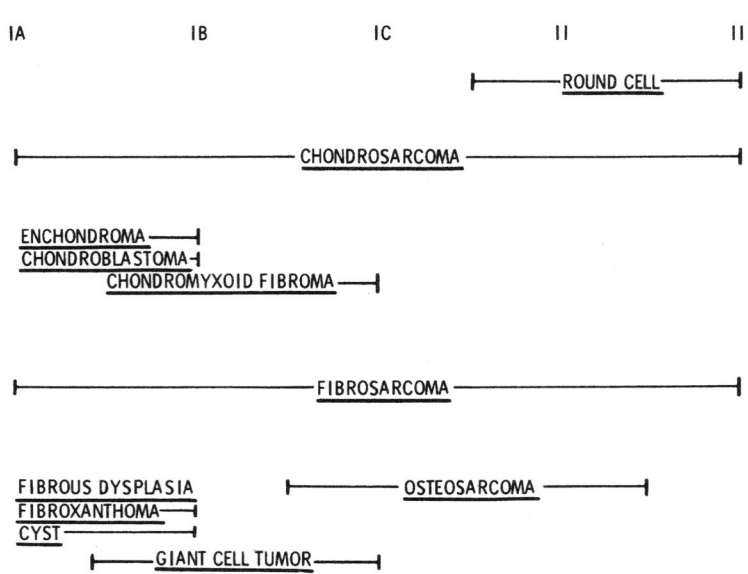

LYTIC PATTERNS
(AGGRESSION INCREASING FROM LEFT TO RIGHT)

This diagram delineates common bone tumors and their typical patterns of bone destruction. IA, Geographic destruction, well-defined, with sclerosis in margin. IB, Geographic destruction, well-defined, but no sclerosis in margin. IC, Geographic destruction with ill-defined margin. II, Motheaten (regionally invasive). III. Permeative (diffusively invasive). Note that most benign tumors occur on the left-hand side, from IA to IC, whereas most malignant tumors occur on the right-hand side, from IC to III. This illustrates the general principle that the biologic activity and probability of malignancy increase from left to right. Chondrosarcoma and fibrosarcoma can present with any of the five patterns. In our experience, they frequently arise in preexisting benign lesions. In such cases, the radiographic pattern may lag behind the histologic activity, producing a radiographic discrepancy (slow-appearing lesions with malignant histology).

Reference
Madewell JE, Ragsdale BD, Sweet DE: Radiologic and pathologic analysis of solitary bone lesions. Part I: Internal margins. Radiol Clin North Am 1981;19:715-748

Gamut D-63-S

RELATIONSHIP OF BIOLOGIC ACTIVITY (GROWTH RATE) TO TYPE OF BONE MARGIN AND PERIOSTEAL REACTION

Growth Rate	Internal Margins	Periosteal Reaction
Slow	Geographic (I) IA IB IC	Solid or Shells Ridged lobulated, or smooth
Intermediate	Motheaten (II)	Codman Triangle Shells or lamellated
Fast	Permeative (III)	Lamellated or spiculated
Fastest	Nonvisible	Spiculated or none

8. Healed or healing benign bone cyst or fibrocystic lesion (eg, nonossifying fibroma {fibroxanthoma}; fibrous cortical defect; osteofibrous dysplasia)
9. Osteoid osteoma
10. Subchondral cyst related to osteoarthritis, inflammatory arthritis or traumatic osteochondral injury

UNCOMMON
1. Chondromyxoid fibroma
2. Clear cell chondrosarcoma
3. Intraosseous ganglion
4. Langerhans cell histiocytosis$_g$ (esp. eosinophilic granuloma—occasionally)
5. Lipoma
6. Liposclerosing myxofibrous tumor (LSMFT)
7. Osteoblastoma
8. Unusual infection (eg, syphilis; yaws; fungal; mycetoma; hydatid disease)

Reference
1. Kransdorf MJ, Murphey MD, Sweet DE: Liposclerosing myxofibrous tumor: A radiologic-pathologic distinct fibro-osseous lesion of bone with marked predilection for the intertrochanteric region of the femur. Radiology 1999; 212:693–698

Gamut D-64

LUCENT LESION OF BONE SURROUNDED BY MARKED SCLEROTIC REACTION OR RIM

COMMON
1. Bone infarct
2. Brodie abscess
3. Chondroblastoma (Codman tumor)
4. Cortical/periosteal desmoid
5. Cystic osteomyelitis (esp. poorly treated bacterial or tuberculous infection)
6. Enchondroma (esp. hand, foot or rib lesion)
7. Fibrous dysplasia (esp. monostotic)

Gamut D-65

SOLITARY WELL-DEMARCATED LYTIC LESION OF BONE

COMMON
+*1. Arthritic or synovial lesion (eg, subchondral cyst related to osteoarthritis, inflammatory arthritis or traumatic osteochondral injury; intraosseous ganglion; amyloidosis; villonodular synovitis)
+*2. Bone cyst
*3. Bone infarct
4. Brown tumor of hyperparathyroidism
*5. Cortical/periosteal desmoid
+*6. Enchondroma

(continued)

*7. Fibrous dysplasia
8. Giant cell tumor
+9. Gouty tophus
*10. Langerhans cell histiocytosis_g (esp. eosinophilic granuloma)
11. Metastasis (esp. from hypernephroma; thyroid carcinoma)
*12. Nonossifying fibroma (fibroxanthoma); fibrous cortical defect
+*13. Osteomyelitis, cystic (esp. poorly treated bacterial; tuberculous; fungal); Brodie abscess

UNCOMMON

1. Adamantinoma (esp. tibia)
+*2. Ameloblastoma (jaws)
+3. Aneurysmal bone cyst
+4. Angiomatous lesion_g (eg, hemangioma; lymphangioma, cystic type)
*5. Bone sarcoma arising in previously benign lesion (eg, chondrosarcoma; fibrosarcoma)
*6. Chondroblastoma (Codman tumor)
+*7. Chondromyxoid fibroma
8. Desmoplastic fibroma
+9. Epidermoid inclusion cyst (phalanx)
+10. Fungus disease (esp. coccidioidomycosis; blastomycosis; histoplasmosis duboisii)
11. Glomus tumor (phalanx)
*12. Granuloma (esp. tuberculous; fungal; foreign body or "thorn")
+13. Hemophilic pseudotumor
+14. Hydatid cyst
+*15. Lipoma
+*16. Liposclerosing myxofibrous tumor (LSMFT)
17. Malignant fibrous histiocytoma; fibrosarcoma
18. Myeloma; plasmacytoma
+19. Myxoma (fibromyxoma)
20. Neurofibroma
21. Osteoblastoma
*22. Osteofibrous dysplasia (esp. tibia)
*23. Osteoid osteoma
+24. Osteosarcoma (telangiectatic variety)
25. Paget's disease
+*26. Periosteal chondroma

*27. Periosteal fibroma
28. Sarcoidosis
*29. Tropical ulcer, benign
*30. Tuberculosis

*Often has sclerotic rim.

+ Has high water content on CT (low attenuation) or MRI (very low signal intensity on T1 and very high signal intensity on T2).

WELL-DEFINED, OFTEN CYST-LIKE, INFECTIOUS LESION OF BONE

1. Brodie abscess (bacterial, usually *Staph. aureus*)
2. Cystic osteomyelitis (esp. poorly treated bacterial infection)
3. Fungus disease (eg, coccidioidomycosis; blastomycosis; histoplasmosis duboisii; mycetoma)
4. Hydatid disease
5. Leprosy (lepromas)
6. Spina ventosa; other cyst-like dactylitis (incl. yaws) (See D-132)
7. Tuberculosis; atypical mycobacterial infections

SOLITARY LESION OF BONE WITH EXPANSILE REMODELING

BENIGN NEOPLASM OF BONE

COMMON

1. Angiomatous lesion_g (eg, hemangioma; lymphangioma)
2. Enchondroma (esp. lesions of hand or foot)
3. Giant cell tumor
4. Nonossifying fibroma (fibroxanthoma)
5. Osteochondroma (esp. with multiple lesions)

UNCOMMON

1. Ameloblastoma (jaws)
2. Chondroblastoma (Codman tumor)
3. Chondromyxoid fibroma
4. Desmoplastic fibroma
5. Lipoma
6. Liposclerosing myxofibrous tumor (LSMFT)
7. Ossifying fibroma (face, jaws)
8. Osteoblastoma
9. Periosteal chondroma or fibroma

MALIGNANT NEOPLASM OF BONE

COMMON

1. Chondrosarcoma
2. Metastasis (esp. from carcinoma of kidney, thyroid, or lung; hepatoma; melanoma)
3. Myeloma; plasmacytoma

UNCOMMON

1. Adamantinoma (esp. tibia)
2. Ameloblastoma (jaws)
3. Hemangioendothelioma; angiosarcoma
4. Lymphoma$_g$ (esp. Burkitt)
5. Malignant fibrous histiocytoma; fibrosarcoma
6. Malignant giant cell tumor
7. Osteosarcoma (esp. telangiectatic)

TUMOR-LIKE LESION OF BONE

COMMON

1. Aneurysmal bone cyst
2. Bone cyst
3. Cortical/periosteal desmoid
4. Fibrous cortical defect
5. Fibrous dysplasia
6. Gouty tophus
7. [Osteoid osteoma]
8. Osteomyelitis (esp. chronic with unusual organism—eg, tuberculous; fungal; yaws)

UNCOMMON

1. Brown tumor of hyperparathyroidism
2. Epidermoid inclusion cyst

3. Gaucher disease; Niemann-Pick disease
4. Hemophilic pseudotumor
5. Hydatid cyst
6. Langerhans cell histiocytosis$_g$ (esp. eosinophilic granuloma)
7. Osteofibrous dysplasia (esp. tibia)

Reference

1. Greenfield GB: Radiology of Bone Diseases. (ed 5) Philadelphia: Lippincott, 1990

Gamut D-68

BONE BLISTER (SOLITARY ECCENTRIC LESION WITH EXPANSILE REMODELING)

COMMON

1. Aneurysmal bone cyst
2. Chondroid lesion (eg, osteochondroma; enchondroma)
3. Giant cell tumor
4. Nonossifying fibroma (fibroxanthoma); fibrous cortical defect

UNCOMMON

1. Angiomatous lesion$_g$ (eg, hemangioma; lymphangioma)
2. Brown tumor of hyperparathyroidism
3. Chondromyxoid fibroma
4. Cortical/periosteal desmoid
5. Desmoplastic fibroma
6. Fibrosarcoma (esp. arising in benign fibrous lesion)
7. Osteofibrous dysplasia (esp. tibia)
8. Gouty tophus
9. Malignant fibrous histiocytoma
10. Metastasis to cortex (esp. lung, breast)
11. Osteoblastoma
12. Osteosarcoma, intracortical
13. Periosteal chondroma or fibroma

Gamut D-69-1

BLOW-OUT LESION OF BONE (SOLITARY LESION WITH MARKED "ANEURYSMAL" EXPANSILE REMODELING) (See D-69-2)

COMMON

1. Aneurysmal bone cyst, primary or secondary
2. Chondrosarcoma
3. Fibrous dysplasia
4. Giant cell tumor
5. Metastatic carcinoma (esp. kidney, thyroid, or lung; hepatoma)
6. Myeloma; plasmacytoma

UNCOMMON

1. Adamantinoma (esp. tibia)
2. Ameloblastoma (jaws)
3. Brown tumor of hyperparathyroidism
4. Burkitt lymphoma
5. Chondromyxoid fibroma
6. Chordoma; parachordoma
7. Desmoplastic fibroma
8. Enchondroma (usually hand or foot lesions)
9. Gouty tophus
10. Hemangioendothelioma; angiosarcoma
11. Hemophilic pseudotumor
12. Hydatid cyst
13. Malignant fibrous histiocytoma; fibrosarcoma
14. Meningocele
15. Nonossifying fibroma associated with neurofibromatosis (type 1) or Jaffe-Campanacci S.
16. Osteoblastoma
17. Osteochondroma
18. Osteofibrous dysplasia (esp. tibia)
19. Osteosarcoma (telangiectatic)
20. Sacrococcygeal teratoma

Gamut D-69-2

LARGE DESTRUCTIVE BONE LESION (OVER 5 CM IN DIAMETER)

COMMON

1. Aneurysmal bone cyst, primary or secondary
2. Angiomatous lesion$_g$ (eg, hemangioma; lymphangioma); hemangioendothelioma; angiosarcoma
3. Bone cyst
4. Bone sarcoma (eg, osteosarcoma; chondrosarcoma; fibrosarcoma; Ewing sarcoma)
5. Enchondroma
6. Fibrous dysplasia
7. Giant cell tumor
8. Langerhans cell histiocytosis$_g$
9. Lymphoma$_g$; Burkitt lymphoma
10. Metastasis
11. Myeloma; plasmacytoma
12. Osteomyelitis; mycetoma
13. Paget's disease

UNCOMMON

1. Adamantinoma (esp. tibia)
2. Ameloblastoma (jaws)
3. Brown tumor of hyperparathyroidism
4. Chondromyxoid fibroma
5. Chordoma; parachordoma
6. Desmoplastic fibroma
7. Gaucher disease
8. Hemophilic pseudotumor
9. Hydatid cyst
10. Lesion arising in spinal canal (eg, meningocele; ependymoma; neurofibroma; sacrococcygeal teratoma)
11. Malignant fibrous histiocytoma
12. Massive osteolysis (Gorham vanishing bone disease)
13. Nonossifying fibroma associated with neurofibromatosis (type 1) or Jaffe-Campanacci S.
14. Osteoblastoma
15. Osteofibrous dysplasia (esp. tibia)

16. [Soft tissue tumor destroying bone (eg, synovial sarcoma)]
17. Syphilis; yaws
18. Tropical ulcer

Gamut D-70

SOLITARY POORLY DEMARCATED OSTEOLYTIC LESION

COMMON

1. Bone sarcoma (esp. Ewing sarcoma; osteosarcoma; chondrosarcoma; fibrosarcoma; angiosarcoma)
2. Langerhans cell histiocytosis$_g$
3. Lymphoma$_g$
4. Metastasis
5. Myeloma; plasmacytoma
6. Osteomyelitis (eg, tuberculous, fungal, bacterial)

UNCOMMON

1. Adamantinoma (esp. tibia)
2. Aneurysmal bone cyst
3. Angiomatous lesion$_g$ (eg, hemangioma; lymphangioma)
4. Brown tumor of hyperparathyroidism
5. Chordoma
6. Fibrous dysplasia
7. Giant cell tumor
8. Hemangioendothelioma
9. Hydatid cyst
10. Malignant fibrous histiocytoma
11. Paget's disease
12. Syphilis; yaws

Gamut D-71

MOTHEATEN OR PERMEATIVE OSTEOLYTIC LESION(S)

COMMON

1. Ewing sarcoma
2. Lymphoma$_g$; leukemia
3. Metastasis (incl. neuroblastoma)
4. Multiple myeloma
5. Osteomyelitis
6. Osteosarcoma

UNCOMMON

1. Adamantinoma (esp. tibia)
2. Chondrosarcoma
3. Giant cell tumor (at margins)
4. Hemangioendothelioma; angiosarcoma
5. Landing-Shirkey disease (multifocal granulomatous osteomyelitis in a compromised child)
6. Langerhans cell histiocytosis$_g$ (esp. eosinophilic granuloma in children)
7. Malignant fibrous histiocytoma; fibrosarcoma
8. Rhabdomyosarcoma
9. Syphilis; yaws

Gamut D-72

OSTEOLYTIC LESION CONTAINING CALCIUM OR BONE DENSITY OR MATRIX

COMMON

*1. Chondrosarcoma
*2. Enchondroma
*3. Fibrous dysplasia
4. Lymphoma$_g$ (reactive osteoid)
5. Metastasis (esp. from breast, thyroid, or mucinous gastrointestinal carcinoma)

(continued)

6. Nonossifying fibroma or bone cyst (healed or heal-ing with sclerosis)
*7. Osteoid osteoma
*8. Osteosarcoma
9. Paget's disease
10. Sequestrum-producing lesions (eg, avascular necro-sis; osteochondrosis dissecans; bone infarct; os-teomyelitis; tropical ulcer; button sequestrum in skull (See A-22)

UNCOMMON
*1. Chondroblastoma (Codman tumor)
*2. Chondromyxoid fibroma (identifiable mineraliza-tion unusual)
3. Ewing sarcoma (reactive bone)
4. Langerhans cell histiocytosis$_g$ (esp. eosinophilic granuloma)
5. Lipoma (metaplastic and reactive bone/cartilage)
6. Liposclerosing myxofibrous tumor (LSMFT) (meta-plastic and reactive bone/cartilage)
7. Malignant fibrous histiocytoma; fibrosarcoma (reac-tive bone or sequestrum)
*8. Osteoblastoma

* Mineralized matrix formation.

Gamut D-73

BONE LESION WITH PROMINENT FLUID-FLUID LEVEL (CT OR MRI)

COMMON
1. Aneurysmal bone cyst, primary (See D-80-S3)
2. Bone cyst (esp. after fracture)
3. Chondroblastoma (Codman tumor)
4. Giant cell tumor
5. Osteoblastoma
6. Osteosarcoma (telangiectatic)

UNCOMMON
1. Brown tumor of hyperparathyroidism
2. Chondromyxoid fibroma

3. Fibrous dysplasia
4. Giant cell granuloma
5. Hemangioma
6. Hemangioendothelioma; hemangiopericytoma
7. Hemophilic pseudotumor
8. Malignant fibrous histiocytoma (MFH); fibrosar-coma
9. Metastasis (esp. renal)
10. Nonossifying fibroma (fibroxanthoma)

Reference
1. Tsai JC, Dalinka MK, Fallon MD, et al: Fluid-fluid level: A nonspecific finding in tumors of bone and soft tissue. Radi-ology 1990;175:779–782

Gamut D-74

MULTIPLE RADIOLUCENT LESIONS OF BONE (See D-107)

COMMON
*1. Arthritis (eg, gout; rheumatoid; subchondral cysts or geodes associated with osteoarthritis, inflammatory arthritis, or traumatic osteochondral injury)
2. Metastases
3. Multiple myeloma
4. Osteomyelitis, multifocal (eg, septic; unusual low virulence organisms—cystic tuberculosis; fungal)
5. Paget's disease

UNCOMMON
*1. Amyloidosis, primary or secondary
2. Angiomatosis (hemangiomatosis; lymphan-giomatosis, cystic type)
3. Brown tumors of hyperparathyroidism
4. Electrical injury
5. Enchondromatosis (Ollier disease); Maffucci S.
6. Fibromatosis (esp. multicentric infantile myofibro-matosis)
*7. Fungus disease (esp. blastomycosis; coccid-ioidomycosis; histoplasmosis duboisii)
8. Gaucher disease; Niemann-Pick disease

9. Hemangioendothelioma; angiosarcoma
*10. Hemophilia; hemophilic pseudotumors
11. Hydatid disease
12. Infantile cortical hyperostosis (Caffey disease)
*13. Jackhammer operator's (driller's) disease of wrists
14. Kaposi sarcoma
15. Landing-Shirkey disease (multifocal granulomatous osteomyelitis in a compromised child)
16. Langerhans cell histiocytosis_g
*17. Leprosy (lepromas)
18. Leukemia; lymphoma_g; Burkitt lymphoma
19. Lipomatosis
*20. Massive osteolysis (Gorham vanishing bone disease)
21. Mastocytosis
22. Membranous lipodystrophy
23. Nonossifying fibromas associated with neurofibromatosis (type 1) or Jaffe-Campanacci S.
24. Osteoglophonic dysplasia
*25. Polycystic osteodysplasia with progressive dementia (hands and feet)
26. Polyostotic fibrous dysplasia (McCune-Albright S.)
*27. Polyvinyl chloride osteolysis
28. Primary bone neoplasms, multiple
29. Radium poisoning
30. Rothmund-Thomson S.
*31. Sarcoidosis
32. Sickle cell disease with bone infarction (esp. hand-foot S.); other dactylitis (See D-132)
*33. Silastic arthropathy
*34. Small particle disease (eg, granulomatous pseudotumors adjacent to joint replacements)
35. Syphilis; yaws
36. Tuberous sclerosis
37. Weber-Christian disease

* Often periarticular.

Reference
1. Greenfield GB: Radiology of Bone Diseases. (ed 5) Philadelphia: Lippincott, 1990

Gamut D-75

WIDESPREAD AREAS OF BONE DESTRUCTION

COMMON
1. Arthritis (esp. rheumatoid; gout)
2. Lymphoma_g; leukemia; Burkitt lymphoma
3. Osteomyelitis (pyogenic; tuberculous)
4. Metastases (esp. carcinomatosis)
5. Multiple myeloma (esp. myelomatosis)
6. Paget's disease

UNCOMMON
1. Angiomatosis (hemangiomatosis; lymphangiomatosis, cystic type)
2. Bone sarcoma, multicentric (eg, Ewing sarcoma; osteosarcoma)
3. Brown tumors of hyperparathyroidism (esp. osteitis fibrosa cystica)
4. Fibromatosis (esp. multicentric infantile myofibromatosis)
5. Fungus disease (eg, blastomycosis; coccidioidomycosis; histoplasmosis duboisii; actinomycosis, nocardiosis—mycetoma)
6. Gaucher disease
7. Hemophilia with pseudotumors
8. Hydatid disease
9. Langerhans cell histiocytosis_g
10. Leprosy
11. Massive osteolysis (Gorham vanishing bone disease)
12. Membranous lipodystrophy
13. Polyostotic fibrous dysplasia (McCune-Albright S.)
14. Sarcoidosis
15. Syphilis; yaws
16. Waldenström macroglobulinemia
17. Weber-Christian disease

Reference
1. Burgener FA, Kormano M: Differential Diagnosis in Conventional Radiology. (ed 2) New York: Thieme Medical Publ, 1991

Gamut D-76

OSTEOLYSIS

COMMON

1. Acro-osteolysis (See D-127)
2. Chronic articular disorder (eg, psoriasis; multicentric reticulohistiocytosis {lipoid dermatoarthritis}; neuroarthropathy)
3. Connective tissue disease (collagen disease)$_g$ (esp. scleroderma)
4. Hyperparathyroidism
5. Trauma

UNCOMMON

1. Ainhum
2. Congenital osteolyses
   a. Multicentric predominantly carpal and tarsal
      i. Multicentric carpal-tarsal osteolysis with and without nephropathy
      ii. Shinohara carpal-tarsal osteolysis
   b. Multicentric predominantly carpal, tarsal, and interphalangeal
      i. Francois S.
      ii. Torg S.
      iii. Winchester S.
      iv. Whyte Hemingway carpal-tarsal phalangeal osteolyses
   c. Predominantly distal phalanges
      i. Giacci familial neurogenic acro-osteolysis
      ii. Hajdu-Cheney S.
      iii. Mandibuloacral dysplasia
   d. Predominantly involving diaphyses and metaphyses
      i. Familial expansile osteolysis
      ii. Juvenile hyaline fibromatosis
3. Calcium pyrophosphate dihydrate crystal deposition disease (CPPD) (unusual neuropathic appearance)
4. Massive osteolysis (Gorham vanishing bone disease)
5. Osteolysis with detritic synovitis
6. Rapidly progressive coxarthrosis
7. Sarcoidosis
8. Thermal injury (eg, burn; frostbite)

References

1. Lachman RS: International Nomenclature and Classification of the Osteochondrodysplasias (1997). Pediatr Radiol 1998:28:737–744
2. Resnick D, Weisman M, Goergen TG, et al: Osteolysis with detritic synovitis: A new syndrome. Arch Intern Med 1978; 138:1003–1005
3. Taybi H, Lachman RS: Radiology of Syndromes, Metabolic Disorders, and Skeletal Dysplasias. (ed 4) St. Louis: Mosby-Year Book Inc, 1996, p 368

Gamut D-77-S1

AGE RANGE OF HIGHEST INCIDENCE OF VARIOUS BONE NEOPLASMS AND TUMOR-LIKE LESIONS

TUMOR	AGE (YEARS)
1. Adamantinoma (esp. tibia)	15–35
2. Aneurysmal bone cyst	10–30
3. Bone cyst	5–20
4. Chondroblastoma (Codman tumor)	10–25
5. Chondromyxoid fibroma	10–30
6. Chondrosarcoma	30–60
7. Chordoma	30–70
8. Cortical/periosteal desmoid	10–20
9. Desmoplastic fibroma	10–40
10. Enchondroma	5–50
11. Ewing sarcoma	5–25
12. Fibrosarcoma	20–70
13. Fibrous dysplasia	2–30
14. Giant cell tumor	20–45
15. Hemangioma	30–70
16. Langerhans cell histiocytosis$_g$	0–15
17. Lymphoma$_g$	15–40
18. Malignant fibrous histiocytoma	20–60
19. Metastasis	40–80
20. Multiple myeloma	40–80
21. Neuroblastoma, metastatic	0–10

TUMOR	AGE (YEARS)
22. Nonossifying fibroma (fibroxanthoma); fibrous cortical defect	5–20
23. Ossifying fibroma (face, jaws)	5–30
24. Osteoblastoma	10–25
25. Osteochondroma	10–25
26. Osteofibrous dysplasia (esp. tibia)	0–15
27. Osteoid osteoma	10–30
28. Osteoma	30–50
29. Osteosarcoma	5–25, 60–75
30. Parosteal sarcoma	30–50

References

1. Greenfield GB: Radiology of Bone Diseases. (ed 5) Philadelphia: Lippincott, 1990
2. Unni KK: Dahlin's Bone Tumors. General Aspects and Data on 11,087 Cases. (ed 5) Philadelphia: Lippincott-Raven, 1996

Gamut D-77-S2

SEX PREDOMINANCE OF VARIOUS BONE LESIONS

	Male Predominance	Ratio*	No Predominance	Female Predominance	Ratio*
Malignant	PNET	>2:1	Adamantinoma	Parosteal osteosarcoma	slight
	Osteosarcoma, telangiectatic	slight			
	Chondrosarcoma	2:1			
	Chordoma	2:1			
	Osteosaarcoma, conventional	slight			
	Ewing sarcoma	slight			
	Myeloma	slight			
	Lymphoma of bone	slight			
	MFH of bone	slight			
Benign	Simple cyst	3:1	Enchondroma	Giant cell tumor	slight
	Osteoid osteoma	3:1	Fibrous dysplasia	Aneurysmal bone cyst	slight
	Osteoblastoma	2:1		Hemangioma	slight
	Osteochondroma	2:1			
	Periosteal chondroma	2:1			
	Chondroblastoma	2:1			
	Chondromyxoid fibroma	2:1			
	Fibrous cortical defect	2:1			
	Nonossifying fibroma	2:1			
	Eosinophilic granuloma	2:1			
	Desmoplastic fibroma	slight			
	Intraosseous lipoma	slight			
	Intraosseous ganglion	slight			

PNET = primitive neuroectodermal tumor; MFH = malignant fibrous histiocytoma

*Ratios are approximate and rounded

Source: Unni KK. Dahlin's Bone Tumors. General Aspects and Data on 11,087 Cases. 5th ed. Philadelphia: Lippincott-Raven, 1996
Fletcher RE, Mills SE. Tumors of the Bones and Joints. Washington DC, Armed Forces Institute of Pathology, 1993

BONE NEOPLASMS CLASSIFIED BY TUMOR MATRIX OR TISSUE OF ORIGIN

CHONDROID (Cartilage-Forming) TUMORS

BENIGN

1. Chondroblastoma (Codman tumor)
2. Chondromyxoid fibroma
3. Enchondroma, incl. enchondromatosis (Ollier disease; Maffucci S.)
4. Osteochondroma, incl. hereditary multiple exostoses (multiple cartilaginous exostoses; osteochondromatosis)
5. Periosteal (juxtacortical) chondroma

MALIGNANT

1. Chondrosarcoma (multiple types) (See D-81-S3)

OSTEOID (Bone-Forming) TUMORS

BENIGN

1. Bone island; enostosis (incl. osteopoikilosis and osteopathia striata)
2. Ossifying fibroma (face, jaws)
3. Osteoblastoma
4. Osteofibrous dysplasia (esp. tibia)
5. Osteoid osteoma
6. Osteoma

MALIGNANT

1. Osteosarcoma (multiple types) (See D-81-S2)

FIBROUS CONNECTIVE TISSUE TUMORS

BENIGN

1. Cortical/periosteal desmoid (cortical avulsive injury)
2. Desmoplastic fibroma
3. Fibromatosis (esp. multicentric infantile myofibromatosis)
4. Fibromyxoma
5. Nonossifying fibroma (fibroxanthoma)
6. Periosteal (juxtacortical) fibroma

MALIGNANT

1. Fibrosarcoma
2. Malignant fibrous histiocytoma

TUMORS OF FATTY TISSUE ORIGIN

BENIGN

1. Lipoma, intraosseous or parosteal
2. Liposclerosing myxofibrous tumor (LSMFT)

MALIGNANT

1. Liposarcoma

TUMORS OF VASCULAR ORIGIN

BENIGN

1. Angiomatosis (hemangiomatosis; lymphangiomatous)
2. Glomus tumor
3. Hemangioma
4. Hemangioendothelioma (benign)
5. Hemangiopericytoma (benign)
6. Lymphangioma
7. Massive osteolysis (Gorham vanishing bone disease)

MALIGNANT

1. Angiosarcoma
2. Hemangioendothelioma (malignant)
3. Hemangiopericytoma (malignant)
4. Kaposi sarcoma

TUMORS OF NEURAL ORIGIN
(RARE IN BONE)
BENIGN
1. Neurilemoma (schwannoma)
2. Neurofibroma (incl. neurofibromatosis)

MALIGNANT
1. Malignant peripheral nerve sheath tumor (MPNST) (neurofibrosarcoma)

GIANT CELL-CONTAINING TUMORS
BENIGN
1. Aneurysmal bone cyst
2. Bone cyst (complicated by fracture)
3. Brown tumor of hyperparathyroidism
4. Chondroblastoma (Codman tumor)
5. Chondromyxoid fibroma
6. Fibrous dysplasia
7. Giant cell granuloma
8. Giant cell tumor (benign)
9. Osteoblastoma
10. Osteofibrous dysplasia (esp. tibia)

MALIGNANT
1. Giant cell tumor (malignant)
2. Malignant fibrous histiocytoma
3. Osteosarcoma

References
1. Edeiken J, Dalinka M, Karasick D: Edeiken's Roentgen Diagnosis of Diseases of Bone. (ed 3) Baltimore: Williams & Wilkins, 1990
2. Resnick D: Diagnosis of Bone and Joint Disorders. (ed 3) Philadelphia: Saunders, 1995
3. Sutton D, Young JWR: A Short Textbook of Clinical Imaging. London: Springer-Verlag, 1990, pp 295–312

BENIGN BONE NEOPLASMS

COMMON
1. Enchondroma
2. Hemangioma
3. Nonossifying fibroma (fibroxanthoma)
4. Osteochondroma
5. [Osteoid osteoma]
6. Osteoma

UNCOMMON
1. Ameloblastoma (jaws)
2. Aneurysmal bone cyst
3. Angiomatosis (hemangiomatosis; lymphangiomatosis, cystic type)
4. Chondroblastoma (Codman tumor)
5. Chondromyxoid fibroma
6. Cortical/periosteal desmoid (cortical avulsive injury)
7. Desmoplastic fibroma
8. Fibromatosis (esp. multicentric infantile myofibromatosis)
9. Fibromyxoma; myxoma
10. Giant cell tumor
11. Glomus tumor
12. Hemangioendothelioma, benign
13. Hemangiopericytoma, benign
14. [Langerhans cell histiocytosis$_g$]
15. Lipoma
16. Liposclerosing myxofibrous tumor (LSMFT)
17. Lymphangioma
18. Neurofibroma; neurilemoma
19. Ossifying fibroma (face, jaws)
20. Osteoblastoma
21. [Osteofibrous dysplasia (esp. tibia)]
22. Periosteal chondroma or fibroma

Gamut D-80

BENIGN TUMOR-LIKE LESIONS OF BONE (NONNEOPLASTIC)
(See D-80-S1 and S2)

COMMON

1. Avascular necrosis
2. Bone cyst
3. Bone infarct
4. Bone island (enostosis)
5. Brown tumor of hyperparathyroidism
6. Cortical/periosteal desmoid (cortical avulsive injury)
7. Fibrous cortical defect
8. Fibrous dysplasia
9. Gouty tophus
10. Langerhans cell histiocytosis
11. Myositis ossificans (parosteal)
12. Osteochondrosis dissecans
13. Osteoid osteoma
14. Osteomyelitis (eg, bacterial; tuberculous; fungal—mycetoma)
15. Paget's disease
16. Stress fracture, healing
17. Subchondral cyst (related to osteoarthritis, inflammatory arthritis, or osteochondral injury)

UNCOMMON

1. Aneurysmal bone cyst (See D-80-S3)
2. Epidermoid; dermoid (skull)
3. Epidermoid inclusion cyst; foreign body or "thorn" granuloma
4. Fibromatosis (esp. multicentric infantile myofibromatosis)
5. Giant cell granuloma
6. Hemophilic pseudotumor
7. Hydatid cyst
8. Intraosseous ganglion
9. Osteofibrous dysplasia (esp. tibia)
10. Plasma cell granuloma
11. Posttraumatic cyst or osteolysis

12. Sarcoidosis
13. Small particle disease (eg, granulomatous pseudo-tumors adjacent to joint replacements) (foreign body reaction)
14. Soft tissue lesion secondarily involving bone (eg, amyloidosis; glomus tumor; giant cell tumor of tendon sheath; pigmented villonodular synovitis)
15. Sternocostoclavicular hyperostosis (SAPHO S.)
16. Xanthomatous lesion (See D-80-S2)

Gamut D-80-S1

BENIGN FIBROCYSTIC LESIONS OF BONE

COMMON

1. Bone cyst
2. Fibrocystic changes of degenerative arthritis (esp. in hip)
3. Fibrous dysplasia, monostotic or polyostotic (Jaffe-Lichtenstein type; McCune-Albright S.)
4. Nonossifying fibroma (fibroxanthoma); fibrous cortical defect

UNCOMMON

1. Ameloblastoma, fibrous type; ameloblastic fibroma (jaws)
2. Cementifying fibroma (jaws)
3. Cherubism (face, jaws), incl. Ramon S.
4. Chondromyxoid fibroma
5. Desmoplastic fibroma
6. Fibrogenesis imperfecta
7. Fibromatosis (esp. multicentric infantile myofibromatosis)
8. Fibromyxoma
9. Foreign body reaction (silastic arthropathy or small particle disease {eg, granulomatous pseudotumors adjacent to joint replacements})
10. Intraosseous ganglion

11. Jaffe-Campanacci S. (disseminated nonossifying fibromas, fractures, kyphoscoliosis)
12. Liposclerosing myxofibrous tumor (LSMFT)
13. Mazabraud S. (fibrous dysplasia and intramuscular myxomas)
14. Ossifying fibroma (face, jaws)
15. Osteofibrous dysplasia (esp. tibia)
16. Xanthoma (xanthofibroma)

Reference
1. Taybi H, Lachman RS: Radiology of Syndromes, Metabolic Disorders, and Skeletal Dysplasias. (ed 4) St. Louis: Mosby-Year Book Inc, 1996, p 183

Gamut D-80-S2

XANTHOMATOUS LESIONS OF BONE

PRIMARY XANTHOMATOUS LESIONS
1. Erdheim-Chester disease (multiple sclerotic lipogranulomatous lesions or xanthofibromas of bone)
2. Xanthoma (xanthofibroma; benign fibrous histiocytoma)
3. Xanthomatosis, cerebrotendinous

SECONDARY XANTHOMATOUS REACTION
1. Aneurysmal bone cyst
2. Bone abscess (Brodie abscess)
3. Bone cyst
4. Langerhans cell histiocytosis$_g$ (esp. eosinophilic granuloma)
5. Fibrous dysplasia
6. Giant cell tumor
7. Nonossifying fibroma (fibroxanthoma)

References
1. Dorfman H: International Skeletal Society Lecture, 1984
2. Resnick D: Diagnosis of Bone and Joint Disorders. (ed 3) Philadelphia: Saunders, 1995

Gamut D-80-S3

LESIONS ASSOCIATED WITH ANEURYSMAL BONE CYST (ABC)

COMMON
1. Chondroblastoma (Codman tumor)
2. Giant cell tumor
3. Osteoblastoma
4. Osteosarcoma, telangiectatic
5. Primary ABC

UNCOMMON
1. Angiomatous lesion (hemangioma; lymphangioma, cystic type)
2. Bone cyst
3. Chondromyxoid fibroma
4. Fibrous dysplasia
5. Giant cell granuloma
6. Hemangioendothelioma
7. Hemangiopericytoma
8. Hemophilic pseudotumor
9. Metastasis (esp. renal or thyroid carcinoma; hepatoma)
10. Nonossifying fibroma (fibroxanthoma)
11. Trauma (ossifying hematoma)

Gamut D-81

PRIMARY MALIGNANT BONE NEOPLASMS

COMMON
1. Chondrosarcoma (See D-81-S3)
2. Ewing sarcoma
3. Fibrosarcoma
4. Lymphoma$_g$ (incl. Burkitt lymphoma; leukemia)
5. Malignant fibrous histiocytoma
6. Multiple myeloma

(continued)

7. Osteosarcoma (See D-81-S2)
8. Undifferentiated sarcoma

UNCOMMON

1. Adamantinoma (esp. tibia)
2. Angiosarcoma
3. Chordoma
4. Giant cell tumor, malignant
5. Hemangioendothelioma, malignant
6. Hemangiopericytoma, malignant (rare)
7. [Kaposi sarcoma (secondary bone involvement)]
8. Liposarcoma (rare)
9. Malignant peripheral nerve sheath tumor (MPNST) (rare)

Gamut D-81-S1

RADIOLOGIC CRITERIA SUGGESTING MALIGNANT BONE NEOPLASM

1. Bone destruction (esp. motheaten or permeative, but may be geographic -particularly with wide transition zone 1C margin) (See D-61-S)
2. Irregular ill-defined margins of lesion ("wide transition zone" between normal and abnormal bone)
3. Cortical erosion or destruction
4. Codman triangle
5. Periosteal lamellation ("onion skin")
6. Periosteal right angle spiculation ("sunburst" or "hair-on-end")
7. Soft tissue mass adjacent to bone destruction
8. Chondroid or osteoid matrix (esp. in extraosseous tissues)
9. Metastasis to distant site

References
1. Madewell JE, Ragsdale BD, Sweet DE: Radiologic and pathologic analysis of solitary bone lesions. Radiol Clin North Am 1981; 19:715–748
2. Nelson SW: Some fundamentals in the radiologic differential diagnosis of solitary bone lesions. Semin Roentgenol 1966; 1:244–267

Gamut D-81-S2

TYPES OF OSTEOSARCOMA

PRIMARY

1. Chondroblastic (chondrogenic)
2. Extraskeletal (eg, soft tissue; renal)
3. Fibroblastic (fibrogenic)
4. Giant cell (osteoclast) rich
5. Gnathic (mandibular)
6. High-grade surface
7. Intracortical
8. Intramedullary, high-grade (central, conventional, or classical)
9. Intramedullary, low-grade (sclerosing osteosarcoma)
10. Mesenchymal
11. Osteosarcomatosis
12. Parosteal (juxtacortical)
13. Periosteal
14. Small-cell
15. Telangiectatic

SECONDARY, ARISING IN OR ASSOCIATION WITH

1. Bone following radiation therapy
2. Bone infarct; osteonecrosis
3. Fibrous dysplasia
4. Fracture (healed)
5. Metallic implants
6. Osteoblastoma
7. Osteogenesis imperfecta
8. Osteomyelitis, chronic
9. Paget's disease
10. Retinoblastoma (esp. familial bilateral type)
11. Rothmund-Thomson S.

References
1. Murphey MD, Robbin MR, McRae GA, Flemming DJ, Temple HT, Kransdorf MJ: The many faces of osteosarcoma. RadioGraphics 1997; 17:1205–1231
2. Murray RO, Jacobson HG, Stoker DJ: The Radiology of Skeletal Disorders. (ed 3) London: Churchill Livingstone, 1990, S49–S52

Gamut D-81-S3

TYPES OF CHONDROSARCOMA

PRIMARY

1. Classical or central (medullary)
2. Clear cell
3. Dedifferentiated
4. Juxtacortical or periosteal
5. Mesenchymal; soft tissue
6. Myxoid; soft tissue

SECONDARY, ARISING IN

1. Bone following radiation therapy
2. Enchondroma (incl. Ollier disease; Maffucci S.)
3. Osteochondroma (incl. hereditary multiple exostoses {multiple cartilaginous exostoses; osteochondromatosis})
4. Other preexisting benign cartilaginous lesion (eg, chondroblastoma (Codman tumor); chondromyxoid fibroma)
5. Paget's disease

Gamut D-81-S4

ROUND CELL LESIONS OF BONE

1. Langerhans cell histiocytosis$_g$ (esp. eosinophilic granuloma)
2. Ewing sarcoma
3. Leukemia; lymphoma$_g$; Burkitt lymphoma
4. Multiple myeloma; plasmacytoma
5. Neuroblastoma
6. Osteomyelitis
*7. Primitive neuroectodermal tumor (PNET)

* Small blue round cell tumor that is identical radiologically with Ewing sarcoma but can often be distinguished histologically, particularly with immunohistochemical studies.

Gamut D-81-S5

FREQUENCY OF PRIMARY MALIGNANT BONE TUMORS*

TYPE OF TUMOR	FREQUENCY
Multiple myeloma	44%
Osteosarcoma (incl. variants)	20%
Chondrosarcoma (incl. variants)	12%
Lymphoma$_g$	8%
Ewing sarcoma	6%
Chordoma	4%
Fibrosarcoma/malignant fibrous histiocytoma	4%
Hemangioendothelioma	1%
Others	1%

* Based on 8,591 primary malignant bone tumors in the Mayo Clinic series.

Reference
1. Unni KK: Dahlin's Bone Tumors. General Aspects and Data on 11,087 Cases. (ed 5) Philadelphia: Lippincott-Raven, 1996

PRECURSORS OF MALIGNANCY IN BONE

Precursor Condition	Comment
Enchondroma	very low risk with solitary lesion, higher risk with multiple lesions
Osteochondroma	very low risk with solitary lesion, higher risk with multiple lesions
Paget's disease	higher risk with more extensive, polyostotic disease
Radiation injury	low risk with 7000 rads or less
Osteomyelitis with chronic sinus tract	long latency period (20+ years)
Bone infarct	rare, 90% or more have multiple infarcts
Fibrous dysplasia	case reports
Metallic implants	case reports
Bone cysts	case reports
Osteogenesis imperfecta	case reports
Genetic predisposition	association with mutant Rb gene and retinoblastoma
Synovial chondromatosis	case reports
Giant cell tumor	rare malignant recurrence after treatment
Osteoblastoma	rare locally aggressive form that does not metastasize
Osteofibrous dysplasia	coexistent with adamantinoma, possibly subsets of of the same disease

MALIGNANT BONE NEOPLASM WITH GROSS DESTRUCTION AND LITTLE OR NO PERIOSTEAL REACTION

COMMON
1. Chondrosarcoma
2. Lymphoma$_g$; leukemia in an adult
3. Malignant fibrous histiocytoma
4. Metastasis
5. Multiple myeloma
6. Osteosarcoma (osteolytic type)

UNCOMMON
1. Adamantinoma (esp. tibia)
2. Angiosarcoma
3. Chordoma
4. Ewing sarcoma
5. Fibrosarcoma
6. Giant cell tumor, malignant
7. Hemangioendothelioma, malignant
8. Hemangiopericytoma, malignant (rare)
9. Liposarcoma (rare)

Gamut D-83

MALIGNANT BONE NEOPLASM WITH MARKED PERIOSTEAL REACTION (MAY BE CONFUSED WITH OSTEOMYELITIS)

1. Burkitt lymphoma
*2. Ewing sarcoma
3. Leukemia in a child
4. Metastasis (esp. neuroblastoma in a child; prostate or gastrointestinal carcinoma in adult)
*5. Osteosarcoma
6. Primitive neuroectodermal tumor (PNET)

* Often onion-skin periosteal reaction.

Gamut D-84

MALIGNANT BONE NEOPLASM WITH MARKED MINERALIZATION RELATIVE TO DESTRUCTION

1. Bone sarcoma or carcinoma superimposed on chronic osteomyelitis or tropical ulcer
2. Bone sarcoma (previously treated) with recurrence
3. Chondrosarcoma (esp. arising in benign cartilaginous lesion)
*4. Ewing sarcoma (esp. lesion in flat bone such as pelvis)
*5. Lymphoma$_g$; leukemia (rarely)
*6. Osteoblastic metastasis
7. Osteosarcoma
8. Parosteal or periosteal osteosarcoma or chondrosarcoma
*9. Primitive neuroectodermal tumor (PNET), esp. lesion in flat bone

* Mineralization represents reactive bone.

Gamut D-85

OSTEOBLASTIC METASTASES

COMMON

1. Carcinoma of breast
2. Carcinoma of prostate
3. Lymphoma$_g$

UNCOMMON

1. Carcinoid, pulmonary
2. Cerebellar medulloblastoma or sarcoma
3. Meningiosarcoma
4. Osteosarcoma (incl. osteosarcomatosis)
5. Other carcinoma (esp. nasopharynx; urinary bladder—transitional cell; stomach, colon, pancreas—mucinous; lung—rarely small cell)
6. Retinoblastoma

Gamut D-86

OSTEOLYTIC METASTASES

COMMON

1. Carcinoma of breast
*2. Carcinoma of kidney (hypernephroma)
3. Carcinoma of lung
4. Leukemia; lymphoma$_g$

UNCOMMON

1. Bone sarcoma (eg, Ewing sarcoma)
*2. Carcinoma of adrenal; pheochromocytoma
3. Carcinoma of gastrointestinal tract (eg, esophagus; stomach; colon; rectum)
4. Carcinoma of prostate
5. Carcinoma of skin (squamous cell)
*6. Carcinoma of thyroid
7. Carcinoma of cervix or uterus
*8. Hepatoma

(continued)

*9. Malignant melanoma
10. Neuroblastoma
11. Other primary neoplasms (eg, urinary bladder; ovary; testis; Wilms tumor)

* Often expansile lytic lesion.

Gamut D-87-S1

RATE OF FREQUENCY OF METASTASES TO BONE FROM VARIOUS PRIMARY CARCINOMAS

1.	Breast (incl. osteoblastic)	35%
2.	Prostate (incl. osteoblastic)	30%
3.	Lung	10%
4.	Kidney	5%
5.	Stomach	2%
6.	Thyroid	2%
7.	Uterus	2%
8.	Colon	1%
9.	Other organs	13%

Reference
1. Greenfield GB: Radiology of Bone Diseases. (ed 5) Philadelphia: Lippincott, 1990

Gamut D-87-S2

DISTRIBUTION OF METASTATIC BONE DISEASE

Axial skeleton (incl. thoracolumbar spine, sacrum and pelvis)	75%
Skull	10%
Upper and lower extremities	11%
Forearm, hand, leg, foot	4%

Reference
1. Greenfield GB: Radiology of Bone Diseases. (ed 5) Philadelphia: Lippincott, 1990

Gamut D-88

PERIOSTEAL OR PAROSTEAL NEOPLASM OR TUMOR-LIKE SURFACE LESION OF BONE

COMMON
1. Cortical/periosteal desmoid (cortical avulsive injury)
2. Myositis ossificans, parosteal (juxtacortical)
3. Osteochondroma (osteocartilaginous exostosis)
4. Osteoid osteoma, subperiosteal
5. Osteosarcoma, parosteal
6. Turret exostosis

UNCOMMON
1. Aneurysmal bone cyst, subperiosteal
2. Bizarre parosteal pseudotumor (BPOP)
3. Chondrosarcoma, periosteal
4. Chondrosarcoma, secondary peripheral in osteochondroma
5. Florid reactive periostitis (ossifying fasciitis; parosteal fasciitis)
6. Ganglion, periosteal or subperiosteal
7. Hemangioma, parosteal
8. Lipoma, parosteal
9. Malignant fibrous histiocytoma; fibrosarcoma
10. Osteoblastoma, subperiosteal
11. Osteoma
12. Osteosarcoma, high-grade surface
13. Osteosarcoma, periosteal
14. Periosteal chondroma
15. Periosteal fibroma
16. Soft tissue tumor in a parosteal location (eg, gouty tophus; synovial sarcoma; giant cell tumor of tendon sheath; glomus tumor; Kaposi sarcoma)

References
1. Dorfman H: Minisymposium on Bone-Surface Lesions Terminology. Presented at International Skeletal Society 18th Annual Refresher Course, San Diego, 1991
2. Greenfield GB: Radiology of Bone Diseases. (ed 5) Philadelphia: Lippincott, 1990
3. Seeger LL, Yao L, Eckardt JJ: Surface lesions of bone. Radiology 1998; 206:17–33

Gamut D-89-S

DIAGRAM OF VARIOUS PERIOSTEAL REACTIONS

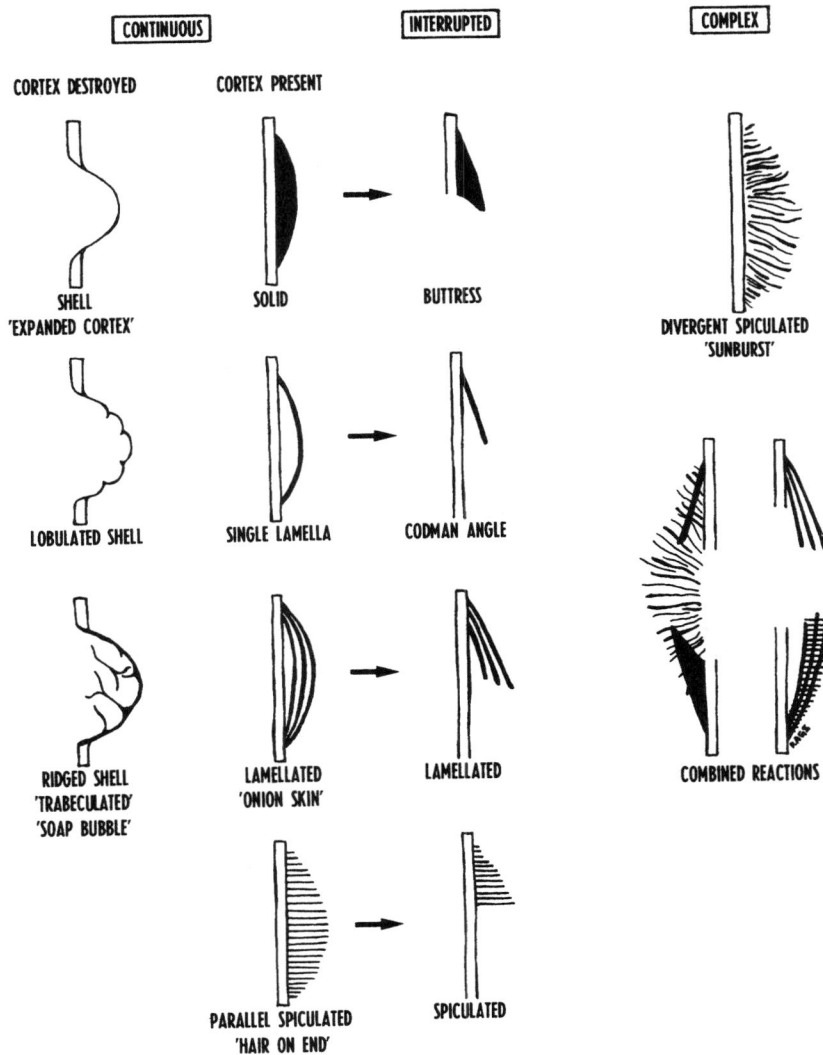

Schematic diagram of periosteal reactions. The arrows indicate that the continuous reactions may be interrupted.

Reference

1. Ragsdale BD, Madewell JE, Sweet DE: Radiologic and pathologic analysis of solitary bone lesions. Part II: Periosteal reactions. Radiol Clin North Am 1981;19: 749–783

Gamut D-90

CODMAN TRIANGLE

COMMON
1. Malignant bone neoplasm, primary (See D-81)

UNCOMMON
1. Aneurysmal bone cyst
2. Healing fracture
3. Metastasis
4. Osteomyelitis (incl. mycetoma)
5. Subperiosteal hemorrhage (eg, hemophilia)

References
1. Edeiken J, Dalinka M, Karasick D: Edeiken's Roentgen Diagnosis of Diseases of Bone. (ed 4) Baltimore: Williams & Wilkins, 1990
2. Greenfield GB: Radiology of Bone Diseases. (ed 5) Philadelphia: Lippincott, 1990
3. Nelson SW: Some fundamentals in the radiologic differential diagnosis of solitary bone lesions. Semin Roentgenol 1966; 1:244–267
4. Ragsdale BD, Madewell JE, Sweet DE: Radiologic and pathologic analysis of solitary bone lesions. Part II: Periosteal reactions. Radiol Clin North Am 1981; 19:749–783

Gamut D-91

PARALLEL SPICULATED ("HAIR-ON-END") OR DIVERGENT SPICULATED ("SUNBURST") PERIOSTEAL REACTION

COMMON
1. Anemia$_g$ (eg, thalassemia or sickle cell disease involving cranial vault with "hair-on-end" pattern)
2. Ewing sarcoma
3. Osteosarcoma

UNCOMMON
1. Adamantinoma (esp. tibia)
2. Bone sarcoma, other (See D-81)
3. Healing fracture (esp. march fracture)
4. Hemangioma (esp. skull)
5. Infantile cortical hyperostosis (Caffey disease)
6. Leukemia
7. Meningioma
8. Metastasis (esp. neuroblastoma metastasis in skull; carcinoma of prostate)
9. Osteomyelitis (incl. mycetoma)
10. Thyroid acropachy

Reference
1. Ragsdale BD, Madewell JE, Sweet DE: Radiologic and pathologic analysis of solitary bone lesions. Part II: Periosteal reactions. Radiol Clin North Am 1981; 19:749–783

Gamut D-92

LOCALIZED PERIOSTEAL REACTION (See D-90 to D-100)

COMMON
1. Arthritis (eg, juvenile rheumatoid; psoriatic; Reiter S.) (See D-232)
2. Dactylitis (See D-132)
3. Fracture, healing with callus; battered child S.
4. Langerhans cell histiocytosis$_g$ (esp. eosinophilic granuloma)
5. Malignant bone neoplasm (esp. Ewing sarcoma; osteosarcoma) (See D-81, D-83)
6. Osteoid osteoma
7. Osteomyelitis (pyogenic; tuberculous; fungal—incl. mycetoma)
8. Reactive periostitis (eg, idiopathic; traumatic)
9. Soft tissue lesion adjacent to bone (eg, diabetic or decubitus ulcer; cellulitis; deep abscess; vascular tumor)
10. Subperiosteal hemorrhage (eg, trauma; hemophilia)

11. Vascular stasis (eg, chronic venous, arterial or lymphatic insufficiency or obstruction)

UNCOMMON

1. Benign bone cyst or neoplasm with expansion or pathologic fracture
2. Bone infarct (esp. in sickle cell disease)
3. Chondroblastoma (Codman tumor) invading metphysis
4. Hypertrophic osteoarthropathy (See D-98)
5. Infantile cortical hyperostosis (Caffey disease)
6. Leukemia; lymphoma$_g$
7. Melorheostosis
8. Metastasis (eg, neuroblastoma)
9. Osteoblastoma
10. Radiation injury
11. Syphilis; yaws
12. Thermal injury (eg, burn; frostbite; electrical)
13. Tropical ulcer ("ivory osteoma")

Gamut D-93

WIDESPREAD OR GENERALIZED PERIOSTEAL REACTION (USUALLY LAYERED OR SOLID AND OFTEN SYMMETRICAL)

COMMON

1. Arthritis (eg, juvenile rheumatoid; psoriatic; Reiter S.) (See D-232)
2. Fractures, traumatic or pathologic; battered child S.
3. Prematurity; physiologic periostitis of newborn (up to 6 months)
4. Vascular stasis (eg, chronic venous, arterial or lymphatic insufficiency or obstruction)

UNCOMMON

1. Acromegaly (hands, feet)
2. Bizarre parosteal pseudotumor (BPOP)

3. Bone infarction, multiple (esp. hand-foot S. in sickle cell disease)
4. Congenital transplacental infection (eg, syphilis; rubella; cytomegalovirus infection)
5. Connective tissue disease (collagen disease)$_g$ with arteritis (eg, lupus erythematosus; polyarteritis nodosa)
6. Copper deficiency, nutritional; Menkes S. (kinky-hair S.)
7. Cushing S. with excess callus
8. Diaphyseal dysplasia (Camurati-Engelmann disease)
9. Fibromatosis (esp. multicentric infantile myofibromatosis)
10. Florid reactive periostitis of the phalanges
11. Fluorosis
12. Gaucher disease; Niemann-Pick disease
13. Hemophilia; Christmas disease
14. Hyperphosphatasia
15. Hypertrophic osteoarthropathy (See D-98)
16. Hypervitaminosis A and D
17. Idiopathic
18. Infantile cortical hyperostosis (Caffey disease)
19. Langerhans cell histiocytosis$_g$
20. Leukemia; lymphoma$_g$
21. Macrodystrophia lipomatosa
22. Mastocytosis (early)
23. Medication induced (eg, Prostaglandin E; methotrexate)
24. Melorheostosis
25. Metastases (eg, neuroblastoma; Ewing sarcoma)
26. Mucolipidosis II (I-cell disease); GM$_1$ gangliosidosis
27. Neurofibromatosis (subperiosteal hemorrhages)
28. Neurogenic disorder$_g$ (eg, congenital insensitivity to pain; spinal cord injury; meningomyelocele; leprosy)
29. Osteomalacia with fractures (eg, Milkman S.; aluminum-induced bone disease)
30. Osteomyelitis, widespread (eg, pyogenic; tuberculous; fungal)
31. Pachydermoperiostosis
32. Renal osteodystrophy (secondary hyperparathyroidism)

(continued)

33. Rickets, healing
34. Scurvy
35. Syphilis; yaws
36. Thermal injury (frostbite; burn; electrical)
37. Thyroid acropachy (hands, feet)
38. Tuberous sclerosis

References
1. Greenfield GB: Radiology of Bone Diseases. (ed 5) Philadelphia: Lippincott, 1990
2. Kozlowski K, Beighton P: Gamut Index of Skeletal Dysplasias. Berlin: Springer-Verlag, 1984, pp 11–13
3. Pineda CJ, Sartoris DJ, Clopton P, Resnick D: Periostitis in hypertrophic osteoarthropathy: relationship to disease duration. AJR 1987;148:773–778
4. Resnick D: Diagnosis of Bone and Joint Disorders. (ed 3) Philadelphia: Saunders, 1995
5. Swischuk LE, John SD: Differential Diagnosis in Pediatric Radiology. (ed 2) Baltimore: Williams & Wilkins, 1995, pp 318–323

Gamut D-94

PERIOSTEAL NEW BONE FORMATION IN A CHILD

COMMON

1. Arthritis (eg, septic; juvenile chronic; juvenile rheumatoid; fungal—mycetoma, *Candida*)
2. Bone sarcoma (eg, Ewing sarcoma; osteosarcoma)
3. Congenital transplacental infection (eg, syphilis; rubella; cytomegalovirus infection)
4. Dactylitis (See D-132)
5. Langerhans cell histiocytosis$_g$ (esp. eosinophilic granuloma)
6. Leukemia; Burkitt lymphoma
7. Metastasis (eg, neuroblastoma; retinoblastoma; embryonal rhabdomyosarcoma)
8. Osteomyelitis (pyogenic; tuberculous; fungal; mycetoma; smallpox—prior to eradication)
9. Prematurity; physiologic periostitis of newborn (up to 6 months)
10. Rickets (all types), healing

11. Sickle cell disease (hand-foot S.)
12. Trauma (eg, callus; traumatic periostitis; battered child S.; stress fracture; osteogenesis imperfecta; campomelic dysplasia)

UNCOMMON

1. Benign bone cyst or neoplasm with expansion or pathologic fracture
2. Copper deficiency, nutritional; Menkes S. (kinky-hair S.)
3. Diaphyseal dysplasia (Camurati-Engelmann disease)
4. Gaucher disease; Niemann-Pick disease
5. Hemophilia; Christmas disease
6. Hyperphosphatasia
7. Hypertrophic osteoarthropathy (See D-98)
8. Hypervitaminosis A and D
9. Idiopathic
10. Infantile cortical hyperostosis (Caffey disease)
11. Infantile multisystem inflammatory disease (NOMID)
12. Medication-induced (eg, Prostaglandin E; methotrexate)
13. Melorheostosis
14. Mucolipidosis II (I-cell disease); GM$_1$ gangliosidosis
15. Osteoid osteoma
16. Pachydermoperiostosis
17. Radiation injury
18. Scurvy
19. Soft tissue lesion adjacent to bone (eg, diabetic or decubitus ulcer; cellulitis; deep abscess; vascular tumor)
20. Thermal injury (eg, burn; frostbite; electrical)
21. Tuberous sclerosis
22. Yaws

References
1. Kozlowski K, Beighton P: Gamut Index of Skeletal Dysplasias. Berlin: Springer-Verlag, 1984, pp 11–13
2. Matzinger MA, Briggs VA, Dunlap HJ, et al: Plain film and CT observations in prostaglandin-induced bone changes. Pediatr Radiol 1992;22:264–266
3. Shopfner CE: Periosteal bone growth in normal infants. AJR 1966;97:154–163

4. Swischuk LE, John SD: Differential Diagnosis in Pediatric Radiology. (ed 2) Baltimore: Williams & Wilkins, 1995, pp 318–326

Gamut D-95-S

CLUES TO THE BATTERED CHILD

SKELETAL INJURIES

HIGH SPECIFICITY

1. Classic metaphyseal lesion (corner fracture; bucket handle fracture; avulsion fracture; metaphyseal infraction)
2. Rib fractures (esp. posterior)
3. Scapular fractures
4. Spinous process fractures
5. Sternal fractures

MODERATE SPECIFICITY

1. Multiple fractures
2. Bilateral fractures
3. Fractures at different stages of healing
4. Epiphyseal separations
5. Vertebral fractures or subluxations
6. Fractures of digits of hands or feet
7. Complex skull fractures

COMMON BUT LOW SPECIFICITY

1. Subperiosteal new bone formation
2. Excessive callus formation
3. Clavicular fractures
4. Fractures of shafts of long bones
5. Simple linear skull fractures

OTHER FEATURES

1. Unsuspected or inadequately or inappropriately explained fractures or other injuries
2. Multiple bruises; healed lacerations; burns

3. Thoracic findings consistent with contusion (eg, focal infiltrate without respiratory infection or fever; pneumothorax; pneumomediastinum; hemothorax; chylothorax)
4. Intramural intestinal hematoma
5. Pneumoperitoneum
6. Pseudocyst of pancreas
7. Solid organ laceration
8. Subdural hematoma
9. Underdevelopment; failure to thrive; poor hygiene
10. Inappropriate affect by the child's caregiver (profound indifference or exaggerated concern)

Reference
1. Kleinman PK: Diagnostic Imaging of Child Abuse. St. Louis: Mosby, 1998

Gamut D-96

EXCESS CALLUS FORMATION

COMMON

1. Steroid therapy; Cushing S.
2. Trauma, unrecognized; battered child S.; stress or march fracture (esp. metatarsal)

UNCOMMON

1. Congenital insensitivity to pain
2. Familial
3. Multiple myeloma (with pathologic fractures)
4. Paralytic disorders$_g$
5. Neuropathic arthropathy (eg, Charcot joint)
6. Osteogenesis imperfecta
7. Renal osteodystrophy (secondary hyperparathyroidism)

Gamut D-97

SCLEROSIS OF BONE WITH PERIOSTEAL REACTION

COMMON

1. Healing fracture with callus
2. Malignant bone neoplasm (eg, Ewing sarcoma; osteosarcoma; chondrosarcoma; lymphoma$_g$)
3. Osteoid osteoma
4. Osteomyelitis, bacterial, subacute to chronic (incl. Garré sclerosing osteomyelitis; Brodie abscess)

UNCOMMON

1. Chondroblastoma (Codman tumor)
2. Infantile cortical hyperostosis (Caffey disease)
3. Melorheostosis
4. Osteoblastic metastasis (esp. prostate)
5. Osteoblastoma
6. Osteomyelitis, unusual/low virulent organism (incl. tuberculosis; fungus disease$_g$—mycetoma; syphilis; yaws)
7. Ribbing disease (hereditary multiple diaphyseal sclerosis)
8. Tropical ulcer
9. Tuberous sclerosis

Gamut D-98

HYPERTROPHIC OSTEOARTHROPATHY

COMMON

1. Carcinoma of lung

UNCOMMON

1. Abscess of lung
2. Arteriovenous fistula of lung
3. Carcinoid, bronchial
4. Chronic gastrointestinal disease (eg, carcinoma; lymphoma; celiac disease; Crohn's disease; ulcerative colitis; Whipple's disease; amebic or bacillary dysentery; juvenile polyposis)
5. Chronic liver disease; cirrhosis (esp. biliary)
6. Chronic pulmonary infection (eg, tuberculosis; fungus disease$_g$; bronchiectasis; empyema; cystic fibrosis {mucoviscidosis})
7. Cyanotic congenital heart disease (clubbing but rarely a periosteal reaction)
8. Emphysema; chronic obstructive pulmonary disease (COPD)
9. Familial
10. Idiopathic
11. Lymphoma of lung
12. Mesothelioma, malignant; localized benign fibrous pleural tumor
13. Metastasis to lung (esp. from osteosarcoma)
14. Nasopharyngeal carcinoma (Schmincke tumor)
15. Pachydermoperiostosis (primary hypertrophic osteoarthropathy)
16. Polyarteritis nodosa
17. Renal osteodystrophy (secondary hyperparathyroidism)
18. Thyroid acropachy

Reference

1. Pineda CJ, Sartoris DJ, Clopton P, Resnick D: Periostitis in hypertrophic osteoarthropathy: Relationship to disease duration. AJR 1987;148:773–778

Gamut D-99

MARKED CORTICAL HYPEROSTOSIS AND/OR THICK, SOLID, WAVY, OR BALLOONED PERIOSTEAL REACTION INVOLVING THE SHAFT OF A BONE

COMMON

1. Fracture (eg, ordinary, stress or march fracture; battered child S.; neurogenic fracture; osteogenesis imperfecta)
2. Osteoid osteoma
3. Osteomyelitis (esp. chronic, low grade, or subperiosteal; Garré sclerosing osteomyelitis; fungus disease—mycetoma)
4. Reactive periostitis (idiopathic—usually due to trauma)
5. Subperiosteal hemorrhage (eg, trauma; hemophilia or other bleeding disorder$_g$; leukemia; scurvy; neurofibromatosis)
6. Venous or lymphatic stasis

UNCOMMON

1. Cellulitis; adjacent soft tissue inflammation
2. Fluorosis
3. Hyperphosphatasia
4. Hypertrophic osteoarthropathy (See D-98)
5. Infantile cortical hyperostosis (Caffey disease)
6. Langerhans cell histiocytosis$_g$
7. Melorheostosis
8. Mucolipidosis II (I-cell disease); GM$_1$ gangliosidosis
9. Osteofibrous dysplasia (esp. tibia)
10. Pachydermoperiostosis
11. Ribbing disease (hereditary multiple diaphyseal sclerosis)
12. Rickets, healing (esp. ribs)
13. Sickle cell disease with bone infarction (esp. hand-foot S.); other dactylitis (See D-132)
14. Syphilis, yaws (healing)
15. Thyroid acropachy
16. Tropical ulcer osteoma
17. Tuberous sclerosis (esp. rib)

Gamut D-100

LOCALIZED CORTICAL THICKENING (ONE OR A FEW BONES) (See D-101)

COMMON

1. Bowed bones (See D-8)
2. Fracture, healing or healed; traumatic periostitis; battered child S.
3. Hypertrophic osteoarthropathy (See D-98)
4. Osteoid osteoma
5. Osteomyelitis with involucrum; Garré sclerosing osteomyelitis; mycetoma; syphilis, yaws (healing)
6. Paget's disease
7. Venous or lymphatic stasis

UNCOMMON

1. Angiomatous lesion$_g$ (eg, hemangioma; angiomatosis)
2. Bone neoplasm (esp. enchondroma; low-grade chondrosarcoma; benign tumor after pathological fracture)
3. Fibrous dysplasia
4. Hypervitaminosis A (esp. ulna)
5. Infantile cortical hyperostosis (Caffey disease)
6. Klippel-Trenaunay S.; Parkes Weber S.
7. Melorheostosis
8. Pachydermoperiostosis
9. Sickle cell disease (eg, with infarction or osteomyelitis)
10. Subperiosteal hemorrhage, old (eg, trauma; hemophilia; scurvy)
11. Thyroid acropachy
12. Tropical ulcer osteoma

Gamut D-101

WIDESPREAD CORTICAL THICKENING

COMMON

1. Conditions in which periosteal new bone has blended with the cortex (esp. widespread osteomyelitis or trauma) (See D-99)
2. Paget's disease

UNCOMMON

1. Acromegaly; gigantism
2. Beckwith-Wiedeman S.
3. Craniodiaphyseal dysplasia (ribs, clavicles)
4. Dentino-osseous dysplasias (esp. trichodentoosseous S.)
5. Dubowitz S.
6. Endosteal hyperostosis (van Buchem and Worth types)
7. Diaphyseal dysplasia (Camurati-Engelmann disease)
8. Erdheim-Chester disease
9. Fluorosis
10. Frontometaphyseal dysplasia
11. Hyperostosis generalisata with striation of bones
12. Hyperphosphatasia
13. Hypertrophic osteoarthropathy (See D-98)
14. Hypervitaminosis A or D
15. Infantile cortical hyperostosis (Caffey disease)
16. Melorheostosis
17. Pachydermoperiostosis
18. Physiologic osteosclerosis of newborn
19. Polyostotic fibrous dysplasia (McCune-Albright S.)
20. Prostaglandin-induced hyperostosis
21. Pyknodysostosis
22. Ribbing disease (hereditary multiple diaphyseal sclerosis)
23. Stanescu dysostosis
24. Tuberous sclerosis
25. Tubular stenosis dysplasia (Kenny-Caffey S.)
26. Weismann-Netter S.

References
1. Greenfield GB: Radiology of Bone Diseases. (ed 5) Philadelphia: Lippincott, 1990
2. Taybi H, Lachman RS: Radiology of Syndromes, Metabolic Disorders, and Skeletal Dysplasias. (ed 4) St. Louis: Mosby-Year Book Inc, 1996, p 1026

Gamut D-102

WIDESPREAD CORTICAL THINNING

COMMON

1. Anemias$_g$
2. Metastatic disease (carcinomatosis); multiple myeloma (myelomatosis)
3. Osteoporosis, all causes (esp. senile; postmenopausal; immobilization; hyperparathyroidism; steroid therapy (See D-43)

UNCOMMON

1. Fibrogenesis imperfecta ossium
2. Gaucher disease; Niemann-Pick disease
3. Mannosidosis; GM_1 gangliosidosis
4. Membranous lipodystrophy
5. Osteogenesis imperfecta (all types)
6. Polyostotic fibrous dysplasia (McCune-Albright S.)
7. Singleton-Merten S.
8. Winchester S.

Reference
1. Taybi H, Lachman RS: Radiology of Syndromes, Metabolic Disorders, and Skeletal Dysplasias. (ed 4) St. Louis: Mosby-Year Book Inc, 1996, p 1026

Gamut D-103

"SPLIT" OR DOUBLE-LAYER CORTEX

COMMON

1. Bone infarct (eg, sickle cell disease)
2. Healing fracture; battered child S.
3. Normal infants, esp. premature (physiologic periostitis of newborn)
4. Osteomyelitis
5. Osteoporosis (esp. disuse; immobilization) (See D-43)
6. Postsurgical removal of intramedullary rod

UNCOMMON

1. Bone graft (local)
2. Gaucher disease
3. Hyperphosphatasia
4. Osteopetrosis
5. Scurvy

Reference
1. Greenfield GB: Radiology of Bone Diseases. (ed 5) Philadelphia: Lippincott, 1990

Gamut D-104

SCALLOPING, EROSION, OR RESORPTION OF THE INNER CORTICAL MARGIN

COMMON

  1. Anemia$_g$ (esp. thalassemia; sickle cell disease)
*2. Bone cyst
*3. Chondroid lesion (eg, enchondroma; chondroblastoma {Codman tumor}; chondromyxoid fibroma; chondrosarcoma; periosteal chondroma)
*4. Fibrous dysplasia
  5. Hyperparathyroidism

6. Langerhans cell histiocytosis$_g$
7. Leukemia; lymphoma$_g$
8. Metastasis
9. Multiple myeloma
*10. Nonossifying fibroma (fibroxanthoma); fibrous cortical defect

UNCOMMON

1. Gaucher disease
2. Malignant fibrous histiocytoma; fibrosarcoma
3. Mastocytosis

* Usually with well-defined, often sclerotic margin.

Reference
1. Greenfield GB: Radiology of Bone Diseases. (ed 5) Philadelphia: Lippincott, 1990

Gamut D-105

DESTRUCTION OR EROSION OF THE EXTERNAL CORTICAL SURFACE OF A BONE (See D-39, D-41)

COMMON

1. Acro-osteolysis (absorption of terminal phalanx) (See D-127)
2. Aneurysm or arteriovenous fistula adjacent to bone (esp. traumatic)
3. Cortical/periosteal desmoid (cortical avulsive injury, esp. lower posterior femur)
4. Gouty tophus
5. Hyperparathyroidism; renal osteodystrophy (secondary hyperparathyroidism)
6. Juxta-articular erosion from rheumatoid or other arthritis or amyloidosis
7. Leukemia; lymphoma$_g$
8. Metastasis (esp. carcinoma of lung; neuroblastoma)
9. Nonossifying fibroma (fibroxanthoma); fibrous cortical defect
10. Primary bone neoplasm

(continued)

11. Soft tissue infection or cellulitis adjacent to bone
12. Soft tissue neoplasm adjacent to bone (eg, hemangioma; neurofibroma; fibroma; lipoma; chondroma; sarcoma)
13. Subperiosteal bone resorption (See D-41)
14. Subperiosteal osteomyelitis; unusual/low virulent organism (eg, syphilis; yaws; tuberculosis; fungus disease—mycetoma)
15. Synovial lesion (eg, giant cell tumor of tendon sheath; pigmented villonodular synovitis; synovial sarcoma)
16. Trauma (eg, tendon avulsion)

UNCOMMON
1. Ainhum
2. Bacillary angiomatosis
3. Foreign body or thorn granuloma
4. Glomus tumor
5. Kaposi sarcoma
6. Periosteal chondroma or fibroma
7. Periosteal or parosteal neoplasm, other (eg, periosteal osteosarcoma; periosteal chondrosarcoma) (See D-88)
8. Squamous cell carcinoma of skin; malignant tropical ulcer
9. Subperiosteal hematoma

Gamut D-106

BONY WHISKERING (PROLIFERATION OF NEW BONE AT TENDON AND LIGAMENT INSERTIONS)

COMMON
1. Ankylosing spondylitis
2. Diffuse idiopathic skeletal hyperostosis (DISH)

UNCOMMON
1. Fluorosis
2. Hypervitaminosis A and D (including cis-retinoic acid and vitamin D-resistant rickets treatment)

3. Hypoparathyroidism
4. Juvenile chronic arthritis
4. Plasma cell dyscrasia (eg, POEMS S.)
5. Psoriatic arthritis
6. Pyoderma gangrenosum
7. Reiter S.
8. Sternocostoclavicular hyperostosis (SAPHO S.)

Reference

1. Resnick D, Greenway GD, Bardwick PA, et al: Plasma-cell dyscrasia with polyneuropathy, organomegaly, endocrinopathy, M-protein, and skin changes: The POEMS syndrome. Radiology 1981; 140:17–22

Gamut D-107-1

POLYOSTOTIC BONE LESIONS IN ADULTS (See D-74)

COMMON
1. Arthritic or synovial-based lesions
2. Bone infarcts; aseptic necroses
3. Fibrous lesions, incl. nonossifying fibromas (fibroxanthomas); polyostotic fibrous dysplasia (McCune-Albright S.)
4. Hyperparathyroidism, primary or secondary (renal osteodystrophy) with brown tumors
5. Metastases
6. Multiple myeloma
7. Osteomyelitis (bacterial; tuberculous; fungal$_g$; smallpox residual)
8. Paget's disease
9. Trauma (fractures; dislocations)

UNCOMMON
1. Acro-osteolysis (See D-127)
2. Amyloidosis
3. Anemia$_g$, primary
4. Angiomatosis (hemangiomatosis; lymphangiomatosis; bacillary angiomatosis)
5. Enchondromatosis (Ollier disease); Maffucci S.

6. Fibromatosis (esp. multicentric infantile myofibromatosis)
7. Gaucher disease; Niemann-Pick disease
8. Hemangioendothelioma; angiosarcoma
9. Hereditary multiple exostoses (multiple cartilaginous exostoses; osteochondromatosis)
10. Hydatid disease
11. Hypertrophic osteoarthropathy (See D-98)
12. Jackhammer operator's (driller's) disease of wrists
13. Kaposi sarcoma
14. Langerhans cell histiocytosis$_g$ (eosinophilic granuloma)
15. Leprosy
16. Leukemia; lymphoma$_g$
17. Mastocytosis
18. Membranous lipodystrophy
19. Mucopolysaccharidoses; mucolipidoses (See J-4)
20. Neurofibromatosis
21. Radium poisoning
22. Sarcoidosis
23. Syphilis; yaws
24. Thyroid acropachy
25. Tuberous sclerosis
26. Weber-Christian disease; pancreatitis with bone lesions

Gamut D-107-2

POLYOSTOTIC BONE LESIONS IN CHILDREN 5–15 YEARS (See D-74)

COMMON

1. Anemia$_g$, primary
2. Fibrous lesions, incl. nonossifying fibromas (fibroxanthomas); fibrous cortical defects; polyostotic fibrous dysplasia (McCune-Albright S.)
3. Hyperparathyroidism, primary or secondary (renal osteodystrophy) with brown tumors

4. Langerhans cell histiocytosis$_g$
5. Leukemia; lymphoma$_g$; Burkitt lymphoma
6. Osteochondrodysplasias and dysostoses (See D-1)
7. Osteomyelitis (bacterial; tuberculous; fungal; smallpox residual)
8. Trauma (fractures; dislocations)

UNCOMMON

1. Angiomatosis (hemangiomatosis; lymphangiomatosis, cystic type)
2. Arthritis (eg, juvenile chronic; juvenile rheumatoid)
3. Bone infarcts (esp. sickle cell disease)
4. Cortical/periosteal desmoids (cortical avulsive injuries—esp. lower posterior femurs)
5. Dactylitis (See D-132)
6. Enchondromatosis (Ollier disease); Maffucci S.
7. Ewing sarcoma
8. Fibromatosis (esp. multicentric infantile myofibromatosis)
9. Gaucher disease; Niemann-Pick disease
10. Hemophilia
11. Hereditary multiple exostoses (multiple cartilaginous exostoses; osteochondromatosis)
12. Hypervitaminosis A and D
13. Landing-Shirkey disease (multifocal granulomatous osteomyelitis in a compromised child)
14. Leprosy
15. Macrodystrophia lipomatosa
16. Mastocytosis
17. Melorheostosis
18. Metastases (incl. neuroblastoma)
19. Mucopolysaccharidoses; mucolipidoses (See J-4)
20. Neurofibromatosis (incl. type 1 with multiple nonossifying fibromas or Jaffe-Campanacci S.)
21. Osteosarcomatosis
22. Pachydermoperiostosis
23. Syphilis; yaws
24. Tuberous sclerosis

Gamut D-107-3

POLYOSTOTIC BONE LESIONS IN INFANTS AND CHILDREN UP TO 5 YEARS (See D-74)

COMMON

1. Anemia$_g$, primary
2. Battered child S.
3. Congenital transplacental infection (toxoplasmosis; rubella; cytomegalovirus infection; herpes; syphilis)
4. Fibrous lesions, incl. nonossifying fibromas (fibroxanthomas); fibrous cortical defects; polyostotic fibrous dysplasia (McCune-Albright S.)
5. Langerhans cell histiocytosis$_g$
6. Leukemia; Burkitt lymphoma
7. Metastases (esp. neuroblastoma)
8. Osteochondrodysplasias and dysostoses (See D-1)
9. Osteomyelitis (bacterial; tuberculous; fungal$_g$)
10. Physiologic periostitis of newborn (up to 6 months)
11. Rickets
12. Trauma (fractures; dislocations)

UNCOMMON

1. Fibromatosis (esp. multicentric infantile myofibromatosis)
2. Hypervitaminosis A
3. Infantile cortical hyperostosis (Caffey disease)
4. Macrodystrophia lipomatosa
5. Mucopolysaccharidoses; mucolipidoses (See J-4)
6. Neurofibromatosis (incl. type 1 with multiple nonossifying fibromas or Jaffe-Campanacci S.)
7. Osteogenesis imperfecta
8. Osteopetrosis
9. Scurvy
10. Tetanus (collapsed vertebrae)
11. Yaws

Gamut D-108-1

MULTIPLE FRACTURES—CONGENITAL SKELETAL DISORDERS WITH INCREASED BONE FRAGILITY

COMMON

1. Enchondromatosis (Ollier disease); Maffucci S.
2. Osteogenesis imperfecta (all types)
3. Polyostotic fibrous dysplasia (McCune-Albright S.)

UNCOMMON

1. Achondrogenesis type I
2. Antley-Bixler S.
3. Cleidocranial dysplasia
4. Congenital insensitivity to pain
5. Cutis laxa
6. Dysosteosclerosis
7. Fibrogenesis imperfecta ossium
8. Geroderma osteodysplastica
9. Juvenile idiopathic osteoporosis
10. Metaphyseal chondrodysplasia (Jansen type)
11. Osteopetrosis
12. Progeria
13. Pyknodysostosis
14. Pyle dysplasia
15. Riley-Day S. (familial dysautonomia)
16. Spondylometaphyseal dysplasia (corner fracture type)
17. Stiff-man S.
18. Thevenard S. (acrodystrophic neuropathy)
19. Trichorhinophalangeal dysplasia, type II (Giedion-Langer S.)
20. Werdnig-Hoffman disease
21. Campomelic dysplasia

References
1. Kozlowski K, Beighton P: Gamut Index of Skeletal Dysplasias. Berlin: Springer-Verlag, 1984, pp 5–6
2. Taybi H, Lachman RS: Radiology of Syndromes, Metabolic Disorders, and Skeletal Dysplasias. (ed 4) St. Louis: Mosby-Year Book Inc, 1996, p 1054

Gamut D-108-2

MULTIPLE FRACTURES—
METABOLIC DISORDERS

COMMON

1. Hyperparathyroidism, primary; osteitis fibrosa cystica
2. Renal osteodystrophy (secondary hyperparathyroidism); renal tubular acidosis
3. Rickets, severe (multiple types); Milkman S.
4. Scurvy (metaphyseal chip fractures)

UNCOMMON

1. Aspartylglucosaminuria
2. Copper deficiency, nutritional; Menkes S. (kinky-hair S.)
3. Cystinosis
4. Gaucher disease; Niemann-Pick disease
5. Glycogen storage disease type I (von Gierke disease)
6. GM_1 gangliosidosis
7. Homocystinuria
8. Hyperphosphatasia
9. Hypophosphatasia
10. Lowe S. (oculocerebrorenal S.)
11. Membranous lipodystrophy
12. Mucolipidosis II (I-cell disease)
13. Oxalosis
14. Wilson disease (hepatolenticular degeneration)

Reference
1. Taybi H, Lachman RS: Radiology of Syndromes, Metabolic Disorders, and Skeletal Dysplasias. (ed 4) St. Louis: Mosby-Year Book Inc, 1996, p 1054

Gamut D-108-3

MULTIPLE FRACTURES—OTHER
SKELETAL DISORDERS IN WHICH
FRACTURES MAY OCCUR

COMMON

1. Metastases (esp. carcinomatosis)
2. Multiple myeloma (esp. myelomatosis)
3. Osteomalacia (See D-44)
4. Osteoporosis (See D-43)
5. Paget's disease
6. Steroid therapy; Cushing S.

UNCOMMON

1. Aluminum-induced bone disease
2. Anemia$_g$, primary (esp. thalassemia)
3. Angiomatosis (hemangiomatosis; lymphangiomatosis, cystic type)
4. Arthrogryposis
5. Langerhans cell histiocytosis$_g$
6. Leukemia
7. Osteomyelitis, diffuse (eg, congenital syphilis)

Gamut D-108-4

MULTIPLE FRACTURES—
SKELETAL FRACTURES IN
OTHERWISE NORMAL BONES

COMMON

1. Trauma; battered child S.

UNCOMMON

1. Seizures; electroshock therapy
2. Tetanus

COMMON SITES OF AVULSION INJURIES

1. Ankle (medial and lateral collateral ligaments)
2. Calcaneus (achilles tendon)
3. Elbow (triceps, collateral ligaments)
4. Fingers (volar plate, mallet finger)
5. Foot (eg, site of external digitorum brevis, peroneus brevis, plantar aponeurosis, and sesamoid of great toe—"turf toe")
6. Greater trochanter of femur (abductors)
7. Iliac crest
8. Iliac spines (anterior superior and inferior)
9. Ischial tuberosity (hamstrings and abductor muscle origins)
10. Knee (esp. cruciate ligament origin or insertion)
11. Lesser trochanter of femur (usually pathologic)
12. Shoulder (esp. greater tuberosity, rotator cuff)
13. Spine (anterior longitudinal ligament C2, clay shoveler's fracture)
14. Symphysis pubis (eg, separation of symphysis or avulsion of fragment inferiorly at insertion of gracilis)
15. Wrist (hook of hamate)

Reference

1. Pavlov H: Avulsion injuries—Presented at the International Skeletal Society 18th Annual Refresher Course, San Diego, 1991

PSEUDOFRACTURES*

COMMON

1. Osteomalacia (concave side of bone) (See D-44)
2. Paget's disease (convex side of bone)
3. Rickets (See D-44)
4. [Spondylolysis]
5. [Stress fracture] (See D-111-S)

UNCOMMON

1. Hyperphosphatasia
2. Hypophosphatasia
3. Idiopathic
4. Neuropathic disorder (eg, leprosy)
5. Osteogenesis imperfecta
6. Osteopetrosis
7. Osteoporosis
8. Polyostotic fibrous dysplasia (McCune-Albright S.)
9. Postoperative (eg, graft donor site)
10. Pyknodysostosis
11. Radiation osteitis
12. Renal osteodystrophy (secondary hyperparathyroidism)
13. Rheumatoid arthritis
14. Steroid therapy; Cushing S.

* Incomplete stress (insufficiency) fractures, presenting as narrow radiolucent bands perpendicular to the bony cortex.

[ ] This condition does not actually cause the gamuted imaging finding, but can produce imaging changes that simulate it.

References

1. Burgener FA, Kormano M: Differential Diagnosis in Conventional Radiology. (ed 2) New York: Thieme Medical Publ, 1991, pp 55–58
2. Greenfield GB: Radiology of Bone Diseases. (ed 5) Philadelphia: Lippincott, 1990
3. Grusd R: Pseudofractures and stress fractures. Semin Roentgenol 1978; 13:81–82
4. Murray RO, Jacobson HG, Stoker DJ: The Radiology of Skeletal Disorders. (ed 3) London: Churchill Livingstone, 1990
5. Schneider R, Kaye JJ: Insufficiency and stress fractures of the long bones occurring in patients with rheumatoid arthritis. Radiology 1975; 116:595–599

Gamut D-110-S

SITES OF PSEUDOFRACTURES (LOOSER'S ZONES, MILKMAN SYNDROME)

1. Femur (neck and shaft)
2. Ischial and pubic rami
3. Scapula, outer margin
4. Clavicle
5. Ribs
6. Other long bones (esp. proximal ulna shaft; distal radius shaft)
7. Metacarpals, metatarsals and phalanges

Reference
1. Burgener FA, Kormano M: Differential Diagnosis in Conventional Radiology. (ed 2) New York: Thieme Medical Publ, 1991, p 58

Gamut D-111-S

STRESS FRACTURE (SITES OF PREDILECTION AND CAUSATIVE ACTIVITIES)

1. Athlete (midtibia-shin splints; pubis)
2. Ball thrower; pitcher (distal humeral shaft; coronoid process of ulna)
3. Ballet dancer (spondylolysis of lumbar vertebra; femoral neck and shaft; midtibia; metatarsals)
4. Bowler (pelvis-obturator ring)
5. Chronic coughing (lower ribs); dyspnea (first rib)
6. Clay-shoveler (cervicodorsal spinous process)
7. Golfer (ribs; hook of hamate)
8. Gymnast (pelvis-obturator ring; femoral shaft)
9. Heavy pack-bearer (first rib)
10. Holding golf club, baseball bat, or tennis racquet (hook of hamate)
11. Hurdler (patella)
12. Javelin-thrower (coronoid process of ulna)
13. Lifting or moving heavy objects; scrubbing floors (spondylolysis of lumbar vertebra)
14. Long-distance runner (femoral neck and shaft; tibia; distal fibular shaft)
15. March fracture (metatarsals and proximal phalanges, esp. of 2nd, 3rd and 4th toes; tarsal navicular; femoral shaft)
16. Parachutist; jumper (dorsolumbar vertebrae; proximal fibula; calcaneus)
17. Pitchfork-handler (ulnar shaft)
18. Postoperative-radical neck dissection (clavicle)
19. Prolonged standing (calcaneus; metatarsals; sesamoids)
20. Stamping on ground (tarsal navicular; metatarsals)
21. Stooping (obturator ring)
22. Tic (clavicle)
23. Trapshooter (coracoid process of scapula)
24. Wheelchair operator (ulnar shaft)

References
1. Burgener FA, Kormano M: Differential Diagnosis in Conventional Radiology. (ed 2) New York: Thieme Medical Publ, 1991, p 54
2. Grusd R: Pseudofractures and stress fractures. Semin Roentgenol 1978; 13:81–82

Gamut D-112

PSEUDOARTHROSIS

COMMON
1. Neurofibromatosis (esp. tibia and fibula; also clavicle and radius)
2. Nonunion fracture in a normal bone
3. Pathologic fracture (eg, neoplasm; cyst; osteomyelitis; postradiation)

UNCOMMON
1. Amniotic band S. (Streeters bands)
2. Ankylosing spondylitis (in fused bamboo spine)
3. Cleidocranial dysplasia (esp. clavicle, femur)

(continued)

4. Congenital (esp. clavicle, tibia, fibula, radius, ulna); proximal femoral focal deficiency
5. Fibrous dysplasia
6. Idiopathic; isolated anomaly; familial
7. Increased bone fragility (eg, osteogenesis imperfecta; osteoporosis; osteomalacia)
8. Kuskokwim S. (clavicle)
9. Osteofibrous dysplasia (esp. tibia)
10. Osteopetrosis

References

1. Bell DF: Congenital forearm pseudoarthrosis: report of six cases and review of the literature. J Pediatr Orthop 1989; 9:438–443
2. Greenfield GB: Radiology of Bone Diseases. (ed 5) Philadelphia: Lippincott, 1990
3. Park WM, Spencer DG, McCall IW, et al: The detection of spinal pseudoarthrosis in ankylosing spondylitis. Br J Radiol 1981; 54:467–472
4. Schatz SL, Kopits SE: Proximal femoral focal deficiency. AJR 1978; 131:289–295
5. Schnall SB, King JD, Marrero G: Congenital pseudoarthrosis of the clavicle: A review of the literature and surgical results of six cases. J Pediatr Orthop 1988; 8:316–321
6. Swischuk LE, John SD: Differential Diagnosis in Pediatric Radiology. (ed 2) Baltimore: Williams & Wilkins, 1995, pp 216–218
7. Taybi H, Lachman RS: Radiology of Syndromes, Metabolic Disorders, and Skeletal Dysplasias. (ed 4) St. Louis: Mosby-Year Book, 1996, pp 1039–1040

Gamut D-113

PENCIL-POINTING OF SHAFT OR END OF BONE (VASCULAR DEOSSIFICATION)*

1. Calcium pyrophosphate dihydrate crystal deposition disease (CPPD)
2. Diabetes
3. Leprosy; other neuropathic arthropathy
4. Massive osteolysis (Gorham vanishing bone disease)
5. Psoriatic arthritis
6. Reiter S.

7. Rheumatoid arthritis
8. Sarcoidosis
9. Septic arthritis

* Results from combination of metaphyseal cutback and epiphyseal articular deossification.

Reference

1. Allman RM, Brower A: Radiological Society of North America Scientific Exhibit, 1982

Gamut D-114

EXOSTOSIS

COMMON

1. [Bunion]
2. [Calcaneal spur] (See D-233)
3. [Fracture fragment; healed avulsion injury]
4. Hereditary multiple exostoses (multiple cartilaginous exostoses; osteochondromatosis)
5. [Hypertrophic spur; degenerative arthritis]
6. [Myositis ossificans (traumatic exostosis)]
7. Osteochondroma (metaphyseal)
8. [Pronounced medial tibial metaphyseal beaks in bowed legs]

UNCOMMON

1. Acrodysostosis (peripheral dysostosis) (proximal tibia)
2. [Acromegaly]
3. Adenosine deaminase deficiency
4. Arteriohepatic S. (Alagille S.)
5. Campomelic dysplasia (calcaneal spur)
6. Chondroectodermal dysplasia (Ellis-van Creveld S.) (tibia, humerus)
7. [Copper deficiency, nutritional; Menkes S. (kinky-hair S.)]
8. [Costoclavicular ligament exostosis—midclavicle]
9. [Fibrodysplasia (myositis) ossificans progressiva]
10. [Fluorosis]
11. Iliac spur with tethered cord-sacral lipoma S.

12. Intracapsular osteochondroma; dysplasia epiphysealis hemimelica (Trevor disease) (esp. knee and ankle epiphyses)
13. [Metachondromatosis (hands, feet, knees)]
14. Nail-patella S. (osteo-onychodysplasia) (iliac horns)
15. Occipital horn S. (Ehlers-Danlos S., type IX)
16. Pachydermoperiostosis
17. Pelvic "digit" or "rib"
18. Posthemorrhagic (eg, hemophilia)
19. Pseudohypoparathyroidism; pseudopseudohypoparathyroidism
20. Radiation injury
21. Short rib-polydactyly S. type II (Majewski) and III
22. Spondyloepimetaphyseal dysplasia with joint laxity
23. Subungual exostosis
24. Supracondylar spur of humerus
25. [Tibia vara (Blount disease)]
26. Trichorhinophalangeal dysplasia, type II (Giedion-Langer S.)
27. Tuberous sclerosis
28. Turner S. (medial tibial condyle)
29. Turret exostosis (phalanx)

[ ] This condition does not actually cause the gamuted imaging finding, but can produce imaging changes that simulate it.

References

1. Greenfield GB: Radiology of Bone Diseases. (ed 5) Philadelphia: Lippincott, 1990
2. Guidera KJ, Scatterwhite Y, Ogden JA, et al: Nail patella syndrome: A review of 44 orthopaedic patients. J Pediatr Orthop 1991; 11:737–742
3. Keret D, Spatz DK, Caro PA, et al: Dysplasia epiphysealis hemimelica: diagnosis and treatment. J Pediatr Orthop 1992; 12:365–372
4. Kozlowski K, Beighton P: Gamut Index of Skeletal Dysplasias. Berlin: Springer-Verlag, 1984, p 14
5. McAlister WH, Siegel MJ, Shackleford GD: A congenital iliac anomaly often associated with sacral lipoma and ipsilateral lower extremity weakness. Skeletal Radiol 1978; 3:161–166
6. Pazzaglia UE, Pedrotti L, Beluffi G, et al: Radiographic findings in hereditary multiple exostoses and a new theory of the pathogenesis of exostoses. Pediatr Radiol 1990; 20:594–597
7. Poznanski AK: The Hand in Radiologic Diagnosis. (ed 2) Philadelphia: WB Saunders, 1984, p 920
8. Swischuk LE, John SD: Differential Diagnosis in Pediatric Radiology. (ed 2) Baltimore: Williams & Wilkins, 1995, pp 232–235
9. Taybi H, Lachman RS: Radiology of Syndromes, Metabolic Disorders, and Skeletal Dysplasias. (ed 4) St. Louis: Mosby-Year Book, 1996, pp 1037, 1044

Gamut D-115

SYNOSTOSIS OF TUBULAR BONES (See D-163, D-166)

1. Acrocephalosyndactyly (Pfeiffer type)
2. Chromosome 4: del(4p) S. (Wolf-Hirschhorn S.)
3. Cloverleaf skull deformity (kleeblattschädel anomaly)
4. Diastrophic dysplasia (metatarsals)
5. Ehlers-Danlos S.
6. Fetal alcohol S.
7. Hereditary multiple exostoses (multiple cartilaginous exostoses; osteochondromatosis)
8. Holt-Oram S.
9. Humeroradial-humeroulnar synostosis (See D-166)
10. Inflammatory periostitis, severe (eg, infantile cortical hyperostosis {Caffey disease})
11. Klinefelter S. (XXY S.)
12. Lenz-Majewski dysplasia
13. Mesomelic dysplasia
14. Multiple synostosis S.
15. Nager acrofacial dysostosis
16. Posttraumatic (esp. following severe bleeding)
17. Radioulnar synostosis (See D-163)
18. Trisomy 18 S.
19. XXXXY S.; XXXXX S.; XXXY S.

References

1. Swischuk LE, John SD: Differential Diagnosis in Pediatric Radiology. (ed 2) Baltimore: Williams & Wilkins, 1995, pp 215–216
2. Taybi H, Lachman RS: Radiology of Syndromes, Metabolic Disorders, and Skeletal Dysplasias. (ed 4) St. Louis: Mosby-Year Book, 1996, p 1042

Gamut D-116

GAS WITHIN BONE
(ESPECIALLY ON CT)

1. Intraosseous ganglion
2. Methylmethacrylate prosthesis
3. Neoplasm (esp. after radiation therapy)
4. Osteomyelitis (gas forming organism)
5. Osteonecrosis
6. Postoperative; posttraumatic
7. Subchondral bone cyst ("vacuum cyst" or pneumatocyst)

References
1. Greenfield GB: Radiology of Bone Diseases. (ed 5) Philadelphia: Lippincott, 1990
2. Ramirez H Jr, Blatt ES, Cable HF, et al: Intraosseous pneumatocysts of the ilium: Findings on radiographs and CT scans. Radiology 1984; 150:503–505

Gamut D-117-1

CONGENITAL THUMB
ABNORMALITIES—ABSENT THUMB

1. Fanconi anemia (pancytopenia-dysmelia S.)
2. Franceschetti S.
3. Holt-Oram S.
4. Phocomelia (eg, thalidomide embryopathy)
5. Poland S. (pectoral muscle aplasia—syndactyly)
6. Rothmund-Thomson S.
7. Seckel S. (bird-headed dwarfism)
8. Trisomy 18 S.
9. Yunis-Varón S.

References
1. Jones KL: Smith's Recognizable Patterns of Human Malformation. Philadelphia: WB Saunders, 1988
2. Poznanski AK: The Hand in Radiologic Diagnosis. (ed 2) Philadelphia: WB Saunders, 1984, p 912

3. Poznanski AK, Garn SM, Holt JF: The thumb in the congenital malformation syndromes. Radiology 1971; 100: 115–129
4. Silverman F (ed): Caffey's Pediatric X-ray Diagnosis. (ed 8) Chicago: Year Book Medical Publ, 1985
5. Swischuk LE, John SD: Differential Diagnosis in Pediatric Radiology. (ed 2) Baltimore: Williams & Wilkins, 1995, pp 270–273
6. Taybi H, Lachman RS: Radiology of Syndromes, Metabolic Disorders, and Skeletal Dysplasias. (ed 4) St. Louis: Mosby-Year Book, 1996, pp 1042–1043

Gamut D-117-2

HYPOPLASTIC THIN
OR SHORT THUMB

1. Acrocephalopolysyndactyly (Carpenter S.)
2. Acrocephalosyndactyly (Apert type)
3. Acrodysostosis (peripheral dysostosis)
4. Aminopterin fetopathy
5. Baller-Gerold S. (craniosynostosis-radial aplasia S.)
6. Brachmann-de Lange S. (de Lange S.)
7. Cephaloskeletal dysplasia (Taybi-Linder S.)
8. Christian S. (adducted thumbs S.)
9. Chromosome 18: del(18q) S.
10. Desbuquois dysplasia
11. Diastrophic dysplasia
12. Dyggve-Melchior-Clausen dysplasia (Smith-McCort S.)
13. Dyssegmental dysplasia
14. Ectodermal dysplasia
15. Familial brachydactyly C or D; hereditary shortness of thumbs
16. Fanconi anemia (pancytopenia-dysmelia S.)
17. Fibrodysplasia (myositis) ossificans progressiva
18. Gorlin S. (nevoid basal cell carcinoma S.)
19. Hand-foot-genital S.
20. Holt-Oram S.
21. Isolated anomaly
22. IVIC S.
23. Juberg-Hayward S.
24. Mesomelic dysplasia (Werner type)

25. Otopalatodigital S. (types I and II)
26. Phocomelia (eg, thalidomide embryopathy)
27. Popliteal pterygium S.
28. Radial hypoplasia syndromes
29. Rubinstein-Taybi S.
30. Smith-Lemli-Opitz S.
31. Symphalangism-surdity S. (symphalangism-brachy-dactyly S. or WL S.)
32. TAR S. (thrombocytopenia-absent radius S.)
33. Trisomy 9p S.
34. Trisomy 18 S.
35. VATER association
36. Werner S.

References
1. Jones KL: Smith's Recognizable Patterns of Human Malformation. Philadelphia: WB Saunders, 1988
2. Poznanski AK: The Hand in Radiologic Diagnosis. (ed 2) Philadelphia: WB Saunders, 1984, p 912
3. Poznanski AK, Garn SM, Holt JF: The thumb in the congenital malformation syndromes. Radiology 1971; 100: 115–129
4. Silverman F (ed): Caffey's Pediatric X-ray Diagnosis. (ed 8) Chicago: Year Book Medical Publ, 1985
5. Swischuk LE, John SD: Differential Diagnosis in Pediatric Radiology. (ed 2) Baltimore: Williams & Wilkins, 1995, pp 270–273
6. Taybi H, Lachman RS: Radiology of Syndromes, Metabolic Disorders, and Skeletal Dysplasias. (ed 4) St. Louis: Mosby-Year Book, 1996, pp 1042–1043

Gamut D-117-3

WIDE THUMB

1. Acrocephalopolysyndactyly (Carpenter S.)
2. Acrocephalosyndactyly (Apert and Pfeiffer types)
3. Acromesomelic dysplasia
4. Diastrophic dysplasia
5. FG syndrome
6. Fibrodysplasia (myositis) ossificans progressiva
7. Frontodigital S.
8. Greig cephalopolysyndactyly S.
9. Hand-foot-genital S.
10. Larsen S.
11. Léri pleonosteosis
12. Meckel S.
13. Otopalatodigital S. (types I and II)
14. Robinow S.
15. Rubinstein-Taybi S.
16. Trisomy 13 S.
17. Weaver-Smith S.

Gamut D-117-4

ENLARGED THUMB

1. Angioma, arteriovenous malformation (Klippel-Trenaunay S.; Parkes Weber S.)
2. Isolated anomaly
3. Lipoma
4. Macrodystrophia lipomatosa
5. Maffucci S.
6. Neurofibromatosis
7. Proteus S.
8. Triphalangeal thumb (eg, Diamond-Blackfan S.)

Gamut D-117-5

ECTOPIC THUMB (ABNORMAL POSITION)

1. Brachmann-de Lange S. (de Lange S.) (proximally placed thumb)
2. Diastrophic dysplasia ("hitchhiker thumb")
3. Freeman-Sheldon S. (whistling face S.) (flexed thumb overlaps palm)
4. Rubinstein-Taybi S. (radially curved or "hitchhiker thumb")

Gamut D-117-6

TRIPHALANGEAL THUMB

1. Aase S.
2. Diamond-Blackfan S.
3. DOOR S.
4. Duane-radial S. (DR S.)
5. Fanconi anemia (pancytopenia-dysmelia S.)
6. Fetal hydantoin S. (Dilantin embryopathy)
7. Goodman S.
8. Holt-Oram S.
9. Hypomelanosis of Ito
10. IVIC S.
11. Juberg-Hayward S.
12. Lacrimo-auriculo-dento-digital S. (LADD S.) (Levy-Hollister S.)
13. Mesomelic dysplasia (Werner type)
14. Normal variant; isolated anomaly
15. Poland S. (pectoral muscle aplasia-syndactyly)
16. Thalidomide embryopathy
17. Townes-Brocks S.
18. Trichorhinophalangeal dysplasia, type II (Giedion-Langer S.)
19. Trisomy 13 S.
20. Trisomy 22 S.
21. VATER association

References

1. Jones KL: Smith's Recognizable Patterns of Human Malformation. Philadelphia: WB Saunders, 1988
2. Poznanski AK: The Hand in Radiologic Diagnosis. (ed 2) Philadelphia: WB Saunders, 1984, p 912
3. Poznanski AK, Garn SM, Holt JF: The thumb in the congenital malformation syndromes. Radiology 1971; 100: 115–129
4. Silverman F (ed): Caffey's Pediatric X-ray Diagnosis. (ed 8) Chicago: Year Book Medical Publ, 1985
5. Swischuk LE, John SD: Differential Diagnosis in Pediatric Radiology. (ed 2) Baltimore: Williams & Wilkins, 1995, pp 270–273
6. Taybi H, Lachman RS: Radiology of Syndromes, Metabolic Disorders, and Skeletal Dysplasias. (ed 4) St. Louis: Mosby-Year Book, 1996, pp 1042–1043

Gamut D-118-S

THUMB APPEARANCE IN VARIOUS SYNDROMES*

	Distal Phalanx				Proximal Phalanx				Metacarpal						
	Cone Epiphysis	Short $\frac{Met\,2}{D1}$	Broad	Triphalangeal Thumb	Short $\frac{Met\,2}{P1}$	Long $\frac{Met\,2}{D1}$	Triangular	Thin Short	Wide $\frac{Met\,2}{Met\,1}$	Long $\frac{Met\,2}{Met\,1}$	Pseudoepiphysis	Clasped Thumb	"Hitchhiker" Thumb	Duplication	Absent Thumb
Apert's and other acrocephalosyndactyly		X	X		X		X						O	O	
Arthrogryposis												X			
Holt-Oram		X		X				X	X						X
Brackmann-de Lange		X							X						
Diastrophic dysplasia		O			O				X					X	
Hand-foot-genital	X	O			O				X	X					
Fibrodysplasia ossificans		X			O	O			X	O					
Otopalatodigital	X	X													
Pancytopenia-dysmelia (Fanconi's anemia)		X						X						O	X
Rubinstein-Taybi		X	X		X	X							X		
Thalidomide embryopathy				X											O
Trisomy 18		O													O

(Modified from Poznanski AK, Garn SM, Holt JF: Radiology 1971;100:115-129)

* O = occasional; X = frequent; P1 = proximal phalanx of thumb; D1 = distal phalanx of thumb

Gamut D-119-1

SHORT DISTAL PHALANX OF THE THUMB—SHORT AND BROAD

1. Acrocephalopolysyndactyly (Carpenter S.)
2. Acrocephalosyndactyly (Apert and Pfeiffer types)
3. Christian S. (adducted thumbs S.)
4. Diastrophic dysplasia
5. Familial brachydactyly A-4 and D
6. Fibrodysplasia (myositis) ossificans progressiva
7. Hand-foot-genital S.
8. Osteodysplasty (Melnick-Needles S.)
9. Otopalatodigital S.
10. Pseudohypoparathyroidism; pseudopseudohypoparathyroidism
11. Robinow S.
12. Rubinstein-Taybi S.

Reference

1. Poznanski AK: The Hand in Radiologic Diagnosis. (ed 2) Philadelphia: WB Saunders, 1984, p 905

Gamut D-119-2

SHORT DISTAL PHALANX OF THE THUMB—THIN AND SMALL

1. Brachmann-de Lange S. (de Lange S.)
2. Fanconi anemia (pancytopenia-dysmelia S.)
3. Fibrodysplasia (myositis) ossificans progressiva
4. Holt-Oram S.
5. Radial hypoplasia syndromes (See D-161)
6. Trisomy 18 S.

Reference
1. Poznanski AK: The Hand in Radiologic Diagnosis. (ed 2) Philadelphia: WB Saunders, 1984, p 905

Gamut D-120

SHORT PROXIMAL PHALANX OF THE THUMB AND/OR OTHER DIGITS

ACQUIRED
1. Arthritis
2. Infection (eg, osteomyelitis; yaws; smallpox residual)
3. Neoplasm
4. Trauma
5. Sickle cell disease

CONGENITAL
1. Acrocephalopolysyndactyly (Carpenter S.)
2. Acrocephalosyndactyly (Apert and Pfeiffer types)
3. Diastrophic dysplasia
4. DOOR S.
5. Familial brachydactyly A-1, A-2, and C
6. Fibrodysplasia (myositis) ossificans progressiva
7. Gorlin S. (nevoid basal cell carcinoma S.)
8. Rubinstein-Taybi S.
9. Trisomy 18 S.

Reference
1. Taybi H, Lachman RS: Radiology of Syndromes, Metabolic Disorders, and Skeletal Dysplasias. (ed 4) St. Louis: Mosby-Year Book, 1996, p 1043

Gamut D-121-1

"DRUMSTICK" DISTAL PHALANGES*

1. Chromosome 5: del(5p) S. (Cri-du-chat S.)
2. Coffin-Lowry S.
3. Holt-Oram S.
4. Normal variant
5. Trisomy 21 (Down S.)
6. Turner S.

* The phalangeal shaft is disproportionately thinned in comparison to the tuft.

References
1. Poznanski AK: The Hand in Radiologic Diagnosis. (ed 2) Philadelphia: WB Saunders, 1984
2. Swischuk LE, John SD: Differential Diagnosis in Pediatric Radiology. (ed 2) Baltimore: Williams & Wilkins, 1995, p 266

Gamut D-121-2

BROAD DISTAL PHALANX OF THE THUMB

1. Acrocephalopolysyndactyly (Carpenter S.)
2. Acrocephalosyndactyly (Apert and Pfeiffer types)
3. Familial brachydactyly B and D
4. Mesomelic dysplasia (Robinow type)
5. Otopalatodigital S.
6. Rubinstein-Taybi S.
7. Syndactyly

Reference
1. Poznanski AK: The Hand in Radiologic Diagnosis. (ed 2) Philadelphia; WB Saunders, 1984, p 901

Gamut D-121-3

BROAD DISTAL PHALANGES
OF OTHER DIGITS

1. Atelosteogenesis (type I)
2. Distal brachydactyly
3. Larsen S.
4. Pachyonychia congenita
5. Warfarin embryopathy

Reference
1. Poznanski AK: The Hand in Radiologic Diagnosis. (ed 2) Philadelphia; WB Saunders, 1984, p 901

Gamut D-121-4

BROAD MIDDLE PHALANGES
OF OTHER DIGITS

1. Achondroplasia (infant)
2. Acrodysostosis (peripheral dysostosis)
3. Acrodysplasia with retinitis pigmentosa and nephropathy (Saldino-Mainzer S.)
4. Acromesomelic dysplasia
5. Campomelic dysplasia
6. Chondrodysplasia punctata (infant)
7. Chondroectodermal dysplasia (Ellis-van Creveld S.) (infant)
8. Familial brachydactyly A-1
9. Frontometaphyseal dysplasia
10. Marshall S.
11. Mucolipidosis III (pseudo-Hurler polydystrophy)
12. Noonan S.
13. Pseudoachondroplasia (pseudoachondroplastic spondyloepiphyseal dysplasia)
14. Trichorhinophalangeal dysplasia, type I (Giedion S.) and II (Giedion-Langer S.)

Reference
1. Poznanski AK: The Hand in Radiologic Diagnosis. (ed 2) Philadelphia; WB Saunders, 1984, p 901

Gamut D-122-1

CONGENITAL ABNORMALITY
OF THE GREAT TOE

COMMON
1. Acrocephalosyndactyly (Apert, Pfeiffer, and Saethre-Chotzen types)
2. Brachmann-de Lange S. (de Lange S.)
3. Fibrodysplasia (myositis) ossificans progressiva
4. Otopalatodigital S.
5. Rubinstein-Taybi S.

UNCOMMON
1. Acrocephalopolysyndactyly (Carpenter S.)
2. Acrocallosal S.
3. Chromosome 4: del (4p) S. (Wolf-Hirschhorn S.)
4. Cleidocranial dysplasia
5. Craniofrontonasal dysplasia
6. Diastrophic dysplasia
7. Femoral hypoplasia—unusual facies S.
8. Freeman-Sheldon S. (whistling face S.)
9. Frontodigital S.
10. Greig cephalopolysyndactyly S.
11. Hand-foot-genital S.
12. Larsen S.
13. Léri pleonosteosis
14. Orofaciodigital syndrome I (Papillon-Leage and Psaume S.) and II (Mohr S.)
15. Popliteal pterygium S.
16. Trisomy 13 S.
17. Trisomy 18 S.
18. XXXXY S.

Reference
1. Poznanski AK: Foot manifestations of the congenital malformation syndromes. Semin Roentgenol 1970; 5:354–366

DUPLICATION OF THE GREAT TOE (HALLUCAL POLYDACTYLY)

1. Acrocallosal S.
2. Acrocephalosyndactyly (Apert, Pfeiffer, and Saethre-Chotzen types)
3. Chromosome 4: del (4p) S. (Wolf-Hirschhorn S.)
4. Craniofrontonasal dysplasia
5. Femoral hypoplasia—unusual facies S.
6. Rubinstein-Taybi S.

References

1. Gorlin RJ, Cohen MM, Jr, Levin LS: Syndromes of the Head and Neck. New York: Oxford Univ Press, 1990, p 678
2. Taybi H, Lachman RS: Radiology of Syndromes, Metabolic Disorders, and Skeletal Dysplasias. (ed 4) St. Louis: Mosby-Year Book, 1996

Gamut D-123

CLINODACTYLY OF THE FIFTH FINGER (INCURVING OF FIFTH DIGIT WITH HYPOPLASTIC SHORT MIDDLE PHALANX)

COMMON

1. Brachmann-de Lange S. (de Lange S.)
2. Ehlers-Danlos S.
3. Familial brachydactyly A1, A2, A3, A4, C
4. Fanconi anemia (pancytopenia-dysmelia S.)
5. Fetal alcohol S.
6. Fibrodysplasia (myositis) ossificans progressiva
7. Hand-foot-genital S.
8. Holt-Oram S.
9. [Kirner deformity (distal phalanx—seen as isolated anomaly or in Brachmann-de Lange S. {de Lange S.} or Silver-Russell S.)]
10. Klinefelter S. (XXY S.)
11. Local disorder (eg, trauma; arthritis; contracture)

12. Marfan S.
13. Metaphyseal chondrodysplasia (Shwachman type)
14. Mitral valve prolapse S.
15. Nail-patella S. (osteo-onychodysplasia)
16. Noonan S.
17. Normal variant; isolated anomaly
18. Oculodento-osseous dysplasia
19. Orofaciodigital syndrome I (Papillon-Leage and Psaume S.) and II (Mohr S.)
20. Otopalatodigital S. (type I)
21. Poland S. (pectoral muscle aplasia—syndactyly)
22. Silver-Russell S.
23. TAR S. (thrombocytopenia-absent radius S.)
24. Trisomy 21 S. (Down S.)
25. Williams S. (idiopathic hypercalcemia)

UNCOMMON

1. Aarskog S.
2. Acrocephalopolysyndactyly (Carpenter S.)
3. Acrocephalosyndactyly (Saethre-Chotzen type)
4. Aminopterin fetopathy
5. Bardet-Biedl S.; Laurence-Moon S.
6. Bloom S.
7. Campomelic dysplasia
8. Cat cry S. (cri du chat S.)
9. Chromosome 4: del(4p) S. (Wolf-Hirschhorn S.)
10. Coffin-Siris S.
11. Cohen S.
12. DOOR S.
13. Dubowitz S.
14. EEC syndrome
15. Fibrochondrogenesis
16. Goltz S. (focal dermal hypoplasia)
17. Goodman S.
18. Hypomelanosis of Ito
19. Lacrimo-auriculo-dento-digital S. (LADD S.) (Levy-Hollister S.)
20. Lenz microphthalmia S.
21. Meckel S.
22. Mesomelic dysplasia (Nievergelt type)
23. Popliteal pterygium S.
24. Prader-Willi S.
25. Rieger S.

26. Roberts S. (pseudothalidomide S.)
27. Robinow S.
28. Rubinstein-Taybi S.
29. Ruvalcaba S. (trichorhinophalangeal S., type III)
30. Seckel S. (bird-headed dwarfism)
31. Symphalangism-surdity S. (symphalangism-brachydactyly S. or WL S.)
32. Treacher Collins S.
33. Trichorhinophalangeal dysplasia, type I (Giedion S.) and II (Giedion-Langer S.)
34. Triploidy
35. Trisomy syndromes (8, 9p, 13, 18)
36. Weill-Marchesani S.
37. XXXX S.; XXXY S.; XXXXX S.; XXXXY S.
38. Zellweger S. (cerebrohepatorenal S.)

[ ] This condition does not actually cause the gamuted imaging finding, but can produce imaging changes that simulate it.

References

1. Edeiken J, Dalinka M, Karasick D: Edeiken's Roentgen Diagnosis of Diseases of Bone. (ed 4) Baltimore: Williams & Wilkins, 1989
2. Jones KL: Smith's Recognizable Patterns of Human Malformation. Philadelphia: WB Saunders, 1988
3. Poznanski AK: The Hand in Radiologic Diagnosis. (ed 2) Philadelphia: WB Saunders, 1984, pp 907, 915
4. Poznanski AK, Pratt GB, Manson G, et al: Clinodactyly, camptodactyly, Kirner's deformity, and other crooked fingers. Radiology 1969; 93:573–582
5. Swischuk LE, John SD: Differential Diagnosis in Pediatric Radiology. (ed 2) Baltimore: Williams & Wilkins, 1995, p 274
6. Taybi H, Lachman RS: Radiology of Syndromes, Metabolic Disorders, and Skeletal Dysplasias. (ed 4) St. Louis: Mosby-Year Book, 1996, p 1025

Gamut D-124

CONGENITAL SYNDROMES WITH ONE OR MORE SHORT MIDDLE PHALANGES (OTHER THAN FIFTH FINGER)

1. Aarskog S.
2. Acrocephalopolysyndactyly (Carpenter S.)
3. Acrocephalosyndactyly (Apert type)
4. Acrodysplasia with retinitis pigmentosa and nephropathy (Saldino-Mainzer S.)
5. Asphyxiating thoracic dysplasia (Jeune S.)
6. Atelosteogenesis
7. Campomelic dysplasia
8. Cleidocranial dysplasia
9. Cloverleaf skull deformity (kleeblattschädel anomaly)
10. Familial brachydactylies A1, A4, B, and C (A2 and A3—second finger)
11. Lacrimo-auriculo-dento-digital S. (LADD S.) (Levy-Hollister S.)
12. Poland S. (pectoral muscle aplasia-syndactyly)
13. Pseudohypoparathyroidism; pseudopseudohypoparathyroidism (second finger)
14. Ruvalcaba S. (trichorhinophalangeal S., type III)
15. Sclerosteosis (second finger)
16. Symphalangism-surdity S. (symphalangism-brachydactyly S. or WL S.)
17. Trichorhinophalangeal dysplasia, type I (Giedion S.) and II (Giedion-Langer S.)

References

1. Poznanski AK: The Hand in Radiologic Diagnosis. (ed 2) Philadelphia: WB Saunders, 1984, p 907
2. Taybi H, Lachman RS: Radiology of Syndromes, Metabolic Disorders, and Skeletal Dysplasias. (ed 4) St. Louis: Mosby-Year Book, 1996

Gamut D-125-1

GENERALIZED SHORT DISTAL PHALANGES OF THE HAND—SHORT AND BROAD

1. Achondroplasia
2. Acrodysostosis (peripheral dysostosis)
3. Acro-osteolysis (eg, frostbite; burn; leprosy; trauma) (See D-127)
4. Asphyxiating thoracic dysplasia (Jeune S.)
5. Cleidocranial dysplasia
6. Coffin-Lowry S.
7. Diastrophic dysplasia
8. DOOR S.
9. Hypochondroplasia
10. Larsen S.
11. Metaphyseal chondrodysplasia (Jansen type)
12. Pachydermoperiostosis
13. Pseudoachondroplasia (pseudoachondroplastic spondyloepiphyseal dysplasia)
14. Pseudohypoparathyroidism; pseudopseudohypoparathyroidism
15. Robinow S.
16. Warfarin embryopathy

Reference
1. Poznanski AK: The Hand in Radiologic Diagnosis. (ed 2) Philadelphia: WB Saunders, 1984, pp 905–906

Gamut D-125-2

GENERALIZED SHORT DISTAL PHALANGES OF THE HAND—THIN AND SMALL

1. Acrocephalopolysyndactyly (Carpenter S.)
2. Acro-osteolysis (eg, frostbite; burn; leprosy; trauma) (See D-127)
3. Asphyxiating thoracic dysplasia (Jeune S.)
4. Chondroectodermal dysplasia (Ellis-van Creveld S.)

5. Christian S. (adducted thumbs S.)
6. Coffin-Siris S.
7. Fetal alcohol S.
8. Fetal hydantoin S. (Dilantin embryopathy)
9. Hypoplastic nails S.
10. Marshall S.
11. Mucolipidosis II (I-cell disease)
12. Opitz trigonocephaly S. (C syndrome)
13. Osteodysplasty (Melnick-Needles S.)
14. Pseudohypoparathyroidism
15. Symphalangism-surdity S. (symphalangism-brachydactyly S. or WL S.)
16. Trisomy 9p S.
17. Trisomy 13 S.
18. Trisomy 18 S.
19. Warfarin embryopathy

Reference
1. Poznanski AK: The Hand in Radiologic Diagnosis. (ed 2) Philadelphia: WB Saunders, 1984, pp 905–906

Gamut D-126

HYPOPLASTIC (SPINDLE-SHAPED OR STUBBY) TERMINAL PHALANGES

COMMON
1. Acro-osteolysis (eg, hyperparathyroidism; frostbite; burn; leprosy; trauma; idiopathic) (See D-127)
2. Brachmann-de Lange S. (de Lange S.)
3. Cleidocranial dysplasia
4. Congenital insensitivity to pain
5. Fanconi anemia (pancytopenia-dysmelia S.)
6. Fibrodysplasia (myositis) ossificans progressiva
7. Holt-Oram S.
8. Normal (foot)
9. Pseudohypoparathyroidism; pseudopseudohypoparathyroidism
10. Pyknodysostosis
11. Spade hand

UNCOMMON

1. Aarskog S.
2. Acrocephalopolysyndactyly (Carpenter S.)
3. Acrocephalosyndactyly (Apert type)
4. Arteriohepatic S. (Alagille S.)
5. Asphyxiating thoracic dysplasia (Jeune S.)
6. Chondroectodermal dysplasia (Ellis-van Creveld S.)
7. Coffin-Lowry S.
8. Coffin-Siris S.
9. Diastrophic dysplasia
10. Ehlers-Danlos S.
11. Epidermolysis bullosa
12. Familial brachydactyly B
13. Fetal hydantoin S. (Dilantin embryopathy)
14. Hand-foot-genital S.
15. Hypoplastic nails S.
16. Larsen S.
17. Osteopetrosis
18. Otopalatodigital S.
19. Progeria
20. Pseudoxanthoma elasticum
21. Rothmund-Thomson S.
22. Rubinstein-Taybi S.
23. Trisomy 13 S.
24. Trisomy 18 S.
25. Warfarin embryopathy

References

1. Brown DM, Bradford DS, Gorlin RJ, et al: The acro-osteolysis syndrome: morphologic and biochemical studies. J Pediatr 1976; 88:573–575
2. Poznanski AK: The Hand in Radiologic Diagnosis. (ed 2) Philadelphia: WB Saunders, 1984, pp 214–215
3. Swischuk LE, John SD: Differential Diagnosis in Pediatric Radiology. (ed 2) Baltimore: Williams & Wilkins, 1995, pp 267–269
4. Taybi H, Lachman RS: Radiology of Syndromes, Metabolic Disorders, and Skeletal Dysplasias. (ed 3) Chicago: Year Book Medical Publ, 1990, pp 464–465

Gamut D-127-1

ACRO-OSTEOLYSIS (EROSION OR DESTRUCTION OF MULTIPLE TERMINAL PHALANGEAL TUFTS)

COMMON

1. Arteriosclerosis obliterans
2. Diabetic gangrene
+*3. Hyperparathyroidism, primary or secondary (renal osteodystrophy)
4. Infection (eg, meningococcemia); osteitis
5. Neuropathic disease (esp. diabetes; leprosy; tabes dorsalis; syringomyelia; meningomyelocele) (See D-150)
6. Psoriatic arthritis
7. Raynaud disease
8. Rheumatoid arthritis; juvenile rheumatoid arthritis (+)
*9. Scleroderma; dermatomyositis; mixed connective tissue disease (MCTD)
10. Thermal injury (eg, burn; frostbite; electrical)
11. Trauma (biomechanical stress; guitar player)

UNCOMMON

1. Amniotic band S. (Streeter bands)
2. Buerger disease (thromboangiitis obliterans)
+3. Cleidocranial dysplasia
4. Clubbing of fingers (See D-133)
+5. Congenital (familial or idiopathic) acro-osteolysis (eg, Hajdu-Cheney S.)
*6. Congenital insensitivity to pain
7. Familial brachydactyly B
8. Farber disease (disseminated lipogranulomatosis)
9. Drug therapy (eg, Dilantin; phenobarbital; ergot reaction)
10. Dysosteosclerosis
11. Ectodermal dysplasia
*12. Ehlers-Danlos S.
*13. Epidermolysis bullosa
*14. Gout
15. Hunger osteopathy

(continued)

16. Hypertrophic osteoarthropathy
17. Lesch-Nyhan S.
18. Mandibuloacral dysplasia
19. Metastasis
20. Multicentric reticulohistiocytosis (lipoid dermatoarthritis)
21. Osteomalacia (eg, malabsorption syndromes)
22. Osteopetrosias
23. Osteopoikilosis
24. Pachydermoperiostosis
25. Papillon-Lefèvre S.
26. Pityriasis rubra
27. Plantar warts
+28. Polyvinyl chloride osteolysis; chemical acro-osteolysis
29. Porphyria
30. Progeria; Werner S.
31. Pseudoxanthoma elasticum
32. Pyknodysostosis
33. Radiation injury
*34. Rothmund-Thomson S.
35. Sarcoidosis
36. Singleton-Merten S.
37. Sjögren S.
38. Snake or scorpion venom
39. Thevenard S.
40. Thrombotic thrombocytopenic purpura
41. Winchester S.

* May be associated with calcification.
+ Band-like resorption of midportion of phalanx.

References

1. Destouet JM, Murphy WA: Acquired acroosteolysis and acronecrosis. Arthritis Rheum 1983; 26:1150–1154
2. Greenfield GB: Radiology of Bone Diseases. (ed 5) Philadelphia: Lippincott, 1990
3. Jones SN, Stoker DJ: Radiology at your fingertips; lesions of the terminal phalanx. Clin Radiol 1988; 39:478–485
4. Kozlowski K, Beighton P: Gamut Index of Skeletal Dysplasias. Berlin: Springer-Verlag, 1984, pp 76–77
5. Moss AA, Mainzer F: Osteopetrosis: An unusual cause of terminal-tuft erosion. Radiology 1970; 97:631–632
6. Poznanski AK: The Hand in Radiologic Diagnosis. (ed 2) Philadelphia: WB Saunders, 1984, p 170
7. Swischuk LE, John SD: Differential Diagnosis in Pediatric Radiology. (ed 2) Baltimore: Williams & Wilkins, 1995, pp 267–269
8. Taybi H, Lachman RS: Radiology of Syndromes, Metabolic Disorders, and Skeletal Dysplasias. (ed 4) St. Louis: Mosby-Year Book, 1996, p 1021

Gamut D-127-2

ACQUIRED ACRO-OSTEOLYSIS CONFINED TO ONE DIGIT

1. Angioma$_g$
2. Carcinoma of nail bed
3. Epidermoid inclusion cyst
4. Fibroma
5. Giant cell tumor of tendon sheath
6. Glomus tumor
7. Infection (eg, osteomyelitis, paronychia)
8. Lymphoma$_g$
9. Metastasis
10. Neurofibroma
11. Subungual exostosis
12. Thermal injury (eg, burn; frostbite; electrical)

Gamut D-127-3

BAND-LIKE DESTRUCTION OR EROSION OF THE MIDPORTION OF A TERMINAL PHALANX

1. Ainhum (usually proximal phalanx)
2. Chemical acro-osteolysis (eg, polyvinyl chloride)
3. Cleidocranial dysplasia
4. Congenital (familial or idiopathic) acro-osteolysis (eg, Hajdu-Cheney S.)
5. Hyperparathyroidism, primary or secondary (renal osteodystrophy)
6. Juvenile rheumatoid arthritis

Reference

1. Burgener FA, Kormano M: Differential Diagnosis in Conventional Radiology. New York: Thieme Medical Publ, 1991, p 280

Gamut D-128

ACRO-OSTEOSCLEROSIS (TERMINAL PHALANGEAL SCLEROSIS)

COMMON

1. Idiopathic, normal variant
2. Rheumatoid arthritis

UNCOMMON

1. Lupus erythematosus
2. Melorheostosis
3. Osteopetrosis
4. Osteopoikilosis
5. Sarcoidosis
6. Scleroderma

References

1. Burgener FA, Kormano M: Differential Diagnosis in Conventional Radiology. New York: Thieme Medical Publ, 1991, p 276
2. Goodman N: The significance of terminal phalangeal osteosclerosis. Radiology 1967; 89:709–712
3. Williams M, Barton E: Terminal phalangeal sclerosis in rheumatoid arthritis. Clin Radiol 1984; 35:237–238

Gamut D-129-1

AMPUTATION OR ABSENCE OF A PHALANX, DIGIT, HAND, OR FOOT—ACQUIRED

COMMON

1. Diabetes
2. Infection; severe osteomyelitis (eg, mycetoma)
3. Leprosy
4. Neurologic disorder
5. Scleroderma
6. Surgical amputation
7. Thermal injury (eg, frostbite; burn; electrical)

8. Trauma; battered child S.
9. Vascular insufficiency (eg, arteriosclerosis; ergot reaction; gangrene)

UNCOMMON

1. Ainhum
2. Congenital insensitivity to pain
3. Constriction (eg, bandages; bands; strings; hair)
4. Disseminated intravascular coagulation (eg, meningococcemia)
5. Lesch-Nyhan S.
6. Psoriasis, severe
7. Psychotic states
8. Radiation, radium injury

References

1. Poznanski AK: The Hand in Radiologic Diagnosis. (ed 2) Philadelphia: WB Saunders, 1984, p 912
2. Swischuk LE, John SD: Differential Diagnosis in Pediatric Radiology. (ed 2) Baltimore: Williams & Wilkins, 1995, pp 276–278

Gamut D-129-2

AMPUTATION OR ABSENCE OF A PHALANX, DIGIT, HAND, OR FOOT—CONGENITAL

COMMON

1. Amniotic band S. (Streeter bands)
2. Thalidomide embryopathy

UNCOMMON

1. Aglossia-adactylia S.; hypoglossia-hypodactylia S.)
2. Aplasia cutis congenita
3. Arthrogryposis (toe)
4. Brachmann-de Lange S. (de Lange S.)
5. Claw hand
6. Fetal hydantoin S. (Dilantin embryopathy)

(continued)

7. Grebe chondrodysplasia (achondrogenesis, Brazilian type)
8. Keratosis palmaris et plantaris familiaris (tylosis)
9. Möbius S.
10. Poland S. (pectoral muscle aplasia—syndactyly)
11. Popliteal pterygium S.
12. Radial and ulnar ray syndromes (See D-161, D-162)
13. Roberts S. (pseudothalidomide S.)

References

1. Poznanski AK: The Hand in Radiologic Diagnosis. (ed 2) Philadelphia: WB Saunders, 1984, p 912
2. Swischuk LE, John SD: Differential Diagnosis in Pediatric Radiology. (ed 2) Baltimore: Williams & Wilkins, 1995, pp 276–278

Gamut D-129-3

SELF-MUTILATION OF DIGITS

1. Congenital insensitivity to pain
2. Congenital sensory neuropathy with or without anhidrosis
3. Diabetic neuropathy
4. Leprosy
5. Lesch-Nyhan S.
6. Psychotic states
7. Riley-Day S. (familial dysautonomia)

Gamut D-130

GANGRENE OF A FINGER OR TOE

COMMON

1. Arteriosclerosis obliterans
2. Arteritis (eg, hypersensitivity angiitis; Kawasaki S.; ergot reaction)
3. Connective tissue disease (collagen disease)$_g$ (eg, scleroderma; polyarteritis nodosa)
4. Diabetes

5. Neuropathic disease$_g$ (eg, leprosy) (See D-150)
6. Trauma, external or postoperative

UNCOMMON

1. Autoimmune disorder; macroglobulinemia (Waldenström macroglobulinemia; tumor-produced globulins)
2. Blood disorder (eg, leukemia; myeloid metaplasia; polycythemia vera)
3. Buerger disease (thromboangiitis obliterans)
4. Constriction (eg, bandage; baby mittens; hair ring or band; ainhum)
5. Disseminated intravascular coagulation (eg, sepsis; meningococcemia)
6. Electrical or chemical injury
7. Iatrogenic (eg, radial artery catheterization)
8. Infection; osteomyelitis
9. Raynaud disease
10. Thermal injury (frostbite; burn)
11. Trench foot
12. Trophic ulcer with underlying destruction

Reference

1. Poznanski AK: The Hand in Radiologic Diagnosis. (ed 2) Philadelphia: WB Saunders, 1984, pp 888–890

Gamut D-131

LYTIC LESION(S) IN A PHALANX (OFTEN CYST-LIKE)

COMMON

*1. Arthritis (esp. gout; rheumatoid arthritis; osteoarthritis)
+*2. Enchondroma
+*3. Osteomyelitis, incl. tuberculosis (spina ventosa)

UNCOMMON

1. Amyloidosis (esp. with renal failure)
2. Aneurysmal bone cyst

3. Angioma$_g$
4. Bone cyst
+5. Carcinoma of skin and nail-bed (incl. keratoacan-thoma)
6. Chondroblastoma (Codman tumor)
7. Chondromyxoid fibroma
8. Chondrosarcoma (slow growing)
+9. Epidermoid inclusion cyst
10. Fibrous dysplasia
11. Ganglion
12. Giant cell tumor
+13. Glomus tumor
14. Hemophilic pseudotumor
*15. Leprosy (leproma)
*16. Lymphoma; leukemia
+*17. Metastasis (esp. lung, breast)
*18. Multiple myeloma
19. Osteoblastoma
20. Osteoid osteoma
21. Periosteal chondroma or fibroma (incl. subun-gual)
*22. Sarcoidosis
*23. Synovial lesion (eg, villonodular synovitis; giant cell tumor of tendon sheath)
+24. Thorn granuloma
+*25. Tuberous sclerosis
*26. Wilson disease (hepatolenticular degeneration)
27. Xanthoma

* May be multiple.
+ Frequent cause of a lytic lesion in the distal phalanx.

Reference
1. Jones SN, Stoker DJ: Radiology at your fingertips; lesions of the terminal phalanx. Clin Radiol 1988; 39:478–485

DACTYLITIS*

COMMON
1. Pyogenic osteomyelitis (esp. *Salmonella*)
2. Sickle cell disease; hand-foot S. (infarction with or without osteomyelitis)
3. Tuberculosis (spina ventosa)

UNCOMMON
1. Atypical mycobacterial infection; BCG vaccination
2. Chronic granulomatous disease of childhood
3. Fungus disease$_g$ (eg, mycetoma; sporotrichosis)
4. Leprosy
5. [Neoplasm (eg, leukemia; metastasis, esp. neuro-blastoma; Ewing sarcoma; angioma; osteoid osteoma)]
6. Pancreatic fat necrosis (with elevated lipase)
7. Phalangeal microgeodic S.
8. Radiation necrosis
9. Sarcoidosis
10. Smallpox—prior to eradication
11. Syphilis; yaws
12. Thermal injury (eg, frostbite; burn; electrical)
13. Tuberous sclerosis

* Varying degrees of bone destruction and expansion, periosteal reaction, and soft tissue swelling involving one or more bones of the hands and/or feet.
[ ] This condition does not actually cause the gamuted imaging finding, but can produce imaging changes that simulate it.

References
1. Bennett OM: Salmonella osteomyelitis and the hand-foot syndrome in sickle cell disease. J Pediatr Orthop 1992; 12:534–538
2. Poznanski K, Beighton P: Gamut Index of Skeletal Dysplasias. Berlin: Springer-Verlag, 1984, pp 607–636
3. Swischuk LE, John SD: Differential Diagnosis in Pediatric Radiology. (ed 2) Baltimore: Williams & Wilkins, 1995, pp 279–280

Gamut D-133

CLUBBING OF THE FINGERS OR TOES

COMMON

1. Alveolar capillary block (eg, pulmonary interstitial fibrosis—sarcoidosis; scleroderma; pneumoconiosis)
2. Bronchogenic carcinoma
3. Cirrhosis
4. Congenital heart disease (esp. chronic cyanotic—tetralogy of Fallot$_g$; also pulmonary stenosis; large PDA or VSD)
5. Emphysema
6. Hypertrophic osteoarthropathy (See D-98)

UNCOMMON

1. Acromegaly
2. Colitis, chronic (eg, ulcerative; Crohn's disease; amebic; tuberculous)
3. Cystic fibrosis (mucoviscidosis)
4. Familial idiopathic osteoarthropathy (Currarino S.)
5. Gastrointestinal disease, chronic (eg, sprue; carcinoma; Cronkite-Canada S.)
6. Hajdu-Cheney S.
7. Hyperthyroidism; thyroid acropachy
8. Hypothyroidism; myxedema
9. Idiopathic
10. Immotile cilia S.
11. Larsen S.
12. Mesothelioma of pleura
13. Pachydermoperiostosis
14. POEMS S.
15. Polycythemia
16. Pulmonary AVMs or telangiectasia (eg, Rendu-Osler-Weber S.)
17. Seckel S. (bird-headed dwarfism)
18. Subacute bacterial endocarditis
19. Urinary tract infection, chronic

References
1. Greenfield GB: Radiology of Bone Diseases. (ed 5) Philadelphia: Lippincott, 1990
2. Swischuk LE, John SD: Differential Diagnosis in Pediatric Radiology. (ed 2) Baltimore: Williams & Wilkins, 1995, p 266
3. Taybi H, Lachman RS: Radiology of Syndromes, Metabolic Disorders, and Skeletal Dysplasias. (ed 4) St. Louis: Mosby-Year Book, 1996, p 1026

Gamut D-134

SYMPHALANGISM (FUSION OF PHALANGES IN A DIGIT)

COMMON

1. Isolated anomaly, esp. PIP joints of fingers ("mark of Shrewsbury") and DIP joints of toes

UNCOMMON

1. Acrocephalosyndactyly S. (Apert and other types)
2. Carpal-tarsal coalition
3. Cushing symphalangism
4. Diastrophic dysplasia
5. Familial brachydactyly B and C
6. Hand-foot-genital S.
7. Multiple synostosis S.
8. Oculodentoosseous dysplasia
9. Popliteal pterygium S.
10. Short rib-polydactyly S. type I (Saldino-Noonan)
11. Symphalangism-surdity S. (symphalangism-brachydactyly S. or WL S.)

References
1. Poznanski AK: The Hand in Radiologic Diagnosis. (ed 2) Philadelphia: WB Saunders, 1984, p 917
2. Poznanski AK: Foot manifestations of the congenital malformation syndromes. Semin Roentgenol 1970; 5:354–366
3. Swischuk LE, John SD: Differential Diagnosis in Pediatric Radiology. (ed 2) Baltimore: Williams & Wilkins, 1995, p 276
4. Taybi H, Lachman RS: Radiology of Syndromes, Metabolic Disorders, and Skeletal Dysplasias. (ed 4) St. Louis: Mosby-Year Book, 1996, p 1041

Gamut D-135

CONTRACTURE OF A DIGIT

1. Ainhum
2. Arthrogryposis (amyoplasia)
3. Camptodactyly (See D-136)
4. Congenital contractural arachnodactyly
5. Congenital or acquired ring contraction, annular band
6. Dupuytren contracture
7. Thermal injury (esp. burn)
8. Volkmann ischemic contracture

Reference

1. Greenfield GB: Radiology of Bone Diseases. (ed 5) Philadelphia: Lippincott, 1990

Gamut D-136

CAMPTODACTYLY (FLEXION DEFORMITY OF ONE OR MORE DIGITS)

ACQUIRED

COMMON

1. Arthritis (esp. rheumatoid)
2. Contracture (eg, Dupuytren; Volkmann)
3. Digital fibroma (esp. in the elderly)
4. Infection
5. Thermal injury (burn; frostbite; electrical)
6. Trauma; fracture

UNCOMMON

1. Ainhum
2. Neoplasm

CONGENITAL

COMMON

1. Arthrogryposis
2. Holt-Oram S.

3. Marfan S.; congenital contractural arachnodactyly
4. Nail-patella S. (osteo-onychodysplasia)
5. Poland S. (pectoral muscle aplasia—syndactyly)
6. Trisomy 18 S.

UNCOMMON

1. Aarskog S.
2. Antley-Bixler S.
3. Arthropathy-camptodactyly S.
4. Camptobrachydactyly
5. Camptodactyly-ankylosis-pulmonary hypoplasia S.
6. Cerebro-oculo-facio-skeletal S. (Pena-Shokeir S. type II)
7. Christian S. (adducted thumbs S.)
8. Craniofrontonasal dysplasia
9. Fetal akinesia deformation sequence (Pena-Shokeir S. type I)
10. Fetal alcohol S.
11. Freeman-Sheldon S. (whistling face S.)
12. Goltz S. (focal dermal hypoplasia)
13. Goodman camptodactyly S., A and B
14. Gordon S. (distal arthrogryposis)
15. Grebe chondrodysplasia (achondrogenesis, Brazilian type)
16. Greig cephalopolysyndactyly S.
17. Isolated absence or hypoplasia of a phalanx
18. Kyphomelic dysplasia
19. Lenz microphthalmia S.
20. Meckel S.
21. Monosomy 21 S.
22. Neu-Laxova S.
23. Noonan S.
24. Oculodentoosseous dysplasia
25. Orofaciodigital syndrome I (Papillon-Leage and Psaume S.)
26. Otopalatodigital S. (type II)
27. Popliteal pterygium S.
28. Pseudodiastrophic dysplasia
29. Roberts S. (pseudothalidomide S.)
30. Spondylocostal dysostosis (Jarcho-Levin S.)
31. Tel Hashomer camptodactyly S.
32. Trisomy 8 S.
33. Trisomy 13 S.

(continued)

34. Weaver-Smith S.
35. Williams S. (idiopathic hypercalcemia)
36. Zellweger S. (cerebrohepatorenal S.)

References

1. Poznanski AK: The Hand in Radiologic Diagnosis. (ed 2) Philadelphia: WB Saunders, 1984, p 916
2. Swischuk LE, John SD: Differential Diagnosis in Pediatric Radiology. (ed 2) Baltimore: Williams & Wilkins, 1995, pp 275–276
3. Taybi H, Lachman RS: Radiology of Syndromes, Metabolic Disorders, and Skeletal Dysplasias. (ed 4) St. Louis: Mosby-Year Book, 1996, p 1024

Gamut D-137

SYNDACTYLY (SOFT TISSUE UNION, WITH OR WITHOUT OSSEOUS UNION, BETWEEN ADJACENT DIGITS)

COMMON

1. Acrocephalopolysyndactyly (Carpenter and other types)
2. Acrocephalosyndactyly (Apert, Pfeiffer, Saethre-Chotzen types)
3. Brachmann-de Lange S. (de Lange S.)
4. Fanconi anemia (pancytopenia-dysmelia S.)
5. Holt-Oram S.
6. Isolated anomaly
7. Oculodentoosseous dysplasia
8. TAR S. (thrombocytopenia-absent radius S.)
9. Thermal injury (esp. burn)
10. Trisomy 13 S.
11. Trisomy 18 S.

UNCOMMON

1. Aarskog S.
2. Acrorenal S.
3. Aminopterin fetopathy
4. Aplasia cutis congenita
5. Arthrogryposis
6. Bardet-Biedl S.; Laurence-Moon S.
7. Bloom S.
8. Chondrodysplasia punctata
9. Chondroectodermal dysplasia (Ellis-van Creveld S.)
10. Cloverleaf skull deformity (kleeblattschädel anomaly)
11. Cohen S.
12. Craniofrontonasal dysplasia
13. DOOR S.
14. Dubowitz S. (toes)
15. EEC syndrome
16. Ehlers-Danlos S.
17. Epidermolysis bullosa
18. Familial brachydactyly A2 and B
19. Fetal hydantoin S. (Dilantin embryopathy)
20. Fibrodysplasia (myositis) ossificans progressiva
21. Fraser S. (cryptophthalmos-syndactyly S.)
22. Goltz S. (focal dermal hypoplasia)
23. Gorlin S. (nevoid basal cell carcinoma S.)
24. Greig cephalopolysyndactyly S.
25. Hallermann-Streiff S. (oculomandibulofacial S.)
26. Hypoglossia-hypodactylia S. (aglossia-adactylia S.)
27. Hypomelanosis of Ito
28. Incontinentia pigmenti
29. Lacrimo-auriculo-dento-digital S. (LADD S.) (Levy-Hollister S.)
30. Lenz microphthalmia S.
31. Meckel S.
32. Mesomelic dysplasia (Werner type)
33. Möbius S.
34. Multiple synostosis S.
35. Nager acrofacial dysostosis
36. Neu-Laxova S.
37. Opitz trigonocephaly S. (C syndrome)
38. Orofaciodigital syndrome I (Papillon-Leage and Psaume S.) and II (Mohr S.)
39. Otopalatodigital S. (types I and II)
40. Pallister-Hall S.
41. Poland S. (pectoral muscle aplasia—syndactyly)
42. Popliteal pterygium S.
43. Prader-Willi S.
44. Roberts S. (pseudothalidomide S.)
45. Robin sequence (Pierre Robin S.)
46. Robinow-Silverman S.
47. Rothmund-Thomson S.

48. Rubinstein-Taybi S.
49. Sclerosteosis
50. Short rib-polydactyly S. type I (Saldino-Noonan)
51. Silver-Russell S.
52. Smith-Lemli-Opitz S.
53. Spondylocostal dysostosis (Jarcho-Levin S.)
54. Trichorhinophalangeal dysplasia, type I (Giedion S.) and II (Giedion-Langer S.)
55. Triploidy (fetal triploidy S.)
56. Trisomy 21 S. (Down S.) (toes)

NOTE: There are over 30 other minor congenital syndromes with syndactyly that are listed in the books by Poznanski and Taybi.

References

1. Jones KL: Smith's Recognizable Patterns of Human Malformation. Philadelphia: WB Saunders, 1988
2. Poznanski AK: The Hand in Radiologic Diagnosis. (ed 2) Philadelphia: WB Saunders, 1984, p 914
3. Swischuk LE, John SD: Differential Diagnosis in Pediatric Radiology. (ed 2) Baltimore: Williams & Wilkins, 1995, pp 276–278
4. Taybi H, Lachman RS: Radiology of Syndromes, Metabolic Disorders, and Skeletal Dysplasias. (ed 4) St. Louis: Mosby-Year Book, 1996, pp 1041–1042

4. Chondrodysplasia punctata
5. Craniofrontonasal dysplasia
6. Diamond-Blackfan S.
7. Dubowitz S.
8. Fibrodysplasia (myositis) ossificans progressiva
9. Grebe chondrodysplasia (achondrogenesis, Brazilian type) (toes)
10. Lacrimo-auriculo-dento-digital S. (LADD S.) (Levy-Hollister S.)
11. Lissencephaly syndromes (congenital agyria)
12. Möbius S.
13. Nager acrofacial dysostosis
14. Poland S. (pectoral muscle aplasia—syndactyly)
15. Prune-belly S. (Eagle-Barrett S.)
16. Rieger S.
17. Short rib-polydactyly S. type II (Majewski)
18. Silver-Russell S.
19. Stickler S. (arthro-ophthalmopathy)
20. Townes-Brocks S. (thumbs)
21. Trisomy 21 S. (Down S.)

Gamut D-138-1

POLYDACTYLY (PREAXIAL—RADIAL SIDE)

COMMON

1. Acrocephalopolysyndactyly (Carpenter and other types)
2. Fanconi anemia (pancytopenia-dysmelia S.)
3. Holt-Oram S.
4. Isolated anomaly
5. VATER association

UNCOMMON

1. Acro-pectoro-vertebral dysplasia
2. Bloom S.
3. Cerebro-renal-digital syndromes

Gamut D-138-2

POLYDACTYLY (POSTAXIAL—ULNAR SIDE)

COMMON

1. Acrocephalopolysyndactyly (Carpenter and other types)
2. Bardet-Biedl S.; Laurence-Moon S.
3. Chondroectodermal dysplasia (Ellis-van Creveld S.)
4. Isolated anomaly
5. Rubinstein-Taybi S.

UNCOMMON

1. Acrocallosal S.
2. Acrorenal S.
3. Asphyxiating thoracic dysplasia (Jeune S.)
4. Biemond S. II
5. Cerebro-renal-digital syndromes

(continued)

6. Goltz S. (focal dermal hypoplasia)
7. Greig cephalopolysyndactyly S.
8. Kaufman-McKusick S. (hereditary hydrometro-colpos)
9. Meckel S.
10. Mesomelic dysplasia (Werner type)
11. Opitz trigonocephaly S. (C syndrome)
12. Orofaciodigital S. II (Mohr S.)
13. Pallister-Hall S.
14. Pseudotrisomy 13 S. (holoprosencephaly-polydactyly S.)
15. Short rib-polydactyly syndromes
16. Smith-Lemli-Opitz S.
17. Trisomy 13 S.
18. Weyers acrodental dysostosis

NOTE: There are over 30 other minor congenital syndromes with poly-dactyly that are listed in the books by Poznanski and Taybi.

References
1. Edeiken J, Dalinka M, Karasick D: Edeiken's Roentgen Diagnosis of Diseases of Bone. (ed 4) Baltimore: Williams & Wilkins, 1989
2. Jones KL: Smith's Recognizable Patterns of Human Malformation. Philadelphia: WB Saunders, 1988
3. Poznanski AK: Foot manifestations of the congenital malformation syndromes. Semin Roentgenol 1970; 5:354–366
4. Poznanski AK: The Hand in Radiologic Diagnosis. (ed 2) Philadelphia: WB Saunders, 1984, pp 266–278
5. Swischuk LE, John SD: Differential Diagnosis in Pediatric Radiology. (ed 2) Baltimore: Williams & Wilkins, 1995, pp 276–278
6. Taybi H, Lachman RS: Radiology of Syndromes, Metabolic Disorders, and Skeletal Dysplasias. (ed 4) St. Louis: Mosby-Year Book, 1996, pp 1038–1039

MACRODACTYLY

COMMON
1. Dactylitis (eg, tuberculosis; hand-foot S. {sickle cell disease})
2. Enchondromatosis (Ollier disease); Maffucci S.
3. Hemangioma
4. Idiopathic (macrodactyly simplex congenita)
5. Klippel-Trenaunay S.; Parkes Weber S.
6. Lymphangioma
7. Macrodystrophia lipomatosa
8. Neurofibromatosis (type 1)
9. Proteus S.

UNCOMMON
1. Duplication
2. Fibrous dysplasia
3. Hemophilic pseudotumor
4. Melorheostosis
5. Neoplasm, other (eg, aneurysmal bone cyst; osteoid osteoma; Ewing sarcoma)
6. Phalangeal microgeodic S.
7. Plexiform neuroma
8. Tuberous sclerosis

References
1. Baruchin AM, Herold ZH, Shmueli G, Lupo L: Macrodystrophia lipomatosa of the foot. J Pediatr Surg 1988; 23:192–194
2. Strickler S: Musculoskeletal manifestations of proteus syndrome: report of two cases with a literature review. J Pediatr Orthop 1992; 12:667–674
3. Swischuk LE, John SD: Differential Diagnosis in Pediatric Radiology. (ed 2) Baltimore: Williams & Wilkins, 1995, p 279
4. Taybi H, Lachman RS: Radiology of Syndromes, Metabolic Disorders, and Skeletal Dysplasias. (ed 4) St. Louis: Mosby-Year Book, 1996, p 1036

Gamut D-140

ARACHNODACTYLY (LONG FINGERS)

COMMON
1. Homocystinuria
2. Marfan S.

UNCOMMON
1. Antley-Bixler S.
2. Cleidocranial dysplasia (long 2nd and 5th metacarpals)
3. Congenital contractural arachnodactyly
4. Ehlers-Danlos S.
5. Frontometaphyseal dysplasia
6. Goodman camptodactyly S. B
7. Gorlin S. (nevoid basal cell carcinoma S.)
8. Ichthyosis syndromes
9. Marden-Walker S.
10. Multiple endocrine neoplasia (MEN) S., type IIB
11. Myotonic dystrophy
12. Rieger S.
13. Sotos S. (cerebral gigantism)
14. Stickler S. (arthro-ophthalmopathy)
15. XYY S.

References
1. Nelle M, Tröger J, Rupprath G, Bettendorf M: Metacarpal index in Marfan's syndrome and in constitutional tall stature. Arch Dis Child 1994; 70:149–150
2. Poznanski AK: The Hand in Radiologic Diagnosis. (ed 2) Philadelphia: WB Saunders, 1984, p 918
3. Taybi H, Lachman RS: Radiology of Syndromes, Metabolic Disorders, and Skeletal Dysplasias. (ed 4) St. Louis: Mosby-Year Book, 1996, p 1021

Gamut D-141

LOCALIZED BRACHYDACTYLY WITH SHORT PHALANGES, METACARPALS OR METATARSALS (EXCLUDING GENERALIZED SHORTENING)

COMMON
1. Acro-osteolysis (eg, congenital; leprosy) (See D-127)
2. Arthritis (esp. juvenile rheumatoid; septic)
3. Congenital syndromes with short metacarpals or metatarsals (See D-143)
4. Congenital syndromes with short phalanges (See D-123–127)
5. Idiopathic; isolated anomaly
6. Osteomyelitis; dactylitis (eg, bacterial, tuberculous, yaws; smallpox residual)
7. Pseudohypoparathyroidism; pseudopseudohypoparathyroidism
8. Sickle cell disease with infarction (hand-foot S.)
9. Trauma (eg, epiphyseal cartilage injury; fracture; thermal—burn, frostbite, electrical)

UNCOMMON
1. Ainhum
2. Amniotic band S. (Streeter bands)
3. Cone-shaped epiphyses (See D-27)
4. Enchondromatosis (Ollier disease)
5. Familial brachydactylies
6. Fibrodysplasia (myositis) ossificans progressiva
7. Gorlin S. (nevoid basal cell carcinoma S.)
8. Kashin-Beck disease (in Manchuria and Russia)
9. Myotonic dystrophy
10. Radiation or radium injury
11. Turner S.

References
1. Edeiken J, Dalinka M, Karasick D.: Edeiken's Roentgen Diagnosis of Diseases of Bone. (ed 4) Baltimore: Williams & Wilkins, 1989

(continued)

2. Greenfield GB: Radiology of Bone Diseases. (ed 5) Philadelphia: Lippincott, 1990
3. Poznanski AK: The Hand in Radiologic Diagnosis. (ed 2) Philadelphia: WB Saunders, 1984
4. Taybi H, Lachman RS: Radiology of Syndromes, Metabolic Disorders, and Skeletal Dysplasias. (ed 4) St. Louis: Mosby-Year Book, 1996, pp 1022–1024

Gamut D-142

CONGENITAL SYNDROMES WITH GENERALIZED BRACHYDACTYLY, SHORT HANDS AND FEET (ACROMELIA); ALSO SPADE HANDS

(Small Square Hands With Shortening of All Bones)

COMMON
1. Achondroplasia
2. Chondroectodermal dysplasia (Ellis-van Creveld S.)
3. Congenital syndromes with short metacarpals or metatarsals (See D-143)
4. Congenital syndromes with short phalanges (See D-123–127)
5. Enchondromatosis (Ollier disease)
6. Hypophosphatasia
7. Hypopituitarism
8. Hypothyroidism, cretinism
9. Mucopolysaccharidoses (eg, Hurler; Hunter; Morquio; Maroteaux-Lamy); mucolipidosis II (I-cell disease) and III (pseudo-Hurler polydystrophy) (See J-4)
10. Pseudohypoparathyroidism; pseudopseudohypoparathyroidism
11. Trisomy 21 S. (Down S.)

UNCOMMON
1. Aarskog S.
2. Achondrogenesis (types I and II)
3. Acrocallosal S.

4. Acrocephalopolysyndactyly (Carpenter and other types)
*5. Acrocephalosyndactyly (Apert and other types)
6. Acro-cranio-facial dysostosis
*7. Acrodysostosis (peripheral dysostosis)
8. Acromesomelic dysplasia
9. Acrorenal S.
*10. Asphyxiating thoracic dysplasia (Jeune S.)
11. Atelosteogenesis
12. Brachmann-de Lange S. (de Lange S.)
*13. Cephaloskeletal dysplasia (Taybi-Linder S.)
14. Chondrodysplasia punctata (brachytelephalangic type)
*15. Diastrophic dysplasia
16. DOOR S.
17. Familial brachdactyly syndromes
18. Fanconi anemia (pancytopenia-dysmelia S.) (esp. thumbs and toes)
19. Fetal alcohol S.
20. Fibrochondrogenesis
21. Goltz S. (focal dermal hypoplasia)
22. Grebe chondrodysplasia (achondrogenesis, Brazilian type)
23. Hand-foot-genital S. (esp. feet)
24. Hanhart S.
25. Hypochondrogenesis
26. Hypochondroplasia
27. Hypoparathyroidism
28. Isolated anomaly
29. Juberg-Hayward S.
30. Keutel S.
31. Larsen S.
*32. Léri pleonosteosis
33. Mesomelic dysplasia (Nievergelt and Werner types)
*34. Metaphyseal chondrodysplasia (McKusick type)
*35. Metatropic dysplasia
36. Möbius S.
37. Neu-Laxova S.
38. Noonan S.
39. Oculo-dento-osseous dysplasia
40. Opitz trigonocephaly S. (C syndrome)
*41. Orofaciodigital syndomes (esp. type I—Papillon-Leage and Psaume S.)

42. Oromandibular-limb hypogenesis syndromes (eg, Hanhart S.)
43. Osteosclerosis-dominant type, Stanescu
*44. Otopalatodigital S. (types I and II)
45. Patterson S.
46. Poland S. (pectoral muscle aplasia-syndactyly)
47. Popliteal pterygium S.
48. Progeria
*49. Pseudoachondroplasia (pseudoachondroplastic spondyloepiphyseal dysplasia)
50. Refsum disease
51. Rothmund-Thomson S.
52. Schneckenbecken dysplasia
*53. Short rib-polydactyly syndromes type I (Saldino-Noonan), II (Majewski) and III
54. Smith-Lemli-Opitz S.
55. Spondyloepimetaphyseal dysplasias (multiple types)
56. Spondylometaphyseal dysplasia (Sedaghatian type)
57. Spondyloperipheral dysplasia
58. Symphalangism-surdity S. (symphalangism-brachydactyly S. or WL S.)
59. TAR S. (thrombocytopenia-absent radius S.)
*60. Thanatophoric dysplasia
61. Trichorhinophalangeal dysplasia, type I (Giedion S.) and II (Giedion-Langer S.)
62. Trisomy 13 S.
63. Trisomy 18 S.
64. Weill-Marchesani S.
65. XXXXX S.; XXXXY S.

* Small square hands with shortening of all bones.
NOTE: There are over 20 other minor congenital syndromes with brachydactyly that are listed in the books by Poznanski and Taybi.

References

1. Felson B (ed): Dwarfs and Other Little People. Semin Roentgenol 1973; 8:257
2. Greenfield GB: Radiology of Bone Diseases. (ed 5) Philadelphia: Lippincott, 1990
3. Jones KL: Smith's Recognizable Patterns of Human Malformation. Philadelphia: WB Saunders, 1988
4. Kozlowski K, Beighton P: Gamut Index of Skeletal Dysplasias, Berlin: Springer-Verlag, 1984, p 72
5. Poznanski AK: The Hand in Radiologic Diagnosis. (ed 2) Philadelphia: WB Saunders, 1984, p 244
6. Swischuk LE, John SD: Differential Diagnosis in Pediatric Radiology. (ed 2) Baltimore: Williams & Wilkins, 1995, p 275
7. Taybi H, Lachman RS: Radiology of Syndromes, Metabolic Disorders, and Skeletal Dysplasias. (ed 4) St. Louis: Mosby-Year Book, 1996, pp 1022–1024

Gamut D-143-1

CONGENITAL SYNDROMES WITH SHORT METACARPALS OR METATARSALS

COMMON

1. Achondroplasia
2. Chondrodysplasia punctata (brachytelephalangic and tibial-metacarpal types)
3. Brachmann-de Lange S. (de Lange S.) (1st metacarpal)
4. Diastrophic dysplasia ("hitchhiker" thumb)
5. Enchondromatosis (Ollier disease)
6. Fibrodysplasia (myositis) ossificans progressiva (thumb and great toe)
7. Gorlin S. (nevoid basal cell carcinoma S.)
8. Holt-Oram S. (esp. thumb)
9. Hypothyroidism; cretinism
10. Idiopathic; isolated anomaly or normal variant
11. Mucopolysaccharidoses (eg, Hurler; Hunter); mucolipidosis II (I-cell disease) (See J-4)
12. Pseudohypoparathyroidism; pseudopseudohypoparathyroidism
13. Radial ray syndromes (1st metacarpal) (See D-161)
14. Rubinstein-Taybi S. (thumb and great toe)
15. Turner S. (4th metacarpal)

UNCOMMON

1. Acrocephalosyndactyly (Saethre-Chotzen type) (4th metacarpal)
2. Acrodysostosis (peripheral dysostosis)
3. Acromesomelic dysplasia
4. Aplasia cutis congenita (absent metacarpals)

(continued)

5. Atelosteogenesis
6. Beckwith-Wiedemann S.
7. Biemond S. I (4th metacarpal)
8. Camptobrachydactyly
9. Cat cry S. (cri du chat S.) (5th metacarpal)
10. Cephaloskeletal dysplasia (Taybi-Linder S.)
11. CHILD S. (ichthyosis-limb reduction S.)
12. Christian S. (adducted thumbs S.) (1st metacarpal)
13. Chromosome 18: del(18q) S. (1st metacarpal)
14. Cockayne S.
15. Coffin-Siris S.
16. Cohen S.
17. Desbuquois dysplasia
18. Diastrophic dysplasia (1st metacarpal)
19. Du Pan S.
20. Dyggve-Melchior-Clausen dysplasia (Smith-McCort S.) (1st metacarpal)
21. Dyschondrosteosis (4th metacarpal)
22. Dyssegmental dysplasia (1st metacarpal)
23. Familial brachydactyly A1, C, E
24. Fanconi anemia (pancytopenia-dysmelia S.) (1st metacarpal)
25. Fetal alcohol S.
26. Goltz S. (focal dermal hypoplasia)
27. Grebe chondrodysplasia (achondrogenesis, Brazilian type)
28. Hand-foot-genital S. (1st metacarpal and metatarsal)
29. Hereditary multiple exostoses (multiple cartilaginous exostoses; osteochondromatosis)
30. Hypochondroplasia
31. Hypoparathyroidism
32. Ichthyosis syndromes
33. Juberg-Hayward S. (1st metacarpal)
34. Larsen S.
35. Megaepiphyseal dwarfism
36. Metaphyseal chondrodysplasia (McKusick type)
37. Multiple epiphyseal dysplasia (Fairbank)
38. Myotonic dystrophy (4th metacarpal)
39. Nager acrofacial dysostosis
40. Omodysplasia (1st metacarpal)
41. Opitz trigonocephaly S. (C syndrome)
42. Osteoglophonic dysplasia
43. Otopalatodigital S. (types I and II) (esp. short thumb and great toe)

44. Pallister-Hall S. (4th metacarpal)
45. Poland S. (pectoral muscle aplasia-syndactyly) (absent 1st or other metacarpals)
46. Pseudodiastrophic dysplasia
47. Refsum disease
48. Robinow S.
49. Rothmund-Thomson S.
50. Short rib-polydactyly syndromes
51. Silver-Russell S. (5th metacarpal)
52. Sjögren-Larsson S.
53. Spondyloepimetaphyseal dysplasia
54. Spondyloperipheral dysplasia
55. Thanatophoric dysplasia
56. Trichorhinophalangeal dysplasia, type I (Giedion S.) and II (Giedion-Langer S.)
57. Trisomy 9p S. (1st metacarpal)
58. Trisomy 18 S. (1st metacarpal)
59. VATER association (1st metacarpal)
60. Weill-Marchesani S.
61. Yunis-Varón S. (absent thumb)

References

1. Kozlowksi K, Beighton P: Gamut Index of Skeletal Dysplasias. Berlin: Springer-Verlag, 1984, pp 72–73
2. Poznanski AK: The Hand in Radiologic Diagnosis. (ed 2) Philadelphia: WB Saunders, 1984, pp 908–909
3. Swischuk LE, John SD: Differential Diagnosis in Pediatric Radiology. (ed 2) Baltimore: Williams & Wilkins, 1995, pp 269–270
4. Taybi H, Lachman RS: Radiology of Syndromes, Metabolic Disorders, and Skeletal Dysplasias. (ed 4) St. Louis: Mosby-Year Book, 1996, pp 1036–1037

Gamut D-143-2

SHORT FIRST METACARPAL OR METATARSAL

COMMON

1. Brachmann-de Lange S. (de Lange S.)
2. Diastrophic dysplasia
3. Dyggve-Melchior-Clausen dysplasia
4. Fanconi anemia (pancytopenia-dysmelia S.)

5. Fibrodysplasia (myositis) ossificans progressiva
6. Holt-Oram S.
7. Idiopathic; isolated anomaly
8. Radial ray syndromes (See D-161)
9. Trisomy 18 S.

UNCOMMON

1. Christian S. (adducted thumbs S.)
2. Chromosome 18: del(18q) S.
3. Dyssegmental dysplasia
4. Hand-foot-genital S.
5. Juberg-Hayward S.
6. Omodysplasia
7. Otopalatodigital S.
8. Poland S. (pectoral muscle aplasia-syndactyly) (thumb may be absent)
9. TAR S. (thrombocytopenia-absent radius S.)
10. Trisomy 9p S.
11. VATER association
12. Yunis-Varón S. (absent thumbs)

References
1. Poznanski AK, Garn SM, Hold JF: The thumb in the congenital malformation syndromes. Radiology 1971; 100:115–129
2. Swischuk LE, John SD: Differential Diagnosis in Pediatric Radiology. (ed 2) Baltimore: Williams & Wilkins, 1995, p 273
3. Taybi H, Lachman RS: Radiology of Syndromes, Metabolic Disorders, and Skeletal Dysplasias. (ed 4) St. Louis: Mosby-Year Book, 1996, p 1036

Gamut D-143-3

SHORT FOURTH METACARPAL*

COMMON

1. Arthritis (esp. juvenile rheumatoid; septic)
2. Idiopathic
3. Osteomyelitis (eg, bacterial, tuberculous, yaws; smallpox residual)
4. Pseudohypoparathyroidism; pseudopseudohypoparathyroidism

5. Sickle cell disease with infarction
6. Trauma; fracture
7. Turner S.

UNCOMMON

1. Biemond S. I
2. Dyschondrosteosis
3. Familial brachydactyly E
4. Gorlin S. (nevoid basal cell carcinoma S.)
5. Multiple epiphyseal dysplasia (Fairbank)
6. Pallister-Hall S.

* Positive metacarpal sign: a line tangential to the heads of the fourth and fifth metacarpals passes through (rather than distal to) the head of the third metacarpal.

References
1. Burgener FA, Kormano M: Differential Diagnosis in Conventional Radiology. New York: Thieme Medical Publ, 1991, p 267
2. Taybi H, Lachman RS: Radiology of Syndromes, Metabolic Disorders, and Skeletal Dysplasias. (ed 4) St. Louis: Mosby-Year Book, 1996, p 1036

Gamut D-144

ACQUIRED DISEASES CAUSING SHORT HANDS AND FEET

1. Acro-osteolysis (See D-127)
2. Hypopituitarism
3. Leprosy
4. Multicentric reticulohistiocytosis (lipoid dermatoarthritis)
5. Osteomyelitis, severe (eg, bacterial; yaws; smallpox residual)
6. Rheumatoid arthritis; arthritis mutilans
7. Sickle cell disease (hand-foot S.)
8. Trauma; surgery; ritual (eg, Chinese bound feet)

Gamut D-145

CONTRACTED HAND (CLAW-HAND)

ACQUIRED

1. Arthritis (esp. rheumatoid)
2. Diabetes
3. Dupuytren contracture
4. Epidermolysis bullosa
5. Leprosy
6. Neoplasm
7. Neurologic disorder $_g$
8. Reflex sympathetic dystrophy (Sudeck's atrophy)
9. Thermal injury (frostbite; burn; electrical)
10. Trauma

CONGENITAL

1. Arthrogryposis
2. Chondrodysplasia punctata
3. Congenital contractural arachnodactyly
4. Diastrophic dysplasia
5. Digitotalar dysmorphism (ulnar drift)
6. EEC syndrome
7. Fetal akinesia deformation sequence (Pena-Shokeir S. type I)
8. Freeman-Sheldon S. (whistling face S.)
9. Gordon S. (distal arthrogryposis)
10. Larsen S.
11. Léri pleonosteosis
12. Mucopolysaccharidoses; mucolipidoses (See J-4); GM$_1$ gangliosidosis
13. Myotonic dystrophy
14. Trisomy 13 S.
15. Trisomy 18 S.

References

1. Poznanski AK: The Hand in Radiologic Diagnosis. (ed 2) Philadelphia: WB Saunders, 1984, p 916
2. Taybi H, Lachman RS: Radiology of Syndromes, Metabolic Disorders, and Skeletal Dysplasias. (ed 4) St. Louis: Mosby-Year Book, 1996, p 1032

Gamut D-146

LARGE HANDS FOR AGE

COMMON

1. Acromegaly; pituitary gigantism
2. Hyperthyroidism, active or treated (eg, thyroid acropachy)
3. Marfan S.
4. Precocious puberty
5. Sotos S. (cerebral gigantism)

UNCOMMON

1. Beckwith-Wiedemann S.
2. Coffin-Lowry S.
3. Congenital total lipodystrophy (lipoatrophic diabetes)
4. Frontometaphyseal dysplasia
5. Pachydermoperiostosis
6. Patterson S.
7. Stickler S. (arthro-ophthalmopathy)

References

1. Poznanski AK: The Hand in Radiologic Diagnosis. (ed 2) Philadelphia: WB Saunders, 1984, p 918
2. Taybi H, Lachman RS: Radiology of Syndromes, Metabolic Disorders, and Skeletal Dysplasias. (ed 4) St. Louis: Mosby-Year Book, 1996, p 1032

Gamut D-147-1

ASYMMETRY IN SIZE OF HAND BONES—SMALL BONES OF ONE HAND (See D-13)

1. Acro-osteolysis (See D-127)
2. Ainhum
3. Amniotic band S. (Streeter bands)
4. Aplasia; hypoplasia

5. Arrested epiphyseal growth
    a. Fracture
    b. Juvenile chronic arthritis (eg, juvenile rheuma-toid arthritis)
    c. Osteomyelitis (eg, septic; yaws; smallpox residual)
    d. Radiation injury
    e. Surgery
    f. Thermal injury (eg, burn; frostbite; electrical)
    g. Wringer injury
6. Chondrodysplasia punctata
7. Paralysis$_g$
8. Poland S. (pectoral muscle aplasia-syndactyly)
9. Warfarin embryopathy

Reference
1. Poznanski AK: The Hand in Radiologic Diagnosis. (ed 2) Philadelphia: WB Saunders, 1984, p 917

Reference
1. Poznanski AK: The Hand in Radiologic Diagnosis. (ed 2) Philadelphia: WB Saunders, 1984, p 917

Gamut D-147-3

GENERALIZED ASYMMETRY IN SIZE OF HAND BONES

1. Beckwith-Wiedemann S.
2. Hemiatrophy (See D-13)
3. Hemihypertrophy (See D-13, D-14)
4. Silver-Russell S.

Reference
1. Poznanski AK: The Hand in Radiologic Diagnosis. (ed 2) Philadelphia: WB Saunders, 1984, p 917

Gamut D-147-2

ASYMMETRY IN SIZE OF HAND BONES—LARGE BONES OF ONE HAND (See D-13, D-14)

1. Bone neoplasm
2. Enchondromatosis (Ollier disease); Maffucci S.
3. Fibrous dysplasia
4. Hyperemia
    a. Hemangioma; arteriovenous fistula
    b. Infection
    c. Juvenile chronic arthritis (eg, juvenile rheuma-toid arthritis)
5. Klippel-Trenaunay S.; Parkes Weber S.
6. Lymphangiectasia
7. Macrodactyly (See D-139)
8. Macrodystrophia lipomatosa
9. Melorheostosis
10. Neurofibromatosis
11. Paget's disease
12. Proteus S.

Gamut D-148

GENERALIZED FAILURE OF MODELING OR TUBULATION IN THE HAND (WIDE OR THICK BONES) (See D-11, D-12)

ACQUIRED

1. Anemia$_g$ (esp. thalassemia; sickle cell disease)
2. Fluorosis
3. Fractures, healed
4. Infarction (eg, hand-foot S.)
5. Infection; osteomyelitis
6. Neoplasm
7. Rickets (healing); biliary rickets in infancy
8. Subperiosteal hemorrhage (eg, hemophilia; osteogenesis imperfecta with trauma)

CONGENITAL

1. Achondroplasia
2. Craniodiaphyseal dysplasia

(continued)

3. Craniometaphyseal dysplasia
4. Diaphyseal dysplasia (Camurati-Engelmann disease)
5. Enchondromatosis (Ollier disease); Maffucci S.
6. Fibrous dysplasia
7. Hyperphosphatasia
8. Melorheostosis
9. Mucolipidoses (See J-4); fucosidosis; mannosidosis; GM_1 gangliosidosis
10. Niemann-Pick disease
11. Oculodento-osseous dysplasia
12. Osteopetrosis
13. Pyle dysplasia
14. Sclerosteosis
15. Singleton-Merten S.

Reference
1. Poznanski AK: The Hand in Radiologic Diagnosis. (ed 2) Philadelphia: WB Saunders, 1984, p 901

Gamut D-149-1

PROXIMAL TAPERING OF SHORT TUBULAR BONES OF THE HANDS AND FEET

1. Brachmann-de Lange S. (de Lange S.)
2. Mucopolysaccharidoses (eg, Hurler; Hunter; Morquio); mucolipidoses (See J-4)

Gamut D-149-2

DISTAL TAPERING OF SHORT TUBULAR BONES OF THE HANDS AND FEET

1. Acro-osteolysis (See D-127)
2. Ainhum
3. Diabetes

4. Epidermolysis bullosa
5. Hyperparathyroidism
6. Leprosy; other neuropathic diseases$_g$
7. Raynaud disease
8. Scleroderma
9. Thermal injury (eg, burn; frostbite; electrical)

Reference
1. Greenfield GB: Radiology of Bone Diseases. (ed 5) Philadelphia: Lippincott, 1990

Gamut D-150

NEUROPATHIC BONE CHANGES (POINTED OR SPINDLED BONES) IN THE HANDS OR FEET

COMMON
1. [Amputation (congenital, traumatic, or surgical)]
2. Arteriosclerosis obliterans; Raynaud disease; Buerger disease (thromboangiitis obliterans)
3. Diabetes
4. Leprosy
5. Psoriatic arthritis
6. Rheumatoid arthritis
7. Scleroderma; dermatomyositis
8. Septic arthritis (pyarthrosis)
9. Spinal cord injury or disease (eg, pernicious anemia; syringomyelia; spina bifida; meningomyelocele; neoplasm)
10. Thermal injury (eg, burn; frostbite; electrical)
11. Trophic ulcer of soft tissue with underlying destruction

UNCOMMON
1. Acrodystrophic neuropathy
2. [Acro-osteolysis] (See D-127)
3. Ainhum
4. Amyloid neuropathy
5. Charcot-Marie-Tooth S.

6. [Clubbing of fingers]
7. Congenital insensitivity to pain
8. Congenital pseudarthrosis
9. Ergot intoxication
10. Hicks S. (familial sensory neural radiculopathy)
11. Idiopathic
12. Malnutrition (alcoholism or nutritional neuropathy)
13. Peripheral nerve injury
14. Porphyria
15. [Pyknodysostosis]
16. Riley-Day S. (familial dysautonomia)
17. Tabes dorsalis
18. Trench foot

[ ] This condition does not actually cause the gamuted imaging finding, but can produce imaging changes that simulate it.

References
1. Gondos B: The pointed tubular bone. Radiology 1972; 105:541–545
2. Greenfield GB: Radiology of Bone Diseases. (ed 5) Philadelphia: Lippincott, 1990
3. Hodgson JR, Pugh DG, Young HH: Roentgenologic aspect of certain lesions of bone: neurotrophic or infectious? Radiology 1948; 50:65–70
4. Kozlowski K, Beighton P: Gamut Index of Skeletal Dysplasias. Berlin: Springer-Verlag, 1984, pp 76–77

Gamut D-151

WELL-DEFINED SOLITARY OR MULTIPLE LUCENT DEFECTS IN BONES OF THE HANDS, WRISTS, FEET, OR ANKLES

COMMON
1. Enchondroma
2. Gout
3. Intraosseous ganglion
4. Osteoarthritis
5. Posttraumatic (eg, avascular necrosis with cystic radiolucency following scaphoid or lunate fracture)
6. Rheumatoid arthritis (adult, juvenile, or sero-negative)

UNCOMMON
1. Amyloidosis (esp. secondary, related to renal failure)
*2. Aneurysmal bone cyst
*3. Bone cyst, developmental cyst
*4. Carcinoma of skin or nail-bed (incl. keratoacanthoma)
*5. Chondroblastoma (Codman tumor)
*6. Chondromyxoid fibroma
7. Enchondromatosis (Ollier disease)
*8. Epidermoid inclusion cyst (distal phalanx)
9. Fibromatosis (esp. multicentric infantile myofibromatosis)
10. Fibrous dysplasia
*11. Giant cell granuloma
*12. Giant cell tumor
13. Glomus tumor (distal phalanx)
14. Granuloma (eg, foreign body; palm thorn)
15. Hemangioma; Maffucci S.
16. Hemochromatosis
17. Hemophilic pseudotumor
18. Jackhammer operator's (driller's) disease of wrists (carpals)
*19. Kienböck disease (lunate necrosis)
20. Langerhans cell histiocytosis$_g$
*21. Lipoma (esp. calcaneus)
22. Metastasis (esp. lung and breast)
23. Mucopolysaccharidosis I-S (Scheie)
24. Multiple myeloma
25. Nonossifying fibroma (fibroxanthoma)
*26. Osteoid osteoma
27. Osteomyelitis (eg, tuberculous; atypical mycobacterial infection; fungal; partially treated bacterial infection)
28. Phalangeal microgeodic S.
29. Sarcoidosis
30. Sickle cell disease (hand-foot S.)
31. Silastic arthropathy
32. Sinus histiocytosis (Rosai Dorfman disease)
*33. Subungual keratoma (distal phalanx)

(continued)

34. Tuberous sclerosis
35. Vascular channels, esp. phalanges
36. Villonodular synovitis
37. Xanthoma; xanthomatosis

* Solitary lesions; all others in this list may be multiple.

Reference
1. Poznanski AK: The Hand in Radiologic Diagnosis. (ed 2) Philadelphia: WB Saunders, 1984, p 919

Gamut D-152

SCLEROTIC FOCUS IN BONES OF THE HANDS OR FEET

COMMON

1. Avascular necrosis (eg, steroid therapy; trauma to scaphoid or lunate)
2. Bone island (enostosis)
3. Enchondroma
4. Healing fracture with callus; florid reactive periostitis
5. Osteomyelitis, chronic; mycetoma

UNCOMMON

1. Arthritis, inflammatory (esp. seronegative psoriatic arthritis or Reiter S.—"ivory phalanx")
2. Bizarre parosteal pseudotumor (BPOP)
3. Bone sarcoma (eg, osteosarcoma; chondrosarcoma; Ewing sarcoma)
4. Connective tissue disease (collagen vascular disease$_g$) (eg, lupus erythematosus; scleroderma)
5. Enchondromatosis (Ollier disease)
6. Fibrous dysplasia
7. Gardner S.
8. Gout (with intraosseous tophus calcification)
9. Hereditary multiple exostoses (multiple cartilaginous exostoses; osteochondromatosis)
10. Infarct (eg, sickle cell disease)
11. Melorheostosis

12. Nonossifying fibroma (fibroxanthoma), healing
13. Osteoblastic metastasis
14. Osteoblastoma
15. Osteochondroma
16. Osteoid osteoma
17. Osteopathia striata (Voorhoeve disease)
18. Osteopoikilosis
19. Paget's disease
20. Sarcoidosis
21. Syphilis
22. Tuberous sclerosis
23. Werner S.
24. Yaws

References
1. Poznanski AK: The Hand in Radiologic Diagnosis. (ed 2) Philadelphia: WB Saunders, 1984, p 899
2. Resnick D: Diagnosis of Bone and Joint Disorders. (ed 3) Philadelphia, WB Saunders, 1995

Gamut D-153

TROPICAL DISEASES INVOLVING THE HANDS AND FEET

COMMON

1. Filariasis; elephantiasis
2. Leprosy
3. Sickle cell dactylitis (hand-foot S.)
4. Tuberculosis
5. Yaws; syphilis

UNCOMMON

1. Ainhum
2. Cysticercosis
3. Guinea worm infection (dracunculiasis)
4. Kaposi sarcoma
5. Loiasis (*Loa loa*)
6. Mycetoma (Madura foot); fungus diseases$_g$
7. Smallpox residual
8. Tropical ulcer (usually tibia)

Reference
1. Palmer PES, Reeder MM: The Imaging of Tropical Diseases, with Epidemiological, Pathological and Clinical Correlation. Heidelberg: Springer-Verlag, 2001

Gamut D-154

CONGENITAL CONDITIONS ASSOCIATED WITH CLUBFOOT, METATARSUS ADDUCTUS, OR OTHER FOOT DEFORMITY

COMMON
1. Faulty intrauterine positioning
2. Idiopathic
*3. Neurologic or neuromuscular disease$_g$ (eg, myotonic dystrophy; meningomyelocele; spina bifida)

UNCOMMON
1. Aarskog S.
2. Aminopterin fetopathy (varus)
3. Amniotic band S. (Streeter bands)
4. Antley-Bixler S.
5. Arthrogryposis
6. Bloom S.
7. Brachmann-de Lange S. (de Lange S.)
8. Caudal dysplasia sequence
9. Cephaloskeletal dysplasia (Taybi-Linder S.)
10. Chondrodysplasia punctata
11. Chondroectodermal dysplasia (Ellis-van Creveld S.) (valgus)
12. Christian S. (adducted thumbs S.)
13. Chromosome 4: del(4p) S. (Wolf-Hirschhorn S.)
14. Chromosome 18: del(18q) S.
15. Desbuquois dysplasia
16. Diastrophic dysplasia
17. Dubowitz S.
18. Ehlers-Danlos S.
19. Femoral hypoplasia—unusual facies S.
20. Fetal akinesia deformation sequence (Pena-Shokeir S. type I)
21. Freeman-Sheldon S. (whistling face S.)
22. Homocystinuria (pes planus or cavus; everted feet)
23. Kniest dysplasia
24. Larsen S.
25. Marfan S. (long great toes; hammer toes)
26. Meckel S.
27. Mesomelic dysplasia (Nievergelt type)
28. Metatropic dysplasia
29. Mietens-Weber S. (pes valgus planus)
30. Möbius S.
31. Mucopolysaccharidoses (eg, Hurler; Hunter; Morquio) (pes planus or cavus; misshapen tarsals) (See J-4)
32. Nager acrofacial dysostosis
33. Nail-patella S. (osteo-onychodysplasia)
34. Neurofibromatosis (pes planus)
35. Noonan S.
36. Otopalatodigital S. (tarsal fusion)
37. Popliteal pterygium S.
38. Potter S. (renal agenesis)
39. Pseudodiastrophic dysplasia
40. Roberts S. (pseudothalidomide S.)
41. Smith-Lemli-Opitz S.
42. Spondyloepimetaphyseal dysplasia with joint laxity
43. TAR S. (thrombocytopenia—absent radius S.)
*44. Trisomy 13 S.
*45. Trisomy 18 S.
46. Weaver-Smith S.
47. XXXXX S.
48. XXXXY S. (pes planus)
49. Zellweger S. (cerebrohepatorenal S.)

* May have vertical talus.

References
1. Jones KL: Smith's Recognizable Patterns of Human Malformation. Philadelphia: WB Saunders, 1988
2. Poznanski AK: Foot manifestations of the congenital malformation syndromes. Semin Roentgenol 1970; 5:354–366
3. Swischuk LE, John SD: Differential Diagnosis in Pediatric Radiology. (ed 2) Baltimore: Williams & Wilkins, 1995, p 213

(continued)

4. Taybi H, Lachman RS: Radiology of Syndromes, Metabolic Disorders, and Skeletal Dysplasias. (ed 4) St. Louis: Mosby-Year Book, 1996, pp 1025–1026

Gamut D-155

LUCENT LESION OF THE CALCANEUS

COMMON

1. Bone cyst
2. Lipoma
3. Osteomyelitis, pyogenic
4. [Pseudocyst (normal thinning of trabeculae)]

UNCOMMON

1. Aneurysmal bone cyst
2. Brown tumor of hyperparathyroidism
3. Chondroblastoma (Codman tumor)
4. Chondromyxoid fibroma
5. Chronic recurrent multifocal osteomyelitis
6. Enchondroma
7. Eosinophilic granuloma
8. Fungal osteomyelitis (eg, mycetoma; cryptococcosis)
9. Giant cell tumor
10. Hemophilic pseudotumor
11. Lymphangioma
12. Metastasis, osteolytic
13. Multiple myeloma
14. Myxoma; fibroma; myxofibroma
15. Sarcoma (eg, fibrosarcoma)

References
1. Kumar R, Matasar K, Stansberry S, et al: The calcaneus: normal and abnormal. Radiographics 1991;11:415–440
2. Resnick D: Diagnosis of Bone and Joint Disorders. (ed 3) Philadelphia: WB Saunders, 1995

Gamut D-156

CONGENITAL SYNDROMES WITH ACCESSORY CARPAL OR TARSAL BONES

1. Anatomic variant
*2. Chondroectodermal dysplasia (Ellis-van Creveld S.)
*3. Diastrophic dysplasia
4. [Dysplasia epiphysealis hemimelica (Trevor disease)]
*5. Familial brachydactyly A1
6. Grebe chondrodysplasia (achondrogenesis, Brazilian type)
7. Hand-foot-genital S.
8. Holt-Oram S.
*9. Larsen S.
*10. Otopalatodigital S.
*11. Stickler S. (arthro-ophthalmopathy)

* Distal carpal row.
[ ] This condition does not actually cause the gamuted imaging finding, but can produce imaging changes that simulate it.

References
1. Kozlowski K, Beighton P: Gamut Index of Skeletal Dysplasias. Berlin: Springer-Verlag, 1984, pp 74–75
2. Poznanski AK: The Hand in Radiologic Diagnosis. (ed 2) Philadelphia: WB Saunders, 1984, pp 196–201

Gamut D-157-1

FRAGMENTED, IRREGULAR, OR SCLEROTIC CARPAL OR TARSAL BONES

COMMON

1. Arthritis (esp. rheumatoid; septic; gout)
2. Avascular necrosis (esp. scaphoid; lunate; tarsal navicular)

3. Infection (eg, mycetoma; osteomyelitis)
4. Normal variant (tarsals)
5. Trauma; postoperative changes

UNCOMMON
1. Chondrodysplasia punctata (all types)
2. Congenital bipartite bone
3. Diastrophic dysplasia
4. Dyggve-Melchior-Clausen dysplasia
5. Dysosteosclerosis
6. Kniest dysplasia
7. Larsen S. (bipartite calcaneus)
8. Melorheostosis
9. Metatropic dysplasia
10. Mixed sclerotic bone dysplasia
11. Morquio S.
12. Mucolipidosis II (I-cell disease); fucosidosis
13. Multiple epiphyseal dysplasia (Fairbank)
14. Osteoglophonic dysplasia
15. Osteolysis with nephropathy; osteolysis without nephropathy (carpal and tarsal osteolysis)
16. Osteopetrosis
17. Osteopoikilosis
18. Parastremmatic dysplasia
19. Pseudorheumatoid dysplasia
20. Seckel S. (bird-headed dwarfism)
21. Spondyloepiphyseal dysplasia (congenita and tarda)
22. Spondylometaphyseal dysplasia (Kozlowski type)
23. Warfarin embryopathy (stippled calcanei)
24. Winchester S.

References
1. Beighton P. Cremin BJ: Sclerosing Bone Dysplasias. Berlin: Springer-Verlag, 1980
2. Swischuk LE, John SD: Differential Diagnosis in Pediatric Radiology. (ed 2) Baltimore: Williams & Wilkins, 1995, pp 281–284
3. Taybi H, Lachman RS: Radiology of Syndromes, Metabolic Disorders, and Skeletal Dysplasias. (ed 4) St. Louis: Mosby-Year Book, 1996, p 1025

Gamut D-157-2

CONGENITAL SYNDROMES WITH SMALL OR DYSPLASTIC CARPAL AND/OR TARSAL BONES

COMMON
1. [Arthritis (esp. rheumatoid)]
2. Arthrogryposis
3. [Avascular necrosis of lunate (Kienbock)]
4. Chondrodysplasia punctata
5. Morquio S.
*6. Multiple epiphyseal dysplasia (Fairbank)
7. Spondyloepiphyseal dysplasia (congenita and tarda)

UNCOMMON
1. Aarskog S.
2. Diastrophic dysplasia
3. Dyggve-Melchior-Clausen dysplasia
*4. Farber disease (disseminated lipogranulomatosis)
5. Frontometaphyseal dysplasia
6. Fucosidosis
7. Gordon S. (distal arthrogryposis)
8. Hypochondrogenesis (esp. calcaneus and talus)
9. Kniest dysplasia
10. Metatropic dysplasia
*11. Osteoglophonic dysplasia
*12. Osteolysis with nephropathy; osteolysis without nephropathy (carpal and tarsal osteolysis)
*13. Parastremmatic dwarfism
14. Pseudoachondroplasia
15. Seckel S. (bird-headed dwarfism)
16. Spondyloepimetaphyseal dysplasia (Strudwick type)
17. Spondylometaphyseal dysplasia (Kozlowski type)
*18. Winchester S.
19. Campomelic dysplasia (talus not ossified)

* With erosions or irregular margins.
[ ] This condition does not actually cause the gamuted imaging finding, but can produce imaging changes that simulate it.

(continued)

References

1. Poznanski AK: The Hand in Radiologic Diagnosis. (ed 2) Philadelphia: WB Saunders, 1984, p 902
2. Taybi H, Lachman RS: Radiology of Syndromes, Metabolic Disorders, and Skeletal Dysplasias. (ed 4) St. Louis: Mosby-Year Book, 1996, p 1025

Gamut D-158

CARPAL AND/OR TARSAL FUSION

COMMON

1. Arthritis (esp. rheumatoid; juvenile chronic; septic; fungal)
2. Arthrogryposis
3. Chondroectodermal dysplasia (Ellis-van Creveld S.) (capitate-hamate)
4. Normal variant, isolated anomaly (esp. triquetrum-lunate, talus-calcaneus, capitate-hamate, trapezium-trapezoid or scaphoid) as in Yoruba tribe of Nigeria
5. Traumatic; surgical

UNCOMMON

1. Acrocephalopolysyndactyly (Carpenter S.)
2. Acrocephalosyndactyly (Apert and Pfeiffer types)
3. Acromegaly
4. Antley-Bixler S.
5. Baller-Gerold S. (craniosynostosis—radial aplasia S.)
6. Chromosomal abnormalities
7. Cleft hand or foot
8. Crouzon S. (craniofacial dysostosis) (calcaneus-cuboid)
9. Diastrophic dysplasia
10. Dyschondrosteosis; Madelung deformity
11. EEC syndrome
12. F syndrome
13. Fetal alcohol S.
14. Frontometaphyseal dysplasia
15. Hand-foot-genital S.
16. Holt-Oram S.
17. Kniest dysplasia
18. LEOPARD S. (multiple lentigenes S.)
19. Mesomelic dysplasia (Nievergelt type)
20. Multiple synostosis S.
21. Osteomyelitis
22. Otopalatodigital S. (type I) (capitate-hamate)
23. Rothmund-Thomson S.
24. Ruvalcaba S. (trichorhinophalangeal S., type III)
25. Scleroderma; dermatomyositis
26. Spondylocarpotarsal fusion S.
27. Symphalangism-surdity S. (symphalangism-brachydactyly S. or WL S.)
28. Thalidomide embryopathy
29. Townes-Brocks S.
30. Turner S.
31. Tylosis (keratosis palmaris et plantaris familiaris)

References

1. Cockshott WP: Carpal fusions. AJR 1963;89:1260–1271
2. Cope JR: Carpal coalition. Clin Radiol 1974; 25:261–266
3. Kozlowski K, Beighton P: Gamut Index of Skeletal Dysplasias. Berlin: Springer-Verlag, 1984, p 74
4. Poznanski AK: Foot manifestations of the congenital malformation syndromes. Semin Roentgenol 1970; 5:354–366
5. Poznanski AK, Holt FF: The carpals in congenital malformation syndromes. AJR 1971; 112:443–459
6. Poznanski AK: The Hand in Radiologic Diagnosis. (ed 2) Philadelphia: WB Saunders, 1984, pp 201–207
7. Swischuk LE, John SD: Differential Diagnosis in Pediatric Radiology. (ed 2) Baltimore: Williams & Wilkins, 1995, pp 280–283
8. Taybi H, Lachman RS: Radiology of Syndromes, Metabolic Disorders, and Skeletal Dysplasias. (ed 4) St. Louis: Mosby-Year Book, 1996, pp 1024–1025

Gamut D-159-1

CONGENITAL SYNDROMES ASSOCIATED WITH A DECREASED CARPAL ANGLE*
(Less than 124°)

1. Dyschondrosteosis
2. Hereditary multiple exostoses (multiple cartilaginous exostoses; osteochondromatosis)
3. Madelung deformity (See D-164-2)
4. Mesomelic dysplasia (Langer type)
5. Mucopolysaccharidoses (esp. Morquio; Hurler) (See J-4)
6. Turner S.

* Normal carpal angle is 131.5° (+ or –7.2°)

References
1. Harper HAS, Poznanski AK, Garn SM: The carpal angle in American populations. Invest Radiol 1974; 9:217–221
2. Poznanski AK: The Hand in Radiologic Diagnosis. (ed 2) Philadelphia: WB Saunders, 1984, pp 193–195
3. Swischuk LE, John SD: Differential Diagnosis in Pediatric Radiology. (ed 2) Baltimore: Williams & Wilkins, 1995, pp 280–281

Gamut D-159-2

CONGENITAL SYNDROMES ASSOCIATED WITH AN INCREASED CARPAL ANGLE*
(Greater than 139°)

1. Arthrogryposis
2. Chondroectodermal dysplasia (Ellis-van Creveld S.)
3. Cleidocranial dysplasia
4. Frontometaphyseal dysplasia
5. Larsen S.
6. Marfan S.
7. Multiple epiphyseal dysplasia (Fairbank)
8. Otopalatodigital S.
9. Pfeiffer-like S.
10. Sotos S. (cerebral gigantism)
11. Stickler S. (arthro-ophthalmopathy)
12. Trichorhinophalangeal dysplasia

* Normal carpal angle is 131.5° (+ or –7.2°).

Reference
1. Poznanski AK: The Hand in Radiologic Diagnosis. (ed 2) Philadelphia: WB Saunders, 1984, pp 193–195

CARPAL ANOMALIES SEEN IN COMMON CONGENITAL SYNDROMES*

	Os Centrale (one or more)	Extra Distal Carpals	Os Triangulare	Irregular Carpal Margins	Abnormally Shaped Scaphoid	Absent or Hypoplastic Scaphoid	Scaphoid Fused to Other Carpals	Abnormally Shaped Capitate	Absent or Hypoplastic Capitate	Some Carpal Fusion	Decreased Carpal Angle	Increased Carpal Angle	Diminution in Size of the Carpus
Arthrogryposis			O		O		O	O		X		X	X
Diastrophic dysplasia		X		X	O		O	O		O		O	X
Dyschondrosteosis										O	X		
Ellis-van Creveld S.		X								X			
Epiphyseal dysplasia				X	O			X	X			X	X
Fanconi's anemia					X	X							
Hand-foot-genital S.	X				X		X			X			
Holt-Oram S.	X		O		X	0	X	O		O			
Homocystinuria								X					
Otopalatodigital S.	O	O			O		O	X		O			O
Symphalangism					O					X			
Turner S.										O	X		

(Modified from Poznanski AK, Holt JF; AJR 1971;112:443-459)

* X = commonly present; O = occasionally present

RADIAL RAY SYNDROMES (HYPOPLASIA OR APLASIA OF THE RADIUS+ AND/OR THUMB AND LATERAL CARPAL BONES)

COMMON

*1. Brachmann-de Lange S. (de Lange S.)
2. Fanconi anemia (pancytopenia-dysmelia S.)
3. Holt-Oram S.
*4. Isolated anomaly
*5. Phocomelia (eg, thalidomide embryopathy)
6. TAR S. (thrombocytopenia—absent radius S.)

UNCOMMON

1. Aase S.
2. Aminopterin fetopathy
3. Baller-Gerold S. (craniosynostosis-radial aplasia S.)
4. de la Chapelle dysplasia

5. Diamond-Blackfan S.
6. Duane-radial dysplasia S. (DR S.)
*7. Dyschondrosteosis
8. Ectodermal dysplasia
9. Facioauriculoradial dysplasia
10. Fetal varicella S.
*11. Ives-Houston S.
12. IVIC S.
13. Juberg-Hayward S.
14. Klippel-Feil S.
15. Lacrimo-auriculo-dento-digital S. (LADD S.) (Levy-Hollister S.)
16. Mesomelic dysplasias
17. Mietens-Weber S.
18. Nager acrofacial dysostosis
19. Poland S. (pectoral muscle aplasia-syndactyly)
*20. Roberts S. (pseudothalidomide S.)
21. Rothmund-Thomson S.
22. Seckel S. (bird-headed dwarfism)
23. Treacher Collins S.
24. Trisomy 18 S.
25. VATER association

* May or must have ulnar hypoplasia or absence as well.
+ Radial hypoplasia may be seen with certain congenital heart diseases; renal anomalies; esophageal, duodenal, or anal atresia; rib anomalies; Klippel-Feil S.; kyphoscoliosis; and hypoplasia or spina bifida of the lumbosacral spine.

References

1. Edeiken J, Dalinka M, Karasick D: Edeiken's Roentgen Diagnosis of Diseases of Bone. (ed 4) Baltimore: Williams & Wilkins, 1989
2. Jones KL: Smith's Recognizable Patterns of Human Malformation. Philadelphia: WB Saunders, 1988
3. Kozlowski K, Beighton P: Gamut Index of Skeletal Dysplasias. Berlin: Springer-Verlag, 1984, p 65
4. Poznanski AK: The Hand in Radiologic Diagnosis. (ed 2) Philadelphia: WB Saunders, 1984, pp 244–248, 911
5. Swischuk LE, John SD: Differential Diagnosis in Pediatric Radiology. (ed 2) Baltimore: Williams & Wilkins, 1995, pp 277–278
6. Taybi H, Lachman RS: Radiology of Syndromes, Metabolic Disorders, and Skeletal Dysplasias. (ed 4) St. Louis: Mosby-Year Book, 1996, pp 1040, 1043

Gamut D-162

ULNAR RAY SYNDROMES (HYPOPLASIA OR APLASIA OF THE ULNA AND/OR FOURTH AND FIFTH FINGERS)

1. Acromesomelic dysplasia
2. Boomerang dysplasia
3. Brachmann-de Lange S. (de Lange S.)
4. Chondrodysplasia punctata (tibial-metacarpal type)
5. de la Chapelle dysplasia
6. Distal osteosclerosis
7. Grebe chondrodysplasia (achondrogenesis, Brazilian type)
8. Hereditary multiple exostoses (multiple cartilaginous exostoses; osteochondromatosis)
9. Klippel-Feil S.—absent ulna
10. Mesomelic dysplasia (Langer, Nievergelt, Rheinhardt-Pfeiffer, Werner types)—ulnofibular dysplasias
11. Miller postaxial acrofacial dysostosis S.
12. Roberts S. (pseudothalidomide S.)
13. Spondyloperipheral dysplasia
14. Ulnar-mammary S.
15. Weyers oligodactyly S.

References

1. Swischuk LE, John SD: Differential Diagnosis in Pediatric Radiology. (ed 2) Baltimore: Williams & Wilkins, 1995, pp 277–278
2. Taybi H, Lachman RS: Radiology of Syndromes, Metabolic Disorders, and Skeletal Dysplasias. (ed 4) St. Louis: Mosby-Year Book, 1996, p 1044

Gamut D-163

RADIOULNAR SYNOSTOSIS

COMMON
1. Ehlers-Danlos S.
2. Hereditary multiple exostoses (multiple cartilaginous exostoses; osteochondromatosis) (distal forearm)
3. Holt-Oram S.
4. Idiopathic; isolated anomaly
5. Trauma (interosseous ligament ossification)

UNCOMMON
1. Acrocephalosyndactyly (Pfeiffer type)
2. Chromosome 4: del(4p) S. (Wolf-Hirschhorn S.)
3. Cloverleaf skull deformity (kleeblattschädel anomaly)
4. Femoral hypoplasia–unusual facies S.
5. Fetal alcohol S.
6. Infantile cortical hyperostosis (Caffey disease)
7. Klinefelter S. (XXY S.)
8. Lacrimo-auriculo-dento-digital S. (LADD S.) (Levy-Hollister S.)
9. Mesomelic dysplasia (Nievergelt type)
10. Multiple synostosis S.
11. Nager acrofacial dysostosis
12. Thalidomide embryopathy
13. Thanatophoric dysplasia
14. Trisomy 18 S.
15. XXXY S.; XXXXX S.; XXXXY S.

References
1. Kozlowski K, Beighton P: Gamut Index of Skeletal Dysplasias. Berlin: Springer-Verlag, 1984, pp 64–65
2. Taybi H, Lachman RS: Radiology of Syndromes, Metabolic Disorders, and Skeletal Dysplasias. (ed 4) St. Louis: Mosby-Year Book, 1996, p 1042

Gamut D-164-1

DEFORMITY OF THE FOREARM

COMMON
1. Galeazzi fracture (fracture of radial shaft with dislocation of distal ulna)
2. Generalized bone growth disturbance (eg, under-constriction or overconstriction of diametaphyses) (See D-10, D-11)
3. Monteggia fracture (fracture of ulnar shaft with dislocation of radial head)
4. Proximal radioulnar dislocation (See D-165)

UNCOMMON
1. Congenital radioulnar synostosis (See D-163)
2. Enchondromatosis (Ollier disease) or Maffucci S. with shortened ulna
3. Hereditary multiple exostoses (multiple cartilaginous exostoses; osteochondromatosis) with short ulna, curved radius, and often radial head dislocation
4. Hypoplasia or aplasia of radius or ulna (radial or ulnar ray syndromes) (See D-161, 162)
5. Isolated anomaly
6. Madelung deformity (See D-164-2).
7. Osteogenesis imperfecta (bowed radius and ulna)
8. Osteomyelitis or smallpox with residual deformity

Reference
1. Burgener FA, Kormano M: Differential Diagnosis in Conventional Radiology. New York: Thieme Medical Publ, 1991, pp 254–255

Gamut D-164-2

DISORDERS ASSOCIATED WITH MADELUNG (OR MADELUNG-LIKE) DEFORMITY*

1. Dyschondrosteosis
2. Enchondromatosis (Ollier disease); Maffucci S.
3. Hereditary multiple exostoses (multiple cartilaginous exostoses; osteochondromatosis)
4. Hurler S. (tilt of distal radius and ulna toward each other)
4. LEOPARD S. (multiple lentigenes S.)
6. Trauma in childhood (pseudo-Madelung deformity)
7. Turner S.

* Premature fusion of ulnar aspect of distal radial epiphysis resulting in (1) ulnar and volar angulation of distal radial articular surface, (2) decreased carpal angle, and (3) dorsal subluxation of distal ulna.

References
1. Kozlowski K, Beighton P: Gamut Index of Skeletal Dysplasias. Berlin: Springer-Verlag, 1984, p 65
2. Poznanski AK: The Hand in Radiologic Diagnosis. (ed 2) Philadelphia: WB Saunders, 1984, p 904
3. Taybi H, Lachman RS: Radiology of Syndromes, Metabolic Disorders, and Skeletal Dysplasias. (ed 4) St. Louis: Mosby-Year Book, 1996, p 1036

Gamut D-165

CONGENITAL SYNDROMES WITH ELBOW ANOMALY (INCLUDING RADIAL HEAD HYPOPLASIA, PROXIMAL RADIOULNAR DISLOCATION, CUBITUS VALGUS)

COMMON

*1. Brachmann-de Lange S. (de Lange S.)
2. Diastrophic dysplasia
*3. Hereditary multiple exostoses (multiple cartilaginous exostoses; osteochondromatosis)
4. Larsen S.
*5. Nail-patella S. (osteo-onychodysplasia)
*6. Neurofibromatosis
+*7. Noonan S.
*8. Otopalatodigital S. (types I and II)
+9. Turner S.

UNCOMMON

1. Aase-Smith S.
2. Acromesomelic dysplasia
3. Aminopterin fetopathy
*4. Campomelic dysplasia
5. Cerebro-costo-mandibular S.
6. Chondroectodermal dysplasia (Ellis-van Creveld S.)
*7. Chromosomal abnormalities (chromosome 18: del(18p) S., chromosome 20: dup(20p) S.)
8. Cleidocranial dysplasia
9. Cloverleaf skull deformity (kleeblattschädel anomaly)
*10. Coffin-Siris S.
*11. Crouzon S. (craniofacial dysostosis)
12. Cutis laxa
+*13. Dyschondrosteosis
14. Enchondromatosis (Ollier disease)
*15. Fanconi anemia (pancytopenia-dysmelia S.)
16. Frontometaphyseal dysplasia

(continued)

*17. Hajdu-Cheney S.
 18. Holt-Oram S.
*19. Humerospinal dysostosis
 20. Idiopathic; isolated anomaly
*21. Klinefelter S. (XXY S.)
+22. Léri pleonosteosis
*23. Mesomelic dysplasia (Nievergelt type)
*24. Mietens-Weber S.
 25. Multiple epiphyseal dysplasia (Fairbank)
 26. Multiple synostosis S.
*27. Occipital horn S.
 28. Oculodento-osseous dysplasia
*29. Opitz trigonocephaly S. (C syndrome)
*30. Seckel S. (bird-headed dwarfism)
*31. Spondyloepimetaphyseal dysplasia with joint laxity
 32. TAR S. (thrombocytopenia—absent radius S.)
 33. Trisomy 8 S.
+34. Trisomy 22 S.
*35. XXXXY S.; XXXXX S.
+36. Zellweger S. (cerebrohepatorenal S.)

* Proximal radioulnar subluxation (dislocation of radial head).
+ Increased carrying angle (cubitus valgus).

References

1. Greenfield GB: Radiology of Bone Diseases. (ed 5) Philadelphia: Lippincott, 1990
2. Jones KL: Smith's Recognizable Patterns of Human Malformation. Philadelphia: WB Saunders, 1988
3. Kozlowski K, Beighton P: Gamut Index of Skeletal Dysplasias. Berlin: Springer-Verlag, 1984, p 66
4. Swischuk LE, John SD: Differential Diagnosis in Pediatric Radiology. (ed 2) Baltimore: Williams & Wilkins, 1995, pp 213, 306
5. Taybi H, Lachman RS: Radiology of Syndromes, Metabolic Disorders, and Skeletal Dysplasias. (ed 4) St. Louis: Mosby-Year Book, 1996, pp 1027–1029

Gamut D-166

RADIOHUMERAL SYNOSTOSIS

1. Acrocephalosyndactyly, Pfeiffer type (Pfeiffer S.)
2. Antley-Bixler S.
3. Femoral hypoplasia—unusual facies S.
4. Lenz-Majewski dysplasia
5. Multiple synostosis S.
6. Roberts S. (pseudothalidomide S.)
7. Smallpox residual
8. Symphalangism-surdity S. (symphalangism-brachydactyly S.; WL S.)

Gamut D-167

DISPLACED ELBOW FAT PAD

COMMON

1. Infection; synovitis
2. Rheumatoid arthritis
3. Trauma with hemorrhage

UNCOMMON

1. Calcium pyrophosphate dihydrate crystal deposition disease (CPPD)
2. Gout
3. Hemophilia
4. Leukemia
5. Metastasis
6. Neuropathic arthropathy (See D-223)
7. Osteoarthritis (usually secondary)
8. Osteochondritis dissecans
9. Osteoid osteoma
10. Synovial osteochondromatosis
11. Synovial sarcoma
12. Villonodular synovitis

Reference

1. Murphy WA, Siegel MJ: Elbow fat pads with new signs and extended differential diagnosis. Radiology 1977; 124: 659–665

Gamut D-168

GROOVED DEFECT, EROSION, OR DEFORMITY OF THE HUMERAL HEAD

COMMON

1. Arthritis (esp. rheumatoid; ankylosing spondylitis; gout; infectious)
2. Avascular necrosis (esp. steroid therapy; sickle cell disease)
3. Chronic dislocation (Hill-Sachs defect)
4. Fracture (esp. of greater tuberosity)

UNCOMMON

1. Arteriovenous fistula, traumatic
2. Erb's palsy with disuse
3. Glenohumeral dysplasia
4. Hemophilia
5. Multicentric reticulohistiocytosis (lipoid dermato-arthritis)
6. Periarthrosis humeroscapularis
7. Pigmented villonodular synovitis
8. Rickets
9. Rotator cuff tear with atrophy and upward sub-luxation
10. Syringomyelia (neuroarthropathy)
11. Tuberculosis

References

1. Hill HA, Sachs MD: The grooved defect of the humeral head. Radiology 1940; 35:690–700
2. Burgener FA, Kormano M: Differential Diagnosis in Conventional Radiology. (ed 2) New York: Thieme Medical Publ, 1991, p 252

Gamut D-169

CONGENITAL SYNDROMES WITH ABNORMAL SCAPULA (USUALLY HYPOPLASIA, ESPECIALLY OF GLENOID)*

COMMON

*1. Acrocephalosyndactyly (Apert type)
2. Campomelic dysplasia
3. Cleidocranial dysplasia
*4. Familial glenoid hypoplasia
*5. Holt-Oram S.
*6. Isolated anomaly; idiopathic
*7. Mucopolysaccharidoses (eg, Hurler S.; Maroteaux-Lamy S.); mucolipidosis II (I-cell disease); fucosidosis; mannosidosis (See J-4)
*8. Nail-patella S. (osteo-onychodysplasia)
9. Sprengel deformity (eg, Klippel-Feil S.)
10. Short rib-polydactyly syndromes

UNCOMMON

1. Achondrogenesis (types 1 and 2)
2. Achondroplasia (flat inferior angle)
3. Antley-Bixler S.
4. CHILD S. (ichthyosis-limb reduction S.)
5. Cloverleaf skull deformity (kleeblattschädel anomaly)
6. de la Chapelle dysplasia
*7. Diastrophic dysplasia
*8. Dyggve-Melchior-Clausen dysplasia
9. Dyssegmental dysplasia
*10. Erb's palsy with disuse
11. Fetal varicella S.
*12. Fibrochondrogenesis
13. Gorlin S. (nevoid basal cell carcinoma S.)
*14. Grant S.
15. Hallermann-Streiff S. (oculomandibulofacial S.)
16. Hypophosphatasia (perinatal lethal form)
17. LEOPARD S. (multiple lentigenes S.)
18. Menkes S. (kinky-hair S.)
*19. Occipital horn S.

(continued)

20. Platyspondylic lethal skeletal dysplasia (PLSD-Luton type)
*21. Poland S. (pectoral muscle aplasia—syndactyly)
22. Proteus S.
23. Scapuloiliac dysostosis
*24. TAR S. (thrombocytopenia—absent radius S.)
25. Thanatophoric dysplasia
*26. Trisomy 8 S.

* Hypoplasia of glenoid fossa.

References
1. Kozlowski K, Beighton P: Gamut Index of Skeletal Dysplasias. Berlin: Springer-Verlag, 1984, p 54
2. Mortier GR, Rimoin DL, Lachman RS: The scapula as a window to the diagnosis of skeletal dysplasias. Pediatr Radiol 1997; 27:447–451
3. Swischuk LE, John SD: Differential Diagnosis in Pediatric Radiology. (ed 2) Baltimore: Williams & Wilkins, 1995, pp 289–290
4. Taybi H, Lachman RS: Radiology of Syndromes, Metabolic Disorders, and Skeletal Dysplasias. (ed 4) St. Louis: Mosby-Year Book, 1996, p 1051

Gamut D-170

LESION OF THE SCAPULA IN AN INFANT OR CHILD

COMMON
*1. Benign bone neoplasm (esp. osteochondroma; also enchondroma; hemangioma; lymphangioma; aneurysmal bone cyst)
2. Congenital syndromes with scapular hypoplasia (See D-169)
3. Fracture (esp. battered child S.)
*4. Langerhans cell histiocytosis$_g$

UNCOMMON
1. Arthritis involving glenohumeral joint (incl. neuro-arthropathy due to syringomyelia)
2. Bone cyst
3. Brachial plexus injury (winged scapula)

4. Erb's palsy with disuse
*5. Fibrous dysplasia
*6. Infantile cortical hyperostosis (Caffey disease)
7. Leukemia; lymphoma$_g$
*8. Malignant fibrous histiocytoma
*9. Metastasis
*10. Osteomyelitis
*11. Sarcoma (esp. Ewing sarcoma)
12. Sprengel deformity (eg, Klippel-Feil S.)

* May cause enlargement or expansion of scapula.

References
1. Hope JW, Gould RJ: Scapular lesions in childhood. AJR 1962;88:496–502
2. Swischuk LE, John SD: Differential Diagnosis in Pediatric Radiology. (ed 2) Baltimore: Williams & Wilkins, 1995, pp 289–290

Gamut D-171

LESION OF THE CLAVICLE IN AN INFANT OR CHILD (See D-172–175)

COMMON
1. Langerhans cell histiocytosis$_g$
2. [Normal rhomboid fossa]
3. Osteomyelitis (incl. chronic recurrent multifocal osteomyelitis)
4. Trauma (fracture; dislocation; battered child S.)

UNCOMMON
1. Benign bone neoplasm (eg, enchondroma; hemangioma)
2. Condensing osteitis of the clavicle
3. Congenital hypoplasia or absence (eg, cleidocranial dysplasia; pyknodysostosis) (See D-172-1)
4. Endosteal hyperostosis (van Buchem and Worth types)
5. Fibrous dysplasia; other fibrocystic lesion
6. Handlebar (hypoplastic, squat) clavicle (See D-172-2)

7. Hyperparathyroidism (esp. secondary)
8. Infantile cortical hyperostosis (Caffey disease)
9. Juvenile chronic arthritis (eg, juvenile rheumatoid arthritis)
10. Leukemia; lymphoma$_g$
11. Malignant bone neoplasm (esp. Ewing sarcoma; osteosarcoma)
12. Metastasis
13. Mucopolysaccharidoses (eg, Hurler S.) (See J-4)
14. Oculodentoosseous dysplasia; craniodiaphyseal dysplasia (expansion of clavicles)
15. Osteodysplasty (Melnick-Needles S.)
16. Osteogenesis imperfecta
17. Osteopetrosis
18. Posttraumatic osteolysis
19. Progeria
20. Pseudoarthrosis, congenital or traumatic
21. Pyle dysplasia
22. Sternocostoclavicular hyperostosis (SAPHO S.)
23. Syphilis
24. Tuberculosis

[ ] This condition does not actually cause the gamuted imaging finding, but can produce imaging changes that simulate it.

Reference
1. Swischuk LE, John SD: Differential Diagnosis in Pediatric Radiology. (ed 2) Baltimore: Williams & Wilkins, 1995, pp 287–289

Gamut D-172-1

APLASTIC, HYPOPLASTIC, OR THIN CLAVICLE

COMMON
1. Cleidocranial dysplasia
2. Holt-Oram S.
*3. Muscular or neuromuscular disorders$_g$ (eg, Werdnig-Hoffman disease)
4. Osteodysplasty (Melnick-Needles S.)
*5. Premature infants
*6. Progeria
7. Pyknodysostosis

UNCOMMON
1. Birth trauma to brachial plexus (unilateral)
2. CHILD S. (ichthyosis-limb reduction S.)
*3. Cockayne S.
4. Coffin-Siris S.
5. Congenital clavicular pseudoarthrosis
*6. Fibrochondrogenesis
7. Fucosidosis
8. Goltz S. (focal dermal hypoplasia)
*9. Larsen S.
10. Mandibuloacral dysplasia
11. Scapuloiliac dysostosis
12. Spondyloepiphyseal dysplasia (delayed ossification)
*13. Trisomy 13 S.
*14. Trisomy 18 S.
*15. Turner S. (thin clavicle laterally)
16. Yunis-Varón S.

* Thin or slender clavicle.

References
1. Jones KL; Smith's Recognizable Patterns of Human Malformation. Philadelphia: WB Saunders, 1988
2. Kozlowski K, Beighton P: Gamut Index of Skeletal Dysplasias. Berlin: Springer-Verlag, 1984, pp 53–54
3. Swischuk LE, John SD: Differential Diagnosis in Pediatric Radiology. (ed 2) Baltimore: Williams & Wilkins, 1995, pp 287–289
4. Taybi H, Lachman RS: Radiology of Syndromes, Metabolic Disorders, and Skeletal Dysplasias. (ed 4) St. Louis: Mosby-Year Book, 1996, pp 1048–1049

Gamut D-172-2

HANDLEBAR (HYPOPLASTIC, SQUAT) CLAVICLE

1. Asphyxiating thoracic dysplasia (Jeune S.)
2. Campomelic dysplasia
3. Diastrophic dysplasia
4. Holt-Oram S.

(continued)

5. Mucopolysaccharidoses (esp. Hurler S.); mucolipidoses (short, thick clavicle)
6. [Normal variant (eg, improper positioning of chest)]
7. TAR S. (thrombocytopenia—absent radius S.)
8. Trisomy 18 S.

[ ] This condition does not actually cause the gamuted imaging finding, but can produce imaging changes that simulate it.

Reference

1. Swischuk LE, John SD: Differential Diagnosis in Pediatric Radiology. (ed 2) Baltimore: Williams & Wilkins, 1995, p 287

Gamut D-173

ELONGATED CLAVICLE

COMMON

1. Trisomy 18 S.

UNCOMMON

1. Atelosteogenesis
2. Fibrochondrogenesis
3. Metatropic dysplasia
4. Pseudodiastrophic dysplasia
5. Schinzel-Giedion S.
6. Schneckenbecken dysplasia

Reference

1. Taybi H, Lachman RS: Radiology of Syndromes, Metabolic Disorders, and Syndromes. (ed 4) St. Louis: Mosby-Year Book Inc., 1996

Gamut D-174-1

BROAD, THICKENED, OR ENLARGED CLAVICLE (See D-174-2)

COMMON

1. Neoplasm, benign (eg, cartilaginous tumor; osteoma) or malignant (eg, osteosarcoma; Ewing sarcoma; metastasis; myeloma)
2. [Normal variant or improper positioning of chest, esp. in a child]
3. Osteomyelitis, chronic productive (incl. *Salmonella; syphilis*)
4. Paget's disease
5. Posttraumatic (healed fracture with callus)

UNCOMMON

1. Copper deficiency, nutritional; Menkes S. (kinky-hair S.)
2. Craniodiaphyseal dysplasia
3. Diaphyseal dysplasia (Camurati-Engelmann disease)
4. Distal osteosclerosis
5. Dysosteosclerosis
6. Endosteal hyperostosis (van Buchem and Worth types)
7. Fibrous dysplasia
8. Holt-Oram S.
9. Hyperphosphatasia
10. Infantile cortical hyperostosis (Caffey disease)
11. Langerhans cell histiocytosis$_g$ (esp. healed)
12. Lenz-Majewski dysplasia
13. Lymphoma$_g$; leukemia
14. Pyle dysplasia
15. Mucolipidoses; fucosidosis; mannosidosis; GM_1 gangliosidosis
16. Mucopolysaccharidoses (esp. Hurler S.)
17. Oculodentoosseous dysplasia
18. Osteodysplasty (Melnick-Needles S.)
19. Sclerosteosis
20. Sternocostoclavicular hyperostosis (SAPHO S.)
21. Winchester S.

[ ] This condition does not actually cause the gamuted imaging finding, but can produce imaging changes that simulate it.

Reference

1. Taybi H, Lachman RS: Radiology of Syndromes, Metabolic Disorders, and Skeletal Dysplasias. (ed 4) St. Louis: Mosby-Year Book, 1996, pp 1048–1049

Gamut D-174-2

SCLEROSIS AND/OR PERIOSTEAL REACTION INVOLVING THE CLAVICLE

COMMON

*1. Arthritis of sternoclavicular or acromioclavicular joint (eg, osteoarthritis; septic arthritis)
2. Bone sarcoma (eg, Ewing sarcoma; osteosarcoma)
3. Fracture with callus
4. Langerhans cell histiocytosis$_g$
5. Metastasis (esp. osteoblastic)
6. Osteomyelitis (incl. *Salmonella;* syphilis; Garré sclerosing osteomyelitis)
7. Paget's disease

UNCOMMON

1. Avascular necrosis
2. Condensing osteitis of the clavicle
3. Endosteal hyperostosis (van Buchem and Worth types)
4. Hypertrophic osteoarthropathy (See D-98)
5. Hypervitaminosis A
6. Infantile cortical hyperostosis (Caffey disease)
7. Leukemia; lymphoma$_g$ (esp. Hodgkin disease)
8. Osteoid osteoma
9. Osteoma
*10. Sternocostoclavicular hyperostosis (SAPHO S.)
*11. Tietze S.

* Involves sternal end of clavicle.

Reference

1. Appell RG, et al: Condensing osteitis of the clavicle in childhood: A rare sclerotic bone lesion. Pediatr Radiol 1983; 13:301–306

Gamut D-175

EROSION, DESTRUCTION, PENCILING, OR DEFECT OF THE OUTER END OF THE CLAVICLE

COMMON

*1. Hyperparathyroidism, primary and secondary (renal osteodystrophy)
2. Metastasis
3. Multiple myeloma
*4. Osteomyelitis (esp. pyogenic; tuberculous)
*5. Posttraumatic osteolysis (esp. weight lifter)
*6. Rheumatoid arthritis
7. Rickets
8. Surgical procedure
9. Trauma (eg, dislocation of acromioclavicular joint; fracture; battered child S.)

UNCOMMON

1. Amyloidosis
2. Congenital syndromes with hypoplasia of the clavicle (eg, cleidocranial dysplasia) (See D-172)
3. Gout
4. Langerhans cell histiocytosis$_g$ (eosinophilic granuloma)
5. Leukemia; lymphoma$_g$ (esp. Hodgkin disease)
6. Mucopolysaccharidoses; mucolipidoses (See J-4)
7. Multicentric reticulohistiocytosis (lipoid dermatoarthritis)
8. Neurogenic osteolysis
9. Primary bone neoplasm (eg, Ewing sarcoma)
*10. Progeria
11. Pyknodysostosis
12. Reiter S.
13. Sarcoidosis
*14. Scleroderma

* Penciled or pointed distal end of clavicle.

References

1. Greenfield GB: Radiology of Bone Diseases. (ed 5) Philadelphia: Lippincott, 1990

(continued)

2. Greenway GD, Danzig LA, Resnick D, et al: The painful shoulder. Med Radiogr Photog 1982; 58:22–67
3. Jacobson HG, Siegelman SS: RSNA Refresher Course Syllabus
4. Swischuk LE, John SD: Differential Diagnosis in Pediatric Radiology. (ed 2) Baltimore: Williams & Wilkins, 1995, pp 288–289

Gamut D-176

TIBIOTALAR TILT

CONGENITAL

UNCOMMON

1. Dysplasia epiphysealis hemimelica (Trevor disease)
2. Endosteal hyperostosis (van Buchem type)
3. Metaphyseal chondrodysplasia (Jansen and other types)
4. Multiple epiphyseal dysplasia (Fairbank)
5. Nail-patella S. (osteo-onychodysplasia)
6. Spondyloepiphyseal dysplasia

DEVELOPMENTAL

COMMON

1. Fibrous dysplasia
2. Neurofibromatosis

UNCOMMON

1. Enchondromatosis (Ollier disease)
2. Hereditary multiple exostoses (multiple cartilaginous exostoses; osteochondromatosis)

ACQUIRED

COMMON

1. Fracture (eg, Salter III or IV fracture of distal tibia; fractured femur with abnormal stress)
2. [Pseudotibiotalar tilt (flexing knee and externally rotating foot during radiography)]
3. Rheumatoid arthritis (esp. juvenile)
4. Tibia vara (Blount disease)

UNCOMMON

1. Avascular necrosis (eg, with chronic renal failure)
2. Bleeding disorder$_g$ with chronic hemarthrosis (esp. hemophilia; leukemia)
3. Cretinism, hypothyroidism
4. Femoral bowing
5. Hypoparathyroidism
6. Hypophosphatasia
7. Osteomyelitis of tibia, chronic (incl. syphilis; yaws; tropical ulcer)
8. Poliomyelitis
9. Rickets
10. Sickle cell disease

[ ] This condition does not actually cause the gamuted imaging finding, but can produce imaging changes that simulate it.

Reference
1. Griffiths H, Wandtke J: Tibiotalar tilt—A new slant. Skeletal Radiol 1981; 6:193–197

Gamut D-177

ISOLATED TIBIAL BOWING

COMMON

1. Absence or hypoplasia of fibula (See D-179)
2. Neurofibromatosis (usually lateral bowing); congenital pseudoarthrosis (usually with fibula)
3. Osteomyelitis (esp. syphilis—saber shin; yaws—boomerang tibia; tropical ulcer)
4. Paget's disease
5. Physiological (idiopathic) anterior or posterior tibial bowing (usually with fibula)
6. Plastic bending or bowing fracture of infancy or childhood
   a. Faulty intrauterine fetal positioning
   b. Greenstick fracture
   c. Weakened tibia (eg, osteogenesis imperfecta; hyperparathyroidism; rickets; hypophosphatasia; hyperphosphatasia; scurvy; leukemia)
7. Tibia vara (Blount disease)

8. Trauma, other (eg, epiphyseal injury; malunited fracture; battered child S.)

UNCOMMON

1. Elongation of fibula (See D-178)
2. Fibrous dysplasia
3. Klippel-Trenaunay S., Parkes Weber S., or limb hypertrophy (See D-14)
4. Weismann-Netter S. (usually with fibula)

References

1. Kozlowski K, Beighton P: Gamut Index of Skeletal Dysplasias. Berlin: Springer-Verlag, 1984, p 67
2. Swischuk LE, John SD: Differential Diagnosis in Pediatric Radiology. (ed 2) Baltimore: Williams & Wilkins, 1995, pp 202–205

Gamut D-178

ELONGATION OF FIBULA

1. Achondroplasia
2. Hypochondroplasia
3. Mesomelic dysplasia
4. Metaphyseal chondrodysplasia (McKusick type)
5. Muscular disorder$_g$
6. Pseudoachondroplasia (pseudoachondroplastic spondyloepiphyseal dysplasia)
7. Spondyloepimetaphyseal dysplasias

Reference

1. Kozlowski K, Beighton P: Gamut Index of Skeletal Dysplasias. Berlin: Springer-Verlag, 1984, p 67

Gamut D-179

APLASIA, HYPOPLASIA, OR SHORTENING OF FIBULA*

1. Atelosteogenesis (types I and III)
2. Campomelic dysplasia
3. Chondroectodermal dysplasia (Ellis-van Creveld S.)
4. Chromosomal abnormalities
5. Cleidocranial dysplasia
6. de la Chapelle dysplasia
7. Du Pan S.
8. Femur-fibula-ulna S.
9. Fibrochondrogenesis
10. Grebe chondrodysplasia (achondrogenesis, Brazilian type)
11. Hereditary multiple exostoses (multiple cartilaginous exostoses; osteochondromatosis)
12. Mesomelic dysplasia (Langer, Nievergelt, Werner types)
13. Mietens-Weber S.
14. Otopalatodigital S. (type II)
15. Proximal femoral focal deficiency
16. Seckel S. (bird-headed dwarfism)
17. Short rib-polydactyly S. type I (Saldino-Noonan)
18. Weyers oligodactyly S.

* Usually seen with tibial hypoplasia, but predominant fibular changes may be seen in above dysplasias. There are over ten other rare syndromes listed in the Taybi-Lachman text.

References

1. Kozlowski K, Beighton P: Gamut Index of Skeletal Dysplasias. Berlin: Springer-Verlag, 1984, p 68
2. Taybi H, Lachman RS: Radiology of Syndromes, Metabolic Disorders, and Skeletal Dysplasias. (ed 4) St. Louis: Mosby-Year Book, 1996, p 1031

Gamut D-180

CONGENITAL SYNDROMES WITH ABSENT, HYPOPLASTIC, DYSPLASTIC, BIPARTITE, OR DISLOCATED PATELLA

COMMON

1. Arthrogryposis (dislocated)
2. Nail-patella S. (osteo-onychodysplasia) (absent or hypoplastic)
3. Neuromuscular disorders$_g$ (esp. cerebral palsy) (fragmented lower pole)
4. Normal variant (bipartite)
5. Sinding-Larsen-Johansson disease (fragmented inferior tip)

UNCOMMON

1. Acrocephalopolysyndactyly (Carpenter S.) (dislocated)
2. Chondrodysplasia punctata (calcific flecks in patella)
3. Diastrophic dysplasia (dislocated, hypoplastic, or multipartite)
4. Familial absence of patella
5. Kuskokwim S. (hypoplastic)
6. Mesomelic dysplasia (Werner type)
7. Multiple epiphyseal dysplasia (Fairbank) (dislocated or bipartite)
8. Neurofibromatosis type I (absent)
9. Popliteal pterygium S. (absent or bipartite)
10. Rubinstein-Taybi S. (dislocated)
11. Seckel S. (bird-headed dwarfism) (absent)
12. Small patella S.
13. Spondyloepimetaphyseal dysplasia
14. Spondyloepiphyseal dysplasia (incl. pseudoachondroplasia)
15. Stickler S. (arthro-ophthalmopathy) (dislocated)
16. Trisomy 8 S. (absent or hypoplastic)
17. Warfarin embryopathy (calcific flecks)
18. Zellweger S. (cerebrohepatorenal S.) (calcific flecks in patella)

References

1. Azouz EM, Kozlowski K: Small patella syndrome: A bone dysplasia to recognize and differentiate from the nail-patella syndrome. Pediatr Radiol 1997; 27:425
2. Braun H-St: Familial aplasia or hypoplasia of the patella. Clin Genet 13:350, 1978
3. Jones KL: Smith's Recognizable Patterns of Human Malformation. Philadelphia: WB Saunders, 1988
4. Kaye JJ, Freiberger RH: Fragmentation of the lower pole of the patella and spastic lower extremities. Radiology 1971; 101:97
5. Kozlowski K, Beighton P: Gamut Index of Skeletal Dysplasias. Berlin: Springer-Verlag, 1984, p 67
6. Rosenthal RK, Levine DB: Fragmentation of the distal pole of the patella in spastic cerebral palsy. J Bone Joint Surg 1977; 59:934–939
7. Swischuk LE, John SD: Differential Diagnosis in Pediatric Radiology. (ed 2) Baltimore: Williams & Wilkins, 1995, pp 284–287
8. Taybi H, Lachman RS: Radiology of Syndromes, Metabolic Disorders, and Skeletal Dysplasias. (ed 4) St. Louis: Mosby-Year Book, 1996, p 1038

Gamut D-181-1

ABNORMAL POSITION OF THE PATELLA—PATELLA ALTA (HIGH PATELLA)

1. Arthritis with joint effusion
2. Chondromalacia of patella
3. Idiopathic; isolated anomaly
4. Neuromuscular disorders$_g$ (eg, poliomyelitis; cerebral palsy)
5. Osgood-Schlatter disease
6. Osteomyelitis of femur
7. Rupture of patellar tendon
8. Sinding-Larsen disease (avascular necrosis of inferior ossification center of patella)
9. Subluxation, recurrent or chronic

References

1. Burgener FA, Kormano M: Differential Diagnosis in Conventional Radiology. New York: Thieme Medical Publ, 1991, pp 229–230

2. Lancourt JE, Cristini JA: Patella alta and patella infera. Their etiological role in patellar dislocation, chondromalacia, and apophysitis of the tibial tubercle. J Bone Joint Surg 1975; 57:1112–1115

Gamut D-181-2

ABNORMAL POSITION OF THE PATELLA—PATELLA BAJA OR PROFUNDA (LOW PATELLA)

1. Achondroplasia; other bone dysplasias
2. Juvenile rheumatoid arthritis
3. Paresis of quadriceps muscle (eg, poliomyelitis)
4. Rupture of quadriceps tendon
5. Surgical transposition of tibial tuberosity

References
1. Burgener FA, Kormano M: Differential Diagnosis in Conventional Radiology. New York: Thieme Medical Publ, 1991, pp 229–230
2. Lancourt JE, Cristini JA: Patella alta and patella infera. Their etiological role in patellar dislocation, chondromalacia, and apophysitis of the tibial tubercle. J Bone Joint Surg 1975; 57:1112–1115

Gamut D-182

LYTIC PATELLAR LESION

COMMON

1. Chondroblastoma (Codman tumor)
2. Dorsal defect of patella
3. Giant cell tumor
4. Subchondral cyst (associated with osteochondritis dissecans or chondromalacia)

UNCOMMON

1. Aneurysmal bone cyst
2. Bone cyst

3. Brown tumor of hyperparathyroidism
4. Enchondroma
5. Gout
6. Hemangioma
7. Intraosseous ganglion
8. Langerhans cell histiocytosis$_g$ (esp. eosinophilic granuloma)
9. Metastasis
10. Multiple myeloma; plasmacytoma
11. Osteoblastoma
12. Osteomyelitis; Brodie abscess; tuberculosis

References
1. Goergen TG, Resnick D, Greenway G, et al: Dorsal defect of the patella (DDP): A characteristic radiographic lesion. Radiology 1979; 130:333–336
2. Haswell DM, Berne AS, Graham CB: The dorsal defect of the patella. Pediatr Radiol 1976; 4:238–242
3. Kransdorf MJ, Moser RP Jr, Vinh TN, et al: Primary tumors of the patella. Skeletal Radiol 1989; 18:365–371

Gamut D-183

ENLARGEMENT OF THE DISTAL FEMORAL INTERCONDYLAR NOTCH

COMMON

1. Hemophilia
2. Juvenile chronic arthritis (esp. juvenile rheumatoid arthritis)

UNCOMMON

1. Diastrophic dysplasia
2. Dysplasia epiphysealis hemimelica (Trevor disease)
3. Metatropic dysplasia
4. Mesomelic dysplasia (Langer type)
5. Mucopolysaccharidoses (Morquio S.; Maroteaux-Lamy S.)
6. Parastremmatic dysplasia
7. Psoriatic arthritis
8. Septic arthritis
9. Tuberculous arthritis

(continued)

Reference

1. Spranger JW, Langer LO, Wiedemann H-R: Bone Dysplasias. Philadelphia: WB Saunders, 1974

Gamut D-184

ENLARGED MEDIAL FEMORAL CONDYLE

1. Brachmann-de Lange S. (de Lange S.)
2. Chondrodystrophies
3. Dyschondrosteosis
4. Posttraumatic
5. Prader-Willi S.
6. Tibia vara (Blount disease)
7. Turner S.
8. Vitamin D-resistant rickets

Reference

1. Swischuk LE, John SD: Differential Diagnosis in Pediatric Radiology. (ed 2) Baltimore: Williams & Wilkins, 1995, p 242

Gamut D-185

GENU VARUM (BOW LEGS)

COMMON

1. Achondroplasia
2. Femoral anteversion
3. Idiopathic; prenatal bowing
*4. Osteoarthritis, primary or secondary (may be associated with medial displacement of femur—genu laxum)
5. Rickets (all causes)
6. Physiologic tibial torsion in infants
*7. Tibia vara (Blount disease)
*8. Trauma (fracture of medial condyle of femur or tibia)

UNCOMMON

1. Acrodysostosis
2. Anadysplasia
3. Campomelic dysplasia
*4. Dysplasia epiphysealis hemimelica (Trevor disease)
*5. Epiphyseal-physeal-metaphyseal injury (trauma; infection; radiation)
6. Fluorosis
7. Hyperparathyroidism
8. Hyperphosphatasia
9. Hypochondroplasia
10. Hypophosphatasia
11. Infantile multisystem inflammatory disease (NOMID)
12. Metaphyseal chondrodysplasia (McKusick, Jansen, Schmid types)
13. Multiple epiphyseal dysplasia (Fairbank)
*14. Neoplasm, localized (eg, osteochondroma; juxta-articular chondroma of lateral aspect of knee)
15. Neurofibromatosis
16. Pseudoachondroplasia (pseudoachondroplastic spondyloepiphyseal dysplasia)
17. Spondyloepimetaphyseal dysplasia
18. Spondyloepiphyseal dysplasia congenita
19. TAR S. (thrombocytopenia—absent radius S.)
20. Thanatophoric dysplasia
21. Turner S.

* Usually or always unilateral.

References

1. Bateson EM: Non-rachitis bow leg and knock-knee deformities in young Jamaican children. Br J Radiol 1966; 39: 92–101
2. Burgener FA, Kormano M: Differential Diagnosis in Conventional Radiology. (ed 2) New York: Thieme Medical Publ, 1991, p 262
3. Currarino G, Kirks DR: Lateral widening of epiphyseal plates in knees of children with bowed legs. AJR 1977; 129:309–312
4. Greenberg LE, Swartz AA: Genu varum and genu valgum: another look. Am J Dis Child 1971; 121:219–221
5. Kozlowski K, Beighton P: Gamut Index of Skeletal Dysplasias. Berlin: Springer-Verlag, 1984, p 66
6. Silverman FN (ed): Caffey's Pediatric X-ray Diagnosis. (ed 9) Chicago: Year Book Medical Publ, 1993, pp 1833–1839

7. Shopfner CE, Coin CG: Genu varus and valgus in children. Radiology 1969; 92:723–732
8. Swischuk LE, John SD: Differential Diagnosis in Pediatric Radiology. (ed 2) Baltimore: Williams & Wilkins, 1995, pp 207–210
9. Taybi H, Lachman RS: Radiology of Syndromes, Metabolic Disorders, and Skeletal Dysplasias. (ed 4) St. Louis: Mosby-Year Book, 1996, p 1032
10. Thompson GH, Carter JR: Late-onset tibia vara (Blount's disease): current concepts. Clin Orthop 1990; 255:24–35

Gamut D-186

GENU VALGUM (KNOCK-KNEES)

COMMON

*1. Arthritis (eg, juvenile rheumatoid arthritis; osteoarthritis involving lateral compartment of knee, primary or secondary to rupture of lateral meniscus or severe rheumatoid arthritis)
2. Pes planus (flat feet)
3. Physiologic
4. Regional muscular weakness from neurologic or neuromuscular disease$_g$

UNCOMMON

1. Acrocephalopolysyndactyly (Carpenter S.)
2. Acrocephalosyndactyly (Apert type)
3. Arthrogryposis
4. Bardet-Biedl S.
5. Chondroectodermal dysplasia (Ellis-van Creveld S.)
6. Cohen S.
7. Diaphyseal dysplasia (Camurati-Engelmann disease)
8. Dyschondrosteosis
*9. Dysplasia epiphysealis hemimelica (Trevor disease)
*10. Epiphyseal-metaphyseal injury (trauma; infection; radiation)
11. Fanconi anemia (pancytopenia-dysmelia S.)
12. Freeman-Sheldon S. (whistling face S.)
13. Frontometaphyseal dysplasia
14. Hajdu-Cheney S.
15. Hereditary multiple exostoses (multiple cartilaginous exostoses; osteochondromatosis)
16. Homocystinuria
17. Hypophosphatasia
18. Mesomelic dysplasia (esp. Langer, Nievergelt types)
19. Metaphyseal chondrodysplasia (Jansen and other types)
20. Mucopolysaccharidoses (eg, Hurler, Morquio) (See J-4)
21. Multiple epiphyseal dysplasia (Fairbank)
22. Nail-patella S. (osteo-onychodysplasia)
*23. Neoplasm, localized (eg, osteochondroma; juxta-articular chondroma of medial aspect of knee)
24. Neurofibromatosis
25. Noonan S.
26. Occipital horn S.
27. Osteodysplasty (Melnick-Needles S.)
28. Otopalatodigital S. (types I and II)
29. Parastremmatic dysplasia
30. Pyle dysplasia
31. Renal osteodystrophy (secondary hyperparathyroidism)
32. Rickets (all types) (with hypotonia—late)
33. Spondyloenchondrodysplasia (enchondromatosis with severe platyspondyly)
34. Spondyloepiphyseal dysplasia congenita (late)
35. Spondylometaphyseal dysplasia (Algerian and Murdoch types)
36. Trisomy 21 S. (Down S.)

* Usually or always unilateral.

References
1. Bateson EM: Non-rachitis bow leg and knock-knee deformities in young Jamaican children. Br J Radiol 1966; 39:92–101
2. Gorlin RT, Cohen MM Jr, Levin LS: Syndromes of the Head and Neck. (ed 3) New York: Oxford University Press, 1990
3. Greenberg LE, Swartz AA: Genu varum and genu valgum: another look. Am J Dis Child 1971; 121:219–221
4. Shopfner CE, Coin CG: Genu varus and valgus in children. Radiology 1969; 92:723–732
5. Swischuk LE, John SD: Differential Diagnosis in Pediatric Radiology. (ed 2) Baltimore: Williams & Wilkins, 1995, pp 207–210

(continued)

6. Taybi H, Lachman RS: Radiology of Syndromes, Metabolic Disorders, and Skeletal Dysplasias. (ed 4) St. Louis: Mosby-Year Book, 1996, pp 1031–1032

Gamut D-187-1

COXA VARA
(UNILATERAL OR BILATERAL)

COMMON

1. Avascular necrosis of femoral head (eg, steroid therapy; sickle cell disease; connective tissue disease (collagen vascular disease)$_g$; Gaucher disease; radiation injury) (See D-48)
2. Legg-Perthes disease (late)
3. Malunited fracture of femoral neck (incl. epiphyseal-physeal-metaphyseal fracture; battered child S.)
4. Paget's disease
5. Rickets (all types); osteomalacia (See D-44)
6. Slipped capital femoral epiphysis (late) (See D-190)

UNCOMMON

1. Congenital (idiopathic) coxa vara (femoral neck defect; hypoplasia of proximal femur {proximal femoral focal deficiency})
2. Congenital syndromes (See D-187-2)
3. Femoral neck lesion; other (eg, osteomyelitis; hydatid disease)
4. Fibrous dysplasia
5. Hyperparathyroidism (esp. secondary—renal osteodystrophy)
6. Hypophosphatasia
7. Hypothyroidism (slipped capital femoral epiphysis)
8. Rheumatoid arthritis (incl. juvenile)

Reference
1. Swischuk LE, John SD: Differential Diagnosis in Pediatric Radiology. (ed 2) Baltimore: Williams & Wilkins, 1995, pp 210–213

Gamut D-187-2

CONGENITAL SYNDROMES
WITH COXA VARA

COMMON

1. Achondroplasia
2. Fibrous dysplasia
3. Multiple epiphyseal dysplasia (Fairbank)
4. Osteogenesis imperfecta
5. Spondyloepiphyseal dysplasia (congenita or tarda)

UNCOMMON

1. Arthrogryposis
2. Cleidocranial dysplasia
3. Congenital (idiopathic) coxa vara (femoral neck defect; hypoplasia of proximal femur {proximal femoral focal deficiency})
4. Cretinism; hypothyroidism
5. Diastrophic dysplasia
6. Dyggve-Melchior-Clausen dysplasia
7. Enchondromatosis (Ollier disease)
8. Femoral hypoplasia—unusual facies S.
9. Frontometaphyseal dysplasia
10. Hereditary multiple exostoses (multiple cartilaginous exostoses; osteochondromatosis)
11. Hyperphosphatasia
12. Hypophosphatasia
13. Kniest dysplasia
14. Metaphyseal chondrodysplasia (Schmid and Shwachman types)
15. Metatropic dysplasia
16. Meyer dysplasia of femoral head
17. Osteodysplasty (Melnick-Needles S.)
18. Osteopetrosis
19. Pseudoachondroplasia (pseudoachondroplastic spondyloepiphyseal dysplasia)
20. Pseudohypoparathyroidism; pseudopseudohypoparathyroidism
21. Schwartz-Jampel S. (chondrodystrophic myotonia)
22. Spondyloepimetaphyseal dysplasias

23. Spondylometaphyseal dysplasia (Kozlowski and corner fracture types)

References

1. Kozlowski K, Beighton P: Gamut Index of Skeletal Dysplasias. Berlin: Springer-Verlag, 1984, pp 58–59
2. Swischuk LE, John SD: Differential Diagnosis in Pediatric Radiology. (ed 2) Baltimore: Williams & Wilkins, 1995, pp 207–210
3. Taybi H, Lachman RS: Radiology of Syndromes, Metabolic Disorders, and Skeletal Dysplasias. (ed 4) St. Louis: Mosby-Year Book, 1996, p 1027

Gamut D-188

COXA VALGA

COMMON

1. Chronic leg injury
2. Chronic muscular hypotonia; paralytic disorder$_g$; neuromuscular disorder$_g$; (eg, meningomyelocele; cerebral palsy; muscular dystrophy; poliomyelitis)
3. Developmental dysplasia of the hip—DDH (congenital hip dysplasia or dislocation), untreated
4. Rheumatoid arthritis (incl. juvenile)

UNCOMMON

1. Acrocephalopolysyndactyly (Carpenter S.)
2. Arthrogryposis
3. Baller-Gerold S. (craniosynostosis-radial aplasia S.)
4. Chromosome 18: del(18q) S.
5. Cleidocranial dysplasia
6. Cockayne S.
7. Coffin-Lowry S.
8. Coffin-Siris S.
9. Dyschondrosteosis
10. Dysplasia epiphysealis hemimelica (Trevor disease)
11. Frontometaphyseal dysplasia
12. Glycogen storage disease type I (von Gierke disease)
13. Hallermann-Streiff S. (oculomandibulofacial S.)
14. Hypoplasia or agenesis of sacrum; caudal dysplasia sequence (caudal regression S.)
15. Mucopolysaccharidoses (eg, Hurler; Hunter; Morquio; Maroteaux-Lamy); mucolipidosis II (I-cell disease) and III (pseudo-Hurler polydystrophy); sialidosis; mannosidosis; fucosidosis (See J-4)
16. Niemann-Pick disease
17. Occipital horn S.
18. Osteodysplasty (Melnick-Needles S.)
19. Otopalatodigital S. (type I)
20. Prader-Willi S.
21. Progeria
22. Pseudohypoparathyroidism
23. Pyknodysostosis
24. Pyle dysplasia
25. Schwartz-Jampel S. (chondrodystrophic myotonia)
26. Spondyloepiphyseal dysplasia with joint laxity
27. Stickler S. (arthro-ophthalmopathy)
28. TAR S. (thrombocytopenia-absent radius S.)
29. Turner S.
30. Weaver S.
31. XXXXY S.; XXXXX S.

References

1. Griffiths GJ, Evans KT, Roberts GM, Lloyd KN: The radiology of the hip joints and pelvis in cerebral palsy. Clin Radiol 1977; 28:187–192
2. Swischuk LE, John SD: Differential Diagnosis in Pediatric Radiology. (ed 2) Baltimore: Williams & Wilkins, 1995, pp 210–213
3. Taybi H, Lachman RS: Radiology of Syndromes, Metabolic Disorders, and Skeletal Dysplasias. (ed 4) St. Louis: Mosby-Year Book, 1996, p 1026

Gamut D-189-1

ABSENT, HYPOPLASTIC, OR DEFORMED PROXIMAL FEMUR

CONGENITAL

1. Amniotic band sequence
2. Atelosteogenesis
3. Boomerang dysplasia
4. Femoral hypoplasia-unusual facies S.
5. Proximal femoral focal dysplasia
6. Roberts S. (pseudothalidomide S.)
7. Thalidomide embryopathy

ACQUIRED

1. Congenital dislocation of the hip (complication of treatment)
2. Fibrous dysplasia, incl. McCune-Albright S.
3. Fracture with secondary deformity, nonunion
4. Hydatid disease
5. Hyperparathyroidism, primary or secondary (renal osteodystrophy)
6. Malignant bone tumor, primary or metastatic
7. Osteomyelitis (esp. meningococcemia)
8. Paget's disease
9. Septic arthritis, severe sequelae

Gamut D-189-2

FEMORAL HEAD DYSPLASIA

COMMON

1. Cretinism; hypothyroidism
2. Legg-Perthes disease
3. Meyer dysplasia of femoral head
4. Multiple epiphyseal dysplasia (Fairbank and Ribbing types)
5. Osteochondritis dissecans (subchondral dysplasia)

UNCOMMON

1. Bardet-Biedl S.
2. Elsbach dysplasia (bilateral hereditary microepiphyseal dysplasia)
3. Geleophysic dysplasia
4. Kniest dysplasia
5. Pseudoachondroplasia (pseudoachondroplastic spondyloepiphyseal dysplasia)
6. Rubinstein-Taybi S.
7. Silver-Russell S.
8. Spondyloepiphyseal dysplasias
9. Trichorhinophalangeal dysplasia, type I (Giedion S.) and II (Giedion-Langer S.)

Gamut D-189-3

FRAGMENTED OR IRREGULAR FEMORAL HEAD

COMMON

1. Arthritis, advanced (eg, rheumatoid; septic; degenerative; posttraumatic; associated with inflammatory bowel disease; gout; neuroarthropathy)
2. Avascular necrosis, all causes (See D-48)
3. Cretinism; hypothyroidism
4. Developmental dysplasia of the hip—DDH (congenital hip dysplasia or dislocation) (complication of treatment)
5. Legg-Perthes disease (osteochondrosis of femoral epiphysis)
6. Meyer dysplasia of femoral head
7. Multiple epiphyseal dysplasia (Fairbank and Ribbing types)
8. Occlusive vascular disease; thromboembolic disease
9. Sickle cell disease
10. Steroid therapy; Cushing S.
11. Traumatic dislocation; fracture of femoral neck; surgical or manipulative trauma

UNCOMMON

1. Acrodysplasia with retinitis pigmentosa and nephropathy (Saldino-Mainzer S.)
2. Adrenogenital S.
3. Behçet S.
4. Chondrodysplasia punctata
5. Diabetes
6. Diastrophic dysplasia
7. Dyggve-Melchior-Clausen dysplasia
8. Dysplasia epiphysealis hemimelica (Trevor disease)
9. Elsbach dysplasia (bilateral hereditary microepiphyseal dysplasia)
10. Enchondromatosis (Ollier disease)
11. Fabry disease
12. Gaucher disease
13. Geleophysic dysplasia
14. Hemophilia; Christmas disease
15. Infection
16. Kniest dysplasia
17. Leukemia
18. Metachondromatosis
19. Metaphyseal chondrodysplasia (McKusick and Shwachman types)
20. Mucopolysaccharidoses (esp. Hurler; Hunter; Morquio; Maroteaux-Lamy); mucolipidosis II (I-cell disease) and III (pseudo-Hurler polydystrophy) (See J-4)
21. Osteochondritis dissecans
22. Pancreatitis, acute or chronic; alcoholism
23. Pseudoachondroplasia (pseudoachondroplastic spondyloepiphyseal dysplasia)
24. Radiation therapy
25. Renal osteodystrophy (secondary hyperparathyroidism); post renal transplantation
26. Rickets (all types)
27. Sarcoidosis
28. Schwartz-Jampel S. (chondrodystrophic myotonia)
29. Slipped capital femoral epiphysis (late)
30. Spondyloepiphyseal dysplasia
31. Spondylometaphyseal dysplasia (Kozlowski type)
32. Stickler S. (arthro-ophthalmopathy)
33. Trichorhinophalangeal dysplasia, type I (Giedion S.) and II (Giedion-Langer S.)
34. Winchester S.

References

1. Greenfield GB: Radiology of Bone Diseases. (ed 5) Philadelphia: Lippincott, 1990
2. Kozlowski K, Beighton P: Gamut Index of Skeletal Dysplasias. Berlin: Springer-Verlag, 1984, pp 57–58
3. Ozonoff MB: Pediatric Orthopedic Radiology. Philadelphia: WB Saunders, 1992, pp 234–276
4. Swischuk LE, John SD: Differential Diagnosis in Pediatric Radiology. (ed 2) Baltimore: Williams & Wilkins, 1995, pp 236–239
5. Taybi H, Lachman RS: Radiology of Syndromes, Metabolic Disorders, and Skeletal Dysplasias. (ed 4) St. Louis: Mosby-Year Book, 1996, pp 1030–1031

Gamut D-190

SLIPPED CAPITAL FEMORAL EPIPHYSIS

COMMON

1. Idiopathic (age 9–17)
2. Renal osteodystrophy (secondary hyperparathyroidism)
3. Trauma

UNCOMMON

1. Congenital (idiopathic) coxa vara (femoral neck defect; hypoplasia of proximal femur)
2. Drug therapy (eg, chemotherapy; chorionic gonadotropin therapy)
3. Gaucher disease
4. Gigantism (hyperpituitarism); rapid growth spurt; growth hormone deficiency and therapy; pituitary tumor
5. Hemophilia
6. Hyperparathyroidism
7. Hypopituitarism
8. Hypothyroidism
9. Marfan S.
10. Metaphyseal chondrodysplasia (esp. Shwachman type)
11. Multiple endocrine neoplasia, type IIB (MEN IIB)
12. Multiple epiphyseal dysplasia (Fairbank)

(continued)

13. Obesity; mechanical stress
14. Pseudohypoparathyroidism; pseudopseudohy-poparathyroidism
15. Radiation therapy
16. Rickets; poor nutrition
17. Schwartz-Jampel S. (chondrodystrophic myotonia)
18. Scurvy
19. Steroid therapy; Cushing S.
20. Syphilis
21. Trisomy 21 S. (Down S.)

References

1. Greenfield GB: Radiology of Bone Diseases. (ed 5) Philadelphia: Lippincott, 1990
2. Steinbach HL, Young DA: The roentgen appearance of pseudohypoparathyroidism (PH) and pseudo-pseudohypoparathyroidism (PPH). AJR 1966; 97:49–66
3. Taybi H, Lachman RS: Radiology of Syndromes, Metabolic Disorders, and Skeletal Dysplasias. (ed 4) St. Louis: Mosby-Year Book, 1996, p 1031

Gamut D-191

PROTRUSIO ACETABULI (UNILATERAL OR BILATERAL)

COMMON

1. Degenerative joint disease, primary (osteoarthritis) or secondary (incl. hemophilia; hemochromatosis)
2. Hyperparathyroidism
3. Normal variant (children age 4–12)
4. Osteomalacia
5. Osteoporosis
6. Paget's disease
7. Primary or idiopathic (Otto pelvis) (eg, coxa vara with retroversion of femoral neck)
8. Renal osteodystrophy (secondary hyperparathyroidism)
9. Rheumatoid arthritis (incl. juvenile)
10. Rickets
11. Trauma (acetabular fracture with medial dislocation of hip)

UNCOMMON

1. Acrodysostosis
2. Arthritis, other (eg, ankylosing spondylitis; juvenile chronic arthritis; gout; psoriatic)
3. Fibrous dysplasia
4. Homocystinuria
5. Hydatid disease
6. Hyperphosphatasia
7. Infectious arthritis (eg, septic; tuberculous)
8. Marfan S.
9. Mucopolysaccharidoses (esp. Morquio S.) (See J-4)
10. Neoplasm involving acetabulum, primary or metastatic (incl. multiple myeloma), with medial dislocation of hip
11. Ochronosis (alkaptonuria)
12. Osteogenesis imperfecta
13. Postsurgical (eg, medial dislocation of femoral head prosthesis following total hip replacement)
14. Radiation therapy (esp. in a child)
15. Sickle cell disease
16. Stickler S. (arthro-ophthalmopathy)
17. Turner S.

References

1. Kuhlman JE, et al: Acetabular protrusion in the Marfan syndrome. Radiology 1987; 164:415–417
2. McEwen C, Poppel MH, Poker N, Jacobson HG: Protrusio acetabuli in rheumatoid arthritis. Radiology 1956; 66:33–40
3. Murray RO, Jacobson HG, Stoker DJ: The Radiology of Skeletal Disorders. (ed 3) London: Churchill Livingstone, 1990
4. Taybi H, Lachman RS: Radiology of Syndromes, Metabolic Disorders, and Skeletal Dysplasias. (ed 4) St. Louis: Mosby-Year Book, 1996, p 1045

Gamut D-192

CONGENITAL SYNDROMES WITH AN ABNORMAL PELVIS
(See D-193 to D-195)

COMMON

1. Achondroplasia (small trident pelvis; short sacroil-iac notches)
2. Mucopolysaccharidoses (eg, Hurler; Morquio) (flared iliac wings; steep acetabular roofs; narrow pelvic inlet; coxa valga)
3. Trisomy 21 S. (Down S.) (hypoplastic, flared iliac wings; decreased acetabular and iliac angles; ischial tapering)

UNCOMMON

1. Achondrogenesis (types I and II) (hypoplastic pelvis; sacral, pubic, ischial bones not ossified; flat acetabula)
2. Arthrogryposis
3. Asphyxiating thoracic dysplasia (Jeune S.) (flared ilia; small trident pelvis)
4. Campomelic dysplasia (narrow pelvis with poor ossification)
5. Caudal dysplasia sequence (caudal regression S.) (caudal hypoplasia or aplasia—narrow pelvis with absence or hypoplasia of sacrum)
6. Cephaloskeletal dysplasia (Taybi-Linder S.) (short iliac wings; flat acetabular angles; narrow sciatic notches)
7. Chondrodysplasia punctata (trapezoid ilium)
8. Chondroectodermal dysplasia (Ellis-van Creveld S.) (trident pelvis)
9. Chromosome 4: del(4p) S. (Wolf-Hirschhorn S.) (small pelvis with underdeveloped pubic rami; increased iliac angles)
10. Cleidocranial dysplasia (wide pubic symphysis)
11. Cockayne S. (small square pelvis)
12. Diastrophic dysplasia (short thick iliac bones)
13. Dyggve-Melchior-Clausen dysplasia (small sciatic notches; serrated iliac crests)

14. Dyssegmental dysplasia (wide flared ilia with small sacrosciatic notches; broad pubis and ischia)
15. Enchondromatosis (Ollier disease)
16. Fibrochondrogenesis (hypoplastic pelvis; squared iliac wings; trident roof)
17. Goltz S. (focal dermal hypoplasia) (hypoplastic pelvis; pubic diastasis)
18. Hereditary multiple exostoses (multiple cartilaginous exostoses; osteochondromatosis)
19. Hypochondrogenesis (hypoplastic iliac wings; flat acetabular roofs; unossified pubic bones; vertical ischia)
20. Hypochondroplasia (small pelvis with short ilia; flat acetabular roofs; small sacroiliac incisura; small sacrum)
21. Kniest dysplasia (trefoil-shaped pelvis; coxa vara; delayed pubic ossification)
22. Marfan S. (wide pelvic cavity; vertical ilia)
23. Metaphyseal chondrodysplasia (Shwachman type) (abnormal acetabula)
24. Metatropic dysplasia (small iliac height and sacro-sciatic notches)
25. Nail-patella S. (osteo-onychodysplasia) (iliac horns)
26. Osteodysplasty (Melnick-Needles S.) (narrow pelvis with flared iliac wings; flat acetabula and tapered ischia)
27. Osteogenesis imperfecta (protrusio acetabuli)
28. Osteopetrosis (alternating bands of increased density)
29. Parastremmatic dysplasia (small sciatic notches; serrated iliac crests)
30. Pelvic "digit" or "rib"
31. Polyostotic fibrous dysplasia (McCune-Albright S.)
32. Rubinstein-Taybi S. (flared ilia; small iliac index)
33. Schneckenbecken dysplasia (small sciatic notches)
34. Spondyloepimetaphyseal dysplasia with joint laxity (also Strudwick type) (small sciatic notches)
35. Spondyloepiphyseal dysplasia congenita (squared ilia; delayed pubic and femoral head ossification)
36. Stickler S. (arthro-ophthalmopathy) (hypoplastic iliac wings; protrusio acetabuli)
37. Thanatophoric dysplasia (squared ilia with small sacrosciatic notches; trident pelvis)

(continued)

38. Trisomy 13 S. (hypoplastic pelvis; low acetabular angles)
39. Trisomy 18 S. (small "antimongoloid" pelvis with vertical ilia; steep acetabular angles)
40. Tuberous sclerosis (patchy sclerotic densities)
41. Weaver S. (small iliac wings)

References
1. Swischuk LE, John SD: Differential Diagnosis in Pediatric Radiology. (ed 2) Baltimore: Williams & Wilkins, 1995, pp 290–294
2. Taybi H, Lachman RS: Radiology of Syndromes, Metabolic Disorders, and Skeletal Dysplasias. (ed 4) St. Louis: Mosby-Year Book, 1996, pp 1044–1045

Gamut D-193-1

ABNORMAL PELVIC CONFIGURATION IN AN INFANT OR CHILD—SMALL SACROILIAC (SCIATIC) NOTCHES

1. Achondroplasia
2. Cephaloskeletal dysplasia (Taybi-Linder S.)
3. Chondroectodermal dysplasia (Ellis-van Creveld S.)
4. Dyggve-Melchior-Clausen dysplasia
5. Dyssegmental dysplasia
6. Hypochondroplasia
7. Metaphyseal chondrodysplasia (Shwachman type)
8. Metatropic dysplasia
9. Parastremmatic dysplasia
10. Schneckenbecken dysplasia
11. Short rib-polydactyly S. type I (Saldino-Noonan)
12. Spondyloepimetaphyseal dysplasia with joint laxity (also Strudwick type)
13. Thanatophoric dysplasia and variants

References
1. Kozlowski K, Beighton P: Gamut Index of Skeletal Dysplasias. Berlin: Springer-Verlag, 1984, pp 56–57
2. Taybi H, Lachman RS: Radiology of Syndromes, Metabolic Disorders, and Skeletal Dysplasias. (ed 4) St. Louis: Mosby-Year Book, 1996, p 1045

Gamut D-193-2

CRENATED OR SERRATED ILIAC CRESTS IN AN INFANT OR CHILD

1. Dyggve-Melchior-Clausen dysplasia
2. Fluorosis
3. Parastremmatic dysplasia

References
1. Kozlowski K, Beighton P: Gamut Index of Skeletal Dysplasias. Berlin: Springer-Verlag, 1984, pp 56–57
2. Taybi H, Lachman RS: Radiology of Syndromes, Metabolic Disorders, and Skeletal Dysplasias. (ed 4) St. Louis: Mosby-Year Book, 1996, p 1044

Gamut D-193-3

NARROW PELVIS IN AN INFANT OR CHILD

1. Campomelic dysplasia
2. Caudal dysplasia sequence (caudal regression S.); sacral agenesis
3. Mucopolysaccharidoses (Hurler; Morquio)
4. Osteodysplasty (Melnick-Needles S.)

Reference
1. Kozlowski K, Beighton P: Gamut Index of Skeletal Dysplasias. Berlin: Springer-Verlag, 1984, pp 56–57

Gamut D-193-4

PELVIC EXOSTOSIS, ILIAC HORN, DIGIT OR RIB IN AN INFANT OR CHILD

1. Avulsion fracture of anterior superior or inferior iliac spine (healed)
2. Exostosis (incl. radiation-induced osteochondroma)
3. Hereditary multiple exostoses (multiple cartilaginous exostoses; osteochondromatosis)
4. Metachondromatosis
5. Nail-patella S. (osteo-onychodysplasia) (iliac horns)
6. Pelvic "digit" or "rib"

References
1. Kozlowski K, Beighton P: Gamut Index of Skeletal Dysplasias. Berlin: Springer-Verlag, 1984, pp 56–57
2. Taybi H, Lachman RS: Radiology of Syndromes, Metabolic Disorders, and Skeletal Dysplasias. (ed 4) St. Louis: Mosby-Year Book, 1996, p 1044

Gamut D-193-5

TRIDENT PELVIS (TRIRADIATE ACETABULUM) IN AN INFANT OR CHILD

1. Asphyxiating thoracic dysplasia (Jeune S.)
2. Chondroectodermal dysplasia (Ellis-van Creveld S.)
3. Fibrochondrogenesis
4. Thanatophoric dysplasia

Reference
1. Kozlowski K, Beighton P: Gamut Index of Skeletal Dysplasias. Berlin: Springer-Verlag, 1984, pp 56–57

Gamut D-194-1

CONGENITAL SYNDROMES WITH FLAT OR DECREASED ACETABULAR ANGLE—TYPE A PELVIS (Small, squared iliac wings and irregular acetabular roofs)

COMMON
1. Achondroplasia

UNCOMMON
1. Achondrogenesis (types I and II)
2. Asphyxiating thoracic dysplasia (Jeune S.)
3. Caudal dysplasia sequence (caudal regression S.); sacral agenesis
4. Cephaloskeletal dysplasia (Taybi-Linder S.)
5. Chondrodysplasia punctata (rhizomelic form)
6. Chondroectodermal dysplasia (Ellis-van Creveld S.)
7. Dyggve-Melchior-Clausen dysplasia
8. Dyssegmental dysplasia
9. Fibrochondrogenesis
10. Hypochondrogenesis
11. Hypochondroplasia
12. Kniest dysplasia
13. Metaphyseal chondrodysplasia (esp. Shwachman type—advanced)
14. Metatropic dysplasia
15. Morquio S.
16. Schneckenbecken dysplasia
17. Short rib-polydactyly S. type I (Saldino-Noonan)
18. Spondyloepimetaphyseal dysplasia
19. Spondyloepiphyseal dysplasia congenita
20. Spondylometaphyseal dysplasia (Kozlowski type)
21. Thanatophoric dysplasia and variants

References
1. Swischuk LE, John SD: Differential Diagnosis in Pediatric Radiology. (ed 2) Baltimore: Williams & Wilkins, 1995, pp 291–293
2. Taybi H, Lachman RS: Radiology of Syndromes, Metabolic Disorders, and Skeletal Dysplasias. (ed 4) St. Louis: Mosby-Year Book, 1996, p 1044

Gamut D-194-2

CONGENITAL SYNDROMES WITH ABNORMAL ACETABULAR ANGLE, USUALLY FLAT OR DECREASED—TYPE B PELVIS
(Iliac wings less hypoplastic, outwardly flared, and more tapered than square)

COMMON

1. Arthrogryposis
*2. Developmental dysplasia of the hip—DDH (congenital hip dysplasia or dislocation)
3. Hypothyroidism; cretinism
4. Trisomy 21 S. (Down S.)

UNCOMMON

1. Acrocephalopolysyndactyly (Carpenter S.)
2. Acrocephalosyndactyly (Waardenburg type)
3. Aminopterin fetopathy
4. Brachmann-de Lange S. (de Lange S.)
5. Cleidocranial dysplasia
6. Cockayne S.
7. Exstrophy of bladder
8. Frontometaphyseal dysplasia
9. Hypophosphatasia
10. Larsen S.
11. Metaphyseal dysplasia (Jansen and other types) (mild)
*12. Mucolipidosis II (I-cell disease) and III (pseudo-Hurler polydystrophy)
*13. Mucopolysaccharidoses (Hurler; Sanfilippo) (See J-4)
14. Nail-patella S. (osteo-onychodysplasia)
15. Osteodysplasty (Melnick-Needles S.)
16. Osteogenesis imperfecta (types II and III)
17. Otopalatodigital S. (type II)
18. Popliteal pterygium S.
19. Prune-belly S. (Eagle-Barrett S.)
20. Rubinstein-Taybi S.
21. Sacral agenesis
22. Stickler S. (arthro-ophthalmopathy)
23. Trisomy 13 S.
*24. Trisomy 18 S.
25. Weissenbacher-Zweymüller phenotype

* Usually have steep acetabular angles.

References

1. Swischuk LE, John SD: Differential Diagnosis in Pediatric Radiology. (ed 2) Baltimore: Williams & Wilkins, 1995, pp 291–293
2. Taybi H, Lachman RS: Radiology of Syndromes, Metabolic Disorders, and Skeletal Dysplasias. (ed 4) St. Louis: Mosby-Year Book, 1996, p 1044

Gamut D-195

CONGENITAL SYNDROMES WITH DELAYED OR DEFECTIVE PELVIC AND/OR PUBIC OSSIFICATION (WIDE SYMPHYSIS)

COMMON

1. Chondrodystrophies (See D-1)
2. Cleidocranial dysplasia
3. Ehlers-Danlos S. (distraction during delivery)
4. Prune-belly S. (Eagle-Barrett S.)
5. Spondyloepiphyseal dysplasia congenita

UNCOMMON

1. Achondrogenesis I and II
2. Asphyxiating thoracic dysplasia (Jeune S.)
3. Atelosteogenesis
4. Boomerang dysplasia
5. Campomelic dysplasia
6. Caudal dysplasia sequence (caudal regression S.)
7. Cephaloskeletal dysplasia (Taybi-Linder S.)
8. Chondrodysplasia punctata
9. Chondroectodermal dysplasia (Ellis-van Creveld S.)
10. Chromosome 4: del(4p) S. (Wolf-Hirschhorn S.)
11. Dyggve-Melchior-Clausen dysplasia
12. Familial pubic diastasis

13. Femoral hypoplasia–unusual facies S.
14. Fraser S. (cryptophthalmos-syndactyly S.)
15. Goltz S. (focal dermal hypoplasia)
16. Hypochondrogenesis
17. Hypophosphatasia, severe
18. Hypothyroidism; cretinism (newborn)
19. Kniest dysplasia
20. Larsen S.
21. Metaphyseal chondrodysplasia (Jansen type)
22. Opsismodysplasia
23. Osteodysplasty (Melnick-Needles S.)
24. Pseudoachondroplasia (pseudoachondroplastic spondyloepiphyseal dysplasia)
25. Schinzel-Giedion S.
26. Sjögren-Larsson S.
27. Spondyloepimetaphyseal dysplasia (Strudwick type)
28. Spondylomegaepiphyseal-metaphyseal dysplasia
29. Thanatophoric variants
30. Trisomy 9p S.

References

1. Kozlowski K, Beighton P: Gamut Index of Skeletal Dysplasias. Berlin: Springer-Verlag, 1984, pp 56–57
2. Swischuk LE, John SD: Differential Diagnosis in Pediatric Radiology. (ed 2) Baltimore: Williams & Wilkins, 1995
3. Taybi H, Lachman RS: Radiology of Syndromes, Metabolic Disorders, and Skeletal Dysplasias. (ed 4) St. Louis: Mosby-Year Book, 1996, p 1045

gression S.); anal atresia; imperforate anus with rectovaginal fistula; urethral duplication
3. Congenital syndromes with pubic hypoplasia (esp. cleidocranial dysplasia; chondrodystrophies; Ehlers-Danlos S.; prune-belly S. {Eagle-Barrett S.}; hypophosphatasia) (See D-195)
4. Diastasis recti
5. Epispadias; hypospadias
6. Exstrophy of bladder
7. Hyperparathyroidism
8. Hypothyroidism
9. Idiopathic
10. Malignant neoplasm, primary or metastatic; lymphoma$_g$; multiple myeloma
11. Osteomyelitis (eg, pyogenic; tuberculous)
12. Osteonecrosis pubis (chronic stress in young athletes)
13. Paraplegia with neurogenic bone resorption (incl. syringomyelia)

References

1. Muecke EC, Currarino G: Congenital widening of the pubic symphysis. AJR 1968; 103:179–185
2. Swischuk LE, John SD: Differential Diagnosis in Pediatric Radiology. (ed 2) Baltimore: Williams & Wilkins, 1995
3. Taybi H, Lachman RS: Radiology of Syndromes, Metabolic Disorders, and Skeletal Dysplasias. (ed 4) St. Louis: Mosby-Year Book, 1996, p 1045

Gamut D-196

WIDENING OF THE PUBIC SYMPHYSIS

COMMON

1. Osteitis pubis, early (after pelvic surgery; parturition)
2. Pregnancy
3. Traumatic dislocation

UNCOMMON

1. Ankylosing spondylitis; rheumatoid arthritis (early)
2. Congenital anorectal, genital, or urinary tract malformation; caudal dysplasia sequence (caudal re-

Gamut D-197

BRIDGING OR FUSION OF THE PUBIC SYMPHYSIS

COMMON

1. Ankylosing spondylitis (late)
2. Degenerative changes; osteoarthritis
3. Idiopathic
4. Infection, healed (eg, tuberculous or pyogenic osteomyelitis)
5. Osteitis pubis, healed
6. Posttraumatic; postparturition

(continued)

UNCOMMON

1. Fluorosis
2. Juvenile chronic arthritis (eg, juvenile rheumatoid arthritis)
3. Myositis ossificans (pseudomarsupial bones)
4. Ochronosis (alkaptonuria)
5. Postradiation therapy
6. Psoriatic arthritis
7. Rheumatoid arthritis (late)
8. Sternocostoclavicular hyperostosis (SAPHO S.)
9. Surgical fusion

References
1. Forrester DM, Brown JC, Nesson JW: The Radiology of Joint Disease. (ed 3) Philadelphia: WB Saunders, 1987
2. Resnick D, Niwayama G: Diagnosis of Bone and Joint Disorders. (ed 2) Philadelphia: WB Saunders, 1988
3. Schwarz G, Schwarz GS: Noninfectious symphysial bridging and pseudomarsupial bones. AJR 1966; 97:687–692

Gamut D-198-1

CONGENITAL SYNDROMES WITH ELEVEN PAIRS OF RIBS

COMMON

1. Campomelic dysplasia
2. [Normal variant]
3. Trisomy 21 S. (Down S.)

UNCOMMON

1. Asphyxiating thoracic dysplasia (Jeune S.)
2. Atelosteogenesis
3. Cleidocranial dysplasia
4. Femoral hypoplasia—unusual facies S.
5. Kyphomelic dysplasia
6. Short rib-polydactyly syndromes
7. Spondylocostal dysostosis (Jarcho-Levin S.)
8. Trisomy 18 S.

[ ] This condition does not actually cause the gamuted imaging finding, but can produce imaging changes that simulate it.

Reference
1. Taybi H, Lachman RS: Radiology of Syndromes, Metabolic Disorders, and Skeletal Dysplasias. (ed 4) St. Louis: Mosby-Year Book, 1996, p 1049

Gamut D-198-2

CONGENITAL SYNDROMES WITH THIRTEEN PAIRS OF RIBS

1. Aarskog S.
2. Alagille S. (arteriohepatic S.)
3. Fetal akinesia deformation sequence (Pena-Shokier S., type I)
4. Holt-Oram S.
5. Idiopathic
6. Incontinentia pigmenti
7. Turner S.

Reference
1. Taybi H, Lachman RS: Radiology of Syndromes, Metabolic Disorders, and Skeletal Dysplasias. (ed 4) St. Louis: Mosby-Year Book, 1996, p 1050

Gamut D-199

THIN, RIBBON-LIKE, OR TWISTED RIBS

COMMON

1. Idiopathic; congenital hypoplasia; cervical rib
2. Intrauterine growth retardation (IUGR)
*3. Neurofibromatosis (type 1)
4. Neuromuscular disorders$_g$ (eg, myotonic dystrophy; myotubular myopathy; hypotonia; Werdnig-Hoffmann disease)
5. Osteoporosis, severe
*6. Regenerated rib (after resection)

UNCOMMON

1. Achondrogenesis (type 1)
2. Aminopterin fetopathy
3. Angiomatosis
4. Antley-Bixler S.
5. Campomelic dysplasia
6. Cockayne S.
7. Contractural arachnodactyly
*8. Gorlin S. (nevoid basal cell carcinoma S.)
9. Hallermann-Streiff S. (oculomandibulofacial S.)
10. Hyperparathyroidism
11. Larsen S.
12. Metaphyseal chondrodysplasia (Jansen type)
13. Morquio S. (posterior portion)
*14. Osteodysplasty (Melnick-Needles S.)
15. Osteogenesis imperfecta (types I, III, IV)
16. Otopalatodigital S. (type II)
17. Paraplegia; poliomyelitis
18. Progeria
19. Rheumatoid arthritis
20. Scleroderma
*21. Spondylocostal dysostosis (Jarcho-Levin S.)
*22. Spondylothoracic dysplasia
23. 3-M syndrome
24. Trisomy 8 S.
25. Trisomy 13 S.
26. Trisomy 18 S.
27. Trisomy 21 S. (Down S.)
28. Turner S.

* Ribs may be twisted.

References
1. Greenfield GB: Radiology of Bone Diseases. (ed 5) Philadelphia: Lippincott, 1990
2. Kozlowski K, Beighton P: Gamut Index of Skeletal Dysplasias. Berlin: Springer-Verlag, 1984, pp 51–52
3. Murray RO, Jacobson HG, Stoker DJ: The Radiology of Skeletal Disorders. (ed 3) London: Churchill Livingstone, 1990
4. Swischuk LE, John SD: Differential Diagnosis in Pediatric Radiology. (ed 2) Baltimore: Williams & Wilkins, 1995, pp 298–300
5. Taybi H, Lachman RS: Radiology of Syndromes, Metabolic Disorders, and Skeletal Dysplasias. (ed 4) St. Louis: Mosby-Year Book, 1996, p 1050

Gamut D-200

WIDE OR THICKENED RIBS

COMMON

1. Achondroplasia
2. Acromegaly
3. Anemia$_g$ (esp. thalassemia; sickle cell disease)
4. Fibrous dysplasia
5. Fluorosis
6. Mucopolysaccharidoses (See J-4)
7. Normal variant
8. Osteomyelitis, healed (eg, actinomycosis)
9. Paget's disease
10. Posttraumatic (healed fractures with callus)
11. Rickets (rosary)

UNCOMMON

1. Adenosine deaminase deficiency with severe combined immunodeficiency and chondro-osseous dysplasia
2. Craniodiaphyseal dysplasia
3. Craniometaphyseal dysplasia
4. Dysosteosclerosis
5. Endosteal hyperostosis (van Buchem and Worth types)
6. Erdheim-Chester disease
7. Freeman-Sheldon S. (whistling face S.)
8. Fryns S.
9. Fucosidosis; mannosidosis; GM$_1$ gangliosidosis
10. GAPO S.
11. Gaucher disease; Niemann-Pick disease
12. Geleophysic dysplasia
13. Gorlin S. (nevoid basal cell carcinoma S.)
14. Hyperphosphatasia
15. Hypochondroplasia
16. Hypophosphatasia (childhood form)
17. Infantile cortical hyperostosis (Caffey's disease)
18. Lenz-Majewski dysplasia
19. Melorheostosis
20. Metaphyseal chondrodysplasia (Schmid type)
21. Mucolipidosis II (I-cell disease) and III (pseudo-Hurler polydystrophy)

(continued)

22. Oculodento-osseous dysplasia
23. Osteogenesis imperfecta (thick bone type II)
24. Osteopetrosis
25. Pachydermoperiostosis
26. Polycythemia
27. Prostaglandin periostosis
28. Proteus S.
29. Pseudoachondroplasia (pseudoachondroplastic spondyloepiphyseal dysplasia)
30. Pyle dysplasia
31. Schinzel-Giedion S.
32. Sclerosteosis
33. Scurvy
34. Sternocostoclavicular hyperostosis (SAPHO S.)
35. Trisomy 8 S.
36. Tuberous sclerosis
37. Weill-Marchesani S.
38. Winchester S.

References
1. Greenfield GB: Radiology of Bone Diseases. (ed 5) Philadelphia: Lippincott, 1990
2. Taybi H, Lachman RS: Radiology of Syndromes, Metabolic Disorders, and Skeletal Dysplasias. (ed 4) St. Louis: Mosby-Year Book, 1996, pp 1050–1051

Gamut D-201

SHORT RIBS* (See F-131)

COMMON

1. Achondroplasia
2. Rickets (all types)

UNCOMMON

1. Achondrogenesis (types I and II)
2. Adenosine deaminase deficiency with severe combined immunodeficiency and chondro-osseous dysplasia
3. Asphyxiating thoracic dysplasia (Jeune S.)
4. Atelosteogenesis
5. Campomelic dysplasia
6. Cerebro-costo-mandibular S.
7. Chondroectodermal dysplasia (Ellis-van Creveld S.)
8. Cleidocranial dysplasia
9. Dysosteosclerosis
10. Dyssegmental dysplasia
11. Enchondromatosis (Ollier disease)
12. Fibrochondrogenesis
13. Hypochondrogenesis
14. Hypophosphatasia
15. Kyphomelic dysplasia
16. Mandibuloacral dysplasia
17. Metaphyseal chondrodysplasia (Jansen type)
18. Metatropic dysplasia
19. Mucolipidosis II (I-cell disease) and III (pseudo-Hurler polydystrophy)
20. Mucopolysaccharidoses (esp. Morquio S.)
21. Osteodysplasty (Melnick-Needles S.)
22. Osteogenesis imperfecta (type II)
23. Otopalatodigital S. (type II)
24. Pseudoachondroplasia (pseudoachondroplastic spondyloepiphyseal dysplasia)
25. Pseudodiastrophic dysplasia
26. Schneckenbecken dysplasia
27. Short rib-polydactyly syndromes
28. Spondylocostal dysostosis (Jarcho-Levin S.)
29. Spondyloepimetaphyseal dysplasias
30. Spondyloepiphyseal dysplasia congenita
31. Thanatophoric dysplasia and variants
32. Weaver S.

* Usually associated with small thorax.

References
1. Greenfield GB: Radiology of Bone Diseases. (ed 5) Philadelphia: Lippincott, 1990
2. Kozlowski K, Beighton P: Gamut Index of Skeletal Dysplasias. Berlin: Springer-Verlag, 1984, pp 50–51
3. Taybi H, Lachman RS: Radiology of Syndromes, Metabolic Disorders, and Skeletal Dysplasias. (ed 4) St. Louis: Mosby-Year Book, 1996, p 1050

Gamut D-202

MULTIPLE SYMMETRICAL ANTERIOR RIB ENLARGEMENT, FLARING, OR CUPPING

COMMON
1. Achondroplasia
2. Normal variant
3. Rickets (all types)
4. Scurvy
5. Thanatophoric dysplasia

UNCOMMON
1. Achondrogenesis (types I and II)
2. Adenosine deaminase deficiency with severe combined immunodeficiency and chondro-osseous dysplasia
3. Asphyxiating thoracic dysplasia (Jeune S.); other narrow thorax-short rib syndromes
4. Copper deficiency, nutritional; Menkes S. (kinky-hair S.)
5. Dyggve-Melchior-Clausen dysplasia
6. Dyssegmental dysplasia
7. Farber disease (disseminated lipogranulomatosis)
8. Fibrochondrogenesis
9. GM_1 gangliosidosis
10. Hypochondrogenesis
11. Hypophosphatasia
12. Kyphomelic dysplasia
13. Leukemia (chloromas)
14. Metaphyseal chondrodysplasia (anadysplasia, Jansen, McKusick, Schmid, Shwachman types)
15. Metatropic dysplasia
16. Osteopetrosis
17. Pseudodiastrophic dysplasia
18. Schneckenbecken dysplasia
19. Short rib-polydactyly syndromes
20. Spondyloepimetaphyseal dysplasia (Strudwick type)
21. Spondyloepiphyseal dysplasia congenita
22. Spondylometaphyseal dysplasia
23. Thalassemia
24. Craniodiaphyseal dysplasia

References
1. Austin JHM: Chloroma; report of a patient with unusual rib lesions. Radiology 1969; 93:671–672
2. Kozlowski K, Beighton P: Gamut Index of Skeletal Dysplasias. Berlin: Springer-Verlag, 1984, p 53
3. Taybi H, Lachman RS: Radiology of Syndromes, Metabolic Disorders, and Skeletal Dysplasias. (ed 4) St. Louis: Mosby-Year Book, 1996, p 1050

Gamut D-203

CLASSIFICATION OF RIB NOTCHING

ARTERIAL
1. High aortic obstruction
   a. Aortitis
   b. Coarctation of aorta
   c. Coarctation of aorta involving left subclavian artery or anomalous right subclavian artery (unilateral)
2. Low aortic obstruction (eg, aortic thrombosis)
3. Subclavian artery obstruction
   a. Blalock-Taussig operation (unilateral)
   b. Pulseless disease (eg, Takayasu's arteritis); advanced arteriosclerosis
4. Pulmonary oligemia
   a. Absent pulmonary artery (unilateral)
   b. Ebstein's anomaly
   c. Emphysema
   d. Pseudotruncus arteriosus
   e. Pulmonary valvular stenosis or atresia
   f. Tetralogy of Fallot

VENOUS
1. Obstruction of superior vena cava, innominate or subclavian vein

ARTERIOVENOUS
1. Arteriovenous fistula of chest wall (intercostal artery—vein)
2. Pulmonary arteriovenous fistula

(continued)

NEUROGENIC

1. Intercostal neurofibroma or neurilemmoma
2. Neurofibromatosis (type 1)
3. Bulbar poliomyelitis; quadriplegia

OSSEOUS

1. Hyperparathyroidism
2. Osteodysplasty (Melnick-Needles syndrome)
3. Thalassemia

MISCELLANEOUS

1. Idiopathic; normal variant
2. Indwelling catheter

References

1. Boone ML, Swenson BE, Felson B: Rib notching: Its many causes. Am J Roentgenol 1964; 91:1075–1088
2. Felson B, Weinstein AW, Spitz HB: Principles of Chest Roentgenology: A Programmed Text. Philadelphia: WB Saunders, 1965, p 197
3. Sutton D (ed): Textbook of Radiology and Imaging. (ed 6) New York: Churchill Livingstone, 1998, p 344

Gamut D-204

RESORPTION OR NOTCHING OF THE SUPERIOR RIB MARGINS

COMMON

1. Connective tissue disease (collagen disease)$_g$ (eg, rheumatoid arthritis; scleroderma; lupus erythematosus)
2. Hyperparathyroidism
3. Localized pressure effect (eg, thoracic drainage tube; rib retractor; intercostal neurofibroma; hereditary multiple exostoses)

UNCOMMON

1. Coarctation of thoracic aorta (superior and inferior margins)

2. Idiopathic
3. Intercostal muscle atrophy in restrictive lung disease
4. Marfan S.
5. Neurofibromatosis (type 1)
6. Osteogenesis imperfecta
7. Paralysis$_g$ (eg, poliomyelitis)
8. Radiation therapy
9. Sjögren S.

References

1. Eisenberg RL: Clinical Imaging: An Atlas of Differential Diagnosis. (ed 3) Philadelphia: Lippincott-Raven, 1997
2. Greenfield GB: Radiology of Bone Diseases. (ed 5) Philadelphia: Lippincott, 1990
3. Sargent EN, Turner AF, Jacobson G: Superior marginal rib defects. AJR 1969; 106:491–505

Gamut D-205

RIB LESION IN A CHILD

CONGENITAL

COMMON

1. Achondroplasia
2. Bifid rib; supernumerary rib; synostosis
3. Cervical rib
4. Coarctation of aorta (rib notching)
5. Hypoplasia or absence of rib
6. Thalassemia; sickle cell disease

UNCOMMON

1. Congenital syndromes and dysplasias, other (See D-1)
2. Gorlin S. (nevoid basal cell carcinoma S.)
3. Mucopolysaccharidoses (eg, Hurler; Morquio) (See J-4)
4. Neurofibromatosis (type 1)
5. Osteopetrosis

INFLAMMATION

COMMON

1. Osteomyelitis (eg, bacterial; tuberculous; fungal$_g$)

UNCOMMON

1. Infantile cortical hyperostosis (Caffey's disease)
2. Granulomatous disease of childhood
3. Hydatid disease

NEOPLASM

COMMON

1. Angiomatous lesion$_g$ (eg, hemangioma; lymphangioma)

UNCOMMON

1. Chondromyxoid fibroma
2. Enchondroma, esp. in enchondromatosis (Ollier disease)
3. Leukemia; lymphoma$_g$
4. Mesenchymal hamartoma of chest wall
5. Metastasis (esp. neuroblastoma)
6. Neurofibroma
7. Nonossifying fibroma, fibroxanthoma (often sclerosing type)
8. Osteoblastoma
9. Osteochondroma
10. Osteoma
11. Sarcoma (eg, Ewing sarcoma; osteosarcoma)

MISCELLANEOUS

COMMON

1. Fibrous dysplasia
2. Langerhans cell histiocytosis$_g$
3. Postoperative (rib removal or regeneration)
4. Rib notching, other causes (See D-203)
5. Rickets (all types) (See D-44)
6. Trauma (eg, fracture; callus)

UNCOMMON

1. Bone cyst
2. Scurvy

SHORT LESION OF A RIB (UNDER 6 CM) (See D-207)

COMMON

1. Angiomatous lesion (hemangioma; lymphangioma); arteriovenous fistula
2. Chondrosarcoma
3. Enchondroma, esp. in enchondromatosis (Ollier disease)
4. Enostosis; bone island
5. Fibrous dysplasia
6. Fracture; callus
7. Langerhans cell histiocytosis$_g$ (esp. eosinophilic granuloma)
8. Metastasis
9. Osteomyelitis (eg, bacterial; tuberculous; fungal$_g$)
10. Plasmacytoma; multiple myeloma

UNCOMMON

1. Aneurysmal bone cyst
2. Bone cyst
3. Bone sarcoma; other (eg, Ewing sarcoma; osteosarcoma)
4. Brown tumor of hyperparathyroidism
5. Chondroblastoma (Codman tumor)
6. Chondromyxoid fibroma
7. Gaucher disease
8. Giant cell tumor
9. Lipoma
10. Lymphoma$_g$ (esp. Hodgkin's)
11. Melorheostosis
12. Mesenchymal hamartoma of chest wall
13. Nonossifying fibroma
14. Osteoblastoma
15. Osteochondroma; exostosis (esp. in hereditary multiple exostoses)
16. Osteoid osteoma
17. Osteoma

Gamut D-207

LONG LESION OF A RIB
(OVER 6 CM—USUALLY EXPANSILE)
(See D-206)

COMMON

1. Bone sarcoma (eg, chondrosarcoma; osteosarcoma; Ewing sarcoma)
2. Fibrous dysplasia
3. Fused or bifid rib (incl. basal cell nevus S.)
4. Metastasis (esp. from carcinoma of breast, prostate, lung, or kidney; neuroblastoma)
5. Osteomyelitis (eg, bacterial; tuberculous; fungal)
6. Plasmacytoma; multiple myeloma
7. Surgical removal; regeneration

UNCOMMON

1. Aneurysmal bone cyst
2. Bone cyst
3. Chondromyxoid fibroma
4. Gaucher disease
5. Hydatid cyst
6. Langerhans cell histiocytosis$_g$ (esp. eosinophilic granuloma)
7. Malignant fibrous histiocytoma; fibrosarcoma
8. Melorheostosis
9. Mesenchymal hamartoma of chest wall
10. Paget's disease

References

1. Jeung MY, Gangi A, Gasser B, et al: Imaging of chest wall disorders. RadioGraphics 1999; 19:617–637
2. Omell GH, Anderson LS, Bramson RT: Chest wall tumors. Radiol Clin North Am 1973; 11:197–214

Gamut D-208

MULTIPLE EXPANDING RIB LESIONS

COMMON

1. Anemia$_g$ (eg, thalassemia; sickle cell disease)
2. Metastases
3. Multiple myeloma
4. Osteomyelitis (esp. fungal; actinomycosis; blastomycosis; coccidioidomycosis; histoplasmosis duboisii)

UNCOMMON

1. Amyloidomas, primary or secondary
2. Angiomatosis (hemangiomatosis; lymphangiomatosis, cystic variety)
3. Brown tumors of hyperparathyroidism
4. Diaphyseal dysplasia (Camurati-Engelmann disease)
5. Enchondromatosis (Ollier disease)
6. Endosteal hyperostosis (van Buchem and Worth types)
7. Gaucher disease
8. Hereditary multiple exostoses (multiple cartilaginous exostoses; osteochondromatosis)
9. Hydatid disease
10. Hypophosphatasia
11. Infantile cortical hyperostosis (Caffey disease)
12. Langerhans cell histiocytosis$_g$
13. Leukemia (chloromas); lymphoma$_g$
14. Mesenchymal hamartomas of chest wall
15. Mucopolysaccharidoses (esp. Hurler; Morquio) (See J-4)
16. Osteogenesis imperfecta
17. Pachydermoperiostosis
18. Paget's disease
19. Polyostotic fibrous dysplasia (McCune-Albright S.)
20. Rickets (rosary)
21. Scurvy

Gamut D-209-1

CONGENITAL STERNAL ABNORMALITY— HYPERSEGMENTATION OR UNDERSEGMENTATION

HYPERSEGMENTATION
1. Trisomy 21 S. (Down S.)

UNDERSEGMENTATION (OFTEN WITH HYPOPLASIA AND PREMATURE FUSION OF STERNUM)
1. Campomelic dysplasia
2. Brachmann-de Lange S. (de Lange S.)
3. Noonan S.
4. Trisomy 18 S.

Reference
1. Swischuk LE, John SD: Differential Diagnosis in Pediatric Radiology. (ed 2) Baltimore: Williams & Wilkins, 1995

Gamut D-209-2

PECTUS CARINATUM (PIGEON BREAST) (Same as F-129)

COMMON
1. Congenital heart disease, esp. cyanotic
2. Ehlers-Danlos S.
3. Fetal alcohol S.
4. Homocystinuria
5. Idiopathic; isolated finding
6. Marfan S.
7. Mucopolysaccharidoses (esp. Morquio S.) (See J-4)
8. Osteogenesis imperfecta

UNCOMMON
1. Asphyxiating thoracic dysplasia (Jeune S.)
2. Coffin-Lowry S.
3. Currarino-Silverman S.

4. Dyggve-Melchior-Clausen dysplasia
5. Hyperphosphatasia
6. LEOPARD S. (multiple lentigenes S.)
7. Noonan S.
8. Prune-belly S. (Eagle-Barrett S.)
9. Ruvalcaba S. (trichorhinophalangeal S., type III)
10. Schwartz-Jampel S. (chondrodystrophic myotonia)
11. Spondyloepimetaphyseal dysplasia (Strudwick type)
12. Spondyloepiphyseal dysplasia congenita
13. 3-M syndrome
14. Undersegmentation or hypoplasia of sternum (See D-209-1)

References
1. Felson B (ed): Dwarfs and other little people. Semin Roentgenol 1973; 8:133–263
2. Swischuk LE, John SD: Differential Diagnosis in Pediatric Radiology. (ed 2) Baltimore: Williams & Wilkins, 1995, p 295
3. Taybi H, Lachman RS: Radiology of Syndromes, Metabolic Disorders, and Skeletal Dysplasias. (ed 4) St. Louis: Mosby, 1996, p 1049

Gamut D-209-3

PECTUS EXCAVATUM (Same as F-130)

COMMON
1. Congenital heart disease
2. Ehlers-Danlos S.
3. Fetal alcohol S.
4. Homocystinuria
5. Idiopathic; isolated finding
6. Marfan S.
7. Myotonic dystrophy
8. Newborn with respiratory distress (eg, infantile respiratory distress S.)
9. Osteogenesis imperfecta
10. Osteomalacia
11. Turner S.

UNCOMMON
1. Aarskog S.
2. Coffin-Lowry S.

(continued)

3. Cowden S. (multiple hamartoma S.)
4. Cutis laxa
5. F syndrome
6. Freeman-Sheldon S. (whistling face S.)
7. Gorlin S. (nevoid basal cell carcinoma S.)
8. LEOPARD S. (multiple lentigenes S.)
9. Mitral valve prolapse syndrome (MVPS)
10. Noonan S.
11. Osteodysplasty (Melnick-Needles S.)
12. Prune-belly S. (Eagle-Barrett S.)
13. 3-M syndrome
14. Trauma with flail chest

References

1. Ebel K-D, et al: Differential Diagnosis in Pediatric Radiology. Stuttgart: Thieme, 1999, p 118
2. Swischuk LE, John SD: Differential Diagnosis in Pediatric Radiology. (ed 2) Baltimore: Williams & Wilkins, 1995, p 295
3. Taybi H, Lachman RS: Radiology of Syndromes, Metabolic Disorders, and Skeletal Dysplasias. (ed 4) St. Louis: Mosby, 1996, p 1049

Gamut D-210

EROSION, SCLEROSIS, AND/OR FUSION OF THE STERNOMANUBRIAL SYNCHONDROSIS OR STERNOCLAVICULAR JOINTS

COMMON

1. Ankylosing spondylitis
2. Degenerative arthritis
3. Posttraumatic; postsurgical
4. Psoriatic arthritis
5. Rheumatoid arthritis (esp. juvenile)

UNCOMMON

1. Congenital fusion anomaly
2. Enteropathic arthritis
3. Fluorosis
4. Infection (pyogenic; tuberculous)
5. Reiter S.
6. Relapsing polychondritis

Reference

1. Burgener FA, Kormano M: Differential Diagnosis in Conventional Radiology. (ed 2) New York: Thieme Medical Publ, 1991, p 224

Gamut D-211

CONGENITAL SYNDROMES WITH LIMITED JOINT MOBILITY OR CONTRACTURES

COMMON

1. Achondroplasia (elbow)
2. Arthrogryposis
3. Bony exostoses or synostoses around a joint (See D-114, D-115)
4. Mucopolysaccharidoses; mucolipidoses (See J-4)
5. Neuromuscular disorders$_g$ (eg, Duchenne muscular dystrophy)
6. Radioulnar synostosis syndromes (See D-163)

UNCOMMON

1. Aase-Smith S.
2. Acrocephalosyndactyly (Apert type)
3. Antley-Bixler S.
4. Aplasia cutis congenita
5. Cerebro-oculo-facio-skeletal S. (Pena-Shokeir S. type II)
6. Chondrodysplasia punctata, severe (Conradi-Hünermann and rhizomelic types)
7. Chondroectodermal dysplasia (Ellis-van Creveld S.)
8. Cockayne S.
9. Contractural arachnodactyly
10. Brachmann-de Lange S. (de Lange S.) (elbow)
11. Diabetes, juvenile
12. Diastrophic dysplasia
13. Dyggve-Melchior-Clausen dysplasia
14. Dyschondrosteosis; Madelung deformity (elbow, wrist)
15. Dysplasia epiphysealis hemimelica (Trevor disease)

16. Dyssegmental dysplasia
17. Fabry disease
18. Familial dwarfism with stiff joints
19. Farber disease (disseminated lipogranulomatosis)
20. Femoral hypoplasia—unusual facies S.
21. Fetal akinesia deformation sequence (Pena-Shokeir S. type I)
22. Fetal alcohol S.
23. Fibrodysplasia (myositis) ossificans progressiva
24. Freeman-Sheldon S. (whistling face S.)
25. Frontometaphyseal dysplasia
26. Geleophysic dysplasia
27. GM$_1$ gangliosidosis
28. Hereditary multiple exostoses (multiple cartilaginous exostoses; osteochondromatosis)
29. Infantile multisystem inflammatory disease (NOMID)
30. Kniest dysplasia
31. Kuskokwim S.
32. Léri's pleonosteosis
33. Macrodystrophia lipomatosa
34. Marden-Walker S.
35. Melorheostosis
36. Mesomelic dysplasia (Nievergelt type)
37. Metaphyseal chondrodysplasia (Jansen and other types)
38. Metatropic dysplasia
39. Mietens-Weber S. (knee)
40. Multiple epiphyseal dysplasia (Fairbank) (hip)
41. Multiple synostosis S.
42. Nail-patella S. (osteo-onychodysplasia)
43. Osteogenesis imperfecta (incl. Bruck S.)
44. Otopalatodigital S. (elbow)
45. Pachydermoperiostosis
46. Parastremmatic dysplasia
47. Popliteal pterygium S.
48. Progeria
49. Progressive pseudorheumatoid chondrodysplasia
50. Pseudoachondroplasia (pseudoachondroplastic spondyloepiphyseal dysplasia)
51. Pseudodiastrophic dysplasia
52. Rigid spine S.
53. Schwartz-Jampel S. (chondrodystrophic myotonia)
54. Seckel S. (bird-headed dwarfism)

55. Spondyloepimetaphyseal dysplasias
56. Spondyloepiphyseal dysplasia tarda
57. Spondylometaphyseal dysplasia
58. Stickler S. (arthro-ophthalmopathy)
59. Symphalangism-surdity S. (symphalangism-brachydactyly S. or WL S.)
60. Trisomy 8 S.
61. Trisomy 13 S. (fingers)
62. Trisomy 18 S.
63. Weill-Marchesani S.
64. Winchester S.
65. XXXXX S.; XXXXY S. (radioulnar synostosis)
66. Zellweger S. (cerebrohepatorenal S.) (third and fifth fingers)

References
1. Jones KL: Smith's Recognizable Patterns of Human Malformation. Philadelphia: WB Saunders, 1988
2. Swischuk LE, John SD: Differential Diagnosis in Pediatric Radiology. (ed 2) Baltimore: Williams & Wilkins, 1995
3. Taybi H, Lachman RS: Radiology of Syndromes, Metabolic Disorders, and Skeletal Dysplasias. (ed 4) St. Louis: Mosby, 1996, pp 1034–1035

Gamut D-212

CONGENITAL SYNDROMES WITH JOINT LAXITY OR HYPERMOBILITY

COMMON
1. Ehlers-Danlos S.
2. Marfan S.
3. Morquio S.
4. Trisomy 21 S. (Down S.)

UNCOMMON
1. Aarskog S.
2. Bannayan-Riley-Ruvalcaba S. (Ruvalcaba-Myhre-Smith S.)
3. Coffin-Lowry S.
4. Coffin-Siris S.
5. Cohen S.

(continued)

6. Cutis laxa
7. Desbuquois dysplasia
8. FG syndrome
9. Geroderma osteodysplastica
10. Goltz S. (focal dermal hypoplasia)
11. Hajdu-Cheney S.
12. Hallermann-Streiff S. (oculomandibulofacial S.)
13. Hypochondroplasia
14. Johanson-Blizzard S.
15. Joint hypermobility S.
16. Larsen S.
17. Lenz-Majewski dysplasia
18. LEOPARD S. (multiple lentigenes S.)
19. Lowe S. (oculocerebrorenal S.)
20. Marfanoid hypermobility S.
21. Metaphyseal chondrodysplasia (McKusick type)
22. Mitral valve prolapse S.
23. Multiple endocrine neoplasia (type IIB)
24. Multiple epiphyseal dysplasia (Fairbank)
25. Nail-patella S. (osteo-onychodysplasia)
26. Osteogenesis imperfecta (types I, III, IV)
27. Osteoporosis-pseudoglioma S.
28. Pseudoachondroplasia (pseudoachondroplastic spondyloepiphyseal dysplasia)
29. Robinow S.
30. Rubinstein-Taybi S.
31. Seckel S. (bird-headed dwarfism)
32. SHORT S.
33. Spondyloepimetaphyseal dysplasias (esp. with joint laxity)
34. Stickler S. (arthro-ophthalmopathy)
35. 3-M syndrome
36. XXXXY S.

References

1. Jones KL: Smith's Recognizable Patterns of Human Malformation. Philadelphia: WB Saunders, 1988
2. Swischuk LE, John SD: Differential Diagnosis in Pediatric Radiology. (ed 2) Baltimore: Williams & Wilkins, 1995
3. Taybi H, Lachman RS: Radiology of Syndromes, Metabolic Disorders, and Skeletal Dysplasias. (ed 4) St. Louis: Mosby, 1996, pp 1033–1034

CONGENITAL SYNDROMES WITH JOINT DISLOCATION OR SUBLUXATION (See D-212)

COMMON

1. Arthrogryposis
2. Congenital dislocation of radial head (See D-165)
3. Developmental dysplasia of the hip—DDH (congenital hip dysplasia or dislocation)
4. Dyschondrosteosis; Madelung deformity (distal ulna)
5. Ehlers-Danlos S.
6. Marfan S.
7. Trisomy 21 S. (Down S.) (hip, elbow)

UNCOMMON

1. Aminopterin fetopathy (hip)
2. Atelosteogenesis
3. Brachmann-de Lange S. (de Lange S.) (elbow)
4. Campomelic dysplasia (hips, radial heads)
5. Cat-eye S. (hip)
6. Coffin-Siris S.
7. Cutis laxa
8. Desbuquois dysplasia
9. Diastrophic dysplasia
10. Fanconi anemia (pancytopenia-dysmelia S.) (hip)
11. Farber disease (disseminated lipogranulomatosis) (hip)
12. Fetal hydantoin S. (Dilantin embryopathy)
13. Fetal trimethadione S.
14. Freeman-Sheldon S. (whistling face S.)
15. Frontometaphyseal dysplasia (radial head)
16. Genu recurvatum (knee)
17. Geroderma osteodysplastica (hip)
18. Hajdu-Cheney S.
19. Humerospinal dysostosis (elbow, knee)
20. Keratosis palmaris et plantaris familiaris (tylosis)
21. Kniest dysplasia (hip)
22. Larsen S. (elbow, knee, hip)
23. Mesomelic dysplasia (Robinow and Werner types)

24. Mucopolysaccharidoses (eg, Morquio S.) (hip, elbow, fingers)
25. Nager acrofacial dysostosis (hip)
26. Nail-patella S. (osteo-onychodysplasia)
27. Neurofibromatosis (type 1)
28. Noonan S. (elbow)
29. Oculodentoosseous dysplasia (hip)
30. Osteogenesis imperfecta (type I)
31. Otopalatodigital S. (types I and II) (elbow)
32. Pallister-Hall S. (radial head)
33. Potter sequence
34. Pseudoachondroplasia (pseudoachondroplastic spondyloepiphyseal dysplasia) (hip)
35. Pseudodiastrophic dysplasia
36. Pterygium syndromes
37. Riley-Day S. (familial dysautonomia) (hip)
38. Seckel S. (bird-headed dwarfism) (hip)
39. Silver-Russell S. (hip, elbow)
40. Spondyloepimetaphyseal dysplasia with joint laxity
41. Stickler S. (arthro-ophthalmopathy)
42. TAR S. (thrombocytopenia-absent radius S.)
43. Trichorhinophalangeal dysplasia, type I (Giedion S.) (radial head, hip)
44. Turner S.
45. XXXXX S. (elbow); XXXXY S. (radial head)

References

1. Jones KL: Smith's Recognizable Patterns of Human Malformation. Philadelphia:WB Saunders, 1988
2. Swischuk LE, John SD: Differential Diagnosis in Pediatric Radiology. (ed 2) Baltimore: Williams & Wilkins, 1995
3. Taybi H, Lachman RS: Radiology of Syndromes, Metabolic Disorders, and Skeletal Dysplasias. (ed 4) St. Louis: Mosby, 1996, p 1033

Gamut D-214

MONOARTICULAR JOINT DISEASE

COMMON

1. Avascular necrosis (See D-48)
2. Gout
*3. Infectious arthritis (eg, septic; tuberculous; fungal$_g$; Lyme disease)
4. Juvenile chronic arthritis (esp. juvenile rheumatoid arthritis)
5. Osteoarthritis, secondary (eg, trauma; excess wear or mechanical stress; deformity or malalignment)

UNCOMMON

1. Amyloidosis
2. Calcium pyrophosphate dihydrate crystal deposition disease (CPPD); other causes of chondrocalcinosis (occasionally)
3. Neuropathic arthropathy (Charcot joint) (See D-223)
4. Pigmented villonodular synovitis
*5. Regional migratory osteoporosis of legs
*6. Reiter S.
*7. Rheumatoid monoarthritis (rare in adults)
8. Sternocostoclavicular hyperostosis (SAPHO S.)
*9. Sympathetic joint effusion (eg, secondary to neoplasm in adjacent bone)
10. Synovial neoplasm (esp. synovial sarcoma), cyst, or other lesion (See D-238)
11. Synovial chondromatosis
*12. Transient osteoporosis of hips
13. Tumoral calcinosis

* Associated with marked periarticular demineralization.

POLYARTICULAR JOINT DISEASE

COMMON

1. Ankylosing spondylitis
2. Chondrocalcinosis (eg, calcium pyrophosphate dihydrate crystal deposition disease {CPPD}) (See D-242)
3. Gout
*4. Juvenile chronic arthritis (esp. juvenile rheumatoid arthritis)
5. Osteoarthritis, primary or secondary (incl. erosive osteoarthritis)
6. Psoriatic arthritis
*7. Reiter S.; Reiter/reactive arthritis
*8. Rheumatoid arthritis

UNCOMMON

1. Acromegaly
*2. AIDS (HIV)—associated arthritis
*3. Amyloidosis
*4. Connective tissue disease (collagen disease)$_g$ (eg, lupus erythematosus; scleroderma; CREST S.; dermatomyositis; mixed connective tissue disease (MCTD); polyarteritis nodosa)
5. Diffuse idiopathic skeletal hyperostosis (DISH)
*6. Enteropathic arthritis (eg, ulcerative colitis; Crohn's disease; Whipple's disease) (esp. sacroiliitis)
7. Familial Mediterranean fever (familial recurrent polyserositis)
8. Hemochromatosis
*9. Hemophilia
*10. Infectious arthritis (eg, septic; tuberculous; fungal$_g$)
11. Jaccoud's arthritis (post-rheumatic fever)
12. Kashin-Beck disease
*13. Lyme disease
14. Multicentric reticulohistiocytosis (lipoid dermatoarthritis)
15. Neuropathic arthropathy (Charcot joint) (See D-223)

16. Ochronosis (alkaptonuria)
*17. Regional migratory osteoporosis of legs
18. Relapsing polychondritis
19. Sarcoidosis
*20. Sjögren S.
21. Smallpox residual (esp. elbows)
22. Sternocostoclavicular hyperostosis (SAPHO S.)
*23. Viral synovitis, transient (eg, rubella; mumps; serum hepatitis)
24. Wilson disease (hepatolenticular degeneration)

* Associated with periarticular demineralization.

ARTHRITIS OCCURRING PREDOMINANTLY IN MEN

1. AIDS (HIV)—associated arthritis
2. Ankylosing spondylitis
3. Diffuse idiopathic skeletal hyperostosis (DISH)
4. Gout
5. Hemophilia
6. Ochronosis (alkaptonuria)
7. Psoriatic arthritis
8. Reiter S.

TRANSIENT ARTHRITIS OR ARTHRALGIAS

1. Behçet S.
2. Connective tissue disease (collagen disease)$_g$ (eg, lupus erythematosus; scleroderma; CREST S.; dermatomyositis; mixed connective tissue disease {MCTD}; polyarteritis nodosa)
3. Enteropathic arthritis (eg, ulcerative colitis; Crohn's disease; Whipple's disease) (esp. sacroiliitis)
4. Jaccoud's arthritis (post-rheumatic fever)

5. Lyme disease
6. Regional migratory osteoporosis of legs
7. Relapsing polychondritis
8. Sarcoidosis
9. Sjögren S.
10. Transient osteoporosis of hips
11. Viral (eg, rubella; mumps; serum hepatitis; AIDS)

* Transient episodes of arthritic symptoms and/or joint effusions that usually subside without residual joint damage.

Reference
1. Eisenberg RL: Clinical Imaging: An Atlas of Differential Diagnosis. (ed 3) Philadelphia: Lippincott-Raven, 1997, p 768

Gamut D-218

RHEUMATOID-LIKE ARTHRITIS

COMMON
1. Ankylosing spondylitis
2. Erosive osteoarthritis, acute
3. Gout
4. Juvenile chronic arthritis (See D-219-S)
5. Lupus erythematosus
6. Psoriatic arthritis
7. Reiter S.; Reiter/reactive arthritis
8. Scleroderma; CREST S.
9. [Sudeck's atrophy]

UNCOMMON
1. Dermatomyositis
2. Enteropathic arthritis (eg, ulcerative colitis; Crohn's disease; Whipple's disease)
3. Hemochromatosis
4. Jaccoud's arthritis (post-rheumatic fever)
5. Mixed connective tissue disease (MCTD)
6. Multicentric reticulohistiocytosis (lipoid dermato-arthritis)
7. Sjögren S.

[ ] This condition does not actually cause the gamuted imaging finding, but can produce imaging changes that simulate it.

Gamut D-219-S

CLASSIFICATION OF JUVENILE CHRONIC ARTHRITIS

1. Juvenile-onset adult type (seropositive) rheumatoid arthritis
2. Juvenile chronic arthritis (eg, juvenile rheumatoid arthritis)
   a. Classic systemic disease (Still's disease)
   b. Polyarticular disease
   c. Pauciarticular or monoarticular disease
3. Juvenile-onset ankylosing spondylitis
4. Psoriatic arthritis
5. Enteropathic arthritis
6. Miscellaneous arthritis

Reference
1. Resnick D, Niwayama G: Diagnosis of Bone and Joint Disorders. Philadelphia: WB Saunders, 1981, p 1009

Gamut D-220

DEGENERATIVE JOINT DISEASE IN A YOUNG ADULT (PREMATURE OSTEOARTHRITIS)

COMMON
1. Acromegaly
2. Avascular necrosis (See D-48)
3. Calcium pyrophosphate dihydrate crystal deposition disease (CPPD)
4. Chondromalacia of patella
5. Developmental dysplasia of the hip—DDH (congenital hip dysplasia or dislocation)
6. Diffuse idiopathic skeletal hyperostosis (DISH; Forestier's disease)
7. Erosive osteoarthritis
8. Gout
9. Hemophilia

(continued)

10. Infectious arthritis (septic; tuberculous; fungal; smallpox residual)
11. Juvenile chronic arthritis
12. Neuropathic arthropathy (Charcot joint)
13. Obesity; mechanical stress; malalignment
14. Rheumatoid arthritis (esp. juvenile)
15. Scoliosis
16. Spondylosis deformans
17. Thermal injury (burn; frostbite; electrical)
18. Trauma; postoperative

UNCOMMON

1. Amyloidosis
2. Congenital bone dysplasias
3. Diabetes, juvenile
4. Ehlers-Danlos S.; other causes of joint laxity and subluxation (See D-212, D-213)
5. Exostosis; intra-articular chondroma; dysplasia epiphysealis hemimelica (Trevor disease)
6. Familial Mediterranean fever (familial recurrent polyserositis)
7. Hemochromatosis
8. Hydroxyapatite deposition disease (HADD)
9. Idiopathic
10. Jackhammer operator's (driller's) disease of wrists
11. Kashin-Beck disease
12. Macrodystrophia lipomatosa
13. Multiple epiphyseal dysplasia (Fairbank)
14. Ochronosis (alkaptonuria)
15. Osteochondritis dissecans
16. Scheuermann disease
17. Slipped capital femoral epiphysis
18. Spondyloepiphyseal dysplasia
19. Wilson disease (hepatolenticular degeneration)

Reference
1. Greenfield GB: Radiology of Bone Diseases. (ed 5) Philadelphia: Lippincott, 1990

SECONDARY OSTEOARTHRITIS OF THE HIP

COMMON

1. Avascular necrosis of femoral head
2. Athletic activity in adolescence; abnormal stress forces
3. Coxa vara, incl. idiopathic (See D-187-1 and -2); Otto pelvis
4. Developmental dysplasia of the hip—DDH (congenital hip dysplasia or dislocation)
5. Fracture; subluxation
6. Legg-Perthes disease
7. Previous arthritis (eg, rheumatoid; septic; tuberculous)
8. Slipped capital femoral epiphysis

UNCOMMON

1. Acetabular dysplasia
2. Acromegaly
3. Endocrine disorders
4. Multiple epiphyseal dysplasia (Fairbank)
5. Obesity
6. Ochronosis (alkaptonuria)

Reference
1. Greenfield GB: Radiology of Bone Diseases. (ed 5) Philadelphia: Lippincott, 1990

LOCAL COMPLICATIONS OF TOTAL HIP, KNEE, OR OTHER JOINT ARTHROPLASTY

COMMON

1. Aseptic loosening; subsidence
2. Chondrolysis (unipolar arthroplasty only)
3. Dislocation
4. Fracture of bone (due to insufficiency or during surgery)
5. Hematoma
6. Heterotopic bone formation (myositis ossificans)
7. Lucent line (fibrous tissue—no loosening)
8. Phlebitis
9. Polyethylene fracture, wear, or dislocation
10. Small particle disease (eg, granulomatous pseudo-tumors adjacent to joint replacements) (foreign body reaction)

UNCOMMON

1. Cement extrusion
2. Fracture of prosthesis or cement
*3. Greater trochanteric bursitis or separation; nonunion of osteotomy
4. Infection
5. Malpositioned prosthetic components
6. Osteolysis, local
**7. Patellar avascular necrosis
8. Prosthesis migration or protrusion
9. Silastic arthropathy
10. Vascular or neurologic impairment

* Hip replacement only.
** Knee replacement only.

References

1. Errico TJ, Fetto JF, Waugh TR: Heterotopic ossification: Incidence and relation to trochanteric osteotomy in 100 total hip arthroplasties. Clin Orthop 1984; 190:138–141
2. Gaskill MF: Local complications of total hip replacements. Semin Roentgenol 1986; 21:3–4
3. Heist KP: Complications of total hip replacement. J Am Osteopath Assoc 1981; 80:356–365
4. Weissman BN: Radiographic evaluation of total joint replacement. In: Kelly WN, Harris ED Jr., Ruddy S, Sledge CB (eds): Textbook of Rheumatology. Philadelphia: WB Saunders, 1994
5. Weissman BN: Imaging of total hip replacement. Radiology 1997; 202:611–623
6. Wiklund I, Romanus B: A comparison of life before and after arthroplasty in patients who had arthrosis of the hip joint. J Bone Joint Imag [A] 1991; 73:765–767

IMAGING FINDINGS SUGGESTING LOOSENING AND/OR INFECTION OF JOINT ARTHROPLASTY

RADIOGRAPHIC FINDINGS

*1. Bone destruction
2. Cement-bone or metal-cement lucency of > 2mm
+3. Cement fracture
+4. Component fracture (metal or polyethylene)
5. Development or widening of cement-bone or metal-cement lucency > 2 years after surgery
*6. Gas formation in or around joint
#7. Increasing metallic bead displacement
*8. Intraarticular effusion with extraarticular extension (by sonography)
9. Migration of prosthetic components
+10. Motion of components (may require stress views or fluoroscopy to demonstrate)
*11. Periosteal reaction
#12. Prominent prosthetic subsidence (> 10mm femoral component)

* More commonly associated with infection.
\+ Highest accuracy in identifying loosening/infection.
\# Ingrowth arthroplasty.

ARTHROGRAPHIC FINDINGS

1. Extension of contrast material in the cement-bone or metal-cement interface

(continued)

*a. In zone 2 (or multiple zones including 2) about acetabulum (90% accuracy)

*b. In zone 1 and/or 3 about acetabulum (57% accuracy)

*c. Greater than 2mm—any zone (95% accuracy)

+d. Below intertrochanteric line (> 90% accuracy including nuclear medicine arthrography)

2. Lymphatic filling
3. Filling defects in surrounding bursa or fistulous tracts indicate infection

* Acetabular component of total hip replacement only.
\+ Femoral component of total hip replacement only.

SCINTIGRAPHIC FINDINGS

1. Diffuse uptake, especially around all components, suggests infection (> 9 months after surgery)
2. Focal uptake about any component (> 6-9 months after surgery—seen in septic or aseptic loosening)
3. Increased gallium uptake compared to that with bone scintigraphy suggests infection but is insensitive
4. Increased labeled WBC uptake (increased sensitivity for infection—can be false positive at femoral stem tip up to 2 years after surgery)

References

1. Weissman BN: Total joint replacement: Fixation of prosthetic components. Syllabus for the Categorical Course on Diagnostic Techniques in the Musculoskeletal System. American College of Radiology, 1986, pp 119–131
2. Weissman BN: Radiographic evaluation of total joint replacement. In: Kelly WN, Harris ED Jr., Ruddy S, Sledge CB (eds): Textbook of Rheumatology. Philadelphia: WB Saunders, 1994
3. Weissman BN: Imaging of total hip replacement. Radiology 1997; 202:611–623
4. Wiklund I, Romanus B: A comparison of life before and after arthroplasty in patients who had arthrosis of the hip joint. J Bone Joint Imag [A] 1991; 73:765–767

NEUROPATHIC ARTHROPATHY (INCLUDING CHARCOT JOINT)

COMMON

1. Diabetic myelopathy or neuropathy
2. Syphilis (tabes dorsalis)
3. Syringomyelia
4. Trauma to spinal cord or brain (eg, hemiplegia; paraplegia)

UNCOMMON

1. Acrodystrophic neuropathy
2. Alcoholism
3. Amyloid neuropathy
4. Calcium pyrophosphate dihydrate crystal deposition disease (CPPD) (rarely)
5. Charcot-Marie-Tooth S.
6. Congenital disease involving spinal cord (eg, meningomyelocele; diastematomyelia; spina bifida vera)
7. Congenital insensitivity to pain
8. Cushing S.; systemic or local steroid therapy
9. Gangrene
10. Inflammatory disease of spinal cord (eg, arachnoiditis; acute myelitis; poliomyelitis)
11. Leprosy
12. Massive osteolysis (Gorham vanishing bone disease) (rarely)
13. Multiple sclerosis; other neurological diseases[g]
14. Myelopathy of pernicious anemia
15. Neoplasm of spinal cord
16. Peripheral nerve injury
17. Post-renal transplantation
18. Riley-Day S. (familial dysautonomia)

References

1. Greenfield GB: Radiology of Bone Diseases. (ed 5) Philadelphia: Lippincott, 1990
2. Peitzman SJ, Miller JL, Ortega L, et al: Charcot arthropathy secondary to amyloid neuropathy. JAMA 1976; 235: 1345–1347
3. Resnick D, Niwayama G: Diagnosis of Bone and Joint Disorders. Philadelphia: WB Saunders, 1981, pp 2422–2447

Gamut D-224-1

BILATERAL SYMMETRICAL SACROILIAC JOINT DISEASE

COMMON
1. Ankylosing spondylitis
2. Inflammatory bowel disease (Crohn's disease; ulcerative colitis; Whipple's disease)
3. Osteitis condensans ilii
4. Osteoarthritis
5. Psoriatic arthritis
6. Reiter/reactive disease
7. Rheumatoid arthritis

UNCOMMON
1. Behçet S.
2. Familial Mediterranean fever
3. Gout
4. Hyperparathyroidism
5. Juvenile rheumatoid arthritis
6. Mixed connective tissue disease (overlap S.)
7. Relapsing polychondritis
8. SAPHO S.

Gamut D-224-2

BILATERAL ASYMMETRICAL SACROILIAC JOINT DISEASE

COMMON
1. Osteoarthritis
2. Psoriatic arthritis
3. Reiter/reactive disease
4. Rheumatoid arthritis

UNCOMMON
1. Behçet S.
2. Familial Mediterranean fever

3. Gout
4. Infection
5. Juvenile rheumatoid arthritis
6. Mixed connective tissue disease (overlap S.)
7. Relapsing polychondritis
8. SAPHO S.

Gamut D-224-3

UNILATERAL SACROILIAC JOINT DISEASE

COMMON
1. Infection
2. Osteoarthritis
3. Psoriatic arthritis
4. Reiter/reactive disease

UNCOMMON
1. Behçet S.
2. Familial Mediterranean fever
3. Gout
4. Juvenile rheumatoid arthritis
5. Mixed connective tissue disease (overlap S.)
6. Relapsing polychondritis
7. Rheumatoid arthritis
8. SAPHO S.

Gamut D-225

NARROWED JOINT SPACE
(Note: Most arthritides cause joint space narrowing in their advanced stages)

COMMON

1. Ankylosing spondylitis
2. Avascular necrosis (See D-48)
3. Degenerative arthritis, primary or secondary (eg, posttraumatic)
4. Erosive osteoarthritis
5. Juvenile chronic arthritis (esp. juvenile rheumatoid arthritis)
6. Other chronic arthritides in their more advanced stages (eg, gout; enteropathic; neuropathic; lupus erythematosus; scleroderma; tuberculous; fungal)
7. Psoriatic arthritis
8. Rheumatoid arthritis
9. Septic arthritis

UNCOMMON

1. Calcium pyrophosphate dihydrate crystal deposition disease (CPPD)
2. Farber disease (disseminated lipogranulomatosis)
3. Hemophilic arthropathy; other bleeding disorders$_g$
4. Pigmented villonodular synovitis
5. Postoperative (eg, repair of slipped capital femoral epiphysis)
6. Reiter S.; Reiter/reactive arthritis
7. Sarcoidosis
8. Smallpox residual
9. Sternocostoclavicular hyperostosis (SAPHO S.)
10. Stickler S. (arthro-ophthalmopathy)
11. Synovial neoplasm (esp. hemangioma)
12. Winchester S.

References

1. Resnick D, Niwyama G: Diagnosis of Bone and Joint Disorders. Philadelphia: WB Saunders, 1981
2. Swischuk LE, John SD: Differential Diagnosis in Pediatric Radiology. (ed 2) Baltimore: Williams & Wilkins, 1995

Gamut D-226

WIDENED JOINT SPACE
(Note: Many arthritides cause joint widening in their early stages)

COMMON

1. Congenital syndromes with joint laxity or subluxation (eg, neuromuscular disorders$_g$) (See D-212, D-213)
2. Developmental dysplasia of the hip (DDH) or other joints
3. Hemarthrosis (eg, trauma; hemophilia or other bleeding disorder)
4. Legg-Perthes disease, early
5. Septic arthritis, early
6. Serous effusion (eg, rheumatoid arthritis; connective tissue disease {collagen disease}$_g$; tuberculous arthritis)
7. Toxic (transient) synovitis, severe
8. Traumatic dislocation

UNCOMMON

1. Acromegaly (cartilage hypertrophy)
2. Inflammatory synovial thickening
   a. Rheumatoid arthritis
   b. Gout
   c. Tuberculous or fungal arthritis
   d. Hemophiliac arthropathy
   e. Farber disease (disseminated lipogranulomatosis)
   f. Pigmented villonodular synovitis
3. Ligamentum teres rupture; retained cartilage fragment (hip)
4. Multicentric reticulohistiocytosis (lipoid dermatoarthritis)
5. Neuropathic arthropathy (atrophic type with bone resorption)
6. Sarcoidosis
7. Synovial chondromatosis
8. Synovial neoplasm (esp. hemangioma)

References
1. Resnick D, Niwyama G: Diagnosis of Bone and Joint Disorders. Philadelphia: WB Saunders, 1981
2. Swischuk LE, John SD: Differential Diagnosis in Pediatric Radiology. (ed 2) Baltimore: Williams & Wilkins, 1995

Gamut D-227

JOINT EFFUSION

COMMON
1. Gout
2. Infectious arthritis (septic; tuberculous; fungal; Lyme disease)
3. Psoriatic arthritis
4. Reiter S.; Reiter/reactive arthritis
5. Rheumatoid arthritis (incl. juvenile)
6. Synovitis (acute or chronic)
7. Trauma with hemorrhage

UNCOMMON
1. Allergic reaction (eg, drugs; insect bite)
2. Bone neoplasm, primary or metastatic
3. Calcium pyrophosphate dihydrate crystal deposition disease (CPPD)
4. Hemophilia or other bleeding disorder$_g$
5. Juvenile chronic arthritis
6. Leukemia; lymphoma$_g$
7. Neuropathic arthropathy (Charcot joint) (See D-223)
8. Pigmented villonodular synovitis
9. Rheumatic fever (acute)
10. Synovial chondromatosis
11. Synovial neoplasm (esp. hemangioma)

References
1. Greenfield GB: Radiology of Bone Diseases. (ed 5) Philadelphia: Lippincott, 1990
2. Oh KS, Ledesma-Medina J, Bender TM: Practical Gamuts and Differential Diagnosis in Pediatric Radiology. Chicago: Year Book Medical Publ, 1982, p 136
3. Resnick D, Niwayama G: Diagnosis of Bone and Joint Disorders. Philadelphia: WB Saunders, 1981

Gamut D-228

ARTHRITIS WITH OSTEOPOROSIS*

COMMON
1. Rheumatoid arthritis (incl. juvenile)
2. Septic arthritis

UNCOMMON
1. AIDS (HIV)-associated arthritis
2. Amyloidosis
3. Dermatomyositis; polymyositis
4. Enteropathic arthritis (eg, ulcerative colitis; Crohn's disease; Whipple's disease)
5. Familial Mediterranean fever (familial recurrent polyserositis)
6. Fungal arthritis; mycetoma
7. Hemophilia
8. Juvenile chronic arthritis
9. Lupus erythematosus (late)
10. Lyme disease
11. Mixed connective tissue disease (MCTD)
12. [Regional migratory osteoporosis of legs]
13. Reiter S. (acute); Reiter/reactive arthritis
14. Scleroderma
15. Sjögren S.
16. [Sudeck's atrophy]
17. Transient osteoporosis of the hips
18. Tuberculous arthritis

* All arthritis in late chronic stages may have osteoporosis.
[ ] This condition does not actually cause the gamuted imaging finding, but can produce imaging changes that simulate it.

Gamut D-229

ARTHRITIS WITH LITTLE OR NO OSTEOPOROSIS*

COMMON

1. Ankylosing spondylitis
2. Calcium pyrophosphate dihydrate crystal deposition disease (CPPD)
3. Diffuse idiopathic skeletal hyperostosis (DISH)
4. Gout
5. Neuropathic arthropathy (Charcot joint) (See D-223)
6. Osteoarthritis (degenerative, traumatic, erosive)
7. Psoriatic arthritis

UNCOMMON

1. Amyloidosis
2. Jaccoud's arthritis (post-rheumatic fever)
3. Lupus erythematosus (early)
4. Multicentric reticulohistiocytosis (lipoid dermato-arthritis)
5. Pigmented villonodular synovitis
6. Reiter S. (chronic or recurrent); Reiter/reactive arthritis
7. Sarcoidosis

* All arthritis in late chronic stages may have osteoporosis.

Gamut D-230

ARTHRITIS WITH MULTIPLE JOINT SUBLUXATIONS (USUALLY ULNAR DEVIATION IN THE HANDS)

COMMON

1. Rheumatoid arthritis

UNCOMMON

*1. Ehlers-Danlos S.
*2. Jaccoud's arthritis (post-rheumatic fever)

*3. Juvenile chronic arthritis
*4. Lupus erythematosus
*5. Mixed connective tissue disease (MCTD)
*6. Neuropathic arthropathy with or without destruction (See D-223)
7. Other advanced arthritis (eg, gout; septic; tuberculous; fungal)
8. Psoriatic arthritis
9. Smallpox residual (elbows)

* Often without associated bone destruction.

Gamut D-231

ARTHRITIS WITH "SWAN-NECK" DEFORMITY*

1. Jaccoud's arthritis (post-rheumatic fever)
2. Lupus erythematosus
3. Mixed connective tissue disease (MCTD)
4. Psoriatic arthritis
5. Rheumatoid arthritis
6. Scleroderma
7. Trauma

* Extension at the PIP joint and flexion at the DIP joint of a finger.

Reference

1. Burgener FA, Kormano M: Differential Diagnosis in Conventional Radiology. New York: Thieme Medical Publ, 1991, p 88

Gamut D-232

ARTHRITIS ASSOCIATED WITH PERIOSTITIS OR OTHER NEW BONE PRODUCTION*

COMMON

1. Ankylosing spondylitis (bony whiskering)
2. Gout (overhanging edges)
3. Juvenile chronic arthritis (esp. juvenile rheumatoid arthritis)
4. Psoriatic arthritis
5. Reiter S.; Reiter/reactive arthritis
6. Rheumatoid (carpus and tarsus)
7. Septic arthritis

UNCOMMON

1. AIDS (HIV)-associated arthritis
2. Enteropathic arthritis (rarely)
3. Fungus disease$_g$; mycetoma
4. Hemophilia
5. Hypertrophic osteoarthropathy
6. Sternocostoclavicular hyperostosis (SAPHO S.)
7. Tuberculosis

* Bone production includes periostitis, whiskering, excrescences and/or osseous ankylosis.

Gamut D-233

CALCANEAL SPUR (PLANTAR SURFACE)

*1. Ankylosing spondylitis
2. Diffuse idiopathic skeletal hyperostosis (DISH)
3. Hypertrophic osteoarthritis (esp. from running or other chronic trauma)
4. Idiopathic
5. Plantar fasciitis
*6. Psoriatic arthritis
*7. Reiter S.; Reiter/reactive arthritis

*8. Rheumatoid arthritis
*9. Sternocostoclavicular hyperostosis (SAPHO S.)

* Usually a fluffy rather than sharp spur.

Gamut D-234

CALCANEAL BONE RESORPTION (PLANTAR OR POSTERIOR SURFACE)

COMMON

1. Psoriatic arthritis
2. Reiter S.
3. Rheumatoid arthritis

UNCOMMON

1. Ankylosing spondylitis
2. Gout
3. Hyperparathyroidism
4. Multicentric reticulohistiocytosis (lipoid dermato-arthritis)
5. Osteomyelitis; decubitus ulcer

Reference

1. Greenfield GB: Radiology of Bone Diseases. (ed 5) Philadelphia: Lippincott, 1990

Gamut D-235

ARTHRITIS WITH SOFT TISSUE NODULES*

COMMON

1. Gout
2. Rheumatoid arthritis (incl. rheumatoid nodulosis)

UNCOMMON

1. Amyloidosis
2. Multicentric reticulohistiocytosis (lipoid derma-toarthritis)

(continued)

3. Pigmented villonodular synovitis
4. Sarcoidosis
5. Xanthomas (esp. with hyperlipidemia)

* Nodular or "lumpy-bumpy" arthritis.

Reference
1. Kinard RE, Vogler JB III, Helms CA: The nodular arthritides: The importance of soft tissue nodules in the evaluation of arthritic conditions. American Roentgen Ray Society Scientific Exhibit, Boston, 1985

Gamut D-236

SOFT TISSUE MASS ABOUT A JOINT

COMMON
1. Aneurysm; arteriovenous fistula
2. Bunion (esp. great toe)
3. Bursal fluid collection; bursitis
4. Calcific tendonitis
5. Fluid or blood in joint
6. Ganglion
7. Gouty tophus
8. Infection (esp. abscess)
9. Myositis ossificans
10. Neuropathic arthropathy (Charcot joint) (See D-223)
11. Osteoarthritis with Heberden/Bouchard nodes or mucoid cyst
12. Periarticular calcification (eg, connective tissue disease$_g$; secondary hyperparathyroidism) (See D-243)
13. Synovial cyst (eg, Baker cyst) (See D-237)
14. Synovial hypertrophy secondary to arthritis
15. Synovial chondromatosis or osteochondromatosis

UNCOMMON
1. Amyloidosis
2. Calcium pyrophosphate dihydrate crystal deposition disease (CPPD) (tophaceous pseudogout)
3. Chondroma, articular or para-articular
4. Hydatid disease

5. Lipoma; lipoma arborescens
6. Meniscal cyst; perilabral cyst
7. Multicentric reticulohistiocytosis (lipoid dermatoarthritis)
8. Myxoma (juxtaarticular type)
9. Neuroma
10. Parosteal sarcoma (esp. osteosarcoma or chondrosarcoma); other parosteal neoplasm (See D-88)
11. Pigmented villonodular synovitis
12. Synovial hemangioma
13. Synovial sarcoma
14. Synovitis, localized nodular (giant cell tumor of tendon sheath; xanthoma)
15. Tumoral calcinosis

Gamut D-237

POPLITEAL (BAKER) CYST

COMMON
1. Chronic joint effusion (any cause)
2. Internal derangement of knee (meniscal tear; cruciate tear; intraarticular loose body)
3. Osteoarthritis
4. Rheumatoid arthritis (incl. juvenile)

UNCOMMON
1. Arthritis, other (eg, septic; gout; calcium pyrophosphate dihydrate crystal deposition disease {CPPD}; lupus erythematosus; Reiter S.)
2. Chondromalacia of patella
3. Granulomatous synovitis (eg, tuberculosis; brucellosis)
4. Idiopathic (esp. in adolescent)
5. Osteochondritis dissecans
6. Pigmented villonodular synovitis
7. Sjögren S.

References
1. Burleson RJ, Bicket WH, Dahlin DC: Popliteal cyst: A clinicopathologic survey. J Bone Joint Surg 1956; 38: 1265–1274

2. Gristina AG, Wilson PD: Popliteal cysts in adults and children: A review of 90 cases. Arch Surg 1964; 88:357–363
3. Moore PT: Popliteal cysts. Semin Roentgenol 1982; 17:3
4. Resnick D, Niwayama O: Diagnosis of Bone and Joint Diseases. Philadelphia: WB Saunders, 1981, pp 1156–1157
5. Weissman BN: Arthrography in arthritis. Radiol Clin North Am 1981; 19:379-392

Gamut D-238

BENIGN SYNOVIAL LESION INVOLVING A MAJOR JOINT

COMMON

1. Ganglion (intraarticular type)
2. Meniscal cyst; perilabral cyst
3. Pigmented villonodular synovitis
4. Synovial chondromatosis or osteochondromatosis
5. Synovial cyst (eg, Baker cyst) (See D-237)
6. Synovial hypertrophy secondary to arthritis or infection
7. Synovitis, localized nodular

UNCOMMON

1. Amyloidosis (esp. secondary associated with renal failure)
2. Intracapsular chondroma
3. Lipoma; lipoma arborescens
4. Synovial hemangioma

Gamut D-239

BONE LESIONS INVOLVING BOTH SIDES OF A JOINT

COMMON

*1. Arthritic cysts or erosions (eg, degenerative arthritic cysts or geodes; gouty, rheumatoid, neuropathic or psoriatic erosions)
*2. Infection (esp. granulomatous-tuberculosis; fungus disease; mycetoma; sarcoidosis)
3. Metastases
4. Multiple myeloma

UNCOMMON

*1. Amyloidosis
2. Angiomatous lesions (esp. hemangiomatosis or lymphangiomatosis, synovial type)
3. Enchondromas; enchondromatosis (Ollier disease); Maffucci S.
*4. Hemophilia
5. Hereditary multiple exostoses (multiple cartilaginous exostoses; osteochondromatosis)
*6. Hydatid disease
*7. Jackhammer operator's disease (driller's disease; vibration S.)
8. Osteopathia striata (Voorhoeve disease)
9. Osteopoikilosis
*10. Pigmented villonodular synovitis
*11. Synovial sarcoma

* With joint involvement.

Gamut D-240

MULTIPLE FILLING DEFECTS IN THE KNEE OR OTHER JOINTS ON ARTHROGRAPHY

COMMON

1. Cartilage or bone fragments from trauma or degenerative joint disease
2. Rheumatoid arthritis
3. Synovial chondromatosis
4. Synovitis (inflammatory, crystal, infectious or nonspecific)

UNCOMMON

1. Blood clots; hemophilic arthritis; other bleeding disorder$_g$
2. Gouty tophi
3. Lipoma arborescens
4. Neoplasm (eg, synovial hemangioma)
5. Pigmented villonodular synovitis
6. Tuberculosis

Reference
1. Burgan DW: Lipoma arborescens of the knee: another cause of filling defects on a knee arthrogram. Radiology 1971; 101:583–584

Gamut D-241

CALCIFIED INTRAARTICULAR (OFTEN LOOSE) BODY IN A JOINT

COMMON

1. [Chondrocalcinosis (eg, calcium pyrophosphate dihydrate crystal deposition disease {CPPD})] (See D-242)
2. Degenerative arthritis with detached osteochondral fragment
3. Meniscus fragmentation with calcification

4. Neuropathic arthropathy (Charcot joint) with debris (See D-223)
5. Osteochondrosis dissecans (osteochondral fragment or "joint mouse")
6. Synovial osteochondromatosis
7. Trauma (eg, acute fracture with avulsed fragment in joint; intraarticular (often loose) bodies from old avulsed bone or cartilage fragments)

UNCOMMON

1. [Dysplasia epiphysealis hemimelica (Trevor disease —unilateral intracapsular chondroma involving knee or ankle)]
2. Rheumatoid arthritis, chronic
3. Sequestrum from osteomyelitis, tuberculosis, or septic arthritis
4. [Synovial sarcoma]
5. Synovitis (other causes)

[ ] This condition does not actually cause the gamuted imaging finding, but can produce imaging changes that simulate it.

Reference
1. Moldofsky PJ, Dalinka MK: Multiple loose bodies in rheumatoid arthritis. Skeletal Radiol 1979; 4:219–222

Gamut D-242

CHONDROCALCINOSIS (CALCIFICATION IN ARTICULAR CARTILAGE)*

COMMON

1. Calcium pyrophosphate dihydrate crystal deposition disease (CPPD)
2. Degenerative or posttraumatic osteoarthritis
3. Hemochromatosis
4. Hyperparathyroidism, primary or esp. secondary (renal osteodystrophy)
5. Idiopathic (2% of normals; 3% of elderly)

UNCOMMON

1. Acromegaly
2. Chronic pyarthrosis; osteomyelitis
3. Diabetes
4. Gout
5. Hydroxyapatite deposition disease (HADD)
6. Hypophosphatasia
7. Ochronosis (alkaptonuria)
8. Oxalosis
9. Pseudoxanthoma elasticum
10. Wilson disease

* Calcium may be calcium pyrophosphate, calcium hydroxyapatite, or calcium orthophosphate.

References

1. Greenfield GB: Radiology of Bone Diseases. (ed 5) Philadelphia: Lippincott, 1990
2. Helms CA, et al: CPPD crystal deposition disease or pseudogout. Radiographics 1982; 2:40
3. Jensen P: Chondrocalcinosis and other calcifications. Radiol Clin North Am 1988; 26:1315–1325
4. Jensen PS, Putman CE: Current concepts with respect to chondrocalcinosis and the pseudogout syndrome. AJR 1975; 123:531–539
5. Moskowitz RW, Garcia F: Chondrocalcinosis articularis (pseudogout syndrome). Arch Intern Med 1973; 132:87–91
6. Murray RO, Jacobson HG, Stoker DJ: The Radiology of Skeletal Disorders. (ed 3) London: Churchill Livingstone, 1990

Gamut D-243

PERIARTICULAR OR INTRAARTICULAR CALCIFICATION
(See D-241, 242)

COMMON

+1. Degenerative arthritis (intraarticular osteochondral fragment or "joint mouse")
2. Calcium pyrophosphate dihydrate crystal deposition disease (CPPD); other causes of chondrocalcinosis (See D-242)
3. Gout

*4. Hyperparathyroidism; renal osteodystrophy (secondary hyperparathyroidism)
5. Myositis ossificans
+6. Neuropathic arthropathy (Charcot joint) (See D-223); paraplegia; paralysis$_g$
+7. Osteochondrosis dissecans (intraarticular osteochondral fragment or "joint mouse")
8. Peritendinitis calcarea (calcific synovitis, bursitis, tendonitis)
+9. Posttraumatic (eg, Pellegrini-Stieda disease; avulsed fracture fragment; meniscus fragmentation with calcification)
10. Scleroderma; CREST S.
+11. Synovial osteochondromatosis
12. Vascular (eg, arteriosclerosis; aneurysm; varix)

UNCOMMON

1. Acromegaly
2. Burn
3. Calcinosis circumscripta, usually with connective tissue disease (collagen disease)$_g$
4. Calcinosis interstitialis universalis
5. Chondrodysplasia punctata
6. Dermatomyositis
7. Diabetes
8. Dysplasia epiphysealis hemimelica (Trevor disease); intracapsular chondroma
9. Fluorosis
10. GM$_1$ gangliosidosis
11. Hematoma, traumatic or spontaneous; hemophilia
+12. Hemochromatosis
*13. Hemodialysis, chronic (therapy for renal failure with 1-α-OHD$_3$)
14. Hydroxyapatite deposition disease (HADD)
15. Hypervitaminosis D
16. Hypoparathyroidism
17. Hypothyroidism (stippling before ossification)
18. Lupus erythematosus
19. Metastatic calcification
*20. Milk-alkali S.
21. Mixed connective tissue disease (MCTD)
22. Multiple endocrine neoplasia (MEN) S. (type IIA)
23. Ochronosis (alkaptonuria)

(continued)

---

24. Osteochondroma; spur
25. Parosteal sarcoma (eg, osteosarcoma; chondrosarcoma)
+26. Rheumatoid arthritis
27. Sarcoidosis
28. Septic arthritis
29. Synovial sarcoma
30. Tuberculous arthritis (healed)
*31. Tumoral calcinosis (bursa)
32. Warfarin embryopathy
33. Werner S.
34. Widespread bone destruction (eg, metastatic disease)
35. Wilson disease
36. Zellweger S. (cerebrohepatorenal S.) (hip)

* May show calcium-fluid levels.
+ Usually intraarticular.

References

1. Greenfield GB: Radiology of Bone Diseases. (ed 5) Philadelphia: Lippincott, 1990
2. Resnick D, Niwayama G: Diagnosis of Bone and Joint Disorders. Philadelphia: WB Saunders, 1981, pp 1588–1591
3. Taybi H, Lachman RS: Radiology of Syndromes, Metabolic Disorders, and Skeletal Dysplasias. (ed 4) St. Louis: Mosby-Year Book, 1996, p 1053

Gamut D-244

SOFT TISSUE OSSIFICATION

COMMON

1. Myositis ossificans (heterotopic bone formation)
2. Paraplegia; other neuropathic states$_g$ with prolonged immobilization
3. Posttraumatic degenerative arthritis with ossified debris and osteochondral bodies in and around a joint (esp. hip, knee, ankle)
4. Surgical scar; post-major joint replacement
5. Synovial osteochondromatosis (joint)

UNCOMMON

1. Burn, severe
2. Chondroma
3. Chondrosarcoma (soft tissue or juxtacortical)
4. Fibrodysplasia (myositis) ossificans progressiva
5. Osteosarcoma (soft tissue or parosteal)

Gamut D-245-1

CALCIFICATION IN THE MUSCLES AND SUBCUTANEOUS TISSUES— SYSTEMIC OR WIDESPREAD (See D-247–249)

COMMON

1. Dermatomyositis
2. Gout; hyperuricemia
3. Hyperparathyroidism; renal osteodystrophy (secondary hyperparathyroidism)
4. Hypervitaminosis D
5. Immobilization osteoporosis (eg, paralysis$_g$; paraplegia; poliomyelitis)
6. Ligamentous or tendonous (eg, DISH; Reiter S.; rheumatoid arthritis; ankylosing spondylitis; psoriatic arthritis; hypervitaminosis A; SAPHO S.) (See D-246-2)
7. Lymph nodes (esp. tuberculosis) (See D-249)
8. Scleroderma; CREST S.; acrosclerosis
9. Vascular—arterial or venous (See D-247)

UNCOMMON

1. Calcinosis universalis
2. Calcium pyrophosphate dihydrate crystal deposition disease (CPPD) (tophaceous pseudogout)
3. Carbon monoxide poisoning
4. Congenital fibromatosis (esp. aponeurotic type)
5. Connective tissue disease (collagen disease)$_g$, other (lupus erythematosus; MCTD; polymyositis)
6. Copper deficiency, nutritional; Menkes S. (kinky-hair S.)

7. Cystic fibrosis (mucoviscidosis) (eg, metastatic calcification)
8. Ehlers-Danlos S.
9. Epidermal nevus S.
10. Epidermolysis bullosa
11. Fat necrosis (pancreatitis; Weber-Christian disease —panniculitis; neonatal subcutaneous fat necrosis-pseudosclerema)
12. Fibrodysplasia (myositis) ossificans progressiva
13. Fibrogenesis imperfecta ossium
14. Fluorosis
15. Gorlin S. (nevoid basal cell carcinoma S.)
16. Homocystinuria (vascular)
17. Hydroxyapatite deposition disease (HADD)
18. Hypoparathyroidism; pseudohypoparathyroidism; pseudopseudohypoparathyroidism
19. Leprosy (nerves)
20. Lipomatosis
21. Maffucci S.
22. Milk-alkali S.
23. Oxalosis
24. Pachydermoperiostosis
25. Parasites (eg, cysticerci; guinea worms; *Loa loa;* hydatid cysts)
26. Porphyria
27. Progeria; Werner S.
28. Pseudoxanthoma elasticum
29. Rothmund-Thomson S.
30. Widespread bone destruction with hypercalcemia (eg, metastases; myeloma; leukemia)
31. Williams S. (idiopathic hypercalcemia)

References

1. Edeiken J, Dalinka M, Karasick D: Edeiken's Roentgen Diagnosis of Diseases of Bone. (ed 4) Baltimore: Williams & Wilkins, 1989
2. Gayler BW, Brogdon BG: Soft tissue calcifications in the extremities in systemic disease. Am J Med Sci 1965; 590–605
3. Greenfield GB: Radiology of Bone Diseases. (ed 5) Philadelphia: Lippincott, 1990
4. Kuhn JP, Rosenstein BJ, Oppenheimer EH: Metastatic calcification in cystic fibrosis. Radiology 1970; 97:59–64
5. Poznanski AK: The Hand in Radiologic Diagnosis. (ed 2) Philadelphia: WB Saunders, 1984, p 866
6. Stewart YL, Herling P, Dalinka MK: Calcification in soft tissues. JAMA 1983; 250:78–81
7. Taybi H, Lachman RS: Radiology of Syndromes, Metabolic Disorders, and Skeletal Dysplasias. (ed 4) St. Louis: Mosby-Year Book, 1996, p 1067
8. Teplick JG, Haskin ME: Roentgenologic Diagnosis. (ed 3) Philadelphia: WB Saunders, 1976

Gamut D-245-2

CALCIFICATION IN THE MUSCLES AND SUBCUTANEOUS TISSUES— LOCALIZED (See D-246–251)

COMMON

1. Calcinosis circumscripta (esp. with scleroderma or other connective tissue disease (collagen disease)$_g$
2. Fracture with avulsed fragment
3. Idiopathic; physiologic
4. Injection or inoculation (eg, calcified sterile abscess or fat necrosis; antibiotic, bismuth, calcium gluconate, insulin, camphorated oil, or quinine injection; BCG vaccination)
5. Ligamentous or tendonous (eg, DISH; Reiter S.; rheumatoid arthritis; ankylosing spondylitis; psoriatic arthritis) (See D-246-2)
6. Lymph nodes (esp. tuberculosis) (See D-249)
7. Myositis ossificans (posttraumatic; postoperative—esp. after total hip or knee replacement; or in paraplegia—esp. around hip); calcified hematoma
8. Peritendinitis calcarea (calcific bursitis or tendonitis)
9. Vascular—arterial or venous (See D-247)

UNCOMMON

1. Epithelioma
2. Foreign body granuloma
3. Healing infection or abscess (eg, tuberculosis; pyogenic myositis or fibrositis)
4. Leprosy (nerves)
5. Melorheostosis

(continued)

6. Neoplasm, benign (eg, hemangioma; lipoma; chondroma; fibromyxoma; leiomyoma; xanthoma)
7. Neoplasm, malignant (eg, soft tissue or parosteal osteosarcoma or chondrosarcoma; malignant fibrous histiocytoma; fibrosarcoma; liposarcoma; synovial sarcoma)
8. Parasite (eg, guinea worm; *Loa loa;* hydatid cyst)
9. Radiation therapy
10. Scar
11. Singleton-Merten S. (subungual; forearm)
12. Thermal injury (eg, burn; frostbite; electrical)
13. Tumoral calcinosis
14. Volkmann ischemic contracture

References
1. Edeiken J, Dalinka M, Karasick D: Edeiken's Roentgen Diagnosis of Diseases of Bone. (ed 4) Baltimore: Williams & Wilkins, 1989
2. Greenfield GB: Radiology of Bone Diseases. (ed 5) Philadelphia: Lippincott, 1990
3. Poznanski AK: The Hand in Radiologic Diagnosis. (ed 2) Philadelphia: WB Saunders, 1984, p. 866
4. Stewart YL, Herling P, Dalinka MK: Calcification in soft tissues. JAMA 1983; 250:78–81
5. Teplick JG, Haskin ME: Roentgenologic Diagnosis. (ed 3) Philadelphia: WB Saunders, 1976

Gamut D-246-1

CALCIFICATION IN A BURSA

1. Bursal osteochondromatosis
2. Calcific bursitis
3. Calcium pyrophosphate dihydrate crystal deposition disease (CPPD) (tophaceous pseudogout)
4. Gout
5. Hyperparathyroidism
6. Hypervitaminosis D
7. Kikuya bursa (Africa)
8. Tumoral calcinosis

Reference
1. Greenfield GB: Radiology of Bone Diseases. (ed 5) Philadelphia: Lippincott, 1990

Gamut D-246-2

CALCIFICATION IN A TENDON OR LIGAMENT

COMMON
1. Ankylosing spondylitis
2. Avulsive trauma (incl. medial collateral ligament of knee {Pellegrini-Stieda disease})
3. Calcium pyrophosphate dihydrate crystal deposition disease (CPPD)
4. Degenerative change, physiologic (eg, Cooper's ligament; ligamentum nuchae)
5. Diffuse idiopathic skeletal hyperostosis (DISH)
6. Idiopathic
7. Peritendinitis calcarea (esp. supraspinatus)
8. Psoriatic arthritis
9. Reiter S.; Reiter/reactive arthritis
10. Sternocostoclavicular hyperostosis (SAPHO S.)

UNCOMMON
1. Calcinosis universalis
2. Fibrodysplasia (myositis) ossificans progressiva
3. Fibromatosis (esp. multicentric infantile myofibromatosis and aponeurotic type)
4. De Quervain's disease (rare)
5. Diabetes
6. Fluorosis
7. Ganglion (rare)
8. Gout
9. Hypervitaminosis A and D (including cis-retinoic acid)
10. Ochronosis (alkaptonuria)
11. Pyoderma gangrenosum
12. Renal osteodystrophy (secondary hyperparathyroidism)
13. Rheumatoid arthritis

Reference
1. Greenfield GB: Radiology of Bone Diseases. (ed 5) Philadelphia: Lippincott, 1990

Gamut D-246-3

CALCIFICATION IN A NERVE

1. Leprosy
2. Neurofibromatosis

Reference
1. Greenfield GB: Radiology of Bone Diseases. (ed 5) Philadelphia: Lippincott, 1990

Gamut D-247

VASCULAR CALCIFICATION

COMMON

1. Aneurysm
2. Arteriosclerosis
3. Hemangioma; arteriovenous malformation
*4. Hyperparathyroidism, primary or secondary (renal osteodystrophy)
5. Mönckeberg's medial sclerosis
6. Phleboliths (eg, normal; varicose veins; hemangioma; Maffucci S.)
7. Premature atherosclerosis
   a. Familial hyperlipemia
   b. Generalized (idiopathic) arterial calcification of infancy
   c. Osteogenesis imperfecta
   d. Progeria
   e. Secondary hyperlipemia
      i. Congenital total lipodystrophy (lipoatrophic diabetes)
      ii. Cushing S.
      iii. Diabetes
      iv. Glycogen storage disease
      v. Hypothyroidism
      vi. Nephrotic S.
      vii. Renal homotransplantation
   f. Werner S.

UNCOMMON

1. Buerger disease (thromboangiitis obliterans)
2. Calcified thrombus (eg, vena cava; portal vein; left atrium; pulmonary artery; peripheral artery; Leriche S.)
3. Cystic fibrosis (mucoviscidosis)
4. Gout; hyperuricemia
5. Homocystinuria
*6. Hypervitaminosis D
7. Hypoparathyroidism
*8. Immobilization
*9. Milk-alkali S.
10. Ochronosis (alkaptonuria)
11. Oxalosis
12. Pseudoxanthoma elasticum
13. Radiation therapy
14. Raynaud disease
*15. Sarcoidosis
16. Takayasu arteritis
17. Thermal injury (eg, burn; frostbite)
*18. Widespread bone destruction (eg, metastatic disease)
*19. Williams S. (idiopathic hypercalcemia)

* Hypercalcemia.

References
1. Taybi H, Lachman RS: Radiology of Syndromes, Metabolic Disorders, and Skeletal Dysplasias. (ed 4) St. Louis: Mosby-Year Book, 1996
2. Teplick JG, Haskin ME: Roentgenologic Diagnosis. (ed 3) Philadelphia: WB Saunders, 1976

CALCIFICATION ABOUT THE FINGERTIPS

COMMON

1. Scleroderma (incl. CREST S.; acrosclerosis)

UNCOMMON

1. Calcinosis circumscripta or universalis
2. Dermatomyositis
3. Epidermolysis bullosa
4. Lupus erythematosus
5. Mixed connective tissue disease (MCTD)
6. Raynaud disease
7. Rothmund-Thomson S.

References

1. Greenfield GB: Radiology of Bone Diseases. (ed 5) Philadelphia: Lippincott, 1990
2. Taybi H, Lachman RS: Radiology of Syndromes, Metabolic Disorders, and Skeletal Dysplasias. (ed 4) St. Louis: Mosby-Year Book, 1996, p 1067

CALCIFICATION IN LYMPH NODES*

COMMON

1. Histoplasmosis
2. Idiopathic
3. Tuberculosis

UNCOMMON

1. BCG vaccination
2. Chronic granulomatous disease of childhood
3. Coccidioidomycosis
4. Filariasis
5. Lymphoma (postradiation therapy)

6. Metastasis from osteosarcoma or other calcifying neoplasm (eg, carcinoma of ovary, thyroid, or colon)
7. Sarcoidosis
8. Silicosis; coal-workers' pneumoconiosis

* Primarily in mediastinal and hilar nodes.

Reference

1. Greenfield GB: Radiology of Bone Diseases. (ed 5) Philadelphia: Lippincott, 1990

SOLITARY LARGE CALCIFIED SOFT TISSUE MASS ADJACENT TO BONE (See D-243–246, D-261)

COMMON

1. Bursal calcification (See D-246-1)
2. Gouty tophus
3. Hyperparathyroidism, primary or secondary (renal osteodystrophy)
4. Lymph nodes (esp. tuberculosis) (See D-249)
5. Myositis ossifans (heterotopic bone formation)
6. Neuropathic arthropathy (Charcot joint) (See D-223)
7. Osteochondroma
8. Synovial osteochondromatosis (usually multiple)
9. Synovial sarcoma
10. Tendon or ligament calcification (esp. peritendinitis calcarea; calcific tendonitis)

UNCOMMON

1. Aneurysm
2. Calcifying aponeurotic fibroma
3. Calcium pyrophosphate dihydrate crystal deposition disease (CPPD) (tophaceous pseudogout)
4. Chondroma (soft tissue)
5. Dracunculiasis (guinea worm infection)
6. Fibromatosis (esp. multicentric infantile myofibromatosis)

7. Ganglion (rarely)
8. Hemangioma
9. Hydatid disease (echinococcal cyst)
10. Hydroxyapatite deposition disease (HADD)
11. Hypervitaminosis D
12. Immobilization (eg, paralysis$_g$; paraplegia; body cast)
13. Lipoma (incl. parosteal type)
14. Malignant fibrous histiocytoma; fibrosarcoma
15. Osteoma or juxtacortical chondroma
16. Parosteal sarcoma (osteosarcoma; chondrosarcoma)
17. Soft tissue sarcoma (osteosarcoma; chondrosarcoma; liposarcoma)
18. Tumoral calcinosis

Gamut D-251

SOFT TISSUE MASS WITH UNDERLYING BONE EROSION OR DESTRUCTION

COMMON

1. Abscess; cellulitis
2. Aneurysm (esp. aorta)
3. Carcinoma of skin or mouth
4. Decubitus ulcer
5. Gouty tophus
6. Rheumatoid arthritis

UNCOMMON

1. Amyloidosis (esp. secondary, associated with chronic renal failure)
2. Angiomatous lesion (hemangioma; lymphangioma; arteriovenous fistula)
3. Bacillary angiomatosis
4. Carcinoma developing in sinus tract of chronic osteomyelitis or tropical ulcer

*5. Chondroma (soft tissue)
*6. Ewing sarcoma / PNET (extraskeletal)
7. Fibromatosis (esp. multicentric infantile myofibromatosis)
8. Fungus disease (eg, actinomycosis; blastomycosis)
9. Ganglion (esp. periosteal type)
10. Glomus tumor
11. Hemophilia or other bleeding disorder$_g$
12. Keratosis palmaris et plantaris familiaris (tylosis)
13. Kaposi sarcoma
*14. Lymph node (benign or malignant)
15. Malignant fibrous histiocytoma; fibrosarcoma
16. Meningioma
17. Multicentric reticulohistiocytosis (lipoid dermatoarthritis)
18. Neurofibroma; neurofibromatosis (type 1)
*19. Neuroma (eg, Morton neuroma of toe)
20. Nodular synovitis; giant cell tumor of tendon sheath
21. Parachordoma
22. Parosteal sarcoma or other neoplasm (See D-88)
23. Pigmented villonodular synovitis
*24. Sarcoidosis
*25. Synovial chondromatosis (incl. bursal/tenosynovial types)
26. Schwannoma (neurilemmoma)
27. Sebaceous or other cyst
28. Soft tissue sarcoma (chondrosarcoma; osteosarcoma)
29. Sternocostoclavicular hyperostosis (SAPHO S.)
30. Surfer's knot
31. Synovial sarcoma
*32. Tumoral calcinosis (primary or secondary associated with renal disease)
*33. Xanthomas (multiple, associated with hyperlipidemia type)

* Rare causes.

MUSCULOSKELETAL LESIONS WITH PROMINENT SURROUNDING EDEMA (CT, MRI)

COMMON

1. Fasciitis
2. Hematoma, acute
3. Infection (osteomyelitis; cellulitis; pyomyositis; abscess)
4. Myositis ossificans
5. Osteoblastoma
6. Osteoid osteoma
7. Popliteal cyst, ruptured
8. Primary bone tumor with pathologic fracture
9. Soft tissue metastasis

UNCOMMON

1. Bursitis
2. Gouty tophus
3. Primary bone or soft tissue sarcoma
4. Synovitis, noninfective

9. Osteosarcoma
10. Pigmented villonodular synovitis

UNCOMMON

1. Amyloid (esp. secondary)
2. Brown tumor of hyperparathyroidism
3. Clear cell sarcoma
4. Extensively mineralized mass
5. Granular cell tumor
6. Granuloma annulare
7. Leiomyoma
8. Malignant fibrous histiocytoma/fibrosarcoma
9. Metastases
10. Multiple myeloma
11. Nodular synovitis (giant cell tumor of tendon sheath)

* Similar to or equal to fat on non-fat suppressed sequences.

Gamut D-253

MUSCULOSKELETAL LESIONS WITH PREDOMINANT LOWER SIGNAL ON T2-WEIGHTED MRI*

COMMON

1. Chronic hematoma
2. Dermatofibrosarcoma protuberans (DFSP)
3. Ewing sarcoma/PNET
4. Fibromatosis
5. Fibrous dysplasia (20–40% of cases)
6. Giant cell tumor
7. Gout
8. Lymphoma

Gamut D-254-S

CLASSIFICATION OF SOFT TISSUE TUMORS

BENIGN	MALIGNANT
Muscle	
Leiomyoma	Leiomyosarcoma
Leiomyoblastoma	Rhabdomyosarcoma
Rhabdomyoma	
Fat	
Lipoma and lipoma variants	Liposarcoma
Lipomatosis	
Lipoblastoma	
Hibernoma	
Fibrolipomatous hamartoma of nerve	
Fibrous Connective Tissue	
Nodular fasciitis	Fibrosarcoma
Proliferative fasciitis	
Proliferative myositis	
Fibroma (tendon sheath)	
Elastofibroma	

BENIGN	MALIGNANT	BENIGN	MALIGNANT

Fibrous Connective Tissue

Ossifying fibromyoid tumor
  of soft parts
Fibromatoses
  Juvenile variants
    Myofibromatosis
      (multicentric infantile
      myofibromatosis)
    Fibromatosis colli
    Fibrous hamartoma of
      infancy
    Infantile fibromatosis
    Infantile digital fibromatosis
    Juvenile aponeurotic
      fibromatosis
  Adult variants
    Aggressive fibromatoses
    Extraabdominal desmoid
    Palmar and plantar fibromatosis
    Penile fibromatosis
    Giant cell fibroblastoma
    Idiopathic retroperitoneal
      fibrosis
    Keloid
    Fibrodysplasia (myositis)
      ossificans progressiva
    Calcifying fibrous pseudotumor

Fibrohistiocytic

Benign fibrous histiocytoma	Malignant fibrous histiocytoma (MFH)

Xanthoma; xanthomatosis — Dermatofibrosarcoma
Atypical fibroxanthoma — protuberans (DFSP)
Angiomatoid fibrous
  histiocytoma

Peripheral Nerve

Neurilemmoma (schwannoma) — Malignant peripheral
Neurofibroma — nerve sheath tumor
Neurofibromatosis — (MPNST)
Traumatic neuroma — Neurofibrosarcoma

Peripheral Nerve

Morton neuroma
Ganglion of nerve sheath

Neural Crest

Granular cell tumor	Malignant granular cell tumor

Melanotic neuroecto- — Neuroblastoma
  dermal tumor — Ganglioneuroblastoma
  of infancy — Malignant pheochromo-
Ganglioneuroma —   cytoma
Pheochromocytoma — Malignant paraganglioma
Paraganglioma — Malignant carotid body tumor
Carotid body tumor — Neuroepithelioma
   — Primitive neuroectodermal
     tumor (PNET)
   — Askin tumor (PNET of chest
     wall)
   — Extraskeletal Ewing sarcoma
   — Clear cell sarcoma

Synovial

Giant cell tumor of tendon sheath	Synovial chondrosarcoma
	Synovial sarcoma

Pigmented villonodular
  synovitis
Synovial cyst; bursitis
Ganglion
Myxoma (juxtaarticular type)
Synovial chondromatosis
Hemangioma (synovial type)
Xanthoma

Angiomatous Lesion (Vascular or Lymphatic)

Hemangioma — Angiosarcoma
Angiomatosis — Kaposi sarcoma
Angiomatous syndromes — Pleomorphic hyalinizing
  (eg, Maffucci S.; —   angiectatic tumor of soft
  Klippel-Trenaunay S.; —   parts
  Parkes Weber S.) — Malignant hemangio-
Hemangioendothelioma —   endothelioma
Hemangiopericytoma — Malignant hemangiopericy-
Glomus tumor —   toma

(continued)

BENIGN	MALIGNANT	BENIGN	MALIGNANT

Angiomatous Lesion (Vascular or Lymphatic)

BENIGN	MALIGNANT
Angiolipoma	Lymphangiosarcoma
Reactive vascular lesions	Lymphoma$_g$
Lymphangioma, cavernous or cystic	(extranodal)
Cystic hygroma	
Adventitial cystic disease	
Castleman disease (giant lymph node hyperplasia)	

Extraskeletal Osseous and Cartilage

BENIGN	MALIGNANT
Soft tissue chondroma	Extraskeletal chondro-
Osteoma	sarcoma
Myositis ossificans (heterotopic bone formation)	Extraskeletal osteo- sarcoma
Fibrodysplasia (myositis) ossificans progressiva	
Melorheostosis	
Giant cell tumor of bone (soft tissue recurrence)	
Bizarre parosteal pseudotumor (BPOP)	

Uncertain or Mixed Histogenesis

BENIGN	MALIGNANT
Benign mesenchymoma	Malignant mesen- chymoma
Myxoma (intramuscular)	Alveolar soft part sarcoma
Granular cell myoblastoma	Malignant granular cell myoblastoma
Skin appendage tumors	Skin appendage tumors
	Epithelioid sarcoma
	Malignant mesothe- lioma
	Parachordoma

Others, Including Neoplasm Mimics

BENIGN	MALIGNANT
Primary bone neoplasm invading soft tissue	Primary bone sarcoma invading soft tissue
Accessory muscle	Malignant teratoma
Amyloidosis	Metastases
Aneurysm and pseudoaneurysm	
Arteriovenous malformation or fistula	
Bursal swelling	
Calcific myonecrosis	
Calcific tendonitis	
Cat scratch disease	
Cellulitis; abscess	
Diabetic muscle ischemia	
Epidermal inclusion cyst	
Fasciitis (necrotizing)	
Fungal or unusual infection	
Gout and tophaceous pseudogout	
Granuloma annulare	
Hematoma	
Hydatid disease	
Myositis (inflammatory and infectious); pyomyositis	
Noma (cancrum oris)	
Rhinoscleroma (scleroma)	
Tendon or muscle injury or tear	
Tumoral calcinosis	

References

1. Greenfield GB: Radiology of Bone Diseases. (ed 4) Philadelphia: Lippincott, 1986, pp 713–714
2. Kransdorf MJ, Murphey MD: Imaging of Soft Tissues. Philadelphia: WB Saunders, 1997

BENIGN SOFT TISSUE TUMORS: INCIDENCE

1.	Lipoma and variants	16%
2.	Benign fibrous histiocytoma	13%
3.	Nodular fasciitis	11%
4.	Fibromatosis	10%
5.	Hemangioma	8%
6.	Giant cell tumor of tendon sheath	5%
7.	Neurilemmoma	5%
8.	Neurofibroma	5%
9.	Fibroma (incl. tendon sheath)	3%
10.	Myxoma	3%
11.	Chondroma	2%
12.	Granular cell tumor	2%
13.	Granuloma annulare	2%
14.	Hemangiopericytoma, benign	2%
15.	Leiomyoma	2%
*16.	Ganglion	1%
17.	Glomus tumor	1%
18.	Lipoblastoma	1%
*19.	Lymphangioma	1%
*20.	Myositis ossificans	1%

* Much lower incidence than reality owing to referral bias.

Reference
1. Kransdorf MJ: Benign soft-tissue tumors in a large referral population: Distribution of diagnosis by age, sex, and location. AJR 1995;164:395–402.

MALIGNANT SOFT TISSUE TUMORS: INCIDENCE

1.	Malignant fibrous histiocytoma (MFH)	24%
2.	Liposarcoma	14%
3.	Sarcoma (unspecified)	12%
4.	Leiomyosarcoma	8%
5.	Dermatofibrosarcoma protuberans (DFSP)	6%
6.	Malignant peripheral nerve sheath tumor (MPNST)	6%
7.	Fibrosarcoma (adult and infantile)	5%
8.	Synovial sarcoma	5%
9.	Angiomatoid MFH	2%
10.	Angiosarcoma	2%
11.	Chondrosarcoma (extraskeletal)	2%
12.	Rhabdomyosarcoma	2%
13.	Alveolar soft part sarcoma	1%
14.	Atypical fibroxanthoma	1%
15.	Clear cell sarcoma	1%
16.	Epithelioid sarcoma	1%
17.	Ewing sarcoma (extraskeletal)	1%
18.	Hemangioendothelioma	1%
19.	Hemangiopericytoma	1%
20.	Kaposi sarcoma	1%
21.	Osteosarcoma (extraskeletal)	1%

Reference
1. Kransdorf MJ: Malignant soft-tissue tumors in a large referral population: Distribution of diagnosis by age, sex and location. AJR 1995;164:129–134

Gamut D-257-S

ROUND CELL LESIONS OF SOFT TISSUE

1. Ewing sarcoma (extraskeletal)
2. Lymphoma$_g$; leukemia
3. Multiple myeloma (extraskeletal)
4. Primitive neuroectodermal tumor (PNET)
5. Rhabdomyosarcoma
6. Synovial sarcoma (poorly differentiated types)

Gamut D-258-1

COMMON SOFT TISSUE TUMORS IN CHILDREN (<16 years of age)

BENIGN

1. Fibromatosis
2. Fibrous histiocytoma
3. Granuloma annulare
4. Hemangioma

MALIGNANT

1. Malignant fibrous histiocytoma (MFH); fibrosarcoma
2. Malignant peripheral nerve sheath tumor (MPNST)
3. Rhabdomyosarcoma
4. Synovial sarcoma

Gamut D-258-2

COMMON SOFT TISSUE TUMORS IN YOUNG ADULTS (16–45 years of age)

BENIGN

1. Benign fibrous histiocytoma
2. Ganglion
3. Hemangioma
4. Lipoma
5. Neurogenic neoplasm (neurilemmoma; neurofibroma)
6. Nodular fasciitis

MALIGNANT

1. Dermatofibrosarcoma protuberans (DFSP)
2. Kaposi sarcoma
3. Liposarcoma
4. Malignant fibrous histiocytoma (MFH); fibrosarcoma
5. Malignant peripheral nerve sheath tumor (MPNST)
6. Synovial sarcoma

Gamut D-258-3

COMMON SOFT TISSUE TUMORS IN OLDER ADULTS (Over 45 years of age)

BENIGN

1. Benign fibrous histiocytoma
2. Ganglion
3. Lipoma
4. Myxoma
5. Neurogenic neoplasm (neurilemmoma; neurofibroma)
6. Nodular fasciitis

MALIGNANT

1. Dermatofibrosarcoma protuberans (DFSP)
2. Kaposi sarcoma
3. Leiomyosarcoma
4. Liposarcoma
5. Malignant fibrous histiocytoma (MFH); fibrosarcoma
6. Malignant peripheral nerve sheath tumor (MPNST)

Gamut D-259-1

SOFT TISSUE TUMORS BY LOCATION: SUBCUTANEOUS

BENIGN

COMMON

1. Angiomatous lesions
2. Benign fibrous histiocytoma
3. Lipoma
4. Myxoma
5. Nodular fasciitis

UNCOMMON

1. Granuloma annulare (children)
2. Neurogenic neoplasm (neurilemmoma; neurofibroma)
3. Skin appendage tumors

MALIGNANT

COMMON

1. Dermatofibrosarcoma protuberans (DFSP)
2. Malignant fibrous histiocytoma (MFH); fibro-sarcoma
3. Metastases (esp. melanoma; carcinoma of breast)

UNCOMMON

1. Kaposi sarcoma
2. Leiomyosarcoma
3. Liposarcoma
4. Lymphoma$_g$
5. Malignant peripheral nerve sheath tumor (MPNST)

Gamut D-259-2

SOFT TISSUE TUMORS BY LOCATION: INTERMUSCULAR

BENIGN

1. Fibromatosis
2. Ganglion; synovial cyst; bursa
3. Lipoma
4. Neurogenic tumor (neurilemmoma; neurofibroma)
5. Nodular fasciitis

MALIGNANT

1. Extraskeletal myxoid chondrosarcoma
2. Leiomyosarcoma
3. Liposarcoma (esp. myxoid and higher grade)
4. Malignant peripheral nerve sheath tumor (MPNST)
5. Synovial sarcoma

Gamut D-259-3

SOFT TISSUE TUMORS BY LOCATION: INTRAMUSCULAR

BENIGN

COMMON

1. Angiomatous lesions
2. Lipoma

UNCOMMON

1. Myxoma
2. Nodular fasciitis

MALIGNANT

COMMON

1. Liposarcoma (low-grade, well-differentiated)
2. Malignant fibrous histiocytoma (MFH); fibrosar-coma

(continued)

UNCOMMON

1. Ewing sarcoma (soft tissue); PNET
2. Leiomyosarcoma
3. Rhabdomyosarcoma

Gamut D-259-4

SOFT TISSUE TUMORS BY LOCATION: INTRAARTICULAR OR JUXTAARTICULAR

COMMON

1. Giant cell tumor of tendon sheath
2. Pigmented villonodular synovitis
3. Synovial chondromatosis
4. Synovial cyst, bursa, or ganglion
5. Tumoral calcinosis

UNCOMMON

1. Lipoma arborescens
2. Soft tissue chondroma (knee)
3. Synovial hemangioma
4. Synovial sarcoma

Gamut D-260

SOFT TISSUE TUMORS THAT CAN BE MULTIFOCAL

COMMON

1. Ganglion
2. Hemangioma, lymphangioma (angiomatosis)
3. Lipoma; lipomatosis; lipoblastomatosis
4. Lymphoma$_g$; leukemia (chloroma); Burkitt's lymphoma
5. Metastases
6. Neurofibroma (with type I neurofibromatosis)

UNCOMMON

1. Angiosarcoma
2. Fibromatosis
3. Glomus tumor
4. Kaposi sarcoma
5. Myxoma associated with fibrous dysplasia (Mazabraud S.)
6. Neurilemmoma
7. Paraganglioma

References

1. Enzinger FM, Weiss SW: Soft Tissue Tumors. (ed 3) St. Louis: Mosby, 1995
2. Kransdorf MJ, Murphey MD: Imaging of Soft Tissue Tumors. Philadelphia: WB Saunders, 1997

Gamut D-261

SOFT TISSUE TUMORS WITH ASSOCIATED CALCIFICATION OR OSSIFICATION

BENIGN

COMMON

1. Hemangioma (phleboliths)
2. Lipoma
3. Myositis ossificans; calcified or ossified hematoma
4. Synovial chondromatosis

UNCOMMON

1. Benign mesenchymoma
2. Calcifying aponeurotic fibroma; myofibromatosis
3. Chondroma (soft tissue)
4. Desmoid tumor (rare)
5. Hemangioendothelioma or hemangiopericytoma (benign)
6. Leiomyoma
7. Neurogenic tumor, benign (eg, schwannoma; neurofibroma)
8. Tumoral calcinosis

MALIGNANT

COMMON

1. Osteosarcoma
2. Synovial sarcoma

UNCOMMON

1. Chondrosarcoma
2. Epithelioid sarcoma
3. Leiomyosarcoma
4. Liposarcoma
5. Malignant fibrous histiocytoma; fibrosarcoma
6. Malignant hemangioepithelioma or hemangiopericytoma
7. Malignant mesenchymoma
8. Malignant peripheral nerve sheath tumor (MPNST) (eg, malignant schwannoma; neurofibrosarcoma)

References

1. Dorfman HD, Bhagavan BS: Malignant fibrous histiocytoma of soft tissue with metaplastic bone and cartilage formation: A new radiologic sign. Skeletal Radiol 1982;9:145–150
2. Murphey MD, Gross TK, Rosenthal HG: Musculoskeletal malignant fibrous histiocytoma: Radiologic-pathologic correlation. RadioGraphics 1994;14:807–826
3. Murphey MD, Smith WS, Smith SE, Kransdorf MJ, Temple RT: Imaging of musculoskeletal neurogenic tumors: Radiologic-pathologic correlation. RadioGraphics 1999;19:1253–1280
4. Pringle J, Stoker DJ: Case report 110: Juvenile aponeurotic fibroma. Skeletal Radiol 1980;5:53–55

Gamut D-262

"CYSTIC" SOFT TISSUE TUMORS (CT, MRI)

1. Bursa
2. Epidermoid cyst
3. Ganglion
4. Mucoid cyst

5. Myxoid benign neurogenic neoplasm (neurilemmoma; neurofibroma)
6. Myxoid sarcoma (liposarcoma; malignant fibrous histiocytoma; malignant peripheral nerve sheath tumor {MPNST}; chondrosarcoma)
7. Myxoma
8. Perilabral cyst (meniscal, shoulder, hip, etc.)
9. Synovial cyst
10. Tropical pyomyositis

Gamut D-263

SOFT TISSUE TUMORS WITH PROMINENT FLUID-FLUID LEVELS (CT, MRI)

COMMON

1. Angiomatoid fibrous histiocytoma
2. Angiosarcoma
3. Hemangioma
4. Hemangioendothelioma, hemangiopericytoma
5. Hematoma
6. Malignant fibrous histiocytoma (MFH)
7. Synovial sarcoma
8. Tumoral calcinosis

UNCOMMON

1. Alveolar soft part sarcoma
2. Benign neurogenic neoplasms (neurilemmoma; neurofibroma)
3. Lymphangioma
4. Malignant peripheral nerve sheath tumor (MPNST)
5. Rhabdomyosarcoma

Reference

1. Tsai JC, Dalinka MK, Fallon MD, et al: Fluid-fluid level: A nonspecific finding in tumors of bone and soft tissue. Radiology 1990;175:779–782

Gamut D-264

SOFT TISSUE TUMORS WITH PROMINENT VISIBLE VASCULARITY* (CT, MRI)

COMMON

1. Angiosarcoma
2. Alveolar soft part sarcoma
+3. Hemangioma
+4. Hemangioendothelioma; hemangiopericytoma
5. Kaposi sarcoma

UNCOMMON

1. Bacillary angiomatosis (esp. in AIDS)
2. Ewing sarcoma (extraskeletal)
3. Malignant fibrous histiocytoma (MFH); fibrosarcoma
4. Paraganglioma
5. Primitive neuroectodermal tumor (PNET)
6. Rhabdomyosarcoma (esp. alveolar type)
7. Synovial sarcoma

* Identifiable vascular channels or spaces.
+ All above lesions show high flow, but these entities (+) may have low flow as well.

Gamut D-265-S1

ENNEKING STAGING OF SARCOMAS OF SOFT TISSUE AND BONE

STAGE	GRADE	EXTENT	METASTASIS
IA	G1	T1	M0
IB	G1	T2	M0
IIA	G2	T1	M0
IIB	G2	T2	M0
III	G1–G2	T1	M1
	G1–G2	T2	M1

Surgical Grade: **G1**: low risk of metastasis, < 25%, **G2**: high risk of metastasis, > 25%
Site: **T1**: intracompartmental, **T2**: extracompartmental
Metastasis: **M0**: no regional or distant metastases, **M1**: regional or distant metastases present

*Modified with permission from Enneking WF, Spanier SS, Goodman MA: A system for the surgical staging of musculoskeletal sarcoma. Clin Orthop 1980;153:106–120

Stage I. Histologically low grade (G₁); well differentiated; few mitoses; moderate nuclear atypia. Tends to recur locally. Radioisotope uptake moderate

IA — Intraosseous or intracompartmental

IB — Extraosseous or extracompartmental: penetrates cortex or compartment boundaries

Stage II. Histologically high grade (G₂); poorly differentiated; high cell-to-matrix ratio; many mitoses; much nuclear atypia, necrosis, neovascularity; permeative. Radioisotope uptake intense. Higher incidence of metastases

IIA — Intraosseous or intracompartmental

IIB — Extraosseous or extracompartmental: penetrates cortex or compartment boundaries

Stage III. Metastases; regional or remote (visceral, lymphatic, or osseous)

D. Bone, Joints, and Soft Tissues

Gamut D-265-S2

*AMERICAN JOINT COMMISSION STAGING PROTOCOL FOR SARCOMAS OF SOFT TISSUE

Stage	G	T	N	M
1A	1	1	0	0
1B	1	2	0	0
IIA	2	1	0	0
IIB	2	2	0	0
IIIA	3–4	1	0	0
IIIB	3–4	2	0	0
IVA	1–4	1–2	1	0
IVB	1–4	1–2	0–1	1

Histologic grade (G)
G1 well differentiated
G2 moderately well differentiated
G3–4 poorly differentiated, undifferentiated

Regional lymph nodes (N)
N0 no regional lymph node metastasis
N1 regional lymph node metastasis

Primary Tumor (T)
T1 tumor 5cm or less in greates dimension
T2 tumor more than 5cm in greatest dimension

Distant metastasis (M)
M0 no distant metastasis

*Modified with permission from Arlen M, Marcone R: Sarcoma management based on a standardized TNM classification. Semin Surg Oncol 1992; 8:98–103

Gamut D-265-S3

*HADJU CLASSIFICATION OF SOFT TISSUE SARCOMAS

Stage	Size (cm)	Site	Grade
0	<5	S	L
1A	<5	S	H
1B	<5	D	L
1C	>5	S	L
IIA	<5	D	H
IIB	>5	S	H
IIC	>5	D	L
III	>5	D	H

Site (S)
S superficial (subcutaneous) to fascia
D deep to fascia

Grade (G)
L low
H high

*Modified with permission from Hadju SI. Pathology of soft tissue tumors. Philadelphia 1979, Lea and Febiger. Based on 8,591 primary malignant bone tumors in the Mayo Clinic series.

Gamut D-266-S

RATES OF RECURRENCE FROM COMMON SOFT TISSUE SARCOMAS

	Local*	Distant*[a]	5-yr survival
1. Angiosarcoma	75%	63%	14%
2. Chondrosarcoma (extraskeletal)	50%	44%	55–85%
3. Dermatofibrosarcoma protuberans	2–75%	5–6%	95–100%
4. Fibrosarcoma (adult)	18–79%	60%	39–60%
5. Leiomyosarcoma	21–60%	10–57%	0–29%
6. Liposarcoma (dedifferentiated)	100%	36–100%[b]	0–64%
7. Liposarcoma (high-grade round cell/pleomorphic)	24–73%	48–90%	56%
8. Liposarcoma (myxoid)	53–70%	40–50%	88%
9. Liposarcoma (well-differentiated)	10–60%	Rare	100%
10. Malignant fibrous histiocytoma	44–66%	23–50%	36–50%
11. Malignant peripheral nerve sheath tumor (MPNST)	40%	65%	40–50%
12. Synovial sarcoma	28–83%	50%	36–64%
13. Rhabdomyosarcoma	26%	20%	55%

* Wide range owing to various initial treatments with higher rates for local excision and lower rates for wide excision.
[a] Cases with a wide range are due to various histologic types or tumor location (i.e., subcutaneous versus retroperitoneal).
[b] Variation owing to size of dedifferentiated focus in well-differentiated liposarcoma.

References
1. Enzinger FM, Weiss SW: Soft Tissue Tumors. (ed 3) St. Louis: Mosby, 1995
2. Kransdorf MJ, Murphey MD: Imaging of Soft Tissue Tumors. Philadelphia: WB Saunders, 1997

Gamut D-267-1

DISEASES AFFECTING MUSCLE TO FAT RATIO
Diminution of Muscle:Cylinder Ratio (Below 0.64) (Decreased Muscle Mass, Often Increased Fat)

COMMON
1. Muscular dystrophy (eg, myotonic dystrophy)
2. Paralysis$_g$ (eg, poliomyelitis; meningomyelocele; brain damage)
3. [Steroid therapy; Cushing S. (increased subcutaneous fat)]

UNCOMMON
1. Amyotonia congenita (Oppenheim's disease)
2. Arthrogryposis
3. Benign congenital hypotonia (Walton)
4. Farber disease (disseminated lipogranulomatosis)
5. Prader-Willi S.
6. Spondyloepiphyseal dysplasia congenita
7. Werdnig-Hoffmann disease (infantile spinal muscular atrophy)

[ ] This condition does not actually cause the gamuted imaging finding, but can produce imaging changes that simulate it.

References
1. Greenfield GB: Radiology of Bone Diseases. (ed 5) Philadelphia: Lippincott, 1990

(continued)

2. Litt RE, Altman DH: Significance of the muscle cylinder ratio in infancy. AJR 1967; 100:80–87
3. Swischuk LE, John SD: Differential Diagnosis in Pediatric Radiology. (ed 2) Baltimore: Williams & Wilkins, 1995, pp 310–312

Gamut D-267-2

DISEASES AFFECTING MUSCLE TO FAT RATIO
Increase of Muscle:Cylinder Ratio (Over 0.72) Diminution in Subcutaneous Fat

COMMON

1. Malnutrition; cachexia; debilitating disease (eg, anorexia nervosa)

UNCOMMON

1. Congenital total lipodystrophy (lipoatrophic diabetes)
2. Diencephalic S.
3. Hyperthyroidism
4. Mucopolysaccharidoses (eg, Hurler; Morquio) (See J-4)
5. Progeria; Werner S.
6. Renal tubular acidosis
7. Scleroderma; dermatomyositis

References
1. Greenfield GB: Radiology of Bone Diseases. (ed 5) Philadelphia: Lippincott, 1990
2. Litt RE, Altman DH: Significance of the muscle cylinder ratio in infancy. AJR 1967; 100:80–87
3. Swischuk LE, John SD: Differential Diagnosis in Pediatric Radiology. (ed 2) Baltimore: Williams & Wilkins, 1995, pp 310–312

Gamut D-267-3

DISEASES AFFECTING MUSCLE TO FAT RATIO
Increase in Muscle Mass; Normal Fat

COMMON

1. Exercise hypertrophy

UNCOMMON

1. Congenital muscular hypertrophy
2. Kocher-Debré-Sémélaigne S.
3. Muscle tumor or infection (pyomyositis)
4. Duchenne muscular dystrophy

References
1. Greenfield GB: Radiology of Bone Diseases. (ed 5) Philadelphia: Lippincott, 1990
2. Swischuk LE, John SD: Differential Diagnosis in Pediatric Radiology. (ed 2) Baltimore: Williams & Wilkins, 1995, pp 310–312

Gamut D-267-4

DISEASES AFFECTING MUSCLE TO FAT RATIO
Increase in Fat; Normal Muscle

COMMON

1. Exogenous obesity
2. Steroid therapy

UNCOMMON

1. Bardet-Biedl S.
2. Cushing S.
3. Prader-Willi S.

References
1. Greenfield GB: Radiology of Bone Diseases. (ed 5) Philadelphia: Lippincott, 1990
2. Swischuk LE, John SD: Differential Diagnosis in Pediatric Radiology. (ed 2) Baltimore: Williams & Wilkins, 1995, pp 310–312

Gamut D-268

THICKENING OF HEEL PAD
(Greater than 23 mm)

COMMON

1. Acromegaly
2. Generalized edema (eg, congestive heart failure; deep vein thrombosis; lymphedema)
3. Infection of soft tissues (eg, mycetoma)
4. Normal variant; genetic (esp. black and Polynesian males)
5. Obesity; high body weight (over 200 pounds)
6. Trauma

UNCOMMON

1. Dilantin (hydontoin) therapy
2. Myxedema; thyroid acropachy
3. Occupational
4. Pachydermoperiostosis

References

1. Greenfield GB: Radiology of Bone Diseases. (ed 5) Philadelphia: Lippincott, 1990
2. Kattan KR: Thickening of the heel pad associated with long-term Dilantin therapy. AJR 1975; 124:52–56
3. Kho KM, Wright AD, Doyle FH: Heel pad thickness in acromegaly. Br J Radiol 1970; 43:119–122

Gamut D-269

SOFT TISSUE EMPHYSEMA OR GAS

1. Gas abscess (pyomyositis from *Staph. aureus*)
2. Gas phlegmon; gas gangrene (*Clostridium* infection)
3. Infiltration of air (eg, tracheostomy; thoracotomy; open wound; hypodermoclysis; drainage tube insertion)
4. Mediastinal emphysema (eg, air-trapping from asthma; bronchial foreign body)

5. Trauma (eg, penetrating knife or gunshot injury; explosion; blunt chest trauma with severe contusion; fractured ribs with lung injury; fractured trachea or bronchi)

References

1. Greenfield GB: Radiology of Bone Diseases. (ed 5) Philadelphia: Lippincott, 1990
2. Swischuk LE, John SD: Differential Diagnosis in Pediatric Radiology. (ed 2) Baltimore: Williams & Wilkins, 1995, p 317

Gamut D-270

SWELLING OF THE SOFT TISSUE INTERSTITIAL MARKINGS
("Reticulation" of Soft Tissues)

COMMON

1. Edema, other causes
2. Heart failure
3. Hemorrhage, spontaneous or traumatic
4. Infection of soft tissues (eg, cellulitis; tuberculosis; fungus disease; mycetoma)
5. Lymphatic obstruction; Milroy disease
6. Myxedema; thyroid acropachy
7. Neoplasm primary in soft tissues (eg, vascular or lymphatic tumor—lymphangioma) or edema secondary to bone neoplasm
8. Nephrosis; nephritis
9. Osteomyelitis
10. Thermal injury (eg, burn; frostbite; electrical)

UNCOMMON

1. Acromegaly
2. Erythroblastosis fetalis
3. Fibrodysplasia (myositis) ossificans progressiva (early)
4. Infantile cortical hyperostosis (Caffey disease)
5. Melorheostosis

(continued)

6. Neurofibromatosis (type 1)
7. Sudeck's atrophy

Reference

1. Greenfield GB: Radiology of Bone Diseases. (ed 5) Philadelphia: Lippincott, 1990

Gamut D-271

LYMPHANGIECTASIA
(Lymphatic Vessel Dysplasia)

COMMON

1. Filariasis; elephantiasis
2. Infection (eg, tuberculosis; histoplasmosis; other fungal disease
3. Neoplasm (lymphoma$_g$; lymphangioma; metastases to lymph nodes; angiosarcoma arising in chronic lymphedema {Stewart-Treves S.})
4. Postoperative
5. Posttraumatic

UNCOMMON

1. Cirrhosis
2. Noonan S.
3. Primary congenital lymphatic dysplasia (isolated)
4. Turner S.

References

1. Brown LR, Reiman HM, Rosenow EC III, et al: Intrathoracic lymphangioma. Mayo Clin Proc 1986; 61:882–892
2. Hoeffel JC, Juncker P, Remy J: Lymphatic vessels dysplasia in Noonan's syndrome. AJR 1980; 134:399–401

Gamut D-272

LYMPHATIC OBSTRUCTION ON LYMPHANGIOGRAM (Lymphedema)

COMMON

1. Filariasis; elephantiasis
2. [High pressure injection of contrast media]
3. Inflammation; lymphadenitis; phlebitis
4. Lymphoma$_g$ (esp. Hodgkin)
5. Metastases to lymph nodes
6. Postoperative (eg, following excision of lymph nodes and damage to lymphatics, esp. radical mastectomy); lymphocyst; lymphocele
7. Trauma (peripheral lymphedema from extensive skin loss or burn; injury to cisterna chyli causing chylothorax)

UNCOMMON

1. Lymphangioma (esp. of thoracic duct)
2. [Primary lymphedema]
   a. Lymphedema congenita (eg, Milroy disease; also seen with Turner S.)
   b. Lymphedema praecox (females, ages 9 to 25)
   c. Lymphedema tarda (after age 35)
3. Radiation therapy

[ ] This condition does not actually cause the gamuted imaging finding, but can produce imaging changes that simulate it.

References

1. Escobar-Prieto A, Gonzalez G, Templeton AW, et al: Lymphatic channel obstruction: Patterns of altered flow dynamics. AJR 1971; 113:366–375
2. Sutton D, Young JWR: A Short Textbook of Clinical Imaging. London: Springer-Verlag, 1990, pp. 253–254

Gamut D-273-S

ROENTGEN SIGNS OF LYMPHATIC CHANNEL OBSTRUCTION

1. Backflow
2. Collateral circulation
3. Dilatation of lymph vessels
4. Extravasation
5. Stasis of lymph flow

Gamut D-274

FILLING DEFECT IN LYMPH NODE ON LYMPHANGIOGRAM

COMMON

1. Granulomatous disease (eg, sarcoidosis; tuberculosis; fungus disease$_g$)
2. Idiopathic
3. Lymphoma$_g$
4. Metastatic neoplasm (eg, carcinoma; melanoma; sarcoma)

UNCOMMON

1. Acute lymphadenitis (abscess)
2. Amyloidosis
3. Fatty replacement
4. Multiple myeloma
5. Normal anatomic hilum
6. Reactive hyperplasia of connective tissue disease (collagen disease)$_g$, esp. rheumatoid arthritis
7. Sjögren S.

References

1. Kuisk H: Technique of Lymphography and Principles of Interpretation. St. Louis: Warren H Green, 1971
2. Wallace S, Jackson L, Dodd GD, Greening RR: Lymphangiographic interpretation. Radiol Clin North Am 1965; 3:467–485

E

Cardiovascular

E

E

CONGENITAL SYNDROMES WITH CONGENITAL HEART DISEASE OR MYOCARDIOPATHY

COMMON

1. Adrenogenital S.; Addison disease (aortic, tricuspid, or mitral insufficiency)
2. Asplenia S. (Ivemark S.); polysplenia S. (complex cyanotic conditions)
3. Chondrodysplasia punctata (rhizomelic type) (VSD; PDA)
4. Chondroectodermal dysplasia (Ellis-van Creveld S.) (septal defects; common atrium)
5. Chronic granulomatous disease of childhood (aortic stenosis)
6. Ehlers-Danlos S. (medial necrosis of aorta; dissecting aneurysm; aortic insufficiency; mitral valve prolapse)
7. Eisenmenger S. (pulmonary hypertension with bidirectional or reversed shunt at the atrial, ventricular, or aortopulmonary level)
8. Fetal alcohol S. (septal defect)
9. Fetal rubella S. (PDA; VSD; PS; pulmonary artery branch stenosis)
10. Friedreich ataxia (myocardiopathy)
11. Gaucher disease; Niemann-Pick disease (mitral stenosis or insufficiency; aortic stenosis; myocardiopathy)
12. Hemochromatosis (myocardiopathy)
13. Hemolytic-uremic S. (cardiomegaly; heart failure)
14. Holt-Oram S. (ASD, VSD)
15. Homocystinuria (medial degeneration of aorta and pulmonary artery causing dilatation; arterial and venous thromboses)
16. Hyperthyroidism (myocardiopathy)
17. Hypothyroidism; cretinism (myocardiopathy)
18. Infant of diabetic mother (cardiomyopathy; idiopathic hypertrophic subaortic stenosis (IHSS)
19. Kartagener S.; immotile cilia S. (dextrocardia or situs inversus; septal defects)
20. Klinefelter S. (XXY S.) (PDA; ASD)

21. Marfan S. (aortic insufficiency; mitral insufficiency secondary to mitral valve prolapse; cystic medial necrosis of aorta or occasionally pulmonary artery; dissecting aneurysm)
22. Mucolipidosis II (I-cell disease) (myocardiopathy) and III (pseudo-Hurler polydystrophy) (valvular disease)
23. Mucopolysaccharidoses (eg, Morquio S.; Maroteaux-Lamy S.; Scheie S.—aortic insufficiency; Hurler S.; Hunter S.—intimal thickening of coronary arteries and valves; myocardiopathy)
24. Myotonic dystrophy (conduction abnormalities; mitral valve prolapse)
25. Neurofibromatosis (PS; aortic stenosis; coarctation of aorta; VSD)
26. Noonan S. (stenosis of pulmonary valve or pulmonary artery branches; ASD; VSD; myocardiopathy; constrictive pericarditis)
27. Osteogenesis imperfecta (aortic or mitral insufficiency)
28. Pseudoxanthoma elasticum (premature atherosclerosis; restrictive myocardiopathy; mitral stenosis or insufficiency; myocardial infarction)
29. Trisomy 21 S. (Down S.) (VSD; AS; AV communis)
30. Tuberous sclerosis (myocardiopathy; rhabdomyoma of heart)
31. Turner S. (coarctation of aorta; aortic stenosis; PS; ASD)
32. Venolobar or scimitar S. (partial APVR)
33. Williams S. (idiopathic hypercalcemia) (supravalvular aortic stenosis; pulmonary artery branch stenoses)

UNCOMMON

1. Aase S. (VSD; coarctation of aorta)
2. Acrocephalopolysyndactyly (Carpenter S.) (PDA)
3. Acrocephalosyndactyly (Apert and other types) (VSD)
4. African myocardiopathy (endomyocardial fibrosis)
5. Aminopterin fetopathy (various)
6. Antley-Bixler S.
7. Aspartylglycosaminuria (myocardiopathy; mitral insufficiency)
8. Bardet-Biedl S. (myocardiopathy; VSD)

(continued)

9. Brachmann-de Lange S. (de Lange S.)
10. Campomelic dysplasia
11. Carcinoid S. (endocardial fibrosis with tricuspid valve lesions; PS)
12. Cardiofacial S. (ASD; VSD; AV canal; PDA; tetralogy; PS; coarctation of aorta)
13. Cardio-facio-cutaneous S. (ASD; PS)
14. Cerebrohepatorenal S. (Zellweger S.) (PDA; septal defects)
15. Chromosome 4: del (4p) S. (Wolf-Hirschhorn S.) (ASD; VSD; PDA)
16. Chromosome 5: del (5p) S. (cat cry S. or cri du chat S.) (ASD; VSD; PDA)
17. Chromosome 18: del (18q) S. (ASD; VSD; PDA)
18. Cutis laxa (coarctation of aorta; pulmonary artery stenoses)
19. Deaf-mutism (PS, mitral insufficiency)
20. Degos S. (myocardiopathy)
21. DiGeorge S. (right aortic arch; coarctation of aorta; tetralogy)
22. Duchenne muscular dystrophy (myocardiopathy)
23. Fabry disease (myocardiopathy)
24. Fanconi anemia (pancytopenia—dysmelia S.) (hypoplastic left heart)
25. Fetal hydantoin S. (Dilantin embryopathy) (various)
26. Glycogen storage disease, type II (Pompe disease) or III (persistence of left supracardinal vein; myocardiopathy)
27. GM_1 gangliosidosis (myocardiopathy)
28. Goltz S. (focal dermal hypoplasia) (aortic stenosis)
29. Gorlin S. (nevoid basal cell carcinoma S.) (cardiac fibroma)
30. Hallermann-Streiff S. (oculo-mandibulo-facial S.) (septal defects; PS; tetralogy)
31. Hyperphosphatasia (cardiomegaly; hypertension)
32. Kawasaki disease (coronary artery aneurysms; pancarditis)
33. Kearns-Sayre S. (myocardiopathy; heart block)
34. Kugelberg-Welander S. (myocardiopathy)
35. LEOPARD S. (multiple lentigenes S.) (PS; aortic stenosis; myocardiopathy)
36. Lutembacher S. (rheumatic mitral stenosis and ASD)
37. Mesomelic dysplasia (Robinow and Werner types) (right-sided lesions; VSD)

38. Neuroacanthocytosis (myocardiopathy)
39. Oculo-auriculo-vertebral spectrum (Goldenhar S.) (PDA; VSD; tetralogy; coarctation of aorta; total APVC; asplenia S.)
40. Prune-belly S. (Eagle-Barrett S.) (PDA; VSD)
41. Refsum S. (AV conduction defect; acute heart failure)
42. Rubinstein-Taybi S. (PDA; VSD)
43. Seckel S. (bird-headed dwarfism) (VSD; PDA)
44. Shone-Edwards complex (parachute mitral valve; subaortic stenosis)
45. Smith-Lemli-Opitz S. (VSD; PDA)
46. Spondyloepimetaphyseal dysplasia with joint laxity (CHD with cor pulmonale)
47. Spondylometaphyseal dysplasia (Sedaghatian type) (myocardiopathy; ASD)
48. Sternal-cardiac malformations association (pectus carinatum; PDA; VSD; ASD; tetralogy; transposition of GV)
49. Sturge-Weber S. (coarctation of aorta)
50. TAR S. (thrombocytopenia—absent radius S.) (ASD; VSD; tetralogy)
51. Thoracoabdominal wall defect S. (dextrocardia; pericardial hernia; left ventricular diverticulum)
52. Treacher Collins S. (VSD; PDA; ASD)
53. Trichorhinophalangeal dysplasia, type I (Giedion S.)
54. Trisomy 13 S. (VSD; ASD; PDA; dextrocardia)
55. Trisomy 18 S. (VSD; PDA; PS; coarctation of aorta)
56. VATER association (tetralogy; VSD)
57. Velocardiofacial S. (VSD; tetralogy; hypoplastic pulmonary arteries)
58. Weill-Marchesani S. (PDA)
59. XXXY S.; XXYY S.; XXXYY S.; XXXXX S. (PDA; ASD; others)
60. Yunis-Varón S. (cleidocranial dysostosis with micrognathia and absent thumbs) (myocardiopathy; tetralogy)

References

1. Elliott LP: Cardiac Imaging in Infants, Children, and Adults. Philadelphia: Lippincott, 1991, pp 111–112
2. Felson B (ed): Dwarfs and other little people. Semin Roentgenol 1973; 8:260
3. Hurst JW, Logue RB, Schlant RC, et al: The Heart. (ed 3) New York: McGraw-Hill, 1974

4. Jones KL: Smith's Recognizable Patterns of Human Malformation. Philadelphia: WB Saunders, 1988
5. Mishkin FS: Lung curve indicating a left-to-right shunt in an infant with a large heart. Semin Nucl Med 1981;11:161–164
6. Moss AJ, Adams FH, Emmanouilides GC: Heart Disease in Infants, Children and Adolescents. (ed 2) Baltimore: Williams & Wilkins, 1977
7. O'Brien KM: Congenital Syndromes with Congenital Heart Disease. Semin Roentgenol 1985; 20:104–105
8. Taybi H, Lachman RS: Radiology of Syndromes, Metabolic Disorders, and Skeletal Dysplasias. (ed 4) St. Louis: Mosby-Year Book, 1996, pp 970–971
9. Wilson JD, et al: Harrison's Principles of Internal Medicine. (ed 12) New York: McGraw-Hill, 1991

Gamut E-2-S

RELATIVE INCIDENCE OF VARIOUS CONGENITAL HEART DISEASES*
(IN ORDER OF DECREASING FREQUENCY)

HEART DISEASE	INCIDENCE
COMMON	
+1. VSD	20–25%
2. PDA	12–15%
3. Tetralogy of Fallot	11–15%
4. Pulmonary stenosis	10–15%
5. ASD	7–14%
6. Transposition of great vessels	5–9%
7. Coarctation of aorta	5–9%
8. Aortic stenosis	3–6%
UNCOMMON	
1. Single ventricle	2–3%
2. Tricuspid atresia	1.2–3%
3. Corrected transposition	1.2–3%
4. Truncus arteriosus	1–3%
5. Atrioventricular canal defect	2%
6. APVC, total	2%
7. Aortic atresia	2%
8. Pulmonary atresia	1–1.7%
9. Ebstein anomaly	1%
10. Endocardial fibroelastosis	>1%

* All others are very rare (less than 1%).
+ Isolated VSD or associated with other complex lesions.

Reference
1. Burgener FA, Kormano M: Differential Diagnosis in Conventional Radiology. (ed 2) New York: Thieme Medical Publ, 1991, p 315

KEY FINDINGS IN NEONATAL CONGENITAL HEART DISEASE

PULMONARY VASCULARITY	CONGESTIVE FAILURE		CYANOSIS	
	Early	Late	Early*	Late
I. INCREASED (SHUNT OR OVERCIRCULATION)				
COMMON				
1. APVC, total (above diaphragm)		+		
2. Coarctation S. (coarctation + VSD and/or PDA)		+		
3. Complete atrioventricular canal		+		+
4. Complete transposition of GV (+ VSD or ASD and/or PDA)			+	
5. Hypoplastic left heart S.$_g$ (eg, aortic atresia with ASD and PDA)	+		+	
6. PDA—preterm infant	+			
7. Persistent fetal circulation			+	
8. Truncus arteriosus		+		+
9. VSD		+		
UNCOMMON				
1. ASD		+		
2. Common atrium		+		
3. Double outlet RV (DORV)		+		+
4. Hemitruncus		+		
5. Peripheral AVM		+		
6. Single ventricle with transposition		+		+
II. PULMONARY VENOUS HYPERTENSION (PVH)				
COMMON				
1. Aortic atresia or severe stenosis	+		+	
2. APVC, total (below diaphragm)	+		+	
3. Coarctation of aorta, severe (preductal)	+		+	
UNCOMMON				
1. Anomalous origin of left coronary artery from pulmonary artery		+		
2. Cardiac tumor (eg, rhabdomyoma)	+			
3. Cor triatriatum		+		
4. Endocardial fibroelastosis		+		
5. Glycogen storage disease II (Pompe)		+		
6. Infant of diabetic mother—myocardiopathy	+	+		
7. Mitral atresia or severe stenosis	+			
8. Myocarditis		+		
9. Pulmonary vein stenosis		+		
III. DECREASED PULMONARY VASCULARITY				
COMMON				
1. Tetralogy of Fallot$_g$			+	
UNCOMMON				
1. Complete transposition with pulmonary atresia + VSD			+	
2. Corrected transposition with pulmonary atresia + VSD			+	
3. DORV with pulmonary atresia + VSD			+	
4. Single ventricle with pulmonary atresia + VSD			+	
5. Tricuspid atresia with pulmonary atresia + VSD			+	

* Birth to one week.

Reference
1. Modified from Tonkin ILD: The Infant with Respiratory Distress. In: Elliott LP (ed): Cardiac Imaging in Infants, Children, and Adults. Philadelphia: Lippincott, 1991, p 777

Gamut E-4

EARLY ONSET (BIRTH TO ONE WEEK) OF HEART FAILURE IN NEONATAL CONGENITAL HEART DISEASE

COMMON

1. APVC, total (below diaphragm)
2. Hypoplastic left heart syndrome$_g$ (eg, severe stenosis or atresia of mitral or aortic or aortic arch valve with ASD and PDA)
3. Patent ductus arteriosus (PDA), preterm infant

UNCOMMON

1. Asphyxia (esp. first day)
2. Coarctation of aorta, severe (preductal)
3. Mitral atresia or severe stenosis
4. Myocardiopathy (eg, infant of diabetic mother)
5. Peripheral arteriovenous malformation

Reference

1. Modified from Tonkin ILD: The Infant with Respiratory Distress. In: Elliott LP (ed): Cardiac Imaging in Infants, Children, and Adults. Philadelphia: Lippincott, 1991, p 777

Gamut E-5

HEART FAILURE IN THE FIRST MONTH OF LIFE

COMMON

1. Coarctation of aorta, severe (preductal) or interruption of aortic arch with VSD and/or PDA
2. Left to right shunt, large (VSD; PDA; atrioventricular (AV) canal defect)
3. Tetralogy of Fallot$_g$, with complete AV canal, anemia, or postoperative shunt
4. Transposition of great vessels, complete

UNCOMMON

1. Arteriovenous fistula or hemangioma (eg, vein of Galen aneurysm, peripheral or pulmonary AVM, cavernous hemangioma of liver or skin)
2. Asphyxia (esp. first day)
3. Asplenia S. (Ivemark S.); polysplenia S. with complete AV canal
4. Common atrium
5. Conduction and rhythm abnormalities (eg, tachycardia, arrhythmia, complete heart block)
6. Cor triatriatum
7. Ebstein anomaly; Uhl anomaly
8. Foramen ovale closure, prenatal
9. Hemitruncus
10. High output state (eg, severe anemia — erythroblastosis; neonatal hyperthyroidism)
11. Hypoplastic left heart S.$_g$ (eg, severe stenosis or atresia of mitral or aortic valve or aortic arch with ASD and PDA)
12. Hypoplastic right heart S.
13. Iatrogenic (fluid overload; sodium chloride poisoning)
14. Increased intracranial pressure leading to pulmonary venous congestion (eg, cerebral injury at birth)
15. Mitral atresia or severe stenosis; mitral insufficiency
16. Myocardiopathy (eg, endocardial fibroelastosis; glycogen storage disease II (Pompe); infant of diabetic mother; myocarditis — rubella, toxoplasmosis, coxsackie virus; myocardial ischemia — neonatal hypoxia; anomalous left coronary artery arising from pulmonary artery)
17. Polycythemia (eg, maternal-fetal hemorrhage; placental and twin-to-twin transfusion)
18. Pulmonary vein atresia or stenosis
19. Single ventricle with transposition; single ventricle with PS
20. Total APVC (esp. below diaphragm)
21. Tricuspid atresia with transposition and no PS
22. Truncus arteriosus (in infants with large left to right shunt)

References

1. Eisenberg RL: Clinical Imaging: An Atlas of Differential Diagnosis. (ed 3) Philadelphia, Lippincott-Raven, 1997, pp 255–259

(continued)

2. Elliott LP: Cardiac Imaging in Infants, Children, and Adults. Philadelphia: Lippincott, 1991

3. Moss AJ, Adams FH, Emmanouilides GC: Heart Disease in Infants, Children and Adolescents. (ed 2) Baltimore: Williams & Wilkins, 1977

4. Swischuk LE: Imaging of the Newborn, Infant and Child. Baltimore: Williams & Wilkins, 1989

5. Taybi H, Lachman RS: Radiology of Syndromes, Metabolic Disorders, and Skeletal Dysplasias. (ed 4) St. Louis: Mosby-Year Book, 1996

Gamut E-6

CARDIOMEGALY AND/OR CARDIAC FAILURE IN A NEONATE, INFANT, OR CHILD

COMMON

1. Anemia (esp. erythroblastosis fetalis; sickle cell disease)
2. Coarctation of aorta, severe (preductal); interruption of aortic arch
3. Left to right shunt, large (VSD; PDA; atrioventricular (AV) canal defect)
4. Myocardiopathy (eg, endocardial fibroelastosis; glycogen storage disease type II (Pompe); infant of diabetic mother; myocarditis — rubella, toxoplasmosis, coxsackie virus; myocardial ischemia — neonatal hypoxia; anomalous left coronary artery arising from pulmonary artery)
5. [Pericardial effusion] (See E-49)
6. Rheumatic mitral insufficiency, with or without mycoarditis
7. Tetralogy of Fallot$_g$, with complete AV canal, anemia, or postoperative shunt
8. Transposition of great vessels with large shunt (VSD; PDA)

UNCOMMON

1. Aortic stenosis or atresia
2. APVC, total

3. Arrhythmia (eg, congenital heart block, paroxysmal tachycardia)
4. Asphyxia (esp. first day)
5. Asplenia S. (Ivemark S.); polysplenia S. with complete AV canal
6. Arteriovenous fistula or hemangioma, pulmonary or peripheral (incl. vein of Galen aneurysm; cavernous hemangioma of liver or skin)
7. Coronary disease (anomalous origin of left coronary artery from pulmonary artery; progeria; aneurysm in Kawasaki disease)
8. Cor triatriatum
9. Double outlet right ventricle (DORV)
10. Ebstein anomaly; Uhl anomaly
11. Endocardial fibroelastosis
12. Foramen ovale closure, prenatal
13. High-output state, other (eg, neonatal hyperthyroidism)
14. Hypoplastic left heart S.$_g$
15. Hypoplastic right heart S.
16. Iatrogenic (eg, fluid overload; sodium chloride poisoning)
17. Increased intracranial pressure (eg, cerebral disease from birth injury)
18. Infant of diabetic mother; neonatal hypoglycemia
19. Mitral atresia or severe stenosis or insufficiency, congenital
20. Neoplasm of heart, primary or metastatic (See E-43)
21. [Pectus excavatum; straight spine S.]
22. Polycythemia (eg, maternal-fetal hemorrhage; placental and twin-to-twin transfusion)
23. [Pulmonary lymphangiectasia]
24. Pulmonary veno-occlusive disease (eg, atresia)
25. Single ventricle
26. Tricuspid atresia
27. Truncus arteriosus

[ ] This condition does not actually cause the gamuted imaging finding, but can produce imaging changes that simulate it.

References

1. Eisenberg RL: Clinical Imaging: An Atlas of Differential Diagnosis. (ed 3) Philadelphia, Lippincott-Raven, 1997, pp 255–259
2. Elliott LP: Cardiac Imaging in Infants, Children, and Adults. Philadelphia: Lippincott, 1991

3. Moss AJ, Adams FH, Emmanouilides GC: Heart Disease in Infants, Children and Adolescents. (ed 2) Baltimore: Williams & Wilkins, 1977
4. Swischuk LE: Imaging of the Newborn, Infant and Child. Baltimore: Williams & Wilkins, 1989
5. Taybi H, Lachman RS: Radiology of Syndromes, Metabolic Disorders, and Skeletal Dysplasias. (ed 4) St. Louis: Mosby-Year Book, 1996

Gamut E-7

LEFT TO RIGHT SHUNT IN CONGENITAL HEART DISEASE

COMMON

1. Atrial septal defect (ASD)
2. Atrioventricular (AV) canal defect, partial or complete
3. Patent ductus arteriosus (PDA)
4. Ventricular septal defect (VSD)

UNCOMMON

1. Aortopulmonary window
2. APVC, total or partial (incl. venolobar S. {scimitar S.})

3. Coronary artery fistula to right heart or pulmonary artery (incl. anomalous origin of left coronary artery from pulmonary artery)
4. Corrected transposition with VSD
5. Hemitruncus (anomalous origin of right pulmonary artery from ascending aorta)
6. Left ventricular-right atrial shunt
7. Ruptured aortic valve cusp with VSD or into right atrium
8. Ruptured sinus of Valsalva aneurysm into right heart
9. Sequestration of lung (eg, drainage to azygos system)
10. Tetralogy of Fallot$_g$, acyanotic ("pink")

References

1. Edwards JE, Carey LS, Neufeld HN, et al: Congenital Heart Disease. Philadelphia: WB Saunders, 1965
2. Elliott LP: Cardiac Imaging in Infants, Children, and Adults. Philadelphia: Lippincott, 1991
3. Felson B (ed): Congenital heart disease, part II. Semin Roentgenol 1985; 20:200
4. Ferencz C, Rubin JD, McCarter RJ, et al: Congenital heart disease: Prevalence at live birth. Am J Epidemiol 1985;121:31–36
5. Mishkin FS: Lung curve indicating a left-to-right shunt in an infant with a large heart. Semin Nucl Med 1981;11:161–164

Gamut E-7-S

DIFFERENTIAL FEATURES OF COMMON LEFT TO RIGHT SHUNTS

	PULM VASC	PULM ART	AORTA	SVC	LV	RV	LA	RA
1. ASD	+	+	−	−	N	+	N	+
2. PDA	+	+	+	N	+	N,+	+	N
3. VSD	+	+	N,−	N	N,+	+	+	N,+

Abbreviations:

+ = increased   PULM VASC = pulmonary vasculature
− = decreased   PULM ART = pulmonary artery segment
N = Normal

Gamut E-8

RIGHT-TO-LEFT SHUNT OR ADMIXTURE LESION IN CONGENITAL HEART DISEASE

COMMON

1. APVC, total (above the diaphragm)
2. Double outlet right ventricle (DORV)
3. Left to right shunt progressing to reversal or high resistance vascularity (Eisenmenger physiology)
4. Tetralogy of Fallot$_g$
5. Transposition of great vessels
6. Tricuspid atresia
7. Truncus arteriosus

UNCOMMON

1. Anomalous systemic venous return to left atrium (eg, via left superior vena cava)
2. Aortic atresia
3. Coarctation of aorta, severe (preductal)
4. Common atrium
5. Ebstein anomaly with ASD
6. Hypoplastic right heart S.
7. Mitral atresia or stenosis (usually with VSD or PDA)
8. Pulmonary arteriovenous malformation
9. Pulmonary stenosis or atresia with intact ventricular septum and ASD (trilogy of Fallot)
10. Pulmonary vein atresia
11. Right pulmonary artery fistula to left atrium

References

1. Crupi G, Macartney FJ, Anderson RH: Persistent truncus arteriosus. Am Cardiol 1977; 40:569–578
2. Edwards JE, Carey LS, Neufeld HN, et al: Congenital Heart Disease. Philadelphia: WB Saunders, 1965
3. Elliott LP: Cardiac Imaging in Infants, Children, and Adults. Philadelphia: Lippincott, 1991
4. Felson B (ed): Congenital heart disease, part 1. Semin Roentgenol 1985; 20:110
5. Ferencz C, Rubin JD, McCarter RJ, et al: Congenital heart disease: Prevalence at live birth. Am J Epidemiol 1985; 121:31–36
6. Lester RG: Radiological concepts in the evaluation of heart disease. Mod Concepts Cardiovasc Dis 1968;37:113–118
7. Moss AJ, Adams FH, Emmanouilides GC: Heart Disease in Infants, Children and Adolescents. (ed 2) Baltimore: Williams & Wilkins, 1977
8. Rees S: Arterial connections of the lung. Clin Radiol 1981;32:1–15

DIFFERENTIAL FEATURES OF MAJOR CYANOTIC CONGENITAL HEART DISEASES

	CARDIAC SIZE	PULM VASC	AORTIC ARCH	EKG
1. Tetralogy of Fallot$_g$, incl. pseudotruncus (40%)*	N,+	−	R(25%)	RVH
2. Transportation of great vessels (15%)	+	+	L	RVH/LVH
3. Tricuspid atresia (10%)	N,+	−	L	LVH
4. Trilogy of Fallot (pulmonary atresia with ASD) (5%)	+	−	L	RVH
5. Truncus arteriosus (10%)	+	+,−	R(25%)	RVH/LVH

Abbreviations:

+ = increased − = decreased N = normal

* The five T's comprise approximately 80% of all cyanotic congenital heart disease.

TIME OF ONSET OF AND DEGREE OF CYANOSIS IN CONGENITAL HEART DISEASE

MARKED CYANOSIS AT BIRTH OR IN FIRST WEEK

1. Asplenia S. (Ivemark S.); polysplenia S.
2. Ebstein anomaly
3. Hypoplastic left heart S.$_g$ (eg, aortic or mitral atresia or severe stenosis; interruption of aortic arch)
4. Hypoplastic right heart S.
5. Persistent fetal circulation
*6. Pulmonary atresia
*7. Tetralogy of Fallot$_g$ with severe pulmonary stenosis or atresia (eg, pseudotruncus arteriosus)
8. Transposition of great vessels, complete

* Associated with pulmonary oligemia.

MILD OR INTERMITTENT CYANOSIS AT BIRTH OR SOON AFTER

1. APVC, total (below the diaphragm)
2. Atrioventricular (AV) canal defect (usually complete)
3. Large left to right shunt with failure
4. Truncus arteriosus

LATE ONSET OF CYANOSIS IN NEONATAL CONGENITAL HEART DISEASE

1. Double outlet right ventricle with pulmonary stenosis
2. Single ventricle with pulmonary stenosis
3. Single ventricle with transposition
4. Tetralogy of Fallot$_g$
5. Tricuspid atresia
6. Trilogy of Fallot

(continued)

References

1. Elliott LP: Cardiac Imaging in Infants, Children, and Adults. Philadelphia: Lippincott, 1991, pp 776–777
2. Felson B (ed): Congenital heart disease, part 1. Semin Roentgenol 1985;20:110
3. Rowe RD, Mehrizi A: The Neonate with Congenital Heart Disease. Major Problems in Clinical Pediatrics. Philadelphia: WB Saunders, 1968, vol 5
4. Modified from Tonkin ILD: The Infant with Respiratory Distress. In: Elliott LP (ed): Cardiac Imaging in Infants, Children, and Adults. Philadelphia: Lippincott, 1991, p 777

Gamut E-10

RIGHT TO LEFT SHUNT AT ATRIAL LEVEL

COMMON

1. APVC, total
2. ASD with severe pulmonary resistance (Eisenmenger physiology)
3. Transposition of great vessels with interatrial communication
4. Tricuspid atresia

UNCOMMON

1. ASD with left superior vena cava to left atrium communication
2. Ebstein anomaly
3. Hypoplasia of right ventricle, isolated
4. Normal newborn with patent foramen ovale
5. Pentalogy of Fallot
6. Pulmonary hypertension, primary, with interatrial communication
7. Pulmonary stenosis or atresia with intact ventricular septum and ASD (trilogy of Fallot)
8. Single atrium
9. Tricuspid stenosis with interatrial communication
10. Uhl anomaly

References

1. Elliott LP: Cardiac Imaging in Infants, Children, and Adults. Philadelphia: Lippincott, 1991

2. Felson B (ed): Congenital heart disease, part 1. Semin Roentgenol 1985:20:110
3. Meszaros WT: Cardiac Roentgenology. Springfield, IL: CC Thomas, 1969
4. Moss AJ, Adams FH, Emmanouilides GC: Heart Disease in Infants, Children and Adolescents. (ed 2) Baltimore: Williams & Wilkins, 1977
5. Swischuk LE: Plain Film Interpretation in Congenital Heart Disease. (ed 2) Baltimore: Williams & Wilkins, 1979

Gamut E-10-S

COMPLICATED ATRIAL LEVEL SHUNTS

I. CONVENTIONAL ASD ASSOCIATED WITH ANOTHER USUALLY INDEPENDENT ANOMALY

1. APVC, partial
2. Lutembacher S. (rheumatic mitral stenosis and ASD)
3. Mitral valve regurgitation or prolapse (MVP); cleft mitral valve
4. Pulmonary stenosis (eg, trilogy of Fallot)
5. Ventricular septal defect (VSD)

II. ATRIAL SEPTUM IS INTACT; SITE OF SHUNT IS DISTAL TO ATRIAL SEPTUM BUT MAY DRAIN INTO RA

1. Coronary artery fistula
2. Left ventricular-right atrial shunt
3. Rupture of posterior aortic sinus aneurysm into RA

III. ASD IS PART OF A DEVELOPMENTAL COMPLEX

1. APVC, total
2. Complete atrioventricular canal defect (AV communis or total endocardial cushion defect)
3. Pentalogy of Fallot

Reference

1. Elliott LP: Cardiac Imaging in Infants, Children, and Adults. Philadelphia: Lippincott, 1991, p 593

Gamut E-11

RIGHT TO LEFT SHUNT AT VENTRICULAR LEVEL

COMMON
1. Complete transposition of great vessels with VSD
2. Tetralogy of Fallot$_g$ with pulmonary atresia
3. VSD with pulmonary hypertension (Eisenmenger physiology)

UNCOMMON
1. Corrected transposition with VSD and predominant PS
2. Double outlet right ventricle (DORV)
3. Single ventricle
4. Truncus arteriosus

References
1. Elliott LP: Cardiac Imaging in Infants, Children, and Adults. Philadelphia: Lippincott, 1991
2. Felson B (ed): Congenital heart disease, part 1. Semin Roentgenol 1985; 20:1103.
3. Meszaros WT: Cardiac Roentgenology. Springfield, IL: CC Thomas, 1969
4. Moss AJ, Adams FH, Emmanouilides GC: Heart Disease in Infants, Children and Adolescents. (ed 2) Baltimore: Williams & Wilkins, 1977

Gamut E-12-S1

CARDIOVASCULAR ANOMALIES ASSOCIATED WITH VSD

VSD AN ESSENTIAL PART OF THE ANOMALY

COMMON
1. Tetralogy of Fallot$_g$ (incl. pseudotruncus)

UNCOMMON
1. Complete atrioventricular canal (AV communis)
2. Double outlet left ventricle
3. Double outlet right ventricle (DORV)
4. Pentalogy of Fallot$_g$ (tetralogy + ASD)
5. S. Truncus arteriosus

VSD FREQUENTLY ASSOCIATED WITH THE ANOMALY

COMMON
1. Atrial septal defect (ASD)
2. Coarctation of aorta
3. Complete transposition of great vessels
4. Patent ductus arteriosus (PDA)
5. Pulmonary stenosis

UNCOMMON
1. APVC
2. Chromosomal abnormalities (eg, trisomy anomalies)
3. Corrected transposition of great vessels
4. Ectopia cordis
5. Interruption of aortic arch
6. Left ventricular outflow tract obstruction
7. Prolapse of right aortic cusp with aortic insufficiency
8. Single ventricle
9. Sinus of Valsalva aneurysm
10. Tricuspid atresia

(continued)

References
1. Edwards JE: The pathology of ventricular septal defect. Semin Roentgenol 1966; 1:2–23
2. Elliott LP: Cardiac Imaging in Infants, Children, and Adults. Philadelphia: Lippincott, 1991, pp 575–576

Gamut E-12-S2

CARDIOVASCULAR ANOMALIES ASSOCIATED WITH COMPLETE ATRIOVENTRICULAR CANAL (CAVC)

1. Asplenia S. (Ivemark S.)
2. Patent ductus arteriosus (PDA)
3. Single ventricle
4. Tetralogy of Fallot$_g$
5. Trisomy 21 S. (Down S.)

References
1. Edwards JE: The pathology of ventricular septal defect. Semin Roentgenol 1966; 1:2–23
2. Elliott LP: Cardiac Imaging in Infants, Children, and Adults. Philadelphia: Lippincott, 1991, pp 575–576

Gamut E-13

RIGHT-TO-LEFT SHUNT AT DUCTUS LEVEL

COMMON
1. Coarctation of aorta, severe (preductal)
2. PDA with severe pulmonary vascular resistance (Eisenmenger physiology)
3. Persistent fetal circulation

UNCOMMON
1. APVC, total
2. Hypoplastic left heart S. (severe stenosis or atresia of mitral valve, aortic valve, or aortic arch)
3. Pulmonary vein atresia

References
1. Elliott LP: Cardiac Imaging in Infants, Children, and Adults. Philadelphia: Lippincott, 1991
2. Meszaros WT: Cardiac Roentgenology. Springfield, IL: CC Thomas, 1969
3. Moss AJ, Adams FH, Emmanouilides GC: Heart Disease in Infants, Children and Adolescents. (ed 2) Baltimore: Williams & Wilkins, 1977

Gamut E-14-S

PULMONARY ARTERIAL VASCULARITY IN COMMON CONGENITAL HEART DISEASES (See E-15–19)

SHUNT VASCULARITY (OVERCIRCULATION) WITH PROMINENT PULMONARY ARTERY SEGMENT

	Incidence
1. VSD	22%
2. PDA	12%
3. ASD	11%
4. APVC, total (above diaphragm)	2%
5. Atrioventricular canal defect	2%
6. Aortopulmonary window	
7. All other left-to-right shunts with normally related great vessels	

SHUNT VASCULARITY WITH FLAT OR CONCAVE PULMONARY ARTERY SEGMENT
*1. Complete transposition of great vessels	6%
*2. Truncus arteriosus (types II and III)	3%
*3. Corrected transposition with VSD	
*4. Single ventricle	
*5. Tricuspid atresia with normally related vessels	

NORMAL VASCULARITY

<table>
<tr><td></td><td></td><td align="right">Incidence</td></tr>
<tr><td>1.</td><td>Pulmonary valvular stenosis</td><td align="right">10%</td></tr>
<tr><td>2.</td><td>Coarctation of aorta</td><td align="right">7%</td></tr>
<tr><td>3.</td><td>Aortic stenosis</td><td align="right">3%</td></tr>
<tr><td>4.</td><td>Corrected (L-loop) transposition of great vessels</td><td align="right"><2%</td></tr>
<tr><td>5.</td><td>Endocardial fibroelastosis</td><td align="right"><2%</td></tr>
<tr><td>6.</td><td>Small left to right shunt</td><td></td></tr>
<tr><td>7.</td><td>Subaortic stenosis</td><td></td></tr>
</table>

DECREASED VASCULARITY

<table>
<tr><td>*1.</td><td>Tetralogy of Fallot$_g$ (incl. pseudotruncus)</td><td align="right">12%</td></tr>
<tr><td>*2.</td><td>Tricuspid atresia or stenosis</td><td align="right">3%</td></tr>
<tr><td>*3.</td><td>Ebstein anomaly; Uhl anomaly</td><td align="right"><2%</td></tr>
<tr><td>*4.</td><td>Pulmonary atresia or severe stenosis with ASD, transposition, or single ventricle (eg, trilogy of Fallot)</td><td align="right">>2%</td></tr>
<tr><td>5.</td><td>Tricuspid insufficiency, congenital (severe)</td><td align="right"><2%</td></tr>
</table>

* Cyanotic lesions.

References

1. Chen JTT: Essentials of Cardiac Roentgenology. Boston: Little, Brown, 1987
2. Gedgaudas E, Moller JH, Castaneda-Zuniga WR, et al: Cardiovascular Radiology. Philadelphia: WB Saunders, 1985
3. Lester RG: Radiological concepts in the evaluation of heart disease. Mod Concepts Cardiovasc Dis 1968;37:113–118
4. Sotomora RF, Edwards JE: Anatomic identification of so called absent pulmonary artery. Circulation 57:624, 1978
5. Swischuk LE: Plain Film Interpretation in Congenital Heart Disease. (ed 2) Baltimore: Williams & Wilkins, 1979

ACYANOTIC CONGENITAL HEART DISEASE WITH NORMAL PULMONARY VASCULARITY*

COMMON

1. Aortic stenosis
2. Coarctation of aorta
3. Pulmonary stenosis
4. Small left-to-right shunts

UNCOMMON

*1. Anomalous origin of left coronary artery from pulmonary artery
*2. Aortic insufficiency
*3. Cor triatriatum
*4. Endocardial fibroelastosis
*5. Hypoplastic left heart S.$_g$
*6. Idiopathic hypertrophic subaortic stenosis (IHSS)
*7. Interruption of aortic arch (usually with VSD and PDA)
*8. Mitral insufficiency
*9. Mitral stenosis
*10. Myocardiopathy (eg, glycogen storage disease; rubella S.; Noonan S.; mucopolysaccharidoses) (See J-4)

* Normal pulmonary vasculature until left-sided heart failure develops in infancy, at which time pulmonary venous hypertension may be noted.

Gamut E-16

ACYANOTIC CONGENITAL HEART DISEASE WITH INCREASED PULMONARY VASCULARITY (SHUNT) (See E-51)

COMMON

1. Atrial septal defect (ASD)
2. Atrioventricular (AV) canal defect, partial or complete
3. Patent ductus arteriosus (PDA)
4. Ventricular septal defect (VSD)

UNCOMMON

1. Aortopulmonary window
2. APVC, partial
3. Coronary artery fistula
4. Ruptured sinus of Valsalva aneurysm (into RV or occasionally RA)

References

1. Chen JTT: Essentials of Cardiac Roentgenology. Boston: Little, Brown, 1987
2. Eisenberg RL: Clinical Imaging. An Atlas of Differential Diagnosis. (ed 3) Philadelphia: Lippincott-Raven, 1997, pp 230–233

Gamut E-17

CYANOTIC CONGENITAL HEART DISEASE WITH INCREASED PULMONARY VASCULARITY (See E-51)

COMMON

1. APVC, total (above diaphragm)
2. Complete transposition of great vessels
3. Truncus arteriosus (types I, II, and III)

UNCOMMON

1. Aortic atresia
2. Common atrium
3. Double outlet right ventricle (DORV); Taussig-Bing anomaly
4. Left-to-right shunt with reversal (Eisenmenger physiology, esp. PDA, VSD, AV canal)
5. Single ventricle without PS
6. Tricuspid atresia without PS

References

1. Chen JTT: Essentials of Cardiac Roentgenology. Boston: Little, Brown, 1987
2. Elliott LP: Cardiac Imaging in Infants, Children, and Adults. Philadelphia: Lippincott, 1991, p 156
3. Gedgaudas E, Moller JH, Castaneda-Zuniga WR, et al: Cardiovascular Radiology. Philadelphia: WB Saunders,1985

Gamut E-18

CYANOTIC CONGENITAL HEART DISEASE WITH PRECAPILLARY HYPERTENSION VASCULARITY (High Vascular Resistance, Eisenmenger Physiology)

COMMON

1. ASD, large
2. Atrioventricular (AV) canal
3. PDA, large
4. VSD (all types), large

UNCOMMON

1. Common atrium
2. Double outlet right ventricle (DORV) without PS
3. Single ventricle without PS
4. Transposition of great vessels, complete or corrected, with VSD or PDA, but without PS
5. Tricuspid atresia without PS
6. Truncus arteriosus (Types I, II, III)

CONGENITAL HEART DISEASE WITH DECREASED PULMONARY VASCULARITY (USUALLY CYANOTIC)

COMMON

1. Tetralogy of Fallot$_g$, incl. pseudotruncus (systemic collateral vasculature)

UNCOMMON

1. Asplenia S. (Ivemark S.)
2. Double outlet right ventricle with PS
3. Ebstein anomaly with ASD
4. Persistent fetal circulation
5. Pulmonary atresia or severe stenosis (isolated anomaly or associated with ASD)
6. Pulmonary stenosis with intact ventricular septum and ASD (trilogy of Fallot)
7. Single ventricle with PS
8. Transposition of great vessels, complete or corrected, with VSD and PS or atresia
9. Tricuspid atresia or stenosis with PS or atresia
10. Tricuspid insufficiency
11. Truncus arteriosus (rarely types II or III)
12. Uhl anomaly (parchment RV)

References
1. Chen JTT: Essentials of Cardiac Roentgenology. Boston: Little, Brown, 1987
2. Elliott LP: Cardiac Imaging in Infants, Children, and Adults. Philadelphia: Lippincott, 1991, p 156
3. Felson B (ed): Congenital heart disease, part I. Semin Roentgenol 1985; 20:110
4. Gedgaudas E, Moller JH, Castaneda-Zuniga WR, et al: Cardiovascular Radiology. Philadelphia: WB Saunders, 1985
5. Lester RG: Radiological concepts in the evaluation of heart disease. Mod Concepts Cardiovasc Dis 1968;37:113–118
6. Schiebler GL, Miller RH, Gessner IH: The triad of cyanosis, decreased pulmonary vascularity and cardiomegaly. Radiol Clin North Am 1968;6:361–365
7. Wesenberg RL: The Newborn Chest. Hagerstown, MD: Harper & Row, 1973

FLAT OR CONCAVE PULMONARY ARTERY SEGMENT IN CONGENITAL HEART DISEASE

COMMON

1. Complete transposition of great vessels
2. Tetralogy of Fallot$_g$ (incl. pseudotruncus)

UNCOMMON

1. Asplenia S. (Ivemark S.)
2. Corrected transposition (pulmonary artery medially positioned)
3. Double outlet right ventricle (DORV) with pulmonary stenosis
4. Hypoplastic right heart S.
5. Pulmonary atresia with intact ventricular septum
6. Single ventricle with transposition of great vessels
7. Tricuspid atresia or stenosis with transposition of great vessels
8. Truncus arteriosus (types II and III)

References
1. Elliott LP: Cardiac Imaging in Infants, Children, and Adults. Philadelphia: Lippincott, 1991.
2. Moss AJ, Adams FH, Emmanouilides GC: Heart Disease in Infants, Children and Adolescents. (ed 2) Baltimore: Williams & Wilkins, 1977
3. Swischuk LE: Plain Film Interpretation in Congenital Heart Disease. (ed 2) Baltimore:Williams & Wilkins, 1979

Gamut E-21-S

VASCULAR RING AND OTHER ANOMALIES OF THE AORTIC ARCH AND BRACHIOCEPHALIC ARTERIES

COMMON

1. Coarctation of aorta
   a. Preductal (infantile—long segment narrowing)
   b. Postductal (adult—short, discrete narrowing)
2. Double aortic arch
3. Left aortic arch with aberrant right subclavian artery (incl. aortic diverticulum)
4. Pseudocoarctation of aorta
5. Right anterior aortic arch (Type I aortic arch) (mirror image branching of major arteries)
6. Right posterior aortic arch (Type II aortic arch)

UNCOMMON

1. Anomalous innominate artery
2. Anomalous left common carotid artery
3. Cervical aortic arch (right or left)
4. Innominate artery compression S.
5. Left aortic arch, right ductus, and right descending aorta
6. Pulmonary sling (left pulmonary artery arising from right pulmonary artery)
7. Right aortic arch, left descending aorta
8. Right aortic arch, right descending aorta, and aberrant or isolated left subclavian artery (Type III aortic arch)

References

1. Baron RL, Gutierrez FR, Sagel SS: CT of anomalies of the mediastinal vessels. AJR 1981;137:571–576
2. Chen JTT: Essentials of Cardiac Roentgenology. Boston: Little, Brown, 1987
3. Edwards JE, Carey LS, Neufeld HN: Congenital Heart Disease: Correlation of Pathologic Anatomy and Angiocardiography. Philadelphia: WB Saunders, 1965
4. Felson B, Palayew MJ: The two types of right aortic arch. Radiology 1963;81:745–759
5. Salomonowitz E, Edwards JE, Hunter DW: The three types of aortic diverticula. AJR 1984;142:673–679
6. Shuford WH, Sybers RG, Weens HS: The angiographic features of double aortic arch. AJR 1972;116:125–140
7. Soulen RL, Donner RM: Advances in noninvasive evaluation of congenital anomalies of the thoracic aorta. Radiol Clin North Am 1985;23:727–736
8. Spindola-Franco H, Fish BG: In Elliott L (ed): Cardiac Imaging in Infants, Children and Adults. Philadelphia: Lippincott, 1991, pp 344–368
9. Stewart JR, Kincaid OW, Edwards JE: An Atlas of Vascular Rings and Related Malformations of the Aortic Arch System. Springfield, IL: CC Thomas, 1964
10. Swischuk LE: Imaging of the Newborn, Infant and Child. Baltimore: Williams & Wilkins, 1989

Gamut E-22

CONGENITAL HEART DISEASE ASSOCIATED WITH ANTERIOR RIGHT AORTIC ARCH (TYPE I—MIRROR IMAGE BRANCHING)

1. Anatomically corrected malposition — 50%*
2. Asplenia S. (Ivemark S.) — 30–40%
3. Pseudotruncus arteriosus (pulmonary atresia with VSD) — 40–50%
4. Tetralogy of Fallot$_g$; — 25%
   "Pink" tetralogy — 15%
5. Transposition of great vessels with VSD and PS — 5–10%
6. Tricuspid atresia — 5%
7. Truncus arteriosus — 25–35%
8. VSD (uncomplicated large) — 2%

* % refers to approximate percentage of all cases of that anomaly with a right aortic arch.

Reference

1. Elliott LP: Cardiac Imaging in Infants, Children, and Adults. Philadelphia: Lippincott, 1991, p 146

POSITIONAL ANOMALIES OF THE THORACIC AORTA AND AORTIC ARCH

	ARCH	DESCENDING L	DESCENDING R	SUBCLAVIAN ARTERY N	SUBCLAVIAN ARTERY ANOMALY	AORTIC DIVER-TICULUM	CONGENITAL HEART DISEASE
Normal	L	+		+		0	rare
Anomalous descending A	L		+			rare	rare
RAA type I	R	rare	+	+	rare	0	com
RAA type II	R	rare	+	rare	com	com	rare
Cervical AA, L	L	rare	com	rare	com	com	rare
Cervical AA, R	R	+		+	com	rare	
Anomalous R subclavian artery	L	+			+	com	rare
Double AA	L&R	+				0	rare

Abbreviations:

N = Normal   A = Aorta   L = Left   com = common

+ = Present   AA = Aortic arch   R = Right

0 = Absent

ANOMALOUS ARTERIAL COMMUNICATION IN THE THORAX

DIRECT COMMUNICATION OF AORTA AND PULMONARY ARTERY

1. Aortopulmonary window
2. PDA
3. Postoperative shunt (eg, Blalock-Taussig; Waterston; Potts)
4. Pseudotruncus
5. Truncus arteriosus

AORTIC OR SYSTEMIC ARTERY ANOMALY

1. Fistula
   a. Aortic—left ventricular tunnel
   b. Brachiocephalic artery to systemic vein (eg, fistula from transverse cervical artery to internal jugular vein)
   c. Coronary artery fistula
   d. Postoperative aortic-cardiac fistula
   e. Ruptured sinus of Valsalva aneurysm into heart
   f. Systemic—pulmonary AV malformation (bronchial, brachiocephalic, or chest wall artery to pulmonary artery, pulmonary vein, or azygos system)
2. Anomalous origin of systemic artery
   a. Left coronary artery from pulmonary artery
   b. Subclavian artery from pulmonary artery

(continued)

PULMONARY ARTERY ANOMALY

1. Fistula
   a. Pulmonary AV malformation
   b. Right pulmonary artery to left atrium fistula
2. Anomalous origin of pulmonary artery
   a. Left pulmonary artery from right pulmonary artery (pulmonary sling)
   b. Left or right pulmonary artery from descending aorta
   c. Left or right pulmonary artery from ascending aorta (hemitruncus)
3. Anomalous artery arising from aorta to supply a lung segment
   a. Sequestration of lung
   b. Venolobar S. (scimitar S.)

References
1. Franken EA, Hurwitz RA: Radiological Society of North America Scientific Exhibit, 1973
2. Spindola-Franco H, Fish BG (eds): Radiology of the Heart: Cardiac Imaging in Infants and Children. New York: Springer-Verlag
3. Viamonte M Jr: Intrathoracic extracardiac shunts. Semin Roentgenol 1967;2:342–367

Gamut E-25-S

ANOMALOUS PULMONARY VENOUS RETURN CONNECTIONS (APVC)

TOTAL (TAPVC)*

1. Left vertical vein	37%
2. Coronary sinus	16%
3. Infracardiac (abdominal)	15%
4. Right SVC	14%
5. Right atrium	11%
6. Mixed	7%

PARTIAL (PAPVC)

1. SVC
2. Azygos vein
3. Right atrium
4. IVC; portal vein; hepatic vein (eg, scimitar S.)
5. Left innominate vein (via vertical vein)
6. Coronary sinus
7. Mixed

* 25% to 30% of patients with TAPVC may have other anomalies, such as VSD, PDA, coarctation or interruption of the aortic arch.

Reference
1. Moes CAF, Freedom RM, Burrows PE: Anomalous pulmonary venous connections. Semin Roentgenol 1985;20: 134–150

Gamut E-26

ABNORMAL CARDIAC POSITION; CARDIAC DISPLACEMENT (Congenital or Acquired)

CONGENITAL

1. Absence of a pulmonary artery
2. Agenesis or hypoplasia of a lobe or lung; venolobar S. (scimitar S.)
3. Asplenia S. or polysplenia S.
4. Congenital absence of left pericardium
5. Dextrocardia, mirror-image type with situs inversus
6. Dextroposition; mesocardia
7. Dextroversion with situs solitus or situs indeterminate
8. Levoversion (levocardia with situs inversus)
9. Pectus excavatum

ACQUIRED

1. Atelectasis; fibrosis of lung
2. Diaphragmatic hernia; elevation of hemidiaphragm
3. Emphysema, unilateral (esp. bullous)
4. Mass lesion (eg, neoplasm; cyst; hematoma; aneurysm)
5. Pleural fluid or thickening; mesothelioma
6. Pneumonectomy with resultant fibrothorax

7. Pneumothorax (tension)
8. Scoliosis (heart shifted to concave side)
9. Technical (rotation of patient)

References
1. Baron RL, Gutierrez FR, Sagel SS: CT of anomalies of the mediastinal vessels. AJR 1981;137:571–577
2. Cooley RN: Editorial: Congenital dextrocardia and the general radiologist. AJR 1972;116:211–214
3. Felson B: Chest Roentgenology. Philadelphia: WB Saunders, Co., 1973
4. Majeski JA, Upshur JK: Asplenia syndrome: A study of congenital anomalies in 16 cases. JAMA 1978;240:1508–1510
5. Stanger P, Rudolph AM, Edwards JE: Cardiac malpositions: An overview based on study of sixty-five necropsy specimens. Circulation 1977;56:159–172
6. Tonkin ILD, Tonkin AK: Visceroatrial situs abnormalities: Sonographic and computed tomographic appearance. AJR 1982;138:509–515
7. Van Praagh R: The importance of segmental situs in the diagnosis of congenital heart disease. Semin Roentgenol 1985; 20:254–271

Gamut E-26-S

TYPES OF DEXTROCARDIA

1. **Situs inversus** (all visceral organs opposite of normal; slightly increased incidence of cardiac anomalies in 5% to 10% of patients)
2. **Dextroposition with situs solitus** (cardiac apex displaced into right hemithorax—eg, hypoplasia of right lung; venolobar S.)
3. **Dextroversion with situs solitus** (anatomic relations are normal, but cardiac apex is in right side of chest—due to abnormal rotation of embryonic cardiac loop)
4. **Dextrocardia with situs ambiguus in asplenia S.** (bilateral right-sidedness—absent spleen; three lobes in each lung; left lobe of liver same size as right lobe; malrotation of bowel; cardiac apex in either hemithorax—cardiac anomalies include common atrium; single ventricle; PS; transposition of great vessels; and TAPVR)

5. **Dextrocardia with situs ambiguus in polysplenia S.** (bilateral left-sidedness—each lung has two lobes; hepatic segment of IVC is absent; cardiac apex is in right hemithorax in 50% of patients—cardiac anomalies include ASD; PAPVR; and interruption of IVC with azygos continuation)

Reference
1. Gedgaudas E, Moller JH, Castaneda-Zuniga WR, Amplatz K: Cardiovascular Radiology. Philadelphia: WB Saunders, 1985, pp 175–181

Gamut E-27

RIGHT ATRIAL ENLARGEMENT

COMMON

1. Left to right shunt into right atrium (eg, ASD; patent foramen ovale; atrioventricular canal defect; total or partial APVR; left ventricular–right atrial shunt; ruptured sinus of Valsalva aneurysm into right atrium)
2. [Pericardial cyst, lipoma, or encapsulated fluid]
3. Pulmonary stenosis
4. Right heart failure, any cause
5. Right ventricular enlargement resulting in atrial enlargement (esp. cor pulmonale; mitral stenosis; chronic left heart failure) (See E-54)
6. Tetralogy of Fallot$_g$; trilogy of Fallot
7. Tricuspid insufficiency (See E-28)

UNCOMMON

1. Congenital or idiopathic right atriomegaly; atrial aneurysm
2. Coronary artery fistula to RA
3. Ebstein anomaly; Uhl anomaly
4. Endocardial fibroelastosis
5. Endomyocardial fibrosis
6. Hypoplastic left heart S.$_g$ (stenosis or atresia of mitral valve, aortic valve, or aortic arch with ASD and PDA)

(continued)

7. Neoplasm of right atrium or ventricle (eg, myxoma) (See E-43)
8. Post-mitral valve replacement
9. Pulmonary atresia (with tricuspid insufficiency)
10. Transposition of great vessels with interatrial communication
11. Tricuspid atresia or stenosis (incl. carcinoid S.)

[ ] This condition does not actually cause the gamuted imaging finding, but can produce imaging changes that simulate it.

References
1. Eisenberg RL: Clinical Imaging: An Atlas of Differential Diagnosis. (ed 3) Philadelphia: Lippincott-Raven, 1997, pp 212–213
2. Gedgaudas E, Moller JH, Castaneda-Zuniga WR, Amplatz K: Cardiovascular Radiology. Philadelphia: WB Saunders, 1985
3. Meszaros WT: Cardiac Roentgenology. Springfield, IL: CC Thomas, 1969
4. Rubin SA, Hightower CW, Flicker S: Giant right atrium after mitral valve replacement: Plain film findings in 15 patients. AJR 1987;149:257–260
5. Swischuk LE, John SD: Differential Diagnosis in Pediatric Radiology (ed 2) Baltimore: Williams & Wilkins, 1995, p 101

Gamut E-28

TRICUSPID INSUFFICIENCY

COMMON

1. Pulmonary hypertension; cor pulmonale
2. Rheumatic heart disease
3. Right ventricular failure with enlargement

UNCOMMON

1. AV canal defect
2. Bacterial endocarditis (esp. in narcotics abuser)
3. Carcinoid S.
4. Ebstein anomaly
5. Endomyocardial fibrosis
6. Myxoma of right atrium
7. Trauma
8. Tricuspid valve prolapse

References
1. Eisenberg RL: Clinical Imaging: An Atlas of Differential Diagnosis. (ed 3) Philadelphia: Lippincott-Raven, 1997, p 212
2. Wilde P, Hartnell GG: Tricuspid insufficiency. In: Sutton D, Young JWR (eds): A Short Textbook of Clinical Imaging. London: Springer-Verlag, 1990, p 176

Gamut E-29

RIGHT VENTRICULAR ENLARGEMENT

COMMON

1. Chronic left heart failure (eg, mitral insufficiency; myocardiopathy) (See E-40)
2. Cor pulmonale; pulmonary arterial hypertension, primary or secondary (eg, COPD; diffuse interstitial fibrosis; pulmonary emboli; Eisenmenger physiology with reversed left-to-right shunt) (See E-54)
3. Left to right shunt (esp. ASD; VSD; PDA) (See E-7)
4. Mitral stenosis, acquired
5. Pseudotruncus arteriosus
6. Pulmonary stenosis with right ventricular failure

UNCOMMON

1. Double outlet right ventricle (DORV)
2. Ebstein anomaly; Uhl anomaly
3. Hypoplastic left heart syndrome$_g$ (stenosis or atresia of mitral valve, aortic valve, or aortic arch with ASD and PDA)
4. Infarction of right ventricle
5. Neoplasm of right ventricle or left atrium (eg, myxoma) (See E-43)
6. Pulmonary atresia (with tricuspid insufficiency)
7. Pulmonary insufficiency; absent pulmonary valve
8. Pulmonary venous obstruction (eg, congenital mitral stenosis; cor triatriatum; veno-occlusive disease) (See E-3-S, E-59)
9. Transposition of great vessels
10. Tricuspid insufficiency

11. Trilogy of Fallot
12. Truncus arteriosus

References

1. Bjornsson J, Edwards WD: Primary pulmonary hypertension: A histopathologic study of 80 cases. Mayo Clin Proc 1985;60:16–25
2. Eisenberg RL: Clinical Imaging: An Atlas of Differential Diagnosis. (ed 3) Philadelphia: Lippincott-Raven, 1997, pp 214–217
3. Gedgaudas E, Moller JH, Castaneda-Zuniga WR, Amplatz K: Cardiovascular Radiology. Philadelphia: WB Saunders, 1985
4. Holmes JC, Fowler NO, Kaplan S: Pulmonary valvular insufficiency. Am J Med 1968;44:851–862
5. Meszaros WT: Cardiac Roentgenology. Springfield, IL: CC Thomas, 1969

Gamut E-30

FILLING DEFECT IN RIGHT VENTRICLE ON ANGIOCARDIOGRAPHY

COMMON

1. Jet of unopacified blood (eg, VSD with left-to-right shunt)
2. Thrombus

UNCOMMON

1. Aneurysm or diverticulum of ventricular septum
2. Anomalous muscle bundle
3. [Bernheim S. (left ventricular hypertrophy encroaching on right ventricle)]
4. Endocardial fibroelastosis (with bulging ventricular septum)
5. Foreign body (eg, catheter)
6. Idiopathic myocardial hypertrophy (eg, IHSS)
7. Neoplasm of heart, primary or metastatic (See E-43)
8. Prolapsed valve

[ ] This condition does not actually cause the gamuted imaging finding, but can produce imaging changes that simulate it.

Gamut E-31

LEFT ATRIAL ENLARGEMENT

COMMON

1. Left ventricular failure
2. Mitral insufficiency (See E-32)
3. Mitral stenosis, congenital or acquired (incl. prolapsed mitral valve)
4. Myocardiopathy (See E-40)
5. PDA; aortopulmonary window
6. VSD

UNCOMMON

1. ASD with late reversal of shunt (Eisenmenger physiology)
2. Atriomegaly, left, congenital or idiopathic (giant left atrium S.)
3. Constrictive pericarditis (See E-48)
4. Coronary artery fistula
5. Double outlet right ventricle (DORV)
6. Endocardial fibroelastosis
7. Mitral anulus anomaly
8. Neoplasm of left atrium (eg, myxoma) (See E-43)
9. Papillary muscle rupture
10. Parachute mitral valve complex
11. Single ventricle (cor triloculare biatriatum)
12. Thrombus in left atrium (esp. ball-valve)
13. Transposition of great vessels
14. Tricuspid atresia
15. Trilogy of Fallot
16. Truncus arteriosus

References

1. Burgener FA, Kormano M: Differential Diagnosis in Conventional Radiology. New York: Thieme Medical Publ, 1991, pp 324–328
2. Eisenberg RL: Clinical Imaging: An Atlas of Differential Diagnosis. (ed 3) Philadelphia: Lippincott-Raven, 1997, pp 214–217
3. Fowler NO: Cardiac Diagnosis and Treatment. (ed 3) Hagerstown, MD: Harper & Row, 1980
4. Gedgaudas E, Moller JH, Castaneda-Zuniga WR, Amplatz K: Cardiovascular Radiology. Philadelphia: WB Saunders, 1985
5. Waller BF: Nonrheumatic causes of pure mitral regurgitation. Practical Card 1985;11:69–84

MITRAL INSUFFICIENCY

COMMON

1. Bacterial endocarditis
2. Functional—left ventricular dilatation (eg, cardiac failure; coarctation of aorta; aortic insufficiency; myocardiopathy)—(See E-40)
3. Mitral valve prolapse
4. Myxomatous degeneration of valve leaflets
5. Papillary muscle rupture or dysfunction (eg, infarction; ischemic heart disease; trauma)
6. Postoperative (eg, mitral valve repair; valvotomy; balloon valvoplasty; dysfunctional prosthetic mitral valve)
7. Rheumatic endocarditis
8. Ruptured chordae tendineae

UNCOMMON

1. Atrioventricular canal defect
2. Congenital valvular insufficiency
3. Corrected transposition (with anomalous left atrioventricular valve)
4. Ehlers-Danlos S.
5. Endocardial fibroelastosis
6. Idiopathic hypertrophic subaortic stenosis (IHSS)
7. Marfan S.
8. Mitral anulus anomaly or calcification
9. Neoplasm (eg, carcinoid, left atrial myxoma) (See E-43)
10. Polychondritis; osteogenesis imperfecta
11. Takayasu arteritis

References

1. Elliott LP: Cardiac Imaging in Infants, Children, and Adults. Philadelphia: Lippincott, 1991, pp 531–541
2. Meszaros WT: Cardiac Roentgenology. Springfield, IL: CC Thomas, 1969
3. Sutton D (ed): Textbook of Radiology and Imaging. (ed 6) New York: Churchill Livingstone, 1998, pp 599–603
4. Waller BF: Nonrheumatic causes of pure mitral regurgitation. Practical Card 1985;11:69–84

EXTRA BUMP ALONG THE UPPER LEFT HEART BORDER (THE THIRD MOGUL)

COMMON

1. Aneurysm of left ventricle
2. Left atrial appendage enlargement (esp. rheumatic or congenital heart disease)
3. [Pericardial adhesion, postoperative (eg, CABG) or other]
4. [Pericardial defect, total or partial, with herniation of left atrial appendage]
5. [Thymus gland; mediastinal mass, esp. thymoma; thymic cyst; germ cell lesion; lymphoma$_g$]

UNCOMMON

1. Coronary artery aneurysm; or AV fistula
2. Corrected transposition or single ventricle with left-sided ascending aorta and rudimentary right ventricle in inverted position
3. Cyst (eg, pericardial; hydatid)
4. Ebstein's anomaly
5. Myocardiopathy (See E-40)
6. Neoplasm of heart or pericardium (See E-43)
7. [Pleural plaque (asbestosis)]
8. Postoperative deformity (eg, pulmonary artery conduit; aneurysm)
9. Right atrial appendage, levoposition
10. Sinus of Valsalva aneurysm (left)
11. Tetralogy of Fallot$_g$ (eg, postoperative dilatation of patch used for correction of infundibular stenosis)

References

1. Daves M: Skiagraphing the mediastinal moguls. New Physician Jan 1970, p 49
2. Swischuk LE: Plain Film Interpretation in Congenital Heart Disease. (ed 2) Baltimore: Williams & Wilkins, 1979
3. Swischuk LE, John SD: Differential Diagnosis in Pediatric Radiology (ed 2) Baltimore: Williams & Wilkins, 1995, p 99

[ ] This condition does not actually cause the gamuted imaging finding, but can produce imaging changes that simulate it.

LEFT VENTRICULAR ENLARGEMENT

COMMON

1. Aortic insufficiency (eg, rheumatic heart disease) (See E-35)
2. Aortic stenosis (rheumatic; congenital—bicuspid aortic valve; degenerative—idiopathic calcific stenosis) when in left ventricular failure
3. Athlete's heart (no disease)
4. Coarctation of aorta when in left ventricular failure
5. Coronary or arteriosclerotic heart disease (incl. myocardial infarction; left ventricular aneurysm) when in left ventricular failure
6. Heart failure (See E-4, E-59)
7. High output heart disease (eg, anemia; thyrotoxicosis; arteriovenous fistula) (See E-39)
8. Hypertension (eg, essential; renal disease; Cushing S.; pheochromocytoma) (See E-37)
9. Mitral insufficiency (See E-32)
10. Myocardiopathy; myocarditis (See E-40)
11. PDA; aortopulmonary window
12. VSD

UNCOMMON

1. Atrioventricular canal defect
2. Double outlet right ventricle (DORV)
3. Endocardial fibroelastosis
4. IHSS (subvalvular aortic stenosis)
5. Neoplasm of left ventricle (See E-43)
6. [Pericardial defect, total or partial]
7. Pulmonary atresia with intact ventricular septum
8. Supravalvular aortic stenosis (eg, Williams S.)
9. Subvalvular left ventricular aneurysm (African)
10. Transposition of great vessels
11. Tricuspid atresia or stenosis
12. Truncus arteriosus

[ ] This condition does not actually cause the gamuted imaging finding, but can produce imaging changes that simulate it.

References

1. Burgener FA, Kormano M: Differential Diagnosis in Conventional Radiology. (ed 2) New York: Thieme Medical Publ, 1991, pp 316–323
2. Eisenberg RL: Clinical Imaging: An Atlas of Differential Diagnosis. (ed 3) Philadelphia: Lippincott-Raven, 1997, pp 220–223
3. Gedgaudas E, Moller JH, Castaneda-Zuniga WR, Amplatz K: Cardiovascular Radiology. Philadelphia: WB Saunders, 1985
4. Meszaros WT: Cardiac Roentgenology. Springfield, IL: CC Thomas, 1969
5. Miller DH, Borer JS: The cardiomyopathies: A pathophysiologic approach to therapeutic management. Arch Intern Med 1983;143:2157–2162
6. Subramanian R, Olson LJ, Edwards WD: Surgical pathology of pure aortic stenosis: A study of 374 cases. Mayo Clin Proc 1984;59:683–690
7. Sutton D (ed): Textbook of Radiology and Imaging. (ed 6) New York: Churchill Livingstone, 1998, pp 605–627

Gamut E-34-S

RADIOLOGIC FINDINGS (PULMONARY VASCULATURE AND LV SIZE) IN COMMON DISEASES WITH LEFT VENTRICULAR STRAIN

PULMONARY VASCULATURE	SIZE OF LEFT VENTRICLE	
	Normal to Slightly Enlarged	Moderately to Markedly Enlarged
Normal	Aortic or subaortic stenosis Coarctation of aorta Hypertension Athlete's heart	Aortic insufficiency Myocardiopathy Hypertension (severe) Pericardial effusion
Venous Congestion	Acute myocardial infarction Mitral stenosis Hypervolemia Constrictive pericarditis	Heart failure Mitral insufficiency Mitral stenosis with aortic and/or tricuspid insufficiency
Arterial and Venous Distention	VSD (large shunt) PDA (large shunt) AV malformations	Complete AV canal Combination of 2 to 3 shunts or valve incompetence

Reference
1. Burgener FA, Kormano M: Differential Diagnosis in Conventional Radiology. Philadelphia: WB Saunders, 1985, p 315 (modified)

Gamut E-35

AORTIC INSUFFICIENCY

COMMON

1. Aortic root dilatation with stretched valve ring (eg, cystic medial necrosis of ascending aorta; aortic ectasia; aneurysm of ascending aorta—esp. dissecting aneurysm; atherosclerosis; hypertension)
2. Congenital valvular deformity (eg, bicuspid or fenestrated aortic valve)
*3. Dissection of aorta (eg, Marfan S.) (See E-64)
4. Rheumatic fever (aortic valvulitis; endocarditis)

UNCOMMON

1. Aneurysm of left ventricle, subvalvular (African)
2. Aortic—left ventricle tunnel
3. Aortic valve stenosis with calcification
4. Aortitis (eg, syphilitic; rheumatic; rheumatoid arthritis; ankylosing spondylitis; Reiter S.; Takayasu arteritis; giant cell idiopathic)
*5. Bacterial endocarditis
6. Behçet S.
7. Blunt chest trauma
8. Connective tissue disease (collagen disease)$_g$
9. Mucopolysaccharidoses (See J-4)
10. Myxomatous aortic valve degeneration
11. Postoperative (eg, after valvotomy for aortic stenosis or balloon valvoplasty)
12. Prosthetic aortic valve dysfunction, degeneration, or thrombosis
*13. Rupture of aortic cusp, traumatic or other

14. Sinus of Valsalva aneurysm, congenital or acquired (eg, syphilitic, dissecting, traumatic, mycotic, atherosclerotic)
15. Supravalvular aortic stenosis (eg, Williams S.)
16. VSD high in septum with prolapsed noncoronary aortic cusp

* Acute aortic insufficiency.

References

1. Fowler NO: Cardiac Diagnosis and Treatment. (ed 3) Hagerstown, MD: Harper & Row, 1980
2. Meszaros WT: Cardiac Roentgenology. Springfield, IL: CC Thomas, 1969
3. Olson LJ, Subramanian R, Edwards WD: Surgical pathology of pure aortic insufficiency: A study of 225 cases. Mayo Clin Proc 1984;59:835–841
4. Subramanian R, Olson LJ, Edwards WD: Surgical pathology of combined aortic stenosis and insufficiency: A study of 213 cases. Mayo Clin Proc 1985;60:247–254
5. Sutton D (ed): Textbook of Radiology and Imaging. (ed 6) New York: Churchill Livingstone, 1998, pp 606–608

Gamut E-36-S

PROSTHETIC VALVE REGURGITATION*

1. Change in size of occluding ball or disc
2. Degeneration of xenograft or homograft
3. Infection
4. Strut fracture
5. Suture line dehiscence
6. Thrombosis of prosthesis

* Best evaluated by 2-D echocardiography, pulsed or color flow Doppler, isotope ventriculography, or MRI.

Reference

1. Wilde P, Hartnell GG: Prosthetic valves. In: Sutton D, Young JWR (eds): A Short Textbook of Clinical Imaging. London: Springer-Verlag, 1990, pp 220–221

Gamut E-37

HYPERTENSION AND HYPERTENSIVE CARDIOVASCULAR DISEASE

COMMON

1. Adrenal disease (eg, adrenocortical adenoma; adrenal carcinoma; pheochromocytoma; adrenogenital S.; aldosteronism; Cushing S.)
2. Essential (idiopathic) hypertension
3. Renal disease (eg, glomerulonephritis; chronic pyelonephritis; renal tumor; renal agenesis or hypoplasia; polycystic kidneys)
4. Renovascular disease (eg, renal artery stenosis; fibromuscular hyperplasia; perirenal hematoma (Page kidney) (See H-59-1, H-59-2)

UNCOMMON

1. Central nervous system disorder (eg, psychogenic; neurogenic; familial dysautonomia (Riley-Day S.)
2. Coarctation of aorta
3. Connective tissue disease (collagen disease)$_g$ (esp. lupus erythematosus; polyarteritis nodosa)
4. Drug therapy (eg, estrogen-containing oral contraceptives)
5. Hyperthyroidism
6. Pituitary disease (eg, acromegaly; Cushing S.)

References

1. Eisenberg RL: Clinical Imaging: An Atlas of Differential Diagnosis. (ed 3) Philadelphia: Lippincott-Raven, 1997, pp 262–265
2. Streiter ML: Gamut: Unilateral renal lesion that may result in hypertension. Semin Roentgenol 1981;16:75–76

Gamut E-38

ISCHEMIC HEART DISEASE

COMMON
1. Coronary atherosclerosis
2. Coronary embolism or thrombosis
3. Coronary spasm
4. Myocardial infarction

UNCOMMON
1. Anemia$_g$
2. Aortic valve stenosis; other left ventricular outflow obstruction
3. Compression of coronary arteries by neoplasm, major vessel, or muscle bridge
4. Coronary artery fistula
5. Kawasaki disease
6. Syphilis
7. Vasculitis (eg, polyarteritis nodosa)

Reference
1. Wilde P, Hartnell GG: Ischemic heart disease. In: Sutton D, Young JWR (eds): A Short Textbook of Clinical Imaging. London: Springer-Verlag, 1990, p 158

Gamut E-38-S

COMPLICATIONS OF MYOCARDIAL INFARCTION REQUIRING RADIOLOGICAL EVALUATION

1. Heart failure
2. Left ventricular aneurysm
3. Pericardial effusion
4. Ruptured interventricular septum
5. Ruptured papillary muscle

Reference
1. Wilde P, Hartnell GG: Ischemic heart disease. In: Sutton D, Young JWR (eds): A Short Textbook of Clinical Imaging. London: Springer-Verlag, 1990, pp 161–163

Gamut E-39

HIGH OUTPUT HEART DISEASE*

COMMON
1. Anemia$_g$ (eg, sickle cell disease; thalassemia; hookworm disease)
2. Hypervolemia (fluid overload; overtransfusion)
3. Pregnancy
4. Thyrotoxicosis

UNCOMMON
1. Athletes, highly trained
2. AV fistula or malformation —peripheral, pulmonary, abdominal (eg, cavernous hemangioma of liver), or cerebral (eg, vein of Galen aneurysm)
3. Beriberi (vitamin B$_1$ deficiency)
4. Leukemia
5. Liver disease (eg, acute liver failure; advanced cirrhosis)
6. Obesity (Pickwickian S.)
7. Paget's disease
8. Polycythemia vera
9. Pyrexia; septic shock

* Also referred to as high-flow syndromes or hyperkinetic circulatory states.

References
1. Eisenberg RL: Clinical Imaging: An Atlas of Differential Diagnosis. (ed 3) Philadelphia: Lippincott-Raven, 1997, pp 260–261
2. Elliott LP: Cardiac Imaging in Infants, Children, and Adults. Philadelphia: Lippincott, 1991, pp 563–564
3. Teplick JG, Haskin ME: Roentgenologic Diagnosis. (ed 3) Philadelphia: WB Saunders Co, 1976
4. Wilson JD, et al: Harrison's Principles of Internal Medicine. (ed 12) New York: McGraw-Hill, 1991

Gamut E-40-1

MYOCARDIOPATHY

COMMON

1. Amyloidosis
2. Anemia_g
3. Connective tissue disease (collagen disease)_g (esp. scleroderma; lupus erythematosus; dermatomyositis; rheumatoid arthritis)
*4. Endocardial fibroelastosis
*5. Hypertrophic cardiomyopathy, primary or secondary (eg, aortic stenosis; IHSS; coarctation of aorta; hypertension)
6. Idiopathic dilated cardiomyopathy
*7. Infectious myocarditis (rheumatic fever; sepsis; diphtheria; Chagas' disease; toxoplasmosis; Coxsackie; rubella; other viral disease)
*8. Ischemia (incl. coronary artery disease; hypoxia)
*9. Nutritional deficiency (eg, beriberi; alcoholism; cirrhosis; starvation)
10. Thyrotoxicosis

UNCOMMON

1. Acromegaly
*2. Anomalous origin of left coronary artery from pulmonary artery
3. Congenital syndromes (eg, glycogen storage disease; Hurler S.) (See E-40-2)
*4. Coronary artery calcification in infants
5. Cushing S.
6. Endomyocardial fibrosis (African myocardiopathy)
7. Familial
8. Hemochromatosis
*9. Leukemia; lymphoma_g
10. Myxedema (hypothyroidism)
*11. Neoplasm, metastatic or primary (eg, fibroma; rhabdomyoma—esp. with tuberous sclerosis) (See E-43)
12. Neuromuscular disorder_g (eg, Friedreich's ataxia; Duchenne's progressive muscular dystrophy)
13. Postpartum

*14. Potassium or magnesium depletion
15. Pseudoxanthoma elasticum
16. Radiation therapy
17. Sarcoidosis
*18. Subvalvular left ventricular aneurysm (African)
*19. Toxicity (eg, drugs, esp. cytotoxic, Adriamycin; chemicals; cobalt—beer drinker's heart)
*20. Uremia

* Seen in infants or young children.

References

1. Eisenberg RL: Clinical Imaging: An Atlas of Differential Diagnosis. (ed 3) Philadelphia: Lippincott-Raven, 1997, p 222
2. Elliott LP: Cardiac Imaging in Infants, Children, and Adults. Philadelphia: Lippincott, 1991, pp 461–481
3. Goodwin JF: Clarification of the cardiomyopathies. Mod Concepts Cardiovasc Dis 1972;41:41–46
4. Gotsman MS, van der Horst RL, Winship WS: The chest radiograph in primary myocardial disease. Radiology 1971;99:1–13
5. Meszaros WT: Cardiac Roentgenology. Springfield, IL: CC Thomas, 1969
6. Miller DH, Borer JS: The cardiomyopathies: A pathophysiologic approach to therapeutic management. Arch Intern Med 1983;143:2157–2162
7. Palmer PES, Cockshott WP: Cardiac Diseases in the Tropics. In: Palmer PES, Reeder MM: The Imaging of Tropical Diseases, With Epidemiological, Pathological, and Clinical Correlation. (ed 2) Heidelberg: Springer-Verlag, 2000
8. Perloff JK: Cardiomyopathy associated with heredofamilial neuromyopathic diseases. Mod Concepts Cardiovasc Dis 1971;40:23–26
9. Rowe RD, Mehrizi A: The Neonate with Congenital Heart Disease. Major Problems in Clinical Pediatrics. Philadelphia: WB Saunders, 1968, vol 5
10. Wilson JD, et al: Harrison's Principles of Internal Medicine. (ed 12) New York: McGraw-Hill, 1991

Gamut E-40-2

CONGENITAL SYNDROMES WITH MYOCARDIOPATHY

COMMON

1. Adrenogenital S. (congenital adrenal hyperplasia)
2. Gaucher disease; Niemann-Pick disease
3. Glycogen storage disease, types II (Pompe) and III
4. Hemochromatosis
5. Hyperthyroidism (congenital)
6. Hypothyroidism; cretinism
7. Mucolipidoses, types II (I-cell disease) and III (pseudo-Hurler polydystrophy)
8. Mucopolysaccharidoses (esp. Hurler S.) (See J-4)
9. Neuromuscular disorder$_g$ (eg, Friedreich ataxia; Duchenne muscular dystrophy; Werdnig-Hoffmann disease; Kugelberg-Welander S.)
10. Noonan S.

UNCOMMON

1. Aspartylglycosaminuria
2. Congenital rubella S.
3. Degos S.
4. Endomyocardial fibrosis (African myocardiopathy)
5. Fabry disease
6. Farber disease (disseminated lipogranulomatosis)
7. GM$_1$ gangliosidosis; fucosidosis; mannosidosis
8. Hemolytic-uremic S.
9. Hyperphosphatasia
10. Kearns-Sayre S.
11. Leigh disease
12. LEOPARD S. (multiple lentigenes S.)
13. Neuroacanthocytosis
14. Polymyositis; dermatomyositis
15. Pseudoxanthoma elasticum
16. Refsum disease
17. Spondylometaphyseal dysplasia (Sedaghatian type)
18. Yunis-Varón S.

Reference
1. Taybi H, Lachman RS: Radiology of Syndromes, Metabolic Disorders, and Skeletal Dysplasias. (ed 4) St. Louis: Mosby-Year Book, 1996, p 970

Gamut E-41

GROSSLY ENLARGED HEART

COMMON

1. Aortic insufficiency
2. Combined valvular disease (esp. mitral and aortic)
3. Heart failure, advanced
4. Large left to right shunt (esp. ASD; VSD; PDA) in various combinations
5. Mitral insufficiency
6. Myocardiopathy (See E-40)
7. Pericardial effusion; hemopericardium

UNCOMMON

1. Complete atrioventricular canal
2. Tricuspid insufficiency (eg, Ebstein anomaly)
3. Valvular atresia (esp. pulmonary)

Gamut E-42

SMALL HEART

COMMON

1. Asthenia
2. Cor pulmonale (AP view)
3. [Emphysema (eg, asthma; senile; cystic fibrosis)]
4. Normal
5. Senile atrophy
6. Wasting disease; cachexia (eg, malnutrition; dehydration; kwashiorkor; tuberculosis; carcinoma; lymphoma$_g$; anorexia nervosa; scleroderma)

UNCOMMON

1. Adrenal insufficiency (Addison's disease)
2. Adrenogenital S.
3. Blood loss, severe
4. Constrictive pericarditis (See E-48)
5. Hypovolemia (eg, burn; dysentery)

[ ] This condition does not actually cause the gamuted imaging finding, but can produce imaging changes that simulate it.

Reference
1. Swischuk LE: Microcardia: An uncommon diagnostic problem. AJR 1968;103:115–118

Gamut E-43

CARDIAC OR PERICARDIAL NEOPLASM OR CYST

COMMON

1. Invasive pulmonary or mediastinal neoplasm (eg, lymphoma$_g$; bronchogenic or esophageal carcinoma; thymoma)
2. Metastasis (eg, from lung; breast; melanoma; lymphoma$_g$; leukemia)
*3. Myxoma (esp. left atrial)
4. Pericardial cyst
5. Rhabdomyoma (esp. with tuberous sclerosis)
6. Sarcoma (eg, rhabdomyosarcoma; fibrosarcoma; liposarcoma; hemangiosarcoma; myxosarcoma; undifferentiated sarcoma)

UNCOMMON

1. Angioma (eg, hemangioma; lymphangioma)
2. Bronchogenic cyst (intrapericardial)
*3. Fibroma (fibrous hamartoma)
4. Hydatid cyst
5. Lipoma
*6. Mesenchymoma, benign or malignant
7. Mesothelioma
8. Pericardial diverticulum
9. Pheochromocytoma
10. Teratoma (intrapericardial)

* May show calcification in tumor.

References
1. Bogren HG, DeMaria AN, Mason DT: Imaging procedures in the detection of cardiac tumors with emphasis on echocardiography: A review. Cardiovasc Intervent Radiol 1980; 3:107–125
2. David GD, Kincaid OW, Hallerman FJ: Roentgen aspects of cardiac tumors. Semin Roentgenol 1969;4:384–394
3. Elliott LP: Cardiac Imaging in Infants, Children, and Adults. Philadelphia: Lippincott, 1991, pp 482–502
4. Gross BH, Glazer GM, Francis IR: CT of intracardiac and intrapericardial masses. AJR 1983;140:903–907
5. Klatte EC, Yune HY: Diagnosis and treatment of pericardial cysts. Radiology 1972;104:541–544
6. McConnell TH: Bony and cartilaginous tumors of the heart and great vessels. Report of an osteosarcoma of the pulmonary artery. Cancer 1970;25:611–617
7. Pinet F, Moderator: Cardiac Tumour Symposium. Ann Radiol 1978;21:315–341
8. Prichard RW: Tumors of the heart: Review of the subject and report of one hundred and fifty cases. Arch Pathol 1951; 51:98–128
9. Sutton D (ed): Textbook of Radiology and Imaging. (ed 6) New York: Churchill Livingstone, 1998, pp 622–623, 667–668
10. Tsuchiya F, Kohno A, Saitoh R, et al: CT findings of atrial myxoma. Radiology 1984;151:139–143
11. Wilde P, Hartnell GG: Cardiac tumors; Pericardial tumors. In: Sutton D, Young JWR (eds): A Short Textbook of Clinical Imaging. London: Springer-Verlag, 1990, pp 217–218, 229–230

Gamut E-44

CALCIFICATION IN THE HEART OR GREAT VESSELS

COMMON

*1. Aneurysm$_g$ of aorta or sinus of Valsalva (See E-63)
*2. Aortic annulus (atherosclerosis; aging; syphilis) or valve (aortic stenosis; infective endocarditis; bicuspid aortic valve)
3. Aortitis (eg, syphilis; Takayasu S.)
4. Atherosclerosis of aorta
*5. Coronary arteriosclerosis; Mönckeberg's medial sclerosis (incl. progeria)
6. Mitral annulus (atherosclerosis; Marfan S.) or valve (rheumatic endocarditis with mitral stenosis)
*7. Myocardial infarction, old; myocardial left ventricular aneurysm
*8. [Pericardial calcification; constrictive pericarditis (See E-45, E-48)]

(continued)

UNCOMMON

1. Alkaptonuria (ochronosis)
2. Aneurysm of left ventricle, subvalvular (African)
*3. Coronary artery aneurysm (eg, Kawasaki S.) (See E-65)
4. Diabetes
*5. Ductus arteriosus or ligamentum arteriosus
*6. Endocardial fibroelastosis
7. Endocardium (eg, jet site from ASD or VSD)
*8. Hydatid cyst
*9. Idiopathic
10. Left atrial wall (rheumatic endocarditis, severe mitral valve disease)
*11. Metastatic calcinosis (eg, hyperparathyroidism; hypervitaminosis D)
*12. Myocardiopathy (eg, IHSS; Hurler S.)
*13. Neoplasm of heart (eg, myxoma, esp. of left atrium; fibroma) (See E-43)
14. Oxalosis
15. Postmyocarditis (esp. rheumatic fever)
16. Pulmonary hypertension
*17. Singleton-Merten S.
18. Thrombus in heart chamber (esp. with myocardial infarct or aneurysm or in Chagas' disease) or in great vessel (eg, aorta; inferior vena cava; pulmonary artery)
*19. Trauma, external or iatrogenic (eg, incision; coronary bypass graft; conduit)

* May occur in children.
[ ] This condition does not actually cause the gamuted imaging finding, but can produce imaging changes that simulate it.

References

1. Arndt RD, Smith LE, Po J, et al: Myocardial calcification of the infant heart following infarction. AJR 1974;122: 133–136
2. Bisset GS III: Gamut: Cardiac and great vessel calcifications in childhood: Semin Roentgenol 1985;20:194–195
3. Eisenberg RL: Clinical Imaging: An Atlas of Differential Diagnosis. (ed 3) Philadelphia: Lippincott-Raven, 1997, p 266–271
4. Kleiner JP, Way GL, Hamaker WR: Intracardiac calcification in a child. Chest 1977;72:517–518
5. Littleton JT, Cady JB: Free-floating calculi in the pericardial cavity. AJR 1978;131:901–903
6. MacGregor JH, Chen JTT, Chiles C, et al: The radiographic distinction between pericardial and myocardial calcifications. AJR 1987;148:675–677
7. Meszaros WT: Cardiac Roentgenology. Springfield, IL: CC Thomas, 1969, p 8
8. Shabetai R: The Pericardium. New York: Grune & Stratton, 1981
9. Shapiro JH, Jacobson HG, Rubinstein BM, et al: Calcifications of the Heart. Springfield, IL: CC Thomas, 1963
10. Shawdon HH, Dinsmore RE: Pericardial calcification: Radiological features and clinical significance in twenty-six patients. Clin Radiol 1967;18:205–214
11. Teplick JG, Haskin ME: Roentgenologic Diagnosis. (ed 3) Philadelphia: WB Saunders, 1976

Gamut E-45

PERICARDIAL CALCIFICATION

COMMON

1. Chronic constrictive pericarditis (esp. tuberculosis) (See E-48)
2. Idiopathic pericarditis
3. Purulent pericarditis

UNCOMMON

1. Asbestos plaques along pericardium
2. Hemopericardium
3. Rheumatic fever

References

1. Elliott LP: Cardiac Imaging in Infants, Children, and Adults. Philadelphia: Lippincott, 1991, pp 377–378, 409
2. Roberts WC, Spray TL: Pericardial heart disease: A study of its causes, consequences, and morphologic features. Cardiovasc Clin 1976;7:11–65

GAS EMBOLISM IN THE HEART OR BLOOD VESSELS (See E-47)

COMMON

1. Fetal death
2. Hyaline membrane disease
3. Intravascular catheterization, cannulation, or therapy (eg, umbilical vein; central venous pressure line; blood transfusion or other infusion; angiography)
4. Postoperative or intraoperative (eg, cardiac bypass; lung resection; biopsy; abdominal aortic graft)
5. Respirator therapy (eg, PEEP)
6. Resuscitation maneuver
7. Trauma, penetrating (eg, laceration; blast; percutaneous high pressure injection; air hose injection)

UNCOMMON

1. Abortion; parturition; vaginal insufflation (eg, cunnilingus; douching)
2. Abscess perforation into vessel
3. ARDS
4. Asthmatic episode
5. Decompression sickness (eg, caisson disease)
6. Dental procedure (root canal treatment; drilling)
7. Emphysematous gastritis; corrosive gastritis
8. Gastrointestinal perforation into vessel (eg, enema; peptic ulcer)
9. Hydrogen peroxide enema
10. Injection of gas (eg, cerebral pneumography; arthrography; Rubin's test; artificial pneumothorax or pneumoperitoneum; suicidal or homicidal attempt)
11. Irrigation (lavage) or drainage of abscess, empyema, or paranasal sinus
12. Malignant neoplasm with invasion of vessel (eg, bronchovascular fistula; esophageal-aortic fistula)
13. Necrotizing enterocolitis; mesenteric infarction; toxic megacolon
14. Sepsis with gas-producing organism (esp. in a diabetic)
15. Thoracentesis; pericardiocentesis; peritoneocentesis (incl. hemodialysis)
16. Whooping cough (pertussis)

References

1. Cholankeril JV, Joshi RR, Cenizal JS, et al: Massive air embolism from the pulmonary artery. Radiology 1982;142:33–34
2. Kizer KW, Goodman PC: Radiographic manifestations of venous air embolism. Radiology 1982;144:35–39
3. Kogutt MS: Systemic air embolism secondary to respiratory therapy in the neonate: Six cases including one survivor. AJR 1978;131:425–429
4. Shook DR, Cram KB, Williams HJ: Pulmonary venous air embolism in hyaline membrane disease. AJR 1975;125:538–542

PNEUMOPERICARDIUM

COMMON

1. Iatrogenic (eg, postoperative; intubation; pericardiocentesis; resuscitation; respiratory therapy; positive pressure ventilation)

UNCOMMON

1. ARDS
2. Congenital absence of the pericardium with pneumothorax
3. Hyaline membrane disease
4. Idiopathic
5. [Intracardiac gas (See E-46)]
6. Perforation from adjacent abscess (esp. amebic), neoplasm, or radiation necrosis; cutaneous fistula
7. Pericarditis due to gas-forming organism
8. Pneumomediastinum or interstitial pulmonary leakage with extension into pericardium
9. Trauma, external (eg, stab wound; tracheal injury)

[ ] This condition does not actually cause the gamuted imaging finding, but can produce imaging changes that simulate it.

Reference

1. Higgins CB, Broderick TW, Edwards DK, et al: The hemodynamic significance of massive pneumopericardium in preterm infants with respiratory distress syndrome. Radiology 1979;133:363–368

Gamut E-48

CONSTRICTIVE PERICARDITIS

COMMON
1. Idiopathic
2. Tuberculosis

UNCOMMON
1. Asbestosis (pleuropericardial); talcosis
2. Histoplasmosis
3. Neoplasm (eg, primary, metastatic, or locally invasive—esp. mesothelioma; invasive thymoma; lymphoma$_g$) (See E-43)
4. Parasitic disease (eg, amebic abscess from liver or lung rupturing into pericardial sac)
5. Postpericardiotomy S.
6. Pyogenic infection (esp. staphylococcal; pneumococcal)
7. Radiation therapy (esp. for lymphoma$_g$; carcinoma of breast)
8. Rheumatic pericarditis
9. Traumatic pericarditis; hemopericardium
10. Uremia; prolonged hemodialysis
11. Viral pericarditis (esp. Coxsackie B)

References
1. Deutsch V, Miller H, Yahini JH, et al: Angiocardiography in constrictive pericarditis. Chest 1974;65:379–387
2. Eisenberg RL: Clinical Imaging: An Atlas of Differential Diagnosis. (ed 3) Philadelphia: Lippincott-Raven, 1997, p 275
3. Elliott LP: Cardiac Imaging in Infants, Children, and Adults. Philadelphia: Lippincott, 1991, pp 373–378
4. Wilson JD, et al: Harrison's Principles of Internal Medicine. (ed 12) New York: McGraw-Hill, 1991

Gamut E-49

PERICARDIAL EFFUSION

COMMON
1. Connective tissue disease (collagen vascular disease)$_g$ (esp, lupus erythematosus; rheumatoid disease; scleroderma; MCTD; polyarteritis arteritis)
2. Heart failure
3. Neoplasm of pericardium or heart, primary or invasive from lung, pleura, or mediastinum (eg, bronchogenic carcinoma; mesothelioma; lymphoma$_g$; invasive thymoma) or metastatic (eg, carcinoma of lung or breast; melanoma) (See E-43)
4. Pericarditis, infectious (viral; Coxsackie; bacterial; amebic; toxoplasmic; tuberculous; histoplasmic; rheumatic)
5. Postmyocardial infarction S. (Dressler S.)
6. Postpericardiotomy S. (incl. coronary artery bypass)
7. Trauma, external or iatrogenic (hemopericardium)
8. Uremia; nephrotic S.

UNCOMMON
1. Amyloidosis; Waldenström's macroglobulinemia; familial Mediterranean fever
2. Anemia$_g$ (eg, thalassemia; erythroblastosis fetalis)
3. Behçet S.
4. Beriberi; hypoalbuminemia
5. Bleeding or clotting disorder$_g$ (eg, hemophilia; thrombocytopenia; hypoprothrombinemia; anticoagulant therapy)
6. Congenital syndromes (eg, Erdheim-Chester S.; Degos S.; Kawasaki S.; Turner S.; Wissler S.; yellow nail S.; arthropathy-camptodactyly S.)
7. Dissecting aneurysm with leakage
8. Drug reaction
9. Endomyocardial fibrosis (African myocardiopathy)
10. Gout
11. Idiopathic
12. Myxedema; hypothyroidism
13. Pancreatitis
14. Polyserositis

15. Radiation therapy (eg, for lymphoma$_g$; carcinoma of breast or lung)
16. Reiter S.; Reiter/reactive arthritis
17. Sarcoidosis
18. Stevens-Johnson S.
19. Superior vena cava obstruction
20. Wegener granulomatosis
21. Whipple's disease

References

1. Agner RC, Gallis HA: Pericarditis: Differential diagnostic considerations. Arch Intern Med 1979;139:407–412
2. Eisenberg RL: Clinical Imaging: An Atlas of Differential Diagnosis. (ed 3) Philadelphia: Lippincott-Raven, 1997, pp 272–274
3. Taybi H, Lachman RS: Radiology of Syndromes, Metabolic Disorders, and Skeletal Dysplasias. (ed 4) St. Louis: Mosby-Year Book, 1996, p 972
4. Teplick JG, Haskin ME: Roentgenologic Diagnosis. (ed 3) Philadelphia: WB Saunders, 1976
5. Wilson JD, et al: Harrison's Principles of Internal Medicine. (ed 12) New York: McGraw-Hill, 1991

Gamut E-50-S

COMMON CARDIAC CONDITIONS DIAGNOSED BY ECHOCARDIOGRAPHY

1. Aortic stenosis or insufficiency
2. Bacterial endocarditis
3. Cardiac tumor (esp. myxoma of LA) (See E-43)
4. IHSS
5. Mitral stenosis or insufficiency
6. Mitral valve prolapse (MVP)
7. Myocardiopathy
8. Pericardial effusion
9. Shunts (with evaluation of flow and direction by pulsed Doppler)

References

1. Duncan W: Color Doppler in Clinical Cardiology. Philadelphia: WB Saunders, 1988

2. Feigenbaum H: Echocardiology. (ed 4) Philadelphia: Lea & Febiger, 1986
3. Goldberg S.: Doppler Echocardiography. (ed 2) Philadelphia: Lea & Febiger, 1988
4. Kisslo J: Doppler Color Flow Imaging. New York: Churchill Livingstone, 1988
5. Seward J, Fajek A, Edwards W, et al: Two Dimensional Echocardiographic Atlas. New York: Springer-Verlag, 1987

Gamut E-51

GENERALIZED PULMONARY ARTERIAL HYPERVASCULARITY (See E-16, 17)

COMMON

1. High output heart disease (See E-39)
2. Left to right shunt (esp. ASD; VSD; partial or complete AV communis; PDA; AP window) (See E-7)

UNCOMMON

1. Aneurysm of sinus of Valsalva rupture
2. Aorta-pulmonary artery fistula (eg, traumatic; postoperative; ruptured aneurysm)
3. Aortic atresia
4. APVC, partial or total
5. Common atrium
6. Cor biloculare
7. Coronary artery fistula
8. Double outlet right ventricle without PS
9. Eisenmenger physiology (reversal of left to right shunt with development of pulmonary hypertension)
10. Pulmonary arteriovenous malformation
11. Single ventricle without PS
12. Taussig-Bing S.
13. Transposition of great vessels with large VSD
14. Tricuspid atresia without PS
15. Truncus arteriosus

References

1. Eisenberg RL: Clinical Imaging: An Atlas of Differential Diagnosis. (ed 3) Philadelphia: Lippincott-Raven, 1997, pp 224-227, 230–233

(continued)

2. Elliott LP: Cardiac Imaging In Infants, Children, and Adults. Philadelphia: Lippincott, 1991, p 156
3. Gedgaudas E, Moller JH, Castaneda-Zuniga WR, Amplatz K: Cardiovascular Radiology. Philadelphia: WB Saunders, 1985
4. Meszaros WT: Cardiac Roentgenology. Springfield, IL: CC Thomas, 1969, p 324
5. Simon M: The pulmonary vasculature in congenital heart disease. Radiol Clin North Am 1968;6:303–318
6. Swischuk LE: Plain Film Interpretation in Congenital Heart Disease. (ed 2) Baltimore: Williams & Wilkins, 1979
7. Teplick JG, Haskin ME: Roentgenologic Diagnosis. (ed 3) Philadelphia: WB Saunders, 1976

Gamut E-52

INCREASED PULMONARY ARTERIAL CIRCULATION TO ONE LUNG

COMMON

1. Air trapping in contralateral lung (eg, Swyer-James S.; bullous emphysema)
2. Arteriovenous malformation (congenital or acquired)
3. Obstruction of contralateral pulmonary artery (eg, thromboembolism; neoplasm; histoplasmic lymphadenopathy)

UNCOMMON

1. Contralateral scimitar S.; hypogenetic lung; pulmonary artery atresia, stenosis, or coarctation
2. Left-to-right shunt with increased flow to one lung (eg, PDA; AV communis)
3. Postoperative cyanotic congenital heart disease (eg, Waterson, Blalock, or Potts procedure)
4. Unilateral origin of a pulmonary artery from the aorta; truncus arteriosus with single pulmonary artery

Reference

1. Chen JTT, Capp MP, Goodrich JK, et al: Roentgen appearance of pulmonary vascularity in the diagnosis of heart disease. AJR 1971;112:559–570

Gamut E-53

PROMINENCE OF THE MAIN PULMONARY ARTERY SEGMENT

COMMON

1. "Aneurysm" of pulmonary artery (See E-55)
2. Cor pulmonale; pulmonary arterial hypertension, primary or secondary (eg, diffuse lung or pulmonary arterial disease; chronic heart disease; obesity) (See E-54)
3. [Enlarged left atrial appendage]
4. Heart failure (See E-4, E-59)
5. High output heart disease (eg, anemia$_g$; thyrotoxicosis; fluid overload) (See E-39)
6. Idiopathic
7. Left to right shunt (eg, ASD, VSD, PDA) (See E-7)
8. [Mediastinal or left hilar mass (eg, bronchogenic carcinoma; metastasis)]
9. Mitral stenosis or insufficiency, acquired or congenital
10. Normal in young adults under 25 (esp. women)
11. Pregnancy
12. Pulmonary thromboembolism
13. Pulmonary valvular stenosis (poststenotic dilatation)
14. [Technical or positional factor (eg, lordotic view; patient rotation; cardiac rotation in left lower lobe collapse; dextroscoliosis; pectus excavatum)]

UNCOMMON

1. Absent pulmonary valve
2. Aortopulmonary fistula, traumatic or postoperative (eg, laceration; ruptured aneurysm; Potts procedure)
3. APVC, partial or total
4. Coarctation of pulmonary artery or its branches
5. Congenital absence of the pericardium
6. Cor triatriatum
7. Double outlet right ventricle
8. Eisenmenger physiology (reversal of left to right shunt with development of pulmonary hypertension)
9. Endomyocardial fibrosis (African myocardiopathy)

10. Hypoplastic left heart S.$_g$ (incl. interrupted aortic arch)
11. Left to right shunt, other (eg, aortopulmonary window; atrioventricular canal defect; coronary artery fistula to right heart or PA)
12. Marfan S.
13. Neoplasm of heart (esp. left atrial myxoma) (See E-43)
14. Parachute mitral valve complex
15. Pulmonary insufficiency
16. Tricuspid atresia without pulmonary stenosis
17. Trilogy of Fallot
18. Truncus arteriosus, type 1

[ ] This condition does not actually cause the gamuted imaging finding, but can produce imaging changes that simulate it.

References

1. Burgener FA, Kormano M: Differential Diagnosis in Conventional Radiology. (ed 2) New York: Thieme Medical Publ, 1991, pp 341–345
2. Eisenberg RL: Clinical Imaging: An Atlas of Differential Diagnosis. (ed 3) Philadelphia: Lippincott-Raven, 1997, pp 248–251
3. Gedgaudas E, Moller JH, Castaneda-Zuniga WR, Amplatz K: Cardiovascular Radiology. Philadelphia: WB Saunders, 1985
4. Meszaros WT: Cardiac Roentgenology. Springfield, IL: CC Thomas, 1969

Gamut E-54

PULMONARY ARTERIAL HYPERTENSION (COR PULMONALE)

CHRONIC HYPOXIA

1. Chest deformity (eg, kyphoscoliosis; thoracoplasty)
2. Chronic upper airway obstruction (eg, enlarged tonsils or adenoids; sleep apnea S.; Crouzon S.; Robin S.)
3. High altitude dwelling
4. Neuromuscular disorder$_g$
5. Obesity (Pickwickian S.)
6. Pleural fibrothorax

DIFFUSE LUNG DISEASE

1. Alveolar microlithiasis
2. Asthma; chronic bronchitis
3. Bronchiolo-alveolar cell carcinoma
4. Bronchiectasis
5. Connective tissue disease (collagen disease)$_g$ (eg, scleroderma; rheumatoid lung; lupus erythematosus; dermatomyositis)
6. Cystic fibrosis (mucoviscidosis)
7. Emphysema (incl. alpha$_1$-antitrypsin deficiency S.)
8. Fat embolism
9. Fungus disease
10. Interstitial fibrosis
11. Langerhans cell histiocytosis$_g$
12. Metastases, lymphangitic or embolic (eg, trophoblastic)
13. Pneumoconiosis
14. Sarcoidosis
15. Tuberculosis

DIFFUSE PULMONARY VASCULAR OR HEART DISEASE

1. Arteritis (eg, polyarteritis nodosa; lupus erythematosus; Takayasu S.; Wegener granulomatosis)
2. Congenital syndromes (eg, cutis laxa; Ehlers-Danlos S.; Marfan S.; osteodysplasty {Melnick-Needles S.}; mucopolysaccharidoses—Hurler; Scheie; Hunter; Maroteaux-Lamy)
3. Hypoplastic left heart S.$_g$
4. [Idiopathic (usually young women)]
5. Left-to-right shunt, chronic (esp. ASD, VSD, PDA—with Eisenmenger physiology (reversal of left to right shunt with development of pulmonary hypertension) (See E-7)
6. Left ventricular failure, chronic
7. Mitral stenosis or insufficiency (longstanding)
8. Primary pulmonary hypertension, idiopathic; pulmonary arteriolar sclerosis
9. Pulmonary artery stenoses or coarctations, multiple (incl. Williams S.; Alagille S. {arteriohepatic dysplasia})

(continued)

10. Pulmonary thromboembolism (eg, multiple pulmonary emboli; intravenous drug abuse; sickle cell disease; polycythemia vera; tumor emboli)
11. Pulmonary venous hypertension (See E-59)
12. Schistosomiasis
13. Tuberous sclerosis
14. Venolobar S. (scimitar S.)
15. Ventriculoatrial shunt for hydrocephalus

[ ] This condition does not actually cause the gamuted imaging finding, but can produce imaging changes that simulate it.

References
1. Fraser RS, Müller NL, Coleman N, Paré PD (eds): Fraser & Paré: Diagnosis of Diseases of the Chest. (ed 4) Philadelphia: WB Saunders, 1999
2. Harvey RM: Pulmonary (arterial) hypertension. In: Clinical Challenges in Cardiopulmonary Medicine, Vol 1. Park Ridge, IL: American College of Chest Physicians
3. Matthay RA, Schwarz MI, Ellis JH Jr, et al: Pulmonary artery hypertension in chronic obstructive pulmonary disease: Determination by chest radiography. Invest Radiol 1981; 16:95–100
4. Meszaros WT: Cardiac Roentgenology. Springfield, IL: CC Thomas, 1969, p 78
5. Taybi H, Lachman RS: Radiology of Syndromes, Metabolic Disorders, and Skeletal Dysplasias. (ed 4) St. Louis: Mosby-Year Book, 1996, p 973
6. Teplick JG, Haskin ME: Roentgenologic Diagnosis. (ed 3) Philadelphia: WB Saunders, 1976

Gamut E-55

PULMONARY ARTERY "ANEURYSM"*

COMMON

1. False aneurysm (external trauma; postoperative)
2. Left to right shunt, large (See E-7)
3. Pulmonary arterial hypertension (eg, emphysema; schistosomiasis) (See E-54)
4. Pulmonary valvular stenosis (poststenotic dilatation)

UNCOMMON

1. Arteriovenous malformation
2. Arteritis (eg, polyarteritis nodosa; Takayasu S.; syphilis)

3. Atherosclerosis
4. Behçet S.
5. Hughes-Stovin S. (venous thrombosis plus pulmonary artery aneurysms)
6. Idiopathic
7. Medial degeneration or necrosis /dissection (eg, Marfan S.; Ehlers-Danlos S.; mucopolysaccharidoses)—(See J-4)
8. Mycotic aneurysm (esp. drug addiction)

* Marked aneurysmal-like dilatation of the main pulmonary artery.

References
1. Reid JM, Stevenson JG: Aneurysm of the pulmonary artery. Dis Chest 1959;36:104–107
2. Viamonte M Jr, LePage JR: Pitfalls in the radiographic evaluation of mediastinal abnormalities. Radiol Clin North Am 1968;6:451–465

Gamut E-56

LOCALIZED ENLARGEMENT OF A PULMONARY VESSEL

COMMON

*1. AV malformation, congenital or acquired (eg, traumatic)
2. Obstructed pulmonary vein or artery (eg, thrombus; neoplasm; granulomatous lesion)
*3. Varix, congenital or acquired (eg, mitral stenosis)

UNCOMMON

*1. Aneurysm of pulmonary artery (eg, polyarteritis nodosa; Takayasu S.; mycotic aneurysm in drug addiction)
2. Anomalous insertion site of pulmonary vein into left atrium
3. Anomalous pulmonary vein (eg, scimitar or venolobar S.); partial APVC
4. Atresia or stenosis of pulmonary vein (veno-occlusive disease)
*5. Bronchial artery dilatation (eg, tetralogy of Fallot$_g$)

6. Cirsoid aneurysm
*7. Coarctation or stenosis of pulmonary artery or its branches (poststenotic dilatation)
8. Sequestration of lung; anomalous pulmonary artery arising from aorta
9. Systemic artery—pulmonary artery shunt (See E-24, E-60)
*10. Telangiectasia (eg, portal hypertension; Osler-Weber-Rendu S.)
11. Tetralogy of Fallot$_g$ with absent pulmonary valve

* Sometimes multiple.

References
1. Ben-Menachem Y, Kuroda K, Kyger ER III, et al: The various forms of pulmonary varices: Report of three new cases and review of the literature. AJR 1975;125:881–889
2. Lundell C, Finck E: Arteriovenous fistulas originating from Rasmussen aneurysms. AJR 1983;140:687–688
3. Rees S: Arterial connections of the lung: The inaugural Keith Jefferson Lecture. Clin Radiol 1981;32:1–15
4. Taybi H, Lachman RS: Radiology of Syndromes, Metabolic Disorders, and Skeletal Dysplasias. (ed 4) St. Louis: Mosby-Year Book, 1996

Gamut E-57

PULMONARY VALVE OR MAIN PULMONARY ARTERY OBSTRUCTION (OFTEN LEADING TO PULMONARY HYPOVASCULARITY)

COMMON
*1. Lymphadenopathy with compression (eg, sarcoidosis; tuberculosis; histoplasmosis)
*2. Metastatic or locally invasive neoplasm with compression or luminal obstruction (esp. bronchogenic carcinoma; hypernephroma; melanoma; invasive thymoma; lymphoma$_g$)
3. Pulmonary valve stenosis or atresia, congenital
*4. Thromboembolism in pulmonary artery

UNCOMMON
*1. Coarctation of pulmonary artery
*2. Compression by aortic aneurysm$_g$
3. Constrictive pericarditis
4. Endocardial fibroelastosis
5. Endomyocardial fibrosis
6. Hypertrophy of the left ventricle encroaching on the right ventricle (Bernheim S.)
7. IHSS (African myocardiopathy)
8. Mediastinal fibrosis
*9. Neoplasm of heart or pulmonary artery (esp. carcinoid; sarcoma; metastasis) (See E-43)
10. Pulmonary stenosis, acquired (eg, rheumatic fever; carcinoid S.)
11. Septal and infundibular hypertrophy from VSD (Gasul S.)
*12. Takayasu S. involving pulmonary artery
13. Tetralogy of Fallot$_g$

* Often unilateral.

References
1. Fowler NO: The Pericardium in Health and Disease. Mount Kisco, NY: Futura Publishing, 1985
2. Jeffery RF, Moller JH, Amplatz K: The dysplastic pulmonary valve: A new roentgenographic entity; with a discussion of the anatomy and radiology of other types of valvular pulmonary stenosis. AJR 1972;114:322–339
3. Singh D, Tan L: Primary arteritis of the pulmonary vessels and the aorta. Singapore Med J 1975;16:57–61

Gamut E-58

GENERALIZED PULMONARY ARTERIAL HYPOVASCULARITY (See E-19)

COMMON
1. Congenital heart disease with right-to-left shunt (eg, tetralogy of Fallot$_g$; pseudotruncus arteriosus; pulmonary atresia with intact ventricular septum {trilogy of Fallot}; tricuspid atresia or stenosis)
2. Emphysema, diffuse or bullous

(continued)

3. Pulmonary hypertension, primary or secondary (eg, schistosomiasis)
4. Right ventricular failure, esp. with marked tricuspid insufficiency

UNCOMMON

1. Compression of pulmonary artery trunk (eg, neoplasm; histoplasmic lymphadenopathy)
2. Ebstein anomaly; Uhl anomaly
3. Hypoventilation
4. Hypovolemia
5. Mechanical obstruction at, or proximal to, tricuspid valve (eg, right atrial myxoma; hypernephroma extending up IVC into RA; tricuspid stenosis)
6. Mitral stenosis (postcapillary hypertension)
7. Myocardiopathy (See E-40)
8. Pericardial tamponade
9. Pulmonary artery stenosis or coarctation
10. Pulmonary valvular atresia or severe stenosis, congenital or acquired (eg, carcinoid S.)
11. Thromboembolism to many small pulmonary arteries (incl. trophoblastic embolic metastases)
12. Vasculitis (eg, polyarteritis nodosa)

References

1. Eisenberg RL: Clinical Imaging: An Atlas of Differential Diagnosis. (ed 3) Philadelphia: Lippincott-Raven, 1997, pp 228–229
2. Felson B: Chest Roentgenology. Philadelphia: WB Saunders, 1973
3. Fraser RS, Müller NL, Coleman N, Paré PD (eds): Fraser & Paré: Diagnosis of Diseases of the Chest. (ed 4) Philadelphia: WB Saunders, 1999
4. Ravin CE, Cooper C: Review of Radiology. Philadelphia: WB Saunders, 1990, p 24
5. Simon M: The pulmonary vasculature in congenital heart disease. Radiol Clin North Am 1968;6:303–318
6. Swischuk LE: Plain Film Interpretation in Congenital Heart Disease. (ed 2) Baltimore: Williams & Wilkins, 1979

PULMONARY VENOUS OBSTRUCTION OR HYPERTENSION (INCREASED VENOUS VASCULARITY OR VASCULAR REDISTRIBUTION) (See E-3)

COMMON

1. Left ventricular failure, any cause (eg, hypertension; myocardial ischemia; aortic stenosis; high output heart disease; myocardiopathy) (See E-37–40)
2. Mitral stenosis or insufficiency

UNCOMMON

1. Airway obstruction (eg, laryngeal)
2. Aortic insufficiency
3. [Basal emphysema or thromboembolism (redistribution)]
4. Coarctation S. (coarctation of aorta with VSD and/or PDA)
5. Hypoplastic left heart S.$_g$; aortic atresia
6. Neoplasm (esp. left atrial myxoma) (See E-43)
7. Obstruction of pulmonary veins
   a. Congenital
      i. APVC, total (below the diaphragm; or above the diaphragm with stenosis of an anomalous venous trunk)
      ii. Atresia or stenosis of the common or individual pulmonary veins
      iii. Cor triatriatum
      iv. Primary pulmonary veno-occlusive disease
   b. Acquired
      i. Constrictive pericarditis (See E-48)
      ii. Mediastinal tumor
      iii. Mediastinitis or mediastinal fibrosis (eg, histoplasmosis)
      iv. Thrombosis of pulmonary veins
8. Parachute mitral valve complex
9. Peripheral AV malformations
10. Thrombus in left atrium (esp. ball-valve)

[ ] This condition does not actually cause the gamuted imaging finding, but can produce imaging changes that simulate it.

References

1. Chen JTT: Essentials of Cardiac Roentgenology. Boston: Little, Brown, 1987
2. Elliott LP: Cardiac Imaging in Infants, Children, and Adults. Philadelphia: Lippincott, 1991, pp 505–509
3. Lester RG: Radiological concepts in the evaluation of heart disease. Mod Concepts Cardiovasc Dis 1968;37:113–118
4. McLoughlin MJ: Cor triatriatum sinister. Clin Radiol 1970;21:287–296
5. Meszaros WT: Cardiac Roentgenology. Springfield, IL: CC Thomas, 1969, p 97
6. Robinson AE, Capp MP, Chen JT, et al: Left-sided obstructive diseases of the heart and great vessels. Semin Roentgenol 1968;3:410–419
7. Shackleford GD, Sacks EJ, Mullins JD, et al: Pulmonary veno-occlusive disease: Case report and review of the literature. AJR 1977;128:643–648

4. Cirrhosis
5. Cystic adenomatoid malformation of the lung
6. Emphysema; chronic bronchitis
7. Infection of chest wall (eg, actinomycosis)
8. Neoplasm of thoracic wall (eg, Hodgkin's disease)
9. Occlusion of pulmonary vein
10. Venolobar S. (scimitar S.)

References

1. Ekstrom D, Weiner M, Baier B: Pulmonary arteriovenous fistula as a complication of trauma. AJR 1978;130:1178–1180
2. Rees S: Arterial connections of the lung: The inaugural Keith Jefferson Lecture. Clin Radiol 1981;32:1–15
3. Tadavarthy SM, Klugman J, Castaneda-Zuniga WR, et al: Systemic-to-pulmonary collaterals in pathological states. Radiology 1982;144:55–59

Gamut E-60

SYSTEMIC TO PULMONARY VASCULAR SHUNT ON ANGIOGRAPHY (See E-24)

COMMON

1. Bronchiectasis
2. Congenital cyanotic heart disease (eg, tetralogy of Fallot$_g$; tricuspid atresia; single ventricle; double outlet right ventricle; complete or corrected transposition of great vessels)
3. Neoplasm of lung (esp. bronchogenic carcinoma)
4. Occlusion of pulmonary artery (eg, thromboembolism; surgical ligation; mediastinal fibrosis or invasive neoplasm; other external compression) (See E-57)
5. Postoperative (eg, Blalock or Potts procedure for tetralogy; Mustard operation for transposition)
6. Sequestration of lung

UNCOMMON

1. Absence or atresia of pulmonary artery
2. Anomalous origin of pulmonary artery (eg, right PA from ascending aorta)
3. AV malformation, congenital or acquired (eg, pulmonary; thoracic wall)

Gamut E-61

SMALL ASCENDING AORTA OR AORTIC ARCH

COMMON

1. [ASD]
2. Coarctation of aorta (long segment infantile type); interrupted aortic arch
3. Decreased cardiac output (eg, endocardial fibroelastosis or other myocardiopathy; small heart; constrictive pericarditis; mitral stenosis) (See E-40, E-42, E-48)
4. [Technical (eg, rotated patient; dextroscoliosis; pectus excavatum)]

UNCOMMON

1. APVC, total
2. Hypoplastic left heart S.$_g$; aortic atresia
3. Supravalvular aortic stenosis (incl. Williams S.)

[ ] This condition does not actually cause the gamuted imaging finding, but can produce imaging changes that simulate it.

(continued)

References

1. Eisenberg RL: Clinical Imaging: An Atlas of Differential Diagnosis. (ed 3) Philadelphia: Lippincott-Raven, 1997, pp 242–243
2. Meszaros WT: Cardiac Roentgenology. Springfield, IL: CC Thomas, 1969, pp 148–149

Gamut E-62

PROMINENT ASCENDING AORTA OR AORTIC ARCH

COMMON

1. Aneurysm of aorta$_g$, incl. dissecting aneurysm (eg, atherosclerosis; hypertension; cystic medial necrosis; Marfan S.; syphilis; mycotic infection; trauma) (See E-63)
2. Aortic arch anomaly (eg, right aortic arch; double aortic arch; cervical aortic arch)
3. Aortic insufficiency (eg, syphilis; infective endocarditis; dissecting aneurysm; Marfan S.) (See E-35)
4. Aortic stenosis (congenital—bicuspid valve; rheumatic; atherosclerotic)
5. Aortitis (eg, syphilitic; giant cell; rheumatoid; Takayasu arteritis, connective tissue disease {collagen vascular disease}, esp. lupus erythematosus)
6. Atherosclerosis (tortuosity, elongation, unfolding, and/or dilatation of aorta)
7. Coarctation of aorta; pseudocoarctation
8. Hypertensive heart disease (See E-37)
9. Medial degeneration of aorta; cystic medial necrosis (eg, Marfan S.; Ehlers-Danlos S.; pseudoxanthoma elasticum; osteogenesis imperfecta) (See E-64, Uncommon no. 3)
10. [Mediastinal mass simulating large aorta (eg, thymoma; lymphoma$_g$; invasive or metastatic carcinoma)]
11. PDA
12. Tetralogy of Fallot$_g$ (incl. pseudotruncus)

UNCOMMON

1. Aneurysm of sinus of Valsalva or coronary artery (See E-65)
2. Aorta—left ventricle tunnel
3. Aortomegaly, idiopathic
4. Aortopulmonary window
5. Corrected transposition with left-sided ascending aorta and PS
6. Pulmonary atresia with intact ventricular septum
7. Tricuspid atresia without transposition
8. Truncus arteriosus

[ ] This condition does not actually cause the gamuted imaging finding, but can produce imaging changes that simulate it.

References

1. Eisenberg RL: Clinical Imaging: An Atlas of Differential Diagnosis. (ed 3) Philadelphia: Lippincott-Raven, 1997, pp 236–241
2. Gedgaudas E, Moller JH, Castaneda-Zuniga WR, Amplatz K: Cardiovascular Radiology. Philadelphia: WB Saunders, 1985
3. Liu YQ: Radiology of aortoarteritis. Radiol Clin North Am 1985;23:671–688
4. Teplick JG, Haskin ME: Roentgenologic Diagnosis. (ed 3) Philadelphia: WB Saunders, 1976

Gamut E-63

ANEURYSM OF AORTA AND OTHER MAJOR ARTERIES

COMMON

1. Atherosclerosis (degenerative)
2. Congenital (esp. cerebral—circle of Willis)
3. Dissecting (See E-64)
4. Trauma (incl. false aneurysm)

UNCOMMON

1. Angiomyolipoma (renal)
2. Cystic medial necrosis with or without Marfan S.
3. "Inflammatory" aneurysm (degenerative abdominal aortic aneurysm with periarterial fibrosis)
4. Kawasaki disease (coronary aneurysm)

5. Mycotic aneurysm (sepsis; bacterial endocarditis; tuberculosis)
6. Necrotizing vasculitis, arteritis (eg, polyarteritis nodosa; lupus erythematosus; Wegener's granulomatosis; drug abuse—esp. methamphetamine; idiopathic aortitis; Takayasu S.; acute pancreatitis; atrial myxoma embolization)
7. Neurofibromatosis
8. Osler-Weber-Rendu S.; AV malformation
9. Poststenotic aneurysm, distal to
   a. Atheromatous stenosis in any vessel
   b. Coarctation in thoracic aorta
   c. Fibromuscular dysplasia (esp. in renal artery)
   d. Subclavian stenosis in thoracic inlet S.
10. Pseudoxanthoma elasticum
11. Syphilis

References
1. Sutton D (ed): Textbook of Radiology and Imaging. (ed 6) New York: Churchill Livingstone, 1998, pp 695–702
2. Taybi H, Lachman RS: Radiology of Syndromes, Metabolic Disorders, and Skeletal Dysplasias. (ed 4) St. Louis: Mosby-Year Book, 1996

Gamut E-64

DISSECTING ANEURYSM OF THE ASCENDING AORTA OR ARCH

COMMON
1. Coarctation of aorta
2. Cystic medial necrosis or degeneration of aorta (esp. Marfan S.)
3. Hypertension

UNCOMMON
1. Aortic stenosis; bicuspid aortic valve
2. Aortitis (eg, collagen disease$_g$, esp. lupus erythematosus)
3. Cystic medial necrosis, other causes:
   a. Cogan S.

b. Cutis laxa
c. Ehlers-Danlos S.
d. Idiopathic
e. Mucopolysaccharidoses (See J-4)
f. Osteogenesis imperfecta
g. Pseudoxanthoma elasticum
h. Relapsing polychondritis
i. Turner S.
4. Iatrogenic (eg, catheterization; intramural injection of contrast medium)
5. Infection (eg, syphilis; bacterial endocarditis—mycotic aneurysm)
6. Postoperative prosthetic aortic valve replacement
7. Pregnancy
8. Trauma

References
1. Dow J, Roebuck EJ, Cole F: Dissecting aneurysms of the aorta. Br J Radiol 1970;39:915–927
2. Earnest F IV, Muhm JR, Sheedy PF II: Roentgenographic findings in thoracic aortic dissection. Mayo Clin Proc 1979;54:43–50
3. Meszaros WT: Cardiac Roentgenology. Springfield, IL: CC Thomas 1969, p 160
4. Sutton D (ed): Textbook of Radiology and Imaging. (ed 6) New York: Churchill Livingstone, 1998, pp 698–701
5. Weissleder R, Rieumont MJ, Wittenburg J: Primer of Diagnostic Imaging. (ed 2) St. Louis: Mosby-Year Book, 1997, pp 614–617

Gamut E-65

ANEURYSM OF CORONARY ARTERY

COMMON
1. Atherosclerosis
2. Congenital

UNCOMMON
1. Connective tissue disease (collagen disease)$_g$
2. Dissection
3. Iatrogenic (eg, catheter or operative injury)
4. Kawasaki S.

(continued)

5. Marfan S.
6. Mucopolysaccharidoses (See J-4)
7. Mycotic (incl. bacterial endocarditis)
8. Necrotizing arteritis
9. Rheumatic heart disease
10. Syphilis
11. Trauma

References
1. Norwood WI, Miller SW: Case Records of the Massachusetts General Hospital. N Engl J Med 1980;303:571–577
2. Wada J, Endo M, Takao A, et al: Mucocutaneous lymph node syndrome. Chest 1980;77:443–446

Gamut E-66

ARTERIAL STENOSIS AND THROMBOSIS

1. Arteritis (eg, Takayasu S.; giant cell; mesenteric; idiopathic aortitis)
2. Atherosclerosis with atheromatous plaque (esp. in internal carotid and vertebral artery origins, coronary, renal, iliac and femoral arteries, and abdominal aorta (with thrombosis = Leriche S.)
3. Buerger's disease (thromboangiitis obliterans)
4. Congenital stenoses (eg, coarctation of thoracic or abdominal aorta, origins of splanchnic or renal arteries, or pulmonary arteries; fibromuscular hyperplasia)
5. Extrinsic compression of artery (eg, thoracic outlet S.; renal artery stenosis due to fibrous band or neurofibromatosis; celiac axis compression S.; popliteal cysts and entrapment)
6. Neoplastic compression or invasion ("cuffing")

Reference
1. Sutton D (ed): Textbook of Radiology and Imaging. (ed 6) New York: Churchill Livingstone, 1998, pp 702–704

Gamut E-67

EMBOLUS

COMMON
1. Atheromatous plaque or ulcer with mural thrombus
2. Bacterial endocarditis
3. Iatrogenic (eg, postendarterectomy; arterial or venous catheterization)
4. Septic
5. Venous thrombosis or thrombophlebitis (incl. paradoxical embolus from venous system through patent foramen ovale to systemic circulation)

UNCOMMON
1. Arterial aneurysm with mural thrombus
2. Atrial fibrillation with left atrial thrombus
3. Chagas' myocardiopathy with intracardiac thrombus
4. Myocardial infarction with left ventricular thrombus
5. Neoplasm (tumor emboli), incl. left atrial myxoma

Gamut E-68

DIGITAL ISCHEMIA AND RAYNAUD'S PHENOMENON

COMMON
1. Atherosclerosis with atheroma
2. Arteritis (incl. Takayasu S.; giant cell)
3. Blood disorder (eg, sickle cell disease; polycythemia; contraceptive pill; cryoagglutination; polyvinylchloride poisoning)
4. Buerger's disease (thromboangiitis obliterans)
5. Connective tissue disease (collagen disease)$_g$ (eg, polyarteritis nodosa; scleroderma; rheumatoid disease)
6. Spastic response to cold in healthy individuals
7. Thromboembolism

UNCOMMON

1. African idiopathic aortitis
2. Ergotism
3. Fibromuscular hyperplasia
4. Thoracic outlet S.
5. Vibratory tools

Reference

1. Sutton D (ed): Textbook of Radiology and Imaging. (ed 6) New York: Churchill Livingstone, 1998, pp 706–709

Gamut E-69

AZYGOS VEIN DILATATION*

COMMON

1. Congenital absence or interruption of infrahepatic segment of inferior vena cava with azygos continuation to SVC (eg, polysplenia S.)
2. Constrictive pericarditis (See E-48)
3. [Enlarged azygos node; mediastinal mass]
4. Heart failure (eg, right ventricular failure secondary to left ventricular failure or mitral stenosis)
5. Normal (expiration, recumbency)
6. Obstruction of inferior vena cava (See E-71)
7. Obstruction of superior vena cava (See E-70)
8. Overhydration
9. Pericardial effusion and tamponade (See E-49)
10. Portal hypertension; splenic or portal vein thrombosis
11. Pregnancy
12. Tricuspid insufficiency (See E-28)

UNCOMMON

1. APVC, total (esp. via the azygos vein)
2. AV malformation (esp. thoracic wall)
3. Idiopathic
4. Mechanical obstruction proximal to or at tricuspid valve (eg, myxoma of RA; hypernephroma extending up IVC into RA; rare tricuspid stenosis)

5. [Right aortic arch with displaced azygos vein]
6. Sequestration of lung (esp. extralobar)
7. Traumatic azygos pseudoaneurysm or AV fistula

* Round or oval density crossing over right main bronchus at the tracheobronchial angle and measuring over 10 mm in diameter on erect PA chest radiograph. Azygos vein decreases in size with inspiration, erect position, or Valsalva maneuver.

[ ] This condition does not actually cause the gamuted imaging finding, but can produce imaging changes that simulate it.

References

1. Eisenberg RL: Clinical Imaging: An Atlas of Differential Diagnosis. (ed 3) Philadelphia: Lippincott-Raven, 1997, p 254
2. Felson B: Chest Roentgenology. Philadelphia: WB Saunders, 1973
3. Fraser RS, Müller NL, Coleman N, Paré PD (eds): Fraser & Paré: Diagnosis of Diseases of the Chest. (ed 4) Philadelphia: WB Saunders, 1999

Gamut E-70

SUPERIOR VENA CAVA DILATATION*

COMMON

1. Bronchogenic carcinoma (eg, superior sulcus)
2. Increased central venous pressure (eg, congestive heart failure; cardiac tamponade from pericardial effusion or constrictive pericarditis)
3. Lymphadenopathy (eg, oat cell carcinoma of lung; histoplasmosis; tuberculosis)
4. Lymphoma$_g$; lymphosarcoma
5. Mediastinal fibrosis or granuloma (eg, histoplasmosis; tuberculosis; ergotrate; radiation therapy; idiopathic)
6. Neoplasm of esophagus, thyroid or mediastinum (eg, goiter; cystic hygroma; thymoma; germ cell tumor)
7. Thrombosis (eg, iatrogenic—broken pacemaker wire; central line catheter; ventriculo-atrial shunt for

(continued)

hydrocephalus; post-tetralogy of Fallot repair; poly-cythemia vera)

UNCOMMON

1. Aneurysm of aorta or great artery$_g$; AV fistula
2. Axillary vein thrombosis with extension
3. Behçet S.
4. Congenital heart disease (eg, tricuspid insufficiency; total APVC)
5. Idiopathic
6. Mediastinal emphysema, severe; tension pneumo-thorax
7. Mediastinitis, acute
8. Myxoma of right atrium
9. Osteomyelitis of clavicle
10. Pneumoconiosis (coal-worker's; silicosis) with con-glomerate mass
11. Postoperative (eg, after surgery for congenital heart disease)
12. Sarcoidosis
13. Trauma (eg, laceration; transection; mediastinal hematoma)

* Well-defined, smooth widening of the right side of the upper medi-astinum.

References
1. Eisenberg RL: Clinical Imaging: An Atlas of Differential Diagnosis. (ed 3) Philadelphia: Lippincott-Raven, 1997, pp 252–253
2. Felson B: Chest Roentgenology. Philadelphia: WB Saunders, 1973
3. Heitzman ER: The Mediastinum: Radiologic Correlation with Anatomy and Pathology. St. Louis: CV Mosby, 1977
4. Mahajan V, Strimlan V, VanOrdstrand HS, et al: Benign superior vena cava syndrome. Chest 1975;68:32–35
5. Mikkelson WJ: Varices of the upper esophagus in superior vena caval obstruction. Radiology 1963;81:945–948
6. Moncada R, Cardella R, Demos TC, et al: Evaluation of superior vena cava syndrome by axial CT and CT phlebography. AJR 1984;143:731–736
7. Scoggin C: Identifying and managing superior vena cava syndrome. J Resp Dis Sept. 1981
8. Shimm DS, Logus MD, Rigsby LC: Evaluating the superior vena cava syndrome. JAMA 1981;245:951–953

OBSTRUCTION OF THE INFERIOR VENA CAVA OR ILIAC VEINS

COMMON

1. Direct tumor invasion of IVC (eg, renal cell carci-noma [hypernephroma]; Wilms' tumor; hepatocellu-lar carcinoma)
2. Extrinsic compression (eg, by lymphadenopathy; retroperitoneal tumor, cyst, hematoma, or abscess; pelvic lymphocele; aortic aneurysm; liver mass or enlarged liver; hydatid cyst)
3. Therapeutic interruption of IVC by ligation or filters (eg, to prevent pulmonary emboli, or as therapy for schistosomiasis)
4. Thromboembolism
5. Transient compression (eg, ascites; pregnancy)

[ ] This condition does not actually cause the gamuted imaging finding, but can produce imaging changes that simulate it.

UNCOMMON

1. Adhesions
2. [Congenital anomaly (eg, absence or hypoplasia of IVC; left-sided or double IVC)]
3. Lymphedema praecox (compression of left common iliac vein by right common iliac artery crossing over it)
4. Pelvic varicosities
5. Posttraumatic; post-radiation therapy
6. Retroperitoneal fibrosis
7. Sarcoma of IVC (eg, leiomyosarcoma; angiosar-coma); lipoma of IVC
8. Web at junction of IVC and right atrium

Reference
1. Sutton D (ed): Textbook of Radiology and Imaging. (ed 6) New York: Churchill Livingstone, 1998, pp 749–752

Gamut E-72-S

ANOMALIES OF THE INFERIOR VENA CAVA

1. Absence of IVC	Failure to form a prerenal cava
2. Azygos continuation, unilateral or bilateral	Persistence of left supracardinal vein
3. Bilateral cavae (common in asplenia S.)	Failure of dominance of right supracardinal vein
4. Circumaortic venous collar	Failure of regression of superior intersupra-cardinal anastomosis
5. Left IVC	Regression of right supracardinal vein
6. Retrocaval ureter	Failure of regression of right posterior cardinal vein

References
1. Mayo J, Gray RR, St. Louis EL, et al: Exhibit, American Roentgen Ray Society Meeting, Boston, 1984
2. Sutton D (ed): Textbook of Radiology and Imaging. (ed 6) New York: Churchill Livingstone, 1998, p 749

Gamut E-73-S

COMPLICATIONS OF CENTRAL VENOUS (SUBCLAVIAN, JUGULAR) OR PULMONARY ARTERY CATHETERIZATION

COMMON

1. Arterial insertion with perforation (esp. subclavian or carotid artery)
2. Catheter embolism; broken, trapped, or occluded catheter
3. Extravascular infusion (eg, mediastinal; intrapleural; subcutaneous)
4. Infection (local or sepsis)
5. Malpositioned or dislodged catheter (eg, in RV, IVC, hepatic vein, jugular vein)
6. Perforation of vessel with hematoma, hemothorax, hydrothorax, hemopericardium, or hemomedi-astinum
7. Pneumothorax
8. Thrombosis (eg, SVC); thrombophlebitis; pulmonary thromboembolism

UNCOMMON

1. Air embolism
2. AV fistula
3. Cardiac (eg, myocardial perforation; tamponade; arrhythmias)
4. Nerve injury (phrenic nerve or brachial plexus)
5. Subcutaneous or mediastinal emphysema
6. Thoracic duct laceration

References
1. Boyd KD, Thomas SJ, Gold J, et al: A prospective study of complications of pulmonary artery catheterization in 500 consecutive patients. Chest 1983;84:245–249
2. Gibson RN, Hennessy OF, Collier N, Hemingway AP: Major complications of central venous catheterization; A report of five cases and a brief review of the literature. Clin Radiol 1985; 36:205–208
3. Henschke CI, Pasternack GS, Herman PG: Maximizing the efficacy of chest radiography in the ICU. Appl Radiol, 1984; 13:139–143
4. Kattan KR: Migration of central venous catheters. AJR 1985;145:727–728
5. Kattan KR, Gutman E, Pantoja E, et al: Tubes, wires and rods seen in chest roentgenograms. CRC Crit Rev Diagn Imag 1984;21:257–287
6. Katz JD, Cronau LH, Barash PG, et al: Pulmonary artery flow-guided catheters in the perioperative period: Indications and complications. JAMA 1977;237:2832–2834
7. Mitchell SE, Clark RA: Complications of central venous catheterization. AJR 1979;133:467–476
8. Wilde P, Hartnell GG: Cardiac tumors; Pericardial tumors. In: Sutton D, Young JWR (eds): A Short Textbook of Clinical Imaging. London: Springer-Verlag, 1990, p 222

F

Chest

F

F

PLEURAL, EXTRAPLEURAL, AND CHEST WALL LESIONS

F

F

ROENTGEN SIGNS OF ALVEOLAR DISEASE (CONSOLIDATION, AIR SPACE PATTERN)

1. Acinar or peribronchiolar nodules
2. Air alveologram and bronchiologram
3. Air bronchogram
4. Butterfly or "bat's wing" distribution
5. Coalescence (early)
6. Fluffy, ill-defined margins
7. Perihilar, diffuse, segmental or lobar distribution
8. Present soon after onset of symptoms; rapid change

References
1. Felson B: A new look at pattern recognition of diffuse pulmonary disease. AJR 1979; 133:183–189
2. Felson B: Chest Roentgenology. Philadelphia: WB Saunders, 1973

LOCALIZED SEGMENTAL OR LOBAR CONSOLIDATION (ALVEOLAR, AIR SPACE) PATTERN, SOLITARY OR MULTIPLE

COMMON

1. Aspiration pneumonia (eg, acute—foreign body in bronchus; chronic—esophageal or neuromuscular disorder$_g$) (See F-7)
2. Atelectasis, incl. round atelectasis (See F-5)
3. Contusion of lung (pulmonary hemorrhage)
4. Obstructive pneumonia (eg, bronchogenic carcinoma; carcinoid; bronchial stenosis; foreign body aspiration; mucus plug; mucoid impaction)
5. Pneumonia, infectious, acute or organizing, lobar or lobular—bronchopneumonia (incl. bacterial—*Streptococcus, Staph. aureus, H. influenzae, E. coli,*

Proteus, Klebsiella, Bacteroides, Yersinia pestis (plague), pseudomonas, tularemia, anthrax, legionella, tuberculous, nocardia, actinomyces; varicella; cytomegalovirus; other viral; mycoplasma; rickettsial; AIDS with secondary infection) (See F-74-S)
6. Pulmonary edema, localized
7. Pulmonary thromboembolism with infarction
8. Round pneumonia
9. Tuberculosis, primary or secondary; atypical mycobacterial infection

UNCOMMON

1. Bronchioloalveolar carcinoma
2. Eosinophilic pneumonia, acute (eg, PIE; Löffler syndrome) or chronic
3. Fungus disease, esp. histoplasmosis; coccidioidomycosis; cryptococcosis (torulosis); blastomycosis; zygomycosis (mucormycosis) (See F-74-S)
4. Lipoid pneumonia$_g$
5. Lung torsion (trauma in children)
6. Lupus erythematosus (lung base)
7. Lymphoma$_g$; pseudolymphoma
8. Mucoid impaction (eg, asthma; hypersensitivity aspergillosis; bronchial obstruction)
9. Parasitic disease* (eg, *Pneumocystis carinii* (late); ascariasis; strongyloidiasis; amebiasis; paragonimiasis)
10. Pneumoconiosis (conglomerate mass of silicosis or coal-worker's pneumoconiosis)
11. Pulmonary hemorrhage (See F-12)
12. Pulmonary sequestration (intralobar)
13. Radiation pneumonitis
14. Sarcoidosis

* Note: These parasitic diseases more often cause a diffuse bronchopeumonia or scattered mixed alveolar and interstitial pattern.

References
1. Eisenberg RL: Clinical Imaging: An Atlas of Differential Diagnosis. (ed 3) Philadelphia: Lippincott-Raven, 1997, pp 4–17
2. Felson B: Chest Roentgenology. Philadelphia, WB Saunders, 1973

(continued)

3. Fraser RG, Paré JAP, Paré PD, Fraser RS: Differential Diagnosis of Diseases of the Chest. Philadelphia, WB Saunders, 1991, pp 11–20, 25–30
4. Fraser RS, Müller NL, Coleman N, Paré PD (eds): Fraser & Paré: Diagnosis of Diseases of the Chest. (ed 4) Philadelphia: WB Saunders, 1999
5. Reed JC: Chest Radiology. Plain Film Patterns and Differential Diagnoses. (ed 4) St. Louis, Mosby-Year Book, 1997, pp 211–225

Gamut F-3

LOBAR ENLARGEMENT (WITH BULGING INTERLOBAR FISSURE)

COMMON

1. Pneumonia (esp. *Klebsiella;* streptococcal; also tuberculous; pseudomonas; staphylococcal; *E. coli; H. influenzae;* plague; actinomycosis; mycoplasma)

UNCOMMON

1. Abscess
2. Bronchogenic carcinoma with obstructive pneumonia (drowned lung); bronchioloalveolar carcinoma
3. [Interlobar fluid]

[ ] This condition does not actually cause the gamuted imaging finding, but can produce imaging changes that simulate it.

References

1. Eisenberg RL: Clinical Imaging: An Atlas of Differential Diagnosis. (ed 3) Philadelphia: Lippincott-Raven, 1997, pp 84–85
2. Felson B: Chest Roentgenology. Philadelphia, WB Saunders, 1973
3. Reed JC: Chest Radiology. Plain Film Patterns and Differential Diagnoses. (ed 4) St. Louis: Mosby-Year Book, 1997, p 213

Gamut F-4

CHRONIC LOBAR CONSOLIDATION

COMMON

1. Bronchogenic carcinoma with obstructive pneumonia ("drowned lung")
2. Pneumonia, slowly resolving or organizing

UNCOMMON

1. Bronchioloalveolar carcinoma
2. Fungus disease (esp. cryptococcosis; zygomycosis; blastomycosis); actinomycosis; nocardiosis (See F-74-S)
3. Lipoid pneumonia$_g$
4. Lymphoma$_g$
5. Radiation pneumonitis
6. Tuberculous pneumonia

Reference

1. Epstein DM, Gefter WB, Miller WT: Lobar bronchiolo-alveolar cell carcinoma. AJR 1982; 139:463–468

Gamut F-5

LOBAR OR SEGMENTAL ATELECTASIS (COLLAPSE, VOLUME LOSS)

COMMON

1. Bronchiectasis
2. Bronchogenic carcinoma
3. Carcinoid
4. Compression atelectasis (eg, pleural effusion; large lung neoplasm; mesothelioma; diaphragmatic hernia; tension pneumothorax; congenital lobar emphysema; bullous emphysema)
5. Contraction atelectasis; pulmonary fibrosis (IPF)
6. Foreign body aspiration (eg, peanut; meat)
7. Mucous plugs, peripheral (eg, anesthesia; postoperative; pneumonia; chronic bronchitis; asthma, em-

physema; bronchiolitis obliterans; tetanus; bulbar paralysis)
8. Postoperative adhesive atelectasis (eg, left lower lobe collapse following CABG or other cardiac or thoracic surgery)

UNCOMMON

1. Amyloidosis
2. Aortic aneurysm
3. Broncholithiasis
4. Bronchomalacia
5. Cardiac enlargement (esp. dilated left atrium—ASD, mitral stenosis) with left lower lobe collapse
6. Cystic fibrosis (mucoviscidosis)
7. Endotracheal tube malposition (too low)
8. Lymphadenopathy, hilar (esp. bronchogenic or metastatic carcinoma; lymphoma$_g$; tuberculosis)
9. Mediastinal tumor
10. Metastatic disease to lymph nodes or endobronchial metastasis (esp. from carcinoma of kidney or breast or melanoma)
11. Middle lobe syndrome (chronic lymphadenopathy or bronchial stenosis due to histoplasmosis; tuberculosis; silicosis)
12. Mucoid impaction (eg, asthma; hypersensitivity bronchopulmonary aspergillosis)
13. Neoplasm of lung, other (eg, sarcoma; hamartoma; myoblastoma)
14. Parasitic disease (*Ascaris* in bronchus)
15. Pertussis
16. Pneumonia, organized
17. Pulmonary thromboembolism with infarction (unusual)
18. Radiation fibrosis; radiation pneumonitis (occasionally)
19. Rounded atelectasis
20. Scoliosis
21. Stricture of bronchus (eg, tuberculosis; histoplasmosis)
22. Trauma (eg, fractured bronchus)
23. Wegener granulomatosis

References

1. Eisenberg RL: Clinical Imaging: An Atlas of Differential Diagnosis. (ed 3) Philadelphia: Lippincott-Raven, 1997, pp 86–91
2. Felson B: Chest Roentgenology. Philadelphia, WB Saunders, 1973
3. Fraser RS, Müller NL, Coleman N, Paré PD (eds): Fraser & Paré: Diagnosis of Diseases of the Chest. (ed 4) Philadelphia: WB Saunders, 1999
4. Reed JC: Chest Radiology. Plain Film Patterns and Differential Diagnoses. (ed 4) St. Louis: Mosby-Year Book, 1997, pp 185–210
5. Teplick JG, Haskins ME: Roentgenologic Diagnosis. (ed 3) Philadelphia: WB Saunders, 1976

Gamut F-6

RECURRENT PNEUMONIA (See F-7)

COMMON

1. Alcoholism or debilitation with aspiration
2. Asthma
3. Bronchial disease, nonneoplastic (eg, bronchiectasis; inflammatory or congenital bronchial stenosis)
4. Cystic fibrosis (mucoviscidosis)
5. Esophageal disease with aspiration (eg, carcinoma; stricture; hiatus hernia; achalasia; scleroderma; Zenker diverticulum)
6. Foreign body in bronchus (esp. in children); mucus plug; broncholith
7. Idiopathic
8. Inadequate drug therapy
9. Neoplasm (eg, carcinoid; bronchogenic carcinoma)
10. Neuromuscular disorder$_g$ with aspiration (eg, brain damage; stroke; myasthenia gravis; paralysis$_g$)
11. Opportunistic infection, esp. *Pneumocystis carinii* pneumonia (eg, in HIV; AIDS; other immunologic disorder$_g$; excess steroid or immunosuppressive usage; chemotherapy; malignancy; cachexia; diabetes)
12. Parasitic disease (eg, ascariasis; strongyloidiasis; paragonimiasis; schistosomiasis; tropical pulmonary eosinophilia (filarial)

(continued)

UNCOMMON

1. Anemia$_g$, primary (esp. sickle cell disease)
2. Choanal atresia; cleft palate
3. Chronic granulomatous disease of childhood
4. Chronic pneumonia resolving by fibrosis (eg, tuberculosis; fungus disease)
5. Chronic sinusitis (incl. Kartagener S.; immotile cilia S.)
6. Connective tissue disease (collagen vascular disease)$_g$ (eg, lupus erythematosus)
7. Eosinophilic pneumonia$_g$ (eg, PIE; Löffler S.)
8. Esophageal bronchus
9. Extrinsic compression of tracheobronchial tree (eg, vascular ring); laryngeal disease
10. Hypersensitivity pneumonitis (extrinsic allergic alveolitis) (eg, farmer's lung; silo-filler's disease with multiple exposures; byssinosis) (See F-69)
11. Pulmonary sequestration (intralobar)
12. Rheumatoid or ankylosing spondylitis
13. Riley-Day S. (familial dysautonomia)
14. Tracheal lesion (See F-81-1)
15. Tracheoesophageal fistula
16. Tracheostomy

Reference

1. Berkmen YM: Aspiration and inhalation pneumonias. Semin Roentgenol 1980; 15:73–84

---

ysis$_g$; quadriplegia; amyotonia congenita; Duchenne muscular dystrophy; Werdnig-Hoffman disease)
5. Tracheoesophageal fistula (H-type or in association with esophageal atresia)

UNCOMMON

1. Choanal atresia; cleft palate
2. Laryngeal disease (incl. congenital wall deficiency; laryngotracheal cleft)
3. Lipoid pneumonia$_g$
4. Micrognathia
5. Riley-Day S. (familial dysautonomia)
6. Tracheal lesion (incl. vascular ring) (See F-81-1)

References

1. Fraser RS, Müller NL, Coleman N, Paré PD (eds): Fraser & Paré: Diagnosis of Diseases of the Chest. (ed 4) Philadelphia: WB Saunders, 1999
2. Gatewood OMB, Vanhoutte JJ: The role of the barium swallow examination in evaluation of pediatric pneumonias. AJR 1966; 97:203–210
3. Hughes RL, Freilich RA, Bytell DE, et al: Aspiration and occult esophageal disorders: Clinical conference in pulmonary disease from Northwestern University Medical School, Chicago. Chest 1981; 80:489–495

Gamut F-7

CHRONIC ASPIRATION PNEUMONIA IN A CHILD (See F-4, 6)

COMMON

1. Debilitation; malnutrition
2. Esophageal disease (eg, esophageal atresia or stenosis; achalasia; chalasia; hiatus hernia)
3. Idiopathic
4. Neuromuscular disorder$_g$ (eg, brain damage; cerebral palsy; meningomyelocele; poliomyelitis; paral-

---

Gamut F-8

ACUTE DISSEMINATED CONSOLIDATION (ALVEOLAR, AIR SPACE) PATTERN (INCL. BILATERAL CENTRAL DENSE OPACIFICATION)

COMMON

1. ARDS; oxygen toxicity
*2. Pneumonia (See F-75-S)
   a. Aspiration
   b. Bacterial (eg, staphylococcal; streptococcal; pseudomonas; plague; *Klebsiella; H. influenzae; E. coli;* legionella; leptospirosis; tuberculous;

atypical mycobacterial); nocardiosis; actinomycosis

  c. Chemical (eg, hydrocarbon)
  d. Eosinophilic$_g$ (eg, Löffler S.; PIE)
  e. Fungal, acute (eg, aspergillosis; histoplasmosis; blastomycosis; zygomycosis)
  f. Lipoid
  g. *Mycoplasma*
  h. Opportunistic or other unusual etiology (esp. *Pneumocystis carinii* or other parasitic)
  i. Rickettsial (eg, Rocky Mountain spotted fever; Q fever)
  j. Viral (eg, chickenpox; measles; influenza; cytomegalovirus; hantavirus) or chlamydial (psittacosis)
3. Pulmonary edema (See F-10)
*4. Respiratory distress S.; transient tachypnea of newborn

UNCOMMON
  1. Embolism (eg, fat; amniotic fluid; pulmonary thromboembolism with infarction, septic or bland)
*2. Hypersensitivity pneumonitis (extrinsic allergic alveolitis)
  3. Pulmonary hemorrhage (See F-12)
*4. Radiation pneumonitis

* Often has a mixed interstitial and alveolar pattern.

References
1. Felson B: A new look at pattern recognition of diffuse pulmonary disease. AJR 1979; 133:183–189
2. Felson B: Chest Roentgenology. Philadelphia: WB Saunders, 1973
3. Fraser RS, Müller NL, Coleman N, Paré PD (eds): Fraser & Paré: Diagnosis of Diseases of the Chest. (ed 4) Philadelphia: WB Saunders, 1999

CHRONIC DISSEMINATED CONSOLIDATION (ALVEOLAR, AIR SPACE) PATTERN

COMMON
  1. Alveolar proteinosis
  2. Bronchioloalveolar carcinoma
  3. Desquamative interstitial pneumonitis (DIP); nonspecific interstitial pneumonitis (NSIP); lymphocytic interstitial pneumonitis (LIP); bronchiolitis oibliterans with organizing pneumonia (BOOP)
  4. Lymphoma$_g$
  5. Obstructive pneumonia (eg, bronchogenic carcinoma "drowned lung"; carcinoid; foreign body)
  6. Recurrent pneumonia (See F-6, F-7)
  7. Sarcoidosis (alveolar phase)

UNCOMMON
  1. Alveolar microlithiasis
  2. Eosinophilic pneumonia, chronic
  3. Fungus disease (eg, aspergillosis)
  4. Lipoid pneumonia$_g$ (eg, mineral oil aspiration)
  5. Metastases, hemorrhagic (eg, choriocarcinoma)
  6. Pulmonary sequestration (intralobar)
  7. Silicoproteinosis (resembles alveolar proteinosis but with acute course)
  8. Tuberculosis; atypical mycobacterial infection

References
1. Felson B: A new look at pattern recognition of diffuse pulmonary disease. AJR 1979; 133:183–189
2. Felson B: Chest Roentgenology. Philadelphia: WB Saunders, 1973
3. Fraser RS, Müller NL, Coleman N, Paré PD (eds): Fraser & Paré: Diagnosis of Diseases of the Chest. (ed 4) Philadelphia: WB Saunders, 1999

Gamut F-10-1

PULMONARY EDEMA

COMMON

*1. Agonal; terminal illness
*2. ARDS (eg, shock lung; respirator lung); cardiopul-
     monary bypass; open heart surgery; sepsis; oxygen
     toxicity
*3. Aspiration of gastric contents (Mendelson S.),
     hydrocarbons, or hypertonic contrast material
*4. Drug reaction (eg, nitrofurantoin; aspirin; hydro-
     chlorothiazide; beta-adrenergic drugs; interleukin-
     2; radiologic contrast media) (See F-73-S)
*5. Heart failure with pulmonary venous hypertension
     (eg, left ventricular failure; mitral stenosis or insuf-
     ficiency; left atrial myxoma or thrombus; thyrotox-
     icosis; myocardiopathy; sickle cell disease; arterio-
     venous fistula; left-to-right shunt; total APVR;
     coarctation of aorta; hypoplastic left heart S.$_g$)
     (See E-3, E-59)
6.   Hypersensitivity pneumonitis (extrinsic allergic
     alveolitis) (eg, farmer's lung; bagassosis)
     (See F-69)
*7. Iatrogenic (incl. hypervolemia; fluid overload;
     overtransfusion, drug overdose)
*8. Inhalation of noxious gas, smoke, paint fumes, sul-
     fur dioxide, beryllium, silica, dinitrogen tetroxide,
     nitrogen dioxide (silo-filler's disease), carbon
     monoxide, fluorocarbons, hydrocarbons, paraquat,
     ammonium, chlorine, hydrogen sulfide, phosgene,
     cadmium (See F-72-S)
9.   Narcotic abuse (esp. heroin; morphine; methadone;
     cocaine)
10. Neurogenic, cerebral (stroke; head trauma;
     epilepsy; intracranial neoplasm; increased intracra-
     nial pressure)
11. Pulmonary thromboembolism with infarction
*12. Renal failure; uremia; acute glomerulonephritis;
     nephrosis
13. Shock (eg, insulin reaction; gram-negative sep-
     ticemia; snake bite; burn; electric shock; anaphy-

lactic reaction to penicillin, blood transfusion, or
radiologic contrast medium)
*14. Trauma, thoracic; contusion of lung; blast injury

UNCOMMON

*1. Amniotic fluid embolism
2.   Connective tissue disease (collagen vascular
     disease)$_g$
*3. Disseminated intravascular coagulation (DIC)
4.   Eclampsia
5.   Fat embolism (incl. oily contrast medium)
*6. Hepatic disease (eg, acute hepatitis)
7.   High altitude
*8. Hypoproteinemia (eg, malabsorption)
*9. Hypoxia, any cause
*10. Near-drowning
11. Pancreatitis, acute
*12. Parasitic disease (eg, malaria; strongyloidiasis)
13. Pericarditis (esp. constrictive)
14. Pheochromocytoma (catecholamine release)
15. Pleural air or fluid aspiration, rapid or excessive;
     rapid reexpansion of lung following treatment for a
     large pneumothorax
*16. [Pneumonia]
17. Pregnancy
18. [Pulmonary hemorrhage (incl. bleeding diathesis$_g$;
     idiopathic hemosiderosis; Goodpasture S.)]
     (See F-12)
*19. [Pulmonary lymphangiectasia]
20. Radiation pneumonitis
*21. Upper airway obstruction (eg, aspirated food;
     foreign body; epiglottitis; croup; hanging;
     suffocation)
*22. Venous or lymphatic obstruction (eg, pulmonary
     vein thrombosis or veno-occlusive disease; block-
     age by mediastinal mass; sclerosing mediastinitis)

* May occur in an infant.
[ ] This condition does not actually cause the gamuted imaging finding,
but can produce imaging changes that simulate it.

References
1. Brodey PA, Fisch AE, Huffaker J: Acute pulmonary edema
    resulting from treatment for premature labor. Radiology
    1981;140:631–633

2. Eisenberg RL: Clinical Imaging: An Atlas of Differential Diagnosis. (ed 3) Philadelphia: Lippincott-Raven, 1997, pp 18–25
3. Fraser RS, Müller NL, Coleman N, Paré PD (eds): Fraser & Paré: Diagnosis of Diseases of the Chest. (ed 4) Philadelphia: WB Saunders, 1999
4. Heitzman ER: The Lung: Radiologic-Pathologic Correlations. (ed 2) St. Louis: CV Mosby, 1984, p 182
5. Reed JC: Chest Radiology. Plain Film Patterns and Differential Diagnoses. (ed 4) St. Louis: Mosby-Year Book, 1997
6. Rigsby C, Swett HA, Sostman HD, et al: Roentgenographic features of drug-induced disease. J Resp Dis 1983;11:60–68

Gamut F-10-2

UNILATERAL PULMONARY EDEMA

COMMON

1. Aspiration, unilateral (eg, water; kerosene; ethyl alcohol; gastric juice)
2. Contralateral disease (eg, emphysema; post-lobectomy; occlusion, absence, or hypoplasia of a pulmonary artery—Swyer-James-McLeod S.; pulmonary arterial thromboembolism)
3. Contusion of one lung
4. Idiopathic
5. Pleural air or fluid aspiration, rapid or excessive; rapid reexpansion of lung following treatment for a large pneumothorax
6. Postural (prolonged lateral decubitus position)

UNCOMMON

1. Bronchial obstruction with "drowned lung" (eg, carcinoid; bronchogenic carcinoma; foreign body in bronchus; mucus plug)
2. Catheter malposition with infusion into pulmonary artery and lung
3. Congenital heart disease (eg, unilateral ductus shunt)
4. Obstruction of pulmonary vein (eg, bronchogenic carcinoma or bronchogenic cyst; unilateral veno-occlusive disease)

5. Postoperative systemic-pulmonary artery shunt (eg, Potts, Blalock-Taussig, or Waterston operation)

References

1. Amjad H, Bigman O, Tabor H: Unilateral pulmonary edema. JAMA 1974; 229:1094–1095
2. Calenoff L, Kruglik GD, Woodruff A: Unilateral pulmonary edema. Radiology 1978;126:19–24
3. Eisenberg RL: Clinical Imaging: An Atlas of Differential Diagnosis. (ed 3) Philadelphia: Lippincott-Raven, 1997, pp 26–29
4. Fraser RS, Müller NL, Coleman N, Paré PD (eds): Fraser & Paré: Diagnosis of Diseases of the Chest. (ed 4) Philadelphia: WB Saunders, 1999

Gamut F-11-1

ADULT RESPIRATORY DISTRESS SYNDROME (ARDS)

COMMON

1. Anaphylactic reaction (eg, penicillin; bee sting; blood transfusion; radiologic contrast media)
2. Multi-system injury or failure
3. Respirator lung (oxygen toxicity)
4. Sepsis (gram-positive or gram-negative septicemia)
5. Shock lung (hemorrhagic, septic, cardiogenic, anaphylactic)
6. Trauma, massive (lung or body)

UNCOMMON

1. Aspiration
2. Disseminated intravascular coagulation (DIC)
3. Electric shock
4. Embolism of fat or amniotic fluid
5. Inhalation of smoke, paint or noxious fumes (eg, phosgene; nitrous oxide)
6. Insulin reaction
7. Narcotics (eg, heroin; methadone); other drugs
8. Near-drowning
9. Near-strangulation
10. Pancreatitis, acute

(continued)

11. Pneumonia, incl. severe viral (eg, varicella)
12. Snake bite

References

1. Dähnert W: Radiology Review Manual. (ed 4) Baltimore: Williams & Wilkins, 1999, pp 377–378
2. Seely JM, Effmann EL: Acute lung injury and acute respiratory distress syndrome in children. Semin Roentgenol 1998;33:163–173

Gamut F-11-2

ACUTE LUNG INJURY AND ARDS IN CHILDREN

1. ARDS (acute respiratory distress syndrome) (eg, sepsis; pneumonia; aspiration; near-drowning; near-strangulation; smoke inhalation; multi-system injury or failure; anaphylaxis)
2. Aspiration
3. Inhalation of smoke, paint or noxious fumes
4. Near-drowning
5. Oxygen toxicity
6. Trauma (eg, pulmonary laceration or contusion)

Reference

1. Seely JM, Effmann EL: Acute lung injury and acute respiratory distress syndrome in children. Semin Roentgenol 1998;33:163–173

Gamut F-12

PULMONARY HEMORRHAGE

COMMON

1. Contusion of lung; blunt trauma
2. Renal disease with or without immunologic abnormality (incl. Goodpasture S.)

UNCOMMON

1. Anticoagulant therapy; other drug-induced bleeding
2. Aspiration from a bleeding pulmonary lesion (eg, arteriovenous malformation bronchogenic carcinoma; vascular metastasis)
3. Bleeding or clotting disorder$_g$ (eg, hemophilia; leukemia; thrombocytopenia; Henoch-Schönlein purpura)
4. Bone marrow transplantation
5. Bronchitis; bronchiectasis
6. Connective tissue disease (collagen vascular disease)$_g$ (esp. lupus erythematosus; polyarteritis nodosa—vasculitis)
7. Disseminated intravascular coagulation (DIC)
8. Drug abuse (esp. heroin)
9. Heart failure
10. Iatrogenic (eg, bronchoscopy; lung biopsy)
11. Idiopathic
12. Idiopathic pulmonary hemosiderosis
13. Infection (eg, Rocky Mountain spotted fever; saprophytic fungal infection; aspergillosis; zygomycosis)
14. Leukocytoclastic vasculitis
15. Mitral stenosis
16. Parasitic disease (eg, malaria; strongyloidiasis)
17. Pulmonary thromboembolism (esp. with infarction)
18. Wegener granulomatosis

References

1. Albelda SM, Gefter WB, Epstein DM, et al: Diffuse pulmonary hemorrhage: A review and classification. Radiology 1985;154:289–297
2. Felson B: Chest Roentgenology. Philadelphia: WB Saunders, 1973
3. Fiegler VW, Siemoneit KD: Pulmonary manifestations in anaphylactoid purpura (Henoch-Schönlein syndrome). Fortschr Röntgenstr 1981;134:269–272
4. Fraser RS, Müller NL, Coleman N, Paré PD (eds): Fraser & Paré: Diagnosis of Diseases of the Chest. (ed 4) Philadelphia: WB Saunders, 1999
5. Herman PG, Balikian JP, Seltzer SE, et al: The pulmonary-renal syndrome. AJR 1978; 130:1141–1148
6. Reed JC: Chest Radiology. Plain Film Patterns and Differential Diagnoses. (ed 4) St. Louis: Mosby-Year Book, 1997
7. Schwartz EE, Teplick JG, Onesti G, et al: Pulmonary hemorrhage in renal disease: Goodpasture's syndrome and other causes. Radiology 1977;122:39–46

Gamut F-13

REVERSE BUTTERFLY PATTERN

COMMON

1. ARDS
2. Contusion of lung
3. Eosinophilic pneumonia (PIE; Löffler syndrome)
4. Pneumonia
5. Sarcoidosis

UNCOMMON

1. Bronchioloalveolar carcinoma
2. Bronchiolitis obliterans with organizing pneumonia (BOOP)
3. Connective tissue disease (collagen vascular disease)$_g$
4. Pulmonary edema, atypical
5. Pulmonary thromboembolism with multiple infarctions
6. Parasitic disease (esp. ascariasis; strongyloidiasis)
7. Radiation pneumonitis

Reference
1. Fraser RS, Müller NL, Coleman N, Paré PD (eds): Fraser & Paré: Diagnosis of Diseases of the Chest. (ed 4) Philadelphia: WB Saunders, 1999
2. Liebow AA, Carrington CB: The eosinophilic pneumonias. Medicine 1969; 48:251–285

Gamut F-14

CONSOLIDATION (ALVEOLAR, AIR SPACE) PATTERN IN A PATIENT WITH LEUKEMIA OR LYMPHOMA

COMMON

1. Bacterial pneumonia
2. Fungus disease (esp. angioinvasive aspergillosis; cryptococcosis (torulosis); histoplasmosis; moniliasis; zygomycosis) (See F-74-S)
3. Lymphomatous or leukemic infiltration
4. *Pneumocystis carinii* pneumonia

UNCOMMON

1. Alveolar proteinosis
2. Cytomegalovirus pneumonia
3. Drug reaction (eg, methotrexate)
4. Leukostasis; leukemia cell lysis
5. Mycoplasma pneumonia
6. Parasitic disease (eg, strongyloidiasis)
7. Pulmonary edema (eg, heart failure)
8. Pulmonary hemorrhage
9. Varicella (chickenpox) pneumonia

References
1. Miller WT, Talbot GH, Epstein DM, et al: Radiographic findings in acquired immune deficiency syndrome. Appl Radiol 1985; May/June:86–95
2. Pennington JE: Dilemma: Pneumonia in the immunocompromised patient. J Resp Dis 1982;3:25–29

Gamut F-15

MULTIFOCAL ILL-DEFINED OPACITIES IN THE LUNGS*

COMMON

1. ARDS; shock lung; respirator lung (See F-11-1, F-11-2)
2. Aspiration pneumonia
3. Bronchopneumonia (esp. staphylococcal; streptococcal; *Pseudomonas; Klebsiella; Legionella; E. coli;* other gram-negative bacteria; melioidosis; nocardiosis) (See F-74-S)
4. Eosinophilic pneumonia, idiopathic (eg, Löffler S.) or secondary to parasitic disease (eg, paragonimiasis; ascariasis; strongyloidiasis; hookworm disease; schistosomiasis; toxocariasis; tropical eosinophilia {filarial})
5. Fungus disease (eg, histoplasmosis; coccidioidomycosis; blastomycosis; candidiasis; actinomycosis;

(continued)

aspergillosis; cryptococcosis (torulosis); zygomycosis; sporotrichosis)

6. Metastases (eg, choriocarcinoma; vascular tumors)
7. Pneumoconiosis (esp. silicosis; coal worker's pneumoconiosis; asbestosis)
8. *Pneumocystis carinii* pneumonia (esp. in AIDS)
9. Pulmonary edema
10. Pulmonary thromboembolism with infarctions; septic emboli
11. Sarcoidosis
12. Tuberculosis; atypical mycobacterial infection (esp. in AIDS)
13. Viral and *Mycoplasma* pneumonias (See F-74-S)

UNCOMMON

1. Amyloidosis; Waldenström macroglobulinemia
2. Arteriovenous fistulas
3. Bronchiolitis obliterans with organizing pneumonia (BOOP)
4. Bronchioloalveolar carcinoma
5. Drug reaction (esp. chemotherapeutic agents) (See F-73-S)
6. Langerhans cell histiocytosis (eosinophilic granuloma)
7. Hypersensitivity pneumonitis (extrinsic allergic alveolitis) (eg, farmer's lung; bagassosis)
8. Kaposi sarcoma (esp. in AIDS)
9. Lung abscesses, multiple
10. Lymphoma_g
11. Neonatal retained fluid S.; bronchopulmonary dysplasia
12. Pneumonia of unusual etiology (eg, lipoid; rickettsial—Q fever, Rocky Mountain spotted fever)
13. Pulmonary hemorrhage (eg, Goodpasture S.; hemolytic-uremic S.; idiopathic pulmonary hemosiderosis)
14. Pulmonary sequestration (intralobar)
15. Radiation therapy (pneumonitis or fibrosis)
16. Usual interstitial pneumonitis (UIP); desquamative interstitial pneumonitis (DIP); lymphocytic interstitial pneumonitis (LIP)
17. Vasculitis (eg, collagen vascular disease_g—esp. polyarteritis nodosa, lupus erythematosus; Wegener

granulomatosis; lymphomatoid granulomatosis; zygomycosis; aspergillosis)

* Not confined to lobar or segmental distribution.

References

1. Heitzmann ER: The Lung: Radiologic-Pathologic Correlations. (ed 2) St. Louis: CV Mosby, 1984
2. Reed JC: Chest Radiology. Plain Film Patterns and Differential Diagnoses. (ed 4) St. Louis: Mosby-Year Book, 1997, pp 249–279

Gamut F-16

DIFFUSE PULMONARY DISEASE WITH A MIXED ALVEOLAR (AIR SPACE) AND INTERSTITIAL (RETICULONODULAR OR SMALL IRREGULAR) PATTERN

COMMON

1. Bronchioloalveolar carcinoma
2. Hypersensitivity pneumonitis (extrinsic allergic alveolitis) (eg, farmer's lung; bagassosis) (See F-69)
3. *Pneumocystis carinii* pneumonia (esp. in AIDS)
4. Pulmonary edema in heart failure or ARDS
5. Sarcoidosis

UNCOMMON

1. Desquamative interstitial pneumonitis (DIP); nonspecific interstitial pneumonitis (NSIP)
2. Drug or poison toxicity (eg, bleomycin; methotrexate; busulfan; Cytoxan; mitomycin; amiodarone; gold)
3. Goodpasture syndrome
4. Pneumonia of unusual etiology (eg, mycoplasma, cytomegalovirus, or
5. *Strongyloides,* esp. in AIDS or other immunocompromised host)
6. Pulmonary hemorrhage, recurrent or chronic (eg, bleeding or clotting disorder_g; idiopathic pulmonary hemosiderosis)

Reference
1. Fraser RG, Paré JAP, Paré PD, Fraser RS: Differential Diagnosis of Diseases of the Chest. Philadelphia: WB Saunders, 1991, pp 85–88

Gamut F-17-S

ROENTGEN PATTERNS OF INTERSTITIAL DISEASE

1. Bronchial disease (eg, peribronchial thickening; mucoid impaction; bronchiectasis)
2. Discrete miliary nodules
3. Honeycomb lung
4. Kerley lines
5. Small irregular shadows (reticular or reticulonodular pattern)
6. Vascular abnormality (incl. pulmonary arterial, pulmonary venous, or bronchial arterial)

References
1. Felson B: A new look at pattern recognition of diffuse pulmonary disease. AJR 1979;133:183–189
2. Felson B: Disseminated interstitial diseases of the lung. Ann Radiol 1966; 9:325–345

Gamut F-18

ACUTE DIFFUSE FINE RETICULAR OPACITIES (KERLEY LINES, ACUTE—A, B, AND C) (See F-19)

COMMON

1. Pneumonia (esp. interstitial—infectious mononucleosis, cytomegalovirus, *H. influenzae; Mycoplasma;* atypical mycobacterial; *Pneumocystis carinii*)
2. Pulmonary edema (esp. heart failure; myocardial infarction; valvular heart disease; renal failure; uremia; fluid overload; drug reaction) (See F-10)

3. Transient tachypnea of the newborn (retained fetal lung fluid); Wilson-Mikity S.; bronchopulmonary dysplasia

UNCOMMON

1. Hypersensitivity pneumonitis (extrinsic allergic alveolitis) (eg, farmer's lung; bagassosis) (See F-69)
2. Hypoproteinemia (eg, cirrhosis; nephrosis; burn; exudative skin disorder)
3. Pulmonary hemorrhage (incl. Henoch-Schönlein purpura) (See F-12)
4. Pulmonary veno-occlusive disease, acute

References
1. Felson B: A new look at pattern recognition of diffuse pulmonary disease. AJR 1979;133:183–189
2. Felson B: Chest Roentgenology. Philadelphia: WB Saunders, 1973
3. Trapnell DH: The differential diagnosis of linear shadows in chest radiographs. Radiol Clin North Am 1973;11:77–92

Gamut F-19

KERLEY LINES, CHRONIC—A, B, AND C (See F-18)

COMMON

1. Bronchogenic carcinoma (lymphangitic spread of tumor)
2. Idiopathic pulmonary fibrosis (IPF) (See F-22)
3. Lymphangitic metastases
4. Pneumoconiosis (esp. silicosis) (See F-70-S)
5. Mitral stenosis

UNCOMMON

1. Alveolar proteinosis (late)
2. Bronchioloalveolar carcinoma
3. Congenital heart disease (eg, total APVR)
4. Connective tissue disease (collagen vascular disease)$_g$ (eg, rheumatoid lung; scleroderma)

(continued)

5. Desquamative interstitial pneumonitis (DIP); lymphocytic interstitial pneumonitis (LIP)
6. Hypersensitivity pneumonitis (extrinsic allergic alveolitis) (eg, farmer's lung; bagassosis) (See F-69)
7. Left atrial neoplasm (esp. myxoma)
8. Lipoid pneumonia$_g$
9. Lymphoma$_g$ (esp. alveolar); leukemia
10. Mediastinal mass with lymphatic obstruction; fibrosing mediastinitis
11. Pulmonary hemorrhage, late (eg, idiopathic pulmonary hemosiderosis) (See F-12)
12. Pulmonary lymphangiectasia
13. Pulmonary lymphangioleiomyomatosis; tuberous sclerosis
14. Pulmonary veno-occlusive disease; pulmonary vein atresia
15. Radiation fibrosis
16. Sarcoidosis
17. Thoracic duct ligation, obstruction, or injury

References

1. Felson B: A new look at pattern recognition of diffuse pulmonary disease. AJR 1979; 133:183–189
2. Felson B: Chest Roentgenology. Philadelphia: WB Saunders, 1973
3. Heitzman ER: The Lung: Radiologic-Pathologic Correlations. (ed 2) St Louis: CV Mosby, 1984
4. Reed JC: Chest Radiology. Plain Film Patterns and Differential Diagnoses. (ed 4) St. Louis: Mosby-Year Book, 1997
5. Trapnell DH: The differential diagnosis of linear shadows in chest radiographs. Radiol Clin North Am 1973;11:77–92

Gamut F-20-1

WIDESPREAD MILIARY NODULES IN THE LUNGS (LESS THAN 5 MM DIAMETER)

COMMON

*1. Fungus disease (esp. histoplasmosis; blastomycosis; coccidioidomycosis; candidiasis) (See F-74-S)
2. Langerhans cell histiocytosis$_g$ (esp. eosinophilic granuloma)

3. [Interstitial fibrosis (eg, early stage or subliminal honeycombing)]
4. Metastases, hematogenous (esp. carcinoma of thyroid; melanoma); lymphangitic carcinomatosis (esp. carcinoma of breast, lung, stomach, pancreas, prostate)
5. Pneumoconiosis (esp. silicosis; coal-worker's pneumoconiosis; asbestosis; siderosis; stannosis; berylliosis) (See F-70-S)
6. Sarcoidosis
*7. Tuberculosis, miliary

UNCOMMON

1. Alveolar microlithiasis
2. Amyloidosis
*3. Bronchiolitis, acute or chronic
*4. Bronchiolitis obliterans (eg, noxious vapors; chemicals) (See F-72-S, 73-S); Asian panbronchiolitis
5. Bronchioloalveolar carcinoma
*6. Fat embolism (esp. oily contrast medium after lymphangiography or hysterosalpingography)
7. Gaucher disease; Niemann-Pick disease
*8. Hypersensitivity pneumonitis (extrinsic allergic alveolitis) (eg, farmer's lung; bagassosis; byssinosis) (See F-69)
9. Lymphocytic interstitial pneumonitis (LIP)
10. Lymphoma$_g$; leukemia
*11. Melioidosis
*12. Parasitic disease (esp. schistosomiasis; tropical pulmonary eosinophilia {filarial})
*13. Pneumonia of unusual etiology (eg, viral—chickenpox, measles, influenza; pertussis; nocardiosis; listeriosis; chlamydia; opportunistic) (See F-74-S, 75-S)
14. Pulmonary hemosiderosis (eg, mitral stenosis; idiopathic)
15. Pulmonary lymphangioleiomyomatosis
*16. Infantile respiratory distress S. (hyaline membrane disease)
17. Tuberous sclerosis

* Usually acute disease.
[ ] This condition does not actually cause the gamuted imaging finding, but can produce imaging changes that simulate it.

References

1. Eisenberg RL: Clinical Imaging: An Atlas of Differential Diagnosis. (ed 3) Philadelphia: Lippincott-Raven, 1997, pp 56-59
2. Felson B: A new look at pattern recognition of diffuse pulmonary disease. AJR 1979;133:183–189
3. James DG, Carstairs LS: Miliary diseases of the lung. Dis Mon. July 1962;1–40
4. Reed JC: Chest Radiology. Plain Film Patterns and Differential Diagnoses. (ed 4) St. Louis: Mosby-Year Book, 1997, pp 280–294

Gamut F-20-2

WIDESPREAD MILIARY NODULES IN THE LUNGS OF A NEONATE OR YOUNG INFANT

*1. Acute bronchiolitis
 2. Langerhans cell histiocytosis (esp. Letterer-Siwe disease)
*3. Pneumonia (esp. *Chlamydia*)
 4. [Pulmonary lymphangiectasia]
*5. Respiratory distress S.
 6. [Total APVR]

* Acute.
[ ] This condition does not actually cause the gamuted imaging finding, but can produce imaging changes that simulate it.

Gamut F-21

WIDESPREAD SMALL IRREGULAR OPACITIES (RETICULAR, NODULAR, OR RETICULONODULAR PATTERN) (See F-22)

COMMON

 1. Chronic bronchitis; COPD
*2. Hypersensitivity pneumonitis (extrinsic allergic alveolitis) (eg, farmer's lung; bagassosis; byssinosis; mushroom-worker's lung) (See F-69)
 3. Idiopathic pulmonary fibrosis (IPF); usual interstitial pneumonitis (UIP) (See F-23-S1)
 4. Interstitial fibrosis or leiomyomatosis (eg, from recurrent infection; chronic aspiration; radiation; lung trauma; prior thromboembolism) (See F-22)
 5. Interstitial pulmonary edema with pulmonary venous hypertension (eg, Kerley lines in chronic mitral valve disease)
 6. Metastases, hematogenous (esp. from thyroid carcinoma; melanoma); lymphangitic carcinomatosis (esp. from carcinoma of breast, lung, larynx, stomach, pancreas, cervix, or prostate); leukemia
 7. Pneumoconiosis (esp. silicosis; coal-worker's pneumoconiosis; asbestosis; talcosis; berylliosis; siderosis; stannosis; baritosis; aluminum pneumoconiosis) (See F-70-S)
*8. Pneumonia of unusual etiology (eg, staphylococcal; salmonella; legionella; melioidosis; measles; chickenpox; cytomegalovirus; echovirus; mycoplasma; *Pneumocystis carinii; Toxoplasma;* other opportunistic) (See F-74-S, 75-S)
 9. Sarcoidosis
10. Tuberculosis; atypical mycobacterial infection

UNCOMMON

 1. Alveolar microlithiasis
 2. Amyloidosis (bronchopulmonary)
*3. Bronchiolitis, acute or chronic with peribronchial cuffing (eg, bronchiolitis obliterans; noxious vapors; Asian panbronchiolitis)

(continued)

4. Bronchioloalveolar carcinoma
5. Connective tissue disease (collagen vascular disease)$_g$ (eg, scleroderma; dermatomyositis; polymyositis; lupus erythematosus)
6. Cystic fibrosis (mucoviscidosis)
7. Desquamative interstitial pneumonitis (DIP); lymphocytic interstitial pneumonitis (LIP); nonspecific interstitial pneumonitis (NSIP)
*8. Drug-induced (esp. nitrofurantoin; busulfan; bleomycin; methotrexate; Cytoxan; amiodarone; methysergide; procainamide) (See F-73-S)
*9. Fat embolism$_g$ (incl. oily contrast medium)
*10. Fungus disease (esp. histoplasmosis; coccidioidomycosis; cryptococcosis {torulosis}; blastomycosis) (See F-74-S)
11. Gaucher disease; Niemann-Pick disease
12. Goodpasture syndrome
13. Idiopathic pulmonary hemosiderosis (late)
14. Langerhans cell histiocytosis (eosinophilic granuloma)
15. Lymphoma$_g$; leukemia
16. Neurofibromatosis
*17. Oxygen toxicity (usually infants)
*18. Parasitic disease (esp. schistosomiasis; ascariasis; tropical pulmonary eosinophilia (filarial); paragonimiasis; toxoplasmosis)
19. Pulmonary lymphangiectasia
20. Pulmonary lymphangioleiomyomatosis; tuberous sclerosis
21. Pulmonary veno-occlusive disease
22. Rheumatoid lung
23. Riley-Day S. (familial dysautonomia)
24. Sjögren S.
25. "Small airways disease"
*26. Thromboembolism of talc in drug addicts or of metallic mercury
*27. Transient tachypnea of the newborn
28. Waldenström macroglobulinemia
29. Wilson-Mikity S.; bronchopulmonary dysplasia

* May be acute.

References

1. Eisenberg RL: Clinical Imaging: An Atlas of Differential Diagnosis. (ed 3) Philadelphia: Lippincott-Raven, 1997, pp 30–39
2. Felson B: A new look at pattern recognition of diffuse pulmonary disease. AJR 1979; 133:183–189
3. Felson B: Chest Roentgenology. Philadelphia: WB Saunders, 1973
4. Fraser RG, Paré JAP, Paré PD, Fraser RS: Differential Diagnosis of Diseases of the Chest. Philadelphia: WB Saunders, 1991, pp 71–84
5. Fraser RS, Müller NL, Coleman N, Paré PD (eds): Fraser & Paré: Diagnosis of Diseases of the Chest. (ed 4) Philadelphia: WB Saunders, 1999
6. Friedman PJ: Idiopathic and autoimmune type III-like reactions: Interstitial fibrosis, vasculitis, and granulomatosis. Semin Roentgenol 1975; 10:43–51
7. Gaensler EA, Carrington CB: Open biopsy for chronic diffuse infiltrative lung disease: Clinical, roentgenographic, and physiological correlations in 502 patients. Ann Thorac Surg 1980; 30:411–426

Gamut F-22

INTERSTITIAL FIBROSIS (INCLUDING HONEYCOMB LUNG—END-STAGE INTERSTITIAL FIBROSIS)

COMMON

*1. Connective tissue disease (collagen vascular disease)$_g$ (esp. scleroderma; also rheumatoid lung; dermatomyositis; polymyositis)
2. [Cystic bronchiectasis (incl. cystic fibrosis and tuberculosis)]
*3. Idiopathic pulmonary fibrosis (IPF); acute interstitial pneumonitis (formerly Hamman-Rich syndrome); usual interstitial pneumonitis (UIP) (See F-23-S1)
*4. Langerhans cell histiocytosis (eosinophilic granuloma)
*5. Pneumoconiosis (esp. silicosis; coal-worker's pneumoconiosis; asbestosis; talcosis; berylliosis; siderosis; stannosis; baritosis; aluminum pneumoconiosis) (See F-70-S)
*6. Sarcoidosis

UNCOMMON

1. Amyloidosis
*2. Ankylosing spondylitis (upper lobes)
*3. Desquamative interstitial pneumonitis (DIP); non-specific interstitial pneumonitis (NSIP)
*4. Drug sensitivity (esp. bleomycin; busulfan; methotrexate; Cytoxan; carmustine; nitrofurantoin; hexamethonium; amiodarone; methysergide; procainamide) (See F-73-S)
*5. Gaucher disease; Niemann-Pick disease
*6. Hypersensitivity pneumonitis (extrinsic allergic alveolitis) (eg, farmer's lung; bagassosis; bird-fancier's lung; air-conditioner lung) (See F-69)
*7. Inhalation of noxious fumes or chemicals, late (eg, silo-filler's disease; sulfur dioxide; cadmium; chlorine; phosgene) (See F-72-S)
*8. Lipoid pneumonia$_g$; chronic aspiration (usually localized in lower lobe)
*9. Neurofibromatosis (rare)
*10. Oxygen toxicity; shock lung; [ARDS]
11. Pulmonary hemorrhage; idiopathic pulmonary hemosiderosis (late) (See F-12)
*12. Pulmonary lymphangioleiomyomatosis; tuberous sclerosis
13. Radiation fibrosis
14. Schistosomiasis

* Can often progress to development of end-stage interstitial fibrosis or honeycomb lung.
[ ] This condition does not actually cause the gamuted imaging finding, but can produce imaging changes that simulate it.

References

1. Carrington CB, Gaensler EA, Couty RE, et al: Natural history and treated course of usual and desquamative interstitial pneumonia. N Engl J Med 1978; 298:801–809
2. Eisenberg RL: Clinical Imaging: An Atlas of Differential Diagnosis. (ed 3) Philadelphia: Lippincott-Raven, 1997, pp 40–43
3. Felson B: A new look at pattern recognition of diffuse pulmonary disease. AJR 1979; 133:183–189
4. Felson B: Chest Roentgenology. Philadelphia: WB Saunders, 1973
5. Fraser RS, Müller NL, Coleman N, Paré PD (eds): Fraser & Paré: Diagnosis of Diseases of the Chest. (ed 4) Philadelphia: WB Saunders, 1999
6. Genereux GP: The end-stage lung: Pathogenesis, pathology, and radiology. Radiology 1975; 116:279–289
7. Heard BE: Pathology of interstitial lung diseases, with particular reference to terminology, classification and trephine lung biopsy. Chest 1976; 69:252–253
8. Lynch JP III: Practice guidelines in idiopathic pulmonary fibrosis. J Resp Dis 1981; 121–131
9. Reed JC: Chest Radiology. Plain Film Patterns and Differential Diagnoses. (ed 4) St. Louis: Mosby-Year Book, 1997, pp 314–327
10. Scadding JG: Diffuse pulmonary alveolar fibrosis. Thorax 1974; 29:271–281
11. Spencer H: Pathology of the Lung (Excluding Pulmonary Tuberculosis). (ed 3) New York: Pergamon Press, 1977

Gamut F-23-S1

SYNONYMS FOR IDIOPATHIC OR USUAL INTERSTITIAL PNEUMONITIS

1. Bronchiolar emphysema
2. Chronic interstitial pneumonitis
3. Diffuse chronic fibrosing interstitial pneumonitis
4. Diffuse interstitial fibrosis
5. Fibrosing (or sclerosing) alveolitis
6. Hamman-Rich syndrome (acute form)
7. Idiopathic pulmonary fibrosis (IPF)
8. Muscular cirrhosis
9. Organizing interstitial pneumonia

Reference

1. Reed JC: Chest Radiology. Plain Film Patterns and Differential Diagnoses. (ed 4) St. Louis: Mosby-Year Book, 1997, p 299

Gamut F-23-S2

ENTITIES THAT CAN PRODUCE HISTOLOGIC CHANGES SIMILAR TO USUAL INTERSTITIAL PNEUMONITIS

1. Connective tissue disease (collagen vascular disease)$_g$ (scleroderma; rheumatoid lung; lupus erythematosus; erythema nodosum)
2. Drug therapy (eg, bleomycin; busulfan; methotrexate; amiodarone)
3. Idiopathic
4. Noxious gases
5. Pneumoconiosis (eg, asbestosis; talcosis)
6. Radiation injury
7. Viral disease

References
1. Gaensler EA, Carrington CB, Coutu RE: Chronic interstitial pneumonias. Clinical Notes on Respiratory Diseases, Vol. 10. New York: American Thoracic Society, 1972, pp 1–16
2. Reed JC: Chest Radiology. Plain Film Patterns and Differential Diagnoses. (ed 4) St. Louis: Mosby-Year Book, 1997, p 299

Gamut F-24

DIFFUSE INTERSTITIAL DISEASE WITH PLEURAL EFFUSION

COMMON
1. Metastatic disease (esp. lymphangitic carcinomatosis)
2. Pneumonia (eg, viral, mycoplasma)
3. Pulmonary edema (eg, heart failure; renal failure)
4. Tuberculosis

UNCOMMON
1. Asbestosis
2. Connective tissue disease (collagen vascular disease)$_g$ (eg, lupus erythematosus; rheumatoid disease)

3. Drug-induced pulmonary disease (eg, nitrofurantoin; hydralazine; procainamide) (See F-73-S)
4. Lymphoma$_g$; leukemia
5. Parasitic disease (eg, paragonimiasis; filariasis—tropical pulmonary eosinophilia)
6. Pulmonary lymphangioleiomyomatosis; tuberous sclerosis; lymphangiomatosis
7. Sarcoidosis
8. Waldenström macroglobulinemia

Reference
1. Fraser RS, Müller NL, Coleman N, Paré PD (eds): Fraser & Paré: Diagnosis of Diseases of the Chest. (ed 4) Philadelphia: WB Saunders, 1999

Gamut F-25

DIFFUSE INTERSTITIAL DISEASE WITH ASSOCIATED LYMPHADENOPATHY

COMMON
1. AIDS (eg, cytomegalovirus or atypical mycobacterial infection; Kaposi sarcoma; lymphoma)
2. Metastatic disease (eg, lymphangitic carcinomatosis)

UNCOMMON
1. Amyloidosis
2. Cystic fibrosis (mucoviscidosis)
3. Drug reaction (eg, hydantoin {Dilantin}; trimethadione; methotrexate)
4. Fungus disease (esp. histoplasmosis; coccidioidomycosis; blastomycosis) (See F-74-S)
5. Hypersensitivity pneumonitis (extrinsic allergic alveolitis) (esp. mushroom-worker's lung—rare in other entities)
6. Langerhans cell histiocytosis (rarely)
7. Lymphoma$_g$; leukemia
8. Parasitic disease (eg, acute schistosomiasis; filariasis-tropical pulmonary eosinophilia) (occasionally)

9. Pneumoconiosis (eg, silicosis; coal-worker's pneumoconiosis; berylliosis)
10. Pulmonary lymphangioleiomyomatosis
11. Sarcoidosis

12. Tuberculosis
13. Viral infection (eg, infectious mononucleosis; chickenpox; measles; cat-scratch fever; ECHO virus; *Mycoplasma*); *Chlamydia*—psittacosis

HIGH-RESOLUTION CT (HRCT) PATTERNS OF CHRONIC INTERSTITIAL LUNG DISEASE (CILD)—SEPTAL THICKENING*

COMMON

1. Pulmonary edema — Smooth, often associated areas of ground-glass opacity

2. Pulmonary fibrosis (eg, idiopathic; drug-induced; connective tissue disease$_g$—esp. scleroderma, rheumatoid lung, dermatomyositis; sarcoidosis; asbestosis; chronic pneumonia; neurofibromatosis) — Irregular thickening with architectural distortion and traction bronchiectasis

3. Lymphangitic carcinomatosis (esp. from carcinoma of breast, lung, stomach, and pancreas; leukemia) — Interstitial nodules ± peribronchovascular and subpleural thickening and effusion

4. Hypersensitivity pneumonitis (extrinsic allergic alveolitis) (eg, farmer's lung, bagassosis) (See F-69) — Immunologic response to inhaled organic antigens; bilateral small nodules, ground-glass opacities, patchy consolidation and septal lines acutely; chronic exposure leads to fibrosis

5. Infection (eg, viral pneumonia; mycoplasma; miliary tuberculosis; miliary histoplasmosis) — Symmetric perihilar interstitial infiltrate; no pleural effusion

6. Sarcoidosis — Widely variable pulmonary patterns including interstitial thickening, 2 to 10 mm nodules, perilymphatic distribution, ± lymphadenopathy

7. Silicosis or coal-worker's pneumoconiosis — Small, upper lobe predominant, frequently calcified nodules and septal thickening; may coalesce to PMF with honeycombing; calcified nodes common

UNCOMMON

1. Alveolar microlithiasis — Calcific interlobular septal thickening; 1 mm punctate calcified nodules (microliths), patchy or diffuse

2. Alveolar proteinosis — Idiopathic overproduction of surfactant by pneumocytes; diffuse airspace disease ± septal thickening; treatment with BAL; predisposed to infection, particularly *Nocardia*

(continued)

3. Kaposi sarcoma	Lower lobe bronchovascular thickening; skin or mucous membrane lesions invariably present; irregular "flame-shaped" nodules; lymphadenopathy; pleural effusions
4. Lymphoma$_g$; leukemia	Uncommon pattern of direct perihilar lymphatic spread
5. Pulmonary lymphangiectasia	Rare; generalized lymphatic dilatation; small effusions
6. Pulmonary lymphangioleiomyomatosis	Rare; extensive septal thickening; pleural effusions; pneumothorax

* Fluid or cellular infiltrates in interlobular septa. Linear opacities (1 to 2 cm) seen best in lung periphery. Visualization of a few peripheral interlobular septa is normal.

Reference

1. Fraser RS, Müller NL, Coleman N, Paré PD (eds): Fraser & Paré: Diagnosis of Diseases of the Chest. (ed 4) Philadelphia: WB Saunders, 1999

Gamut F-27

GROUND-GLASS OPACITIES ON HRCT*

COMMON

1. Hypersensitivity pneumonitis (extrinsic allergic alveolitis) (eg, farmer's lung, bagassosis) (See F-69)	Immunologic response to inhaled organic antigens; acute or subacute phase shows diffuse or lower lung zone predominance; often associated with diffuse centrilobular nodules, ground-glass opacities, patchy consolidation and septal lines acutely; chronic exposure leads to fibrosis
2. Nonspecific interstitial pneumonia (NSIP) (idiopathic or associated with collagen vascular disease$_g$ or AIDS)	Patchy or diffuse; mild, if any, fibrosis; may have areas of consolidation
3. Acute interstitial pneumonia (AIP)	Patchy or diffuse; often associated with reticulation or consolidation; consolidation involves predominantly dependent lung regions
4. Idiopathic pulmonary fibrosis (IPF) and active phase	Usually in association with predominantly peripheral lower lung zone interstitial fibrosis
5. Pulmonary hemorrhage (eg, bronchitis; bronchiectasis; pulmonary thromboembolism; bronchogenic carcinoma; contusion of lung; vasculitis—Wegener granulomatosis, Goodpasture S., lupus erythematosis; aspergilloma; anticoagulation; bleeding diathesis; arteriovenous malformation; DIC; vascular metastases	Focal or diffuse

6. Connective tissue disease$_g$ (esp.lupus erythematosus; scleroderma) | In association with interstitial fibrosis, hemorrhage or pneumonia

7. Sarcoidosis | Widely variable pulmonary involvement + adenopathy, including interstitial, nodular, and occasional alveolar pattern; peribroncho-vascular nodules on HRCT

8. BOOP | Usually associated with typically peripheral or peribronchial consolidation

9. Bronchiolitis obliterans | Small airway inflammation or fibrosis; air trapping on expiration; areas with ground-glass opacity have increased vascularity due to blood flow redistribution (mosaic perfusion)

10. Infection

   a. *Pneumocystis carinii* pneumonia | Common AIDS infection; perihilar interstitial or ground-glass pattern early; airspace, nodules, cysts, and pneumothorax when advanced; effusion and adenopathy rare; BAL usually diagnostic

   b. Viral (esp. cytomegalovirus in immunocompromised patients) | Often associated with consolidation

   c. Bacterial | Usually in association with consolidation

   d. Tuberculosis; atypical mycobacterial infection | Usually in association with centrilobular nodules and branching linear opacities ("tree-in-bud")

UNCOMMON

1. Alveolar proteinosis | Idiopathic overproduction of surfactant by pneumocytes; diffuse, symmetric airspace disease ± septal thickening; treatment with BAL; predisposing to infection, particularly *Nocardia*

2. Desquamative interstitial pneumonitis (DIP) | Lower lung zone and peripheral predominance; mild, if any, fibrosis

3. Eosinophilic pneumonia | Usually associated consolidation

4. Langerhans cell histiocytosis (eosinophilic granuloma) | Upper lobe-predominant interstitial disease with a variable combination of small nodules and cysts; fibrosis and pneumothorax may develop

5. Lymphocytic interstitial pneumonitis (LIP) | Idiopathic condition in children with AIDS or adults with Sjögren syndrome or multicentric Castleman disease; septal thickening and ill-defined nodules

* Partial airspace filling or alveolar septal inflammation that does not obscure vessels. Typically represents an active, acute, and reversible disease process.

References
1. Müller NL: Lecture at 16th Masters Diagnostic Radiology Conference, Kauai, Hawaii, 1999
2. Fraser RS, Müller NL, Coleman N, Paré PD (eds): Fraser & Paré: Diagnosis of Diseases of the Chest. (ed 4) Philadelphia: WB Saunders, 1999

Gamut F-28

CHRONIC AIRSPACE CONSOLIDATION ON HRCT

1. Bronchiolitis obliterans with organizing pneumonia (BOOP)
2. Bronchioloalveolar carcinoma
3. Chronic eosinophilic pneumonia
4. Lymphoma$_g$
5. Sarcoidosis (alveolar phase)

References

1. Müller N: Lecture at Eleventh Masters Diagnostic Radiology Conference, Kauai, Hawaii, 1992
2. Fraser RS, Müller NL, Coleman N, Paré PD (eds): Fraser & Paré: Diagnosis of Diseases of the Chest. (ed 4) Philadelphia: WB Saunders, 1999

Gamut F-29

PERIBRONCHOVASCULAR INTERSTITAL THICKENING ON HRCT

COMMON

1. Pulmonary edema	Smooth interstitial thickening with cardiomegaly and pleural effusions
2. Sarcoidosis	Widely variable pulmonary patterns including interstitial thickening and peribronchovascular nodules ± lymphadenopathy
3. Lymphangitic carcinomatosis (esp. carcinoma of breast, lung, stomach and pancreas; leukemia)	Interstitial nodules ± peribronchovascular and subpleural thickening and effusion; local spread of lung cancer or hematogenous spread of breast cancer are most common
4. Hypersensitivity pneumonitis (extrinsic allergic alveolitis) (See F-69)	Immunologic response to inhaled organic antigens; bilateral small nodules, ground-glass opacities, patchy consolidation and septal lines acutely that clear over weeks; chronic exposure leads to fibrosis
5. Interstitial fibrosis (idiopathic pulmonary fibrosis—IPF)	Reticular pattern and associated traction bronchiectasis
6. Pneumoconiosis (silicosis; coal worker's pneumoconiosis; stannosis; siderosis)	Small, upper lobe predominant, frequently calcified 2 to 5 mm nodules and septal thickening; may coalesce to PMF; calcified nodes common
7. Asbestosis	Basilar reticular pattern, often associated with pleural plaques or thickening and pleural calcification

UNCOMMON

1. Berylliosis	Pattern resembles sarcoidosis
2. Connective tissue disease$_g$ (esp. scleroderma; dermatomyositis; rheumatoid lung)	Reticular pattern

3. Kaposi sarcoma — Bronchovascular thickening; skin or mucous membrane lesions invariably present; irregular "flame-shaped" nodules; lymphadenopathy; pleural effusions

4. Lymphoma$_g$; leukemia — Smooth or nodular; usually associated with mediastinal adenopathy ± unilateral hilar adenopathy

References
1. Müller NL: Lecture at 16th Masters Diagnostic Radiology Conference, Kauai, Hawaii, 1999
2. Fraser RS, Müller NL, Coleman N, Paré PD (eds): Fraser & Paré: Diagnosis of Diseases of the Chest. (ed 4) Philadelphia: WB Saunders,1999

Gamut F-30

INCREASED LUNG LUCENCY (USUALLY CYSTIC PATTERN) ON HRCT

COMMON

1. Bronchiectasis — Tram-tracks; cystic lesions

2. Bronchiolitis obliterans — Peripheral attenuation of vessels; hyperinflation. HRCT shows mosaic pattern of perfusion (Note: Does *not* show a cystic pattern on HRCT)

3. Emphysema — Centrilobular, paraseptal, panacinar, bullous

4. Interstitial fibrosis, end-stage (eg, idiopathic pulmonary fibrosis (IPF); scleroderma; rheumatoid lung) — Honeycomb pattern

5. Pneumatocele — Traumatic or post-infectious (esp. in *Pneumocystis carinii* or staphylococcal pneumonia)

UNCOMMON

1. Langerhans cell histiocytosis (eosinophilic granuloma) — Cystic lesions; nodules; involves mainly mid and upper lung zones

2. Pulmonary lymphangioleiomyomatosis — Cystic lesions on high-resolution CT

Reference
1. Fraser RS, Müller NL, Coleman N, Paré PD (eds): Fraser & Paré: Diagnosis of Diseases of the Chest. (ed 4) Philadelphia: WB Saunders, 1999

Gamut F-31

UPPER LUNG DISEASE ON HRCT

COMMON

1. Cystic fibrosis   Bronchiectasis;
   (mucoviscidosis)   hyperinflation
2. Sarcoidosis   Nodules; fibrosis;
                             lyrnphadenopathy
3. Silicosis and coal   Nodules or
   worker's pneumoconiosis   conglomerate masses
4. Tuberculosis   Nodules, cavitation,
                             consolidation and
                             scarring

UNCOMMON

1. Ankylosing spondylitis   Upper lobe fibrosis
2. Talcosis   Intravenous drug abuse;
                            small nodules, con-
                            glomerate masses,
                            centrilobular emphy-
                            sema

Reference
1. Fraser RS, Müller NL, Coleman N, Paré PD (eds): Fraser &
   Paré: Diagnosis of Diseases of the Chest. (ed 4) Philadelphia: WB Saunders,1999

Gamut F-32

LOWER LUNG DISEASE ON HRCT

COMMON

1. Asbestosis   Reticulation, honey-
                            combing; pleural
                            thickening
2. Aspiration pneumonia   Dependent lung zones
3. Connective tissue disease$_g$ Reticulation and
   (esp. scleroderma;   honeycombing
   rheumatoid lung;
   dermatomyositis)
4. Idiopathic pulmonary   Reticulation and
   fibrosis (IPF)   honeycombing
5. Lymphangitic   Septal lines; pleural
   carcinomatosis   effusion; lymph-
                            adenopathy

UNCOMMON

1. Hypersensitivity   Centrilobular nodules;
   pneumonitis (extrinsic   ground-glass attenua-
   allergic alveolitis)   tion; reticulation
2. Lipoid pneumonia   Dependent lung zones.
                            HRCT shows areas
                            with fat attenuation

Reference
1. Fraser RS, Müller NL, Coleman N, Paré PD (eds): Fraser &
   Paré: Diagnosis of Diseases of the Chest. (ed 4) Philadelphia: WB Saunders, 1999

SMALL NODULAR OPACITIES ON HRCT*

COMMON

1. Asbestosis — Subpleural nodules; interstitial fibrosis predominantly in lower lung zones; pleural thickening ± plaques

2. Bronchiolitis (eg, respiratory, cellular, infectious, and panbronchiolitis) — Small airway inflammation; ground-glass attenuation, small centrilobular nodules, and "tree-in-bud"'opacities on HRCT; expiratory images may show air trapping

3. Bronchopneumonia (eg, *Pseudomonas; Staphylococcus; Streptococcus; Klebsiella;* bacillary angiomatosis; anaerobes; *Mycoplasma; Legionella; Nocardia; Actinomyces;* tuberculous; viral; fungal— histoplasmosis, aspergillosis; lipoid— chronic oil aspiration) — Ill-defined focal consolidation

4. Granulomatous disease, old (esp. histoplasmosis; tuberculosis) — Often calcified

5. Mycobacterial infection (esp. miliary tuberculosis) — Transbronchial or hematogenous spread

6. Lymphangitic carcinomatosis (esp. from carcinoma of breast, lung, stomach, and pancreas; leukemia) — Interstitial nodules ± peribronchovascular and subpleural thickening and effusion

7. Pulmonary metastases — Smooth, round, various size; predominantly lower lobe and peripheral nodules; ill-defined if hemorrhagic

8. Sarcoidosis — Widely variable pulmonary patterns ± adenopathy, including interstitial thickening and ill-defined nodules; characteristic peribronchovascular nodules on HRCT

9. Silicosis and coal worker's pneumoconiosis — Small, upper lobe- and posterior-predominant; frequently calcified nodules and septal thickening; may coalesce to PMF; calcified nodes common

UNCOMMON

1. Amyloidosis — Variable patterns, including interstitial disease and solitary or multiple nodules, ± calcification or cavitation

2. Bronchioloalveolar cell carcinoma — Can present as focal or multifocal consolidation, nodules, or a mass

3. Follicular bronchiolitis (lymphoid hyperplasia) — Centrilobular nodules; peribronchial nodules; patchy ground-glass opacities

4. Hypersensitivity pneumonitis (extrinsic allergic alveolitis) (See F-69) — Immunologic response to inhaled organic antigens such as moldy hay or bird droppings; patterns include bilateral small nodules, ground-glass opacities, patchy consolidation, and septal lines

(continued)

5. Lymphoma$_g$ (esp. recurrent non-Hodgkin)	Almost always mediastinal adenopathy; nodules ± air bronchograms
6. Lymphocytic interstitial pneumonitis (LIP)	Idiopathic pseudolymphomatous condition in children with AIDS or adults with Sjögren syndrome or multicentric Castleman disease; septal thickening and ill-defined centrilobular, peribronchovascular, and septal nodules
6. Langerhans cell histiocytosis (eosinophilic granuloma)	Upper lobe-predominant interstitial disease with a variable combination of small nodules and cysts; fibrosis and pneumothorax may develop

* Usually interstitial.

References

1. Müller NL: Lecture at 16th Masters Diagnostic Radiology Conference, Kauai, Hawaii, 1999
2. Fraser RS, Müller NL, Coleman N, Paré PD (eds): Fraser & Paré: Diagnosis of Diseases of the Chest. (ed 4) Philadelphia: WB Saunders, 1999

Gamut F-34-1

SMALL NODULE DISTRIBUTION ON HRCT—PERILYMPHATIC
(Peribronchovascular, Septal, and Subpleural)

COMMON

1. Lymphangitic carcinomatosis (esp. from carcinoma of breast, lung, stomach and pancreas; leukemia)	Interstitial nodular thickening (beaded septa) ± peribronchovascular and subpleural thickening and pleural effusion
2. Sarcoidosis	Widely variable pulmonary patterns ± adenopathy, including 2–10 mm peribronchovascular and subpleural nodules
3. Silicosis and coal worker's pneumoconiosis	Upper lobe- and posterior-predominant; frequently calcified 2–5 mm nodules and septal thickening; may coalesce to PMF; calcified nodes common

UNCOMMON

1. Amyloidosis	Solitary or multiple nodules ± calcification or cavitation
2. Follicular bronchiolitis (lymphoid hyperplasia)	Centrilobular nodules; peribronchial nodules; patchy ground-glass opacities
3. Lymphocytic interstitial pneumonitis (LIP)	Idiopathic pseudolymphomatous condition in children with AIDS; septal thickening and ill-defined nodules
4. Lymphoma$_g$; leukemia	Usually associated mediastinal adenopathy ± unilateral hilar adenopathy

Gamut F-34-2

SMALL NODULE DISTRIBUTION ON HRCT—Randomly or Evenly Distributed Throughout Lung

1. Miliary tuberculosis	Typically very ill or immunocompromised patient
2. Pulmonary metastases	Smooth, round, variable size; peripheral and lower lobe predominance; hemorrhagic nodules ill defined

Gamut F-34-3

SMALL NODULE DISTRIBUTION ON HRCT—Centrilobular

COMMON

1. Bronchiolitis	Ground-glass and "tree-in-bud" opacities. Expiratory images may show air trapping in involved regions
2. Bronchopneumonia due to viruses, mycoplasma, bacteria or *Aspergillus*	Ill-defined nodules and ground-glass attenuation; bronchiectasis
3. Cystic fibrosis (mucoviscidosis)	Hyperinflation; bronchiectasis; mucus plugging; allergic bronchopulmonary aspergillosis; asthma
4. Silicosis and coal worker's pneumoconiosis	Upper lobe- and posterior-predominant, frequently calcified 2–5 mm nodules and septal thickening; may coalesce to PMF; calcified nodes common
5. Tuberculosis; atypical mycobacterial infection	Endobronchial spread with "tree-in-bud" pattern

UNCOMMON

1. Bronchioloalveolar cell carcinoma	Can present as focal or multifocal consolidation, nodules, or a mass
2. Follicular bronchiolitis (lymphoid hyperplasia)	Centrilobular nodules; peribronchial nodules; patchy ground-glass opacities
3. Hypersensitivity pneumonitis (extrinsic allergic alveolitis)	Ill-defined nodules and ground-glass opacities; patchy consolidation, and septal lines
4. Langerhans cell histiocytosis (eosinophilic granuloma)	Upper lobe-predominant interstitial disease with a variable combination of small nodules and cysts; interstitial fibrosis and pneumothorax may develop

References

1. Müller N: Lecture at 16th Masters Diagnostic Radiology Conference, Kauai, Hawaii, 1999
2. Fraser RS, Müller NL, Coleman N, Paré PD (eds): Fraser & Paré: Diagnosis of Diseases of the Chest. (ed 4) Philadelphia: WB Saunders, 1999

Gamut F-35-S

WORLD HEALTH ORGANIZATION 1982—HISTOLOGIC CLASSIFICATION OF LUNG NEOPLASMS (SLIGHTLY MODIFIED)

I. EPITHELIAL NEOPLASMS

A. BENIGN
1. Papillomas
   a. Squamous cell papilloma
   b. Transitional papilloma
2. Adenomas
   a. Pleomorphic adenoma (mixed tumor)
   b. Monomorphic adenoma
   c. Others

B. DYSPLASIA
1. Carcinoma in situ

C. MALIGNANT
1. Squamous cell carcinoma (epidermoid carcinoma)
   a. Variant
      i. Spindle cell (squamous) carcinoma
2. Small cell carcinoma
   a. Oat cell carcinoma
   b. Intermediate cell type
   c. Combined oat cell carcinoma
3. Adenocarcinoma
   a. Acinar adenocarcinoma
   b. Papillary adenocarcinoma
   c. Bronchiolo-alveolar carcinoma
   d. Solid carcinoma with mucus formation
4. Large cell carcinoma
   a. Variants
      i. Giant cell carcinoma
      ii. Clear cell carcinoma
5. Adenosquamous carcinoma
6. Carcinoid
7. Bronchial gland carcinomas
   a. Adenoid cystic carcinoma
   b. Mucoepidermoid carcinoma
   c. Others
8. Others

II. SOFT TISSUE NEOPLASMS

III. MESOTHELIAL NEOPLASMS

A. LOCALIZED FIBROUS PLEURAL TUMOR

B. MALIGNANT MESOTHELIOMA
1. Epithelial
2. Fibrous (spindle cell)
3. Biphasic

IV. MISCELLANEOUS NEOPLASMS

A. BENIGN
1. Hamartoma

B. MALIGNANT
1. Carcinosarcoma
2. Blastoma
3. Melanoma
4. Lymphoma$_g$
5. Others

V. SECONDARY NEOPLASMS

VI. UNCLASSIFIED NEOPLASMS

VII. NEOPLASM-LIKE LESIONS
1. Inflammatory pseudotumor
2. Langerhans cell histiocytosis$_g$ (eosinophilic granuloma)
3. Lymphoproliferative lesions
4. Tumorlet
5. Others

Reference
1. World Health Organization histological typing of lung tumours. Am J Clin Pathol 1982; 77:123–136.

CHEST TUMORS IN INFANTS, CHILDREN, AND ADOLESCENTS

LUNGS

COMMON
1. [Inflammatory pseudotumor (eg, plasma cell granuloma; sclerosing hemangioma)]
2. Metastatic tumor (esp. Wilms' tumor; osteosarcoma)

UNCOMMON
1. Askin tumor
2. Bronchogenic carcinoma
3. Carcinoid; cylindroma; mucoepidermoid carcinoma; pleomorphic adenoma
4. Hamartoma
5. Metastatic tumor, other (eg, Ewing sarcoma; rhabdomyosarcoma; lymphoma$_g$; leukemia; hepatoblastoma; neuroblastoma; germ cell tumor; carcinoma of thyroid; laryngeal papillomatosis)
6. Pulmonary blastoma
7. Spindle cell tumor (eg, leiomyoma; neurofibroma)

MEDIASTINUM (See Gamuts F-86 to F-91)

HEART

1. Metastatic tumor (eg, lymphoma; neuroblastoma; Wilms' tumor; sarcomas; hepatoblastoma)
2. Primary tumor (eg, rhabdomyoma; fibroma; lipoma; myxoma—esp. atrial; teratoma; rhabdomyosarcoma; other sarcomas; hemangiopericytoma)

[ ] This condition does not actually cause the gamuted imaging finding, but can produce imaging changes that simulate it.

Gamut F-37

SOLITARY PULMONARY NODULE (UNDER 4 CM DIAMETER)

COMMON
1. Carcinoid$_g$
*2. Carcinoma, bronchogenic (incl. bronchioloalveolar)
3. [Chest wall lesion (skin tumor; nipple shadow; rib lesion); artifact; foreign body]
*4. Fungus disease (esp. histoplasmosis; rarely coccidioidomycosis) (See F-74-S)
5. Hamartoma
6. Idiopathic (incl. postinflammatory scar)
*7. Metastasis (esp. from sarcoma; melanoma; carcinoma of breast, colon, kidney, testis)
8. Round pneumonia (eg, atypical viral; pneumococcal; streptococcal; legionella; nocardia)
*9. Tuberculoma

UNCOMMON
*1. Abscess of lung
*2. Amyloidoma
3. Blood vessel (eg, normal vessel seen end-on near hilum; arteriovenous malformation; varix; pulmonary artery aneurysm; anomalous pulmonary vein)
*4. Bulla, fluid-filled (infected)
*5. Cyst, fluid-filled (bronchial; bronchiectatic)
6. [Diaphragmatic hernia, localized]
7. [Encapsulated pleural fluid; interlobar effusion; fibrin ball]
8. [Extramedullary hematopoiesis; splenosis]
*9. Fungus ball (esp. *Aspergillus*)
10. Granuloma, other (eg, paraffinoma; sarcoidosis)
11. Gumma
*12. Hematoma
*13. Inflammatory pseudotumor; organized pneumonia
14. Lipoid pneumonia$_g$ (paraffinoma)
15. [Localized fibrous tumor of pleura; mesothelioma]
16. Lymph node, intrapulmonary; giant lymph node hyperplasia (Castleman disease)

(continued)

*17. Lymphoma$_g$
*18. [Mediastinal mass]
19. Mucoid impaction (eg, obstructive; *Aspergillus* hypersensitivity; asthma); mucocele (bronchial atresia)
20. Mucus plug (eg, cystic fibrosis {mucoviscidosis})
21. Neoplasm, benign (eg, spindle cell tumor$_g$)
*22. Parasitic disease (eg, hydatid cyst; paragonimiasis; *Dirofilaria immitis*)
23. Plasmacytoma, pulmonary
24. [Pleural plaque (eg, asbestos related pleural disease)]
25. Pneumoconiosis (conglomerate mass from silicosis or coal-worker's pneumoconiosis; also asbestosis; talcosis) (See F-70-S)
*26. Pulmonary infarct
*27. Pulmonary sequestration (intralobar)
*28. Rheumatoid nodule
29. Rounded atelectasis
30. Sarcoma of lung (eg, leiomyosarcoma; rhabdomyosarcoma); pulmonary blastoma
*31. Wegener granulomatosis$_g$

* May show cystic appearance or cavitation.
[ ] This condition does not actually cause the gamuted imaging finding, but can produce imaging changes that simulate it.

References

1. Felson B: Chest Roentgenology. Philadelphia: WB Saunders, 1973
2. Fraser RG, Pare JAP, Pare PD, Fraser RS: Differential Diagnosis of Diseases of the Chest. Philadelphia: WB Saunders, 1991, pp 39–48
3. Fraser RS, Müller NL, Coleman N, Paré PD (eds): Fraser & Paré: Diagnosis of Diseases of the Chest. (ed 4) Philadelphia: WB Saunders, 1999
4. Reed JC: Chest Radiology. Plain Film Patterns and Differential Diagnoses. (ed 4) St. Louis: Mosby-Year Book, 1997, pp 328–345
5. Reeder MM, Hochholzer L, Evans RG: RPC of the Month from the AFIP: Amyloid tumor of the lung. Radiology 1969;93:1369–1375
6. Siegelman SS, Zerhouni EA, Leo FP, et al: CT of the solitary pulmonary nodule. AJR 1980; 135:1–13
7. Steele JD: The Solitary Pulmonary Nodule. Springfield, IL: CC Thomas, 1964
8. Theodore AC, Snider GL: When a routine exam reveals a solitary pulmonary nodule. J Resp Dis 1984; 15–25
9. Toomes H, Delphendahl A, Manke H-G, et al: The coin lesion of the lung. A review of 955 resected coin lesions. Cancer 1983; 51:534–537

Gamut F-38

SOLITARY PULMONARY MASS (GREATER THAN 4 CM DIAMETER)

COMMON

*1. Abscess of lung (pyogenic or amebic)
*2. Carcinoma of lung (bronchogenic or bronchioloalveolar)
*3. Metastasis (esp. from sarcoma; melanoma; carcinoma of breast, colon, kidney, testis)
4. Round pneumonia

UNCOMMON

*1. Adenomatoid malformation (fluid-filled)
*2. Amyloidosis
3. Arteriovenous malformation
*4. Bulla (fluid-filled)
5. Carcinoid$_g$
6. [Chest wall lesion (eg, lipoma; rib lesion); breast implant or prosthesis]
*7. Cyst, fluid-filled (eg, bronchial; bronchiectatic) *
8. [Diaphragmatic hernia]
9. [Encapsulated pleural fluid; interlobar effusion; fibrin ball]
*10. Fungus ball (esp. *Aspergillus*)
*11. Fungus disease (eg, cryptococcosis (torulosis); blastomycosis; histoplasmosis; coccidioidomycosis); actinomycosis, nocardiosis (See F-74-S)
12. Giant lymph node hyperplasia (Castleman disease)
*13. Granuloma (esp. tuberculoma; fungal)
14. Hamartoma
*15. Hematoma of lung
*16. Hydatid cyst
*17. Inflammatory pseudotumor$_g$; organized pneumonia
18. Lipoid pneumonia$_g$ (paraffinoma)
19. [Localized fibrous tumor of pleura; mesothelioma]

*20. Lymphoma$_g$
*21. [Mediastinal mass]
22. Neoplasm, benign (eg, spindle cell tumor$_g$)
23. Plasmacytoma, pulmonary
24. [Pleural plaque (eg, asbestos-related pleural disease)]
25. Pneumoconiosis (conglomerate mass from silicosis or coal-worker's pneumoconiosis; also asbestosis) (See F-70-S)
26. Pulmonary blastoma
*27. Pulmonary infarct
*28. Pulmonary sequestration (intralobar)
29. Radiation pneumonitis (nodular)
30. Rounded atelectasis
31. Sarcoma of lung (eg, leiomyosarcoma; rhabdomyosarcoma);
*32. Wegener granulomatosis$_g$

* May have cystic appearance or cavitation.
[ ] This condition does not actually cause the gamuted imaging finding, but can produce imaging changes that simulate it.

References

1. Felson B: Chest Roentgenology. Philadelphia: WB Saunders, 1973
2. Fraser RG, Pare JAP, Pare PD, Fraser RS: Differential Diagnosis of Diseases of the Chest. Philadelphia: WB Saunders, 1991, pp 49–58
3. Fraser RS, Müller NL, Coleman N, Paré PD (eds): Fraser & Paré: Diagnosis of Diseases of the Chest. (ed 4) Philadelphia: WB Saunders, 1999
4. Reed JC: Chest Radiology. Plain Film Patterns and Differential Diagnoses. (ed 4) St. Louis: Mosby-New York, 1997
5. Reeder MM, Hochholzer L, Evans RG: RPC of the Month from the AFIP: Amyloid tumor of the lung. Radiology 1969;93:1369–1375
6. Steele JD: The Solitary Pulmonary Nodule. Springfield, IL: CC Thomas, 1964

Gamut F-39

SUPERIOR SULCUS LESION

COMMON

1. [Artifact (eg, hair braid)]
2. Bulla or bleb
3. Fracture of rib, clavicle, or spine (incl. hematoma and callus)
4. Hemorrhage, extrapleural (eg, trauma; rupture of aorta or other great vessel)
5. Iatrogenic (esp. subclavian catheter perforation)
6. Metastasis
7. Neoplasm, benign (esp. lipoma; schwannoma; neurofibroma)
8. Neoplasm, malignant (esp. bronchogenic carcinoma—Pancoast tumor; rarely liposarcoma)
9. Neoplasm of rib, clavicle, or spine
10. [Normal variant; apical cap; subclavian artery]
11. Pleural thickening or fluid (eg, tuberculosis)
12. Pneumothorax (apical)

UNCOMMON

1. Abscess, esp. extrapleural with osteomyelitis of rib
2. Arteriovenous fistula
3. Cervical lesion with extension (eg, infection; thyroid goiter or neoplasm)
4. Dilated great vessel (eg, subclavian artery with coarctation of aorta)
5. Localized fibrous tumor of the pleura; mesothelioma
6. Lymphoma$_g$
7. Mediastinal fat extension (eg, steroid lipomatosis)
8. Radiation reaction (esp. therapy for carcinoma of breast)
9. Spinal fluid leakage (eg, neoplasm; fracture; avulsion of nerve root)
10. Spinal lesion extension (eg, tuberculosis; metastasis)

[ ] This condition does not actually cause the gamuted imaging finding, but can produce imaging changes that simulate it.

(continued)

References
1. Gondos B: The left apical cap (Letter to the editor). Radiology 1982;142:254
2. McLoud TC, Isler RJ, Novelline RA, et al: Review: the apical cap. AJR 1981;137:299–306

Gamut F-40

MASS-LIKE PERIHILAR OR CENTRAL PULMONARY OPACITY OR LESION RADIATING FROM THE HILUM

COMMON

1. Bronchogenic carcinoma
2. Lymphadenopathy, hilar (See F-103, 104)
3. Lymphoma$_g$
4. Metastasis
5. Pneumonia (incl. chronic aspiration)
6. Pulmonary edema (See F-10)
7. Tuberculosis

UNCOMMON

1. Alveolar proteinosis (rarely)
2. Fungus disease (esp. actinomycosis; blastomycosis)
3. Lipoid pneumonia$_g$
4. Pneumoconiosis (conglomerate mass of silicosis or coal-worker's pneumoconiosis)
5. Pulmonary hemorrhage (eg, bleeding or clotting disorder$_g$; hemolytic-uremic S.) (See F-12)

Gamut F-41

SHAGGY PULMONARY NODULE OR MASS WITH FUZZY BORDERS, SOLITARY OR MULTIPLE

COMMON

1. Abscess of lung; infected bulla or cyst
2. Carcinoma of lung (bronchogenic; bronchioloalveolar)
3. Fungus disease (eg, histoplasmosis; coccidioidomycosis; blastomycosis; cryptococcosis (torulosis); actinomycosis; nocardiosis (See F-74-S)
4. Metastasis (esp. choriocarcinoma)
5. Pneumoconiosis with conglomerate mass (eg, silicosis; coal-worker's pneumoconiosis; asbestosis; talcosis)
6. Pulmonary infarct, bland or septic
7. Round pneumonia
8. Tuberculosis

UNCOMMON

1. Amyloidosis
2. Hematoma of lung (esp. traumatic)
3. Inflammatory pseudotumor$_g$
4. Lipoid pneumonia$_g$
5. Lymphoma$_g$
6. Parasitic disease (esp. amebic abscess; complicated hydatid cyst; paragonimiasis)
7. Postoperative scar
8. Pulmonary sequestration (intralobar)
9. Radiation-treated carcinoma
10. Rheumatoid nodule
11. Rounded atelectasis
12. Sarcoidosis ("alveolar" pattern)
13. Wegener granulomatosis$_g$

Reference
1. Fraser RS, Müller NL, Coleman N, Paré PD (eds): Fraser & Paré: Diagnosis of Diseases of the Chest. (ed 4) Philadelphia: WB Saunders, 1999

Gamut F-42

MULTIPLE DISCRETE PULMONARY NODULES OR MASSES (NONMILIARY)

COMMON

1. Bronchioloalveolar carcinoma
2. [Chest wall lesions (neurofibromatosis; nipple shadows; rib lesions); foreign bodies; artifacts]
*3. Fungus disease (esp. histoplasmosis; coccidioidomycosis) (See F-74-S)
*4. Metastases
*5. Tuberculosis

UNCOMMON

1. Abscesses of lung (usually staphylococcal); bacillary angiomatosis (*Bartomella henselae*)
*2. Amyloidosis
3. Arteriovenous malformations or fistulas; varices; pulmonary arterial coarctations
4. Bronchiectatic cysts, fluid-filled
5. [Encapsulated pleural effusions]
6. Gaucher disease; Niemann-Pick disease
*7. Hamartomas (incl. Carney's triad)
8. Hematomas of lung
9. Hydatid cysts
10. Kaposi sarcoma
11. Langerhans cell histiocytosis (eosinophilic granuloma)
*12. Leiomyomatosis (benign metastasizing leiomyomas)
13. Lipoid pneumonia_g
14. Lymphoma_g
15. Measles, atypical with round nodule complexes
16. Melioidosis
17. Mucoid impactions (esp. allergic bronchopulmonary aspergillosis)
18. Mucus plugs (eg, cystic fibrosis {mucoviscidosis})
19. Multiple myeloma (plasmacytomas)
20. Papillomatosis of lung
*21. Paragonimiasis
22. Pneumoconiosis (eg, conglomerate masses in silicosis or coal-worker's pneumoconiosis; asbestosis; talcosis; stannosis; berylliosis)
23. Polyarteritis nodosa
*24. Pulmonary hemosiderosis with ossification (eg, mitral stenosis)
25. Pulmonary infarcts
26. Rheumatoid nodules (incl. Caplan S.)
27. Sarcoidosis
28. Septic emboli
29. Wegener granulomatosis_g

* May be calcified.
[ ] This condition does not actually cause the gamuted imaging finding, but can produce imaging changes that simulate it.

Gamut F-43-1

SHARPLY DEFINED CAVITARY LESION(S) OF THE LUNG—THIN-WALLED

	NUMBER
COMMON	
1. Abscess of lung (bacterial, fungal, septic, amebic, opportunistic)	SM
2. Bronchogenic carcinoma	S
3. Bulla; bleb	SM
4. Cystic bronchiectasis	M
5. Fungus disease (esp. coccidioidomycosis) (See F-74-S); fungus ball (esp. *Aspergillus*)	SM
	S
6. Honeycomb lung (See F-22)	M
7. Metastasis	SM
8. Pneumatocele (esp. staphylococcal or hydrocarbon pneumonia; traumatic) (See F-48)	SM
9. *Pneumocystis carinii* pneumonia (esp. in AIDS)	SM
10. Tuberculosis (incl. granuloma)	SM
UNCOMMON	
1. Amyloidosis	SM
2. Behçet syndrome	M
3. Cyst (eg, bronchial)	S

(continued)

 4. Cystic adenomatoid malformation M
 5. Cystic fibrosis (mucoviscidosis) M
 6. [Diaphragmatic hernia] S
 7. Langerhans cell histiocytosis$_g$ M
 8. Hydatid cyst SM
 9. [Hydropneumothorax, encapsulated SM
    (incl. interlobar bronchopleural fistula);
    loculated pneumothorax]
10. Inflammatory pseudotumor$_g$ S
11. Lymphoma$_g$ (esp. Hodgkin lymphoma) SM
12. Melioidosis SM
13. Papillomatosis of lung M
14. Parasitic disease, other SM
    (esp. paragonimiasis)
15. [Plombage, lucite] M
16. Polyarteritis nodosa; lupus M
    erythematosus
17. Pulmonary infarct SM
18. Pulmonary sequestration (intralobar) SM
19. Rheumatoid nodule SM
20. Sarcoidosis (cystic) M
21. Septic embolus SM
22. Traumatic lung cyst (hematoma; SM
    laceration)
23. Wegener granulomatosis$_g$ SM

[ ] This condition does not actually cause the gamuted imaging finding, but can produce imaging changes that simulate it.

References

 1. Castaneda-Zuniga WR, Hogan MT: Cavitary pulmonary nodules in systemic lupus erythematosus. Radiology 1976; 118:45–48
 2. Felson B: Chest Roentgenology. Philadelphia: WB Saunders, 1973
 3. Fraser RG, Paré JAP, Paré PD, Fraser RS: Differential Diagnosis of Diseases of the Chest. Philadelphia: WB Saunders, 1991, pp 31–38
 4. Fraser RS, Müller NL, Coleman N, Paré PD (eds): Fraser & Paré: Diagnosis of Diseases of the Chest. (ed 4) Philadelphia: WB Saunders, 1999
 5. Godwin JD, Webb WR, Savoca CJ, et al: Multiple, thin-walled cystic lesions of the lung. AJR 1980;135:593–604
 6. Woodring JH, Fried AM: Significance of wall thickness in solitary cavities of the lung: A follow-up study. AJR 1983; 140:473–474

Gamut F-43-2

SHARPLY DEFINED CAVITARY LESION(S) OF THE LUNG— THICK-WALLED

COMMON	NUMBER
1. Abscess of lung (bacterial— staphylococcal, *klebsiella* pseudomonas, proteus; fungal; septic; amebic; opportunistic)	SM
2. Bronchogenic carcinoma	S
3. Cystic bronchiectasis	M
4. Fungus disease (esp. coccidioido-mycosis) (See F-74-S)	SM
5. Metastasis	SM
6. Tuberculosis (incl. granuloma)	SM

UNCOMMON

1. Amyloidosis	SM
2. Cystic adenomatoid malformation	M
3. Cystic fibrosis (mucoviscidosis)	M
4. Hydatid cyst	SM
5. [Hydropneumothorax, encapsulated (incl. interlobar bronchopleural fistula); loculated pneumothorax]	SM
6. Inflammatory pseudotumor$_g$	S
7. Lymphoma$_g$ (esp. Hodgkin lymphoma)	SM
8. Melioidosis	SM
9. Papillomatosis of lung	M
10. Parasitic disease, other (esp. para-gonimiasis, dirofilariasis)	SM
11. Pneumoconiosis (silicosis or coal-worker's pneumoconiosis with conglomerate mass)	S
12. Pneumonia, cavitating	SM
13. Pulmonary infarct	SM
14. Pulmonary sequestration (intralobar)	SM
15. Rheumatoid nodule	SM
16. Septic embolus	SM
17. Traumatic lung cyst (hematoma; laceration)	SM
18. Wegener granulomatosis$_g$	SM

[ ] This condition does not actually cause the gamuted imaging finding, but can produce imaging changes that simulate it.

References

1. Felson B: Chest Roentgenology. Philadelphia: WB Saunders, 1973
2. Fraser RG, Paré JAP, Paré PD, Fraser RS: Differential Diagnosis of Diseases of the Chest. Philadelphia: WB Saunders, 1991, pp 31–38
3. Fraser RS, Müller NL, Coleman N, Paré PD (eds): Fraser & Paré: Diagnosis of Diseases of the Chest. (ed 4) Philadelphia: WB Saunders, 1999
4. Woodring JH, Fried AM: Significance of wall thickness in solitary cavities of the lung: A follow-up study. AJR 1983; 140:473–474

Gamut F-44

CYST-LIKE OR CAVITARY PULMONARY LESION(S) IN AN INFANT OR CHILD

COMMON

1. Abscess of lung (eg, bacterial or amebic)
2. Bronchopulmonary dysplasia (sequel to RDS—ventilator lung); Wilson-Mikity S.; interstitial pulmonary emphysema
3. Cystic bronchiectasis (eg, cystic fibrosis {mucoviscidosis})
4. Pneumatocele (See F-48)
5. Pneumonia with cavitation (eg, staphylococcus; pseudomonas; *Klebsiella; S. pneumoniae;* bacteroides; mycoplasma; cold agglutinin; or opportunistic—*Pneumocystis carinii* in AIDS; *Aspergillus; Candida;* zygomycosis)
6. Pulmonary sequestration (intralobar)
7. Tuberculosis

UNCOMMON

1. Bronchial or bronchogenic cyst
2. Bulla; bleb
3. [Congenital lobar emphysema]
4. Cystic adenomatoid malformation

5. [Diaphragmatic or paraesophageal hiatal hernia]
6. [Eventration with elevation of air-filled stomach]
7. Fungus disease (esp. coccidioidomycosis) (See F-74-S); fungus ball (esp. *Aspergillus*)
8. Honeycomb lung (eg, Langerhans cell histiocytosis$_g$)
9. Kartagener S. with bronchiectasis
10. Lymphoma$_g$ (eg, Hodgkin disease)
11. Metastasis
12. Mounier-Kuhn S. (tracheobronchomegaly)
13. Papillomatosis (laryngeal or tracheobronchial with spread to lungs)
14. Parasitic disease (esp. hydatid disease; paragonimiasis) (See F-74-S)
15. [Pneumothorax, loculated]
16. Pulmonary blastoma
17. Rheumatoid nodules with cavitation
18. Septic embolus
19. Traumatic lung cyst (laceration of lung)
20. Williams-Campbell S. with saccular bronchiectasis

[ ] This condition does not actually cause the gamuted imaging finding, but can produce imaging changes that simulate it.

References

1. Coussement AM, Gooding GA: Cavitating pulmonary metastatic disease in children. AJR 1973;117:833–839
2. Ebel KD, Blickman H, Willich E, Richter E: Differential Diagnosis in Pediatric Radiology. New York: Thieme, 1999, pp 82–90
3. Godwin JD, Webb WR, Savoca CJ, et al: Multiple, thin-walled cystic lesions of the lung. AJR 1980;135:593–604
4. Kaufman HJ, Mahboubi S: Unusual air distribution patterns in prematures on positive pressure ventilation. Ann Radiol 1975;18:431–438

Gamut F-45

SOLITARY CAVITARY PULMONARY LESION (CYST, NODULE, OR MASS) WITH A SHARP OUTLINE (See F-43-2)

COMMON

1. Abscess (eg, bacterial or amebic)
2. Bronchogenic carcinoma
3. Bulla; bleb
4. Fungus disease (esp. coccidioidomycosis)
5. Metastasis
6. Opportunistic infection (esp. fungus such as *Crypto-coccus; Candida;* zygomycosis; fungus ball—esp. *Aspergillus*) (See F-75-S)
7. Pneumatocele (See F-48)
8. Tuberculosis

UNCOMMON

1. Amyloidosis
2. Behçet syndrome
3. Cyst (bronchial or traumatic)
4. Granuloma
5. Hamartoma
6. Hydatid cyst
7. [Hydropneumothorax, encapsulated]
8. Lymphoma$_g$ (esp. Hodgkin disease)
9. Parasitic disease, other (eg, paragonimiasis; dirofilariasis immitis)
10. Pulmonary blastoma
11. Pulmonary infarct
12. Rheumatoid nodule
13. Sequestration of lung (intralobar)
14. Wegener granulomatosis$_g$

[ ] This condition does not actually cause the gamuted imaging finding, but can produce imaging changes that simulate it.

References

1. Lubbers DL: Gamut: Solitary pulmonary nodule with cavitation. Semin Roentgenol 1984;19:160–161
2. Woodring JH, Fried AM: Significance of wall thickness in solitary cavities of the lung: A follow-up study. AJR 1983; 140:473–474

Gamut F-46

SOLITARY CAVITARY LESION OF THE LUNG WITH A SHAGGY (IRREGULAR OR SPICULATED) OUTLINE

COMMON

1. Abscess (bacterial; amebic; opportunistic infection)
2. Carcinoma (bronchogenic; bronchioloalveolar)
3. Fungus disease (esp. coccidioidomycosis) (See F-74-S)
4. Metastasis
5. Pneumatocele, infected (See F-48)
6. Pulmonary infarct
7. Sequestration of lung (intralobar)
8. Tuberculosis

UNCOMMON

1. [Diaphragmatic hernia]
2. Granuloma (incl. idiopathic)
3. Hematoma
4. [Hydropneumothorax, encapsulated]
5. Lymphoma$_g$ (esp. Hodgkin disease)
6. Parasitic disease (eg, hydatid cyst—esp. infected; *Paragonimus* cyst)
7. Pneumoconiosis (conglomerate mass of silicosis or coal-worker's pneumoconiosis)
8. Pneumonia, localized (eg, staphylococcal; *Klebsiella;* aspiration)
9. Rheumatoid nodule
10. Wegener granulomatosis$_g$

[ ] This condition does not actually cause the gamuted imaging finding, but can produce imaging changes that simulate it.

Gamut F-47-S

PREDISPOSING FACTORS FOR A LUNG ABSCESS

DEPRESSED GAG REFLEX

1. Alcoholism
2. Anesthesia; postoperative state
3. Cerebral disease (eg, stroke; neoplasm)
4. Debilitation
5. Drug abuse
6. Epilepsy; other convulsive disorders
7. Intubation (eg, indwelling nasogastric tube)

UPPER AIRWAY INFECTION

1. Gingivitis
2. Tonsillitis

ESOPHAGOGASTRIC DISEASE WITH ASPIRATION

1. Achalasia
2. Chalasia (gastroesophageal regurgitation)
3. Other esophageal disease (eg, scleroderma)
4. Peptic disease
5. Tracheoesophageal fistula

PULMONARY DISEASE

1. Actinomycosis; nocardiosis
2. Bronchiectasis
3. Bronchogenic carcinoma
4. Cystic fibrosis (mucoviscidosis)
5. Foreign body (eg, peanut in bronchus)
6. Fungus disease (eg, blastomycosis; aspergillosis; coccidioidomycosis; cryptococcosis; zygomycosis) (See F-74-S)
7. Immotile cilia S.; Kartagener S.
8. Immunosuppression; opportunistic infection (See F-75-S)
9. Parasitic disease (esp. amebiasis; hydatid disease) (See F-74-S)

10. Pneumonia (esp. staphylococcal; *Klebsiella; E. coli;* pseudomonas; proteus; aspiration)
11. Sequestration of lung (intralobar)
12. Tuberculosis

MISCELLANEOUS

1. Antitrypsinase deficiency
2. Sickle cell disease

Reference
1. Arms RA, Dines DE, Tinstman TC: Aspiration pneumonia. Chest 1974; 65:136–139

Gamut F-48

PNEUMATOCELE

1. Hemorrhage in lung with interstitial emphysema
2. Hydrocarbon aspiration$_g$
3. Hyperimmunoglobulinemia E syndrome (Buckley S. or Job S.)
4. Pneumonia (eg, staphylococcal; pneumococcal; *Klebsiella; E. coli;* legionella; *H. influenzae;* viral; *Pneumocystis carinii*)
5. Pulmonary infarct
6. Respirator therapy
7. Trauma (contusion, laceration or hematoma of lung)
8. Tuberculosis

References
1. Albelda SM, Gefter WB, Kelley MA, et al: Ventilator-induced subpleural air cysts: Clinical, radiographic, and pathologic significance. Am Rev Respir Dis 1983;127:360–365
2. Dines DE: Diagnostic significance of pneumatocele of the lung. JAMA 1968;204:79–82
3. Fagan CJ, Swischuk LE: Traumatic lung and paramediastinal pneumatoceles. Radiology 1976;120:11–18

MULTIPLE LUCENT OR CAVITARY LESIONS OF THE LUNG (See F-43, 44)

COMMON

1. Bronchiectasis
2. Bullae; blebs
3. Fungus disease (esp. coccidioidomycosis) (See F-74-S)
4. Honeycomb lung (end-stage interstitial fibrosis) (See F-22)
5. [Hydropneumothorax, encapsulated; pneumothorax, loculated]
6. Metastases, necrotic
7. Opportunistic infection (esp. *Pneumocystis carinii;* fungus disease; pseudomonas) (See F-75-S)
8. Pneumatoceles (See F-48)
9. Pulmonary thromboembolism with infarcts
10. Septic emboli or abscesses (eg, narcotic addiction)
11. Tuberculosis (incl. atypical mycobacterial infection)

UNCOMMON

1. Abscesses (usually staphylococcal)
2. Amyloidosis
3. Carcinoma of lung, primary multicentric
4. Cystic adenomatoid malformation
5. [Diaphragmatic hernia]
6. Granulomas
7. Hydatid cysts
8. Langerhans cell histiocytosis (eosinophilic granuloma)
9. Lymphoma$_g$ (eg, Hodgkin disease); lymphomatoid granulomatosis
10. Melioidosis
11. Papillomatosis (laryngeal or tracheobronchial with spread to lungs)
12. Paragonimiasis
13. Pneumoconiosis (coal-worker's pneumoconiosis or silicosis with conglomerate masses; progressive massive fibrosis)

14. Pulmonary lymphangioleiomyomatosis; tuberous sclerosis
15. Rheumatoid nodules
16. Sarcoidosis (cystic form)
17. Wegener granulomatosis$_g$; pulmonary angiitis and granulomatosis

[ ] This condition does not actually cause the gamuted imaging finding, but can produce imaging changes that simulate it.

References

1. Felson B: Chest Roentgenology. Philadelphia: WB Saunders, 1973
2. Fraser RG, Paré JAP, Paré PD, Fraser RS: Differential Diagnosis of Diseases of the Chest. Philadelphia: WB Saunders, 1991, pp 31–38, 59–64
3. Fraser RS, Müller NL, Coleman N, Paré PD (eds): Fraser & Paré: Diagnosis of Diseases of the Chest. (ed 4) Philadelphia: WB Saunders, 1999
4. Godwin JD, Webb WR, Savoca CJ, et al: Multiple, thin-walled cystic lesions of the lung. AJR 1980;135:593–604

EXTENSIVE PULMONARY OPACITY WITH CAVITATION (DESTRUCTIVE PATTERN) (See F-46)

COMMON

1. Abscess of lung, acute or chronic (eg, bacterial; amebic; aspiration)
2. Bronchial obstruction with distal abscess (eg, from bronchogenic carcinoma; carcinoid; lymphadenopathy; foreign body; bronchial stricture)
3. [Bronchiectasis, esp. cystic]
4. Bronchogenic carcinoma
5. Fungus disease, primary (eg, blastomycosis; coccidioidomycosis; cryptococcosis; zygomycosis) or opportunistic (*Aspergillus; Candida*) (See F-74-S)
6. Pneumonia (esp. *Pneumocystis carinii; Staphylococcus aureus; Klebsiella*)
7. Sepsis

8. Traumatic laceration of lung
9. Tuberculosis (incl. atypical mycobacterial infection)

UNCOMMON

1. Actinomycosis; nocardiosis
2. Gangrene of lung; infarcted pneumonia (esp. *Klebsiella*)
3. Pulmonary thromboembolism with infarction
4. Lymphoma$_g$ (esp. Hodgkin disease)
5. Melioidosis
6. Metastatic disease
7. Paragonimiasis
8. Sequestration of lung (intralobar)
9. Wegener granulomatosis$_g$

[ ] This condition does not actually cause the gamuted imaging finding, but can produce imaging changes that simulate it.

References

1. Fraser RS, Müller NL, Coleman N, Paré PD (eds): Fraser & Paré: Diagnosis of Diseases of the Chest. (ed 4) Philadelphia: WB Saunders, 1999
2. Godwin JD, Webb WR, Savoca CJ, et al: Multiple, thin-walled cystic lesions of the lung. AJR 1980;135:593–604
3. O'Reilly GV, Dee PH, Otteni GV: Gangrene of the lung: Successful medical management of three patients. Radiology 1978;126:575–579

Gamut F-51

MASS IN A PULMONARY CAVITY (MENISCUS OR BULL'S-EYE SIGN), MOBILE OR FIXED

COMMON

*1. Fungus ball (esp. *Aspergillus;* rarely *Cryptococcus; Candida;* Coccidioides)
*2. Hydatid cyst

UNCOMMON

*1. Abscess with inspissated pus
*2. Blood clot in a tuberculous cavity, pulmonary infarct, or laceration of lung

*3. Gangrene of lung; infarcted lung in cavity (esp. *Klebsiella;* angioinvasive fungal disease)
4. Neoplasm (bronchogenic carcinoma; pulmonary blastoma; sarcoma; metastasis)
5. Opportunistic infection (esp. fungus disease; *Pseudomonas;* nocardia)
*6. Paragonimiasis (worm in cyst—corona sign)

* Usually mobile.

References

1. Braman SS: Case records of the Massachusetts General Hospital. N Engl J Med 1983;310:178–187
2. Felson B: Chest Roentgenology. Philadelphia: WB Saunders, 1973
3. Fraser RS, Müller NL, Coleman N, Paré PD (eds): Fraser & Paré: Diagnosis of Diseases of the Chest. (ed 4) Philadelphia: WB Saunders, 1999
4. Reeder MM: RPC of the Month from the AFIP: Hydatid cyst of the lung. Radiology 1970;94:429–437

Gamut F-52

INCREASED RADIOLUCENCY OF BOTH LUNGS (BILATERAL HYPERINFLATION)

COMMON

1. Asthma
2. Bronchiolitis, acute diffuse of infants (usually viral)
3. Bronchitis, acute or chronic
4. Bronchopulmonary dysplasia sequela (eg, respirator lung)
5. Bullous emphysema, advanced ("vanishing lung" disease)
6. Congenital heart disease (esp. cyanotic—right-to-left shunts, esp. tetralogy of Fallot, pseudotruncus arteriosus; right heart obstruction; Eisenmenger physiology) (See E-8, E-18, E-19)
7. Cystic fibrosis (mucoviscidosis)
8. Emphysema, chronic obstructive (COPD)
9. Hyperventilation (eg, air hunger—metabolic disturbance; acidosis; dehydration; gastroenteritis)
10. Kyphosis (eg, senile "emphysema")

(continued)

11. Normal profound inspiration (eg, athlete; horn player)
12. Pectoral muscle absence, congenital (Poland syndrome) or surgical (bilateral mastectomy) or atrophy (eg, polio)
13. Pulmonary hypertension, primary or secondary
14. [Technical factors: overpenetrated film; thin patient]
15. Tracheal or laryngeal obstruction, stenosis, or compression (eg, foreign body; vascular ring; tumor—carcinoma, adenoid cystic carcinoma {cylindroma}, papilloma, hemangioma, cyst; mediastinal neoplasm, cyst, or lymphadenopathy; tracheobronchomegaly; tracheomalacia; cutis laxa; congenital, posttraumatic, postintubation or tracheostomy stenosis; saber-sheath trachea; relapsing polychondritis) (See F-81-1, 83)

UNCOMMON

1. Bronchiolitis obliterans
2. Bronchiolitis, other (eg, thermal; graft versus host disease)
3. Bronchopneumonia, infantile diffuse, with hyperinflation (eg, measles, influenza, pertussis)
4. Immunologic disorder$_g$; antitrypsin deficiency
5. Pulmonary thromboembolism, central or widespread
6. Tracheoesophageal fistula

[ ] This condition does not actually cause the gamuted imaging finding, but can produce imaging changes that simulate it.

References

1. Ebel KD, Blickman H, Willich E, Richter E: Differential Diagnosis in Pediatric Radiology. New York: Thieme, 1999, pp 14–17
2. Eisenberg RL: Clinical Imaging: An Atlas of Differential Diagnosis. (ed 3) Philadelphia: Lippincott-Raven, 1997
3. Felson B: Chest Roentgenology. Philadelphia: WB Saunders, 1973
4. Reed JC: Chest Radiology. Plain Film Patterns and Differential Diagnoses. (ed 4) St. Louis: Mosby-Year Book, 1997, pp 373–389
5. Swischuk LE, John SD: Differential Diagnosis in Pediatric Radiology. (ed 2) Baltimore: Williams & Wilkins, 1995, pp 1–6
6. Thurlbeck WM, Simon G: Radiographic appearance of the chest in emphysema. AJR 1978;130:427–440

UNILATERAL HYPERLUCENT SEGMENT, LOBE, LUNG, OR HEMITHORAX (See F-52)

COMMON

1. Compensatory distention of adjacent lobe or lung (secondary to lobar atelectasis, agenesis or hypoplasia, or lobectomy or shunting procedure)
2. [Contralateral increased density (eg, chest wall hemihypertrophy; pleural effusion)]
3. Emphysema, bullous or diffuse; large bulla
4. Emphysema, obstructive endobronchial with air trapping (eg, bronchial foreign body, stricture, atresia, granuloma; broncholith; mucus plug or mucoid impaction; neoplasm—bronchogenic carcinoma, carcinoid, endobronchial metastasis)
5. Normal variant
6. Pectoral muscle absence, congenital (eg, Poland syndrome) or surgical (mastectomy) or atrophy (eg, polio)
7. Pneumothorax
8. Scoliosis
9. [Technical factors: heel effect; lateral decubitus film; positioning (eg, patient rotation); grid cutoff]

UNCOMMON

1. Congenital lobar emphysema (See F-54)
2. Cystic adenomatoid malformation
3. [Diaphragmatic hernia]
4. Extrabronchial obstruction or compression (eg, mediastinal mass; hilar lymphadenopathy—tuberculosis, histoplasmosis, sarcoidosis, lymphoma, metastatic disease; anomalous vessels)
5. Pneumatocele (eg, staphylococcal pneumonia; hydrocarbon inhalation) (See F-48)
*6. Pulmonary artery atresia, hypoplasia, coarctation, branch stenosis or anomalous origin (eg, "pulmonary sling" with left PA arising from right PA)
*7. Pulmonary artery compression by inflammatory process or neoplasm

*8. Pulmonary sequestration (intralobar)
*9. Pulmonary vein atresia or stenosis
10. Pulmonary thromboembolism
*11. Swyer-James S.; bronchiolitis obliterans
*12. Venolobar S. (scimitar S.)

* Small hyperlucent hemithorax, especially in children.
[ ] This condition does not actually cause the gamuted imaging finding, but can produce imaging changes that simulate it.

References

1. Ebel KD, Blickman H, Willich E, Richter E: Differential Diagnosis in Pediatric Radiology. New York: Thieme, 1999, pp 18–27
2. Felson B: Chest Roentgenology. Philadelphia: WB Saunders, 1973
3. Gaensler EA: Unilateral hyperlucent lung. In: Simon M, Potchen J, LeMay M: Frontiers of Pulmonary Radiology. New York: Grune & Stratton, 1969
4. Reed JC: Chest Radiology. Plain Film Patterns and Differential Diagnoses. (ed 4) St. Louis: Mosby-Year Book, 1997, pp 373–389
5. Reid L, Simon G: Unilateral lung transradiancy. Thorax 1962; 17:230–239
6. Swischuk LE, John SD: Differential Diagnosis in Pediatric Radiology. (ed 2) Baltimore: Williams & Wilkins, 1995, pp 17–29

Gamut F-54

CONGENITAL LOBAR EMPHYSEMA (LOBAR AIR TRAPPING)

COMMON

1. Bronchial cartilage ring anomaly with partial collapse and air trapping (cartilage absence, hypoplasia, or malacia)
2. Idiopathic

UNCOMMON

1. Bronchial atresia (segmental)
2. Bronchial kinking; lobar torsion
3. Extrinsic pressure on bronchus (eg, bronchogenic cyst)

4. Foreign body in bronchus
5. Mucosal flap or enlarged fold in bronchus
6. Neoplasm of bronchus
7. Patent ductus arteriosus
8. Postinflammatory cyst
9. Pulmonary sling with left PA arising from right PA

References

1. Cremin BJ, Movsowitz H: Lobar emphysema in infants. Br J Radiol 1971;44:692–6962.
2. Fraser RS, Müller NL, Coleman N, Paré PD (eds): Fraser & Paré: Diagnosis of Diseases of the Chest. (ed 4) Philadelphia: WB Saunders, 1999

Gamut F-55

NEONATAL RESPIRATORY DISTRESS

COMMON

1. Aspiration of meconium or amniotic fluid
2. Congenital heart disease (esp. cyanotic)
3. Diaphragmatic hernia
4. Hyaline membrane disease (incl. its sequel—bronchopulmonary dysplasia)
5. Pneumonia
6. Pulmonary immaturity
7. Respirator therapy (eg, PEEP); shock lung; Wilson-Mikity S.
8. Transient tachypnea of the newborn (retained fetal alveolar fluid)

UNCOMMON

1. Choanal atresia
2. Congenital lobar emphysema
3. Cystic adenomatoid malformation
4. Eventration or paralysis of diaphragm
5. Laryngeal atresia
6. Neuromuscular disorder$_g$ (eg, Werdnig-Hoffmann disease)
7. Overly medicated mother
8. Persistent fetal circulation

(continued)

9. Pierre Robin S. (Robin sequence)
10. Pneumothorax; chylothorax
11. Pulmonary edema
12. Pulmonary hemorrhage
13. Pulmonary hypoplasia or agenesis (eg, asphyxiating thoracic dysplasia {Jeune S.}; short ribpolydactyly syndromes)
14. Pulmonary lymphangiectasia
15. Tracheoesophageal fistula
16. Vascular ring

References
1. Silverman FN, Kuhn JP (eds): Caffey's Pediatric X-ray Diagnosis. (ed 9) St. Louis: CV Mosby, 1993
2. Swischuk LE, John SD: Differential Diagnosis in Pediatric Radiology. (ed 2) Baltimore: Williams & Wilkins, 1995
3. Wesenberg RL: The Newborn Chest. Hagerstown, MD: Harper & Row, 1973

Gamut F-56

BUBBLY LUNGS IN INFANTS AND CHILDREN

COMMON

1. Bronchiectasis, cylindical or saccular (esp. cystic fibrosis; severe infections; chronic foreign bodies)
+2. Bronchopulmonary dysplasia
*3. Pulmonary interstitial emphysema from positive pressure ventilation

UNCOMMON

1. Cystic adenomatoid malformation
*2. Infantile respiratory distress S. (hyaline membrane disease) (tiny bubbles)
+3. Wilson-Mikity S.

* From overdistention of terminal bronchioles and alveolar ducts.
+ From uneven pattern of alveolar aeration.

Reference
1. Swischuk LE, John SD: Differential Diagnosis in Pediatric Radiology. (ed 2) Baltimore: Williams & Wilkins, 1995, pp 54–55

Gamut F-57

BILATERAL UNDERAERATION (Esp. in Children)

COMMON

1. Abdominal distention (eg, ascites; mass)
2. Poor inspiration

UNCOMMON

1. Bilateral eventration of diaphragm
2. Cheyne-Stokes breathing in neonate
3. Diaphragmatic paralysis (eg, polio; phrenic nerve injury or paralysis)
4. Inspiratory airway obstruction (eg, tracheal or laryngeal obstruction, stenosis, or compression) (See no. 15 in F-52)
5. Maternal oversedation in neonate
6. Neurologic disorder$_g$
7. Primary muscle disorder$_g$
8. Pulmonary hypoplasia in neonate

Reference
1. Swischuk LE, John SD: Differential Diagnosis in Pediatric Radiology. (ed 2) Baltimore: Williams & Wilkins, 1995, p 6.

Gamut F-58

ASYMMETRY OF LUNG SIZE

COMMON

1. Atelectasis (eg, bronchogenic carcinoma; carcinoid; foreign body or mucus plug in bronchus)
2. Displacement of hemidiaphragm by subphrenic mass or abscess, hepatomegaly, splenomegaly, distended stomach or colon
3. Emphysema, unilateral or asymmetrical (eg, bullous emphysema; ball-valve obstruction)
4. Eventration of hemidiaphragm
5. Phrenic nerve paralysis

6. Pleural effusion or malignancy, diffuse unilateral or asymmetrical (eg, mesothelioma; metastatic adeno-carcinoma; invasive thymoma)
7. Postoperative lobectomy or partial lung resection; fibrothorax
8. Pulmonary fibrosis, unilateral (eg, healed tuberculo-sis; postradiation)

UNCOMMON
1. Bronchial atresia or stenosis
2. Congenital lobar emphysema
3. Cystic adenomatoid malformation
4. Diaphragmatic hernia
5. Hypoplastic lung or pulmonary artery
6. Lung transplantation
7. Swyer-James S.
8. Thoracoplasty
9. Venolobar S. (scimitar S.)

Gamut F-59

LOCALIZED CHRONIC PULMONARY INFILTRATE

COMMON
1. Abscess of lung (bacterial, fungal, amebic)
2. Aspiration pneumonia, chronic (eg, neurologic or neuromuscular disorder$_g$; pharyngeal or esophageal disease—Zenker's diverticulum; achalasia; chalasia; hiatus hernia; esophageal atresia; tracheoesophageal fistula; scleroderma; carcinoma of esophagus) (See F-7)
3. Bronchial obstruction (eg, carcinoid; bronchogenic carcinoma; foreign body; stricture; mucus plug; mucoid impaction—*Aspergillus* sensitivity, asthma)
4. Bronchiectasis (See F-80)
5. Infection, esp. untreated or antibiotic resistant (eg, tuberculosis; fungus disease; *Klebsiella; Mycoplasma*)

6. Opportunistic infection (eg, in immune deficiency disorder$_g$; AIDS; steroid or immunosuppressive therapy) (See F-77)
7. Pneumonia, organized; inflammatory pseudotumor

UNCOMMON
1. Alveolar proteinosis
2. Bronchioloalveolar carcinoma
3. Cystic fibrosis (mucoviscidosis)
4. Foreign body in pulmonary tissue (eg, splinter, needle); lycoperdonosis
5. Idiopathic pulmonary fibrosis (IPF)
6. Lipoid pneumonia
7. Lymphoma$_g$
8. Parasitic disease (esp. amebiasis; paragonimiasis; ascariasis) (See F-74-S)
9. Pulmonary hemorrhage, late or recurrent (eg, hemo-philia; idiopathic pulmonary hemosiderosis)
10. Pulmonary sequestration (intralobar)
11. Radiation pneumonitis or fibrosis

References
1. Fraser RS, Müller NL, Coleman N, Paré PD (eds): Fraser & Paré: Diagnosis of Diseases of the Chest. (ed 4) Philadel-phia: WB Saunders, 1999
2. Swischuk LE, John SD: Differential Diagnosis in Pediatric Radiology. (ed 2) Baltimore: Williams & Wilkins, 1995

Gamut F-60

UNILATERAL DIFFUSE LUNG DISEASE

COMMON
*1. Aspiration, acute or chronic
2. Bronchiectasis (incl. destroyed lung of tubercu-losis)
*3. Contusion of lung
*4. Fungus disease (See F-74-S)
5. Metastases, esp. lymphangitic
6. Neoplasm, malignant (esp. bronchioloalveolar carcinoma)

(continued)

*7. Pneumonia (incl. opportunistic)
*8. Pulmonary edema (See F-10)
  9. Radiation therapy (eg, for breast or lung carcinoma)
*10. Tuberculosis

UNCOMMON

*1. Atelectasis, entire lung, central obstructive or nonobstructive (eg, postoperative, traumatic)
 2. Cystic adenomatoid malformation
 3. Cysts (esp. hydatid)
 4. Esophageal lung, congenital
 5. Lymphoma$_g$
*6. Pulmonary gangrene
*7. Pulmonary infarcts; septic emboli

* May be acute.

References
1. Fraser RS, Müller NL, Coleman N, Paré PD (eds): Fraser & Paré: Diagnosis of Diseases of the Chest. (ed 4) Philadelphia: WB Saunders, 1999
2. Youngberg AS: Unilateral diffuse lung opacity. Differential diagnosis with emphasis on lymphangitic spread of cancer. Radiology 1977;123:277–281

Gamut F-61

BILATERAL BASILAR PULMONARY DISEASE

COMMON

1. Asbestosis
2. Aspiration pneumonia (incl. hydrocarbon) (see F-7)
3. Atelectasis (eg, immobilization; splinting; post-cardiac surgery—usually unilateral LLL)
4. Bronchiectasis (often secondary to chronic pneumonia)
5. Connective tissue disease$_g$ (collagen vascular disease) (eg, scleroderma; rheumatoid lung; dermatomyositis; lupus erythematosus; Sjögren syndrome)

6. Interstitial fibrosis$_g$ [esp. idiopathic pulmonary fibrosis (IPF)]
7. Pulmonary edema (See F-10)
8. Viral pneumonia

UNCOMMON

 1. Alveolar proteinosis
 2. Bronchiolitis obliterans with organizing pneumonia (BOOP)
 3. Chemotherapy, other drugs (eg, methotrexate; busulfan; bleomycin; amiodarone; nitrofurantoin; BCNU—carmustine; methysergide; cyclophosphamide; procainamide) (See F-73-S)
 4. Desquamative interstitial pneumonitis (DIP); lymphocytic interstitial pneumonitis (LIP)
 5. Kaposi sarcoma
 6. Lipoid pneumonia$_g$
 7. Lymphomatoid granulomatosis
 8. Metastases (esp. lymphangitic)
 9. Neurofibromatosis
10. Nonspecific interstitial pneumonitis (NSIP) and nonspecific interstitial pulmonary fibrosis (NIPF)

References
1. Berkman YM: Aspiration and inhalation pneumonias. Semin Roentgenol 1980; 15:73–84
2. Fraser RS, Müller NL, Coleman N, Paré PD (eds): Fraser & Paré: Diagnosis of Diseases of the Chest. (ed 4) Philadelphia: WB Saunders, 1999

Gamut F-62

RETROCARDIAC LESION

COMMON

1. Aortic aneurysm or ectasia
2. Atelectasis of lower lobe
3. Diaphragmatic hernia (eg, hiatal; Bochdalek; traumatic)
4. Esophageal lesion (eg, carcinoma; leiomyoma; varices; achalasia)

5. Granuloma of lung (eg, tuberculoma; fungus disease, esp. histoplasmoma)
6. Left atrial enlargement
7. Lymphadenopathy (eg, inflammatory; lymphoma; metastatic disease)
8. Mediastinal lesion, middle or posterior (eg, bronchogenic cyst; lymphadenopathy; neurogenic tumor; thoracic kidney; extramedullary hematopoiesis) (See F-89, F-90)
9. Neoplasm of lung (eg, bronchogenic carcinoma; bronchioloalveolar carcinoma; carcinoid; hamartoma; metastasis)
10. Pleural effusion
11. Pneumonia or other disease in lower lobe (eg, aspiration pneumonia; tuberculosis; fungus disease; abscess of lung; bronchiectasis—esp. cystic)
12. Pulmonary infarct
13. Pulmonary sequestration (intralobar)
14. Spinal lesion (eg, osteoarthritic spurring; fracture; osteomyelitis; discogenic disease; hemangioma, sarcoma, myeloma or other primary or metastatic neoplasm); paraspinal abscess, hematoma, adenopathy or neoplasm)

UNCOMMON

1. Azygos vein dilatation
2. Cardiac tumor or aneurysm (esp. left ventricular)
3. Cystic adenomatoid malformation
4. Hydatid cyst
5. Neoplasm of pleura (eg, mesothelioma; localized fibrous tumor of pleura; metastasis)

Gamut F-63

BLURRING OF THE HEART BORDER ON PA CHEST FILM

COMMON

1. Idiopathic
2. Infiltrate or edema in left lingula, right middle lobe, or anterior segment of an upper lobe

3. Mediastinal lesion, anterior (eg, thymoma; thymic cyst; thymolipoma; teratoma; lymphoma$_g$; pericardial cyst; lipoma; mediastinitis; fibrosis) (See F-88)
4. Normal or congested blood vessels (esp. right heart border)
5. Pericardial fat pad
6. Pleural fluid
7. Pleuropericardial adhesion; postinfarction myocardial scar
8. Pneumoconiosis (esp. asbestosis) (See F-70-S)

UNCOMMON

1. Hernia (hepatic or Morgagni)
2. Pectus excavatum; funnel breast
3. Pericarditis (constrictive)
4. Venolobar S. (scimitar S.)

Reference
1. Felson B: Chest Roentgenology. Philadelphia: WB Saunders, 1973

Gamut F-64

SUBPLEURAL OR PERIPHERAL LESION ARISING IN LUNG (See F-125)

COMMON

1. Asbestosis
2. Carcinoma of lung (esp. Pancoast tumor)
3. Eosinophilic pneumonia (Löffler syndrome; PIE)
4. Granuloma (eg, tuberculosis; histoplasmosis; coccidioidomycosis)
5. Metastasis
6. Pulmonary infarct
7. Rounded atelectasis

UNCOMMON

1. Actinomycosis; nocardiosis
2. Fungus disease (eg, cryptococcosis {torulosis})
3. Inflammatory pseudotumor$_g$; organized pneumonia

(continued)

4. Lymphoma$_g$
5. [Mesothelioma; localized fibrous tumor of pleura]
6. Pulmonary sequestration (intralobar)
7. Rheumatoid nodule
8. Wegener granulomatosis$_g$

Reference

1. Reed JC: Chest Radiology. Plain Film Patterns and Differential Diagnoses. (ed 4) St. Louis: Mosby-Year Book, 1997

[ ] This condition does not actually cause the gamuted imaging finding, but can produce imaging changes that simulate it.

Gamut F-65

LONG LINEAR OR CURVILINEAR SHADOW(S) IN THE LUNG

COMMON

1. Azygos lobe (rarely hemiazygos lobe on left)
2. Bronchial wall thickening, enlarged bronchus (eg, chronic bronchitis, bronchiectasis—"tram lines")
3. Bulla, pneumatocele, or thin-walled cavity (partially visible)
4. Interlobar fissure, normal or thickened or fluid-filled; accessory fissure
5. Kerley lines
6. Linear (plate-like, discoid) atelectasis, transverse or vertical (Fleischner line)
7. Lymphangitic carcinomatosis
8. Pneumothorax (edge of lung)
9. Pulmonary artery or vein (eg, scimitar syndrome; arteriovenous malformation; other anomalous vessel)
10. Scar (linear)
11. [Skin fold; artifact]

UNCOMMON

1. Bronchial artery (eg, cyanotic congenital heart disease)
2. Mucoid impaction in bronchus

3. Paragonimiasis (with worm burrows or bronchiectasis)
4. [Pleural band or scar]

[ ] This condition does not actually cause the gamuted imaging finding, but can produce imaging changes that simulate it.

References

1. Fleischner F, Hampton AD, Castleman B: Linear shadows in the lung (interlobar pleuritis, atelectasis and healed infarction). AJR 1941;46:610–618
2. Fraser RS, Müller NL, Coleman N, Paré PD (eds): Fraser & Paré: Diagnosis of Diseases of the Chest. (ed 4) Philadelphia: WB Saunders, 1999
3. Simon G: Further observations on the long line shadow across a lower zone of the lung. Br J Radiol 1970;43:327–332
4. Sutton D: Textbook of Radiology and Imaging. (ed 6) New York: Churchill Livingstone, 1998, pp 321–323
5. Trapnell DH: The differential diagnosis of linear shadows in chest radiographs. Radiol Clin North Am 1973;11:77–92

Gamut F-66

COMBINED SKIN AND WIDESPREAD LUNG OR PLEURAL DISORDER

COMMON

1. Chickenpox; measles
2. Connective tissue disease (collagen vascular disease)$_g$ (esp. scleroderma; lupus erythematosus, rheumatoid arthritis, dermatomyositis)
3. Immunologic disorder$_g$; congenital or acquired (esp. AIDS)
4. Malignant neoplasm of skin with metastasis (eg, melanoma; squamous cell carcinoma)
5. Radiation therapy
6. Sarcoidosis

UNCOMMON

1. Acanthosis nigricans
2. Amyloidosis
3. Bleeding or clotting disorder$_g$
4. Burn

5. Cutis laxa
6. Drug reaction; chemotherapy
7. Ectodermal dysplasia
8. Ehlers-Danlos S.
9. Erythema nodosum; erythema multiforme
10. Fungus disease (eg, candidiasis; blastomycosis) (See F-74-S)
11. Kaposi sarcoma
12. Langerhans cell histiocytosis$_g$
13. Lymphoma; leukemia; mycosis fungoides
14. Melioidosis
15. Neurofibromatosis
16. Osler-Weber-Rendu S. (familial telangiectasia)
17. Parasitic disease (eg, amebiasis; acute schistosomiasis; strongyloidiasis)
18. Progeria
19. Tuberous sclerosis
20. Wegener granulomatosis$_g$
21. Yellow nail S.

References

1. Fraser RS, Müller NL, Coleman N, Paré PD (eds): Fraser & Paré: Diagnosis of Diseases of the Chest. (ed 4) Philadelphia: WB Saunders, 1999
2. Ruben EG, Siegelman SS: The Lungs in Systemic Diseases. Springfield, IL: CC Thomas, 1969
3. Taybi H, Lachman RS: Radiology of Syndromes, Metabolic Disorders, and Skeletal Dysplasias. (ed 4) St. Louis: Mosby-Year Book, 1996

Gamut F-67

COMBINED LUNG AND BONE DISORDER

COMMON

1. Bronchogenic carcinoma with thoracic or extra-thoracic bone metastasis
2. Connective tissue disease (collagen disease)$_g$ (esp. scleroderma; dermatomyositis)
3. Immunologic disorder$_g$ (esp. AIDS; chronic granulomatous disease of childhood)
4. Infection (eg, osteomyelitis and pneumonia; septic emboli)
5. Langerhans cell histiocytosis$_g$ (eosinophilic granuloma)
6. Lymphoma$_g$; leukemia
7. Metastatic disease
8. Rheumatoid arthritis
9. Sarcoidosis
10. Sickle cell disease; other primary anemia
11. Trauma
12. Tuberculosis (incl. atypical mycobacterial infection)

UNCOMMON

1. Actinomycosis; nocardiosis
2. Amyloidosis; plasma cell dyscrasia
3. Ankylosing spondylitis
4. Asphyxiating thoracic dysplasia (Jeune S.) and other congenital bone dysplasias (eg, thanatophoric dysplasia; chondroectodermal dysplasia {Ellis-van Creveld S.})
5. Cystic fibrosis (mucoviscidosis)
6. Drug addiction (sepsis)
7. Ehlers-Danlos S.; Marfan S.; homocystinuria; cutis laxa
8. Farber's disease (disseminated lipogranulomatosis)
9. Fat embolism (traumatic)
10. Fungus disease (esp. blastomycosis; coccidioidomycosis; histoplasmosis) (See F-74-S)
11. Gaucher disease; Niemann-Pick disease
12. Hyperparathyroidism
13. Melioidosis
14. Multiple myeloma
15. Neurofibromatosis
16. Parasitic disease (esp. hydatid disease—*Echinococcus granulosus*)
17. Radiation fibrosis and osteitis
18. Rubella S.
19. Steroid therapy
20. Tuberous sclerosis
21. Wegener granulomatosis$_g$

(continued)

References

1. Edeiken J, Dalinka M, Karasick D: Edeiken's Roentgen Diagnosis of Diseases of Bone. (ed 4) Baltimore: Williams & Wilkins, 1989
2. Fraser RS, Müller NL, Coleman N, Paré PD (eds): Fraser & Paré: Diagnosis of Diseases of the Chest. (ed 4) Philadelphia: WB Saunders, 1999
3. Garrett MK: Gamut: Combined lung and bone disorder. Semin Roentgenol 1985; 20:323–324
4. Murray RO, Jacobson HG, Stoker DJ: The Radiology of Skeletal Disorders. (ed 3) London: Churchill Livingstone, 1990
5. Taybi H, Lachman RS: Radiology of Syndromes, Metabolic Disorders, and Skeletal Dysplasias. (ed 4) St. Louis: Mosby-Year Book, 1996

Gamut F-68

PULMONARY DISEASE WITH EOSINOPHILIA

COMMON

1. Asthma (incl. allergic granulomatosis)
2. Drug reaction (eg, penicillin; sulfonamides; isoniazid; nitrofurantoin; nonsteroid anti-inflammatory drug—NSAID; aminosalicylic acid) (See F-73-S)
3. Eosinophilic leukemia; Hodgkin's disease
4. Eosinophilic pneumonia, idiopathic acute (Löffler S.) or chronic
5. Hypersensitivity bronchopulmonary aspergillosis (mucoid impaction)
6. Parasitic disease (eg, ascariasis; paragonimiasis; strongyloidiasis; tropical pulmonary eosinophilia (filarial); schistosomiasis; ancylostomiasis; visceral larval migrans; dirofilariasis immitis) (See F-74-S)
7. PIE (pulmonary infiltrate with eosinophilia)

UNCOMMON

1. Bacterial infection (eg, brucellosis)
2. Carcinoma (esp. bronchogenic)

3. Connective tissue disease (collagen vascular disease)$_g$ (esp. polyarteritis nodosa)
4. Desquamative interstitial pneumonitis (DIP)
5. Fungus disease (esp. coccidioidomycosis) (See F-74-S)
6. Hypereosinophilic S.
7. Hypersensitivity pneumonitis (extrinsic allergic alveolitis) (eg, farmer's lung; bagassosis) (See F-69)
8. Langerhans cell histiocytosis$_g$ (eosinophilic granuloma)
9. Rheumatoid lung
10. Sarcoidosis
11. Tuberculosis
12. Wegener granulomatosis$_g$

References

1. Eisenberg RL: Clinical Imaging. An Atlas of Differential Diagnosis. (ed 3) Philadelphia: Lippincott-Raven, 1997
2. Fraser RS, Müller NL, Coleman N, Paré PD (eds): Fraser & Paré: Diagnosis of Diseases of the Chest. (ed 4) Philadelphia: WB Saunders, 1999
3. Heitzman ER: The Lung: Radiologic-Pathologic Correlations. (ed 2) St. Louis: CV Mosby, 1984, pp 241, 276
4. Liebow AA, Carrington CB: The eosinophilic pneumonias. Medicine 1969;48:251–285
5. Schatz M, Wasserman S, Patterson R: The eosinophil and the lung. Arch Intern Med 1982;142:1515–1519

Gamut F-69

HYPERSENSITIVITY PNEUMONITIS (EXTRINSIC ALLERGIC ALVEOLITIS {EAA}, ORGANIC DUST DISEASE)

COMMON

1. Bagassosis (sugarcane)
2. Byssinosis (cotton)
3. Farmer's lung (moldy hay, wheat dust, tabacosis)
4. Humidifier lung; air-conditioner lung
5. Pigeon-breeder's lung; bird-fancier's lung; budgerigar lung; ostrich feather lung

UNCOMMON

1. Auto-worker's lung (machine operator's lung)
2. Basement shower EAA
3. Black fat tobacco smoker's lung
4. Building-associated EAA
5. Castor bean lung
6. Cave explorer's lung
7. Cheese brusher's lung
8. Coffee-worker's lung
9. Detergent-worker's lung
10. Fish meal-worker's lung
11. Fog-fever
12. Furrier's lung
13. Green coffee-worker's disease
14. Hemp dust inhalation disease
15. Hot-tub lung
16. Isocyanate-associated EAA
17. Japanese summer-type EAA
18. Malt worker's pneumonia
19. Maple bark stripper's disease
20. Mushroom-worker's lung; lycoperdonosis (puff-ball fungus spores from mushrooms)
21. Organophosphate insecticide inhalation
22. Paprika splitter's lung
23. Pituitary snuff-taker's lung
24. Prawn-worker's lung
25. Sequoiosis
26. Starch sprayer's lung
27. Suberosis (cork)
28. Thatched roof dust disease
29. Thesaurosis (hair spray)
30. Wheat weevil disease
31. Wood pulp-worker's lung

References

1. Fink JN: Organic dust-induced hypersensitvity pneumonitis. J Occup Med 1973;15:245–247
2. Fraser RS, Müller NL, Coleman N, Paré PD (eds): Fraser & Paré: Diagnosis of Diseases of the Chest. (ed 4) Philadelphia: WB Saunders, 1999
3. Webb WR, Möller NL, Naidich DP: High Resolution CT of the Lung. (ed 3) Philadelphia: Lippincott, Williams & Wilkins, 2001

Gamut F-70-S

INORGANIC DUSTS THAT CAUSE PNEUMOCONIOSIS

COMMON

1. Asbestos
2. Coal
3. Silica

UNCOMMON

1. Aluminum, bauxite (Shaver's disease)
2. Antimony
3. Barium sulfate (baritosis)
4. Beryllium
5. Cadmium
6. Carcinogens (arsenic; chromate; uranium; thorium; plutonium; radioactive ore; radon)
7. Cement dust
8. Cerium (arc lamp)
9. Cobalt and tungsten carbide ("hard metal")
10. Diatomaceous earth
11. Fuller's earth
12. Graphite
13. Iron (siderosis)
14. Kaolin (clay)
15. Manganese
16. Mica
17. Osmium
18. Platinum
19. Polyvinyl chloride
20. Silicon carbide
21. Silver; ferric oxide + silver (argyrosiderosis)
22. Synthetic mineral fibers
23. Talc (incl. drug abuse)
24. Tin oxide (stannosis)
25. Titanium dioxide (rutile)
26. Vanadium
27. Volcanic dust
28. Zeolites (Erionite)
29. Zirconium

(continued)

References

1. Fraser RS, Müller NL, Coleman N, Paré PD (eds): Fraser & Paré: Diagnosis of Diseases of the Chest. (ed 4) Philadelphia: WB Saunders, 1999
2. Lapp NL: Lung disease secondary to inhalation of nonfibrous minerals. Clin Chest Med 1981;2:219–233
3. Morgan WKC, Seaton A: Occupational Lung Diseases. Philadelphia: WB Saunders, 1975, p 241
4. Ostiguy GL: Summary of task force report on occupational respiratory disease (pneumoconiosis). Can Med Assoc J 1979;121:414–421
5. Sander OA: The nonfibrogenic (benign) pneumoconioses. Semin Roentgenol 1967;2:312–321

Gamut F-71-S

ILO 1980 INTERNATIONAL CLASSIFICATION OF RADIOGRAPHS OF THE PNEUMOCONIOSES: SUMMARY OF DETAILS OF CLASSIFICATION (INTERNATIONAL LABOUR OFFICE, GENEVA)

Features		Codes	Definitions
TECHNICAL QUALITY		1	Good.
		2	Acceptable, with no technical defect likely to impair classification of the radiograph for pneumoconiosis.
		3	Poor, with some technical defect but still acceptable for classification purposes.
		4	Unacceptable.
PARENCHYMAL ABNORMALITIES *Small Opacities*	*Profusion*		The category of profusion is based on assessment of the concentration of opacities by comparison with the *standard radiographs.*
		0/- 0/0 0/1	Category 0—small opacities absent or less profuse than the lower limit of category 1.
		1/0 1/1 1/2	Category 1, 2, and 3—represent increasing profusion of small opacities as defined by the corresponding standard radiographs.
		2/1 2/2 2/3 3/2 3/3 3/+	
	Extent	RU RM RL	The zones in which the opacities are seen are recorded. The right (R) and left (L) thorax are both divided into three zones—upper (U), middle (M), and lower (L).
		LU LM LL	The category of profusion is determined by considering the profusion as a whole over the affected zones of the lung and by comparing this with the standard radiographs.

Gamut F-71-S Continued

Features		Codes	Definitions
	Shape and Size rounded	p/p q/q r/r	The letters p, q, and r denote the presence of small rounded opacities. Three sizes are defined by the appearances on standard radiographs. p = diameter up to about 1.5 mm. q = diameter exceeding about 1.5 mm and up to about 3 mm. r = diameter exceeding about 3 mm and up to about 10 mm.
	irregular	s/s t/t u/u	The letters s, t, and u denote the presence of small irregular opacities. Three sizes are defined by the appearances on standard radiographs. s = width up to 1.5 mm. t = width exceeding about 1.5 mm and up to about 3 mm. u = width exceeding 3 mm and up to about 10 mm.
	mixed	p/s p/t p/u p/q p/r q/s q/t q/u q/p q/r r/s r/t r/u r/p r/q s/p s/q s/r s/t s/u t/p t/q t/r t/s t/u u/p u/q u/r u/s u/t	For mixed shapes (or sizes) of small opacities the predominant shape and size is recorded first. The presence of a significant number of another shape and size is recorded after the oblique stroke.
Large Opacities		A B C	The categories are defined in terms of the *dimensions* of the opacities. Category A—an opacity having a greatest diameter exceeding about 10 mm and up to and including 50 mm, or several opacities each greater than about 10 mm, the sum of whose greatest diameters does not exceed about 50 mm. Category B—one or more opacities larger or more numerous than those in category A whose combined area does not exceed the equivalent of the right upper zone. Category C—one or more opacities whose combined area exceeds the equivalent of the right upper zone.
PLEURAL ABNORMALITIES *Pleural Thickening* *Chest Wall*	Type		Two types of pleural thickening of the chest wall are recognized: circumscribed (plaques) and diffuse. Both types may occur together.
	Site	R L	Pleural thickening of the chest wall is recorded separately for the right and left thorax.
	Width	a b c	For pleural thickening seen along the lateral chest wall the measurement of *maximum width* is made from the inner line of the chest wall to the inner margin of the shadow seen most sharply at the parenchymal-pleural boundary. The maximum width usually occurs at the inner margin of the rib shadow at its outermost point. a = maximum width up to about 5 mm. b = maximum width over about 5 mm and up to about 10 mm. c = maximum width over about 10 mm.

(continued)

Gamut F-71-S Continued

Features			Codes	Definitions
		Face on	Y N	The presence of pleural thickening seen face on is recorded even if it can be seen also in profile. If pleural thickening is seen face on only, width cannot usually be measured.
		Extent	1 2 3	Extent of pleural thickening is defined in terms of the *maximum length* of pleural involvement, or as the sum of maximum lengths, whether seen in profile or face on. 1 = total length equivalent up to one-quarter of the projection of the lateral chest wall. 2 = total length exceeding one-quarter but not one-half of the projection of the lateral chest wall. 3 = total length exceeding one-half of the projection of the lateral chest wall.
	Diaphragm	Presence	Y N	A plaque involving the diaphragmatic pleura is recorded as present (Y) or absent (N), separately for the right and left thorax.
		Site	R L	
	Costophrenic Angle Obliteration	Presence	Y N	The presence (Y) or absence (N) of costophrenic angle obliteration is recorded separately from thickening over other areas, for the right (R) and left (L) thorax. The lower limit for this obliteration is defined by a *standard radiograph*.
		Site	R L	If the thickening extends up the chest wall then both costophrenic angle obliteration and pleural thickening should be recorded.
	Pleural Calcification			The site and extent of pleural calcification are recorded separately for the two lungs, and the extent defined in terms of *dimensions*.
		Site chest wall diaphragm other	R L R L R L	"Other" includes calcification of the mediastinal and pericardial pleura.
		Extent	1 2 3	1 = an area of calcified pleura with greatest diameter up to about 20 mm, or a number of such areas the sum of whose greatest diameters does not exceed about 20 mm.
				2 = an area of calcified pleura with greatest diameter exceeding about 20 mm and up to about 100 mm, or a number of such areas the sum of whose greatest diameters exceeds about 20 mm but does not exceed about 100 mm.
				3 = an area of calcified pleura with greatest diameter exceeding about 100 mm, or a number of such areas whose sum of greatest diameter exceeds about 100 mm.
SYMBOLS				It is to be taken that the definition of each of the symbols is preceded by an appropriate word or phrase such as "suspect," "changes suggestive of," or "opacities suggestive of," etc.
			ax	–coalescence of small pneumoconiotic opacities
			bu	–bulla(e)
			ca	–cancer of lung or pleura
			cn	–calcification in small pneumoconiotic opacities
			co	–abnormality of cardiac size or shape

Gamut F-71-S Continued

Features		Codes	Definitions
		cp	–cor pulmonale
		cv	–cavity
		di	–marked distortion of the intrathoracic organs
		ef	–effusion
		em	–definite emphysema
		es	–eggshell calcification of hilar or mediastinal lymph nodes
		fr	–fractured rib(s)
		hi	–enlargement of hilar or mediastinal lymph nodes
		ho	–honeycomb lung
		id	–ill-defined diaphragm
		ih	–ill-defined heart outline
		kl	–septal (Kerley) lines
		od	-other significant abnormality
		pi	-pleural thickening in the interlobar fissure or mediastinum
		px	-pneumothorax
		rp	-rheumatoid pneumoconiosis
		tb	-tuberculosis
COMMENT	Presence	Y N	Comments should be recorded pertaining to the classification of the radiograph, particularly if some other cause is thought to be responsible for a shadow that could be thought by others to have been due to pneumoconiosis, also to identify radiographs for which the technical quality may have affected the reading material.

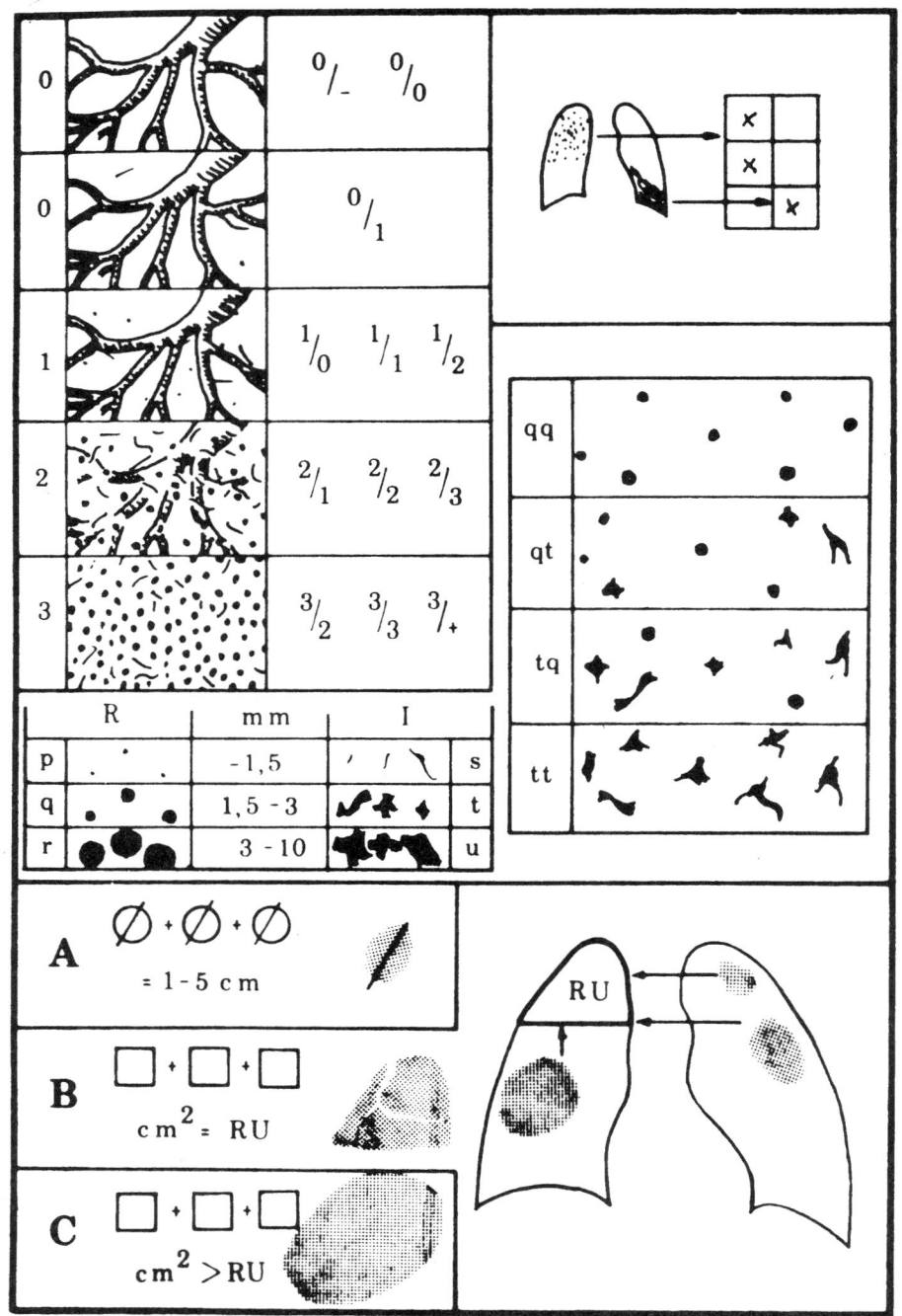

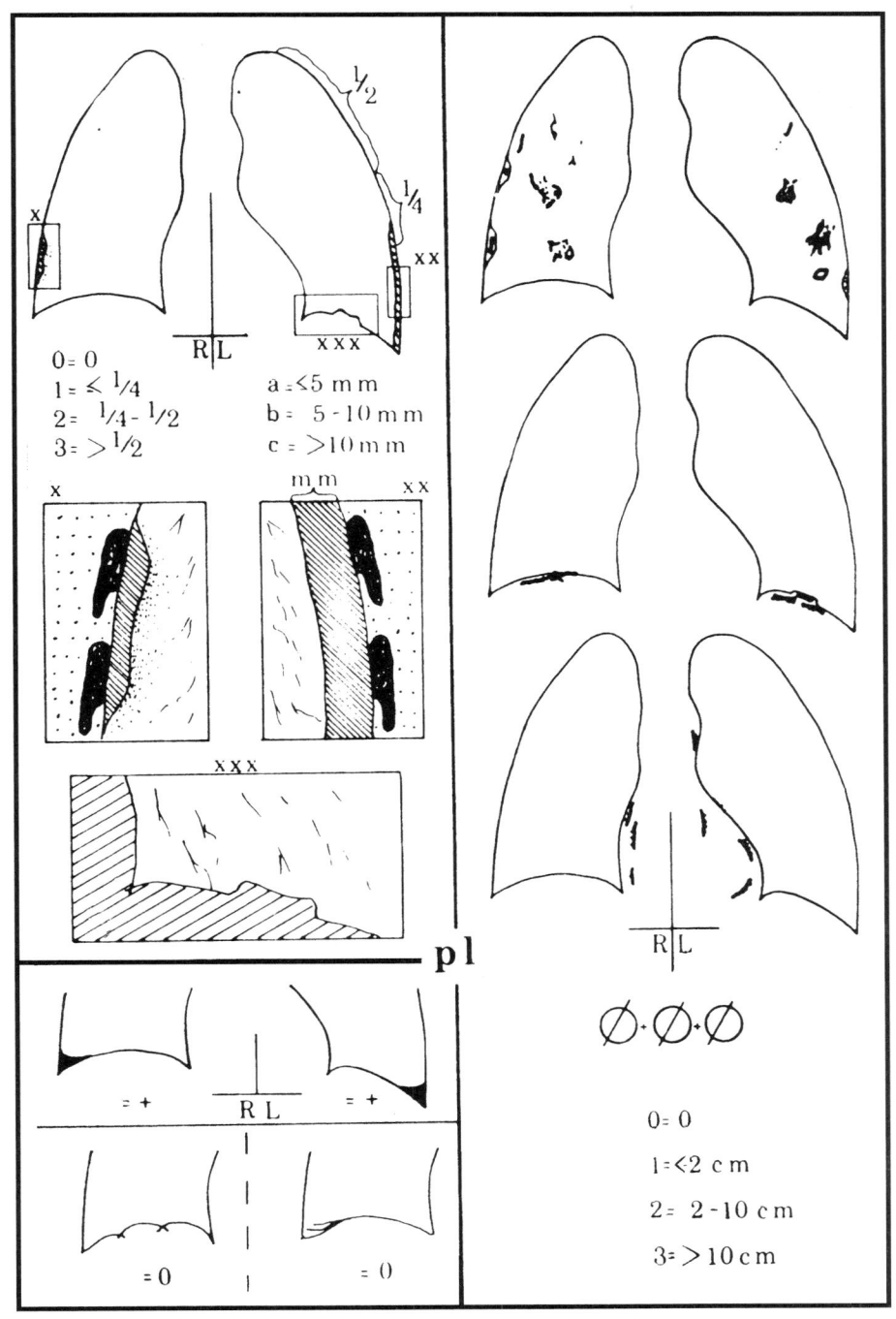

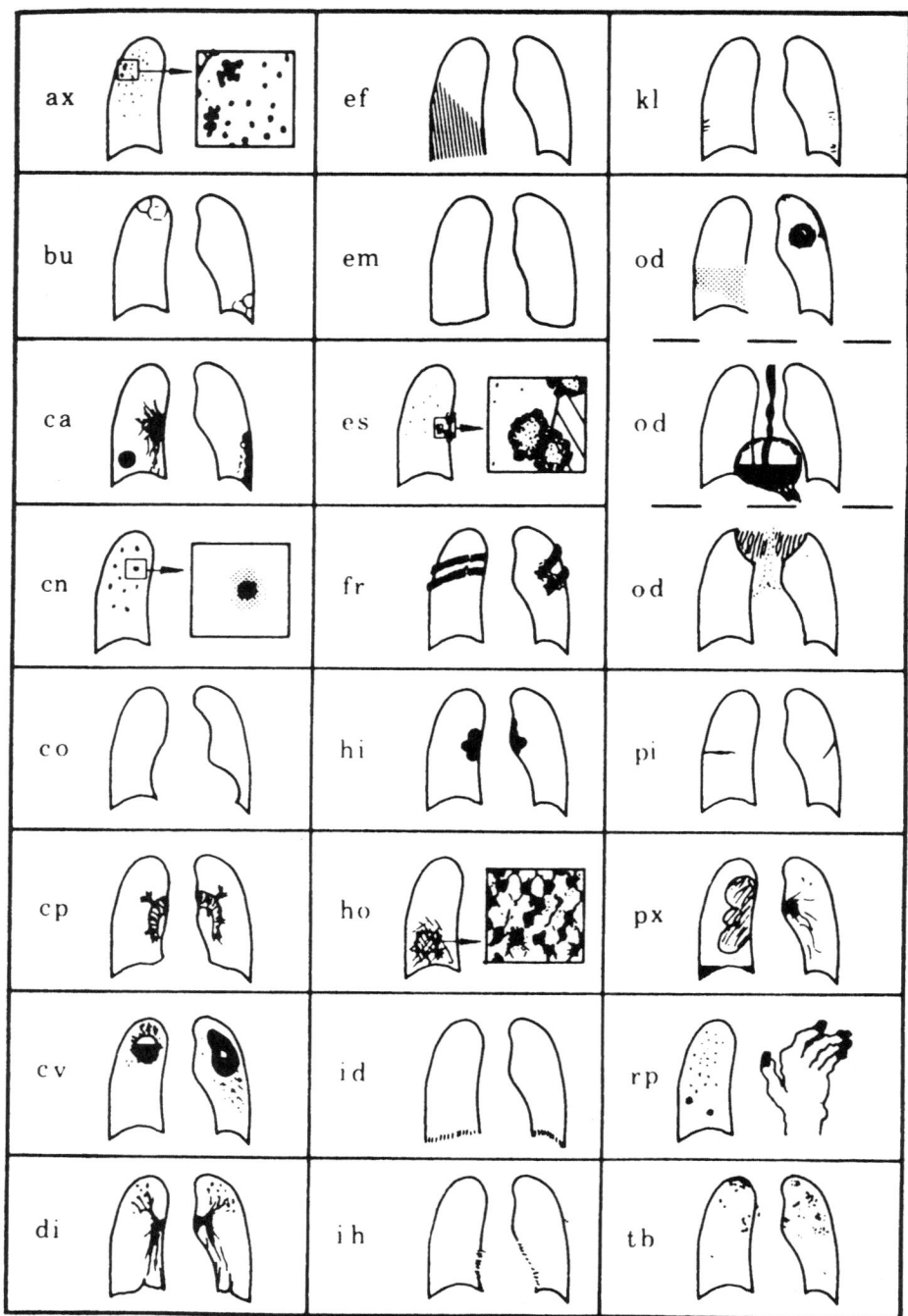

Gamut F-72-S

NOXIOUS VAPORS THAT CAUSE PULMONARY DAMAGE

HALOGENS
1. Bromine
2. Chlorine

HALOGENATED HYDROCARBONS
1. Carbon tetrachloride
2. Chloropicrin
3. Methyl bromide
4. Methyl chloride
5. Trichloroethylene

OXIDES OF NITROGEN
1. Nitric oxide (electric arc welding)
2. Nitrogen dioxide (silo-filler's disease)

IRRITANT GASES
1. Ammonia
2. Hydrogen fluoride
3. Hydrogen sulfide
4. Lewisite
5. Mustard gas
6. Nickel carbonyl
7. Phosgene
8. Sulfur dioxide

OTHERS
1. Acetone
2. Acrolein
3. Hair spray (thesaurosis)
4. Insecticides
5. Isoamyl acetate
6. Oxygen (high concentration)
7. Ozone
8. Smoke

References
1. Fraser RS, Müller NL, Coleman N, Paré PD (eds): Fraser & Paré: Diagnosis of Diseases of the Chest. (ed 4) Philadelphia: WB Saunders, 1999
2. Putman CE, Loke J, Matthay PA, et al: Radiologic manifestations of acute smoke inhalation. AJR 1977;129:865–870
3. Teixidor HS, Rubin E, Novick GS, et al: Smoke inhalation: Radiologic manifestations. Radiology 1984;149:383–387

Gamut F-73-S

DRUGS OR CHEMICALS THAT CAN INDUCE LUNG DISEASE

ANTIBIOTICS
1. Ampicillin
2. Cephalosporin
3. Ethambutol
4. Griseofulvin
5. Isoniazid (INH)
6. Nitrofurantoin
7. Para-aminosalicylic acid (PAS)
8. Penicillin
9. Pyrimethamine
10. Sulfonamides
11. Tetracycline and minocycline

CHEMOTHERAPEUTIC AGENTS
1. 5-Fluoruracil
2. 6-Mercaptopuran
3. Azathioprine
4. Bleomycin
5. Busulfan
6. Chlorambucil
7. Cyclophosphamide (Cytoxan)
8. Cyclosporin A
9. Cytosine arabinoside
10. Etoposide
11. Fludarabine
12. Hormonal agents (tamoxifen; nilutomide)
13. Hydroxyurea

(continued)

14. Ifosphamide
15. Interleukin
16. L-Asparaginase
17. Melphalan
18. Methotrexate
19. Mitomycin
20. Nitrosoureas
21. Peplomycin
22. Procarbazine
23. Vinca alkaloids

ANALGESICS

1. Acetylsalicylic acid
2. Codeine
3. Colchicine
4. Mesalamine

NARCOTICS AND SEDATIVES

1. Bromocarbamide
2. Buprenorphine
3. Chlordiazepoxide (Librium)
4. Codeine
5. Ethchlorvynol (Placidyl)
6. Febarbamate
7. Heroin
8. Methadone
9. Naloxone
10. Paraldehyde
11. Propoxyphene (Darvon)

ANTICONVULSANTS

1. Carbamazepine
2. Hydantoin (Dilantin)
3. Trimethadione

ANTICOAGULANTS

1. Coumadin
2. Quinidine
3. Warfarin

ANTIHYPERTENSIVES

1. Hexamethonium
2. Hydrochlorothiazide; hydralazine

MISCELLANEOUS AGENTS

1. 5-Aminosalycilic acid
2. Amiodarone
3. Amitriptyline
4. Beclomethasone diproprionate aerosol
5. Beta-adrenergic blocking agents (beta-blockers)
6. Beta$_2$ sympathomimetics with corticosteroids
7. Chlorpromazine
8. Chlorpropamide
9. Clomipramine
10. Cocaine
11. Desferioxamine
12. Diproprionate aerosol
13. Ergotamine and derivatives (bromocriptine; mesulergine)
14. Fluoxetine hydrochloride (Prozac)
15. Gold
16. Imipramine
17. Lidocaine
18. Marijuana
19. Mesalamine
20. Methacrylate
21. Methysergide (Sansert)
22. Mineral oil
23. Neocarzinostatin
24. Penicillamine
25. Phenothiazines
26. Procainamide (Pronestyl)
27. Propylthiouracil
28. Sulfasalazine
29. Sympathetic drugs (terbutaline; ritodrine; isoxsuprine)
30. Tocainide
31. Trimipramine
32. Verapamil

References

1. Batist G, Andrews JL Jr: Pulmonary toxicity of antineo-plastic drugs. JAMA 1981; 246:1449–1453
2. Cooper JAD Jr., Matthay RA: Drug-induced pulmonary disease. In: Bone RC (ed): Disease-a-Month. Chicago, IL: Year Book Med Publ, 1987, vol 33

3. Fraser RS, Müller NL, Coleman N, Paré PD (eds): Fraser & Paré: Diagnosis of Diseases of the Chest. (ed 4) Philadelphia: WB Saunders, 1999

4. Morrison DA, Goldman AL: Radiographic patterns of drug-induced lung disease. Radiology 1979;131:299–304

5. Rigsby CM, Sostman HD, Matthay RA: Drug-induced lung disease. In: Flenley DC, Petty TL (eds): Recent Advances in Respiratory Medicine. New York: Churchill Livingstone, 1983, pp 131–158

6. Rosenow EC III: The spectrum of drug-induced pulmonary disease. Ann Intern Med 1972;97:977–991

7. Rosenow EC III, Wilson WR, Cockerill RF III: Pulmonary disease in the immunocompromised host. Mayo Clin Proc 1985;60:473–487

8. Weiss RB, Muggia FM: Cytotoxic drug-induced pulmonary disease: Update 1980. Am J Med 1980;8:259–266

Gamut F-74-S

PULMONARY PATHOGENIC MICROORGANISMS

BACTERIAL, VIRAL, RICKETTSIAL

1. *Actinobacillus actinomycetemcomitans*
2. Actinomyces species*
3. Adenoviruses
4. Aerobacter species
5. Aeromonas species
6. *Bacillus anthracis*
7. Bacteroides species
8. *Bartonella henselae*
9. *Bordetella pertussis*
10. Brucella species
11. *Burkholderia (Pseudomonas) cepacia, mallei, pseudomallei*
12. *Chlamydia pneumoniae, trachomatis,* and *psittaci*
13. *Chromobacterium violaceum*
14. Clostridium species
15. *Corynebacterium pseudodiphtheriticum*
16. *Coxiella burnetii*
17. Coxsackie virus
18. Cytomegalovirus
19. ECHO viruses
20. *Eikenella corrodens*
21. Enterobacter-serratia species
22. Epstein-Barr virus
23. *Escherichia coli*
24. Eubacterium species
25. *Francisella tularensis*
26. *Haemophilus influenzae, parainfluenza*
27. Hanta virus
28. Herpes simplex
29. Herpes zoster
30. Influenza viruses
31. *Klebsiella pneumoniae, oxytoca*
32. Legionella species
33. Leptospira organisms
34. *Listeria monocytogenes*
35. Morganella species
36. *Mycobacterium tuberculosis* (also atypical mycobacteria)
37. *Mycoplasma pneumoniae*
38. *Neisseria meningitides*
39. Parainfluenza virus
40. Nocardia species*
41. *Pasteurella multocida*
42. *Peptococcus*
43. *Peptostreptococcus*
44. Proteus species
45. *Pseudomonas aeruginosa; Ps. cepacia*
46. Respiratory syncytial virus
47. *Rhodococcus (corynebacterium) equi*
48. *Rickettsia tsutsugamushi*
49. Rubeola virus
50. Salmonella species
51. *Staphylococcus aureus* and *epidermidis*
52. *Streptococcus (Diplococcus) pneumoniae* and *pyogenes*
53. *Treponema pallidum*
54. *Tropheryma whippleii*
55. Viellonella species
56. *Yersinia pestis (Pasteurella pestis)*

PARASITIC

1. *Ancylostoma duodenale*
2. Armillifer species
3. *Ascaris lumbricoides*

(continued)

4. Babesia species
5. *Cysticercus cellulosae*
6. Dirofilaria species (esp. *Dirofilaria immitis*)
7. *Echinococcus granulosus; E. multilocularis*
8. *Entamoeba histolytica*
9. Filaria species
10. Hartmanella-Acanthamoeba species
11. Microsporidia species
12. *Necator americanus*
13. Paragonimus species (esp. *P. westermani*)
14. *Pneumocystis carinii*
15. *Schistosoma mansoni, haematobium, japonicum*
16. *Strongyloides stercoralis*
17. Toxocara species (esp. *T. cani, T. cati*)
18. *Toxoplasma gondii*

MYCOTIC (FUNGAL)

1. Aspergillus species
2. *Blastomyces dermatitidis*
3. Candida species (moniliasis)
4. *Chrysosporium parvum (Emmonsia crescens)*
5. *Coccidioides immitis*
6. *Cryptococcus neoformans*
7. Geotrichum species
8. *Histoplasma capsulatum*
9. *Paracoccidioides brasiliensis*
10. *Penicillium marneffei*
11. Phycomycetes (zygomycosis)
12. *Pseudoallescheria boydii*
13. *Sporothrix schenckii*
14. *Torulopsis glabrata*

* Actinomyces and Nocardia species, formerly listed as fungal organisms, have been reclassified as bacteria.

Reference
1. Fraser RS, Müller NL, Coleman N, Paré PD (eds): Fraser & Paré: Diagnosis of Diseases of the Chest. (ed 4) Philadelphia: WB Saunders, 1999

Gamut F-75-S

COMMON PULMONARY OPPORTUNISTIC ORGANISMS

1. Chickenpox (varicella) virus
2. Cytomegalovirus
3. Fungus (esp. *Aspergillus; Mucormycetes; Candida; Cryptococcus*)
4. Herpes
5. *Mycobacterium tuberculosis* (incl. atypical mycobacterial infection)
6. Nocardia species
7. Parasites (esp. *Strongyloides stercoralis; Toxoplasma; Cryptosporidium*) (See F-74-S)
8. *Pneumocystis carinii*
9. Pseudomonas species; other pyogens (esp. *Staphylococcus aureus; Streptococcus; Legionella*)

Reference
1. Fraser RS, Müller NL, Coleman N, Paré PD (eds): Fraser & Paré: Diagnosis of Diseases of the Chest. (ed 4) Philadelphia: WB Saunders, 1999

Gamut F-76-S

CONDITIONS THAT PREDISPOSE TO OPPORTUNISTIC PULMONARY INFECTION

COMMON

1. Antibiotic therapy
2. Debilitating disease (eg, lymphoma$_g$; leukemia; carcinoma; myeloma; other malignant neoplasm; parasitic disease; renal failure; tuberculosis; cystic fibrosis)
3. Diabetes
4. Drug therapy (eg, steroids; chemotherapeutic agents)
5. Immune deficiency disorder$_g$ (incl. AIDS; granulomatous disease of childhood)

6. Malnutrition; alcoholism; senility
7. Organ transplantation
8. Prematurity
9. Radiation therapy

UNCOMMON

1. Connective tissue disease (collagen vascular disease)$_g$
2. Foreign material (eg, catheter; prosthesis)
3. Myeloid metaplasia; severe anemia$_g$

References
1. Fraser RS, Müller NL, Coleman N, Paré PD (eds): Fraser & Paré: Diagnosis of Diseases of the Chest. (ed 4) Philadelphia: WB Saunders, 1999
2. Pagani JJ, Libshitz HI: Opportunistic fungal pneumonia in cancer patients. AJR 1981;137:1033–1039
3. Roberts SR Jr: Immunology and the lung: An overview. Semin Roentgenol 1975;10:7–19
4. Rosenow EC III, Wilson WR, Cockerill FR III: Pulmonary disease in the immunocompromised host (Part I). Mayo Clinic Proc 1985;60:473–487

Gamut F-77

PULMONARY DISEASE IN AIDS OR OTHER IMMUNOCOMPROMISED PATIENTS

COMMON

1. ARDS
2. Drug-induced lung disease (See F-73-S)
3. Infantile respiratory distress syndrome; oxygen toxicity
4. Neoplasm, malignant (eg, bronchogenic carcinoma; metastasis; recurrent; Kaposi sarcoma; lymphoma$_g$
5. Opportunistic infection (esp. *Pneumocystis carinii* pneumonia; strongyloidiasis; toxoplasmosis; cytomegalovirus infection; fungus disease; *Rhodococcus equi;* bacillary angiomatosis) (See F-75-S)
6. Pulmonary thromboembolism and infarction

7. Tuberculosis and atypical mycobacterial infections
8. Unrelated disease

UNCOMMON

1. Alveolar proteinosis
2. Aspiration pneumonia
3. Graft-versus-host disease
4. Lymphangiography reaction
5. Lymphocytic interstitial pneumonitis (LIP)
6. Nonspecific interstitial pneumonitis (NSIP)
7. Primary pulmonary hypertension
8. Pulmonary edema due to heart failure or noncardiogenic (eg, leukoagglutination)
9. Pulmonary hemorrhage
10. Radiation injury

References
1. Fraser RS, Müller NL, Coleman N, Paré PD (eds): Fraser & Paré: Diagnosis of Diseases of the Chest. (ed 4) Philadelphia: WB Saunders, 1999
2. Pagani JJ, Libshitz HI: Opportunistic fungal pneumonia in cancer patients. AJR 1981;137:1033–1039
3. Rosenow EC III, Wilson WR, Cockerill FR III: Pulmonary disease in the immunocompromised host (Part I). Mayo Clinic Proc 1985;62:473–487

Gamut F-78

BRONCHIAL LESION

COMMON

1. Absent bronchus (congenital; surgical)
2. Bronchiectasis (See F-80)
3. Bronchogenic carcinoma
4. Broncholith
5. Carcinoid
6. Extrinsic pressure (eg, lymphadenopathy; mediastinal mass; pulmonary sling; other vascular anomaly; enlarged left atrium)
7. Foreign body
8. Metastasis, endobronchial (esp. renal cell or breast carcinoma; melanoma)

(continued)

9. Mucoid impaction; mucus plug (eg, aspergillosis; obstructing neoplasm) (See F-79)
10. Stricture, inflammatory (incl. tuberculosis; fungus disease)

UNCOMMON

1. Adenoid cystic carcinoma (cylindroma)
2. Amyloidosis
3. Bronchopleural fistula
4. Cyst (retention or other)
5. Fracture or laceration of bronchus
6. Hematoma
7. Iatrogenic (eg, misdirected endotracheal tube)
8. Inflammatory pseudotumor$_g$
9. Neoplasm, other (eg, hamartoma; lipoma; spindle cell tumor$_g$; angioma; granular cell myoblastoma; osteoma; chondrosarcoma; lymphoma$_g$)
10. Parasite (*Ascaris; Paragonimus*)
11. Pneumoconiosis (conglomerate mass) (See F-70-S)
12. Polyp; papilloma
13. Sarcoidosis
14. Scleroma (rhinoscleroma)
15. Tracheopathia osteoplastica
16. Wegener granulomatosis$_g$

References
1. Caldarola VT, Harrison EG Jr, Clagett OT, et al: Benign tumors and tumorlike conditions of the trachea and bronchi. Ann Oto Rhino Laryngol 1964;73:1042–1061
2. Felson B: Neoplasms of the trachea and main stem bronchus. Semin Roentgenol 1983;18:23–37
3. Fraser RS, Müller NL, Coleman N, Paré PD (eds): Fraser & Paré: Diagnosis of Diseases of the Chest. (ed 4) Philadelphia: WB Saunders, 1999

Gamut F-79

MUCOID IMPACTION IN A BRONCHUS

COMMON

1. *Aspergillus* sensitivity
2. Asthma; other allergic states

3. Bronchogenic carcinoma
4. Carcinoid; metastasis; other endobronchial neoplasm
5. Idiopathic (esp. elderly female)
6. Stricture or granuloma (incl. tuberculosis; fungus disease)

UNCOMMON

1. Bronchial atresia
2. Bronchial cyst
3. Broncholith
4. Cystic fibrosis (mucoviscidosis)

References
1. Felson B: Mucoid impaction in segmental bronchial obstruction. Radiology 1979;133:9–16
2. Fraser RS, Müller NL, Coleman N, Paré PD (eds): Fraser & Paré: Diagnosis of Diseases of the Chest. (ed 4) Philadelphia: WB Saunders, 1999
3. Laforet EG: Mucoid impaction of a stem bronchus. J Thorac Cardiovasc Surg 1974;68:309–312

Gamut F-80

CAUSES OF BRONCHIECTASIS

COMMON

1. Chronic aspiration
2. Chronic bronchitis
3. Cystic fibrosis (mucoviscidosis)
4. Foreign body
5. Idiopathic
6. Obstructing bronchial lesion (eg, carcinoma; carcinoid; stricture; broncholithiasis) (See F-78)
7. Postinfection (eg, pneumonia; whooping cough; measles; Swyer-James S.; allergic bronchopulmonary aspergillosis; paragonimiasis)
8. Pulmonary fibrosis (traction bronchiectasis) (eg, idiopathic {IPF}; radiation therapy; sarcoidosis)
9. Tuberculosis

UNCOMMON

1. Bronchial compression (eg, lymphadenopathy) or poststenotic constriction
2. Bronchiolitis obliterans
3. Connective tissue disease_g (esp. rheumatoid disease)
4. Dyskinetic cilia S.; Kartagener S.
5. Fungus disease (See F-74-S)
6. Immunologic disorder_g (eg, agammaglobulinemia; chronic granulomatous disease of childhood; AIDS; alpha1-antitrypsin deficiency; Chédiak-Higashi S.; Wiskott-Aldrich S.)
7. Inhalation of noxious fumes, smoke, chemicals
8. Mucoid impaction, mucus plugs (eg, obstructing neoplasm; aspergillosis; asthma; postoperative) (See F-79)
9. Riley-Day S. (familial dysautonomia)
10. Tracheobronchomegaly (Mounier-Kuhn S.)
11. Williams-Campbell S. (bronchial cartilage deficiency)
12. Yellow nail S.
13. Young S.

References
1. Fraser RS, Müller NL, Coleman N, Paré PD (eds): Fraser & Paré: Diagnosis of Diseases of the Chest. (ed 4) Philadelphia: WB Saunders, 1999
2. Taybi H, Lachman RS: Radiology of Syndromes, Metabolic Disorders, and Skeletal Dysplasias. (ed 4) St. Louis: Mosby-Year Book, 1996, p 1020

Gamut F-80-S

TYPES OF BRONCHIECTASIS

1. Bronchiolectasis
2. Central
3. Cylindrical, fusiform, tubular
4. Cystic, saccular
5. Reversible (pseudobronchiectasis)
6. Traction
7. Varicose, ampullary

Gamut F-81-1

INTRATRACHEAL MASS OR NODULE, SOLITARY OR MULTIPLE

COMMON

1. [Endotracheal tube; tracheostomy; foreign body]
2. [Extrinsic mass (eg, esophageal lesion; pulmonary or mediastinal mass; anomalous vessel)]
3. Neoplasm, malignant, primary (incl. squamous cell carcinoma; adenoid cystic carcinoma {cylindroma}; mucoepidermoid carcinoma; pleomorphic adenoma; carcinoid; sarcoma)
*4. Neoplasm, malignant, secondary (esp. invasive from thyroid, larynx, esophagus, or lung malignancy; metastatic from carcinoma of kidney, colon or breast, or melanoma)
5. [Stricture or stenosis (eg, congenital; inflammatory; burn; posttraumatic; postoperative; intubation)]

UNCOMMON

*1. Amyloidosis
2. Cyst; mucocele
3. Ectopic endotracheal thymus
*4. Granuloma (idiopathic; tuberculosis; fungus disease)
*5. Inspissated mucus (eg, asthma)
6. Lymphoma_g (esp. chloroma)
7. Neoplasm, benign (eg, spindle cell tumor_g {esp. fibroma; leiomyoma}; chondroma; hamartoma; hemangioma; granular cell myoblastoma; histiocytoma; lipoma; angioma; schwannoma; xanthoma)
*8. Papilloma (esp. laryngotracheal papillomatosis)
9. Plasmacytoma; extramedullary myeloma
10. Polyp; pseudopolyp
*11. Relapsing polychondritis
12. Sarcoidosis
13. Scleroma (rhinoscleroma)
14. Storage diseases
15. Thyroid tissue, ectopic, normal or neoplastic (intratracheal)

(continued)

16. Tracheomalacia
*17. Tracheopathia osteoplastica
18. Trauma (eg, laceration; fracture; hematoma)
19. [Web]
20. Wegener granulomatosis$_g$

* May be multiple.
[ ] This condition does not actually cause the gamuted imaging finding, but can produce imaging changes that simulate it.

References

1. Felson B: Neoplasms of the trachea and main stem bronchi.
   Semin Roentgenol 1983;18:23–37
2. Fleming RJ, Medina J, Seaman WB: Roentgenographic aspects of tracheal tumors. Radiology 1962;79:628–636
3. Fraser RS, Müller NL, Coleman N, Paré PD (eds): Fraser &
   Paré: Diagnosis of Diseases of the Chest. (ed 4) Philadelphia: WB Saunders, 1999
4. Kushner DC, Harris GBC: Obstructing lesions of the larynx
   and trachea in infants and children. Radiol Clin North Am
   1978;16:181–194
5. Weber AL, Grillo HC: Tracheal tumors: A radiological, clinical, and pathological evaluation of 84 cases. Radiol Clin
   North Am 1978;16:227–246

Gamut F-81-2

PEDUNCULATED INTRATRACHEAL MASS

1. Benign tumor (eg, hamartoma; chrondroma; lipoma)
2. Hemangioma
3. Inspissated mucus
4. Metastasis to tracheal mucosa (esp. from renal cell
   carcinoma; melanoma)
5. Polyp (eg, inflammatory; antrochoanal); papilloma
6. Postintubation tracheal granuloma in neonate

References

1. Fraser RS, Müller NL, Coleman N, Paré PD (eds): Fraser &
   Paré: Diagnosis of Diseases of the Chest. (ed 4) Philadelphia: WB Saunders, 1999
2. MacMahon H, O'Connell DJ, Cimochowski GE: Pedunculated endotracheal metastasis. AJR 1978;131:713–714

Gamut F-82

TRACHEAL ENLARGEMENT*

COMMON

1. Cystic fibrosis (mucoviscidosis)
2. Pulmonary fibrosis (esp. post-radiation therapy)

UNCOMMON

1. Immunoglobulin deficiency
2. Ehlers-Danlos S.
3. Relapsing polychondritis
4. Tracheobronchomegaly (Mounier-Kuhn S.)
5. Tracheocele

*Trachea > 26mm in men and > 23mm in women.

Reference

1. Slone RM, Fisher AJ: Pocket Guide to Body CT Differential Diagnosis. New York, McGraw-Hill, 1999, p 26

Gamut F-83

DIFFUSE TRACHEAL NARROWING
(See B-122)

COMMON

1. Croup
2. Extrinsic mass in superior or middle mediastinum
   (eg, intrathoracic goiter; carcinoma of esophagus;
   hematoma; bronchogenic cyst; lymphadenopathy;
   lymphoma$_g$; metastasis) (See F-86, 89)
3. [Normal in infants (expiratory collapse—"floppy
   trachea")]
4. Saber-sheath trachea (advanced emphysema)
5. Stricture, stenosis (eg, congenital; inflammatory;
   burn; chemical; traumatic; radiation; postoperative;
   post-tracheostomy; postintubation)

UNCOMMON

1. Amyloidosis
2. Bronchogenic carcinoma (squamous cell; small cell)
3. Cartilage deficiency (eg, tracheomalacia; traumatic; congenital)
4. Congenital (primary) tracheal stenosis
5. Inflammation, other (tuberculosis; sarcoidosis; epidermolysis bullosa)
6. Juvenile xanthogranuloma
7. Mediastinitis, chronic fibrosing
8. Neoplasm, benign (eg, hemangioma)
9. Neoplasm, malignant (eg, squamous cell carcinoma; adenoid cystic carcinoma {cylindroma}; lymphoma$_g$)
10. Papillomatosis
11. Relapsing polychondritis
12. Scleroma (rhinoscleroma—*Klebsiella rhinoscleromatis* infection)
13. Tracheomalacia (eg, congenital; postoperative; postintubation; post-tracheostomy)
14. Tracheopathia osteoplastica
15. Vascular ring$_g$ (eg, right aortic arch with aberrant left subclavian artery; double aortic arch)
16. Wegener granulomatosis$_g$

[ ] This condition does not actually cause the gamuted imaging finding, but can produce imaging changes that simulate it.

References

1. Ebel K-D, Blickman H, Willich E, Richter E: Differential Diagnosis in Pediatric Radiology. Stuttgart: Thieme, 1999, p 9
2. Fraser RS, Müller NL, Coleman N, Paré PD (eds): Fraser & Paré: Diagnosis of Diseases of the Chest. (ed 4) Philadelphia: WB Saunders, 1999
3. Hemmingsson A, Lindgren PG: Roentgenologic examination of tracheal stenosis. Acta Radiol 1978;19:753–765
4. Slone RM, Fisher AJ: Pocket Guide to Body CT Differential Diagnosis. New York: McGraw-Hill, 1999, pp 23–25

ANTERIOR DISPLACEMENT OF THE TRACHEA

COMMON

1. Aortic aneurysm
2. Duplication cyst$_g$ (eg, bronchogenic; tracheal; enteric; neurenteric)
3. Lymphadenopathy
4. Middle mediastinal mass, other (eg, hematoma; abscess; neurinoma) (See F-89)
5. Neoplasm of esophagus, malignant (esp. carcinoma)
6. [Normal in infants (buckling in expiration)]
7. Thyroid mass (eg, adenoma; goiter; carcinoma; thyroiditis; cyst)
8. [Tracheal lesion] (See F-81-1)
9. Vascular ring$_g$; anomalous vessels (eg, right aortic arch; double aortic arch; aberrant right subclavian artery)

UNCOMMON

1. Achalasia or other esophageal dilatation
2. Lymphangioma (cystic hygroma)
3. Neoplasm of esophagus, benign (eg, gastrointestinal stromal tumor$_g$, esp. leiomyoma)
4. Posterior mediastinal mass (esp. neurogenic tumor) (See F-90)
5. Zenker's diverticulum

[ ] This condition does not actually cause the gamuted imaging finding, but can produce imaging changes that simulate it.

References

1. Berkmen YM: The trachea: The blind spot in the chest. Radiol Clin North Am 1984;22:539–562
2. Ebel K-D, Blickman H, Willich E, Richter E: Differential Diagnosis in Pediatric Radiology. Stuttgart: Thieme, 1999, p 6
3. Fraser RS, Müller NL, Coleman N, Paré PD (eds): Fraser & Paré: Diagnosis of Diseases of the Chest. (ed 4) Philadelphia: WB Saunders, 1999
4. Raider L: The retrotracheal triangle. Chest 1973;63:835–838

WIDENING OF THE RIGHT TRACHEAL STRIPE (5 MM OR OVER)

COMMON

1. Carcinoma of the lung or esophagus
2. Diffuse tracheal narrowing (eg, tracheostomy; postintubation; edema; posttraumatic stenosis; relapsing polychondritis) (See F-83)
3. Hemorrhage (eg, trauma; bleeding disorder$_g$)
4. Lymph node enlargement (eg, sarcoidosis; metastasis; lymphoma$_g$; tuberculosis; histoplasmosis)
5. Normal variant
6. Pleural effusion (free or encapsulated); pleural fibrosis
7. Postoperative (eg, mediastinal or cardiac surgery; mediastinoscopy; right radical neck dissection)
8. Radiation edema or fibrosis
9. Thyroid mass (eg, intrathoracic goiter or carcinoma)
10. Tracheal mass (eg, squamous cell carcinoma; adenoid cystic carcinoma {cylindroma}; fibroma; hemangioma) (See F-81-1)

UNCOMMON

1. Atelectasis of right upper lobe
2. Mediastinitis$_g$; mediastinal abscess
3. Mesothelioma
4. Schwannoma of right vagus or phrenic nerve
5. Tracheobronchitis, viral or other
6. Wegener granulomatosis$_g$

References

1. Felson B: Neoplasms of the trachea and main stem bronchus. Semin Roentgenol 1983;18:23–37
2. Fraser RS, Müller NL, Coleman N, Paré PD (eds): Fraser & Paré: Diagnosis of Diseases of the Chest. (ed 4) Philadelphia: WB Saunders, 1999
3. Savoca CJ, Austin JHM, Goldberg HI: The right paratracheal stripe. Radiology 1977;122:295–301
4. Woodring JH, Pulmano CM, Stevens RK: The right paratracheal stripe in blunt chest trauma. Radiology 1982;143: 605–608

SUPERIOR MEDIASTINAL OR THORACIC INLET MASS

COMMON

1. Aortic dilatation or aneurysm of arch; cervical aorta or high arch
2. [Artifact (eg, hair braid)]
3. [Atelectasis of upper lobe]
4. Brachiocephalic vessel ectasia or elongation
5. Esophageal dilatation
6. Hemorrhage, traumatic or spontaneous (eg, bleeding disorder$_g$)
7. Lymphadenopathy, inflammatory or metastatic (eg, carcinoma of lung, breast, or head and neck) (See F-103)
8. Lymphoma$_g$ (esp. nodular sclerosing Hodgkins); leukemia
9. Right aortic arch, other arch anomaly or vascular ring (See E-21-S)
10. Superior vena cava obstruction (See E-70)
11. Thymic lesion (eg, normal ("rebound hyperplasia") or enlarged—benign or invasive thymoma; thymic cyst; thymic carcinoma) (See F-95)
12. Thyroid mass (eg, intrathoracic goiter, adenoma, carcinoma)
13. Zenker's diverticulum

UNCOMMON

1. Anomalous left superior vena cava
2. APVR, total
3. Arteriovenous fistula of head, neck, or thorax, with dilated great vessels
4. Cyst, mediastinal (eg, thymic; duplication {bronchogenic; enteric; neurenteric}; hydatid)
5. Lymphangioma (cystic hygroma)
6. Fat deposition (eg, obesity; steroid therapy; Cushing S.) (See F-91-1)
7. Germ cell tumor (esp. teratoma)

8. Mediastinitis$_g$
9. Parathyroid adenoma or carcinoma

[ ] This condition does not actually cause the gamuted imaging finding, but can produce imaging changes that stimulate it.

References

1. Baron RL, Levitt RG, Sagel SS, et al: Computed tomography in the evaluation of mediastinal widening. Radiology 1981; 13:107–113.
2. Siegel MJ, Sagel SS, Reed K: The value of computed tomography in the diagnosis and management of pediatric mediastinal abnormalities. Radiology 1986; 142:149–155.
3. Swischuk LE, John SD: Differential Diagnosis in Pediatric Radiology. (ed 2) Baltimore: Williams & Wilkins, 1995.

Gamut F-87

SUPERIOR MEDIASTINAL WIDENING IN INFANTS AND CHILDREN

COMMON

1. [Artifact (eg, hair braids)]
2. [Atelectasis of upper lobe]
3. Cyst, mediastinal (eg, thymic; teratoma; hydatid; duplication$_g$—bronchogenic; enteric; neurenteric)
4. Esophageal dilatation
5. Fat deposition; lipomatosis (eg, obesity; steroid therapy; Cushing S.) (See F-91-1)
6. Hemorrhage, traumatic or spontaneous (eg, bleeding disorder$_g$)
7. Lymphadenopathy (See F-103)
8. Lymphoma$_g$; leukemia
9. Mediastinitis, acute$_g$; mediastinal abscess (See F-102)
10. Mediastinal tumor (eg, teratoma; mixed germ cell tumor; thymoma; neuroblastoma)
11. Right aortic arch; other arch anomaly or vascular ring (See E-21-S); aortic dilatation
12. Thymus, normal ("hyperplasia") or enlarged; thymic rebound, posttreatment (See F-95)

UNCOMMON

1. Anomalous left superior vena cava
2. Aortic elongation (eg, pseudocoarction)—cervical aorta or high arch
3. APVR, total, above the diaphragm ("snowman" or "figure 8")
4. Arteriovenous fistula of head, neck, or thorax—with dilated great vessels
5. Azygos vein dilatation (See E-69)
6. Lymphangioma (cystic hygroma)
7. Superior vena cava enlargement (eg, obstruction; normal variant) (See E-70)
8. Thyroid mass (eg, thyroiditis; intrathoracic goiter; thyroid carcinoma) (See B-103-1)
9. Zenker's diverticulum

[ ] This condition does not actually cause the gamuted imaging finding but can produce imaging changes that stimulate it.

References

1. Baron RL, Levitt RG, Sagel SS, et al: Computed tomography in the evaluation of mediastinal widening. Radiology 1981; 13:107–113
2. Cohen M, Hill CA, Cangir A, Sullivan MP: Thymic rebound after treatment of childhood tumors. AJR 1980; 135:151–156
3. Siegel MJ, Sagel SS, Reed K: The value of computed tomography in the diagnosis and management of pediatric mediastinal abnormalities. Radiology 1986; 142:149–155
4. Silverman FN (ed): Caffey's Pediatric X-ray Diagnosis. (ed 9) Chicago: Year Book Medical Publ, 1992
5. Swischuk LE: Differential Diagnosis in Pediatric Radiology. (ed 2) Baltimore: Williams & Wilkins, 1996

Gamut F-88

ANTERIOR MEDIASTINAL LESION

Anterior to a curved vertical line along posterior border of heart and anterior margin of trachea; on CT or MRI, alongside and anterior to heart and great vessels

COMMON

*1. Aneurysm of ascending aorta or sinus of Valsalva
 2. [Bone lesion, esp. sternum (eg, metastasis; myeloma; sarcoma; osteomyelitis)]

(continued)

3. [Cardiac enlargement]
4. [Diaphragmatic lump, mogul, or eventration]
5. Fat deposition (eg, normal epicardial fat pad; Cushing S.; obesity; steroid therapy; hibernoma; lipomatosis)
*6. Germ cell tumor (eg, teratoma; seminoma; choriocarcinoma; embryonal cell carcinoma; endodermal sinus {yolk sac} tumor; mixed germ cell tumors)
7. Hematoma, hemorrhage (eg, traumatic; bleeding disorder$_g$)
8. Hernia (eg, Morgagni; hepatic; intrapericardial)
9. Innominate or brachiocephalic artery dilatation, buckling or aneurysm
10. Lymphoma$_g$ (esp. nodular sclerosing Hodgkin's); leukemia
11. Pericardial cyst
12. Pericardial disease (eg, effusion; neoplasm; defect)
13. Superior vena cava dilatation (See E-)
*14. Thymic lesion (eg, benign thymoma; invasive thymoma; thymic carcinoma; thymic carcinoid; thymic cyst; lymphoid hyperplasia; thymolipoma; lymphoma or leukemia arising in thymus)
15. Thymus, normal ("hyperplasia")
*16. Thyroid mass (intrathoracic adenomatous goiter; carcinoma)

UNCOMMON

1. Anomalous left superior vena cava
*2. Bronchogenic cyst
*3. Cardiac lesion (eg, tumor; aneurysm)
4. Fluid collection (eg, postoperative; perforated central venous catheter)
*5. Lymphadenopathy (eg, sarcoidosis; tuberculosis; histoplasmosis; giant lymph node hyperplasia {Castleman disease})
6. Lymphangioma (cystic hygroma)
7. Hydatid cyst
8. Lymphangiomatosis
9. Mediastinitis$_g$, acute; mediastinal abscess (See F-102)
*10. Mediastinitis, fibrosing (esp. histoplasmosis; idiopathic)
11. Metastasis

*12. Neoplasm, other (eg, gastrointestinal stromal tumor$_g$, fibroma, schwannoma, lipoma, and their sarcomatous counterparts; hemangioma; epithelioid hemangioendothelioma; hemangiopericytoma; angiosarcoma; benign and malignant fibrous histiocytoma; mesothelioma)
13. Parathyroid adenoma or carcinoma

* May show calcification.
[ ] This condition does not actually cause the gamuted imaging finding, but can produce imaging changes that simulate it.

References

1. Felson B: Chest Roentgenology. Philadelphia: WB Saunders, 1973
2. Fraser RS, Müller NL, Coleman N, Paré PD (eds): Fraser & Paré: Diagnosis of Diseases of the Chest. (ed 4) Philadelphia: WB Saunders, 1999
3. Heitzman ER: The Mediastinum: Radiologic Correlations with Anatomy and Pathology. St. Louis: CV Mosby, 1977
4. Reed JC: Chest Radiology. Plain Film Patterns and Differential Diagnoses. (ed 4) St. Louis: Mosby-Year Book, 1997
5. Rosenow EC III, Hurley BT: Disorders of the thymus. a review. Arch Intern Med 1984;144:763–770
6. Silverman FN (ed): Caffey's Pediatric X-Ray Diagnosis. (ed 8) Chicago: Year Book Medical Publ, 1985
7. Strollo DC, Rosado de Christenson M, Jett JR: Primary mediastinal tumors. Part 1. Tumors of the anterior mediastinum. Chest 1997;112:511–522

Gamut F-89

MIDDLE MEDIASTINAL LESION

Between anterior and posterior mediastinum on plain film, CT, or MRI (See F-88, F-90–93)

COMMON

*1. Aneurysm$_g$ of aorta or major artery (incl. traumatic; infectious); aortic dissection; pseudocoarctation of aorta
2. Azygos vein or SVC dilatation (See E-69, E-70)
3. Bronchogenic carcinoma (squamous cell; small cell; large cell; adenocarcinoma)
*4. Duplication cyst$_g$ (eg, bronchogenic; tracheal; enteric)

5. Esophageal lesion (eg, Zenker or other diverticulum; carcinoma; gastrointestinal stromal tumor$_g$, esp. leiomyoma)
6. Hiatal hernia
7. Innominate or brachiocephalic artery tortuosity or buckling
*8. Lymphadenopathy (eg, metastasis—esp. bronchogenic carcinoma; lymphoma$_g$; leukemia; tuberculosis; histoplasmosis; sarcoidosis; pneumoconiosis—esp. silicosis; giant lymph node hyperplasia {Castleman disease}) (See F-103)
9. Mediastinitis, fibrosing (esp. histoplasmosis; idiopathic)
10. Megaesophagus (eg, achalasia; scleroderma; Chagas' disease; stricture; neoplasm)
11. Pulmonary artery dilatation (See E-53)
12. Right-sided or double aortic arch; vascular ring$_g$ (See E-21-S)
*13. Thyroid mass (intrathoracic goiter; thyroid carcinoma)
14. Varices, mediastinal or esophageal

UNCOMMON

1. Extramedullary hematopoiesis
2. Fluid collection (eg, postoperative; perforated central venous catheter; ascites extending through esophageal hiatus)
3. Lymphangioma (cystic hygroma)
4. Mediastinal hematoma or hemorrhage
5. Mediastinitis$_g$, acute; mediastinal abscess (See F-102)
6. Neoplasm, mediastinal (eg, gastrointestinal stromal tumor$_g$, lipoma, and their sarcomatous counterparts; hemangioma; mesothelioma)
7. Schwannoma of vagus or phrenic nerve
8. Pancreatic pseudocyst
9. Paraganglioma, aorticopulmonary (chemodectoma)
10. Parathyroid adenoma or carcinoma
11. Thymic neoplasm
12. Tracheal tumor (eg, squamous cell carcinoma; adenoid cystic carcinoma {cylindroma}; chondrosarcoma; plasmacytoma; metastasis) (See F-81-1)
13. Tracheobronchomegaly (Mounier-Kuhn S.)

14. Vascular lesion, other (eg, azygos continuation of IVC; left superior vena cava; aberrant right subclavian artery; left superior intercostal vein dilatation; angiosarcoma of pulmonary artery; partial APVR; aberrant left pulmonary artery)

* May show calcification.
[ ] This condition does not actually cause the gamuted imaging finding, but can produce imaging changes that simulate it.

References

1. Daniel RA Jr, Diveley WL, Edwards WH, et al: Mediastinal tumors. Ann Surg 1960;151:783–795
2. Felson B: Chest Roentgenology. Philadelphia: WB Saunders, 1973
3. Fraser RS, Müller NL, Coleman N, Paré PD (eds): Fraser & Paré: Diagnosis of Diseases of the Chest. (ed 4) Philadelphia: WB Saunders, 1999
4. Heitzman ER: The Mediastinum: Radiology Correlations with Anatomy and Pathology. St. Louis: CV Mosby, 1977.
5. Reed JC: Chest Radiology. Plain Film Patterns and Differential Diagnoses. (ed 4) St. Louis: Mosby Year Book, 1997
6. Reed JC, Sobonya RE: Morphologic analysis of foregut cysts in the thorax. AJR 1974;120:851–860
7. Silverman FN (ed): Caffey's Pediatric X-Ray Diagnosis. (ed 8) Chicago: Year Book Medical Publ, 1985
8. Strollo DC, Rosado de Christenson M, Rett JR. Primary mediastinal tumors. Part II. Tumors of the middle and posterior mediastinum. Chest 1997;112:1344–1357

Gamut F-90

POSTERIOR MEDIASTINAL LESION

In paravertebral region on plain film, CT, or MRI (See F-89, 91, 92)

COMMON

*1. Aneurysm of descending aorta (incl. traumatic; infectious); aortic dissection
*2. Neurogenic neoplasm$_g$ arising from cord, nerve root, or sympathetic ganglia
   a. Peripheral nerve tumor, benign or malignant (neurofibroma; schwannoma; malignant tumor of nerve sheath origin)

(continued)

b. Autonomic ganglia tumor (ganglioneuroma; ganglioneuroblastoma; neuroblastoma)

*3. Spinal disease; paraspinal lesion, other (eg, tuberculosis; suppurative spondylitis; abscess; osteomyelitis; fracture)

4. Spinal neoplasm (osteosarcoma*; Ewing sarcoma; hemangioma; aneurysmal bone cyst; giant cell tumor; metastasis)

UNCOMMON

*1. Duplication cyst$_g$ (eg, enteric; neurenteric; bronchogenic)

2. Extramedullary hematopoiesis (esp. sickle cell disease; thalassemia)

*3. Hematoma or hemorrhage, mediastinal or paraspinal (eg, vertebral fracture); loculated hemothorax

4. Hernia (eg, Bochdalek; traumatic)

5. Hydatid cyst

*6. Lymphadenopathy (eg, lymphoma$_g$; metastatic bronchogenic carcinoma; sarcoidosis; tuberculosis; giant lymph node hyperplasia {Castleman disease})

7. Mediastinal varices

8. Mediastinitis$_g$, acute; mediastinal abscess (See F-102)

9. Mediastinitis, fibrosing (esp. histoplasmosis; idiopathic)

10. Meningomyelocele or meningocele (lateral or anterior)

11. Neoplasm, other (eg, fibroma; leiomyoma; lipoma; hemangioma; mesothelioma; plasmacytoma; thymoma)

12. Pancreatic pseudocyst

13. Paraganglioma (eg, pheochromocytoma; chemodectoma; glomus tumor)

*14. Pleural thickening or loculated fluid; empyema

15. Pulmonary sequestration (extralobar)

16. Retroperitoneal mass extending into posterior mediastinum (eg, metastasis; teratoma; sarcoma)

*17. Teratoma (occasionally occur here)

18. Thoracic duct cyst or neoplasm

19. Thoracic kidney (high in retroperitoneum)

*20. Thyroid tumor or goiter (intrathoracic)

* May show calcification.

References

1. Felson B: Chest Roentgenology. Philadelphia: WB Saunders, 1973
2. Fraser RS, Müller NL, Coleman N, Paré PD (eds): Fraser & Paré: Diagnosis of Diseases of the Chest. (ed 4) Philadelphia: WB Saunders, 1999
3. Heitzman ER: The Mediastinum: Radiology Correlations with Anatomy and Pathology. St. Louis: CV Mosby, 1977
4. Reed JC: Chest Radiology. Plain Film Patterns and Differential Diagnosis. (ed 4) St. Louis: Mosby Year Book, 1997
5. Strollo DC, Rosado de Christenson M, Jett JR: Primary mediastinal tumors. Part II. Tumors of the middle and posterior mediastinum. Chest 1997; 112:1344-1357

Gamut F-91-1

CT OF MEDIASTINAL LESIONS—WITH FAT ATTENUATION (−20 TO −130 HU)

COMMON

1. Hernia (eg, omental; mesenteric)

*2. Lipoma

3. Lipomatosis (Cushing S.; steroid therapy; obesity; diabetes)

4. Normal fat (epicardial fat pad; intrapericardial fat)

UNCOMMON

1. Angiomyolipoma

2. Extramedullary hematopoiesis

3. Liposarcoma

*4. Teratoma (mature)

*5. Thymolipoma

* May show calcification.

References

1. Chalaoui J, Sylvestre J, Dussault, et al: Thoracic fatty lesions: Some usual and unusual appearances. J Can Assoc Radiol 1981;32:197–201

2. Eisenberg RL: Clinical Imaging: An Atlas of Differential Diagnosis. (ed 3) Philadelphia: Lippincott-Raven, 1997
3. Fraser RS, Müller NL, Coleman N, Paré PD (eds): Fraser & Paré: Diagnosis of Diseases of the Chest. (ed 4) Philadelphia: WB Saunders, 1999
4. Mendez G Jr, Isikoff MB, Isikoff SK, et al: Fatty tumors of the thorax demonstrated by CT. AJR 1979;133:207–212
5. Moeller KH, Rosado de Christenson ML, Templeton PA: Mediastinal mature teratoma: Imaging features. AJR 1997; 169:985–990
6. Naidich DP, Zerhouni EA, Siegelman SS, Kuhn JP (eds): Computed Tomography and Magnetic Resonance of the Thorax. (ed 2) New York: Raven Press, 1991 pp 60–136
7. Rosado de Christenson ML, Pugatch RD, Moran CA, Galobardes J: Thymolipoma: Analysis of 27 cases. Radiology 1994;193:121–126
8. Strollo DC, Rosado de Christenson ML, Jett JR: Primary mediastinal tumors. Part I. Tumors of the anterior mediastinum. Chest 1997;112:511–522

3. Lymphangioma (cystic hygroma)
4. Lymphocele
5. Meningocele; myelomeningocele
6. Pancreatic pseudocyst

* May show calcification.

References

1. Eisenberg RL: Clinical Imaging: An Atlas of Differential Diagnosis. (ed 3) Philadelphia: Lippincott-Raven, 1997
2. Fraser RS, Müller NL, Coleman N, Paré PD (eds): Fraser & Paré: Diagnosis of Diseases of the Chest. (ed 4) Philadelphia: WB Saunders, 1999
3. Kirejczyk WM, McAdams HP, Rosado de Christenson ML, Matsumoto S: Bronchogenic cysts: Imaging features in 53 cases (Abs). Radiology 1995;197(P) Suppl: 366
4. Mendelson DS, Rose JS, Efremidis SC, et al: Bronchogenic cysts with high CT numbers. AJR 1983;140:463–465
5. Moeller KH, Rosado de Christenson ML, Templeton PA: Mediastinal mature teratoma: Imaging features. AJR 1997; 169:985–990
6. Naidich DP, Zerhouni EA, Siegelman SS, Kuhn JP (eds): Computed Tomography and Magnetic Resonance of the Thorax. (ed 2) New York: Raven Press, 1991, pp 60–136
7. Perusse KR, McAdams HP, Earls JP, Peller PJ: Posttraumatic thoracic lymphocele. RadioGraphics 1994;14:192–195
8. Pugatch RD, Braver JH, Robbins AH, et al: CT diagnosis of pericardial cysts. AJR 1978; 131:515–516
9. Shafer K, Rosado de Christenson ML, Patz CF, et al: Thoracic lymphangioma in adults: CT and MR imaging features. AJR 1994;162:283–289
10. Strollo DC, Rosado de Christenson ML, Jett JR: Primary mediastinal tumors. Part I. Tumors of the anterior mediastinum. Chest 1997;112:511–522
11. Strollo DC, Rosado de Christenson ML, Jett JR: Primary mediastinal tumors. Part II. Tumors of the middle and posterior mediastinum. Chest 1997;112:1344–1357

Gamut F-91-2

CT OF MEDIASTINAL LESIONS—WITH WATER ATTENUATION (0–15 HU)

COMMON

*1. Cyst (eg, pericardial; bronchogenic; enteric; neurenteric; thymic; hydatid)
*2. Cystic neoplasm (thymoma; teratoma; lymphoma$_g$; neurogenic tumor)
 3. Esophageal dilatation, fluid-filled (eg, achalasia; scleroderma; obstruction from tumor or stricture; post-vagotomy S.; Chagas' disease; diverticulum)
 4. Hiatal hernia
*5. Paraspinal abscess
 6. Pericardial effusion

UNCOMMON

1. Esophagectomy with gastric or colon interposition
2. Fluid collection; other (eg, seroma from trauma or surgery; perforated central venous catheter; loculated paramediastinal pleural effusion; ascites extending through esophageal hiatus)

Gamut F-91-3

CT OF MEDIASTINAL LESIONS—WITH SOFT TISSUE ATTENUATION (15–40 HU)

COMMON

*1. Cyst (bronchogenic; enteric; mature hydatid; other)
 2. Esophageal neoplasm (eg, leiomyoma; carcinoma)

(continued)

*3. Hematoma; hemorrhage (mediastinal or paraspinal)
4. Hernia, solid organ or bowel (eg, hepatic; Morgagni; hiatal; Bochdalek)
*5. Lymphadenopathy (metastatic; granulomatous; Castleman disease) (See F-103)
6. Lymphoma$_g$
*7. Mediastinal (substernal) goiter; thyroid neoplasm (esp. carcinoma)
8. Mediastinitis, acute; mediastinal abscess (See F-102); fibrosing mediastinitis
9. Metastasis
*10. Neurogenic tumor$_g$
*11. Spinal lesion (eg, infectious spondylitis; neoplasm; fracture with hematoma; paraspinal abscess)
12. Thoracic kidney
13. Thymic enlargement (normal; hyperplasia; thymitis)
*14. Thymic lesion (eg, thymoma, benign or invasive; carcinoid; carcinoma)
*15. Vascular lesion or abnormality (eg, aortic aneurysm, dilatation, or tortuosity (See F-92)

UNCOMMON
*1. Cardiac neoplasm (eg, fibroma; sarcoma)
2. Extramedullary hematopoiesis
*3. Germ cell neoplasm (teratoma; seminoma; nonseminomatous malignant germ cell neoplasm)
*4. Hemangioma
5. Lymphangioma (cystic hygroma)
6. Mesothelioma; localized fibrous tumor of pleura
7. Paraganglioma
8. Parathyroid adenoma or carcinoma
9. Pulmonary sequestration (extralobar)
10. Sarcoma
11. Spindle cell tumor$_g$

* May show calcification.

References
1. Eisenberg RL: Clinical Imaging: An Atlas of Differential Diagnosis. (ed 3) Philadelphia: Lippincott-Raven, 1997
2. Fraser RS, Müller NL, Coleman N, Paré PD (eds): Fraser & Paré: Diagnosis of Diseases of the Chest. (ed 4) Philadelphia: WB Saunders, 1999
3. Kirejczyk WM, McAdams HP, Rosado de Christenson ML, Matsumoto S: Bronchogenic cysts: Imaging features in 53 cases (Abs). Radiology 1995;197(P) Suppl: 366
4. Mendelson DS, Rose JS, Efremidis SC, et al: Bronchogenic cysts with high CT numbers. AJR 1983;140:463–465
5. Naidich DP, Zerhouni EA, Siegelman SS, Kuhn JP (eds): Computed Tomography and Magnetic Resonance of the Thorax. (ed 2) New York: Raven Press, 1991, pp 60–136
6. Shafer K, Rosado de Christenson ML, Patz CF, et al: Thoracic lymphangioma in adults: CT and MR imaging features. AJR 1994;162:283–289
7. Strollo DC, Rosado de Christenson ML, Jett JR: Primary mediastinal tumors. Part I. Tumors of the anterior mediastinum. Chest 1997;112:511–522
8. Strollo DC, Rosado de Christenson ML, Jett JR: Primary mediastinal tumors. Part II. Tumors of the middle and posterior mediastinum. Chest 1997;112:1344–1357

Gamut F-91-4

CT OF MEDIASTINAL LESIONS—WITH CALCIFICATION

COMMON
1. Aneurysm; atherosclerosis; other vascular lesion
2. Lymphadenopathy (eg, tuberculosis; histoplasmosis; sarcoidosis; silicosis; amyloidosis; Castleman disease)
3. Mediastinal (substernal) goiter

UNCOMMON
1. Abscess, old
2. Cyst (bronchogenic; foregut; thymic)
3. Hemangioma (phleboliths)
4. Hematoma, old
5. Lipoma
6. Lymphoma$_g$ (post-radiation therapy)
7. Neurogenic tumor$_g$ (eg, neurilemmoma; ganglioneuroma; neuroblastoma)
8. Teratoma
9. Thymic lesion (eg, thymoma; thymolipoma)

References

1. Eisenberg RL: Clinical Imaging: An Atlas of Differential Diagnosis. (ed 3) Philadelphia: Lippincott-Raven, 1997
2. Fraser RS, Müller NL, Coleman N, Paré PD (eds): Fraser & Paré: Diagnosis of Diseases of the Chest. (ed 4) Philadelphia: WB Saunders, 1999
3. Kirejczyk WM, McAdams HP, Rosado de Christenson ML, Matsumoto S: Bronchogenic cysts: Imaging features in 53 cases (Abs). Radiology 1995;197(P) Suppl: 366
4. McAdams HP, Rosado de Christenson ML, Moran CA: Mediastinal hemangioma: Radiographic and CT features in 14 patients. Radiology 1994;193:389–402
5. McAdams HP, Rosado de Christenson ML, Fishback NF, Templeton PA: Castleman disease of the thorax: Radiologic features with clinical and histopathologic correlation. Radiology 1998;209:221–228
6. Mendelson DS, Rose JS, Efremidis SC, et al: Bronchogenic cysts with high CT numbers. AJR 1983;140:463–465
7. Moeller KH, Rosado de Christenson ML, Templeton PA: Mediastinal mature teratoma: Imaging features. AJR 1997;169:985–990
8. Naidich DP, Zerhouni EA, Siegelman SS, Kuhn JP (eds): Computed Tomography and Magnetic Resonance of the Thorax. (ed 2) New York: Raven Press, 1991, pp 60–136
9. Strollo DC, Rosado de Christenson ML, Jett JR: Primary mediastinal tumors. Part I. Tumors of the anterior mediastinum. Chest 1997;112:511–522
10. Strollo DC, Rosado de Christenson ML, Jett JR: Primary mediastinal tumors. Part II. Tumors of the middle and posterior mediastinum. Chest 1997;112:1344–1357

Gamut F-91-5

CT OF MEDIASTINAL LESIONS— VASCULAR OR ENHANCING LESIONS

COMMON

*1. Aneurysm, aortic or other vessel; aortic dissection
2. Anomalies of aortic arch and subclavian artery; pulmonary sling (See E-21-S)
3. Azygos vein dilatation
4. Mediastinal goiter; thyroid neoplasm
5. Vessels (varices; collaterals; ectatic or dilated vessels; vascular anomalies)

UNCOMMON

1. Carcinoid tumor
*2. Hemangioma
3. Localized fibrous tumor of pleura
*4. Lymphadenopathy (tuberculous; metastatic; Castleman disease)
*5. Mediastinal tumor; other
*6. Paraganglioma; pheochromocytoma
7. Parathyroid adenoma

* May show calcification.

References

1. Eisenberg RL: Clinical Imaging: An Atlas of Differential Diagnosis. (ed 3) Philadelphia: Lippincott-Raven, 1997
2. Fraser RS, Müller NL, Coleman N, Paré PD (eds): Fraser & Paré: Diagnosis of Diseases of the Chest. (ed 4) Philadelphia: WB Saunders, 1999
3. McAdams HP, Rosado de Christenson ML, Moran CA: Mediastinal hemangioma: Radiographic and CT features in 14 patients. Radiology 1994;193:389–402
4. McAdams HP, Rosado de Christenson ML, Fishback NF, Templeton PA: Castleman disease of the thorax: Radiologic features with clinical and histopathologic correlation. Radiology 1998;209:221–228
5. Naidich DP, Zerhouni EA, Siegelman SS, Kuhn JP (eds): Computed Tomography and Magnetic Resonance of the Thorax. (ed 2) New York: Raven Press, 1991, pp 60–136
6. Strollo DC, Rosado de Christenson ML, Jett JR: Primary mediastinal tumors. Part I. Tumors of the anterior mediastinum. Chest 1997;112:511–522
7. Strollo DC, Rosado de Christenson ML, Jett JR: Primary mediastinal tumors. Part II. Tumors of the middle and posterior mediastinum. Chest 1997;112:1344–1357

Gamut F-92

AORTIC AND VENOUS ABNORMALITIES IN THE MEDIASTINUM
(Esp. on CT, MRI or Angiography)
(See E-21-S, E-61–65, E-69–70, F-91-S)

COMMON

1. Aneurysm of aorta$_g$ (eg, atherosclerotic; traumatic; infectious)
2. Atherosclerosis of aorta and brachiocephalic vessels
3. Coarctation of aorta
4. Dissection of aorta
5. High aortic arch
6. Right anterior aortic arch (Type I) with mirror-image branching
7. Superior vena cava dilatation or obstruction (See E-70)

UNCOMMON

1. Aneurysm or fistula of coronary artery
2. Aneurysm of sinus of Valsalva (incl. rupture into heart)
3. Anomalous artery arising from aorta to supply a lung segment
   a. Pulmonary sequestration
   b. Venolobar S. (scimitar S.)
4. Aortic diverticulum or nipple
5. Aortomegaly (idiopathic)
6. Aortopulmonary window
7. APVR, total ("snow man")
8. Azygos continuation of interrupted inferior vena cava
9. Circumflex or cervical left aortic arch with right descending aorta
10. Circumflex right aortic arch with left descending aorta
11. Corrected transposition of great vessels
12. Cystic medial necrosis of aorta (eg, Marfan S.)
13. Double aortic arch

14. Left aortic arch with aberrant right subclavian artery
15. Necrotizing vasculitis, arteritis (eg, polyarteritis nodosa; lupus erythematosus; Wegener granulomatosis; syphilis; drug abuse—esp. metamphetamine)
16. Patent ductus arteriosus (ligamentum arteriosus)
17. Persistent left superior vena cava
18. Postoperative shunt (eg, Blalock-Taussig; Waterston; Potts)
19. Pseudocoarctation of aortic arch
20. Right posterior aortic arch (Type II) with aberrant left subclavian artery
21. Subvalvular aortic aneurysm (African)
22. Takayasu arteritis
23. Transposition of great vessels
24. Truncus arteriosus

Reference
1. Burgener FA, Kormano M: Differential Diagnosis in Computed Tomography. New York: Thieme, 1996, pp 236–237

Gamut F-93

CYSTIC MEDIASTINAL LESION
(Plain Film, CT, or MRI)

COMMON

1. Duplication cyst$_g$ (eg, bronchogenic; tracheal; enteric; neurenteric)
2. [Hernia, diaphragmatic (containing fluid-filled viscus), esp. hiatal]
3. Pericardial cyst
4. [Pericardial effusion, loculated]

UNCOMMON

1. Cyst, indeterminate or idiopathic
2. [Esophageal diverticulum (fluid-filled)]
3. Granulomatous lymphadenitis (esp. histoplasmic)
4. Hydatid cyst
5. Lymphangioma (cystic hygroma)
6. Lymphocele

7. Mediastinal goiter (intrathoracic thyroid)
8. Mediastinal tumor with cystic degeneration (eg, cystic thymoma; lymphoma$_g$; neurogenic tumor)
9. Meningocele (lateral or anterior); myelo-meningocele
10. Pancreatic pseudocyst
11. Teratoma (mature)
12. Thymic cyst (acquired, congenital)

[ ] This condition does not actually cause the gamuted imaging finding, but can produce imaging changes that simulate it.

References

1. Feigin DS, Fenoglio JJ, McAllister HA, et al: Pericardial cysts. A radiologic-pathologic correlation and review. Radiology 1977;125:15–20
2. Fraser RS, Müller NL, Coleman N, Paré PD (eds): Fraser & Paré: Diagnosis of Diseases of the Chest. (ed 4) Philadelphia: WB Saunders, 1999
3. Kirejczyk WM, McAdams HP, Rosado de Christenson ML, Matsumoto S: Bronchogenic cysts: Imaging features in 53 cases (Abs). Radiology 1995;197(P) Suppl: 366
4. Moeller KH, Rosado de Christenson ML, Templeton PA: Mediastinal mature teratoma: Imaging features. AJR 1997; 169:985–990
5. Naidich DP, Zerhouni EA, Siegelman SS, Kuhn JP (eds): Computed Tomography and Magnetic Resonance of the Thorax. (ed 2) New York: Raven Press, 1991, pp 60–136
6. Ochsner JL, Ochsner SF: Congenital cysts of the mediastinum: 20-year experience with 42 cases. Ann Surg 1966; 163:909–920
7. Perusse KR, McAdams HP, Earls JP, Peller PJ: Posttraumatic thoracic lymphocele. RadioGraphics 1994;14:192–195
8. Shafer K, Rosado de Christenson ML, Patz CF, et al: Thoracic lymphangioma in adults: CT and MR imaging features. AJR 1994;162:283–289
9. Strollo DC, Rosado de Christenson ML, Jett JR: Primary mediastinal tumors. Part I. Tumors of the anterior mediastinum. Chest 1997;112:511–522
10. Strollo DC, Rosado de Christenson ML, Jett JR: Primary mediastinal tumors. Part II. Tumors of the middle and posterior mediastinum. Chest 1997;112:1344–1357
11. Sullivan MA: Case of the day. Case 5: Mediastinal cyst. AJR 1982;138:1202–1203

RETROSTERNAL MASS OR SWELLING

COMMON

1. Anterior mediastinal lesion (eg, thymoma; thymic cyst; thymolipoma; mature teratoma; malignant germ cell neoplasm; pericardial cyst or lipoma; hematoma; Morgagni hernia) (See F-88)
2. Bone lesion (eg, osteomyelitis; neoplasm, primary or secondary)
3. Fat; lipomatosis (eg, pericardial fat pad; adiposity; Cushing S.; steroid therapy)
4. Hemorrhage, traumatic (esp. sternal fracture) or bleeding disorder$_g$
5. Lymphoma$_g$ (esp. nodular sclerosing Hodgkin's)
6. Metastasis to sternum, soft tissues, or lymph nodes (esp. from breast carcinoma)
7. Normal (eg, prominent costal cartilage junction; slight obliquity; internal thoracis muscle; retrosternal line; interface of anterior margin of left lung)
8. Pleural fluid loculation
9. Postoperative (esp. median sternotomy; mediastinal surgery)
10. Thymus, normal (infant) or enlarged (hyperplasia; thymitis; thymic rebound following treatment or stress) (See F-95)

UNCOMMON

1. [Atelectasis of upper lobe]
2. Chest wall lesion with mediastinal involvement, inflammatory or neoplastic (eg, spindle cell tumor$_g$; lipoma; soft tissue myeloma)
3. Clavicle dislocation, posterior (sternal end)
4. Collateral blood vessels (eg, coarctation of aorta; inferior or superior vena cava obstruction; portal hypertension with internal mammary varices)
5. Lymphadenopathy, neoplastic or granulomatous (eg, tuberculosis; histoplasmosis) (See F-103)
6. Mediastinitis, acute$_g$; mediastinal abscess (See F-102)
7. Mesothelioma; localized fibrous tumor of pleura

(continued)

8. [Pericardial fibrosis (constrictive pericarditis)]
9. Venolobar S. (scimitar S.)

[ ] This condition does not actually cause the gamuted imaging finding, but can produce imaging changes that simulate it.

References

1. Jemelin C, Candardjis G: Retrosternal soft tissue: Quantitative evaluation and clinical interest. Landmarks between normal and pathological aspects. Radiology 1973;109:7–11
2. Pfister RC, Oh KS, Ferrucci JT Jr: Retrosternal density: A radiological evaluation of the retrosternal mediastinal space. Radiology 1970;96:317–324
3. Silverman FN (ed): Caffey's Pediatric X-ray Diagnosis. (ed 9) Chicago: Year Book Medical Publ, 1992
4. Whalen JP, Meyers MA, Oliphant M, et al: The retrosternal line: A new sign of an anterior mediastinal mass. AJR 1973; 117:861–872

Gamut F-95

THYMIC ENLARGEMENT

COMMON

1. Lymphoma$_g$ (esp. nodular sclerosing Hodgkin's disease); leukemia
2. Normal newborn or infant thymus
3. Thymic hyperplasia; thymitis
4. Thymic rebound following treatment or stress
5. Thymoma, benign or invasive

UNCOMMON

1. Germ cell neoplasm
2. Hyperthyroidism
3. Progeria
4. Thymic carcinoid
5. Thymic carcinoma
6. Thymic cyst
7. Thymolipoma

Reference

1. Baron RL, Lee JKT, Sagel SS, et al: Computed tomography of the abnormal thymus. Radiology 1982;142:127–134

Gamut F-96

SMALL OR ABSENT THYMUS IN AN INFANT

COMMON

1. Immunologic disorder$_g$ (eg, agammaglobulinemia; dysgammaglobulinemia; AIDS)
2. Stress from serious illness (eg, burn; birth trauma; sepsis; debilitation; anemia)

UNCOMMON

1. Adrenal hyperplasia, congenital
2. Chemotherapy (eg, nitrogen mustard; Cytoxan)
3. Congenital heart disease, esp. cyanotic (eg, complete transposition of great vessels)
4. Graft-versus-host disease
5. Radiation therapy
6. Steroid therapy
7. Thymic agenesis (DiGeorge S.)
8. Trisomy 8q S.
9. Trisomy 18 S.
10. Zellweger S. (cerebrohepatorenal S.)

References

1. Rose JS, Levin DC, Goldstein S: Congenital absence of the pulmonary valve associated with congenital aplasia of the thymus (DiGeorge's syndrome). AJR 1974;122:97–102
2. Taybi H, Lachman RS: Radiology of Syndromes, Metabolic Disorders, and Skeletal Dysplasias. (ed 4) St. Louis: Mosby-Year Book, 1996

Gamut F-97

RIGHT ANTERIOR CARDIOPHRENIC ANGLE LESION

COMMON

1. Epicardial fat pad
2. Hiatal hernia; esophagectomy with gastric or colon interposition

3. [Localized paralysis of right hemidiaphragm ("partial eventration")] (See F-136–137)
4. Morgagni hernia (gut or omentum)
5. Pericardial cyst or diverticulum
6. Pleural effusion (loculated); pleural adhesions
7. [Right atrial dilatation] (See E-27)
8. Right middle lobe disease (eg, neoplasm, esp. bronchogenic carcinoma; pneumonia; atelectasis)

UNCOMMON

1. Cardiac aneurysm or neoplasm
2. [Congenital absence of pericardium]
3. Diaphragmatic neoplasm or rupture (See F-138)
4. Herniation of liver, traumatic or congenital ("ectopic lobe")
5. Hydatid cyst (cardiac, pericardial, or pulmonary)
6. Localized fibrous tumor of pleura
7. Lymphadenopathy, juxtapericardial (esp. lymphoma$_g$)
8. Mediastinal tumor, anterior (eg, thymoma; thymic carcinoma; thymic cyst; thymolipoma; mature teratoma; malignant germ cell neoplasm) (See F-88)
9. Mesothelioma (pleural or pericardial)
10. Metastasis
11. Pericardial effusion (encapsulated)
12. Pulmonary sequestration (extralobar)

[ ] This condition does not actually cause the gamuted imaging finding, but can produce imaging changes that simulate it.

References
1. Castellino RA, Blank N: Adenopathy of the cardiophrenic angle (diaphragmatic) lymph nodes. AJR 1972;114:509–515
2. Felson B: Chest Roentgenology. Philadelphia: WB Saunders,1973
3. Fraser RS, Müller NL, Coleman N, Paré PD (eds): Fraser & Paré: Diagnosis of Diseases of the Chest. (ed 4) Philadelphia: WB Saunders, 1999

ABNORMALITY OF THE AZYGOESOPHAGEAL RECESS (ESP. ON CT)

COMMON

1. Azygos vein dilatation (eg, obstruction of SVC or IVC; azygos continuation of IVC)
2. Carcinoma of esophagus
3. Descending aorta dilatation
4. Duplication cyst$_g$ (esp. bronchogenic; enteric)
5. Esophageal dilatation, any cause (esp. achalasia; obstructing neoplasm)
6. Left atrial enlargement
7. Lymphadenopathy, esp. subcarinal and para-esophageal nodes (eg, carcinoma of lung; metastatic disease; lymphoma$_g$; AIDS; tuberculosis; histoplasmosis; sarcoidosis; Castleman disease) (See F-103)

UNCOMMON

1. Esophageal varices
2. Pleural effusion or thickening
3. Pleural tumor (mesothelioma or metastasis; localized fibrous tumor of pleura)
4. Pulmonary lesion (eg, consolidation; atelectasis)

References
1. Eisenberg RL: Clinical imaging: An Atlas of Differential Diagnosis. (ed 3) Philadelphia: Lippincott-Raven, 1997, pp 134–137
2. Heitzman ER: The Mediastinum: Radiologic Correlation with Anatomy and Pathology. St. Louis: CV Mosby, 1977
3. Lund G, Lien HH: Abnormalities of the azygo-esophageal recess at computed tomography. Acta Radiol (Diagn) 1983:24:3–10

Gamut F-99

DISPLACEMENT OF THE THORACIC PARASPINAL LINE (See F-90)

COMMON

1. Aortic disease (eg, aneurysm; ectasia; laceration)
2. [Left atrial enlargement]
3. Neoplasm of spine, primary (See C-38-S, C-39) or metastatic
4. Osteophytes
5. Paraspinal hemorrhage or hematoma (eg, spine fracture; bleeding or clotting disorder$_g$)
6. [Pleural effusion, encapsulated, but may be free on supine film]
7. Posterior mediastinal mass (See F-90)
8. Tuberculous or other infectious spondylitis

UNCOMMON

1. Azygos vein dilatation
2. Esophageal dilatation or neoplasm
3. Extramedullary hematopoiesis
4. Lymphoma$_g$; other lymphadenopathy
5. Mediastinal edema or hemorrhage (eg, cirrhosis; nephrosis; trauma; bleeding disorder$_g$)
6. Neurogenic tumor$_g$ (eg, schwannoma; neurofibroma; ganglioneuroma; ganglioneuroblastoma; neuroblastoma)
7. Spinal disease, other
8. Varices (mediastinal; esophageal)

[ ] This condition does not actually cause the gamuted imaging finding, but can produce imaging changes that simulate it.

Gamut F-100-S

INTRATHORACIC EXTRAMEDULLARY HEMATOPOIESIS

COMMON

1. Anemia$_g$, primary hemolytic (esp. thalassemia)

UNCOMMON

1. Aplastic anemia; bone marrow injury (eg, benzene; radiation)
2. Carcinomatosis
3. Cyanotic congenital heart disease
4. Erythroblastosis fetalis
5. Erythroleukemia (Di Guglielmo syndrome)
6. Iron deficiency anemia
7. Leukemia; lymphoma$_g$
8. Myelofibrosis; myelosclerosis
9. Paget's disease
10. Pernicious anemia
11. Polycythemia vera
12. Thrombocythemia
13. Thrombocytopenic purpura

References

1. Bree RL, Neiman HL, Hodak JA, et al: Extramedullary hematopoiesis in the spinal epidural space. J Can Assoc Radiol 1974; 25:297–299
2. Samuels MA, Schiller AL, Richardson EP Jr: Paget's disease of bone, paraparesis, and a paravertebral mass. N Engl J Med 1981;304:1411–1421

Gamut F-101-1

MEDIASTINAL WIDENING (See F-101-2, F-102)

COMMON

1. Achalasia; Chagas' disease
2. Fibrosing mediastinitis (esp. histoplasmosis; idiopathic)

3. Hematoma or hemorrhage (eg, sternal or vertebral fractures; venous and arterial tears; aortic transection; penetrating trauma from knife or gunshot wound; postoperative; malposition of vascular catheter with vessel injury)

4. Hiatal hernia (large); pericardial hernia

5. Lymphadenopathy (eg, metastatic disease—esp. from carcinoma of lung or esophagus); lymphoma; tuberculosis; histoplasmosis; giant lymph node hyperplasia (Castleman disease) (See F-103)

6. Mediastinal cyst (eg, thymic, bronchogenic, enteric or neurenteric cyst; hydatid cyst)

7. Mediastinal tumor (eg, thymoma; thymic carcinoma; thymolipoma; teratoma; lymphoma$_g$; intrathoracic goiter; neurogenic tumor)

8. Mediastinitis, acute; mediastinal abscess (See F-102)

9. [Technical factors (eg, expiration or poor inspiration; rotation; AP supine or lordotic film)]

10. Vascular abnormality (eg, dilated or tortuous aorta; aneurysm, dissection or coarctation of aorta; left superior vena cava; dilated superior vena cava)

UNCOMMON

1. Allergic edema of mediastinum

2. Chylomediastinum (eg, thoracic duct obstruction or laceration)

3. Extension of extrathoracic lesion (eg, pharyngeal or abdominal abscess; pancreatitis; pancreatic pseudocyst)

4. Extramedullary hematopoiesis

5. Lipomatosis (eg, obesity; steroid therapy; Cushing S.; normal variant)

6. Pleural disease adjacent to mediastinum (eg, effusion; metastatic disease; mesothelioma)

[ ] This condition does not actually cause the gamuted imaging finding, but can produce imaging changes that simulate it.

Reference

1. Reed JC: Chest Radiology. Plain Film Patterns and Differential Diagnoses. (ed 4) St. Louis: Mosby-Year Book, 1997

Gamut F-102-1

ACUTE DIFFUSE MEDIASTINAL WIDENING

TECHNICAL

1. [Radiograph obtained in expiration or poor inspiration, with patient rotated or in supine or lordotic position, or with short target-film distance]

HEMORRHAGE

1. Aneurysm (ruptured)

2. Aortic dissection

3. Bleeding or clotting disorder$_g$

4. Idiopathic

5. Postoperative

6. Trauma to heart, aorta, or other great vessel; sternal or vertebral fracture

LYMPH ACCUMULATION

1. Lymphangioma with rupture

2. Postthoracotomy lymphocele

3. Thoracic duct obstruction or laceration

EDEMA

1. Heart failure

2. Leakage from clysis (catheter malposition)

3. Postoperative

4. Superior vena cava obstruction

INFLAMMATION, SUPPURATION (EG, ACUTE MEDIASTINITIS) (See F-102)

1. Drug abuse

2. Esophageal perforation

3. Opportunistic infection (esp. in AIDS)

4. Osteomyelitis

5. Pancreatitis; subphrenic abscess (upward extension)

6. Pharyngitis; tonsillitis; parotitis; dental infection (downward extension)

7. Pulmonary or pleural infection

(continued)

LYMPHADENOPATHY

1. Acute leukemia; lymphoma$_g$
2. Anthrax
3. Bacterial infection, other
4. Fungus disease (esp. histoplasmosis; coccidioidomycosis)
5. Infectious mononucleosis
6. Lymphadenitis, acute
7. Plague
8. Sarcoidosis
9. Tuberculosis
10. Tularemia

PNEUMOMEDIASTINUM

1. Spontaneous
2. Traumatic
3. Other (See F-110)

[ ] This condition does not actually cause the gamuted imaging finding, but can produce imaging changes that simulate it.

References

1. Enquist RW, Blanck RR, Butler RH: Nontraumatic mediastinitis. JAMA 1976;236:1048–1049
2. Forrest JV, Shackelford GD, Bramson RT, et al: Acute mediastinal widening. AJR 1973;117:881–885

Gamut F-102-2

ACUTE MEDIASTINITIS OR MEDIASTINAL ABSCESS

COMMON

1. Esophageal perforation (eg, carcinoma; trauma; Boerhaave S.)
2. Histoplasmosis or other fungus disease (eg, coccidioidomycosis); actinomycosis (See F-74-S)
3. Iatrogenic (eg, postoperative; endoscopic trauma; dilatation of esophageal stricture)
4. [Sclerosing or fibrosing mediastinitis, chronic (esp. histoplasmosis; idiopathic)]
5. Tuberculosis

UNCOMMON

1. Drug abuse
2. Opportunistic infection (eg, atypical mycobacterial infection), esp. in AIDS
3. Osteomyelitis of sternum or spine
4. Pancreatitis; pancreatic pseudocyst; subphrenic abscess (upward extension)
5. Pharyngeal abscess; tonsillitis; dental infection (downward extension)
6. Pleural infection; empyema
7. Pneumonia; lung abscess
8. Trauma with tracheal or bronchial rupture

[ ] This condition does not actually cause the gamuted imaging finding, but can produce imaging changes that simulate it.

Reference

1. Reed JC: Chest Radiology. Plain Film Patterns and Differential Diagnoses. (ed 4) St. Louis: Mosby-Year Book, 1997

Gamut F-103

MEDIASTINAL AND/OR HILAR LYMPH NODE ENLARGEMENT

COMMON

1. AIDS (eg, *Pneumocystis carinii, Mycoplasma pneumoniae;* cytomegalovirus, or atypical mycobacterial infection; bacillary angiomatosis; Kaposi sarcoma; lymphoma)
2. Bronchogenic carcinoma
3. [Expiratory or supine film]
4. Fungus disease (esp. histoplasmosis; coccidioidomycosis; blastomycosis) (See F-74-S)
5. [Heart disease with pulmonary artery enlargement (eg, left to right shunt, heart failure; high output heart disease; pulmonary arterial or venous hypertension; cor pulmonale; valvular pulmonary stenosis; absent pulmonary valve; transposition of great vessels; truncus arteriosus; TAPVR below diaphragm; left atrial myxoma; aortic aneurysm]
6. Lymphoma$_g$; leukemia

7. Metastatic disease (esp. bronchogenic squamous or small cell carcinoma; carcinoma of head and neck, breast, kidney, testis; carcinoid; invasive thymoma; malignant teratoma; lymphangitic carcinomatosis; mesothelioma)
8. Pneumoconiosis (esp. coal-worker's pneumoconiosis; silicosis; berylliosis) (See F-70-S)
9. Sarcoidosis
10. Tuberculosis, primary

UNCOMMON

1. Amyloidosis; plasma cell dyscrasia (eg, Waldenström macroglobulinemia; heavy chain disease)
2. Aspiration, chronic (eg, tracheo-esophageal fistula; achalasia; neurologic disorders$_g$)
3. Connective tissue disease (collagen vascular disease)$_g$ (esp. rheumatoid arthritis; lupus erythematosus; mixed—MCTD)
4. Cystic fibrosis (mucoviscidosis)
5. Drug reaction (eg, hydantoin {Dilantin}; trimethadione; methotrexate)
6. Erythema nodosum
7. Giant lymph node hyperplasia (Castleman disease)
8. Hypersensitivity pneumonitis (extrinsic allergic alveolitis, esp. mushroom-worker's lung—rare in other entities) (See F-69)
9. Langerhans cell histiocytosis$_g$
10. Lymphadenitis, idiopathic or other infectious (eg, tularemia; pertussis; plague; anthrax; brucellosis; lung abscess)
11. [Mediastinal mass; prominent right or persistent left superior vena cava]
12. Parasitic disease (eg, occasionally in tropical eosinophilia {filarial}; acute schistosomiasis)
13. [Polycythemia vera]
14. Pulmonary lymphangioleiomyomatosis (rarely)
15. [Pulmonary thromboembolism]
16. Reactive airways disease in children
17. Recurrent childhood pneumonia
18. Sinus histiocytosis

19. Viral infection (eg, psittacosis; infectious mononucleosis; chickenpox; rubeola; cat-scratch fever; ECHO virus; mycoplasma) (See F-74-S)
20. Wegener granulomatosis$_g$

[ ] This condition does not actually cause the gamuted imaging finding, but can produce imaging changes that simulate it.

References

1. Ebel K-D, Blickman H, Willich E, Richter E: Differential Diagnosis in Pediatric Radiology. Stuttgart: Thieme, 1999, pp 98–99
2. Felson B: Chest Roentgenology. Philadelphia: WB Saunders, 1973
3. Fraser RS, Müller NL, Coleman N, Paré PD (eds): Fraser & Paré: Diagnosis of Diseases of the Chest. (ed 4) Philadelphia: WB Saunders, 1999
4. Heitzman ER: The Mediastinum: Radiologic Correlation with Anatomy and Pathology. St. Louis: CV Mosby, 1977
5. Reed JC: Chest Radiology. Plain Film Patterns and Differential Diagnoses. (ed 4) St. Louis: Mosby-Year Book, 1997
6. Teplick JG, Haskin ME: Roentgenologic Diagnosis. (ed 3) Philadelphia: WB Saunders, 1976

Gamut F-104

MARKED HILAR LYMPHADENOPATHY

COMMON

1. Lymphadenitis, infectious (incl. AIDS; tuberculosis; histoplasmosis; plague; tularemia; idiopathic)
2. Lymphoma$_g$; lymphosarcoma
3. Metastatic disease (esp. undifferentiated or small cell carcinoma of lung)
4. Sarcoidosis

UNCOMMON

1. Drug reaction (esp. hydantoin {Dilantin})
2. Erythema nodosum
3. Giant lymph node hyperplasia (Castleman disease)

BILATERAL HILAR ENLARGEMENT
(See F-103)

COMMON

1. Congenital heart disease (eg, left to right shunts—ASD, VSD, PDA; cyanotic admixture lesions; truncus arteriosus, type I)
2. Lymphadenopathy (esp. tuberculosis; histoplasmosis; bronchogenic carcinoma; lymphoma$_g$; sarcoidosis; silicosis; Castleman disease) (See F-103)
3. Pulmonary arterial hypertension, primary or secondary (eg, COPD; Eisenmenger S.; multiple pulmonary artery stenoses or coarctations; schistosomiasis)
4. Pulmonary thromboembolism
5. Pulmonary venous hypertension (eg, heart failure; mitral stenosis)

UNCOMMON

1. Polycythemia

Reference

1. Eisenberg RL: Clinical Imaging: An Atlas of Differential Diagnosis. (ed 3) Philadelphia: Lippincott-Raven, 1997, pp 70–71

UNILATERAL HILAR ENLARGEMENT

COMMON

1. Bronchogenic carcinoma (squamous cell; small cell)
2. Carcinoid
3. Fungus disease (esp. histoplasmosis; coccidioidomycosis; blastomycosis; sporotrichosis) (See F-74-S)
4. Lymphadenopathy, other infectious (eg, bacterial or viral pneumonia; lung abscess; tularemia; plague; actinomycosis; pertussis; mycoplasma; psittacosis; infectious mononucleosis; AIDS) (See F-103)
5. Lymphoma$_g$; leukemia
6. Metastatic disease (eg, from carcinoma of lung, breast, head and neck, kidney, or testis)
7. [Normal prominence of main pulmonary artery under age 25, esp. in women]
8. [Pneumonia in superior segment of a lower lobe; atelectasis in RUL or RML]
9. [Pulmonary stenosis, valvular (poststenotic dilatation of left pulmonary artery)]
10. [Rotation of patient during radiography; scoliosis]
11. Tuberculosis, primary

UNCOMMON

1. Aneurysm of pulmonary artery
2. Arteriovenous malformation
3. Bronchioloalveolar carcinoma
4. Coarctation of a central pulmonary artery (poststenotic dilatation)
5. Cystic fibrosis (mucoviscidosis)
6. [Mediastinal mass superimposed on hilum (eg, thymoma; thymic cyst; bronchogenic cyst; germ cell neoplasm; neurogenic tumor$_g$)]
7. Obstructed, hypoplastic, or absent contralateral pulmonary artery (eg, neoplasm; histoplasmosis; embolus; Swyer-James S.; congenital absence of pulmonary artery or valve)
8. Pericardial defect
9. Postoperative systemic-pulmonary shunt in CHD (Blalock-Taussig; Waterston-Cooley; Potts-Smith procedures)
10. Pulmonary thromboembolus lodged in a main pulmonary artery
11. Sarcoidosis (usually bilateral)

[ ] This condition does not actually cause the gamuted imaging finding, but can produce imaging changes that simulate it.

References

1. Felson B: Chest Roentgenology. Philadelphia: WB Saunders, 1973
2. Fraser RS, Müller NL, Coleman N, Paré PD (eds): Fraser & Paré: Diagnosis of Diseases of the Chest. (ed 4) Philadelphia: WB Saunders, 1999

3. Heitzman ER: The Mediastinum: Radiologic Correlation with Anatomy and Pathology. St. Louis: CV Mosby, 1977

Gamut F-107

UNILATERAL SMALL HILAR SHADOW

COMMON

1. Air trapping, unilateral (eg, bronchial foreign body, neoplasm, stricture)
2. Hyperaeration, unilateral
3. Lobar atelectasis with hilum displaced behind heart
4. Normal variant (esp. left side)
5. Postoperative (eg, lobectomy)
6. Rotation of patient (scoliosis; poor positioning)

UNCOMMON

1. Central pulmonary artery obstruction, unilateral (eg, neoplasm; thromboembolism; fibrosing mediastinitis)
2. Congenital absence (proximal interruption), hypoplasia, or coarctation of pulmonary artery
3. Congenital lobar emphysema (neonatal lobar hyperinflation) (See F-54)
4. Pulmonary agenesis, aplasia or hypoplasia
5. Swyer-James syndrome

References

1. Felson B: Chest Roentgenology. Philadelphia: WB Saunders, 1973
2. Fraser RS, Müller NL, Coleman N, Paré PD (eds): Fraser & Paré: Diagnosis of Diseases of the Chest. (ed 4) Philadelphia: WB Saunders, 1999
3. White RI Jr, Kaufman SL, Donner MW: Angiographic diagnosis of venous thromboembolism revisited. Ann Radiol 1980;23:312–315

Gamut F-108

UNILATERAL OR BILATERAL HILAR DISPLACEMENT

COMMON

1. Atelectasis
2. Bronchiectasis (See F-80)
3. Bronchogenic carcinoma
4. Emphysema
5. Lobectomy
6. Mediastinal mass
7. Pneumoconiosis, esp. with conglomerate mass (eg, silicosis; coal-worker's pneumoconiosis; asbestosis) (See F-70-S)
8. Pneumothorax (See F-111)
9. Tuberculosis, fungus disease, or other chronic pulmonary inflammatory process

UNCOMMON

1. Absent or anomalous pulmonary artery
2. Bronchial atresia
3. Congenital lobar emphysema
4. Cystic adenomatoid malformation
5. Diaphragmatic hernia
6. Lobar agenesis
7. Lobar torsion
8. Radiation fibrosis
9. Sarcoidosis (fibrotic)
10. Sequestration of lung (intralobar)
11. Swyer-James syndrome

References

1. Felson B: Chest Roentgenology. Philadelphia: WB Saunders, 1973
2. Fraser RS, Müller NL, Coleman N, Paré PD (eds): Fraser & Paré: Diagnosis of Diseases of the Chest. (ed 4) Philadelphia: WB Saunders, 1999

Gamut F-109

MEDIASTINAL SHIFT

COMMON

1. Atelectasis
2. Emphysema, unilateral (esp. bullous)
3. Mediastinal, pleural or pulmonary mass, large unilateral (eg, invasive thymoma; teratoma; thymolipoma; mesothelioma; bronchogenic carcinoma)
4. Pectus excavatum
5. Pleural effusion, large unilateral
6. Pneumothorax with tension
7. Postoperative (eg, lobectomy; pneumonectomy)
8. [Scoliosis]

UNCOMMON

1. Bronchiolitis obliterans (incl. Swyer-James S.)
2. Bronchogenic cyst (air-filled in children)
3. Congenital lobar emphysema (infants)
4. Cystic adenomatoid malformation (infants)
5. Diaphragmatic hernia, large
6. Foreign body (eg, peanut) occluding a large bronchus (esp. in a child on expiratory film)
7. Hypoplasia or agenesis of one lung
8. Partial absence of pericardium (cardiac shift)
9. Pulmonary interstitial emphysema (eg, PEEP)

[ ] This condition does not actually cause the gamuted imaging finding, but can produce imaging changes that simulate it.

References

1. Eisenberg RL: Clinical Imaging: An Atlas of Differential Diagnosis. (ed 3) Philadelphia: Lippincott-Raven, 1997
2. Reed JC: Chest Radiology. Plain Film Patterns and Differential Diagnoses. (ed 4) St. Louis: Mosby-Year Book, 1997

Gamut F-110

PNEUMOMEDIASTINUM

COMMON

1. Asthma
2. Barotrauma (overinflation during anesthesia or respiratory therapy, including ARDS; intermittent positive pressure ventilation (PEEP), esp. in newborns)
3. Birth trauma (newborn)
4. [Esophageal air in normal or dilated esophagus]
5. [Hiatal hernia]
6. Iatrogenic (eg, surgical procedure; sternotomy; esophagectomy; tracheostomy; endoscopy; intubation; needle biopsy of lung or kidney; pericardial drainage; retroperitoneal or other gas insufflation)
7. [Pneumopericardium; pneumothorax]
8. Respiratory distress syndrome, infantile or adult
9. Sudden increase in intrathoracic pressure associated with tear of lung parenchyma (eg, cough paroxysm; pertussis; vomiting; resuscitation; Heimlich maneuver; marijuana smoking enhancement; cocaine abuse; convulsion)
10. Trauma to upper or lower respiratory tract or chest wall (incl. blunt or penetrating trauma; stab or gunshot wound; foreign body; rib fracture with pulmonary laceration; fractured bronchus)

UNCOMMON

1. [Abscess, mediastinal]
2. Anorexia nervosa
3. Bronchial dehiscence after lung transplant
4. Caisson disease
5. [Colon interposition, postesophagectomy]
6. Cystic fibrosis (mucoviscidosis)
7. Diabetic ketoacidosis
8. [Esophageal diverticulum; communicating duplication cyst$_g$]
9. Esophageal perforation (eg, carcinoma; dilatation; Boerhaave S.; endoscopy; prolonged vomiting with Mallory-Weiss S.)

10. Extension of air from the neck; subcutaneous emphysema (eg, facial fracture; dental drilling; surgical procedure—neck dissection)
11. High altitude exercise
12. Infection with gas-forming organism (esp. in diabetic)
13. Parturition
14. Pneumoperitoneum; pneumoretroperitoneum (retroperitoneal perforation of gastrointestinal tract with upward extension of gas)
15. Rupture of trachea or main bronchus following bronchoscopy or blunt chest trauma
16. "Spontaneous" (eg, ruptured bulla)
17. Tracheal or esophageal fistula (eg, neoplasm; infection)

[ ] This condition does not actually cause the gamuted imaging finding, but can produce imaging changes that simulate it.

References
1. Eisenberg RL: Clinical Imaging: An Atlas of Differential Diagnosis. (ed 3) Philadelphia: Lippincott-Raven, 1997
2. Felson B: The mediastinum. Semin Roentgenol 1969;4:41–58
3. Fraser RS, Müller NL, Coleman N, Paré PD (eds): Fraser & Paré: Diagnosis of Diseases of the Chest. (ed 4) Philadelphia: WB Saunders, 1999.
4. Gray JM, Hanson GC: Mediastinal emphysema; Aetiology, diagnosis, and treatment. Thorax 1966;21:325–332
5. Munsell WP: Pneumomediastinum: A report of 28 cases and review of the literature. JAMA 1967;202:129–133
6. Sutton D: Textbook of Radiology and Imaging. (ed 6) New York: Churchill Livingstone, 1998, p 373

Gamut F-111

PNEUMOTHORAX

COMMON

1. ARDS
2. [Artifact (eg, skin fold)]
3. Bronchopleural fistula (eg, postoperative; tuberculosis; fungus disease; amebiasis; suppurative pneumonia; lung abscess; empyema; radiation therapy) (See F-112)
4. Cystic fibrosis (mucoviscidosis)
5. [Giant bulla]
6. Iatrogenic (eg, surgical procedure; thoracotomy; endoscopy; thoracentesis; percutaneous or transbronchial biopsy; resuscitation; tracheotomy; subclavian puncture; central line or pacemaker insertion; barotrauma—overinflation with positive pressure ventilation during anesthesia or respirator therapy)
7. Mediastinal emphysema with pleural leak
8. Obstructive emphysema (eg. foreign body; neoplasm)
9. Pneumonia (esp. *Pneumocystis carinii* in AIDS or necrotizing staphylococcal pneumonia)
10. Respiratory distress syndrome (esp. after PEEP therapy); pulmonary interstitial emphysema; meconium aspiration (neonates)
11. Primary "spontaneous" (eg, ruptured bulla)
12. Trauma (eg, rib fracture; blunt or penetrating chest injury; tracheobronchial injury)
13. Wilson-Mikity S.

UNCOMMON

1. Asthma
2. Drug therapy (esp. cytotoxic chemotherapy)
3. Endometriosis (catamenial)
4. Esophageal rupture (eg, endoscopy; carcinoma; Boerhaave S.)
5. Honeycomb lung, interstitial pulmonary fibrosis (esp. sarcoidosis; Langerhans cell histiocytosis$_g$—eosinophilic granuloma; pneumoconiosis—bauxite {Shaver's disease}; familial fibrocystic dysplasia—familial form of IPF) (See F-22)
6. Idiopathic pulmonary hemosiderosis
7. Marfan S.; Ehlers-Danlos S.; cutis laxa
8. Metastasis (esp. osteosarcoma or other sarcomas; carcinoma of pancreas or adrenals; Wilms' tumor)
9. Neoplasm, malignant (eg, bronchogenic carcinoma)
10. Noxious gases (See F-72-S)
11. Parasitic disease (esp. paragonimiasis; ruptured pulmonary hydatid cyst or amebic abscess)
12. Parturition

(continued)

13. Pneumatocele or cyst rupture (eg, staphylococcal pneumonia)
14. Pneumoperitoneum with extension through diaphragm
15. Pulmonary lymphangioleiomyomatosis; tuberous sclerosis
16. Pulmonary thromboembolism with infarction
17. Renal agenesis (Potter S.); intrauterine anuria
18. Tuberculosis (cavitary)
19. Whooping cough (pertussis)

[ ] This condition does not actually cause the gamuted imaging finding, but can produce imaging changes that simulate it.

References
1. Felson B: Chest Roentgenology. Philadelphia: WB Saunders, 1973
2. Fraser RS, Müller NL, Coleman N, Paré PD (eds): Fraser & Paré: Diagnosis of Diseases of the Chest. (ed 4) Philadelphia: WB Saunders, 1999
3. Lee CY, DiLoreto PC, Beaudoin J: Catamenial pneumothorax. Obstet Gynecol 1974; 44:407–411
4. Lote K, Dahl O, Vigander T: Pneumothorax during combination chemotherapy. Cancer 1981;47:1743–1745

Gamut F-112

BRONCHOPLEURAL FISTULA

COMMON
1. Empyema
2. Iatrogenic (eg, intubation; therapeutic pneumothorax; needle, brush or other biopsy)
3. Lung abscess; suppurative or necrotizing pneumonia
4. Neoplasm, malignant (esp. carcinoma of lung or esophagus)
5. Postoperative (eg, lobectomy; pneumonectomy; local resection; thoracoplasty; intubation)
6. Trauma to lung, pleura, or chest wall
7. Tuberculosis

UNCOMMON
1. Fungus disease (see F-74-S)

2. Metastatic disease (esp. sarcoma)
3. Parasitic disease (esp. ameblasis)
4. Pneumothorax (spontaneous)
5. Pulmonary infarct
6. Radiation pneumonitis

References
1. Felson B: Chest Roentgenology. Philadelphia: WB Saunders, 1973
2. Friedman PJ, Hellekant CAG: Radiologic recognition of bronchopleural fistula. Radiology 1977;124:289–295
3. Lams P: Radiographic signs in post-pneumonectomy bronchopleural fistula. J Can Assoc Radiol 1980;31:178–180

Gamut F-113

PLEURAL EFFUSION WITH NORMAL LUNGS (See F-114)

COMMON
1. Abscess, subphrenic or hepatic (eg, amebic; pyogenic)
2. Asbestos-related pleural disease
3. Ascites with permeation through diaphragm (eg, cirrhosis; Meigs S.; peritoneal metastases; extension of retroperitoneal urine collection; peritoneal dialysis)
4. Connective tissue disease (collagen vascular disease)$_g$ (esp. lupus erythematosus; rheumatoid disease)
5. Heart failure (esp. posttreatment)
6. Idiopathic
7. Infection (eg, bacterial; rheumatic fever; viral; infectious mononucleosis; mycoplasma; fungal; actinomycosis; nocardiosis) (See F-74-S)
8. Lymphoma$_g$, mediastinal or retroperitoneal; leukemia
9. Metastasis to pleura (esp. from breast, pancreas, GI tract, ovary, kidney)
10. Normal, physiologic (up to 5 cc); pregnancy
11. Postmyocardial infarction S. (Dressler S.); postpericardiotomy S.

12. Postoperative, following thoracic, cardiac, abdominal, or retroperitoneal surgery (eg, splenectomy; renal surgery)
13. Pulmonary thromboembolism
14. Trauma to chest wall (eg, rib fracture; blunt or penetrating injury) or great vessels (hemothorax)
15. Tuberculosis

UNCOMMON

1. Bleeding or clotting disorder$_g$
2. Chest wall neoplasm (eg, Ewing sarcoma; osteosarcoma; chondrosarcoma)
3. Chylothorax (eg, lymphedema; Milroy's disease; trauma to thoracic duct) (See F-120)
4. Drug reaction (eg, methysergide; nitrofurantoin, busulfan; methotrexate; bromcriptine, procarbazine; also lupus reaction from hydantoin {Dilantin}, hydralazine, isoniazid, procainamide, propylthiouracil)
5. Empyema from retropharyngeal or neck abscess, or in postpneumonectomy space
6. Esophageal rupture or fistula
7. Familial Mediterranean fever (familial recurrent polyscrositis)
8. Hypoproteinemia (incl. hepatic failure)
9. Iatrogenic (eg, fluid overload; ventriculopleural or other shunt; improperly inserted intravenous catheter; instillation of medication)
10. Mesothelioma
11. Multiple myeloma
12. Myxedema
13. Pancreatitis; pancreatic pseudocyst, abscess, or neoplasm
14. Parasitic disease (eg, amebiasis; filariasis; malaria; paragonimiasis)
15. Pericarditis (eg, viral; tuberculous; metastatic; idiopathic; constrictive)
16. Pleural fistula (eg, gastric; esophageal; bronchopleural)
17. Radiation therapy
18. Renal disease (eg, renal failure; nephrosis; pyelonephritis; acute glomerulonephritis; hydronephrosis; uremic pleuritis; hemolytic-uremic S.)

References

1. Baron RL, Stark DD, McClennan BL: Intrathoracic extension of retroperitoneal urine collection. AJR 1981;137:37–41
2. Bierman SM, Reuter KL, Hunter RE: Meigs syndrome and ovarian fibroma: CT findings. J Comput Assist Tomogr 1990;144:833–834
3. Eisenberg RL: Clinical Imaging: An Atlas of Differential Diagnosis. (ed 3) Philadelphia: Lippincott-Raven, 1997
4. Fraser RS, Müller NL, Coleman N, Paré PD (eds): Fraser & Paré: Diagnosis of Diseases of the Chest. (ed 4) Philadelphia: WB Saunders, 1999
5. Reed JC: Chest Radiology. Plain Film Patterns and Differential Diagnoses. (ed 4) St. Louis: Mosby-Year Book, 1997
6. Rosenow EC III: The spectrum of drug-induced pulmonary disease. Ann Intern Med 1972;97:977–991
7. Storey DD, Dines DE, Coles DT: Pleural effusion: A diagnostic dilemma. JAMA 1976;236:2183–2186
8. Teplick JG, Haskin ME: Roentgenologic Diagnosis. (ed 3) Philadelphia: WB Saunders, 1976

Gamut F-114

PLEURAL EFFUSION WITH ASSOCIATED PULMONARY, CARDIAC, OR MEDIASTINAL DISEASE

COMMON

1. Abscess, lung or subphrenic
2. ARDS; shock lung; ventilator lung
3. Bronchogenic carcinoma
4. Heart failure
5. Infection, other (eg, rheumatic fever; fungal; actinomycosis; nocardiosis; bacillary angiomatosis; mycoplasma; viral)
6. Lymphoma$_g$; leukemia
7. Metastatic disease, hematogenous or lymphangitic (esp. from carcinoma of lung, breast, pancreas, GI tract, or kidney; osteosarcoma and other sarcomas; Wilms' tumor)
8. Parasitic disease (eg, malaria; amebiasis; hydatid disease; paragonimiasis) (See F-74-S)
9. Pneumonia (esp. bacterial, usually with empyema—staphylococcal; streptococcal; *Klebsiella;* plague; tularemia) (See F-74-S)

(continued)

10. Postoperative (eg, pneumonectomy; left effusion post-cardiac surgery)
11. Pulmonary thromboembolism and infarction
12. Trauma with hemothorax or chylothorax (esp. laceration of lung; rib fracture; knife or gunshot wound; pulmonary or mediastinal hematoma; aortic rupture; esophageal perforation)
13. Tuberculosis

UNCOMMON

1. Asbestos exposure (usually with asbestos-related pleural disease and/or asbestosis)
2. Bronchopleural fistula
3. Churg-Strauss S.
4. Connective tissue disease (collagen vascular disease)$_g$ (esp. lupus erythematosus; rheumatoid disease)
5. Dressler S. (recent myocardial infarction or cardiac surgery)
6. Drug-induced pulmonary disease, usually diffuse interstitial (eg, nitrofurantoin; hydralazine; procainamide) (See F-73-S)
7. Eosinophilic lung disease$_g$ (eg, Löffler S.)
8. Esophageal rupture or fistula
9. Iatrogenic (eg, fluid overload; ventriculopleural or other shunt; improperly inserted intravenous catheter; instillation of medication)
10. Lymphomatoid granulomatosis
11. Malignant neoplasm, other (eg, bronchioloalveolar carcinoma; mesothelioma; multiple myeloma; rib or chest wall sarcoma; Askin tumor)
12. Obstruction of superior vena cava or azygos vein
13. Pericarditis (eg, viral; tuberculous; metastatic; idiopathic; constrictive)
14. Pulmonary lymphangioleiomyomatosis; tuberous sclerosis
15. Pulmonary lymphangiomatosis
16. Radiation therapy
17. Sarcoidosis
18. Uremia (with pulmonary edema)
19. Waldenström macroglobulinemia
20. Wegener granulomatosis$_g$

References

1. Eisenberg RL: Clinical Imaging: An Atlas of Differential Diagnosis. (ed 3) Philadelphia: Lippincott-Raven, 1997
2. Fraser RS, Müller NL, Coleman N, Paré PD (eds): Fraser & Paré: Diagnosis of Diseases of the Chest. (ed 4) Philadelphia: WB Saunders, 1999
3. Frazier AA, Rosado de Christenson ML, Galvin JR, Fleming MV: Pulmonary angiitis and granulomatosis. RadioGraphics 1998;18:687–710
4. Miller BH, Rosado de Christenson ML, Mason AC, et al: Malignant pleural mesothelioma: Radiologic-Pathologic Correlation. RadioGraphics 1996;16:613–644
5. Reed JC: Chest Radiology. Plain Film Patterns and Differential Diagnoses. (ed 4) St. Louis: Mosby-Year Book, 1997
6. Storey DD, Dines DE, Coles DT: Pleural effusion. A diagnostic dilemma. JAMA 1976;236:2183–2186
7. Teplick JG, Haskin ME: Roentgenologic Diagnosis. (ed 3) Philadelphia: WB Saunders, 1976

Gamut F-115

SMALL PLEURAL EFFUSION WITH SUBSEGMENTAL ATELECTASIS

1. Abdominal disease (eg, subphrenic abscess; amebiasis; pancreatitis; neoplasm)
2. Ascites
3. Postoperative (eg, thoracotomy—esp. CABG; splenectomy; renal surgery)
4. Pulmonary infarct
5. Trauma (eg, rib fractures)

Reference

1. Reed JC: Chest Radiology. Plain Film Patterns and Differential Diagnoses. (ed 4) St. Louis: Mosby-Year Book, 1997

Gamut F-116

PLEURAL EFFUSION WITH ENLARGED HEART

1. Connective tissue disease (collagen vascular disease)$_g$ (esp. lupus erythematosus; rheumatoid disease)
2. Heart failure
3. Malignant neoplasm with direct or metastatic extension to pleura, pericardium and/or heart (eg, mesothelioma; invasive thymoma; malignant germ cell neoplasm; carcinoma of lung, breast or esophagus; lymphoma$_g$)
4. Myocardiopathy
5. Myocarditis or pericarditis with pleuritis (eg, tuberculosis; rheumatic fever, viral infection)
6. Postpericardiotomy S. (esp. CABG); Dressler S.
7. Pulmonary thromboembolism, usually with infarction

Reference
1. Reed JC: Chest Radiology. Plain Film Patterns and Differential Diagnoses. (ed 4) St. Louis: Mosby-Year Book, 1997

Gamut F-117

PLEURAL EFFUSION ASSOCIATED WITH ABDOMINAL DISEASE

COMMON
1. Abdominal neoplasm, primary or secondary (eg, peritoneal metastases)
2. Ascites with permeation through diaphragm (eg, cirrhosis)
3. Meigs S.
4. Pancreatitis
5. Renal disease (eg, nephrotic S.; acute glomerulonephritis; uremia; dialysis; urinoma)
6. Subphrenic abscess; perinephric abscess

7. Trauma, abdominal (eg, knife or gunshot wound; ruptured diaphragm)

UNCOMMON
1. Amebic liver abscess
2. Aneurysm$_g$, thoracoabdominal, with rupture
3. Diaphragmatic hernia, incarcerated
4. Hemolytic-uremic S.
5. Lipoma or liposarcoma, thoracoabdominal
6. Lymphoma$_g$
7. Ovarian hyperstimulation S.

References
1. Fraser RS, Müller NL, Coleman N, Paré PD (eds): Fraser & Paré: Diagnosis of Diseases of the Chest. (ed 4) Philadelphia: WB Saunders, 1999
2. Lieberman FL, Peters RL: Cirrhotic hydrothorax: Further evidence that an acquired diaphragmatic defect is at fault. Arch Intern Med 1970;125:114–117

Gamut F-118-S1

PLEURAL EFFUSION CONTAINING EOSINOPHILS

COMMON
1. Eosinophilic lung disease$_g$ (esp. Löffler S.)
2. Hodgkin's lymphoma
3. Idiopathic
4. Parasitic disease (eg, paragonimiasis; amebiasis; strongyloidiasis) (See F-74-S)

UNCOMMON
1. Asthma
2. Churg-Strauss S.
3. Cirrhosis
4. Connective tissue disease (collagen vascular disease)$_g$ (eg, rheumatoid disease; lupus erythematosus; polyarteritis nodosa)
5. Drug reaction (See F-73-S); pulmonary granulomatosis in addicts

(continued)

6. Foreign material injection (oil; iodine; protein)
7. Infection (eg, fungus) (See F-74-S)
8. Leukemia (eosinophilic)
9. Malignant neoplasm
10. Pulmonary infarct
11. Trauma (blood, lymph)
12. Wegener granulomatosis$_g$

References
1. Frazier AA, Rosado de Christenson ML, Galvin JR, Fleming MV: Pulmonary angiitis and granulomatosis. Radio-Graphics 1998;18:687–710
2. Light RW, Erozan YS, Ball WC Jr: Cells in pleural fluid: Their value in differential diagnosis. Arch Intern Med 1973;132:854–860

Gamut F-118-S2

TYPE OF PLEURAL FLUID— TRANSUDATE (Protein < 3 g/dl)

COMMON
1. Cirrhosis
2. Fluid overload
3. Heart failure
4. Renal failure; uremia

UNCOMMON
1. Ascites
2. Constrictive pericarditis
3. Hypoproteinemia
4. Myxedema
5. Nephrotic syndrome
6. Peritoneal dialysis
7. Superior vena cava obstruction (eg, bronchogenic carcinoma; fibrosing mediastinitis) (See E-70)

Reference
1. Slone RM, Fisher AJ: Pocket Guide to Body CT Differential Diagnosis. New York, McGraw-Hill, 1999, pp 131–132

Gamut F-118-S3

TYPE OF PLEURAL FLUID—EXUDATE (Protein > 3 g/dl)

COMMON
1. Lymphoma$_g$; leukemia
2. Metastases to pleura (esp. bronchogenic carcinoma)
3. Pneumonia (esp. bacterial); lung abscess
4. Pulmonary thromboembolism
5. Tuberculosis

UNCOMMON
1. Connective tissue disorder (collagen vascular disease)$_g$, esp. lupus erythematosus
2. Dressler S. (recent cardiac surgery or myocardial infarction)
3. Drug reaction
4. Fungus disease
5. Meigs' S. (benign ovarian fibroma)
6. Mesothelioma
7. Pericardial disease
8. Postpartum
9. Subphrenic abscess

Reference
1. Slone RM, Fisher AJ: Pocket Guide to Body CT Differential Diagnosis. New York: McGraw-Hill, 1999, p 132

Gamut F-119

HEMOTHORAX

COMMON
1. Iatrogenic (eg, thoracentesis; lung biopsy; chest tube or central venous catheter placement)
2. Malignancy (eg, bronchogenic carcinoma; pleural metastases; mesothelioma)
3. Trauma to chest (eg, rib fracture; lacerated intercostal vessel; contusion)

UNCOMMON

1. Catamenial (eg, endometriosis)
2. Bleeding or clotting disorder$_g$ (eg, anticoagulation therapy; hemophilia)
3. Dissecting aortic aneurysm
4. Extramedullary hematopoiesis
5. Pleural adhesion tear

Reference
1. Slone RM, Fisher AJ: Pocket Guide to Body CT Differential Diagnosis. New York: McGraw-Hill, 1999, p 133

Gamut F-120

CHYLOTHORAX (LYMPHOTHORAX)*

COMMON

1. Iatrogenic (esp. surgical or catheter injury to thoracic duct; surgery for congenital heart disease)
2. Idiopathic; spontaneous
3. Neoplasm involving thoracic duct or mediastinum (eg, metastatic disease; lymphoma$_g$; carcinoma of esophagus or lung; intrathoracic thyroid)
4. Trauma to thoracic duct

UNCOMMON

1. Aneurysm of thoracic duct with rupture
2. Cirrhosis
3. Congenital anomaly (eg, atresia or fistula of thoracic duct; yellow nail S.; Noonan S.; congenital lymphangiectasia)
4. Fibrosing mediastinitis
5. Filariasis; elephantiasis
6. Lymphadenopathy (eg, tuberculous; fungal; other infection) (See F-103)
7. Lymphangioma (cystic hygroma)
8. Neonatal
9. Nephrosis
10. Nonneoplastic mass compressing the thoracic duct (eg, aortic aneurysm$_g$; spinal disease)

11. Pulmonary lymphangioleiomyomatosis; tuberous sclerosis
12. Pulmonary lymphangiomatosis
13. Thromboembolism of left subclavian or innominate vein, or superior vena cava (central venous obstruction)

* Effusion with high lipid content—may be less dense than water on CT.

References
1. Bower GC: Chylothorax: Observations in 20 cases. Chest 1964; 46:464–468
2. Freundlich IM: The role of lymphangiography in chylothorax. A report of six nontraumatic cases. AJR 1975;125: 617–627
3. Hesseling PG, Hoffman H: Chylothorax: A review of the literature and report of 3 cases. S Afr Med J 1981;60:675–678
4. Hughes RL, Mintzer RA, Hidvagi DF, et al: The management of chylothorax. Chest 1979;76:212–218
5. Swensen SJ, Hartman TE, Mayo JR, et al: Diffuse pulmonary lymphangiomatosis: CT findings. J Comput Assist Tomogr 1995;19:348–352

Gamut F-121

MASSIVE PLEURAL EFFUSION

COMMON

1. Ascites (leaky diaphragm)
2. Empyema
3. Heart failure
4. Hemothorax (eg, traumatic; bleeding disorder$_g$; catamenial)
5. Malignant intrathoracic neoplasm (eg, carcinoma, blastoma or sarcoma of lung; lymphoma$_g$; mesothelioma; neuroblastoma; teratoma)
6. Metastatic disease (eg, carcinoma of lung, esp. adenocarcinoma)
7. Nephrosis; acute glomerulonephritis
8. Postoperative
9. Subphrenic or liver abscess or neoplasm
10. Tuberculosis

(continued)

UNCOMMON

1. Actinomycosis; nocardiosis (empyema)
2. Amebiasis
3. Chylothorax (See F-120)
4. Fungus disease (See F-74-S)
5. Iatrogenic (eg, perforation by venous catheter)
6. Idiopathic
7. Pancreatitis
8. Perforation of esophagus or stomach
9. Polyserositis
10. Pulmonary thromboembolism with infarction

References
1. Liberson M: Diagnostic significance of the mediastinal profile in massive unilateral pleural effusions. Am Rev Resp Dis 1963;88:176–180
2. Swischuk LE, John SD: Differential Diagnosis in Pediatric Radiology. (ed 2) Baltimore: Williams & Wilkins, 1995, pp 11–15

Gamut F-122

OPACIFICATION OF ONE HEMITHORAX

COMMON

1. Atelectasis of one lung
2. Consolidation of one lung (eg, pneumonia)
3. Pleural effusion, massive hydrothorax; empyema; hemothorax; chylothorax (See F-119–121)
4. Postpneumonectomy fibrothorax; thoracoplasty
5. [Rotoscoliosis, advanced]

UNCOMMON

1. Agenesis of one lung
2. [Artifact due to faulty radiographic technique (eg, malpositioned filter)]
3. Cardiomegaly, massive
4. Cystic adenomatoid malformation (type III)
5. Diaphragmatic hernia (congenital or traumatic)
6. Eventration of diaphragm
7. Fibrosis of lung or pleura

8. Hematoma of chest wall
9. Mediastinal or pulmonary mass, huge
10. Mesothelioma
11. Metastatic disease to pleura (esp. from adenocarcinoma of ipsilateral lung or from osteosarcoma)

[ ] This condition does not actually cause the gamuted imaging finding, but can produce imaging changes that simulate it.

References
1. Liberson M: Diagnostic significance of the mediastinal profile in massive unilateral pleural effusions. Am Rev Resp Dis 1963;88:176–180
2. Swischuk LE, John SD: Differential Diagnosis in Pediatric Radiology. (ed 2) Baltimore: Williams & Wilkins, 1995, pp 11–15

Gamut F-123-1

PLEURAL THICKENING

COMMON

1. Asbestos-related pleural disease: pleural plaque; talcosis
2. Bronchogenic carcinoma (esp. Pancoast tumor)
3. Empyema, prior
4. [Extrathoracic musculature; lateral pleural stripe; apical pleural capping; extrapleural fat deposition]
5. Metastatic disease
6. Pleural effusion, organized; pleural fibrosis; prior pleuritis or localized effusion, incl. prior interlobar fluid
7. Postoperative; prior drainage via catheter tubes
8. Rib lesion (eg, fracture; osteomyelitis; neoplasm; metastasis)
9. Trauma (old hemothorax)
10. Tuberculosis; atypical mycobacterial infection

UNCOMMON

1. Actinomycosis; nocardiosis
2. Chylothorax, prior
3. Connective tissue disease (collagen vascular disease)$_g$ (esp. rheumatoid disease)
4. Fungus disease (See F-74-S)

5. Invasive thymoma with pleural involvement
6. Lymphoma$_g$; leukemia
7. Melioidosis
8. Mesothelioma
9. Parasitic disease (eg, paragonimiasis; amebiasis; ruptured hydatid cyst)
10. Pulmonary lymphangiomatosis
11. Pulmonary or mediastinal fibrosis, advanced
12. Rounded atelectasis
13. Sarcoidosis
14. Splenosis
15. Subpleural collaterals in pulmonary venous or arterial atresia

[ ] This condition does not actually cause the gamuted imaging finding, but can produce imaging changes that simulate it.

References
1. Ebel K-D, Blickman H, Willich E, Richter E: Differential Diagnosis in Pediatric Radiology. Stuttgart: Thieme, 1999, pp 113–115
2. Miller BH, Rosado de Christenson ML, McAdams HP, Fishback NF: Thoracic sarcoidosis: Radiologic-Pathologic Correlation. RadioGraphics 1995;15:421–437
3. Reed JC: Chest Radiology. Plain Film Patterns and Differential Diagnoses. (ed 4) St. Louis: Mosby-Year Book, 1997

Gamut F-123-2

NODULAR OR TUMOR-LIKE PLEURAL THICKENING

COMMON
1. Mesothelioma, malignant pleural
2. Metastatic disease (usually from adenocarcinoma of ipsilateral lung; occasionally from carcinoma of breast, ovary, prostate, gastrointestinal tract, or kidney)

UNCOMMON
1. Invasive thymoma with pleural involvement
2. Lymphoma$_g$

Gamut F-124

PLEURAL CALCIFICATION

COMMON
1. Asbestos-related pleural disease with plaques
2. Empyema, prior
3. Hemothorax, old
4. Idiopathic
5. Tuberculosis (esp. tuberculous empyema)

UNCOMMON
1. [Alveolar microlithiasis]
2. Calcifying fibrous pseudotumor of pleura
3. Histoplasmosis
4. Hyperparathyroidism, primary or secondary (renal osteodystrophy); chronic hemodialysis
5. [Mineral oil aspiration]
6. Neoplasm (eg, osteosarcoma; rarely mesothelioma)
7. Oleothorax (extrapleural plombage); pleurodesis with talc
8. Parasitic disease (esp. pentastomiasis—*Armillifer* infection); cysticercosis
9. Pleural effusion, chronic
10. Pneumoconiosis, other (mica; talc; other silicates; tin; barium)
11. Pulmonary lymphangiomatosis

[ ] This condition does not actually cause the gamuted imaging finding, but can produce imaging changes that simulate it.

References
1. Nichols DM, Johnson MA: Calcification in a pleural mesothelioma. J Can Assoc Radiol 1983;34:311–313
2. Reed JC: Chest Radiology. Plain Film Patterns and Differential Diagnoses. (ed 4) St. Louis: Mosby-Year Book, 1997
3. Watanabe T, Kobayashi T: Pleural calcification: A type of "metastatic calcification" in chronic renal failure. Br J Radiol 1983;56:93–98

Gamut F-125-1

PLEURAL MASS (See also F-126)

COMMON

1. Empyema
2. [Extrapleural tumor (eg, lipoma; liposarcoma; desmoid; neurofibroma; schwannoma)] (See F-126)
3. Hematoma
4. Lymphoma$_g$
*5. Mesothelioma
*6. Metastatic disease (esp. from adenocarcinoma of lung; also carcinoma of breast, prostate, ovary, pancreas, GI tract)
7. [Pancoast or superior sulcus tumor]
*8. Pleural fluid (loculated or interlobar)
*9. Pleural plaque (asbestos-related pleural disease)
10. Pleural thickening, localized (eg, prior infection, hemorrhage, or surgery)
11. [Rib or chest wall lesion (eg, callus; bone sarcoma; myeloma; metastasis)]

UNCOMMON

1. Cyst (eg, mesothelial; hydatid)
2. Fibrin ball
*3. Invasive thymoma with pleural involvement
4. Localized fibrous tumor of pleura
5. [Mediastinal mass (along mediastinal pleura)]
*6. Splenosis

* Often multiple lesions.
[ ] This condition does not actually cause the gamuted imaging finding, but can produce imaging changes that simulate it.

References
1. Berne AS, Heitzman ER: The roentgenologic signs of pedunculated pleural tumors. AJR 1962;87:892–895
2. Reed JC: Chest Radiology. Plain Film Patterns and Differential Diagnoses. (ed 4) St. Louis: Mosby-Year Book, 1997
3. Reeder MM: Gamut: Pleural-based lesion arising from the lung, pleura or chest wall. Semin Roentgenol 1977;12: 261–262

Gamut F-125-2

MULTIPLE PLEURAL MASSES

COMMON

1. Loculated pleural effusions (eg, postoperative; tuberculosis)
2. Metastases to pleura (eg, from ipsilateral carcinoma of lung; breast; prostate)
3. Pleural plaques (asbestos-related pleural disease)

UNCOMMON

1. Endometriosis
2. Invasive thymoma
3. Localized fibrous tumor of pleura (usually solitary)
4. Lymphoma$_g$
5. Mesothelioma
6. Parasitic disease (eg, paragonimiasis or amebiasis with loculated effusions; pentastomiasis or cysticercosis with calcifications; hydatid disease)
7. Splenosis (thoracic)

Reference
1. Slone RM, Fisher AJ: Pocket Guide to Body CT Differential Diagnosis. New York: McGraw-Hill, 1999, pp 146–147

Gamut F-126

EXTRAPLEURAL OR CHEST WALL LESION (ESP. ON CT, MRI) (INCL. THOSE ASSOCIATED WITH RIB DESTRUCTION) (See F-125-1)

COMMON

*1. Abscess; osteomyelitis of rib, sternum, or spine (eg, pyogenic infection; tuberculosis; actinomycosis; nocardiosis; blastomycosis; aspergillosis)
2. [Asbestos-related pleural disease]
*3. Benign bone lesion (eg, cyst; aneurysmal bone cyst; fibrous dysplasia; enchondroma; osteochon-

droma; angioma; giant cell tumor; chondromyxoid fibroma; brown tumor of hyperparathyroidism)
*4. Bone sarcoma (eg, Ewing sarcoma; osteosarcoma; chondrosarcoma; fibrosarcoma)
*5. Chest wall invasion by bronchogenic carcinoma (eg, Pancoast tumor) or breast carcinoma
*6. Fracture of rib, sternum or spine (esp. with callus or hematoma)
*7. Hematoma
8. Lipoma (subcutaneous, extrapleural intrathoracic, transmural)
*9. Lymphoma$_g$
10. [Mediastinal mass]
*11. Metastasis to rib, chest wall, soft tissue, or spine (esp. from carcinoma of prostate, breast, lung)
*12. Multiple myeloma
13. [Superimposed density, esp. breast or breast implant; nipple; hair braids; artifact; skin lesion (eg, mole; neurofibroma); extrathoracic muscles; retrosternal soft tissue band]
*14. Postoperative (eg, soft tissue deformity; pleurectomy; plombage)

UNCOMMON

*1. Chronic empyema with associated malignancy (eg, lymphoma; sarcoma; mesothelioma)
2. Desmoid tumor, extraabdominal (aggressive fibromatosis)
*3. Empyema necessitatis (esp. tuberculous)
*4. Extramedullary hematopoiesis (esp. thalassemia)
*5. Hydatid disease
*6. Langerhans cell histiocytosis$_g$ (esp. eosinophilic granuloma)
7. Liposarcoma
8. [Lobar agenesis with extrapleural tissue plane anteriorly on lateral view]
9. Lymphangioma (cystic hygroma)
*10. Malignant fibrous histiocytoma
*11. Massive osteolysis (Gorham's vanishing bone disease)
*12. Mesenchymal hamartoma of chest wall
*13. Mesothelioma
14. Muscle tumor (esp. rhabdomyosarcoma)

*15. Neurogenic tumor (eg, schwannoma; neurofibroma; malignant peripheral nerve sheath tumor; neuroblastoma; Askin tumor)
*16. Pleural-based lesion eroding rib (See F-125-1)
17. Spindle cell tumor$_g$; fibroma
*18. Vascular tumor (eg, hemangioma; arteriovenous malformation; hemangiopericytoma; angiosarcoma)

* May be associated with erosion or destruction of rib, sternum, or spine.
[ ] This condition does not actually cause the gamuted imaging finding, but can produce imaging changes that simulate it.

References
1. Felson B: Chest Roentgenology. Philadelphia: WB Saunders, 1973
2. Hachiya J (Tokyo): Lecture at Eleventh Masters Diagnostic Radiology Conference, Kauai, Hawaii, 1992
3. Omell GH, Anderson LS, Bramson RT: Chest wall tumors. Radiol Clin North Am 1973;11:197–214
4. Reed JC: Chest Radiology. Plain Film Patterns and Differential Diagnoses. (ed 4) St. Louis: Mosby-Year Book, 1997
5. Reeder MM: Gamut: Pleural-based lesion arising from lung, pleura, or chest wall. Semin Roentgenol 1977;12:261–262

Gamut F-127

AXILLARY MASS (CT, MRI)

COMMON

1. Lymphoma$_g$; leukemia
2. Metastatic disease (esp. from carcinoma of breast; also lung, kidney and head and neck tumors)

UNCOMMON

1. Desmoid tumor
2. Empyema necessitans
3. Lipoma
4. Lymphadenopathy, other (eg, sarcoidosis; tuberculosis; plague; toxoplasmosis; cat-scratch fever)
5. Lymphangioma
6. Primary malignancy of axilla

Reference
1. Eisenberg RL: Clinical Imaging: An Atlas of Differential Diagnosis. (ed 3) Philadelphia: Lippincott-Raven, 1997, pp 202–204

PEDIATRIC CHEST WALL OR RIB CAGE LESION, OSSEOUS OR SOFT TISSUE (ESP. ON CT, MRI)

CHEST WALL (RIB CAGE)—Benign Bone Tumors

COMMON
1. Aneurysmal bone cyst
2. Enchondroma
3. [Fibrous dysplasia]

UNCOMMON
1. Chondroblastoma (Codman tumor)
2. Mesenchymal hamartoma
3. Osteoblastoma
4. Osteochondroma

CHEST WALL (RIB CAGE)—Malignant Bone Tumors

COMMON
1. Ewing sarcoma
2. Metastasis (eg, neuroblastoma; leukemia)
3. Osteosarcoma

UNCOMMON
1. Askin tumor (primitive neuroectodermal tumor{PNET})
2. Chondrosarcoma
3. Lymphoma$_g$ (primary)
4. Metastases, other (eg, Ewing sarcoma; Wilms' tumor; rhabdomyosarcoma; retinoblastoma; osteosaraoma; lymphoma; medulloblastoma)

CHEST WALL—Benign Soft Tissue Tumors

COMMON
1. Hemangioma; lymphangioma

UNCOMMON
1. Desmoid
2. Hamartoma
3. Neurofibroma
4. Venous malformation

CHEST WALL—Malignant Soft Tissue Tumors

COMMON
1. Rhabdomyosarcoma

UNCOMMON
1. Askin tumor (primitive neuroectodermal tumor {PNET}); may be same as extraosseous Ewing sarcoma
2. Lymphoma
3. Pleuropulmonary blastoma

References
1. Hartman GE, Shochat SJ: Primary pulmonary neoplasms of childhood: a review. Ann Thorac Surg 1983;36:108–119
2. Meyer JS, Nicotra JJ: Tumors of the pediatric chest. Semin Roentgenol 1998;33:187–198

Gamut F-129

CONGENITAL SYNDROMES WITH PECTUS CARINATUM (PIGEON BREAST) (Same as D-209-2)

COMMON
1. Congenital heart disease (esp. cyanotic)
2. Ehlers-Danlos S.
3. Fetal alcohol S.

4. Homocystinuria
5. Idiopathic; isolated finding
6. Marfan S.
7. Mucopolysaccharidoses (esp. Morquio S.)
8. Osteogenesis imperfecta
9. [Rickets]
10. Undersegmentation or hypoplasia of sternum (See D-209-1)

UNCOMMON

1. Asphyxiating thoracic dysplasia (Jeune S.)
2. Coffin-Lowry S.
3. Currarino-Silverman S.
4. Dyggve-Melchior-Clausen dysplasia (Smith-McCort S.)
5. Hyperphosphatasia
6. LEOPARD S. (multiple lentigenes S.)
7. Noonan S.
8. Prune-belly S. (Eagle-Barrett S.)
9. Schwartz-Jampel S. (osteochondromuscular dystrophy)
10. Spondyloepimetaphyseal dysplasia (Strudwick type)
11. Spondyloepiphyseal dysplasia congenita
12. 3-M syndrome

[ ] This condition does not actually cause the gamuted imaging finding, but can produce imaging changes that simulate it.

References

1. Felson B (ed): Dwarfs and other little people. Semin Roentgenol 1973;8:133–263
2. Swischuk LE, John SD: Differential Diagnosis in Pediatric Radiology. (ed 2) Baltimore: Williams & Wilkins, 1995
3. Taybi H, Lachman RS: Radiology of Syndromes, Metabolic Disorders, and Skeletal Dysplasias. (ed 4) St. Louis: Mosby-Year Book, 1996, p 1049

Gamut F-130

CONGENITAL SYNDROMES WITH PECTUS EXCAVATUM (FUNNEL CHEST) (Same as D-209-3)

COMMON

1. Congenital heart disease
2. Ehlers-Danlos S.

3. Fetal alcohol S.
4. Homocystinuria
5. Idiopathic; isolated finding
6. Marfan S.
7. [Mitral valve prolapse syndrome (MVPS)]
8. Myotonic dystrophy
9. [Newborn with respiratory distress]
10. Osteogenesis imperfecta
11. Turner S.

UNCOMMON

1. Aarskog S.
2. Coffin-Lowry S.
3. Cowden S. (multiple hamartoma S.)
4. Cutis laxa
5. F syndrome
6. Freeman-Sheldon S. (whistling face S.)
7. Gorlin S. (nevoid basal cell carcinoma S.)
8. LEOPARD S. (multiple lentigenes S.)
9. Noonan S.
10. Osteodysplasty (Melnick-Needles S.)
11. Prune-belly S. (Eagle-Barrett S.)
12. 3-M syndrome

[ ] This condition does not actually cause the gamuted imaging finding, but can produce imaging changes that simulate it.

References

1. Ebel K-D, Blickman H, Willich E, Richter E: Differential Diagnosis in Pediatric Radiology. Stuttgart: Thieme, 1999, p 118
2. Swischuk LE, John SD: Differential Diagnosis in Pediatric Radiology. (ed 2) Baltimore: Williams & Wilkins, 1995
3. Taybi H, Lachman RS: Radiology of Syndromes, Metabolic Disorders, and Skeletal Dysplasias. (ed 4) St. Louis: Mosby-Year Book, 1996, p 1049

Gamut F-131

CONGENITAL SYNDROMES WITH A SHORT, NARROW THORACIC CAGE

COMMON

1. Achondroplasia (esp. homozygous)
2. Asphyxiating thoracic dysplasia (Jeune S.)

(continued)

3. Chondroectodermal dysplasia (Ellis-van Creveld S.)
4. Cleidocranial dysplasia
5. Metaphyseal chondrodysplasia (Jansen type)
6. Pulmonary hypoplasia, unilateral or bilateral; venolobar S. (scimitar S.)
7. Short rib-polydactyly syndromes (types I {Saldino-Noonan} and II {Majewski})
8. Thanatophoric dysplasia; thanatophoric variants
9. Trisomy 21 S. (Down S.) (bell-shaped thorax)

UNCOMMON

1. Achondrogenesis; hypochondrogenesis
2. Antley-Bixler S.
3. Atelosteogenesis
4. Barnes S.
5. Campomelic dysplasia
6. Cerebro-costo-mandibular S.
7. Diastrophic dysplasia
8. Dyssegmental dysplasia
9. Fibrochondrogenesis
10. Hypophosphatasia
11. Lethal osteosclerotic skeletal dysplasias (many types)
12. Metatropic dysplasia
13. Noonan S.
14. Osteodysplasty (Melnick-Needles S.)
15. Osteogenesis imperfecta
16. Progeria
17. Pseudoachondroplasia
18. Shwachman-Diamond S.
19. Spondylocostal dysostosis (Jarcho-Levin S.)
20. Spondyloepimetaphyseal dysplasia with joint laxity
21. Spondyloepiphyseal dysplasia congenita

References
1. Felson B (ed): Dwarfs and other little people. Semin Roentgenol 1973;8:133–263
2. Taybi H, Lachman RS: Radiology of Syndromes, Metabolic Disorders, and Skeletal Dysplasias. (ed 4) St. Louis: Mosby-Year Book, 1996, p 1051

FETAL OR NEONATAL CHEST ANOMALIES OR MALFORMATIONS (US, PLAIN FILM)

1. Congenital heart defects
2. Congenital lobar emphysema
3. Congenital syndromes with thoracic malformation (eg, asphyxiating thoracic dysplasia {Jeune S.}; thanatophoric dysplasia; achondrogenesis; spondylocostal dysostoses {Jarcho-Levin S.}; chondroectodermal dysplasia (Ellis-van Creveld S.) (See F-129–131)
4. Cystic adenomatoid malformation
5. Developmental (duplication) cyst (eg, bronchogenic; enteric; neurenteric)
6. Diaphragmatic hernia (congenital)
7. Esophageal atresia; tracheoesophageal fistula
8. Fetal hydrothorax
9. Laryngotracheal or bronchial atresia
10. Lymphangioma (cystic hygroma)
11. Pulmonary lymphangiectasia
12. Pulmonary hypoplasia
13. Pulmonary sequestration
14. Tracheal bronchus

Reference
1. Hubbard AM, Crombleholme TM: Anomalies and malformations affecting the fetal/neonatal chest. Semin Roentgenol 1998;33:117–125.

FLAT OR DEPRESSED DIAPHRAGM (UNILATERAL OR BILATERAL)

UNILATERAL

1. Intrathoracic mass (large unilateral)
2. Pleural effusion, hemothorax, chylothorax, empyema

3. Obstructive emphysema (COPD)
4. Tension pneumothorax

BILATERAL

COMMON

1. Asthma
2. COPD
3. Viral infection (incl. bronchiolitis in infants)

UNCOMMON

1. Air hunger (eg, severe congenital heart disease)
2. Hyperaeration with acidosis and dehydration
3. Obstructive emphysema, other causes (eg, cystic fibrosis {mucoviscidosis}; alpha-1 antitrypsin deficiency; cutis laxa; central or bilateral foreign bodies; vascular rings and anomalies; intratracheal lesions; paratracheal masses and cysts)
4. Pleural effusion, hemothorax, chylothorax (bilateral)
5. Tension pneumothorax (bilateral)

Reference
1. Swischuk LE, John SD: Differential Diagnosis in Pediatric Radiology. (ed 2) Baltimore: Williams & Wilkins, 1995, pp 109–111

9. [Subpulmonic pleural effusion, bilateral]
10. Trauma (incl. bilateral rib fractures with guarding)

UNCOMMON

1. [Diaphragmatic hernia, large]
2. Eventration, bilateral
3. Foreign body (laryngotracheal)
4. Lobar atelectasis, bilateral
5. Lupus erythematosus
6. Neuromuscular disease$_g$ (eg, poliomyelitis; myotonic dystrophy)
7. Pleural disease, bilateral
8. Pulmonary thromboembolism with infarction, bilateral
9. Subphrenic abscess, bilateral

[ ] This condition does not actually cause the gamuted imaging finding, but can produce imaging changes that simulate it.

References
1. Felson B: Chest Roentgenology. Philadelphia: WB Saunders, 1973
2. Swischuk LE, John SD: Differential Diagnosis in Pediatric Radiology. (ed 2) Baltimore: Williams & Wilkins, 1995, pp 109–111
3. Wexler HA, Poole CA: Neonatal diaphragmatic dysfunction. AJR 1976;127:617–622

Gamut F-134

BILATERAL ELEVATED DIAPHRAGM

COMMON

1. Abdominal neoplasm or cyst (eg, huge ovarian)
2. Ascites; peritoneal hemorrhage or lavage; peritonitis
3. Expiratory or poor inspiratory film
4. Hepatomegaly and splenomegaly
5. Obesity
6. Pneumoperitoneum
7. Postmyocardial infarction S. (Dressler S.); post-pericardiotomy S.
8. Pregnancy

Gamut F-135

UNILATERAL ELEVATED HEMIDIAPHRAGM

COMMON

1. Atelectasis
2. Distended stomach or splenic flexure of colon
3. Eventration
4. Idiopathic; normal variant
5. Inflammatory disease in abdomen (eg, subphrenic, perinephric, hepatic, or splenic abscess; pancreatitis; cholecystitis; perforated ulcer)
6. Interposition of colon between liver and right hemidiaphragm (Chilaiditi S.)

(continued)

7. [Normal lateral decubitus view (dependent side)]
8. Paralysis (eg, phrenic nerve palsy or paralysis, esp. from bronchogenic carcinoma; primary or metastatic mediastinal malignancy; extrinsic pressure from intrathoracic goiter or aortic aneurysm; trauma; iatrogenic-surgical transection) (See F-136)
9. Pleural disease (eg, acute pleurisy; fibrosis; old empyema, hemothorax or pleural tuberculosis; mesothelioma)
10. Postoperative (eg, lobectomy; pneumonectomy); postpericardiotomy S. (post-CABG)
11. Ruptured spleen or liver (esp. subphrenic hematoma)
12. Scoliosis (on side of concavity)
13. Splinting of diaphragm or guarding from acute process (eg, fractured rib; chest wall trauma; pulmonary infarct; pneumonia)
14. Subphrenic mass (eg, enlargement, tumor, cyst, or abscess of liver or spleen; carcinoma of stomach)
15. [Subpulmonic pleural effusion]
16. Trauma to phrenic nerve, thorax, cervical spine, or brachial plexus

UNCOMMON

1. [Diaphragmatic cyst or tumor, intrinsic or adjacent (eg, mesothelioma; metastasis; localized fibrous tumor of pleura; lipoma)]
2. [Diaphragmatic hernia (Morgagni; Bochdalek; traumatic; large hiatal)]
3. [Emphysema of contralateral lung]
4. Hydatid cyst of liver or spleen
5. Hypoplasia or agenesis of one lung
6. Neurologic or neuromuscular disease$_g$ (eg, polio; Erb's palsy; hemiplegia)
7. Retroperitoneal neoplasm
8. Thoracic kidney
9. Traumatic rupture of diaphragm
10. Venolobar S. (scimitar S.) (incl. accessory diaphragm)

[ ] This condition does not actually cause the gamuted imaging finding, but can produce imaging changes that simulate it.

References

1. Anderson LS, Forrest JV: Tumors of the diaphragm. AJR 1973;119:259–265
2. Felson B: Chest Roentgenology. Philadelphia: WB Saunders, 1973
3. Guenter CA, Whitelaw WA: The role of diaphragm function in disease. Arch Intern Med 1979;139:806–808
4. Reed JC: Chest Radiology. Plain Film Patterns and Differential Diagnoses. (ed 4) St. Louis: Mosby-Year Book, 1997
5. Swischuk LE, John SD: Differential Diagnosis in Pediatric Radiology. (ed 2) Baltimore: Williams & Wilkins, 1995, p 109

Gamut F-136

PARALYZED OR FIXED HEMIDIAPHRAGM

COMMON

1. Eventration
2. Phrenic nerve paralysis (See F-137)
3. Pleural disease, chronic (eg, tuberculosis; empyema; hemothorax)
4. Subphrenic inflammatory disease (eg, subphrenic, perinephric, hepatic, or splenic abscess; pancreatitis; cholecystitis; perforated ulcer)

UNCOMMON

1. Birth trauma (Erb's palsy)
2. Diaphragmatic hernia (esp. traumatic)
3. Fibrosing mediastinitis (esp. histoplasmosis; idiopathic)
4. Gastric dilatation, severe
5. Idiopathic
6. Muscle disease$_g$ (eg, amyotonia congenita)
7. Neoplasm of diaphragm, primary or secondary (incl. mesothelioma)
8. Neuromuscular disorder$_g$ (eg, poliomyelitis; Guillain-Barré S.; hemiplegia)
9. Pneumonia
10. Pulmonary infarct
11. Radiation therapy

References

1. Alexander G: Diaphragm movements and the diagnosis of diaphragmatic paralysis. Clin Radiol 1966;17:79–83
2. Simon G, Bonnell J, Kazantzis G, et al: Some radiological observations on the range of movement of the diaphragm. Clin Radiol 1969;20:231–233

Gamut F-137

PHRENIC NERVE PARALYSIS OR DYSFUNCTION

COMMON

1. Iatrogenic (eg, surgical injury; chest tube; therapeutic avulsion or injection; subclavian vein puncture)
2. Infection (eg, tuberculosis; fungus disease; abscess)
3. Neoplastic invasion or compression (esp. carcinoma of lung)

UNCOMMON

1. Aneurysm$_g$, aortic or other
2. Birth trauma (Erb's palsy)
3. Herpes zoster
4. Neuritis, peripheral (eg, diabetic neuropathy)
5. Neurologic disease$_g$ (eg, hemiplegia; encephalitis; polio; Guillain-Barré S.)
6. Pneumonia
7. Trauma

Reference

1. Prasad S, Athreya BH: Transient paralysis of the phrenic nerve associated with head injury. JAMA 1976;236:2532–2533

Gamut F-138

SEGMENTAL OR LOCALIZED ELEVATION (SCALLOPING), MOGUL OR MASS OF A HEMIDIAPHRAGM

COMMON

1. Abscess of liver, lung, or pleura (esp. amebic)
2. Asbestos-related pleural disease (pleural plaque)
3. Atelectasis of an upper lobe
4. Eventration (localized)
5. Hernia (eg, hepatic; Morgagni; Bochdalek; traumatic)
6. Normal scalloping
7. Pleural mass adjacent to diaphragm, other (eg, mesothelioma; localized fibrous tumor of pleura; lipoma; liposarcoma)
8. Subphrenic, hepatic or splenic abscess, neoplasm or cyst
9. Thoracic kidney

UNCOMMON

1. Cyst (eg, hydatid; bronchogenic)
2. Neoplasm of diaphragm (eg, fibroma; myoma; cystic teratoma)
3. Pulmonary sequestration (extralobar)
4. Segmental paralysis of phrenic nerve (See F-137)
5. Venolobar syndrome (scimitar S.) (pulmonary hypoplasia)

References

1. Kattan KR, Eyler WR, Felson B: The juxtaphrenic peak in upper lobe collapse. Semin Roentgenol 1980;15:187–193
2. Rivero HJ, Bowen AD, Bender TM, et al: Radiological evaluation of diaphragm and juxtadiaphragmatic lesions. Scientific exhibit, American Roentgen Ray Society, Boston, 1985
3. Yen HC, Halton KP, Gray CE: Anatomic variations and abnormalities in the diaphragm seen with US. RadioGraphics 1990;10:1019–1030

Gamut F-139

JUXTADIAPHRAGMATIC LESIONS IN CHILDREN

COMMON

1. Lymphoma$_g$; other lymphadenopathy
2. Neurogenic neoplasm$_g$ (eg, neurofibroma; ganglioneuroma; ganglioneuroblastoma; neuro-blastoma)
3. Pleural effusion, free or loculated, benign or malignant; empyema
4. Pleural thickening

UNCOMMON

1. Diaphragmatic hernia (hiatal; Morgagni; Bochdalek; traumatic)
2. Cyst (pericardial; bronchogenic; hydatid)
3. Germ cell neoplasm, benign or malignant (esp. teratoma)
4. Hemangiopericytoma
5. Sarcoma (esp. Ewing sarcoma; also liposarcoma; osteosarcoma; rhabdomyosarcoma)

Reference
1. Rivero HJ, Bowen AD, Bender TM, et al: Radiological evaluation of diaphragm and juxtadiaphragmatic lesions. Scientific exhibit, American Roentgen Ray Society Meeting, Boston, 1985

Gamut F-140

SOLITARY THORACIC CALCIFICATION

COMMON

1. Asbestos related pleural disease; asbestos pleural plaque
2. Cardiovascular (eg, arteriosclerosis; aneurysm$_g$; mitral or aortic valve; coronary artery; intracardiac myxoma or thrombus; ligamentum arteriosum; old myocardial infarct) (See E-44)

3. Chest wall (esp. rib callus; costal cartilage calcification)
4. Granuloma (eg, tuberculosis; histoplasmosis, other fungus disease; nonspecific)
5. Lymphadenopathy (eg, tuberculosis; histoplasmosis; sarcoidosis; silicosis)
6. Mediastinal neoplasm or cyst (eg, mature teratoma; bronchogenic cyst; hemangioma; thymoma, intrathoracic thyroid; neurogenic neoplasm—schwannoma; ganglioneuroma; neuroblastoma)
7. Pericardial (eg, calcific pericarditis) (See E-45)
8. Pleural, other (eg, old empyema or hemothorax; tuberculosis) (See F-124)

UNCOMMON

1. Abscess of lung, chronic
2. Amyloidoma
3. Bronchogenic carcinoma engulfing a granuloma
4. Broncholith
5. Carcinoid.
6. Chest wall, other (eg, myositis ossificans; neoplasm of rib, breast, or chest wall; parasitic infection—guinea worm)
7. [Foreign body]
8. Fungus ball (mycetoma)
9. Hamartoma
10. Hematoma, old
11. Idiopathic
12. Lymphoma, treated; other necrotic or treated neoplasm
13. Measles pneumonia, atypical with nodular complex
14. Metastasis (See F-142)
15. Mucoid impaction
16. Neoplasm of lung, other rare (eg, leiomyosarcoma; intrapulmonary teratoma)
17. Pneumonia, organized; inflammatory pseudotumor (plasma cell granuloma—rarely)
18. Pulmonary artery aneurysm or hypertension
19. Pulmonary thromboembolism
20. Thrombus in IVC or SVC
21. Varix or hemangioma of lung (phleboliths)

[ ] This condition does not actually cause the gamuted imaging finding, but can produce imaging changes that simulate it.

References
1. Agrons GA, Rosado de Christenson ML, Kirejczyk WM, et al: Pulmonary inflammatory pseudotumor. Radiologic features. Radiology 1998;206:511–518
2. Felson B: Chest Roentgenology. Philadelphia: WB Saunders, 1973
3. Felson B: Thoracic calcifications. Chest 1969;56:330–343
4. Salzman E: Lung Calcifications in X-ray Diagnosis. Springfield: CC Thomas, 1968
5. Swischuk LE, John SD: Differential Diagnosis in Pediatric Radiology. (ed 2) Baltimore: Williams & Wilkins, 1995, pp 47–50

Gamut F-141

MULTIFOCAL OR WIDESPREAD THORACIC CALCIFICATIONS

COMMON

1. Chest wall (eg, costal cartilages; rib fractures with callus)
2. Fungus disease, nodal and parenchymal (esp. histoplasmosis; coccidioidomycosis; candidiasis—late)
3. Lymphadenopathy (eg, tuberculosis; histoplasmosis; sarcoidosis; silicosis)
4. Pleural (eg, asbestos-related pleural disease; talcosis; tuberculosis; old empyema or hemothorax)) (See F-124)
5. Silicosis; coal-worker's pneumoconiosis
6. Tracheobronchial cartilage (physiologic)
7. Tuberculosis (not miliary)
8. Vascular (diffuse/extensive atherosclerosis)

UNCOMMON

1. Alveolar microlithiasis
2. Amyloidosis
3. [Bronchography; lymphangiography]
4. Broncholithiasis
5. Chickenpox pneumonia, healed
6. [Foreign bodies]
7. Hamartomas of lung, multiple (incl. Carney's triad)
8. Idiopathic pulmonary ossification (osteopathia)
9. Lymphoma$_g$ after radiation therapy
10. Metastases (See F-142)
11. Metastatic calcification (metabolic calcinosis) (eg, hyperparathyroidism, primary or secondary {renal osteodystrophy with renal failure; uremia; hemodialysis}; hypervitaminosis D; milk-alkali syndrome; excessive calcium administration)
12. Parasitic disease in lung, pleura, thoracic muscles, or subcutaneous tissues (eg, paragonimiasis; pentastomiasis—*Armillifer* infection; dracunculiasis—guinea worm infection; cysticercosis)
13. Pseudoxanthoma elasticum
14. Pulmonary artery atherosclerosis (eg, pulmonary hypertension; Eisenmenger complex)
15. Pulmonary hemosiderosis (mitral stenosis; idiopathic {Ceelen S.}, esp. on CT)
16. Rheumatoid nodules
17. Sarcoidosis
18. [Tin, barium, or antimony pneumoconiosis]
19. Tracheopathia osteoplastica

[ ] This condition does not actually cause the gamuted imaging finding, but can produce imaging changes that simulate it.

References
1. Bein ME, Lee DBN, Mink JH, et al: Unusual case of metastatic pulmonary calcification. AJR 1979;132:812–816
2. Cohen AM, Maxon HR, Goldsmith RE, et al: Metastatic pulmonary calcification in primary hyperparathyroidism. Arch Intern Med 1977;137:520–522
3. Ebel K-D, Blickman H, Willich E, Richter E: Differential Diagnosis in Pediatric Radiology. Stuttgart: Thieme, 1999, pp 91–95
4. Eisenberg RL: Clinical Imaging: An Atlas of Differential Diagnosis. (ed 3) Philadelphia: Lippincott-Raven, 1997
5. Felson B: Thoracic calcifications. Chest 1969;56:330–343
6. Felson B, Schwarz J, Lukin RR, et al: Idiopathic pulmonary ossification. Radiology 1984;153:303–310
7. Salzman E: Lung Calcifications in X-ray Diagnosis. Springfield: CC Thomas, 1968

Gamut F-142

CALCIFIED PULMONARY METASTASES

COMMON

1. Chondrosarcoma
2. Mucinous (colloid) adenocarcinoma (eg, colon; breast)
3. Osteosarcoma
4. Papillary (psammomatous) adenocarcinoma (eg, ovary; thyroid)

UNCOMMON

1. Cystosarcoma phylloides
2. Dystrophic calcification in metastatic foci (esp. post-radiation or chemotherapy)
3. Epithelioid hemangioendothelioma
4. Germ cell neoplasm
5. Leiomyomatosis (benign metastasizing leiomyomas)
6. Medullary carcinoma of thyroid
7. Mesenchymoma, malignant
8. Synovial sarcoma

References

1. Greenfield GB: Radiology of Bone Diseases. (ed 5) Philadelphia: Lippincott, 1990
2. Maile CW, Rodan BA, Godwin JD, Chen JT, Ravin CE: Calcification in pulmonary metastases. Br J Radiol 1982; 55:108–113
3. Samuels T, Kerenyi N, Hamilton P: Cystosarcoma phylloides: Calcified pulmonary metastases detected by computed tomography. Can Assoc Radiol J 1990;41:217–218
4. Yousem SA, Hochholzer L: Unusual thoracic manifestations of epitheliold hemangioendothelioma. Arch Pathol Lab Med 1987;111:459–463

Gamut F-143

EGGSHELL CALCIFICATIONS IN THE CHEST (ESP. MEDIASTINAL LYMPH NODES)

COMMON

1. Aneurysm of great vessels
*2. Idiopathic
*3. Silicosis; coal-worker's pneumoconiosis

UNCOMMON

*1. Amyloidosis
*2. Fungus disease (esp. histoplasmosis) (See F-74-S)
*3. Hodgkin's lymphoma, treated
4. Pulmonary artery calcification in chronic pulmonary hypertension (eg, atrial septal defect (ASD); cor pulmonale)
*5. Sarcoidosis
*6. Tuberculosis

* Primarily in mediastinal or hilar lymph nodes.

References

1. Felson B: Chest Roentgenology. Philadelphia: WB Saunders, 1973
2. Fraser RS, Müller NL, Coleman N, Paré PD (eds): Fraser & Paré: Diagnosis of Diseases of the Chest. (ed 4) Philadelphia: WB Saunders, 1999
3. Gross GH, Schneider HJ, Proto AV: Eggshell calcification of lymph nodes: An update. AJR 1980;135:1265–1268
4. Jacobson G, Felson B, Pendergrass EP, et al: Eggshell calcifications in coal and metal miners. Semin Roentgenol 1967;2:276–282

Gastrointestinal Tract
and Abdomen

G

G

G

G

G

G

G

G

G

G

Gamut G-1

RETENTION OF BARIUM IN THE HYPOPHARYNX (ESP. CRICOPHARYNGEAL ACHALASIA) (ROENTGEN COUNTERPART OF DYSPHAGIA)

COMMON

1. Connective tissue disease (collagen vascular disease)$_g$ (esp. scleroderma; dermatomyositis)
2. Cricopharyngeal achalasia (minor to severe muscular incoordination)
3. Esophageal obstruction (eg, achalasia; carcinoma)
4. Muscular disorder$_g$ (eg, myasthenia gravis; myotonic dystrophy; steroid or thyrotoxic myopathy; oculopharyngeal myopathy)
5. Neurologic disorder$_g$ (eg, stroke; bulbar or pseudobulbar palsy; bulbar poliomyelitis; high unilateral cervical vagotomy; multiple sclerosis; parkinsonism; amyotrophic lateral sclerosis; syringomyelia; Riley-Day S. (familial dysautonomia); peripheral or central cranial nerve palsy; diphtheria; tetanus)
6. Postradiation therapy for pharyngeal or neck malignancy
7. Zenker's diverticulum

UNCOMMON

1. Abscess; cellulitis (esp. pharyngeal; peritonsillar)
2. Esophageal web (eg, congenital; Plummer-Vinson S.)
3. Foreign body
4. Hematoma of neck
5. Lymphadenopathy, cervical
6. [Pseudodefect from total laryngectomy]
7. Stricture (eg, lye)
8. Thyroid neoplasm

[ ] This condition does not actually cause the gamuted imaging finding, but can produce imaging changes that simulate it.

References
1. Eisenberg RL: Gastrointestinal Radiology: A Pattern Approach. (ed 3) Philadelphia: Lippincott, 1996, pp 5–8
2. Felson B: Chest Roentgenology. Philadelphia: WB Saunders, 1973
3. Jones B: Functional abnormalities of the pharynx. In: Gore RM, Levine MS: Textbook of Gastrointestinal Radiology. (ed 2) Philadelphia: WB Saunders, 2000, pp 316–328
4. Rubesin SE: Pharynx. In: Levine MS, Rubesin SE, Laufer I: Double Contrast Gastrointestinal Radiology. (ed 3) Philadelphia: WB Saunders, 2000, pp 61–91

Gamut G-2

ESOPHAGEAL MOTILITY DISORDER (APERISTALSIS, TERTIARY CONTRACTIONS, SPASM, AND OTHER FORMS)

COMMON

+*1. Achalasia (cardiospasm) (See G-3)
  2. Chalasia (infantile gastroesophageal regurgitation)
  3. Cricopharyngeal achalasia
+4. Diffuse esophageal spasm, idiopathic
+*5. Esophagitis (eg, reflux or peptic; radiation; caustic; monilial; herpes; viral)
+6. Neurologic disorder$_g$ (eg, stroke; peripheral or central cranial nerve palsy; pseudobulbar palsy; bulbar poliomyelitis; syringomyelia; high unilateral cervical vagotomy; multiple sclerosis; parkinsonism; amyotrophic lateral sclerosis; cerebral disease; Riley-Day S. {familial dysautonomia})
+7. Obstructive lesion, extrinsic or intrinsic (eg, Schatzki ring; stricture; esophageal neoplasm; foreign body; web; mediastinal tumor, cyst, or lymphadenopathy; mediastinitis)
+*8. Postsurgical repair of esophageal atresia, tracheoesophageal fistula, or hiatal hernia
+9. Presbyesophagus
*10. Scleroderma
  11. Zenker's diverticulum

UNCOMMON

1. Alcoholic neuropathy
*2. Amyloidosis

(continued)

3. Behçet S.
*4. Chagas' disease
5. Congenital syndromes (eg, Ehlers-Danlos S.; cutis laxa; G syndrome)
*6. Connective tissue disease (collagen vascular disease)$_g$, other (eg, dermatomyositis; polymyositis; mixed connective tissue disease {MCTD}; lupus erythematosus; rheumatoid arthritis)
*7. Crohn's disease
+8. Diabetic neuropathy
*9. Drug reaction (atropine; curare; Pro-Banthine)
+10. Hypertensive lower esophageal sphincter
11. Iatrogenic (eg, postvagotomy S.; sclerotherapy for varices)
12. Intramural diverticulosis of esophagus
+13. Muscular disorder$_g$ (esp. myasthenia gravis; oculopharyngeal myopathy; muscular or myotonic dystrophy; steroid or thyrotoxic myopathy)
+14. Neoplasm, infiltrative (eg, diffuse esophageal carcinoma; leukemia)
+15. Nutcracker esophagus
16. Paraneoplastic S.
17. Thyroid disease (myxedema; thyrotoxicosis)
18. Tylosis (keratosis palmaris et plantaris familiaris)

* Esophagus may be aperistaltic.
\+ Tertiary contractions often present.

References

1. Aly YA: Digital radiography in the evaluation of oesophageal motility disorders. Clin Radiol 2000;55:561–568
2. Bennett JR, Hendricks TR: Diffuse esophageal spasm: A disorder with more than one cause. Gastroenterology 1970; 59:273–279
3. Clouse RE, Diamant NE: Motor physiology and motor disorders of the esophagus. In: Feldman M, Scharschmidt BF, Sleisenger MH: Gastrointestinal and Liver Disease. (ed 6) Philadelphia: WB Saunders, 2000, pp 61–91
4. Eisenberg RL: Gastrointestinal Radiology: A Pattern Approach (ed 3). Philadelphia: Lippincott, 1996, pp 3–24
5. Gelfand DW: Gastrointestinal Radiology. New York: Churchill Livingstone, 1984, p 170
6. Hurwitz AL, Duranceau A, Haddad JK: Disorders of Esophageal Motility, vol 16. In: Smith LH Jr (ed): Major Problems in Internal Medicine series. Philadelphia: WB Saunders, 1979
7. Merhar G: Disorders of esophageal motility. Semin Roentgenol 1981;16:162–163
8. Ogle SJ, Kirk CJC, Bailey RJ, et al: Esophageal function in cirrhotic patients undergoing injection sclerotherapy for esophageal varices. Digestion 1978;18:178–185
9. Ott DJ: Esophageal motility disorders. Semin Roentgenol 1994;29:321–331
10. Ott DJ: Motility disorders of the esophagus. In: Gore RM, Levine MS: Textbook of Gastrointestinal Radiology. (ed 2) Philadelphia: WB Saunders, 2000, pp 316–328
11. Simeone JF, Burrell M, Toffler R, et al: Aperistalsis and esophagitis. Radiology 1977; 123:9–14
12. Teplick JG, Haskin NM: Roentgenologic Diagnosis. (ed. 3) Philadelphia: WB Saunders, 1976
13. Zboralske FF, Dodds WJ: Roentgenographic diagnosis of primary disorders of esophageal motility. Radiol Clin North Am 1969;7:147–162

Gamut G-3

ACHALASIA (CARDIOSPASM) OF THE ESOPHAGUS

COMMON
1. [Carcinoma, esophageal or gastric]
2. Idiopathic
3. [Stricture from esophagitis]

UNCOMMON
1. Amyloidosis
2. Cerebrovascular accident (stroke)
3. Chagas' disease
4. Chronic idiopathic intestinal pseudo-obstruction
5. Connective tissue disease (collagen disease)$_g$ (esp. scleroderma)
6. Diabetic neuropathy
7. Drug reaction (esp. atropine; Pro-Banthine)
8. Hypertensive lower esophageal sphincter
9. Iatrogenic (eg, vagotomy)
10. Nerve destruction (myenteric plexus, sympathetic, or vagus), esp. by neoplasm

[ ] This condition does not actually cause the gamuted imaging finding, but can produce imaging changes that simulate it.

References
1. Eisenberg RL: Gastrointestinal Radiology: A Pattern Approach (ed 3). Philadelphia: Lippincott, 1996, pp 11–19
2. Gelfand DW: Gastrointestinal Radiology. New York: Churchill Livingstone, 1984, p 170
3. Ott DJ: Motility disorders of the esophagus. In: Gore RM, Levine MS: Textbook of Gastrointestinal Radiology. (ed 2) Philadelphia: WB Saunders, 2000, pp 316–328
4. Woodfield CA, Levine MS, Rubesin SE, et al: Diagnosis of primary versus secondary achalasia: reassessment of clinical and radiographic criteria. AJR 2000;175:727–731

Gamut G-4

AIR IN THE ESOPHAGUS

COMMON
1. Achalasia (See G-3)
2. Infant respiratory distress syndrome (hyaline membrane disease)
3. Normal
4. Respirator therapy; intubation
5. Scleroderma

UNCOMMON
1. Caustic esophagitis
2. Chagas' disease
3. Diverticulum, esophageal
4. Gastroesophageal regurgitation, infantile or adult
5. Hypertensive lower esophageal sphincter
6. Obstruction of esophagus (eg, neoplasm of esophagus; mediastinal tumor, cyst, or lymphadenopathy; mediastinitis)
7. Postoperative (eg, esophageal or pulmonary surgery)

References
1. Meredith HC, Anderson RJ, Vujic I: Another look at the segmental air esophagram. AJR 1960;136:23–26
2. Ott DJ: Motility disorders of the esophagus. In: Gore RM, Levine MS: Textbook of Gastrointestinal Radiology. (ed 2) Philadelphia: WB Saunders, 2000, pp 316–328

Gamut G-5

EXTRINSIC IMPRESSION ON THE CERVICAL ESOPHAGUS

COMMON
1. Cricopharyngeal muscle
2. [Esophageal web]
3. Lymph node enlargement
4. Osteophyte of cervical spine
5. Pharyngeal venous plexus (postcricoid impression)
6. Soft tissue abscess or hematoma (esp. retrolaryngeal)
7. Thyroid mass (eg, goiter; adenoma; carcinoma; thyroiditis)

UNCOMMON
1. Aneurysm or buckling of carotid or innominate artery
2. Cervical spine lesion, other (eg, osteomyelitis; neoplasm; anteriorly herniated disk)
3. Ectopic gastric mucosa
4. Parathyroid tumor (eg, adenoma; carcinoma)
5. [Gastrointestinal stromal tumor$_g$ (esp. leiomyoma) or lipoma of esophagus]
6. Tracheal or laryngeal neoplasm

[ ] This condition does not actually cause the gamuted imaging finding, but can produce imaging changes that simulate it.

References
1. Gelfand DW: Gastrointestinal Radiology. New York: Churchill Livingstone, 1984
2. Eisenberg RL: Clinical Imaging: An Atlas of Differential Diagnosis. (ed 3) Philadelphia: Lippincott-Raven, 1997, pp 284–285

Gamut G-6

EXTRINSIC IMPRESSION ON THE THORACIC ESOPHAGUS

COMMON

1. Cardiac enlargement (esp. left atrium)
2. Duplication cyst (bronchogenic or enteric)
3. Hiatal hernia (esp. paraesophageal)
4. Mediastinal lymphadenopathy (eg, metastasis; lymphoma$_g$; tuberculosis; histoplasmosis; sarcoidosis)
5. Mediastinal mass (eg, tumor; cyst; mediastinitis)
6. Normal structure (left main stem bronchus; aortic knob; confluence of left pulmonary veins)
7. Pericardial lesion (eg, effusion; cyst; tumor) (See E-43)
8. Pleuropulmonary fibrosis at lung apex, esp. tuberculosis (pseudoimpression)
9. Pulmonary mass (esp. carcinoma of lung)
10. Vascular impression, abnormal (eg, aortic aneurysm or tortuosity; coarctation of aorta; right, cervical, or double aortic arch; truncus arteriosus; aberrant right or left subclavian artery; pulmonary sling) (See G-7)

UNCOMMON

1. Neurinoma of vagus or phrenic nerve
2. Spinal abnormality (eg, kyphosis; scoliosis; osteophyte; DISH; neoplasm; osteomyelitis)
3. Tracheal neoplasm (See B-111, F-81-1)

References

1. Gelfand DW: Gastrointestinal Radiology. New York: Churchill Livingstone, 1984, p 190
2. Eisenberg RL: Clinical Imaging: An Atlas of Differential Diagnosis. (ed 3) Philadelphia: Lippincott-Raven, 1996, pp 286–291

Gamut G-7

EXTRINSIC VASCULAR IMPRESSION ON THE ESOPHAGUS (See E-18)

COMMON

1. Aberrant right or left subclavian artery
2. Aortic abnormality, acquired (eg, aneurysm; tortuosity)
3. Aortic knob
4. Coarctation of aorta
5. Right aortic arch (esp. posterior or type II aortic arch)

UNCOMMON

1. Anomalous innominate artery
2. Aortic diverticulum
3. APVC, total (below diaphragm)
4. Arteriovenous malformation
5. Azygos or hemiazygos vein dilatation
6. Cervical aortic arch
7. Corrected transposition (medially placed pulmonary artery)
8. Double aortic arch
9. Enlarged "bronchial" artery (incl. truncus arteriosus; absent main pulmonary artery)
10. Pulmonary artery "sling" (anomalous origin of left pulmonary artery)
11. Pulmonary vein confluence draining into back of left atrium
12. Sequestration of lung (anomalous artery from aorta)

References

1. Birnholz JC, Ferrucci JT, Wyman SM: Roentgen features of dysphagia aortica. Radiology 1974;111:93–99
2. Levine MS, Laufer I: Esophagus. In: Levine MS, Rubesin SE, Laufer I: Double Contrast Gastrointestinal Radiology. (ed 3) Philadelphia: WB Saunders, 2000, pp 90–125

Gamut G-8

TRACHEOESOPHAGEAL OR ESOPHAGOBRONCHIAL FISTULA

COMMON
1. Carcinoma of esophagus, lung or trachea
2. Congenital, with or without esophageal atresia

UNCOMMON
1. Abscess, pulmonary or mediastinal
2. Actinomycosis
3. Behçet S.
4. Caustic esophagitis (esp. lye)
5. Crohn's disease
6. Diverticulum of esophagus, perforated
7. Esophageal lung (sequestration)
8. Granulomatous lymphadenitis (esp. histoplasmosis; tuberculosis; syphilis)
9. Infected pulmonary or mediastinal cyst or sequestration of lung
10. Lymphoma$_g$
11. Radiation therapy
12. Rupture of esophagus, "spontaneous" or traumatic (eg, foreign body; missile), or iatrogenic (surgery; instrumentation)

References
1. Cameron DC: Non-malignant oesophago-bronchial fistulae in the adult: Case reports and review of the literature. Australas Radiol 1983; 27:143–153
2. DeBacker AI, De Schepper AM, Vaneerdeweg W: Esophagobronchial fistula following redo Nissen fundoplication. Abdom Imaging 2000;25:116–118
3. Eisenberg RL: Gastrointestinal Radiology: A Pattern Approach. (ed 3) Philadelphia: Lippincott, 1996, pp 131–139
4. Ramakantan R, Shah P: Tuberculous fistulas of the pharynx and esophagus. Gastrointest Radiol 1990;15:145–152
5. Spalding AR, Burney DP, Richie RE: Acquired benign bronchoesophageal fistulas in the adult. Ann Thorac Surg 1979; 28:378–383

Gamut G-9

DOUBLE-BARREL ESOPHAGUS*

COMMON
1. Dissecting intramural hematoma or hemorrhage
   a. Severe vomiting (eg, Boerhaave S. with esophageal perforation, or Mallory-Weiss S. with esophageal tear)
   b. Trauma
   c. Instrumentation (eg, nasogastric intubation; endoscopy)
   d. Ingestion of sharp foreign body
   e. Spontaneous (eg, bleeding diathesis)

UNCOMMON
1. Esophageal duplication
2. Crohn's disease
3. Intraluminal diverticulum
4. Intramural abscess (eg, postendoscopy or foreign body perforation)
5. Intramural pseudodiverticulosis

* Barium opacification of an intramural dissecting channel separated from the normal esophageal lumen by an intervening radiolucent mucosal stripe.

References
1. Canon CL, Levine MS, Cherukuri R, et al: Intramural tracking: a feature of esophageal intramural pseudodiverticulosis. AJR 2000;175:371–374
2. Eisenberg RL: Gastrointestinal Radiology. A Pattern Approach. (ed 3) Philadelphia: Lippincott, 1996, pp 140–145
3. Ghahremani GG: Esophageal trauma. Semin Roentgenol 1994;24:387–400
4. Levine MS: Other esophagitides. In: Gore RM, Levine MS: Textbook of Gastrointestinal Radiology. (ed 2) Philadelphia: WB Saunders, 2000, pp 364–386

Gamut G-10-1

DIVERTICULUM OF THE ESOPHAGUS— UPPER THIRD

COMMON
1. Zenker's diverticulum (pulsion type, posterior wall)

UNCOMMON
1. Killian-Jamieson diverticulum
2. Lateral pharyngeal pouch (pharyngocele), congenital or acquired (eg, glass blower; trumpet player)
3. Traction diverticulum (esp. after upper lobectomy, laryngectomy, or neck infection)

References
1. Eisenberg RL: Gastrointestinal Radiology: A Pattern Approach. (ed 3) Philadelphia: Lippincott, 1996, pp 119–124
2. Rubesin SE: Structural abnormalities of the pharynx. In: Gore RM, Levine MS: Textbook of Gastrointestinal Radiology. (ed 2) Philadelphia: WB Saunders, 2000, pp 227–255

Gamut G-10-2

DIVERTICULUM OF THE ESOPHAGUS— MIDDLE THIRD

COMMON
1. Acquired pulsion diverticulum due to esophageal dysmotility
2. Traction diverticulum (esp. from adherent granulomatous lymph node)

UNCOMMON
1. Congenital pulsion diverticulum (interaortico-bronchial)
2. [Neurenteric or duplication cyst, communicating]

[ ] This condition does not actually cause the gamuted imaging finding, but can produce imaging changes that simulate it.

References
1. Eisenberg RL: Gastrointestinal Radiology: A Pattern Approach. (ed 3) Philadelphia: Lippincott, 1996, pp 119–124
2. Levine MS: Miscellaneous abnormalities of the esophagus. In: Gore RM, Levine MS: Textbook of Gastrointestinal Radiology. (ed 2) Philadelphia: WB Saunders, 2000, pp 465–483

Gamut-10-3

DIVERTICULUM OF THE ESOPHAGUS— LOWER THIRD

1. Epiphrenic ("lower Zenker's")
2. [Mucosal tear, spontaneous (Mallory-Weiss S.) or postinstrumentation]
3. [Penetrating peptic ulcer]
4. Postoperative (eg, for achalasia)

[ ] This condition does not actually cause the gamuted imaging finding, but can produce imaging changes that simulate it.

References
1. Bruggeman LL, Seaman WB: Epiphrenic diverticula: An analysis of 80 cases. AJR 1973; 119:266–276
2. Eisenberg RL: Gastrointestinal Radiology: A Pattern Approach. (ed 2) Philadelphia: Lippincott, 1996, pp 119–124
3. Kreel L: Outline of Radiology. New York: Appleton-Century-Crofts, 1971, pp 110–112
4. Reeders JW, Joosten FB, Rosenbusch G: Radiology of the esophagus. Radiologe 2000;40:479–493

Gamut G-10-4

DIVERTICULA OF THE ESOPHAGUS— DIFFUSE

1. Intramural diverticulosis
2. [Pseudodiverticulosis, esp. with *Candida* or herpes esophagitis]

[ ] This condition does not actually cause the gamuted imaging finding, but can produce imaging changes that simulate it.

References

1. Eisenberg RL: Gastrointestinal Radiology: A Pattern Approach. (ed 2) Philadelphia: Lippincott, 1996, pp 119–124
2. Graham DY, Goyal RK, Sparkman J, et al: Diffuse intramural esophageal diverticulosis. Gastroenterology 1975; 68:781–785.
3. Levine MS, Moolten DN, Herlinger H, Laufer I: Esophageal intramural pseudodiverticulosis: a reevaluation. AJR 1986;147:1165–1170
4. Levine MS: Other esophagitides. In: Gore RM, Levine MS: Textbook of Gastrointestinal Radiology. (ed 2) Philadelphia: WB Saunders, 2000, pp 364–386

9. Prolapsed gastric fold
10. Sarcoma (eg, leiomyosarcoma; Kaposi sarcoma)
11. Ulcer with edema (See G-14)
12. Villous adenoma

References

1. Eisenberg RL: Gastrointestinal Radiology: A Pattern Approach. (ed 3) Philadelphia: Lippincott, 1996, pp 98–118
2. Gelfand DW: Gastrointestinal Radiology. New York: Churchill Livingstone, 1984, p 182
3. Levine MS: Esophagus: Differential diagnosis. In: Gore RM, Levine MS: Textbook of Gastrointestinal Radiology. (ed 2) Philadelphia: WB Saunders, 2000, pp 509–511
4. Styles RA, Gibb SP, Tarshis A, et al: Esophagogastric polyps: Radiographic and endoscopic findings. Radiology 1985;154:307–311

Gamut G-11

SOLITARY INTRAMURAL OR INTRALUMINAL FILLING DEFECT OF THE ESOPHAGUS

COMMON

1. Air bubble; meat impaction; coin; other foreign body
2. Carcinoma of esophagus or stomach
3. Extrinsic lesion invading the esophageal wall (eg, carcinoma of lung; granulomatous lymph node)
4. Gastrointestinal stromal tumor$_g$ (esp. leiomyoma)
5. Papilloma, squamous
6. Plaque-like lesion (eg, candidiasis—usually multiple) (See G-17)
7. Polyp$_g$ (eg, adenomatous; fibrovascular; inflammatory esophagogastric)
8. Varix

UNCOMMON

1. Abscess
2. Angioma
3. Duplication cyst (bronchogenic or enteric)
4. Hematoma, intramural
5. Lipoma
6. Lymphoma$_g$; leukemia
7. Melanoma
8. Metastasis

Gamut G-12

LOCALIZED CONSTRICTION OR NARROWING OF THE ESOPHAGUS

COMMON

1. Achalasia (cardiospasm)
2. Congenital atresia or stenosis, with or without T-E fistula
3. Duplication cyst (eg, bronchogenic cyst; gastro-enteric cyst; neurenteric cyst)
4. Extrinsic pressure (eg, aortic knob; left main stem bronchus; aortic aneurysm or tortuosity, right aortic arch) (See G-5 to G-7)
5. Lower esophageal ring (Schatzki ring)
6. Neoplasm, benign (esp. gastrointestinal stromal tumor$_g$—leiomyoma; lipoma)
7. Neoplasm, malignant (esp. carcinoma or leiomyosarcoma of esophagus or gastric cardia)
8. Physiologic (muscular ring; inferior esophageal sphincter; normal sling fibers of diaphragm)
9. Postoperative (fundoplication; repair of hiatal hernia or esophageal atresia); postgastrectomy alkaline reflux esophagitis
10. Spasm, localized (eg, lower esophageal spasm)

(continued)

11. Stricture (eg, peptic or reflux esophagitis; corrosive esophagitis—lye; oral medication; postradiation; nasogastric intubation; Barrett esophagus; congenital)
12. Web or diaphragm of esophagus

UNCOMMON

1. Benign mucous membrane pemphigoid
2. Cartilaginous ring (tracheobronchial rest)
3. Chronic granulomatous disease of childhood
4. Crohn's disease
5. Epidermolysis bullosa
6. Graft-versus-host disease
7. Hemorrhage in distal esophagus with adherent thrombus (eg, Mallory-Weiss S.; varices)
8. Hiatal hernia (esp. with short esophagus)
9. Infectious or inflammatory esophagitis (eg, candidiasis; herpes simplex; tuberculosis; histoplasmosis; actinomycosis; syphilis; eosinophilic esophagitis; Behçet S.)
10. Intramural esophageal pseudodiverticulosis
11. Lymphoma$_g$
12. Metastasis or direct spread from adjacent malignancy
13. Peptic esophageal ulcer
14. Postinstrumentation stricture (eg, nasogastric intubation; endoscopic perforation)
15. Sclerotherapy of esophageal varices
16. Tylosis (keratosis palmaris et plantaris familiaris)
17. Zollinger-Ellison S.

References

1. Eisenberg RL: Gastrointestinal Radiology: A Pattern Approach. (ed 3) Philadelphia: Lippincott, 1996, pp 70–97
2. Gelfand DW: Gastrointestinal Radiology. New York: Churchill Livingstone, 1984, p 188
3. Levine MS: Esophagus: Differential diagnosis. In: Gore RM, Levine MS: Textbook of Gastrointestinal Radiology. (ed 2) Philadelphia: WB Saunders, 2000, pp 509–511
4. Picus D, Frank PH: Eosinophilic esophagitis. AJR 1981; 136:1001–1003
5. Rohl L, Aksglaede K, Fundi-Jensen P, et al: Esophageal rings and strictures. Acta Radiol 2000;41:275–279

Gamut G-13

THICKENING OF THE ESOPHAGEAL WALL (CT, US, MRI)

COMMON

1. Carcinoma (squamous cell carcinoma in proximal 4/5; adenocarcinoma in distal fifth)
2. Corrosive esophagitis (eg, lye; oral medication)
3. Duplication cyst (eg, bronchogenic cyst; gastroenteric cyst; neurenteric cyst)
4. Infectious or inflammatory esophagitis (eg, candidiasis; herpes simplex; tuberculosis; histoplasmosis; actinomycosis; syphilis; eosinophilic esophagitis; Behçet S.)
5. Metastasis or direct spread from adjacent malignancy
6. Neoplasm, other (esp. gastrointestinal stromal tumor$_g$—leiomyoma; leiomyosarcoma); lipoma
7. Postoperative (fundoplication; repair of hiatal hernia or esophageal atresia)
8. Reflux esophagitis (incl. Zollinger-Ellison S.; postgastrectomy alkaline reflux esophagitis)
9. Varices

UNCOMMON

1. Barrett esophagus
2. Benign mucous membrane pemphigoid
3. Chronic granulomatous disease of childhood
4. Crohn's disease
5. Epidermolysis bullosa
6. Hemorrhage or hematoma involving esophagus
7. [Hiatal hernia (esp. with short esophagus)]
8. Intramural esophageal pseudodiverticulosis
9. Lymphoma$_g$
10. Papillomatosis of esophagus
11. Peptic esophageal ulcer with edema
12. Tylosis (keratosis palmaris et plantaris familiaris)

[ ] This condition does not actually cause the gamuted imaging finding, but can produce imaging changes that simulate it.

References

1. Halpert RD, Feczko PJ: Gastrointestinal Radiology: The Requisites. (ed 2) St. Louis: Mosby-Year Book, 1999

2. Levine MS: Esophagus: Differential diagnosis. In: Gore RM, Levine MS: Textbook of Gastrointestinal Radiology. (ed 2) Philadelphia: WB Saunders, 2000, pp 509–513

Gamut G-14

ESOPHAGEAL ULCERATION(S)

COMMON

1. Barrett esophagus
2. Carcinoma of esophagus
3. Corrosive esophagitis
4. Drug-induced esophagitis (eg, potassium chloride; tetracycline; quinidine; ascorbic acid; ferrous sulfate; bromide)
5. Intubation esophagitis
6. Opportunistic esophagitis (esp. *Candida;* herpes; cytomegalovirus)
7. Reflux or peptic esophagitis (eg, hiatal hernia; vomiting; chalasia; scleroderma; pregnancy; surgery)

UNCOMMON

1. Alcoholic esophagitis, acute
2. Behçet syndrome
3. Benign mucous pemphigoid
4. Eosinophilic esophagitis
5. Epidermolysis bullosa
6. Granulomatous esophagitis (eg, tuberculosis; histoplasmosis; syphilis; Crohn's disease)
7. Human immunodeficiency virus (HIV) infection
8. [Intramural esophageal pseudodiverticulosis]
9. Lymphoma$_g$
10. Metastasis
11. Radiation esophagitis
12. Sclerotherapy of esophageal varices

[ ] This condition does not actually cause the gamuted imaging finding, but can produce imaging changes that simulate it.

References

1. Berkovich GY, Levine MS, Miller WT: CT findings in patients with esophagitis. AJR 2000;175:1431–1434
2. Collazzo LA, Levine MS, Rubesin SE, et al: Acute radiation esophagitis: radiographic findings. AJR 1997;169:1067–1070

3. Eisenberg RL: Gastrointestinal Radiology: A Pattern Approach. (ed 3) Philadelphia: Lippincott, 1996, pp 45–69
4. Frager D, Kotler DP, Baer J. Idiopathic esophageal ulceration in the acquired immunodeficiency syndrome. Abdom Imaging 1994;19:2
5. Levine MS, Caroline D, Thompson JJ, et al: Adenocarcinoma of the esophagus: Relationship to Barrett mucosa. Radiology 1984;150:305–309
6. Levine MS: Esophagus: Differential diagnosis. In: Gore RM, Levine MS: Textbook of Gastrointestinal Radiology. (ed 2) Philadelphia: WB Saunders, 2000, pp 509–511
7. Sam JW, Levine MS, Rubesin SE, et al: The "foamy" esophagus: a radiographic sign of Candida esophagitis. AJR 2000;174:999–1002

Gamut G-15

TRANSVERSE MUCOSAL FOLDS IN THE ESOPHAGUS

COMMON

1. Esophagitis (eg, reflux; candidiasis)
2. Normal (feline esophagus)
3. Scleroderma
4. [Tertiary contractions]

UNCOMMON

1. Achalasia
2. Corrosive esophagitis
3. [Linear transverse ulcerations]

[ ] This condition does not actually cause the gamuted imaging finding, but can produce imaging changes that simulate it.

References

1. Levine MS, Goldstein HM: Fixed transverse folds in the esophagus: a sign of reflux esophagitis. AJR 1984;143:275–278
2. Levine MS: Infectious esophagitis. Semin Roentgenol 1994;24:341–350
3. Reeder JD, Kramer SS, Dudgeon DL: Transverse esophageal folds: Association with corrosive injury. Radiology 1985;159:303–304
4. Reeders JW, Joosten FB, Rosenbusch G: Radiology of the esophagus. Radiologe 2000;40:479–493

Gamut G-16

WIDESPREAD IRREGULAR OR NODULAR ESOPHAGEAL MUCOSA

COMMON

1. [Artifacts (esp. air bubbles)]
2. Corrosive esophagitis
3. Glycogenic acanthosis
4. Intubation esophagitis
5. Opportunistic esophagitis (eg, *Candida;* herpes; cytomegalovirus)
6. Peptic esophagitis (incl. Barrett type)
7. Reflux esophagitis (eg, hiatal hernia; chalasia; scleroderma)
8. Varices

UNCOMMON

1. Acanthosis nigricans
2. Behçet S.
3. Carcinoma, superficial spreading type
4. Cowden S. (multiple hamartoma S.)
5. Crohn's disease
6. Diverticulosis, intramural; pseudodiverticulosis
7. Ectopic sebaceous glands
8. Eosinophilic esophagitis
9. Epidermolysis bullosa
10. Esophagitis cystica
11. [Feline esophagus]
12. Granulomatous esophagitis (eg, tuberculosis; histoplasmosis; syphilis)
13. Hirsute esophagus ("skin tube" esophagus created during reconstructive surgery of pharynx and esophagus)
14. Leukoplakia
15. Lymph follicles
16. Lymphoma$_g$
17. Papillomatosis of esophagus
18. Pemphigus; bullous pemphigoid
19. Radiation esophagitis
20. Scleroderma

[ ] This condition does not actually cause the gamuted imaging finding, but can produce imaging changes that simulate it.

References

1. Gelfand DW: Gastrointestinal Radiology. New York: Churchill Livingstone, 1984, p 173
2. Itai Y, Kogure T, Okuyama Y: Radiological manifestations of oesophageal involvement in acanthosis nigricans. Br J Radiol 1976:49:592–593
3. Itai Y, Kogure T, Okuyama Y, et al: Diffuse finely nodular lesions of the esophagus. AJR 1977;128:563–566
4. Levine MS: Esophagus: Differential diagnosis. In: Gore RM, Levine MS: Textbook of Gastrointestinal Radiology. (ed 2) Philadelphia: WB Saunders, 2000, pp 509–511
5. Meyers C, Durkin MG, Love L: Radiographic findings in herpetic esophagitis. Radiology 1976;119:21–22

Gamut G-17

ESOPHAGEAL PLAQUES

COMMON

1. Candidiasis (moniliasis)

UNCOMMON

1. Acanthosis nigricans
2. Barrett esophagus
3. Carcinoma, early or superficial spreading
4. Corrosive esophagitis
5. Crohn's disease
6. Leukoplakia
7. Reflux esophagitis
8. Tuberculosis
9. Viral esophagitis (herpes; cytomegalovirus)

References

1. Graziani L, Bearzi I, Romagnoli A, et al: Significance of diffuse granularity and nodularity of the esophageal mucosa at double-contrast radiography. Gastrointest Radiol 1985;10: 1–8
2. Reeders JW, Joosten FB, Rosenbusch G: Radiology of the esophagus. Radiologe 2000;40:479–493

Gamut G-18

ESOPHAGEAL VARICES

COMMON

1. Portal hypertension (esp. cirrhosis; portal vein thrombosis; schistosomiasis) (See G-191)
*2. Superior vena cava obstruction (downhill varices) (esp. bronchogenic carcinoma, mediastinal tumor or fibrosis; retrosternal goiter) (See E-70)

UNCOMMON

1. Arteriovenous malformation
2. Idiopathic
3. Noncirrhotic liver disease (eg, primary or metastatic carcinoma of liver; heart failure)
*4. Postsurgical (resection of retrosternal tumor)
5. [Varicoid lesions of esophagus (esp. varicoid carcinoma; lymphoma; esophagitis)] (See G-16)

* Varices may be confined to upper esophagus.
[ ] This condition does not actually cause the gamuted imaging finding, but can produce imaging changes that simulate it.

References
1. Baron RL, Gore RM: Diffuse liver disease. In: Gore RM, Levine MS: Textbook of Gastrointestinal Radiology. (ed 2) Philadelphia: WB Saunders, 2000, pp 1590–1638
2. Felson B, Lessure AP: "Downhill" varices of the esophagus. Dis Chest 1964;46:740
3. Eisenberg RL: Gastrointestinal Radiology: A Pattern Approach (ed 3). Philadelphia: Lippincott, 1996, pp 125–130
4. Reeders JW, Joosten FB, Rosenbusch G: Radiology of the esophagus. Radiologe 2000;40:479–493

Gamut G-19

ESOPHAGEAL LESION IN A CHILD

COMMON

1. Atresia
2. Chalasia (infantile gastroesophageal regurgitation)
3. Duplication cyst (enteric; neurenteric; bronchogenic)
4. Esophagitis (corrosive; reflux; peptic; radiation; infectious; intubation; instrumentation)
5. Extrinsic compression (See G-5-7)
6. Foreign body (esp. coin)
7. Hiatal hernia (esp. with short esophagus)
8. Opportunistic esophagitis (eg, *Candida;* herpes; cytomegalovirus)
9. Postsurgical repair of esophageal atresia, tracheoesophageal fistula, or hiatal hernia
10. Stricture (eg, congenital or secondary to esophagitis)
11. Vascular impression (eg, right aortic arch; double aortic arch; cervical aortic arch; aberrant right or left subclavian artery; pulmonary sling) (See G-7)

UNCOMMON

1. Achalasia
2. Congenital syndromes (eg, Riley-Day S. {familial dysautonomia}; Ehlers-Danlos S.)
3. Diverticulum (See G-10)
4. Epidermolysis bullosa
5. Metastasis
6. Neoplasm, benign or malignant (incl. lymphoma$_g$)
7. Pemphigus
8. Peptic ulcer; Barrett esophagus
9. Trauma
10. Varices
11. Web; diaphragm; Schatzki ring

References
1. Fernbach SK, Zawin JK: Diseases of the pediatric esophagus. In: Gore RM, Levine MS: Textbook of Gastrointestinal Radiology. (ed 2) Philadelphia: WB Saunders, 2000, pp 2074–2089
2. Silverman FN, (ed:) Caffey's Pediatric X-ray Diagnosis: An Integrated Imaging Approach. (ed 8) Chicago: Year Book Medical Publ, 1985
3. Swischuk LE, John SD: Differential Diagnosis in Pediatric Radiology. (ed 2) Baltimore: Williams & Wilkins, 1995, pp 175–176

Gamut G-20

ABNORMAL POSITION OF THE STOMACH (ROTATION OR DISPLACEMENT)

COMMON

1. Cascade stomach
2. Displacement by enlarged adjacent organ (eg, liver; spleen; left kidney; pancreas; aorta) or by adjacent mass, or lesser sac abscess or hernia
3. Eventration or paralysis of left hemidiaphragm
4. Hernia (eg, hiatal; paraesophageal; Morgagni; Bochdalek; traumatic; intrapericardial)
5. Inversion of left hemidiaphragm (pleural effusion; thoracic mass)
6. Obesity; emphysema (anterior displacement)

UNCOMMON

1. Absent hemidiaphragm
2. "Upside-down" stomach
3. Volvulus (organoaxial or mesenteroaxial)

References
1. Burgener FA, Kormano M: Differential Diagnosis in Conventional Radiology. (ed 2) New York: Thieme Medical Publ, 1991, pp 568–571
2. Kreel L: Outline of Radiology. New York: Appleton-Century-Crofts, 1971, pp 133–134

Gamut G-21

FILLING DEFECT(S) IN THE STOMACH (INTRALUMINAL, MUCOSAL, OR INTRAMURAL)

COMMON

*1. Adenomatous polyp (eg, in chronic atrophic gastritis; familial polyposis of colon; Cronkhite-Canada S.)
*2. [Areae gastricae]

3. Bezoar
*4. Blood clot; intramural hematoma
5. Carcinoma
6. Ectopic pancreas
7. [Extrinsic mass (eg, from spleen, liver, pancreas, kidney, colon)]
*8. Foreign body (eg, coin)
9. Giant rugal fold; hypertrophied prepyloric antral fold
*10. Hyperplastic polyp
*11. Leiomyoma, other gastrointestinal stromal tumor_g
*12. Lymphoma_g
*13. Metastasis (esp. melanoma; Kaposi sarcoma; carcinoma of lung or breast)
*14. Neoplasm, other (eg, carcinoid; tubular adenoma; angioma; lipoma; villous adenoma; plasmacytoma)
*15. Peptic ulcer
16. Postoperative defect (eg, suture granuloma; fundoplication)
17. Sarcoma (esp. leiomyosarcoma)
*18. Varix

UNCOMMON

*1. Amyloidosis
*2. Candidiasis
3. [Double pylorus]
4. Duplication cyst
*5. Fundic gland polyposis
6. Gallstone
7. Granuloma with eosinophils (inflammatory fibroid polyp)
*8. Hamartoma (eg, Peutz-Jeghers S. (alimentary tract polyposis); Cowden S. (multiple hamartoma S.); Ruvalcaba-Myhre-Smith S.)
9. Jejunogastric intussusception
*10. Lymphoid hyperplasia; pseudolymphoma
*11. Parasites (esp. *Ascaris; Anisakis*)
12. Prolapse of esophageal mucosa
*13. Thickened folds simulating nodules or filling defects (eg, Ménétrier's disease; Crohn's disease;

tuberculosis; sarcoidosis; eosinophilic gastritis)
(See G-26)
14. Tumefactive extramedullary hematopoiesis

* May be multiple.
[ ] This condition does not actually cause the gamuted imaging finding, but can produce imaging changes that simulate it.

References
1. Cherukuri R, Levine MS, Furth EE, et al: Giant hyperplastic polyps in the stomach: radiographic findings in seven patients. AJR 2000;175:1445–1448
2. Eisenberg RL: Gastrointestinal Radiology: A Pattern Approach. (ed 3) Philadelphia: Lippincott, 1996, pp 243–278
3. Gelfand DW: Gastrointestinal Radiology. New York: Churchill Livingstone, 1984, pp 221, 229
4. Lau CF, Hui PK, Mak KL, et al: Gastric polypoid lesions. Am J Gastroenterol 1998:93:2559–2564
5. Levine MS: Benign tumors of the stomach and duodenum. In: Gore RM, Levine MS: Textbook of Gastrointestinal Radiology. (ed 2) Philadelphia: WB Saunders, 2000, pp 575–600
6. Park SH, Han JK, Kim TK, et al: Unusual gastric tumors: radiologic-pathologic correlation. RadioGraphics 1999;19: 1435–1436

Gamut G-22

FILLING DEFECT IN A GASTRIC REMNANT

COMMON
1. Bezoar
2. Postoperative deformity or defect (eg, suture granuloma; scar; prolapse; mural inversion)
3. Ulcer (esp. marginal ulcer)

UNCOMMON
1. Carcinoma (recurrent; gastric stump)
2. Gastritis, postoperative (incl. bile reflux gastritis)
3. Gastrojejunal mucosal prolapse (antegrade prolapse into efferent or afferent loop)
4. Jejunogastric intussusception (usually efferent loop in Billroth II anastamosis)

5. Lymphoma (gastric stump)
6. Polyp$_g$ (esp. hyperplastic)

References
1. Eisenberg RL: Gastrointestinal Radiology: A Pattern Approach. (ed 3) Philadelphia: Lippincott, 1996, pp 279–288
2. Smith CH, Gore RM: Postoperative stomach and duodenum. In: Gore RM, Levine MS: Textbook of Gastrointestinal Radiology. (ed 2) Philadelphia: WB Saunders, 2000, pp 682–697

Gamut G-23

LESION INVOLVING THE GASTRIC FUNDUS (INTRINSIC OR EXTRINSIC)

COMMON
1. Bezoar
2. Carcinoma of stomach (adenocarcinoma) or esophagus (squamous cell)
3. Diverticulum of fundus
4. Extragastric malignancy (eg, carcinoma of tail or body of pancreas or splenic flexure of colon; liver, kidney, or adrenal neoplasm; lymphoma$_g$ or metastases involving adjacent nodes)
5. Extrinsic pressure from normal or enlarged structure (eg, liver; spleen; splenic flexure of colon; left kidney; heart; aortic aneurysm)
6. Giant rugal folds (incl. Ménétrier's disease)
7. Hiatal hernia with esophagogastric herniation
8. Leiomyoma; neurofibroma; other gastrointestinal stromal tumor$_g$; lipoma
9. Lymphoma$_g$
10. Peptic ulcer
11. Polyp$_g$ (esp. hyperplastic or adenomatous)
12. Postsurgical deformity (eg, Nissen repair of hiatal hernia with fundoplication; postsplenectomy)
13. Varices (eg, cirrhosis; schistosomiasis); portal hypertensive gastropathy

(continued)

UNCOMMON

1. Hematoma, intramural or extrinsic
2. Sarcoma (esp. leiomyosarcoma)
3. Splenosis following splenectomy
4. Subphrenic abscess

References

1. Chang R, Levine MS, Ginsberg GG, et al: Portal hypertensive gastropathy: radiographic findings in eight patients. AJR 2000;175:1609–1612
2. Eisenberg RL: Gastrointestinal Radiology: A Pattern Approach. (ed 3) Philadelphia: Lippincott, 1996, pp 305–316
3. Gore RM, Levine MS, Ghahremani GG, et al: Gastric cancer: radiologic diagnosis. Radiol Clin North Am 1997;35: 311–331

Gamut G-24

GASTRIC ULCERATION

COMMON

1. Carcinoma of stomach
*2. Gastritis (eg, alcohol; aspirin; anti-inflammatory drugs)
3. Lymphoma$_g$
4. Marginal ulcer (postsubtotal gastrectomy)
5. Peptic ulcer

UNCOMMON

1. [Ectopic pancreas (duct)]
2. Carcinoid
3. Chemotherapy (hepatic arterial infusion)
4. Corrosive gastritis
*5. Crohn's disease
6. *Cryptosporidium* antritis
7. Eosinophilic gastritis
8. Kaposi sarcoma
9. Ménétrier's disease (giant hypertrophic gastritis)
10. Metastasis (often bull's-eye lesion, esp. melanoma) (See G-105)
11. Pseudolymphoma

12. Radiation therapy
13. Gastrointestinal stromal tumor$_g$, benign or malignant (esp. leiomyoma; leiomyosarcoma; neurofibroma)
14. Suture line ulceration (esp. after gastric surgery for morbid obesity)
15. Tuberculosis

* May cause aphthoid ulcerations.
[ ] This condition does not actually cause the gamuted imaging finding, but can produce imaging changes that simulate it.

References

1. Eisenberg RL: Gastrointestinal Radiology: A Pattern Approach. (ed 3) Philadelphia: Lippincott, 1996, pp 181–203
2. Gelfand DW: Gastrointestinal Radiology. New York: Churchill Livingstone, 1984, p 216
3. Levine MS: Peptic ulcers. In: Gore RM, Levine MS: Textbook of Gastrointestinal Radiology. (ed 2) Philadelphia: WB Saunders, 2000, pp 509–513

Gamut G-25

EROSIVE GASTRITIS*

COMMON

1. Acute gastritis (eg, alcohol abuse)
2. Crohn's disease
3. Drugs (eg, aspirin; NSAID; steroids)
4. *Helicobacter pylori* infection
5. Idiopathic
6. [Normal areae gastricae]
7. Peptic ulcer; hyperacidity

UNCOMMON

1. Corrosive gastritis
2. *Cryptosporidium* antritis
3. [Lymphoma]
4. Opportunistic infection (eg, candidiasis; herpes simplex; cytomegalovirus)
5. Postoperative gastritis

6. Radiation therapy
7. Zollinger-Ellison S.; multiple endocrine neoplasia (MEN) S.

* Superficial erosions or aphthoid ulcerations seen especially with double contrast technique.
[ ] This condition does not actually cause the gamuted imaging finding, but can produce imaging changes that simulate it.

References
1. Eisenberg RL: Gastrointestinal Radiology: A Pattern Approach. (ed 3) Philadelphia: Lippincott, 1996, pp 204–207
2. Levine MS: Inflammatory conditions of the stomach and duodenum. In: Gore RM, Levine MS: Textbook of Gastrointestinal Radiology. (ed 2) Philadelphia: WB Saunders, 2000, pp 546–574
3. McLean AM, Paul RE Jr, Philips E: Chronic erosive gastritis—Clinical and radiologic features. J Can Assoc Radiol 1982;33:158–162

Gamut G-26

LARGE GASTRIC FOLDS (LOCAL OR WIDESPREAD); ALSO THICKENING OF THE STOMACH WALL ON CT, US, OR MRI

COMMON
1. Carcinoma
2. Gastritis (esp. hypertrophic; alcoholic; antral; *Helicobacter pylori*)
3. Lymphoma$_g$
4. Ménétrier's disease (giant hypertrophic gastritis)
5. Normal variant (hyperrugosity of fundus and greater curvature)
6. Pancreatitis, acute
7. Peptic ulcer disease; hyperacidity
8. Postoperative stomach
9. Varices (eg, cirrhosis; schistosomiasis); portal hypertensive gastropathy

UNCOMMON
1. Amyloidosis
2. Diffuse cystic gastric disease

3. Drug related gastritis (eg, aspirin; NSAID); chemotherapy toxicity
4. [Food retention]
5. Gastritis, other (eg, eosinophilic, corrosive, phlegmonous, or postradiation)
6. Granulomatous infiltration of stomach wall (eg, Crohn's disease; sarcoidosis; tuberculosis; histoplasmosis; actinomycosis; syphilis)
7. Infectious gastritis, other (eg, botulism; dysentery; diphtheria; candidiasis, cryptosporidiosis or cytomegalovirus—esp. in AIDS)
8. Metastasis; extension from carcinoma of pancreas
9. Neoplasm, other (eg, gastrointestinal stromal tumor$_g$—esp. leiomyoma, leiomyosarcoma; carcinoid; Kaposi sarcoma)
10. Parasitic disease (esp. strongyloidiasis; anisakiasis; schistosomiasis with varices)
11. Polyposis of stomach (See G-21, G-106)
12. Pseudolymphoma
13. Zollinger-Ellison S.; multiple endocrine neoplasia (MEN) S. (See J-5)

[ ] This condition does not actually cause the gamuted imaging finding, but can produce imaging changes that simulate it.

References
1. Chang MS, Levine MS, Ginsberg GG, et al: Portal hypertensive gastropathy: radiographic findings in eight patients. AJR 2000;175:1609–1612
2. Eisenberg RL: Gastrointestinal Radiology: A Pattern Approach. (ed 3) Philadelphia: Lippincott, 1996, pp 227–242
3. Farman J, Lerner ME, Ng C, et al: Cytomegalovirus gastritis. Gastrointest Radiol 1992;17:202
4. Levine MS: Stomach and duodenum: Differential diagnosis. In: Gore RM, Levine MS: Textbook of Gastrointestinal Radiology. (ed 2) Philadelphia: WB Saunders, 2000, pp 698–703
5. Levine MS, Laufer I: Stomach. In: Levine MS, Rubesin SE, Laufer I: Double Contrast Gastrointestinal Radiology. (ed 3) Philadelphia: WB Saunders, 2000, pp 149–203
6. Reese DF, Hodgson JR, Dockerty MB: Giant hypertrophy of the gastric mucosa (Ménétrier's disease): Correlation of the roentgenographic, pathologic and clinical findings. AJR 1962;88:619–626
7. Sato T, Sakai Y, Ishiguro S, Furukawa H: Radiologic manifestations of early gastric lymphoma. AJR 1986;146:513–517

LINITIS PLASTICA PATTERN OF THE STOMACH (See G-28)

COMMON

1. Carcinoma of stomach
2. Peptic ulcer (acute ulcer with spasm; chronic ulcer with fibrosis)
3. Stenosing antral gastritis

UNCOMMON

1. Amyloidosis
2. Chemotherapy (hepatic arterial infusion)
3. Corrosive gastritis (esp. acids; ferrous sulfate)
4. Eosinophilic gastritis
5. [Extrinsic mass compressing stomach (esp. marked hepatomegaly)]
6. Granulomatous infiltration of stomach wall (eg, Crohn's disease; sarcoidosis; tuberculosis; histoplasmosis; actinomycosis; syphilis)
7. Idiopathic gastritis
8. Intramural gastric hematoma
9. Lymphoma$_g$ (esp. Hodgkins disease and non-Hodgkins lymphoma)
10. Metastasis (esp. breast carcinoma); direct extension from carcinoma of pancreas or transverse colon; omental "cakes"
11. Opportunistic infection, esp. in AIDS (eg, cytomegalovirus; *Cryptosporidium* gastritis)
12. Parasitic disease (eg, strongyloidiasis; schistosomiasis)
13. Perigastric adhesions
14. Phlegmonous gastritis
15. Postoperative (eg, gastroplasty)
16. Postradiation or postfreezing gastritis
17. Pseudolymphoma

[ ] This condition does not actually cause the gamuted imaging finding, but can produce imaging changes that simulate it.

References

1. Balthazar EJ, Rosenberg H, Davidian MM: Scirrhous carcinoma of the pyloric channel and distal antrum. AJR 1980; 134:669–673
2. Eisenberg RL: Gastrointestinal Radiology: A Pattern Approach. (ed 3) Philadelphia: Lippincott, 1996, pp 208–226
3. Gelfand DW: Gastrointestinal Radiology. New York: Churchill Livingstone, 1984, p 229
4. Lagasse JP, Causse X, Legoux JL, et al: Cytomegalovirus gastritis simulating cancer of the linitis plastica type on endoscopic ultrasonography. Endoscopy 1998;30:S101–102
5. Levine MS: Stomach and duodenum: Differential diagnosis. In: Gore RM, Levine MS: Textbook of Gastrointestinal Radiology. (ed 2) Philadelphia: WB Saunders, 2000, pp 698–702
6. Levine MS, Laufer I: Tumors of the stomach. In: Levine MS, Rubesin SE, Laufer I: Double Contrast Gastrointestinal Radiology. (ed 3) Philadelphia: WB Saunders, 2000, pp 204–238

NARROWING OR DEFORMITY OF THE GASTRIC ANTRUM (See G-27)

COMMON

1. Antral gastritis
2. Carcinoma of stomach
3. Hypertrophic pyloric stenosis (infantile, adult)
4. Pancreatitis; carcinoma of pancreas; pseudocyst
5. Peptic ulcer scarring
6. Prolapse of gastric mucosa or polyp$_g$
7. Pylorospasm

UNCOMMON

1. Aberrant pancreatic tissue
2. Adhesions
3. Amyloidosis
4. Antral diaphragm or web
5. Congenital peritoneal bands (Ladd's bands)
6. Corrosive gastritis
7. *Cryptosporidium* antritis
8. Duplication cyst of stomach
9. Eosinophilic gastritis
10. Gastroenterostomy
11. Granulomatous disease of infancy (neutrophil dysfunction)

12. Granulomatous infiltration of stomach wall (eg, Crohn's disease; sarcoidosis; tuberculosis; histoplasmosis; actinomycosis; syphilis)
13. Lymphoma$_g$
14. Metastasis
15. Parasitic disease (esp. strongyloidiasis; schistosomiasis; anisakiasis)
16. Peptic ulcer perforation (walled off)
17. Radiation therapy

References
1. Gelfand DW: Gastrointestinal Radiology. New York: Churchill Livingstone, 1984, p 229
2. Levine MS: Stomach and duodenum: Differential diagnosis. In: Gore RM, Levine MS: Textbook of Gastrointestinal Radiology. (ed 2) Philadelphia: WB Saunders, 2000, pp 698–702
3. Teplick JG, Haskin ME: Roentgenologic Diagnosis. (ed 3) Philadelphia: WB Saunders, 1976

Gamut G-29

COMBINED GASTRIC ANTRAL AND DUODENAL DISEASE

COMMON
1. Carcinoma of stomach extending to involve duodenum
2. Involvement of stomach and duodenum from adjacent malignancy (esp. carcinoma of pancreas) or pancreatitis
3. Lymphoma$_g$
4. Peptic ulcer disease (incl. Zollinger-Ellison S.)
5. Prolapse of gastric mucosa, inflamed antral-pyloric fold, or polyp$_g$ into duodenal bulb

UNCOMMON
1. Crohn's disease
2. Eosinophilic gastroenteritis
3. Ménétrier's disease

4. Parasitic disease (eg, strongyloidiasis; schistosomiasis)
5. Tuberculosis

Reference
1. Eisenberg RL: Gastrointestinal Radiology: A Pattern Approach. (ed 3) Philadelphia: Lippincott 1996, pp 324–328
2. Levine MS: Inflammatory conditions of the stomach and duodenum. In: Gore RM, Levine MS: Textbook of Gastrointestinal Radiology. (ed 2) Philadelphia: WB Saunders, 2000, pp 546–574

Gamut G-30

GASTRIC OUTLET OBSTRUCTION

COMMON
1. Extrinsic compression (eg, pancreatic, renal, retroperitoneal, duodenal, or colonic lesion)
2. Neoplasm, esp. malignant (eg, carcinoma of gastric antrum or head of pancreas; lymphoma$_g$)
3. Peptic ulcer disease (eg, antral, pyloric, or duodenal)
4. [Physiologic (eg, gastric atony with poor peristalsis and emptying; post-drug therapy; gastric distention)] (See G-31)
5. Prepyloric inflammation, scarring or stricture (eg, corrosive gastritis; Crohn's disease; tuberculosis; sarcoidosis; syphilis; amyloidosis)
6. Pyloric hypertrophy, adult or infantile (hypertrophic pyloric stenosis)
7. Pylorospasm

UNCOMMON
1. Annular pancreas
2. Bezoar
3. Diaphragm or web, antral or duodenal
4. Gastric duplication
5. Hematoma, intramural
6. Intussusception, gastroduodenal
7. Pancreatitis; cholecystitis

(continued)

8. Prolapsed antral mucosa or polyp_g
9. [Proximal small bowel obstruction]
10. Volvulus (with or without hiatal hernia)

[ ] This condition does not actually cause the gamuted imaging finding, but can produce imaging changes that simulate it.

References
1. Eisenberg RL: Gastrointestinal Radiology: A Pattern Approach. (ed 3) Philadelphia: Lippincott, 1996, pp 289–298
2. Teplick JG, Haskin ME: Roentgenologic Diagnosis. (ed 3) Philadelphia: WB Saunders, 1976

Gamut G-31

DILATATION OF THE STOMACH WITHOUT OBSTRUCTION

COMMON

1. Aerophagia; emotional distress; hyperventilation; crying
2. Carbonated beverages; bicarbonate of soda; double contrast; gas pills
3. Coma (uremic or hepatic)
4. Diabetic gastropathy (gastric paresis)
5. Drug therapy (eg, Atropine; morphine; ganglion-blocking agent; Pro-Banthine)
6. Gastritis, acute
7. Iatrogenic (intubation; oxygen tube in esophagus)
8. Immobilization (eg, body cast; paraplegia)
9. Inflammation, acute (eg, pancreatitis; cholecystitis; subphrenic abscess; septicemia)
10. Pain (eg, colic due to renal, ureteral, or biliary stone; porphyria; lead poisoning; sickle cell crisis; migraine)
11. Peritonitis (eg, perforated appendix or peptic ulcer)
12. Postoperative, recent (incl. vagotomy)
13. Small bowel obstruction, proximal
14. Traumatic gastric ileus (eg, spine fracture; ruptured spleen; retroperitoneal hematoma; renal injury)

UNCOMMON

1. Chagas' disease
2. Electrolyte or acid-base imbalance (eg, hypercalcemia; hypocalcemia; hypokalemia; uremia; insulin shock; diabetic ketoacidosis)
3. Idiopathic
4. Muscular disorder_g (esp. muscular dystrophy)
5. Myxedema (hypothyroidism)
6. Neurologic disorder_g (eg, brain tumor; cerebral palsy; bulbar poliomyelitis; tabes dorsalis)
7. Scleroderma; dermatomyositis
8. Tracheoesophageal fistula with esophageal atresia

References
1. Eisenberg RL: Gastrointestinal Radiology: A Pattern Approach. (ed 3) Philadelphia: Lippincott, 1996, pp 300–304
2. Marie I, Levesque H, Ducrotté P, et al: Gastric involvement in systemic sclerosis. Am J Gastroenterol 2001:96: 77–81

Gamut G-32

INTERSTITIAL EMPHYSEMA OF THE STOMACH

COMMON

1. Emphysematous or phlegmonous gastritis (gas-forming organism, esp. in diabetic or alcoholic)
2. Traumatic or iatrogenic emphysema (eg, gastroscopy; intubation; recent surgery; respiratory therapy—esp. PEEP)

UNCOMMON

1. Corrosive gastritis
2. Distention of stomach (eg, bicarbonate of soda; oxygen tube in esophagus) (See G-31)
3. Gastric outlet obstruction (eg, malignancy; volvulus; prepyloric inflammation or stricture) (See G-30)
4. Ischemic gastritis; infarction

5. Necrotizing gastroenterocolitis
6. Peptic ulcer with intramural perforation
7. Perforated appendicitis
8. Pneumatosis cystoides
9. Pneumomediastinum (eg, from emphysema or asthma)

References

1. Eisenberg RL: Gastrointestinal Radiology: A Pattern Approach. (ed 3) Philadelphia: Lippincott, 1996, pp 320–323
2. Tuck JS, Boobis LH: Case report: Interstitial emphysema of the stomach due to perforated appendicitis. Clin Radiol 1987;38:315-317
3. Vaughn BF: Emphysema of the stomach with portal vein gas. Australas Radiol 1972;16:377-378

11. Tuberculosis
12. Typhoid fever

References

1. Alexander ES, Weinberg S, Clark RA, et al: Fistulas and sinus tracts: Radiographic evaluation, management, and outcome. Gastrointest Radiol 1982;7:135–140
2. Laufer I, Joffe N, Stolberg H: Unusual causes of gastrocolic fistula. Gastrointest Radiol 1977;2:21–25
3. Levine MS: Inflammatory conditions of the stomach and duodenum. In: Gore RM, Levine MS: Textbook of Gastrointestinal Radiology. (ed 2) Philadelphia: WB Saunders, 2000, pp 546–574

Gamut G-33

GASTROCOLIC OR GASTRODUODENOCOLIC FISTULA

COMMON

1. Carcinoma of colon, stomach, pancreas, or kidney
2. Pancreatitis; pancreatic abscess
3. Peptic ulcer, perforated (incl. aspirin or NSAID-induced greater curvature ulcer)
4. Postoperative (eg, gastrostomy; retained sponge)
5. Trauma with gastric, duodenal, or colonic perforation

UNCOMMON

1. Actinomycosis
2. Amebic colitis
3. Biliary tract perforation (eg, calculus)
4. Crohn's disease
5. Diverticulum, perforated (eg, colonic, duodenal)
6. Foreign body
7. Idiopathic
8. Lymphoma$_g$
9. Marginal ulcer
10. Metastatic disease

Gamut G-34

INCREASED RETROGASTRIC OR RETRODUODENAL SPACE

COMMON

1. Ascites
2. Hepatomegaly, marked (esp. caudate lobe)
3. Normal variant
4. Obesity
5. Pancreatic mass (esp. carcinoma; pancreatitis; abscess; pseudocyst; cystadenoma) (See G-213, 214)
6. Renal or adrenal mass (eg, renal cell carcinoma (hypernephroma); renal cyst; hydronephrosis; adenoma or carcinoma of adrenal gland; pheochromocytoma; neuroblastoma; Wilms' tumor; perinephric abscess or hematoma) (See H-38–44, H-118)
7. Retroperitoneal mass (eg, sarcoma; lymphoma$_g$; metastasis; lymphadenopathy; tuberculosis; cyst; abscess; hematoma)

UNCOMMON

1. Aortic aneurysm
2. Choledochal cyst
3. Gastrointestinal stromal tumor$_g$ of posterior wall of stomach (esp. leiomyoma; leiomyosarcoma)
4. Herniation of omentum (eg, Morgagni hernia)

(continued)

5. Postoperative
6. Retroperitoneal edema, cellulitis, urinary leakage
7. Retroperitoneal fibrosis

Reference
1. Eisenberg RL: Gastrointestinal Radiology: A Pattern Approach (ed 3). Philadelphia: Lippincott, 1996, pp 317–319

Gamut G-35

EXTRINSIC INDENTATION ON THE DUODENUM (See G-36)

COMMON

1. Coloduodenal apposition
2. Colon lesion (esp. carcinoma of hepatic flexure or transverse colon; amebic pericolic abscess or ameboma)
3. Common duct dilatation or neoplasm (See G-130, G-134)
4. Duodenal diverticulitis or abscess (esp. with giant duodenal diverticulum)
5. Gallbladder, normal or enlarged (eg, hydrops; carcinoma; "Courvoisier gallbladder")
6. Hematoma, intramural or mesenteric
7. Hepatic enlargement (esp. caudate lobe) (eg, liver abscess; hepatocellular carcinoma {hepatoma}) (See G-141)
8. Renal or adrenal mass (eg, renal cell carcinoma {hypernephroma}; renal cyst; hydronephrosis; adenoma or carcinoma of adrenal gland; pheochromocytoma; neuroblastoma; Wilms' tumor; perinephric abscess or hematoma) (See H-38–44, 118)
9. Lymph node enlargement (eg, metastasis; lymphoma$_g$; tuberculosis)
10. Pancreatic mass (eg, carcinoma; pseudocyst; pancreatitis; abscess; annular pancreas) (See G-213, 214)
11. Papilla of Vater enlargement (See G-138)
12. [Postbulbar peptic ulcer]

13. Retroperitoneal mass (eg, sarcoma; lymphadenopathy; abscess; cyst)
14. Superior mesenteric artery compression (See G-44)

UNCOMMON

1. Aortic aneurysm
2. Choledochal cyst
3. Congenital peritoneal bands (Ladd's bands)
4. Gastric neoplasm (esp. leiomyosarcoma; carcinoma)
5. Idiopathic
6. Mesenteric or celiac artery collaterals
7. Pericholecystic abscess
8. Varices, duodenal or retroperitoneal

[ ] This condition does not actually cause the gamuted imaging finding, but can produce imaging changes that simulate it.

Reference
1. Eisenberg RL: Gastrointestinal Radiology: A Pattern Approach. (ed 3) Philadelphia: Lippincott, 1996, pp 365–369

Gamut G-36

WIDENING OF THE DUODENAL C-LOOP (See G-35)

COMMON

1. Normal variant
2. Pancreatic mass (eg, acute or chronic pancreatitis; abscess; pseudocyst; carcinoma; cystadenoma; cystadenocarcinoma) (See G-213, 214)

UNCOMMON

1. Aortic aneurysm
2. Choledochal cyst
3. Duodenal diverticulitis
4. Duodenal hematoma
5. Gastrointestinal stromal tumor$_g$ of duodenum (esp. leiomyosarcoma)
6. Mesenteric or celiac artery collaterals

7. Mesenteric or omental mass (eg, metastasis; hematoma; cystic lymphangioma)
8. Neoplasm of stomach, colon, or kidney (esp. with spread to head of pancreas)
9. Parasitic disease (eg, strongyloidiasis; amebiasis with pericolic abscess)
10. Retroperitoneal lymphadenopathy (eg, metastasis; lymphoma$_g$; tuberculosis; sarcoidosis)
11. Retroperitoneal cyst or neoplasm, primary or metastatic

Reference

1. Eisenberg RL: Gastrointestinal Radiology: A Pattern Approach. (ed 3) Philadelphia: Lippincott, 1996, pp 348–364

Gamut G-37

SOLITARY INTRINSIC DUODENAL MASS

COMMON

1. Ectopic pancreas
2. Metastasis (esp. hypernephroma; melanoma)
3. Neoplasm, primary (Brunner's gland adenoma; leiomyoma; neurofibroma; lipoma; myxoma; hamartoma; hemangioma; lymphangioma; islet cell tumor; carcinoid; villous adenoma)
4. Normal variant (eg, redundant duodenal fold; flexure "defect"; normal papilla of Vater)
5. Pancreatic lesion, attached or invading (esp. carcinoma of pancreas; pancreatitis; pseudocyst) (See G-213, 214)
6. Papilla of Vater enlargement (See G-138)
7. Peptic ulcer with edema or deformity
8. Polyp$_g$
9. Prolapsed gastric mucosa or polyp

UNCOMMON

1. Abscess, juxtaduodenal
2. Blood clot
3. Carcinoma of duodenum or ampulla

4. Cyst (eg, duplication; choledochal—choledochocele)
5. Foreign body in lumen (eg, fruit pit)
6. Gallstone impaction at papilla
7. Intraluminal diverticulum
8. Intramural hematoma
9. Intussusception, gastroduodenal
10. Lymphoma$_g$
11. Mesenteric or celiac artery collateral
12. Parasite (eg, *Ascaris*)
13. Postoperative defect; stitch abscess; prolapsed gastrostomy tube
14. Sarcoma (gastrointestinal stromal tumor$_g$, esp. leiomyosarcoma; Kaposi sarcoma)
15. Varix

References

1. Eisenberg RL: Gastrointestinal Radiology: A Pattern Approach. (ed 3) Philadelphia: Lippincott, 1996, pp 370–396
2. Gelfand DW: Gastrointestinal Radiology. New York: Churchill Livingstone, 1984, p 254
3. Levine MS: Benign tumors of the stomach and duodenum. In: Gore RM, Levine MS: Textbook of Gastrointestinal Radiology. (ed 2) Philadelphia: WB Saunders, 2000, pp 575–600

Gamut G-38

MULTIPLE OR DIFFUSE FILLING DEFECTS IN THE DUODENUM

COMMON

1. Brunner's gland hyperplasia
2. Heterotopic gastric mucosa
3. Metastases (esp. malignant melanoma)
4. Nodular, thickened, or edematous folds (incl. nonerosive duodenitis) (See G-40)
5. Prolapsed gastric mucosa

(continued)

UNCOMMON

1. Ascariasis
2. Blood clots
3. Crohn's disease (cobblestone pattern)
4. Cronkhite-Canada S.
5. Foreign bodies in lumen (eg, fruit pits)
6. Lymphoma$_g$; Kaposi sarcoma; other bull's-eye lesions (See G-105)
7. Mastocytosis
8. Mesenteric or celiac artery collaterals
9. Nodular lymphoid hyperplasia (esp. in dysgamma-globulinemia)
10. Polyps$_g$ (adenomatous or hamartomatous)
11. Varices

Reference

1. Glick SN, Gohel VK, Laufer I: Mucosal surface patterns of the duodenal bulb. Radiology 1984;150:317–322
2. Levine MS, Laufer I, Stevenson G: Duodenum. In: Levine MS, Rubesin SE, Laufer I: Double Contrast Gastrointestinal Radiology. (ed 3) Philadelphia: WB Saunders, 2000, pp 239-274

Gamut G-39

DIMINISHED OR ABSENT FOLD PATTERN IN THE DUODENUM AND SMALL BOWEL

COMMON

1. Crohn's disease
2. Scleroderma
3. Small bowel obstruction or ileus
4. Sprue

UNCOMMON

1. Amyloidosis
2. Cystic fibrosis (mucoviscidosis)
3. Strongyloidiasis, chronic

Gamut G-40

NODULAR OR THICKENED FOLDS IN THE DUODENUM; ALSO THICKENING OF THE DUODENAL WALL ON CT, US, OR MRI

COMMON

1. Brunner's gland hyperplasia
2. Cystic fibrosis (mucoviscidosis)
3. Duodenitis
4. Edema (eg, hypoproteinemia; cirrhosis; nephrotic S.; uremia; chronic dialysis; angioneurotic edema; heart failure)
5. Metastatic disease or direct invasion from adjacent neoplasm (esp. carcinoma of pancreas, stomach, or colon)
6. Normal variant
7. Pancreatitis, acute or chronic
8. Parasitic disease (esp. giardiasis; strongyloidiasis; hookworm disease; intestinal capillariasis)
9. Peptic ulcer disease
10. Zollinger-Ellison S.; multiple endocrine neoplasia (MEN) S. (See J-5)

UNCOMMON

1. AIDS-related infection (eg, *Cryptosporidium;* cytomegalovirus; atypical mycobacterial infection) or neoplasm (eg, Kaposi sarcoma; lymphoma$_g$)
2. Amyloidosis
3. Cholecystitis
4. Corrosive disease
5. Crohn's disease
6. Cronkhite-Canada S.
7. Drug therapy (eg, Pro-Banthine); chemotherapy toxicity
8. Duodenal diverticulitis
9. Ectopic gastric mucosa
10. Eosinophilic enteritis
11. Intestinal lymphangiectasia
12. Intramural hemorrhage (eg, trauma; hemophilia or other bleeding disorder$_g$; anticoagulant therapy)

13. Ischemia; vasculitis (eg, connective tissue disease (collagen vascular disease)$_g$; Henoch-Schönlein purpura)
14. Neoplasm, primary (eg, carcinoma; lymphoma$_g$; Kaposi sarcoma; gastrointestinal stromal tumor$_g$— esp. leiomyoma, leiomyosarcoma, or neurofibroma; lipoma; carcinoid)
15. Mastocytosis
16. Ménétrier's disease
17. Mesenteric or celiac artery collaterals following occlusion of main trunks
18. Nodular lymphoid hyperplasia (esp. in dysgamma-globulinemia)
19. Postoperative
20. Radiation injury, acute or chronic
21. Sprue; celiac disease
22. Tuberculosis
23. Varices
24. Whipple's disease

References

1. Eisenberg RL: Gastrointestinal Radiology: A Pattern Approach. (ed 3) Philadelphia: Lippincott, 1996, pp 337–347
2. Glick SN, Gohel VK, Laufer I: Mucosal surface patterns of the duodenal bulb. Radiology 1984;150:317–322
3. Halpert RD, Feczko PJ: Gastrointestinal Radiology: The Requisites. (ed 2) St. Louis: Mosby-Year Book, 1999
4. Levine MS, Laufer I, Stevenson G: Duodenum. In: Levine MS, Rubesin SE, Laufer I: Double Contrast Gastrointestinal Radiology. (ed 3) Philadelphia: WB Saunders, 2000, pp 239–274
5. Levine MS: Stomach and duodenum: Differential diagnosis. In: Gore RM, Levine MS: Textbook of Gastrointestinal Radiology. (ed 2) Philadelphia: WB Saunders, 2000, pp 698–703
6. Rubesin SE, Herlinger H: Small bowel: Differential diagnosis. In: Gore RM, Levine MS: Textbook of Gastrointestinal Radiology. (ed 2) Philadelphia: WB Saunders, 2000, pp 884–891

POSTBULBAR DUODENAL ULCERATION

COMMON

1. [Diverticulum]
2. Neoplasm, malignant, extrinsic (eg, invasion from pancreas, colon, right kidney, or gallbladder)
3. Peptic ulcer
4. Zollinger-Ellison S.

UNCOMMON

1. Aorticoduodenal fistula (esp. aortic graft)
2. Carcinoma of duodenum
3. Ectopic pancreas
4. Fistula, duodenocolic or other (See G-107)
5. Gastrointestinal stromal tumor$_g$ (esp. leiomyoma; leiomyosarcoma; neurofibroma)
6. Granulomatous disease (eg, Crohn's disease; tuberculosis)
7. Intramural duodenal pseudodiverticulosis
8. Lymphoma$_g$
9. Metastasis (eg, melanoma; Kaposi sarcoma)
10. Parasitic disease (eg, strongyloidiasis)

[ ] This condition does not actually cause the gamuted imaging finding, but can produce imaging changes that simulate it

References

1. Eisenberg RL: Gastrointestinal Radiology: A Pattern Approach (ed 3). Philadelphia: Lippincott, 1996, pp 331–336
2. Gelfand DW: Gastrointestinal Radiology. New York: Churchill Livingstone, 1984, p 243
3. Solomon DJ, Kottler RE: Duodenal intramural pseudodiverticulosis. Gastrointest Radiol 1992;17:217

Gamut G-42

DUODENAL NARROWING OR OBSTRUCTION (See G-43, 44)

COMMON

1. Congenital atresia, esp. with trisomy 21 S. (Down S.), stenosis, diaphragm or web
2. Extrinsic mass (eg, mesenteric or para-aortic lymphadenopathy; invasive neoplasm from pancreas, kidney, or colon; aortic aneurysm; choledochal cyst)
3. Pancreatitis, acute or chronic; pseudocyst
4. Postbulbar duodenal ulcer or scar
5. Superior mesenteric artery syndrome (See G-44)

UNCOMMON

1. Adhesions
2. Annular pancreas
3. Aorticoduodenal fistula
4. Cholecystitis
5. Congenital peritoneal bands (Ladd's bands)
6. Duplication cyst
7. Gallstone impaction
8. Hematoma (intramural or extrinsic)
9. Inflammatory disease of duodenum (eg, Crohn's disease; tuberculosis; strongyloidiasis; giardiasis with spasm)
10. Internal hernia (eg, paraduodenal)
11. Intraluminal diverticulum
12. Midgut volvulus with malrotation
13. Neoplasm of duodenum, primary (esp. carcinoma; leiomyosarcoma) or metastatic; also Burkitt lymphoma
14. Preduodenal portal vein
15. Prolapsed gastric lesion (eg, polyp$_g$)
16. Pseudo-obstruction, idiopathic
17. Stricture (eg, traumatic; radiation)

Gamut G-43

DUODENAL OBSTRUCTION IN AN INFANT (DOUBLE BUBBLE SIGN)

COMMON

1. Annular pancreas
2. Congenital peritoneal bands (Ladd's bands)
3. Duodenal atresia or stenosis, esp. with trisomy 21 S. (Down S.)
4. Midgut volvulus with malrotation

UNCOMMON

1. Choledochal cyst
2. Diaphragm or web; intraluminal diverticulum
3. Duplication cyst
4. Intramural hematoma
5. Preduodenal portal vein
6. Retroperitoneal tumor (eg, teratoma) or lymphadenopathy

References

1. Kassner EG, Sutton AL, DeGroot TJ: Bile duct anomalies associated with duodenal atresia; paradoxical presence of small bowel gas. AJR 1972;116:577–583
2. Silverman FN (ed): Caffey's Pediatric X-ray Diagnosis: An Integrated Imaging Approach. (ed 8) Chicago: Year Book Medical Publ, 1985
3. Swischuk LE: Imaging of the Newborn, Infant, and Young Child. (ed 3) Baltimore: Williams & Wilkins, 1989
4. Teele RL, Share JC: Diseases of the pediatric stomach and duodenum. In: Gore RM, Levine MS: Textbook of Gastrointestinal Radiology. (ed 2) Philadelphia: WB Saunders, 2000, pp 2090–2107

Gamut G-44

SUPERIOR MESENTERIC ARTERY SYNDROME (BAND-LIKE CONSTRICTION OF TRANSVERSE DUODENUM)

COMMON

1. Immobilization or prolonged bed rest (eg, post-surgery; severe burn; body cast)
2. Normal variant
3. Pancreatic mass; pancreatitis
4. Scleroderma; dermatomyositis; lupus erythematosus
5. Severe weight loss with loss of retroperitoneal fat

UNCOMMON

1. Adhesions; congenital peritoneal bands (Ladd's bands)
2. Aortic aneurysm; postrepair aorticoduodenal fistula
3. Chronic idiopathic intestinal pseudo-obstruction
4. Internal hernia, paraduodenal
5. Loss of abdominal muscle tone (eg, multiple pregnancies)
6. Retroperitoneal inflammatory or neoplastic disease
7. Small vascular (aorticomesenteric) angle
8. Thickening of root of mesentery (eg, Crohn's disease; pancreatitis; tuberculosis; metastatic disease; other lymphadenopathy)

References

1. Anderson JR, Earnshaw PM, Fraser GM: Extrinsic compression of the third part of the duodenum. Clin Radiol 1982;33:75–81
2. Eisenberg RL: Gastrointestinal Radiology: A Pattern Approach. (ed 3) Philadelphia: Lippincott, 1996, pp 411–417
3. Wallace RG, Howard WB: Acute superior mesenteric artery syndrome in the severely burned patient. Radiology 1970;94:307–310

Gamut G-45

DUODENAL DILATATION WITHOUT OBSTRUCTION

COMMON

1. Drug therapy (eg, Pro-Banthine; atropine; morphine; Lomotil)
2. Idiopathic
3. Ileus, localized (eg, acute pancreatitis; cholecystitis; peptic ulcer disease; severe trauma or burn)
4. Immobilization (eg, body cast; burn; paraplegia)
5. Normal variant
6. Postoperative (incl. vagotomy)
7. Scleroderma; dermatomyositis; lupus erythematosus

UNCOMMON

1. Chagas' disease (aganglionosis)
2. Diabetes (incl. acidosis; coma; insulin shock)
3. Emotional state alteration; hyperventilation; aerophagia
4. Pain (eg, lead colic; tabetic crisis; porphyria)
5. Sprue; other malabsorption syndromes
6. Thiamine deficiency neuropathy
7. Zollinger-Ellison S.

Reference

1. Levine MS: Stomach and duodenum: Differential diagnosis. In: Gore RM, Levine MS: Textbook of Gastrointestinal Radiology. (ed 2) Philadelphia: WB Saunders, 2000, pp 698–702

Gamut G-46

ABNORMAL POSITION OF SMALL BOWEL LOOPS

COMMON

1. Anterior abdominal hernia (eg, umbilical; ventral; postoperative incisional)
2. Inguinal or femoral hernia

(continued)

3. Lesser sac hernia
4. Malrotation (incl. midgut volvulus)
5. Paraduodenal hernia (right or esp. left)

UNCOMMON

1. Diaphragmatic hernia
2. Internal hernias (pericecal; small bowel mesentery; sigmoid mesentery; pelvic [broad ligament])
3. Obturator hernia (esp. on right)
4. Omphalocele; Cantrell S.
5. Spigelian hernia

References

1. Burgener FA, Kormano M: Differential Diagnosis in Conventional Radiology. (ed 2) New York: Thieme Medical Publ, 1991, pp 576 577
2. Eisenberg RL: Gastrointestinal Radiology: A Pattern Approach. (ed 3) Philadelphia: Lippincott,1996, pp 909–924

Gamut G-47

SEPARATION OR DISPLACEMENT OF SMALL BOWEL LOOPS

COMMON

1. Abscess, intraperitoneal (eg, appendiceal; diverticular; interloop)
2. Adhesions
3. Ascites or other peritoneal fluid (eg, cirrhosis; congestive heart failure; peritoneal carcinomatosis)
4. Bladder enlargement
5. Crohn's disease
6. Intestinal neoplasm, primary (eg, carcinoid or carcinoma of small bowel)
7. Lymphadenopathy in mesentery or retroperitoneum
8. Mesenteric mass (eg, cyst; leiomyosarcoma; lipomatosis; lymphangioma) (See G-228, 229)
9. Metastatic disease to mesentery, bowel, peritoneum, or retroperitoneal nodes
10. Neoplasm or cyst in abdomen, pelvis or retroperitoneum, other (eg, gastrointestinal stromal tumor$_g$;

ovarian cyst or tumor; retroperitoneal sarcoma; renal mass; pancreatic pseudocyst; hydatid cyst; mesothelioma; plexiform neurofibroma)
11. Peritonitis (eg, bacterial; tuberculous; typhoid fever)
12. Postoperative (eg, resection)

UNCOMMON

1. Amyloidosis
2. Graft-versus-host disease
3. Hematoma or hemorrhage (trauma or bleeding disorder$_g$ involving abdominal wall, mesentery, or bowel wall)
4. Hernia (internal; retroperitoneal)
5. Lymphoma$_g$
6. Mesenteric infarction
7. Mesenteritis (eg, retractile); Weber-Christian disease
8. Radiation enteritis
9. Tuberculosis
10. Whipple's disease

References

1. Burgener FA, Kormano M: Differential Diagnosis in Conventional Radiology. (ed 2) New York: Thieme Medical Publ, 1991, pp 574–577
2. Eisenberg RL: Gastrointestinal Radiology: A Pattern Approach. (ed 3) Philadelphia: Lippincott, 1996, pp 529–540

Gamut G-48

SOLITARY MASS IN THE SMALL BOWEL WITH PRESERVED MUCOSA

COMMON

1. Benign neoplasm (eg, adenoma; angioma; hamartoma; lipoma; leiomyoma, neurofibroma or other gastrointestinal stromal tumor$_g$)
2. Carcinoid (esp. in ileum)
3. Food particle; fruit pit; bezoar; enterolith; pill; foreign body
4. Polyp$_g$ (eg, adenomatous; hamartomatous; inflammatory fibroid)

UNCOMMON

1. Carcinoma, early or atypical (usually destroys mucosa)
2. Cyst (eg, duplication)
3. Endometrial implant
4. Gallstone
5. Heterotopic gastric mucosa; ectopic pancreas
6. Intraluminal diverticulum
7. Intramural hematoma; blood clot
8. Inverted Meckel's diverticulum
9. Lymphoma$_g$
10. Meconium ileus (cystic fibrosis {mucoviscidosis})
11. Metastasis (esp. melanoma)
12. Parasite (eg, *Ascaris* bolus; tapeworm—*Taenia aginata* or *T. solium; Anisakis* with ileocecal phlegmon)
13. Sarcoma (eg, leiomyosarcoma; Kaposi sarcoma)
14. Varix

Reference

1. Eisenberg RL: Gastrointestinal Radiology: A Pattern Approach. (ed 3) Philadelphia: Lippincott, 1996, pp 493–506.

Gamut G-49-S1

BENIGN TUMORS OF THE SMALL BOWEL

1. Adenoma
2. Carcinoid
3. Fibroma
4. Gastrointestinal stromal tumor$_g$ (esp. leiomyoma; neurofibroma)
5. Hamartoma (Peutz-Jeghers S.)
6. Hemangioma; lymphangioma
7. Lipoma

References

1. Eisenberg RL: Gastrointestinal Radiology: A Pattern Approach. (ed 3) Philadelphia: Lippincott, 1996, pp 493–506
2. Good CA: Tumors of the small intestine. AJR 1963; 89:685–705

Gamut G-49-S2

MALIGNANT TUMORS OF THE SMALL BOWEL

1. Adenocarcinoma
2. Carcinoid
3. Gastrointestinal stromal tumor (esp. leiomyosarcoma)
4. Kaposi sarcoma
5. Lymphoma$_g$
6. Metastasis (esp. melanoma)

References

1. Eisenberg RL: Gastrointestinal Radiology: A Pattern Approach. (ed 3) Philadelphia: Lippincott, 1996, pp 493–506
2. Good CA: Tumors of the small intestine. AJR 1963; 89: 685–705
3. Maglinte DDT, Kelvin FM, Herlinger H: Malignant tumors of the small bowel. In: Gore RM, Levine MS: Textbook of Gastrointestinal Radiology. (ed 2) Philadelphia: WB Saunders, 2000, pp 792–814

Gamut G-50

MULTIPLE INTRALUMINAL, MUCOSAL, OR INTRAMURAL FILLING DEFECTS IN THE SMALL BOWEL

COMMON

1. Brunner's gland hyperplasia (duodenum)
2. Food particles; seeds; foreign bodies; pills
3. Meconium ileus (cystic fibrosis (mucoviscidosis)
4. Metastases (esp. melanoma; carcinoma of breast, lung, or ovary; Kaposi sarcoma)
5. Nodular lymphoid hyperplasia (esp. in dysgamma-globulinemia)
6. Parasites (ascarids; tapeworms—*Taenia saginata*)
7. Polyposis syndromes (esp. Peutz-Jeghers S.; Gardner S.; Cronkhite-Canada S.,) (See G-106)

(continued)

UNCOMMON

1. Amyloidosis
2. Behçet S.
3. Benign neoplasms (eg, hemangiomas; lipomas; leiomyomas, neurofibromas and other gastrointestinal stromal tumors$_g$)
4. Blood clots
5. Carcinoids
6. Crohn's disease (cobblestone pattern)
7. Gallstones
8. Hyperplastic Peyer's patches in ileum (typhoid fever)
9. Lymphoma$_g$
10. Mastocytosis (duodenum)
11. Varices

References

1. Eisenberg RL: Gastrointestinal Imaging: A Pattern Approach (ed 3). Philadelphia: Lippincott, 1996, pp 507–517
2. Rubesin SE, Herlinger H: Small bowel: Differential diagnosis. In: Gore RM, Levine MS: Textbook of Gastrointestinal Radiology. (ed 2) Philadelphia: WB Saunders, 2000, pp 884–891

Gamut G-51-1

SMALL BOWEL DIVERTICULUM

COMMON

1. Duodenal diverticulum

UNCOMMON

1. Diverticulosis of small bowel (esp. jejunal diverticulosis)
2. Giant duodenal diverticulum
3. Jejunal diverticulum
4. Ileal diverticulum
5. Meckel's diverticulum

Reference

1. Eisenberg RL: Gastrointestinal Radiology: A Pattern Approach. (ed 3) Philadelphia: Lippincott, 1996, pp 541–551

Gamut G-51-2

SMALL BOWEL PSEUDODIVERTICULUM

COMMON

1. Chronic duodenal ulcer disease with pseudo-diverticular outpouchings
2. Crohn's disease (pseudodiverticula; fistulae)

UNCOMMON

1. Communicating ileal duplication
2. [Giant duodenal ulcer]
3. Intraluminal duodenal diverticulum
4. [Lymphoma ("aneurysmal" dilatation)]
5. Scleroderma

[ ] This condition does not actually cause the gamuted imaging finding, but can produce imaging changes that simulate it.

Reference

1. Eisenberg RL: Gastrointestinal Radiology: A Pattern Approach. (ed 3) Philadelphia: Lippincott, 1996, pp 541–551

Gamut G-52

THICKENING OF THE SMALL BOWEL WALL, GENERALIZED OR LOCALIZED (BARIUM, US, CT, MRI)

COMMON

1. Crohn's disease
2. Edema (eg, heart failure; constrictive pericarditis; angioneurotic edema; portal hypertension)
3. Eosinophilic enteritis; amyloidosis (fold thickening may be regular in early stages of these diseases)
4. Hemorrhage, intramural (eg, trauma; anticoagulant therapy; hemophilia; other bleeding or clotting disorder$_g$; vasculitis; Henoch-Schönlein purpura)

5. Hypoproteinemia (eg, cirrhosis; Budd-Chiari S.; nephrosis; malnutrition; burn; dysproteinemia)
6. Intestinal lymphangiectasia, primary or secondary (eg, mesenteric neoplasm)
7. Ischemic bowel disease or infarction (eg, atherosclerosis; thromboembolism; vasculitis; polyarteritis nodosa; hypotension)
8. Metastatic disease (esp. malignant melanoma; carcinoma of breast, lung or ovary; Kaposi sarcoma)
9. Neoplasm, primary (eg, carcinoma; carcinoid; lipoma; gastrointestinal stromal tumor$_g$— leiomyoma; leiomyosarcoma)
10. Opportunistic infection, esp, in AIDS (eg, *Cryptosporidium; Campylobacter fetus [jejuni]; Candida; Mycobacterium avium-intracellulare;* cytomegalovirus)
11. Parasitic disease (giardiasis; strongyloidiasis; intestinal capillariasis; hookworm disease; schistosomiasis); terminal ileum—amebiasis; anisakiasis; angiostrongyliasis costaricensis)
12. Peptic ulcer; Zollinger-Ellison S.; multiple endocrine neoplasia (MEN) S. (See J-5)

UNCOMMON

1. A-beta-lipoproteinemia
2. Alpha chain disease
3. Amyloidosis
4. Behçet disease
5. Cystic fibrosis (mucoviscidosis)
6. Enterocolitis (eg, typhoid fever; *Yersinia*)
7. Eosinophilic enteritis
8. Graft-versus-host disease
9. Infections, other (eg, *E. coli; Vibrio;* histoplasmosis)
10. Interloop abscess
11. Intestinal lymphangiectasia, primary or secondary (eg, mesenteric neoplasm)
12. Lymphoma$_g$; leukemic infiltration; pseudolymphoma
13. Mastocytosis
14. Menetrier's disease (stomach and duodenum)
15. Pancreatitis
16. Radiation enteropathy, acute or chronic
17. Tuberculous enteritis or peritonitis

18. Waldenström's macroglobulinemia
19. Whipple's disease
20. Xanthomatosis

References

1. Berk RN, Wall SD, McArdle CB, et al: Cryptosporidiosis of the stomach and small intestine in patients with AIDS. AJR 1984;143:549–554
2. Chen MYM, Ott DJ, Gelfand DW: Radiologic interpretation of diffuse small bowel diseases. Appl Radiol Sept 1990; 30–37
3. Eisenberg RL: Gastrointestinal Radiology: A Pattern Approach (ed 3). Philadelphia: Lippincott, 1996, pp 478–492
4. Goldberg HI, Sheft DJ: Abnormalities in small intestine contour and caliber. Radiol Clin North Am 1976;14: 461–475
5. Halpert RD, Feczko PJ: Gastrointestinal Radiology: The Requisites. (ed 2) St. Louis: Mosby-Year Book, 1999
6. Olmsted WW, Reagin DE: Pathophysiology of enlargment of the small bowel fold. AJR 1976;127:423–428
7. Rubesin SE, Herlinger H: Small bowel: Differential diagnosis. In: Gore RM, Levine MS: Textbook of Gastrointestinal Radiology. (ed 2) Philadelphia: WB Saunders, 2000, pp 884–891

Gamut G-53

MUCOSAL DESTRUCTION OF THE SMALL BOWEL WITH OR WITHOUT STRICTURE (LOCAL OR WIDESPREAD)

COMMON

*1. Crohn's disease; other nonspecific enteritis
*2. Lymphoma$_g$

UNCOMMON

1. [Abscess, interloop]
2. [Adhesions]
*3. Amyloidosis
4. Carcinoid
5. Carcinoma
*6. Eosinophilic enteritis

(continued)

7. Fungus disease$_g$ (eg, histoplasmosis; actinomycosis)
*8. Mastocytosis
*9. Metastatic disease (esp. from melanoma; carcinoma of breast, lung, ovary, uterus, pancreas, or GI tract)
10. [Pancreatitis]
*11. Parasitic disease (giardiasis; strongyloidiasis; intestinal capillariasis; hookworm disease; schistosomiasis; also amebiasis, anisakiasis, angiostrongyliasis costaricensis in terminal ileum)
12. Potassium enteritis
*13. Radiation enteritis
14. Sarcoma (eg, leiomyosarcoma; Kaposi sarcoma)
*15. Scleroderma
*16. Tuberculosis
17. Typhoid fever
18. Ulcerative colitis ("backwash ileitis")
19. Vascular occlusion; ischemia
20. *Yersinia* enterocolitis

* May be widespread.
[ ] This condition does not actually cause the gamuted imaging finding, but can produce imaging changes that simulate it.

References
1. Gelfand DW: Gastrointestinal Radiology. New York: Churchill Livingstone, 1984, p 284
2. Papadopoulos VD, Nolan DJ: Carcinoma of the small intestine. Clin Radiol 1985;36:409 413
3. Palmer PES, Reeder MM: The Imaging of Tropical Diseases. Heidelberg: Springer-Verlag, 2001

Gamut G-54

REGULAR THICKENING OF SMALL BOWEL FOLDS (> 3 mm)

1. Angioneurotic edema
2. Eosinophilic enteritis; amyloidosis (fold thickening may be regular in early stages of these diseases)
3. Heart failure; constrictive pericarditis

4. Hypoproteinemia (eg, cirrhosis; Budd-Chiari S.; nephrosis; malnutrition; burn; dysproteinemia; A-beta-lipoproteinemia)
5. Hemorrhage, intramural (eg, trauma; anticoagulant therapy; hemophilia; other bleeding or clotting disorder$_g$; vasculitis; Henoch-Schönlein purpura)
6. Infection (eg, giardiasis; typhoid fever)
7. Intestinal lymphangiectasia, primary or secondary (eg, mesenteric neoplasm)
8. Ischemic bowel disease or infarction (eg, atherosclerosis; thromboembolism; vasculitis; polyarteritis nodosa; hypotension)
9. Radiation enteropathy
10. Xanthomatosis

References
1. Eisenberg RL: Gastrointestinal Radiology: A Pattern Approach (ed 3). Philadelphia: Lippincott, 1996, pp 468 477
2. Goldberg HI, Sheft DJ: Abnormalities in small intestine contour and caliber. Radiol Clin North Am 1976;14:461–475
3. Olmsted WW, Reagin DE: Pathophysiology of enlargement of the small bowel fold. AJR 1976;127:423–428
4. Rubesin SE, Herlinger H: Small bowel: Differential diagnosis. In: Gore RM, Levine MS: Textbook of Gastrointestinal Radiology. (ed 2) Philadelphia: WB Saunders, 2000, pp 884–891

Gamut G-55

GENERALIZED IRREGULAR OR DISTORTED SMALL BOWEL FOLDS

COMMON

1. Crohn's disease
2. Opportunistic infection, esp, in AIDS (eg, *Cryptosporidium, Candida, Mycobacterium avium-intercellulare,* cytomegalovirus)
3. Parasitic disease (giardiasis; strongyloidiasis; intestinal capillariasis; hookworm disease; schistosomiasis); terminal ileum—amebiasis; anisakiasis; angiostrongyliasis costaricensis

4. Peptic ulcer; Zollinger-Ellison S.; multiple endocrine neoplasia (MEN) S. (See J-5)

UNCOMMON

1. A-beta-lipoproteinemia
2. Alpha chain disease
3. Amyloidosis
4. Cystic fibrosis (mucoviscidosis)
5. Enterocolitis (eg, typhoid fever; *Yersinia)*
6. Eosinophilic enteritis
7. Infections, other (eg, *Campylobacter fetus [jejuni]; Shigella; E. coli; Vibrio;* histoplasmosis)
8. Interloop abscess
9. Intestinal lymphangiectasia, primary or secondary (eg, mesenteric neoplasm)
10. Lymphoma$_g$; pseudolymphoma
11. Mastocytosis
12. Ménétrier's disease (stomach and duodenum)
13. Pancreatitis
14. Radiation injury, acute or chronic
15. Tuberculous enteritis or peritonitis
16. Waldenström's macroglobulinemia
17. Whipple's disease

References

1. Berk RN, Wall SD, McArdle CB, et al: Cryptosporidiosis of the stomach and small intestine in patients with AIDS. AJR 1984;143:549–554
2. Chen MYM, Ott DJ, Gelfand DW: Radiologic interpretation of diffuse small bowel diseases. Appl Radiol Sept 1990;30–37
3. Eisenberg RL: Gastrointestinal Radiology: A Pattern Approach (ed 3). Philadelphia: Lippincott, 1996, pp 478–492
4. Goldberg HI, Sheft DJ: Abnormalities in small intestine contour and caliber. Radiol Clin North Am 1976;14: 461–475
5. Olmsted WW, Reagin DE: Pathophysiology of enlargment of the small bowel fold. AJR 1976;127:423–428
6. Palmer PES, Reeder MM: The Imaging of Tropical Diseases. Heidelberg: Springer-Verlag, 2001

SIMULTANEOUS FOLD THICKENING OF THE STOMACH AND SMALL BOWEL

COMMON

1. Crohn's disease
2. Zollinger-Ellison S.; peptic ulcer disease

UNCOMMON

1. Amyloidosis
2. Eosinophilic gastroenteritis
3. Gastric varices with hypoproteinemia
4. Lymphoma$_g$; pseudolymphoma
5. Ménétrier's disease
6. Opportunistic infection, esp, in AIDS (eg, *Crypto-sporidium; Candida; Mycobacterium avium-intercellulare;* cytomegalovirus)
7. Pancreatitis
8. Parasitic disease (eg, strongyloidiasis; schistosomiasis; anisakiasis)
9. Tuberculosis
10. Whipple's disease

Reference

1. Eisenberg RL: Clinical Imaging: An Atlas of Differential Diagnosis. (ed 3) Philadelphia: Lippincott-Raven, 1997, pp 384–385

MALABSORPTION PATTERN IN THE SMALL BOWEL

COMMON

1. Blind loop S. (See G-58)
2. Crohn's disease
3. Cystic fibrosis (mucoviscidosis)
4. Pancreatic disease (insufficiency; chronic pancreatitis; carcinoma; gastrinoma)

(continued)

5. Parasitic disease (giardiasis; hookworm disease; strongyloidiasis; schistosomiasis japonica; intestinal capillariasis)
6. Postoperative (eg, postgastrectomy steatorrhea; gastroileostomy; short bowel S.; pancreatectomy)
7. Sprue, tropical or nontropical (celiac disease)
8. Steatorrhea, idiopathic

UNCOMMON

1. A-beta-lipoproteinemia
2. Acrodermatitis enteropathica
3. Acute bacterial infection
4. AIDS
5. Allergy (eg, angioneurotic edema)
6. Amyloidosis
7. Bile duct obstruction
8. Carcinoid syndrome
9. Chronic granulomatous disease of childhood
10. Cronkhite-Canada S.
11. Diabetes
12. Disaccharidosis (eg, lactase deficiency)
13. Drug therapy (eg, antimetabolites)
14. Ehlers-Danlos S.
15. Emotional states; anorexia nervosa
16. Eosinophilic gastroenteritis
17. Fistula (See G-107)
18. Henoch-Schönlein purpura
19. Hepatobiliary disease (eg, biliary cirrhosis; biliary atresia)
20. Hypoparathyroidism
21. Hypopituitarism
22. Hypothyroidism (cretinism); hyperthyroidism
23. Immunologic disorder$_g$
24. Intestinal lymphangiectasia
25. Ischemia of intestine, chronic
26. Jejunal diverticulosis
27. Johanson-Blizzard S.
28. Lymphoma$_g$
29. Mastocytosis
30. Metastases, peritoneal
31. Multiple endocrine neoplasia (MEN) S. (eg, gastrinoma; pancreatic non-beta islet cell tumor (VIPoma) or hyperplasia) (See J-5)
32. Nephrotic syndrome
33. Nutritional deficiency (kwashiorkor; pellagra)
34. Protein-losing enteropathy
35. Radiation gastroenteritis
36. Scleroderma; dermatomyositis
37. Tuberculous peritonitis
38. Waldenström's macroglobulinemia; alpha chain disease
39. Whipple's disease
40. Wolman's disease (familial xanthomatosis)
41. Zollinger-Ellison S.

References

1. Herlinger H: Malabsorption. In: Gore RM, Levine MS: Textbook of Gastrointestinal Radiology. (ed 2) Philadelphia: WB Saunders, 2000, pp 759–784
2. Meyer B, Cerda JJ: Malabsorption: Pathophysiologic considerations and diagnosis. Compr Ther 1985;11:49–54
3. Riley SA, Marsh MN: Maldigestion and malabsorption. In: Feldman M, Scharschmidt BF, Sleisenger MH: Gastrointestinal and Liver Disease. (ed 6) Philadelphia: WB Saunders, 2000, pp 1501–1522
4. Taybi H, Lachman RS: Radiology of Syndromes, Metabolic Disorders, and Skeletal Dysplasias. (ed 4) St. Louis: Mosby-Year Book, 1996, pp 963–964
5. Teplick JG, Haskin ME: Roentgenologic Diagnosis. (ed 3) Philadelphia: WB Saunders, 1976

Gamut G-58

BLIND LOOP SYNDROME

COMMON

1. Postoperative (eg, side-to-side anastomosis; gastroileostomy; bypass procedure; short bowel syndrome)
2. Small bowel stricture with proximal dilatation

UNCOMMON

1. Diverticulosis of small bowel (esp. jejunum)
2. Duplication of intestine
3. Meckel's diverticulum, large

4. Sluggish transit (eg, myxedema; cretinism; scleroderma)

Reference

1. Challacombe DN, Richardson JM, Edkins S, et al: Ileal blind loop in childhood. Am J Dis Child 1974;123:719–723

Gamut G-59

SMALL BOWEL DILATATION WITH THICKENED MUCOSAL FOLD PATTERN

COMMON

1. Crohn's disease
2. Infectious enteritis, esp. in AIDS (eg, cryptosporidiosis; cytomegalovirus; *Candida; Salmonella; Mycobacterium avium-intracellulare)*
3. Mesenteric infarction (venous or embolic arterial) or advanced ischemia (atherosclerosis)
4. Metastatic disease to bowel wall or mesentery
5. Zollinger-Ellison S.

UNCOMMON

1. A-beta-lipoproteinemia; A-alpha-lipoproteinemia
2. Amyloidosis
3. Compensatory dilatation of remaining bowel after extensive small bowel resection
4. Hypoalbuminemia (eg, cirrhosis; nephrotic S.)
5. Lymphoma$_g$
6. Parasitic disease (eg, thickened folds with malabsorption and dilated loops can be seen in strongyloidiasis, hookworm disease, intestinal capillariasis, and schistosomiasis japonica)
7. Radiation enteritis
8. Tropical sprue
9. Tuberculosis

Reference

1. Eisenberg RL: Gastrointestinal Radiology: A Pattern Approach. (ed 3) Philadelphia: Lippincott, 1996, pp 464–467

Gamut G-60

SMALL BOWEL DILATATION WITH NORMAL FOLD PATTERN

COMMON

1. Adynamic ("paralytic") ileus
2. Drug effect (esp. anticholinergics)
3. Mechanical obstruction
4. Mesenteric ischemia (eg, atherosclerosis; lupus erythematosus)
5. Postvagotomy; gastrectomy (dumping syndrome)
6. Sprue (esp. nontropical); celiac disease; other malabsorption syndromes (See G-57)

UNCOMMON

1. Amyloidosis
2. Chagas' disease
3. Chronic idiopathic intestinal pseudo-obstruction
4. Hypokalemia (esp. in diabetic)
5. Lactase deficiency
6. Scleroderma; dermatomyositis

References

1. Chen MYM, Ott DJ, Gelfand DW: Radiologic interpretation of diffuse small bowel diseases. Appl Radiol Sept 1990; 30–37
2. Eisenberg RL: Gastrointestinal Radiology: A Pattern Approach. (ed 3) Philadelphia: Lippincott, 1996, pp 453–463

Gamut G-61

ACUTE NONOBSTRUCTIVE SMALL BOWEL DISTENTION ("PARALYTIC ILEUS")

COMMON

1. Drug effect (eg, atropine; morphine; barbiturates; Lomotil; Pro-Banthine; hexamethonium; L-dopa)
2. Electrolyte imbalance (eg, hypokalemia; hypochloremia; calcium or magnesium abnormality)

(continued)

3. Gastroenteritis, acute; food poisoning
4. Pain in abdomen (eg, renal, ureteral, or common bile duct stone; torsion of uterine fibroid or ovarian cyst or tumor; lead colic; sickle cell crisis; tabetic crisis; porphyria)
5. Peritonitis, acute
6. Pneumonia; other acute thoracic disease (eg, myocardial infarction; heart failure)
7. Postoperative (abdominal or pelvic surgery)
8. Retroperitoneal hemorrhage
9. "Sentinel loop," localized ileus (eg, acute cholecystitis; appendicitis; acute pancreatitis; acute diverticulitis) (See G-80)
10. Shock; gram-negative septicemia; hypoxia
11. Trauma (esp. spine or lower rib; abdominal contusion; intramural hematoma)
12. Vascular occlusion (eg, mesenteric infarction)

UNCOMMON

1. Adrenal insufficiency
2. Aerophagia; assisted respiration
3. Ceroidosis (malabsorption with prolonged vitamin E depletion)
4. Chronic idiopathic intestinal pseudo-obstruction
5. Diabetic acidosis; insulin shock
6. Enterocolitis (eg, typhoid fever; *Yersinia*)
7. Hypoparathyroidism
8. Hypothyroidism
9. Interloop abscess
10. Myotonic dystrophy; muscular dystrophy
11. Neonatal adynamic ileus (eg, septicemia; hypoxia-induced vasculitis; infantile respiratory distress S.; intestinal infection; peritonitis; mesenteric thrombosis)
12. Neonatal necrotizing enterocolitis
13. Renal failure; uremia; acute glomerulonephritis
14. Urinary retention

References

1. Burgener FA, Kormano M: Differential Diagnosis in Conventional Radiology. (ed 2) New York: Thieme Medical Publ, 1991, pp 601–602
2. Eisenberg RL: Gastrointestinal Radiology: A Pattern Approach. (ed 3) Philadelphia: Lippincott, 1996, pp 442–452

Gamut G-62

CHRONIC NONOBSTRUCTIVE SMALL BOWEL DISTENTION

COMMON

1. Ascites
2. Connective tissue disease (collagen disease)$_g$ (esp. scleroderma)
3. Neurologic or muscular disorder$_g$ (eg, parkinsonism; myotonic dystrophy; tabes; spinal cord lesion)
4. Sprue, tropical or nontropical (celiac disease)
5. Vagotomy

UNCOMMON

1. Adrenal insufficiency
2. Allergic enterocolitis
3. Amyloidosis
4. Ceroidosis (prolonged malabsorption and vitamin E depletion)
5. Chronic idiopathic intestinal pseudo-obstruction
6. Congenital short intestine
7. Cystic fibrosis (mucoviscidosis)
8. Diabetes with hypokalemia
9. Disaccharidase deficiency (eg, lactase deficiency)
10. Drug effect (eg, Lomotil; morphine)
11. Eosinophilic gastroenteritis
12. Hypoparathyroidism
13. Hypoproteinemia (eg, cirrhosis; nephrosis; malnutrition; burn; A-beta-lipoproteinemia)
14. Intestinal lymphangiectasia
15. Jejunal diverticulosis
16. Lymphoma$_g$
17. Malrotation; internal hernia
18. Mesenteritis
19. Myxedema; hypothyroidism
20. Parasitic disease (esp. Chagas' disease; chronic strongyloidiasis; schistosomiasis japonica)
21. Postoperative (eg, gastrectomy; colectomy; intestinal bypass)
22. Renal failure; uremia; peritoneal dialysis
23. Vascular insufficiency (mesenteric ischemia); vasculitis (eg, lupus erythematosus; polyarteritis nodosa)

24. Waldenström's macroglobulinemia
25. Whipple's disease

References
1. Eisenberg RL: Clinical Imaging: An Atlas of Differential Diagnosis. (ed 3) Philadelphia: Lippincott-Raven, 1997, pp 358–361
2. Rubesin SE, Herlinger H: Small bowel: Differential diagnosis. In: Gore RM, Levine MS: Textbook of Gastrointestinal Radiology. (ed 2) Philadelphia: WB Saunders, 2000, pp 884–891
3. Seaman WB: Motor dysfunction of the gastrointestinal tract. AJR 1972;116:235-244

Gamut G-63

TERMINAL ILEUM LESION

COMMON

1. Appendicitis
2. Carcinoid
3. Crohn's disease
4. Intussusception
5. Mass, extrinsic (eg, ovarian or other pelvic neoplasm; aneurysm of iliac artery)
6. Meconium ileus (cystic fibrosis {mucoviscidosis})
7. Nodular lymphoid hyperplasia; normal lymphoid follicles

UNCOMMON

1. Diverticulitis
2. Endometrial implant
3. Food particles; foreign body; gallstone
4. Fungus disease (eg, actinomycosis; histoplasmosis)
5. Intramural hematoma
6. Laxative abuse
7. Meckel's diverticulum
8. Mesenteric infarction; ischemic enteritis
9. Metastasis (esp. from gastric, colonic or ovarian neoplasm)
10. Neoplasm, benign or malignant (eg, gastrointestinal stromal tumor$_g$; carcinoma; sarcoma; lymphoma$_g$)

11. Parasitic disease
    a. Intraluminal worms (eg, *Ascaris;* tapeworm—*Taenia saginata*)
    b. Inflammatory changes (eg, schistosomiasis; amebiasis; strongyloidiasis; rarely giardiasis; intestinal capillariasis; anisakiasis; angiostrongyliasis costaricensis)
12. Polyp$_g$ (See G-106)
13. Radiation enteritis
14. Tuberculosis
15. Typhoid fever
16. Ulcerative colitis ("backwash ileitis")
17. *Yersinia* enterocolitis

References
1. Calenoff L: Rare ileocecal lesions. AJR 1970;110:343–351
2. Gelfand DW: Gastrointestinal Radiology. New York: Churchill Livingstone, 1984, p 335
3. Herlinger H, Ekberg OT: Other inflammatory conditions of the small bowel. In: Gore RM, Levine MS: Textbook of Gastrointestinal Radiology. (ed 2) Philadelphia: WB Saunders, 2000, pp 704–725
4. Jeffree MA, et al: Primary carcinoid tumors of the ileum: the radiological appearances. Clin Radiol 1984;35:451–455
5. Marshak RH, Lindner AE, Maklansky D: Radiology of the Colon. Philadelphia: WB Saunders, 1980
6. Williams RH, Dixit JK: Filling defect in terminal ileum due to an aneurysm of right common iliac artery. South Med J 1975;68:783–785

Gamut G-64-S

NONDIAPHRAGMATIC HERNIAS

COMMON

1. Femoral
2. Incisional
3. Inguinal
4. Umbilical (incl. omphalocele)
5. Ventral

UNCOMMON

1. Lesser sac (foramen of Winslow)
2. Lumbar

(continued)

3. Mesenteric (small bowel; sigmoid)
4. Obturator
5. Paracecal
6. Paraduodenal
7. Pelvic (broad ligament)
8. Perineal
9. Retroperitoneal
10. Sciatic
11. Spigelian

Reference

1. Eisenberg RL: Gastrointestinal Radiology: A Pattern Approach. (ed 3) Philadelphia: Lippincott, 1996, pp 909–924

Gamut G-65

ABNORMALITIES OF BOWEL ROTATION

COMMON

1. Malrotation
2. Midgut volvulus with malrotation
3. Mobile cecum (high or midline)
4. Nonrotation

UNCOMMON

1. Exomphalos
2. Extroversion of cloaca
3. Paraduodenal hernia
4. Reverse rotation

References

1. Gaines PA, Saunders AJ, Drake D: Midgut malrotation diagnosed by ultrasound. 1987; 38:51–53
2. Houston CS, Wittenborg MH: Roentgen evaluation of anomalies of rotation and fixation of the bowel in children. Radiology 1965;84:1–17
3. Javors BR: Applied embryology of the gastrointestinal tract. In: Gore RM, Levine MS: Textbook of Gastrointestinal Radiology. (ed 2) Philadelphia: WB Saunders, 2000, p 2020

Gamut G-66

CONGENITAL SYNDROMES ASSOCIATED WITH INTESTINAL MALROTATION

1. Abdominal heterotaxy
2. Asplenia or polysplenia S.
3. Brachmann-de Lange S.
4. Cantrell S.
5. Coffin-Siris S.
6. FG syndrome
7. Mobile cecum S.
8. Prune-belly S. (Eagle-Barrett S.)
9. Trisomy 13 S.
10. Trisomy 18 S.
11. Trisomy 21 S. (Down S.)

References

1. Fernbach SK: Neonatal gastrointestinal radiology. In: Gore RM, Levine MS: Textbook of Gastrointestinal Radiology. (ed 2) Philadelphia: WB Saunders, 2000, pp 2042–2074
2. Jones KL: Smith's Recognizable Patterns of Human Malformation. Philadelphia: WB Saunders, 1988
3. Taybi H, Lachman RS: Radiology of Syndromes, Metabolic Disorders, and Skeletal Dysplasias. (ed 4) St. Louis: Mosby-Year Book, 1996, p 964

Gamut G-67

APHTHOID ULCERS IN THE SMALL BOWEL OR COLON*

COMMON

1. Crohn's disease

UNCOMMON

1. Amebiasis
2. [Artifacts (eg, fecal debris; flocculated barium; innominate grooves of colon)]
3. Behçet S.

4. Candidiasis
5. Cytomegalovirus infection of ileum and colon (also esophagus and stomach)
6. Ischemic colitis
7. [Lymphoid hyperplasia of colon]
8. Salmonellosis
9. Tuberculosis
10. *Yersinia* enterocolitis

* Tiny discrete central ulcer containing barium surrounded by a halo of edematous mucosa, best seen on air-contrast examination.
[ ] This condition does not actually cause the gamuted imaging finding, but can produce imaging changes that simulate it.

References
1. Eisenberg RL: Gastrointestinal Radiology: A Pattern Approach. (ed 3) Philadelphia: Lippincott, 1996
2. Gedgaudas-McClees EK: Aphthoid ulcerations in ileocecal candidiasis. AJR 1983; 141:973–977
3. Gore RM: Inflammatory disease. In: Margulis AR: Modern Imaging of the Alimentary Tube. New York: Springer-Verlag, 1998, pp 185-216
4. Simpkins KC: Aphthoid ulcers in Crohn's colitis. Clin Radiol 1977;28:601-608

Gamut G-68

INNUMERABLE TINY NODULES (SAND-LIKE OR GRANULAR LUCENCIES SMALLER THAN 5 MM) IN THE SMALL BOWEL OR COLON

COMMON
1. Crohn's disease ("cobblestone" pattern)
2. [Food particles; seeds; air bubbles]
3. Nodular lymphoid hyperplasia (eg, dysgamma-globulinemia)
4. Normal lymphoid follicles
5. Polyposis syndromes (esp. Cronkhite-Canada S.) (See G-106)

UNCOMMON
1. A-beta-lipoproteinemia
2. Amyloidosis

3. Cystic fibrosis (mucoviscidosis)
4. Eosinophilic enteritis
5. Histoplasmosis
6. Hyperplastic Peyer's patches (eg, typhoid fever)
7. Intestinal lymphangiectasia
8. Lymphoma$_g$
9. Mastocytosis
10. Mycobacterial enteritis
11. Ulcerative colitis
12. Waldenström's macroglobulinemia; heavy chain disease
13. Whipple's disease
14. *Yersinia* enterocolitis

[ ] This condition does not actually cause the gamuted imaging finding, but can produce imaging changes that simulate it.

References
1. Eisenberg RL: Gastrointestinal Radiology: A Pattern Approach. (ed 3) Philadelphia: Lippincott, 1996, pp 518–524
2. Kenney PJ, Koehler RE, Shackelford GD: The clinical significance of large lymphoid follicles of the colon. Radiology 1982;142:41–46
3. Reeder MM: RPC of the Month from the AFIP: Nodular lymphoid hyperplasia of the small intestine. Radiology 1969;93:427–433
4. Rubesin SE, Herlinger H: Small bowel: Differential diagnosis. In: Gore RM, Levine MS: Textbook of Gastrointestinal Radiology. (ed 2) Philadelphia: WB Saunders, 2000, pp 884–890

Gamut G-69

MESENTERIC VASCULAR COMPROMISE (INTESTINAL ISCHEMIA OR INFARCTION)

COMMON
1. Arterial thromboembolism (eg, secondary to myocardial infarction; rheumatic heart disease; atrial fibrillation)
2. Arteriosclerosis
3. Digitalis toxicity

(continued)

4. Heart failure
5. Iatrogenic (eg, catheter arteriography; drug instillation)
6. Idiopathic (normal vessels)
7. Intestinal obstruction (esp. strangulation)
8. Peritoneal band or adhesion
9. Septicemia (eg, drug abuse; bacterial endocarditis)
10. Vascular compression by extrinsic mass
11. Venous thrombosis

UNCOMMON

1. Abdominal or pelvic inflammatory disease
2. Arteritis (eg, Takayasu's arteritis; polyarteritis nodosa)
3. Coarctation of aorta (esp. postoperative)
4. Dissecting aneurysm
5. Fibromuscular hyperplasia of mesenteric artery
6. Polycythemia
7. Postoperative (esp. surgical ligation)
8. Radiation injury
9. Transient ischemia of children
10. Trauma to the intestine or its vessels

References
1. Kaufman SL, Harrington DP, Siegelman SS: Superior mesenteric artery embolization: An angiography emergency. Radiology 1977;124:625–630
2. Smith SL, Tutton RH, Ochsner SF: Roentgenographic aspects of intestinal ischemia. AJR 1972;116:249–255
3. Szucs RA, Wolf EL, Gramm HF, et al: Miscellaneous abnormalities of the colon. In: Gore RM, Levine MS: Textbook of Gastrointestinal Radiology. (ed 2) Philadelphia: WB Saunders, 2000, pp 1084–1122

Gamut G-70

GAS IN THE BOWEL WALL (PNEUMATOSIS INTESTINALIS)

COMMON

1. Colitis (eg, ulcerative; tuberculous; amebic; Crohn's disease)
2. Necrosis of the intestine
   a. Necrotizing enterocolitis (esp. in premature or debilitated infants)
   b. Mesenteric thrombosis with infarction
   c. Gangrenous, pseudomembranous, or other enterocolitis
   d. Strangulated hernia, volvulus, or other intestinal obstruction
   e. Primary infection of bowel wall
   f. Ingestion of corrosives
3. Primary, idiopathic (pneumatosis cystoides intestinalis)
4. Toxic megacolon (See G-94)

UNCOMMON

1. Adynamic ileus (esp. postoperative)
2. Air hose injury of rectum ("goose")
3. Colonic irrigation; hydrogen peroxide enema
4. Congenital obstruction (eg, atresia; stenosis; web; diaphragm; imperforate anus; meconium plug)
5. Connective tissue disease (collagen disease)$_g$ (esp. scleroderma)
6. Diabetes with gas-forming organism
7. Graft-versus-host disease (esp. involving cecum)
8. Hirschsprung's disease or other megacolon (See G-93)
9. Iatrogenic (eg, endoscopy; colonoscopy; catheter jejunostomy; umbilical artery catheterization)
10. Idiopathic
11. Leukemia
12. Malabsorption (eg, sprue)
13. Obstructive pulmonary disease, esp. with coughing (eg, emphysema; bullous disease; asthma; chronic bronchitis)

14. Perforated jejunal diverticulum
15. Pneumomediastinum with abdominal extension of air
16. Postoperative (esp. jejunoileal bypass; postoperative intramural leakage)
17. Pyloroduodenal obstruction (eg, peptic ulcer, esp. with intramural perforation; pyloric stenosis)
18. Steroid and other immunosuppressive therapy
19. Trauma to gut

References

1. Bryk D: Unusual causes of small-bowel pneumatosis: Perforated duodenal ulcer and perforated jejunal diverticula. Radiology 1973;106:299–302
2. Eisenberg RL: Gastrointestinal Radiology: A Pattern Approach. (ed 3) Philadelphia: Lippincott, 1996, pp 925–937
3. Felson B: Abdominal gas: A roentgen approach. Ann NY Acad Sci 1968;150:141–161
4. Gupta A: Pneumatosis intestinalis in children. Br J Radiol 1978; 51:589–595
5. Keats TE, Smith TH: Benign pneumatosis intestinalis in childhood leukemia. AJR 1974;122;150–152
6. Marshak RH, Lindner AE, Maklansky D: Pneumatosis cystoides coli. Gastrointest Radiol 1977;2:85–89
7. Mueller CF, et al: Pneumatosis intestinalis in collagen disorders. AJR 1972;115:300–305
8. Naggar CZ: Pneumatosis intestinalis following common upper-respiratory-tract infection. JAMA 1976;235;2221–2222
9. Shallal JA, Van Heerden JA, Bartholomew LG, et al: Pneumatosis cystoides intestinalis. Mayo Clin Proc 1974;49:180–184
10. Strain JD, Rudikoff JC, Moore EE, et al: Pneumatosis intestinalis associated with intracatheter jejunostomy feeding. AJR 1982;139:107–109

Gamut G-71-1

SMALL AND LARGE BOWEL WALL THICKENING: HOMOGENEOUS ATTENUATION ON POSTCONTRAST CT

COMMON

1. Carcinoma of small bowel and/or colon
2. Lymphoma$_g$
3. Submucosal hemorrhage or hematoma

UNCOMMON

1. Crohn's disease, chronic
2. Infarcted bowel
3. [Pseudothickening related to incomplete distention and residual fluid]
4. Radiation injury, chronic

[ ] This condition does not actually cause the gamuted imaging finding, but can produce imaging changes that simulate it.

Reference

1. Macari M, Baltazar EJ: CT of bowel wall thickening: Significance and pitfalls of interpretation. AJR 2001;176:1105–1116

Gamut G-71-2

SMALL AND LARGE BOWEL WALL THICKENING: HETEROGENEOUS (STRATIFIED OR MIXED) ATTENUATION ON POSTCONTRAST CT

STRATIFIED ATTENUATION*

COMMON

1. Bowel edema related to cirrhosis or hypoproteinemia
2. Crohn's disease
3. Henoch-Schönlein purpura
4. Infectious enterocolitis
5. Ischemia
6. Lupus erythematosus
7. Radiation injury
8. Ulcerative colitis
9. Vasculitis

UNCOMMON

1. Infiltrating scirrhous carcinoma (usually colon or rectum)
2. Pneumatosis
3. [Residual fluid and contrast material]
4. Submucosal fat deposition

(continued)

MIXED ATTENUATION+

1. Carcinoma (esp. mucinous adenocarcinoma)
2. Gastrointestinal stromal tumor_g

* Alternating (stratified) layers of attenuation in a thickened bowel segment may take the form of a double halo or a target configuration. The double halo sign represents an inner low-attenuation (edema) ring surrounded by an outer higher attenuation ring on postcontrast CT. In the target sign, inner and outer layers of high attenuation surrround a central area of decreased (edema) attenuation. The high attenuation in these signs is related to hyperemia.

+ The grossly thickened bowel wall has several irregular zones of lower attenuation haphazardly located next to areas of higher attenuation. These findings are related to ischemia and necrosis and are seen in high-grade, poorly differentiated neoplasms such as adenocarcinoma and stromal cell tumors.

[ ] This condition does not actually cause the gamuted imaging finding, but can produce imaging changes that simulate it.

Reference

1. Macari M, Baltazar EJ: CT of bowel wall thickening: Significance and pitfalls of interpretation. AJR 2001;176: 1105–1116

Gamut G-72-1

MILD THICKENING (< 2 CM) OF BOWEL WALL ON POSTCONTRAST CT

COMMON

1. Bowel edema in cirrhosis
2. Crohn's disease
3. Infectious enterocolitis
4. Ischemia
5. Radiation injury
6. Submucosal hemorrhage
7. Ulcerative colitis

UNCOMMON

1. Adenocarcinoma
2. Lymphoma_g

Reference

1. Macari M, Baltazar EJ: CT of bowel wall thickening: Significance and pitfalls of interpretation. AJR 2001;176: 1105–1116

Gamut G-72-2

MARKED THICKENING (> 2 CM) OF BOWEL WALL ON POSTCONTRAST CT

COMMON

1. Carcinoma
2. Colitis, severe
3. Gastrointestinal stromal tumor_g
4. Lupus erythematosus
5. Lymphoma_g
6. Metastatic disease involving bowel wall

UNCOMMON

1. Crohn's disease
2. Cytomegalovirus infection
3. Histoplasmosis
4. Submucosal hemorrhage
5. Tuberculosis

Reference

1. Macari M, Baltazar EJ: CT of bowel wall thickening: Significance and pitfalls of interpretation. AJR 2001;176: 1105–1116

Gamut G-73

SYMMETRIC VERSUS ASYMMETRIC THICKENING OF BOWEL WALL ON POSTCONTRAST CT

SYMMETRIC

1. Bowel edema in cirrhosis
2. Crohn's disease
3. Infectious enterocolitis
4. Ischemia
5. Lymphoma_g
6. Radiation injury
7. Submucosal hemorrhage
8. Ulcerative colitis

ASYMMETRIC
1. Carcinoma
2. Gastrointestinal stromal tumor$_g$

Reference
1. Macari M, Baltazar EJ: CT of bowel wall thickening: Significance and pitfalls of interpretation. AJR 2001;176: 1105–1116

Gamut G-74-1

FOCAL BOWEL WALL THICKENING (< 10 CM) ON POSTCONTRAST CT

COMMON
1. Carcinoma (esp. adenocarcinoma)
2. Appendicitis
3. Diverticulitis

UNCOMMON
1. Crohn's disease
2. Lymphoma$_g$
3. Tuberculosis

Reference
1. Macari M, Baltazar EJ: CT of bowel wall thickening: Significance and pitfalls of interpretation. AJR 2001;176: 1105–1116

Gamut G-74-2

SEGMENTAL BOWEL WALL THICKENING (10–30 CM) ON POSTCONTRAST CT

COMMON
1. Carcinoma (eg, mucinous or colloid carcinoma of colon; scirrhous carcinoma of colon or rectum)
2. Crohn's disease
3. Infectious ileitis
4. Ischemia
5. Lymphoma$_g$
6. Radiation injury
7. Submucosal hemorrhage

UNCOMMON
1. Lupus erythematosus

Reference
1. Macari M, Baltazar EJ: CT of bowel wall thickening: Significance and pitfalls of interpretation. AJR 2001;176: 1105–1116

Gamut G-74-3

DIFFUSE BOWEL WALL THICKENING ON POSTCONTRAST CT

COMMON
1. Edema from cirrhosis or hypoproteinemia
2. Infectious enterocolitis
3. Lupus erythematosus
4. Ulcerative colitis

(continued)

UNCOMMON

1. Ischemia
2. Pseudomembranous colitis

Reference

1. Macari M, Baltazar EJ: CT of bowel wall thickening: Significance and pitfalls of interpretation. AJR 2001;176: 1105–1116

Gamut G-75

RESIDUAL INTESTINAL BARIUM AFTER GASTROINTESTINAL STUDY (MORE THAN ONE WEEK)

COMMON

1. Barium in appendix or diverticula of small bowel or colon
2. Fecal impaction
3. Gastric obstruction
4. Nonobstructive ileus (See G-61)

UNCOMMON

1. Aganglionosis of colon (eg, Hirschsprung disease; Chagas' disease)
2. Blind loop syndrome (See G-58)
3. [Calcification (esp. milk of calcium)]
4. Cryptosporidiosis
5. Drug effect (eg, morphine)
6. Duplication of intestine
7. Hypothyroidism (eg, myxedema; cretinism)
8. Meckel's diverticulum
9. [Medication, opaque]
10. Perforation of intestine
11. Postoperative (eg, side-to-side anastomosis; gastro-ileostomy; bypass procedure)
12. Scleroderma
13. Stricture of intestine

[ ] This condition does not actually cause the gamuted imaging finding, but can produce imaging changes that simulate it.

Gamut G-76

INTESTINAL OBSTRUCTION IN A NEWBORN*

COMMON

1. Congenital stenosis or atresia of stomach, duodenum, small bowel, colon, rectum*, or anus (imperforate anus)*
 2. Hernia, incarcerated, internal or external (eg, inguinal, femoral, umbilical, diaphragmatic, mesenteric defects)
*3. Hirschsprung disease
 4. Malrotation with midgut volvulus
*5. Meconium ileus (cystic fibrosis {mucoviscidosis})
*6. Meconium plug S.
*7. Small left colon S.

UNCOMMON

 1. Apple peel intestinal atresia
 2. Choledochal cyst
 3. Congenital peritoneal bands (Ladd's bands)
 4. Inspissated milk S.
 5. Intestinal duplication
 6. Intraluminal diaphragm or web
 7. Intramural hematoma (eg, trauma)
*8. Intussusception (rare in newborn)
 9. Meconium peritonitis (eg, meconium ileus)
*10. Megacystis-microcolon-intestinal hypoperistalsis S. (Berdon S.)
11. Neoplasm (usually distention without obstruction)
12. [Paralytic ileus (eg, from drugs given during labor)]
13. Preduodenal portal vein
14. Segmental dilatation of ileum

* Low intestinal obstruction in a newborn.
[ ] This condition does not actually cause the gamuted imaging finding, but can produce imaging changes that simulate it.

References

1. Carty H, Brereton RJ: The distended neonate. Clin Radiol 1983;34:367–380

2. Fernbach SK: Neonatal gastrointestinal radiology. In: Gore RM, Levine MS: Textbook of Gastrointestinal Radiology. (ed 2) Philadelphia: WB Saunders, 2000, pp 2042–2074
3. Silverman FN (ed): Caffey's Pediatric X-ray Diagnosis: An Integrated Imaging Approach. (ed 8) Chicago: Year Book Medical Publ, 1985
4. Swischuk LE: Radiology of the Newborn, Infant, and Young Child. (ed 3) Baltimore: Williams & Wilkins, 1989
5. Taybi H, Lachman RS: Radiology of Syndromes, Metabolic Disorders, and Skeletal Dysplasias. (ed 4) St. Louis: Mosby-Year Book, 1996, p 963

Gamut G-77

INTESTINAL OBSTRUCTION IN A CHILD (See G-76)

COMMON

1. Adhesions (inflammatory; postoperative); congenital peritoneal bands (Ladd's bands)
2. Appendicitis (esp. perforated)
3. Hernia, incarcerated (internal or external)
4. Hirschsprung disease
5. Intussusception (eg, ameboma; intestinal duplication; Henoch-Schönlein purpura; idiopathic; Meckel's diverticulum; polyp$_g$; lymphoma$_g$; other neoplasm)

UNCOMMON

1. Cast S. (cast treatment for scoliosis causing superior mesenteric artery S.)
2. Chronic granulomatous disease of childhood
3. Crohn's disease
4. Cystic fibrosis (mucoviscidosis)
5. Familial Mediterranean fever
6. Fecal impaction
7. Foreign body; bezoar
8. Kawasaki S.
9. Neoplasm, benign or malignant (eg, gastrointestinal stromal tumor$_g$; lymphoma$_g$; sarcoma)
10. Neurofibromatosis I (von Recklinghausen disease)
11. Parasitic disease (esp. *Ascaris* bolus; ameboma)

12. [Pseudo-obstruction, idiopathic]
13. Stenosis, congenital (eg, duodenum; small bowel; rectum)
14. Tuberculous enteritis
15. Volvulus, midgut or other

[ ] This condition does not actually cause the gamuted imaging finding, but can produce imaging changes that simulate it.

References
1. Silverman FN (ed): Caffey's Pediatric X-ray Diagnosis: An Integrated Imaging Approach. (ed 8) Chicago: Year Book Medical Publ, 1985
2. Swischuk LE, John SD: Differential Diagnosis in Pediatric Radiology. (ed 2) Baltimore: Williams & Wilkins, 1995
3. Taybi H, Lachman RS: Radiology of Syndromes, Metabolic Disorders, and Skeletal Dysplasias. (ed 4) St. Louis: Mosby-Year Book, 1996, p 963

Gamut G-78

INTESTINAL OBSTRUCTION IN AN ADULT

COMMON

1. Abscess, abdominal$_g$ (eg, periappendiceal; tubovarian)
2. Adhesions (inflammatory; postoperative); congenital peritoneal bands (Ladd's bands)
3. Carcinoma of colon, rectum, or rarely, small bowel
4. Crohn's disease
5. Diverticulitis (esp. colonic)
6. Fecal impaction
7. Hernia, incarcerated, internal or external (See G-64-S)
8. Intussusception
9. Metastatic disease (esp. melanoma; carcinoma of ovary, breast, lung; peritoneal carcinomatosis) or invasion of bowel by adjacent pelvic or abdominal malignancy
10. Stricture (eg, neoplastic; inflammatory—lymphogranuloma venereum; radiation; potassium-induced; ischemic; posttraumatic; postoperative)
11. Volvulus (esp. cecal or sigmoid)

(continued)

UNCOMMON

1. Amyloidosis
2. Bezoar; enterolith; foreign body
3. Endometriosis
4. Extrinsic pressure from large adjacent neoplasm, distended bladder, or pregnant uterus
5. Familial Mediterranean fever
6. Gallstone ileus
7. Granulomatous disease (eg, actinomycosis; tuberculosis)
8. Hirschsprung disease
9. [Immobilization; Cast S.]
10. Intestinal duplication
11. [Intestinal pseudo-obstruction, idiopathic] (See G-79)
12. Intramural hematoma
13. Lymphoma$_g$
14. Neoplasm, other (gastrointestinal stromal tumor$_g$— esp. leiomyoma; carcinoid; sarcoma); cyst
15. Neurofibromatosis I (von Recklinghausen disease)
16. Parasitic disease (*Ascaris* bolus; amebiasis; Chagas' disease; schistosomiasis)
17. Retractile mesenteritis
18. [Spasm (eg, sickle cell crisis; plumbism; porphyria; tabes; diabetic ketosis; potassium deficiency)]
19. Superior mesenteric artery S.
20. Ulcerative colitis, chronic
21. Vascular occlusion (arterial or venous); mesenteric infarction; ischemic colitis (See G-69)

[ ] This condition does not actually cause the gamuted imaging finding, but can produce imaging changes that simulate it.

References
1. Eisenberg RL: Gastrointestinal Radiology: A Pattern Approach. (ed 3) Philadelphia: Lippincott, 1996, pp 421–441, 748–767
2. Herlinger H, Rubesin SE, Morris JB: Small bowel obstruction. In: Gore RM, Levine MS: Textbook of Gastrointestinal Radiology. (ed 2) Philadelphia: WB Saunders, 2000, pp 815–837

INTESTINAL PSEUDO-OBSTRUCTION (OGILVIE SYNDROME); BOWEL OBSTRUCTION IN THE ABSENCE OF MECHANICAL BLOCKAGE

COMMON

1. Idiopathic ("primary")
2. Paralytic ileus (eg, trauma; hypokalemia; pneumonia; myocardial infarction; pancreatitis; sickle cell crisis)

UNCOMMON

1. Amyloidosis
2. Celiac disease; sprue
3. Ceroidosis (prolonged malabsorption and vitamin E depletion)
4. Connective tissue disorder (collagen disease)$_g$
5. Diverticulosis of small bowel
6. Drug reaction (eg, phenothiazine; antidepressant; anti-Parkinsonism drugs; morphine)
7. Endocrine disorder (eg, myxedema; diabetes; hypoparathyroidism; pheochromocytoma)
8. Enteric muscle disorder (eg, myotonic dystrophy; scleroderma)
9. Jejunoileal bypass
10. Neonatal adynamic ileus
11. Neurologic disorder (eg, parkinsonism, stroke, paralysis, brain damage)
12. Parasitic disease (eg, Chagas' disease; chronic strongyloidiasis)
13. Pelvic surgery (eg, hysterectomy)
14. Porphyria, acute intermittent
15. Retractile mesenteritis
16. Urinary retention
17. Vitamin D deficiency

References
1. Eisenberg RL: Gastrointestinal Radiology: A Pattern Approach. (ed 3) Philadelphia: Lippincott, 1996, pp 447–452

2. Gilchrist AM, Mills JOM, Russell CFJ: Acute large bowel pseudo-obstruction. Clin Radiol 1985;36:401–404
3. Spechler SJ, Nath BJ: Case records of the Massachusetts General Hospital, Case 43. N Engl J Med 1985;313:1070–1079

SENTINEL LOOP (LOCALIZED DILATATION OF SMALL AND/OR LARGE BOWEL)

COMMON

1. Acute appendicitis (right lower quadrant)
2. Acute cholecystitis (right upper quadrant)
3. Acute diverticulitis (left lower quadrant)
4. Acute pancreatitis (upper or mid-abdomen)
5. Acute ureteral colic (stone)
6. Infarction or ischemia of bowel
7. "Paralytic ileus" (See G-61)
8. Perforated peptic ulcer (upper abdomen)
9. [Small bowel obstruction, early or incomplete]

UNCOMMON

1. Abdominal trauma
2. Drug effect
3. Gastroenteritis
4. [Normal variant]
5. [Volvulus]

[ ] This condition does not actually cause the gamuted imaging finding, but can produce imaging changes that simulate it.

References

1. Baker SR, Cho KC: The Abdominal Plain Film with Correlative Imaging. Norwalk, CT: Appleton & Lange, 1998
2. Eisenberg RL: Gastrointestinal Radiology: A Pattern Approach. (ed 3) Philadelphia: Lippincott, 1996, p 447

APPENDICEAL LESION OR MASS ADJACENT TO APPENDIX

COMMON

1. Appendiceal abscess
2. Appendiceal fecalith (calculus)
3. Appendicitis, acute or resolving
4. Carcinoid
5. Ileocecal valve, normal or prolapsed
6. Postoperative (eg, inverted stump; surgical deformity; adhesions)

UNCOMMON

1. [Appendix hernia]
2. Crohn's disease
3. [Diverticulum]
4. Endometrial implant
5. Extrinsic mass
6. Foreign body
7. Invagination or intussusception of appendix
8. Mucocele
9. Myxoglobulosis
10. Neoplasm, benign (eg, gastrointestinal stromal tumor$_g$; lipoma; polyp$_g$)
11. Neoplasm, malignant, primary (eg, carcinoma; lymphoma$_g$) or metastatic implant or extension
12. Parasitic disease (eg, amebiasis; trichuriasis; ascariasis; anisakiasis; schistosomiasis; angiostrongyliasis costaricensis)
13. Tuberculosis
14. Typhoid fever
15. Ulcerative colitis
16. *Yersinia* enterocolitis

[ ] This condition does not actually cause the gamuted imaging finding, but can produce imaging changes that simulate it.

References

1. Balthazar EJ: Diseases of the appendix. In: Gore RM, Levine MS: Textbook of Gastrointestinal Radiology. (ed 2) Philadelphia: WB Saunders, 2000, pp 1123–1150

(continued)

2. Govoni AF: Radiology of para and pericecal lesions. Rev Interamer Radiol 1984; 9:181–185
3. Jeffrey RB, Jr. Chapter 19. Gastrointestinal tract and peritoneal cavity. In: McGahan JP, Goldberg BB (eds): Diagnostic Ultrasound. Philadelphia: Lippincott-Raven, 1997
4. Wolverson MK, Jagannadharao B, Sundaram M, et al: CT as a primary diagnostic method in evaluating intraabdominal abscess. AJR 1979;133:1089–1095

Gamut G-82-S

CONGENITAL ANOMALIES AND VARIATIONS OF THE APPENDIX

COMMON

1. Abnormal length (under 2 cm or over 25 cm)
2. Abnormal location (eg, retrocecal appendix; malposition or malrotation of cecum)
3. Abnormal origin (eg, close to or far from ileocecal valve; high on cecum)

UNCOMMON

1. Absence of appendix
2. Double appendix
3. Primitive appendix (very thin lumen)

References
1. Balthazar EJ, Gade M: The normal and abnormal development of the appendix. Radiology 1976;121:599–604.
2. Balthazar EJ: The appendix. In: Gore RM, Levine MS: Textbook of Gastrointestinal Radiology. (ed 2) Philadelphia: WB Saunders, 2000, pp 1123–1150

Gamut G-83

SOLITARY FILLING DEFECT IN THE COLON

COMMON

1. Carcinoma
2. Diverticulitis; pericolic abscess (See G-89)
3. Fecal mass or impaction
4. Intussusception; ileal prolapse
5. Polyp$_g$ (esp. adenomatous; hyperplastic; juvenile; or hamartomatous) (See G-84-S)

UNCOMMON

1. Amyloidoma
2. Carcinoid
3. Crohn's disease
4. Cyst (duplication or other)
5. Endometrioma
6. Extramedullary plasmacytoma
7. Foreign body; gallstone; food particle; bezoar
8. Intramural hematoma
9. Inverted colonic diverticulum
10. Lymphoma$_g$
11. Metastasis (incl. invasive neoplasm)
12. Mucormycoma
13. Neoplasm, benign (eg, lipoma; hemangioma; leiomyoma or other gastrointestinal stromal tumor$_g$)
14. Parasitic disease (esp. ameboma; schistosomal granuloma; helminthoma; anisakiasis, *Ascaris* bolus)
15. Periappendiceal abscess
16. Postoperative (eg, anastomosis; suture granuloma)
17. Pseudopolyp, "giant" type (in ulcerative colitis)
18. Pseudotumor (eg, fibrous band; adhesion)
19. Sarcoma (incl. Kaposi)
20. Solitary rectal ulcer syndrome
21. Tuberculoma
22. Varix; hemorrhoid
23. Villous adenoma

References
1. Eisenberg RL: Gastrointestinal Radiology: A Pattern Approach. (ed 3) Philadelphia: Lippincott, 1996, pp 683–717

2. Gelfand DW: Gastrointestinal Radiology. New York: Churchill Livingstone, 1984, p 325
3. Rubesin SE, Saul SH, Laufer I: Carpet lesions of the colon. Radiographics 1985;5:537–552

Gamut G-84-S

CLASSIFICATION OF COLONIC TUMORS AND TUMOR-LIKE LESIONS

I. EPITHELIAL TUMORS

BENIGN—ADENOMA

1. Tubular
2. Villous
3. Tubulovillous

MALIGNANT

1. Adenocarcinoma
2. Adenoacanthoma
3. Adenosquamous carcinoma
4. Squamous cell carcinoma
5. Basaloid (cloacogenic) carcinoma
6. Carcinosarcoma

II. NEUROENDOCRINE TUMORS

1. Adenocarcinoid tumor
2. Carcinoid tumor

III. NONEPITHELIAL TUMORS

BENIGN

1. Smooth-muscle tumor
2. Neurilemmoma
3. Lipoma
4. Vascular tumor

IV. HEMATOPOIETIC AND LYMPHOID TUMORS

V. UNCLASSIFIED TUMORS

VI. SECONDARY (METASTATIC) TUMORS

VII. NONNEOPLASTIC (TUMOR-LIKE) LESIONS

HAMARTOMA

1. Peutz-Jeghers polyp
2. Juvenile polyp

HETEROTOPIA

1. Colitis cystica profunda
2. Hyperplastic polyp
3. Lymphoid polyp
4. Inflammatory polyp

References
1. Fengolio-Preiser CM: Gastrointestinal Pathology (ed 2) Philadelphia: Lippincott-Raven, 1999
2. Olmsted WW, Ros PR, Sobin LH, et al: The solitary colonic polyp: Radiologic-histologic differentiation and significance. Radiology 1986;160:9–16

Gamut G-85

ANNULAR ("APPLE CORE" OR "NAPKIN RING") LESION OF THE COLON

COMMON

1. Carcinoma

UNCOMMON

1. Ameboma
2. [Circular muscle contraction (colonic "sphincter")]
3. Diverticulitis (esp. with submucosal abscess)
4. Helminthoma
5. Lymphoma$_g$
6. Stricture, chronic localized (eg, Crohn's disease; ulcerative colitis; ischemic colitis; lymphogranuloma venereum)
7. Tuberculoma
8. Villous adenoma

[ ] This condition does not actually cause the gamuted imaging finding, but can produce imaging changes that simulate it.

(continued)

References

1. Eisenberg RL: Gastrointestinal Radiology: A Pattern Approach (ed 3). Philadelphia: Lippincott, 1996, pp 640–682
2. Gore RM: Colon: Differential diagnosis. In: Gore RM, Levine MS: Textbook of Gastrointestinal Radiology. (ed 2) Philadelphia: WB Saunders, 2000, pp 1159–1165

Gamut G-86

SEGMENTAL NARROWING OF THE COLON

COMMON

1. Abscess or other extrinsic inflammatory process (eg, pericolic) (See G-89)
2. Carcinoma (esp. "apple-core" adenocarcinoma or scirrhous)
3. [Circular muscle contraction or spasm, usually transient]
4. Crohn's disease
5. Diverticulitis
6. Endometriosis
7. Ischemic colitis (See G-69)
8. Postoperative deformity (eg, adhesion; narrow anastomosis)
9. Ulcerative colitis

UNCOMMON

1. Actinomycosis
2. Adhesive bands
3. Amyloidosis
4. Carcinoid
5. Carcinoma developing in ulcerative colitis or Crohn's disease or adjacent to ureterosigmoidostomy stoma
6. Cathartic colon; caustic colitis
7. Colitis, other (eg, herpes; cytomegalovirus; fungal)
8. Foreign body perforation with pericolic abscess
9. Intramural hematoma
10. Lymphogranuloma venereum
11. Lymphoma$_g$

12. Metastatic disease (eg, hematogenous or lymphangitic spread; peritoneal seeding; or direct extension to colon)
13. Neoplasm of colon, benign (eg, lipoma, gastrointestinal stromal tumor$_g$)
14. Neoplasm, extrinsic (eg, pancreatic; ovarian; renal)
15. Pancreatitis with direct spread to transverse colon or splenic flexure
16. Parasitic disease (eg, amebiasis/ameboma; schistosomiasis; helminthoma; strongyloidiasis; angiostrongyliasis costaricensis)
17. Pelvic lipomatosis
18. Radiation fibrosis
19. Retractile mesenteritis
20. Sarcoma (incl. Kaposi)
21. Stricture, idiopathic
22. Tuberculosis
23. Typhlitis
24. Ulcer of colon (esp. solitary rectal ulcer syndrome)

[ ] This condition does not actually cause the gamuted imaging finding, but can produce imaging changes that simulate it.

References

1. Eisenberg RL: Gastrointestinal Radiology: A Pattern Approach. (ed 3) Philadelphia: Lippincott, 1996, pp 640–682
2. Gore RM: Colon: Differential diagnosis. In: Gore RM, Levine MS: Textbook of Gastrointestinal Radiology. (ed 2) Philadelphia: WB Saunders, 2000, pp 1159–1165
3. McDonald JB, Middleton PJ: Tuberculosis of the colon simulating carcinoma. Radiology 1976;118:293–294
4. Simpkins KC, Young AC: The differential diagnosis of large bowel strictures. Clin Radiol 1971;22:449–457
5. Twersky J, Himmelfarb E: Right colonic adhesions. Radiology 1976;120:37–40

Gamut G-87

MULTIPLE FILLING DEFECTS IN THE COLON

COMMON

1. Artifacts (eg, feces; air bubbles; corn or other food particles; mucus strands or globules; oil droplets; foreign bodies)
2. [Diverticulosis]

3. Normal lymphoid follicles
4. Polyposis, familial
5. Polyps$_g$ (See G-84-S)
6. Pseudopolyps (esp. in ulcerative colitis)

UNCOMMON

1. Amebomas
2. Amyloidosis
3. Bannayan-Riley-Ruvalcaba S.
4. Carcinomas, multiple
5. Colitis cystica profunda
6. Colitis, other types (eg, pseudomembranous; ischemic; *Yersinia;* cytomegalovirus; Behçet S.)
7. Cowden S. (multiple hamartoma S.)
8. Cronkhite-Canada S.
9. Cystic fibrosis (mucoviscidosis)
10. Endometriosis
11. Gardner S.
12. Hemangiomas
13. Juvenile polyposis
14. Lipomatous polyposis
15. Lymphoma$_g$; leukemic infiltration
16. Malakoplakia
17. Metastases
18. Neurofibromatosis
19. Nodular lymphoid hyperplasia (if over 4 mm in size, may be due to AIDS with lymphoid hyperplasia); lymphoid polyps
20. Parasites, intraluminal (eg, *Ascaris; Trichuris*)
21. Peutz-Jeghers S. (alimentary tract polyposis)
22. Pneumatosis cystoides intestinalis
23. Polyposis syndromes, other (See G-106)
24. Schistosomiasis (inflammatory polyps)
25. Turcot S.
26. Urticaria, incl. hives, blebs, submucosal edema (secondary to chronic ischemia; colon obstruction; herpes zoster or *Yersinia* colitis; Chagas' disease)
27. Varices; hemorrhoids

[ ] This condition does not actually cause the gamuted imaging finding, but can produce imaging changes that simulate it.

References

1. Danoff DM, Nisenbarum BL, Stewart WB, et al: Segmental polypoid lipomatosis of the colon. AJR 1977;128:858–860
2. Eisenberg RL: Gastrointestinal Radiology: A Pattern Approach. (ed 3) Philadelphia: Lippincott, 1996, pp 718–747
3. Gelfand DW: Gastrointestinal Radiology. New York: Churchill Livingstone, 1984, p 329
4. Taybi H, Lachman RS: Radiology of Syndromes, Metabolic Disorders, and Skeletal Dysplasias. (ed 4) St. Louis: Mosby-Year Book, 1996, p 964
5. Teplick JG, Haskin ME: Roentgenologic Diagnosis. (ed 3) Philadelphia: WB Saunders, 1976
6. Wolfson JJ, Goldstein G, Krivit W, et al: Lymphoid hyperplasia of the large intestine associated with dysgammaglobulinemia: Report of a case. AJR 1970;108:610–614
7. Yousefzadeh DK: Urticaria of the colon. Radiology 1979;132:315–316

Gamut G-88

COLITIS (ULCERATION, EDEMA, SPASM); ALSO THICKENING OF THE COLON WALL ON CT, US, OR MRI

COMMON

1. Amebiasis
2. Carcinoma, esp. scirrhous or mucinous adenocarcinoma
3. Crohn's disease
4. Diverticulitis
5. *Helicobacter fetus* colitis
6. Ischemic colitis (See G-69)
7. Ulcerative colitis

UNCOMMON

1. Actinomycosis
2. Amyloidosis
3. Bacillary dysentery (shigellosis)
4. Behçet S.
5. Bowel edema from cirrhosis, protein loss, portal hypertension
6. Cathartic colon; enema abuse (caustic colitis)
7. Chronic granulomatous disease of childhood
8. Colitis cystica profunda
9. Collagenous colitis

(continued)

10. Drug therapy (esp. steroids; NSAIDs; antibiotics; chemotherapeutic agents; cimetidine; anti-fungal flucytosine; gold; methyldopa)
11. Fungus disease (eg, histoplasmosis; mucormycosis; candidiasis)
12. Graft-versus-host disease
13. Lymphogranuloma venereum (chlamydia infection)
14. Lymphoma$_g$; leukemic infiltration (diffuse)
15. Mercury poisoning
16. Metastatic disease
17. Neoplasm, other (eg, gastrointestinal stromal tumor$_g$; Kaposi sarcoma)
18. Nonspecific benign ulceration of colon
19. Pancreatitis with involvement of transverse colon or splenic flexure
20. Parasitic disease, other (esp. schistosomiasis; strongyloidiasis; helminthoma; Chagas' disease; anisakiasis and angiostrongyliasis costaricensis—ileocecal region)
21. Postoperative colitis (incl. diversion colitis in isolated segment after proximal colostomy or ileostomy; postrectal biopsy ulceration)
22. Proctitis (nonspecific; chemical—paraldehyde; in male homosexuals, often due to gonorrhea, lymphogranuloma venereum, or herpes simplex)
23. Pseudomembranous or necrotizing colitis (eg, *Clostridium difficile* infection, esp. after antibiotic therapy; postoperative; or proximal to colon obstruction)
24. Radiation colitis
25. *Salmonella* colitis
26. Solitary rectal ulcer S.
27. Staphylococcal colitis (eg, after oral tetracycline therapy)
28. Stercoral colitis (in obstruction)
29. Tuberculosis
30. Typhlitis
31. Uremic colitis; hemolytic-uremic S.
32. Urticaria ("colon hives" secondary to chronic ischemia; colon obstruction; herpes zoster or *Yersinia* colitis; Chagas' disease)
33. Viral infection (eg, herpes simplex-anorectal herpes; herpes zoster; cytomegalovirus—esp. in AIDS; rotavirus)
34. *Yersinia* colitis

References

1. Eisenberg RL: Gastrointestinal Radiology: A Pattern Approach. (ed 3) Philadelphia: Lippincott, 1996, pp 601–639
2. Gelfand DW: Gastrointestinal Radiology. New York: Churchill Livingstone, 1984, p 315
3. Gore RM: Inflammatory disease. In: Margulis AR: Modern Imaging of the Alimentary Tube. New York: Springer-Verlag, 1998, pp 185–216
4. Gore RM: Colon: Differential diagnosis. In: Gore RM, Levine MS: Textbook of Gastrointestinal Radiology. (ed 2) Philadelphia: WB Saunders, 2000, pp 1159–1165
5. Halpert RD, Feczko PJ: Gastrointestinal Radiology; The Requisites. (ed 2) St. Louis: Mosby-Year Book, 1999
6. Marshak RH, Lindner AE, Maklansky D: Radiology of the Colon. Philadelphia: WB Saunders, 1980
7. Miller VE, Han SY, Witten DM: Reticular mosaic (urticarial) pattern of the colonic mucosa in *Yersinia* colitis. Radiology 1983;146:307–308
8. Palmer PES, Reeder MM: The Imaging of Tropical Diseases. (ed 2) Heidelberg: Springer-Verlag, 2001
9. Teplick JG, Haskin ME: Roentgenologic Diagnosis. (ed 3) Philadelphia: WB Saunders, 1976

Gamut G-89

PERICOLIC ABSCESS

COMMON

1. Appendicitis
2. Crohn's disease
3. Diverticulitis
4. Neoplasm of colon, perforated primary (esp. carcinoma) or metastatic
5. Pancreatitis
6. Trauma, external or iatrogenic (eg, enema)
7. Tubo-ovarian abscess

UNCOMMON

1. Actinomycosis
2. Foreign body perforation
3. Idiopathic
4. Ischemic colitis

5. Lymphogranuloma venereum (*Chlamydia* infection)
6. Parasitic disease (esp. amebiasis; schistosomiasis; helminthoma; anisakiasis or angiostrongyliasis costaricensis—ileocecal region)
7. Postoperative (eg, suture leak; talc granuloma)
8. Renal infection or abscess
9. Tuberculosis
10. Ulcerative colitis

References
1. Ryan JM, Mueller PR: Abdominal abscess. In: Gore RM, Levine MS: Textbook of Gastrointestinal Radiology. (ed 2) Philadelphia: WB Saunders, 2000, pp 1234–1249
2. Wolverson MK, Jagannadharao B, Sundaram M, et al: CT as a primary diagnostic method in evaluating intraabdominal abscess. AJR 1979;133:1089–1095

Gamut G-90

DOUBLE TRACKING OF BARIUM IN THE DISTAL COLON*

COMMON
1. Crohn's disease
2. Diverticulitis

UNCOMMON
1. Carcinoma of colon

* Barium in an extraluminal sinus tract paralleling the bowel lumen.

Reference
1. Eisenberg RL: Gastrointestinal Radiology: A Pattern Approach. (ed 3) Philadelphia: Lippincott, 1996, pp 784–787

Gamut G-91

SMOOTH COLON

COMMON
1. Cathartic or enema abuse
2. Chronic obstruction (eg, megacolon; Chagas' disease)
3. Ischemic colitis, late (See G-69)
4. Ulcerative colitis, chronic

UNCOMMON
1. Amyloidosis
2. Bacillary dysentery, chronic (shigellosis)
3. Carcinoma, scirrhous
4. Lymphogranuloma venereum, late (*Chlamydia* infection)
5. Lymphoma$_g$
6. Parasitic disease, late (eg, schistosomiasis; strongyloidiasis; amebic stricture)
7. Radiation colitis, late

References
1. Caroline DF, Evers K: Colitis: radiographic features and differentiation of idiopathic inflammatory bowel disease. Radiol Clin North Am 1987;25:47–63
2. Kim SK, Gerle RD, Rozanski R: Cathartic colitis. AJR 1978;130:825–829

Gamut G-92

COLONIC DISTENTION WITHOUT OBSTRUCTION

COMMON
1. Acute nonobstructive distention, "paralytic ileus" (eg, postoperative; peritonitis; appendicitis; pancreatitis; typhoid fever) (See G-61)
*2. Chronic constipation; cathartic abuse
3. Electrolyte imbalance (hypokalemia; hypochloremia; calcium abnormality)

(continued)

*4. Functional megacolon (psychogenic; idiopathic)
*5. Hirschsprung's disease
 6. Mesenteric infarction (See G-69)
 7. Shock; septicemia; hypoxia
 8. Toxic megacolon (See G-94)
 9. Trauma (esp. spine or lower rib injury; intramural hematoma)
10. Ureteral colic

UNCOMMON

*1. Aerophagia
*2. Amyloidosis; familial Mediterranean fever (familial recurrent polyserositis)
*3. Ceroidosis (vitamin E depletion)
*4. Chagas' disease
*5. Connective tissue disease (collagen disease)$_g$ (esp. scleroderma; polyarteritis nodosa)
*6. Cystic fibrosis (mucoviscidosis)
*7. Drug therapy (eg, Pro-Banthine; hexamethonium; chlorpromazin; benztropine; morphine; L-dopa; atropine)
*8. Endocrine disturbance (eg, adrenal insufficiency; multiple endocrine neoplasia (MEN) S.; hypothyroidism; hypoparathyroidism)
 9. Functional (eg, diabetic coma; lead colic; sickle cell crisis; tabes; porphyria; pheochromocytoma)
10. Idiopathic intestinal pseudo-obstruction
11. Kawasaki disease
*12. Muscular, neurologic, or psychiatric disorder$_g$ (eg, amyotonia congenita {Oppenheim's disease}; multiple sclerosis; parkinsonism, Riley-Day S. {familial dysautonomia}; senility; schizophrenia; brain damage; paralysis)
13. Neurofibromatosis (esp. plexiform)
14. Pneumonia or other acute thoracic disease (eg, myocardial infarction; heart failure)
*15. Renal failure; uremia; urinary retention
16. Retroperitoneal hemorrhage
17. Spinal cord lesion; paraplegia
*18. Sprue

* Chronic.

References

1. Baker DA, Morin ME, Tan A, et al: Colonic ileus. Indication for prompt decompression. JAMA 1979; 241:2633–2634
2. Baker SR, Cho KC: The Abdominal Plain Film with Correlative Imaging. Norwalk, CT: Appleton & Lange, 1998
3. Bode WE, Beart RW, Spencer RJ, et al: Colonoscopic decompression for acute pseudoobstruction of the colon (Ogilvie's syndrome): Report of 22 cases and review of the literature. Am J Surg 1984;147:243–254
4. Gilchrist AM, Mills JOM, Russell CFJ: Acute large-bowel pseudo-obstruction. Clin Radiol 1985;36:401–404
5. Meyers MA: Colonic ileus. Gastrointest Radiol 1977;2: 37–40
6. Passail G, Benacerraf R: Acute pseudobstruction of the colon. Ann Radiol 1979; 22:508–514
7. Vanek VW, Al-Salti M: Acute pseudoobstruction of the colon (Ogilvie's syndrome): An analysis of 400 cases. Dis Colon Rectum 1986; 29:203–210

Gamut G-93

MEGACOLON

COMMON

1. Distal obstructing lesion (esp. carcinoma)
*2. Functional (psychogenic; idiopathic)
*3. Hirschsprung disease
*4. Imperforate anus; colon or rectal atresia; anal stenosis
*5. Nonobstructive distention ("paralytic ileus")
6. Scleroderma; dermatomyositis
*7. Toxic megacolon (See G-94)

UNCOMMON

*1. Aerophagia
2. Amyloidosis
3. Chagas' disease
*4. Chronic idiopathic intestinal pseudo-obstruction
*5. Cystic fibrosis (mucoviscidosis); meconium plug S. (dilated colon proximal to plug)
6. Diabetes
*7. Drug therapy (esp. Pro-Banthine; phenothiazine; anti-Parkinsonism agents)

*8. Duplication
*9. Fetal cytomegalovirus infection
*10. Hypothyroidism (esp. myxedema; cretinism)
*11. Immobilization, prolonged (eg, cast S.)
*12. Multiple endocrine neoplasia (MEN) S. (See J-5)
*13. Muscular disorder$_g$ (eg, muscular dystrophy)
*14. Neurologic disorder$_g$ (eg, plexiform neurofibromatosis; meningomyelocele; spina bifida; paralysis; neuronal intestinal dysplasia; Parkinsonism, brain damage)
15. Obstruction of colon from chronic stricture (eg, lymphogranuloma venereum or other rectal stricture; Crohn's disease; postoperative scarring; post-necrotizing enterocolitis*)
*16. Purgative abuse
*17. Riley-Day S. (familial dysautonomia)
*18. Sacrococcygeal teratoma; other pelvic neoplasm
*19. Small left colon S. (dilated colon proximally)
*20. Sotos S. (cerebral gigantism)
*21. Steatorrhea; celiac disease; sprue

* Megacolon in an infant or child.

References
1. Gelfand DW: Gastrointestinal Radiology. New York: Churchill Livingstone, 1984, p 304
2. Messmer JM: Gas and soft tissue abnormalities. In: Gore RM, Levine MS: Textbook of Gastrointestinal Radiology. (ed 2) Philadelphia: WB Saunders, 2000, pp 157–177
3. Solano Jr FX, Starling RC, Levey GS: Myxedema megacolon. Arch Intern Med 1985;145:231
4. Taybi H, Lachman RS: Radiology of Syndromes, Metabolic Disorders, and Skeletal Dysplasias. (ed 4) St. Louis: Mosby-Year Book, 1996, p 964

Gamut G-94

TOXIC MEGACOLON

COMMON
1. Ulcerative colitis

UNCOMMON
1. Amebic colitis
2. Bacillary dysentery, acute (shigellosis)
3. Behçet S.
4. Cholera
5. Crohn's disease
6. Enterocolitis, other (necrotizing; pseudomembranous; hemorrhagic)
7. *Helicobacter fetus* colitis
8. Hirschsprung disease
9. Ischemic colitis
10. Strongyloidiasis
11. Typhoid fever

References
1. Eisenberg RL: Gastrointestinal Radiology: A Pattern Approach. (ed 3) Philadelphia: Lippincott, 1996, pp 768–772
2. Gelfand DW: Gastrointestinal Radiology. New York: Churchill Livingstone, 1984, p 308

Gamut G-95-1

COLON OF REDUCED CALIBER (MICROCOLON) IN A NEWBORN

1. "Apple peel" intestinal atresia S.
2. Berdon S. (megacystis-microcolon-intestinal hypoperistalsis S.)
3. Colon atresia (microcolon to point of atresia)
4. Congenital ileal stenosis, web
5. Distal jejunal atresia (occas. total microcolon of disuse)
6. Hirschsprung disease (aganglionic distal segment may be small)
7. Ileal atresia (total microcolon of disuse)
8. Meconium ileus, esp. with cystic fibrosis {mucoviscidosis} (total microcolon of disuse)
9. Meconium plug S. (entire colon may be slightly small)
10. Microcolon of prematurity
11. Small left colon S. (rectum normal, colon small to splenic flexure)
12. Total aganglionosis coli (entire colon may be slightly small—question mark colon)

(continued)

Reference

1. Taybi H, Lachman RS: Radiology of Syndromes, Metabolic Disorders, and Skeletal Dysplasias. (ed 4) St. Louis: Mosby-Year Book, 1996, p 964

Gamut G-95-2

MECONIUM PLUG IN A NEWBORN

1. Cystic fibrosis (mucoviscidosis) with meconium ileus
2. Hirschsprung disease
3. Meconium plug S.
4. Small left colon S.

References

1. Fernbach SK: Neonatal gastrointestinal radiology. In: Gore RM, Levine MS: Textbook of Gastrointestinal Radiology. (ed 2) Philadelphia: WB Saunders, 2000, pp 2042–2073
2. Taybi H, Lachman RS: Radiology of Syndromes, Metabolic Disorders, and Skeletal Dysplasias. (ed 4) St. Louis: Mosby-Year Book, 1996, p 964

Gamut G-96

CECAL LESION

COMMON

1. Amebiasis
2. Appendiceal stump or lesion (See G-81)
3. Carcinoma
4. Crohn's disease
5. [Fecal matter; pill; food particle; foreign body]
6. Ileocecal valve, normal or fatty ("lipoma"); ileocecal prolapse
7. Ileocecal intussusception (eg, idiopathic; lymphoma; Meckel's diverticulum; appendix)
8. Polyp$_g$
9. Ulcerative colitis
10. Volvulus

UNCOMMON

1. Actinomycosis
2. Benign neoplasm (esp. villous adenoma; angioma; gastrointestinal stromal tumor$_g$; lipoma)
3. Carcinoid
4. Cathartic abuse
5. Cecal diaphragm, web, or adhesion
6. Cytomegalovirus infection (esp. in AIDS)
7. Diverticulosis; diverticulitis
8. Duplication
9. Endometriosis
10. Enterolith
11. Foreign body perforation
12. [Gallstone]
13. Ileus of cecum
14. Lymphoma$_g$ (incl. Burkitt lymphoma)
15. Metastasis (esp. colon, stomach, pancreas, ovary)
16. Parasitic disease, other (eg, schistosomiasis; strongyloidiasis; ascariasis; trichuriasis; anisakiasis; helminthoma; angiostrongyliasis costaricensis)
17. Pneumatosis cystoides intestinalis
18. Tuberculosis
19. Typhlitis
20. Typhoid fever
21. Ulcer, solitary
22. *Yersinia* enterocolitis

[ ] This condition does not actually cause the gamuted imaging finding, but can produce imaging changes that simulate it.

References

1. Eisenberg RL: Gastrointestinal Radiology: A Pattern Approach. (ed 3) Philadelphia: Lippincott, 1996, pp 555–598
2. Felson B, Wiot JF: Case of the Day. Springfield, IL: CC Thomas, 1967, p3
3. Felson B, Wiot JF: Some interesting right lower quadrant entities: Myxoglobulosis of the appendix, ileal prolapse, diverticulitis, lymphoma, endometriosis. Radiol Clin North Am 1969;7:83–95
4. Govoni AF: Radiology of para and pericecal lesions. Rev Interamer Radiol 1984;9:181–185
5. Margolies MN, Welch CE: Case records of the Massachusetts General Hospital. Case 38–1976. N Engl J Med 1976; 295:666–670
6. Szucs RA, Wolf EL, Gramm HF, et al: Miscellaneous abnormalities of the colon. In: Gore RM, Levine MS: Textbook of Gastrointestinal Radiology. (ed 2) Philadelphia: WB Saunders, 2000, pp 1089–1122

Gamut G-97

CONICAL OR CONTRACTED CECUM

COMMON
1. Amebiasis
2. Appendicitis; appendiceal abscess
3. Crohn's disease

UNCOMMON
1. Actinomycosis; South American blastomycosis
2. Anisakiasis; angiostrongyliasis costaricensis
3. Carcinoma
4. Cathartic abuse
5. Cytomegalovirus colitis (esp. in AIDS)
6. Diverticulitis of cecum (esp. following perforation)
7. Idiopathic
8. Lymphoma$_g$; leukemia (esp. in children after treatment)
9. Metastatic disease (eg, from carcinoma of stomach, colon, pancreas, ovary)
10. Radiation therapy
11. Tuberculosis (Stierlin sign)
12. Typhlitis
13. Typhoid fever
14. Ulcerative colitis
15. *Yersinia* enterocolitis

References
1. Eisenberg RL: Gastrointestinal Radiology: A Pattern Approach. (ed 3) Philadelphia: Lippincott, 1996, pp 589–598
2. Gore RM: Colon: Differential diagnosis. In: Gore RM, Levine MS: Textbook of Gastrointestinal Radiology. (ed 2) Philadelphia: WB Saunders, 2000, pp 1159–1165
3. Kreel L: Outline of Radiology. New York: Appleton-Century-Crofts, 1971, p 158

Gamut G-98

ENLARGEMENT OF THE ILEOCECAL VALVE

COMMON
1. Amebiasis
2. Crohn's disease
3. Fatty infiltration (lipomatosis)
4. Intussusception
5. Neoplasm, benign or malignant (esp. villous adenoma; polyp$_g$; lipoma; carcinoid; adenocarcinoma; lymphoma$_g$)
6. Normal variant ("hypertrophy")

UNCOMMON
1. Actinomycosis
2. Anisakiasis
3. Cathartic abuse
4. Foreign body, impacted
5. Gallstone, impacted
6. Ileocolic prolapse
7. Intramural hematoma
8. Lymphoid hyperplasia
9. Tuberculosis
10. Typhoid fever
11. Ulcerative colitis
12. *Yersinia* enterocolitis

Reference
1. Eisenberg RL: Gastrointestinal Radiology: A Pattern Approach. (ed 3) Philadelphia: Lippincott, 1996, pp 555–565

Gamut G-99

ANTERIOR INDENTATION ON THE RECTOSIGMOID JUNCTION

COMMON

1. Abscess, pelvic (eg, bacterial; PID; amebiasis; schistosomiasis; LGV)
2. Ascites (in erect position)
3. Carcinoma of ovary, cervix, uterus, bladder, or rectosigmoid colon
4. Endometriosis
5. Extrinsic pelvic neoplasm, other (eg, teratoma; dermoid or other ovarian cyst; uterine fibroid)
6. Metastasis, peritoneal (Blumer shelf) (esp. from carcinoma of colon, stomach, pancreas, ovary)

UNCOMMON

1. Aneurysm of internal iliac artery
2. Hematoma
3. Hydatid cyst
4. Lymphocele
5. Lymphoma$_g$; other lymphadenopathy
6. Pelvic lipomatosis
7. Postsurgical sling repair for rectal prolapse
8. Rectovaginal fistula (eg, LGV) (See G-101)
9. Retroperitoneal fibrosis
10. Urinoma
11. Vaginal lesion (eg, carcinoma; hematocolpos)

Reference

1. Schulman A, Fataar S: Extrinsic stretching, narrowing, and anterior indentation of the rectosigmoid junction. Clin Radiol 1979;30:463–469

Gamut G-100

RECTAL DISEASE ON BARIUM ENEMA

COMMON

1. Abscess
2. Carcinoma (adenocarcinoma; scirrhous; cloacogenic; anal)
3. Congenital anomaly (eg, Hirschsprung disease; imperforate anus)
4. Crohn's disease
5. Endometriosis
6. Metastasis; invasion from adjacent neoplasm
7. Polyp$_g$
8. Prolapse
9. Radiation proctitis
10. Trauma (sexual; iatrogenic; puerperal or other)
11. Ulcerative colitis
12. Villous adenoma

UNCOMMON

1. Actinomycosis
2. Amyloidosis
3. Bacillary dysentery (shigellosis)
4. Carcinoid
5. Colitis cystica profunda
6. Diverticulitis
7. Ischemic colitis
8. Lymphogranuloma venereum (*Chlamydia* infection)
9. Lymphoma$_g$
10. Neoplasm, benign (eg, gastrointestinal stromal tumor$_g$; lipoma; angioma)
11. Opportunistic infection (eg, herpes)
12. Parasitic disease (esp. amebiasis; schistosomiasis; trichuriasis; Chagas' disease)
13. Pelvic lipomatosis
14. Pneumatosis cystoides intestinalis
15. Proctitis (idiopathic; gonorrheal; chemical—paraldehyde)
16. Retroperitoneal fibrosis

17. Solitary rectal ulcer syndrome
18. Tuberculosis
19. Varices; hemorrhoids

Reference
1. Hama Y, Okizuka H, Odajima K, et al: Gastrointestinal stromal tumor of the rectum. Eur Radiol 2001;11:216–219

Gamut G-101

RECTOVAGINAL FISTULA

COMMON
1. Crohn's disease
2. Diverticulitis
3. Lymphogranuloma venereum (*Chlamydia* infection)
4. Neoplasm, malignant (eg, carcinoma of rectum, cervix, or vagina; other pelvic carcinoma)
5. Radiation therapy
6. Trauma (external; sexual; puerperal; iatrogenic)

UNCOMMON
1. Abscess (eg, appendiceal; tubovarian; perirectal)
2. Actinomycosis
3. Endometriosis
4. Foreign body perforation
5. Imperforate anus or other cloacal anomaly
6. Metastasis
7. Schistosomiasis
8. Tuberculosis
9. Ulcerative colitis

Reference
1. Greenall MJ, Levine AW, Nolan DJ: Complications of diverticular disease: a review of the barium enema findings. Gastrointest Radiol 1983;8:353–361

Gamut G-102

INCREASED RETRORECTAL OR PRESACRAL SPACE (See C-50)

COMMON
1. Abscess, presacral or pelvic (eg, perforated colon from diverticulitis or carcinoma; tubovarian or periappendiceal abscess)
2. Carcinoma of rectum (esp. adenocarcinoma; also scirrhous; cloacogenic; anal)
3. Crohn's disease
4. Diverticulitis
5. Extrinsic soft tissue mass (incl. ovarian cyst or neoplasm; dermoid; teratoma; enteric duplication cyst; tail gut cyst; lipoma)
6. Hematoma (eg, sacral fracture)
7. Lymphadenopathy
8. Metastatic or invasive malignant neoplasm (eg, from bladder, prostate, ovary, cervix)
9. Normal variant
10. Postoperative (eg, resection of rectosigmoid)
11. Radiation proctitis or fibrosis
12. Sacral or coccygeal lesion (eg, metastasis; myeloma; chordoma; osteosarcoma; chondrosarcoma; giant cell tumor; neurofibroma; sacrococcygeal teratoma; hydatid cyst)
13. Trauma (external; sexual; puerperal; iatrogenic—instrumentation)
14. Ulcerative colitis
15. Urinoma

UNCOMMON
1. Amebiasis
2. Amyloidosis of colon
3. Anterior sacral meningocele
4. Colitis cystica profunda; pneumatosis intestinalis
5. Cushing S. (fat deposition)
6. Endometriosis
7. Hemorrhoidal injection
8. Inferior vena cava obstruction (pelvic edema)
9. Inguinal hernia with rectal traction

(continued)

10. Ischemic colitis (See G-69)
11. Lymphocele
12. Lymphogranuloma venereum (*Chlamydia* infection)
13. Lymphoma$_g$ of rectum or retrorectal soft tissues
14. Neoplasm, benign, of soft tissues or rectum (incl. hemangioma; hemangioendothelioma; gastrointestinal stromal tumor$_g$; lipoma)
15. Pelvic lipomatosis
16. Pneumoretroperitoneum
17. Proctitis (idiopathic; traumatic; gonorrheal; chemical—paraldehyde)
18. Retroperitoneal fibrosis
19. Sarcoma (eg, rhabdomyosarcoma)
20. Schistosomiasis
21. Tuberculosis

References

1. Burgener FA, Kormano M: Differential Diagnosis in Conventional Radiology. (ed 2) New York: Thieme Medical Publ, 1991, pp 584–585
2. Eisenberg RL: Clinical Imaging: An Atlas of Differential Diagnosis. (ed 3) Philadelphia: Lippincott-Raven, 1997, pp 420–421
3. Swischuk LE, John SD: Differential Diagnosis in Pediatric Radiology. (ed 2) Baltimore: Williams & Wilkins, 1995, pp 145–146
4. Teplick SK, Stark P, Clark RE, Metz JR, Shapiro JH: The retrorectal space. Clin Radiol 1978;29:177–184

Gamut G-103

"THUMBPRINTING" OF THE GASTROINTESTINAL TRACT (MULTIPLE INTRAMURAL DEFECTS)

COMMON

1. Crohn's disease
2. Diverticulitis
3. Ischemic colitis with hemorrhage into bowel wall (See G-69)
4. Ulcerative colitis

UNCOMMON

1. Amyloidosis
2. Angioneurotic edema
3. Carcinoid S.
4. Cytomegalovirus colitis in AIDS
5. Endometriosis
6. Hemolytic-uremic S. (ischemic enterocolitis preceding onset of renal failure in infants)
7. Intramural hematoma or hemorrhage (eg, trauma; hemophilia or other bleeding diathesis; anticoagulant therapy)
8. Lymphoma$_g$
9. Metastasis, mural or peritoneal
10. Parasitic disease (esp. amebiasis; strongyloidiasis; schistosomiasis; anisakiasis)
11. Pericolic abscess (See G-89)
12. Pneumatosis cystoides intestinalis
13. Pseudomembranous or necrotizing colitis
14. Retractile mesenteritis, other mesenteric or peritoneal lesion (See G-228 to G-231)
15. Toxic megacolon (See G-94)
16. Typhlitis
17. Urticaria ("colon hives" secondary to chronic ischemia; colon obstruction; herpes zoster or *Yersinia* colitis; Chagas' disease)

References

1. Eisenberg RL: Gastrointestinal Radiology: A Pattern Approach. (ed 3) Philadelphia: Lippincott, 1996, pp 773–783
2. Marshak RH, Lindner AE, Maklansky D: Radiology of the Colon. Philadelphia: WB Saunders, 1980
3. Schwartz S, Boley SJ, Schultz L, et al: A survey of vascular diseases of the small intestine. Semin Radiol 1966;1:178–218

Gamut G-104

INTRAMURAL HEMATOMA OF THE GASTROINTESTINAL TRACT

COMMON
1. Anticoagulant therapy
2. Hemophilia; Christmas disease; other bleeding or clotting disorder$_g$
3. Trauma

UNCOMMON
1. Connective tissue disease (collagen vascular disease)$_g$ (esp. polyarteritis nodosa)
2. Drug therapy (eg, cytotoxin)
3. Henoch-Schönlein purpura
4. Idiopathic thrombocytopenic purpura
5. Leukemia

Reference
1. Felson B, Levin EJ: Intramural hematoma of the duodenum: A diagnostic roentgen sign. Radiology 1954; 63:823–830.

Gamut G-105

BULL'S-EYE LESION (SOLITARY OR MULTIPLE NODULES IN THE GASTROINTESTINAL TRACT WITH LARGE CENTRAL ULCERATION)

COMMON
*1. Gastrointestinal stromal tumor$_g$ (esp. leiomyoma; leiomyosarcoma; neurofibroma)
*2. Lymphoma$_g$
*3. Metastatic melanoma
*4. Peptic ulcer

UNCOMMON
1. Amyloid tumor
2. Carcinoid

3. Carcinoma
4. Ectopic pancreas
5. Eosinophilic granuloma
*6. Kaposi sarcoma
*7. Metastases (esp. from kidney; pancreas; breast; lung)

* May be multiple.

References
1. Balthazar EJ, Megibow A, Bryk D, et al: Gastric carcinoid tumors: Radiographic features in eight cases. AJR 1982; 139:1123–1127
2. Cavanagh RC, Buchignani JS Jr, Rulon DB: Metastatic melanoma of the small intestine. Radiology 1971;101: 195–200
3. Eisenberg RL: Gastrointestinal Radiology: A Pattern Approach. (ed 3) Philadelphia: Lippincott, 1996, pp 903–908
4. Marshak RH, Lindner AE: Polypoid lesions of the stomach. Semin Roentgenol 1971; 6:151–167
5. Pandarinath GS, Levine SM, Sorokin JJ, et al: Selective massive amyloidosis of the small intestine mimicking multiple tumors. Radiology 1978;129:609–610
6. Pomerantz H, Margolin HN: Metastases to the gastrointestinal tract from malignant melanoma. AJR 1962;88: 712–717
7. Wolf BS: Observations on roentgen features of benign and malignant gastric ulcers. Semin Roentgenol 1971;6: 140–150

Gamut G-106

POLYPOSIS SYNDROMES

1. Behçet S.
2. Blue rubber bleb nevus S.
3. Cowden S. (multiple hamartoma S.)
4. Cronkhite-Canada S.
5. Familial adenomatous polyposis (eg, familial polyposis; Gardner S.)
6. Juvenile polyposis of infancy; generalized juvenile polyposis
7. Lipomatous polyposis
8. Peutz-Jeghers S. (alimentary tract polyposis)
9. [Polyps, multiple adenomatous]

(continued)

10. Ruvalcaba-Myhre-Smith S.
11. Turcot S.

[ ] This condition does not actually cause the gamuted imaging finding, but can produce imaging changes that simulate it.

References
1. Buck JL, Harned RK: Polyposis syndromes. In: Gore RM, Levine MS: Textbook of Gastrointestinal Radiology. (ed 2) Philadelphia: WB Saunders, 2000, pp 1075–1088
2. Dodds WJ: Clinical and roentgen features of the intestinal polyposis syndromes. Gastrointest Radiol 1976;1:127–142
3. Itzkowitz SH, Kim YS: Colon polyps and polyposis syndromes. In: Feldman M, Scharschmidt BF, Sleisenger MH: Gastrointestinal and Liver Diseases. (ed 6) Philadelphia: WB Saunders, 2000, pp 1865–1905
4. Taybi H, Lachman RS: Radiology of Syndromes, Metabolic Disorders, and Skeletal Dysplasias. (ed 4) St. Louis: Mosby-Year Book, 1996, p 964

Gamut G-107

INTERNAL OR EXTERNAL FISTULA INVOLVING THE GASTROINTESTINAL TRACT

COMMON

1. Abscess$_g$ (eg, appendiceal; perirenal)
2. Carcinoma; other malignant neoplasm, primary or metastatic
3. Crohn's disease
4. Diverticulitis
5. Postoperative (eg, surgical complication; dehiscence; ileostomy; colostomy; gastrostomy)

UNCOMMON

1. Actinomycosis
2. Amebiasis
3. Biliary-enteric fistula (See G-139)
4. Colovesical fistula (esp. diverticulitis; malignancy)
5. Duodenal-renal fistula (eg, tuberculosis; pyelonephritis; duodenal ulcer)
6. Entero-ovarian fistula

7. Foreign body (eg, pin; bone; toothpick)
8. Infarction; ischemic colitis (See G-69)
9. Lymphoma$_g$
10. Peptic ulcer; marginal ulcer
11. Pancreatic fistula (pancreatitis; ruptured pseudocyst; posttraumatic; postsurgical; external drainage of pseudocyst)
12. Prosthetic aortic graft
13. Radiation therapy
14. Rectovaginal, pelvic, or perineal fistula (esp. pelvic inflammatory disease; lymphogranuloma venereum; diverticulitis; Crohn's disease; malignancy) (See G-101)
15. Schistosomiasis
16. Trauma, external or iatrogenic (eg, enema)
17. Tuberculosis
18. Ulcerative colitis

References
1. Eisenberg RL: Gastrointestinal Radiology: A Pattern Approach (ed 3). Philadelphia: Lippincott, 1996, pp 971–981
2. Gore RM, Calenoff L, Rogers LF: Roentgenographic manifestations of ischemic colitis. JAMA 1979;241:1171–1173

Gamut G-108

NONVISUALIZATION OF THE GALLBLADDER (US, CT, NM)

COMMON

1. [Calcified gallbladder wall (porcelain gallbladder); milk of calcium bile]
2. Cholecystitis (acute or chronic; gangrenous; emphysematous)
3. Contracted gallbladder (esp. postprandial)
4. Prior cholecystectomy
5. Technical factors, esp. on ultrasound (eg, gallbladder obscured by gas; obese patient or thin patient with superficial gallbladder)

UNCOMMON

1. [Anomalous position of gallbladder (eg, ectopic gallbladder; situs inversus)]
2. Biliary atresia
3. Carcinoma of gallbladder
4. Compression by adjacent mass
5. Congenital absence or hypoplasia
6. Fibrosis of gallbladder
7. Hepatization of the gallbladder (sludge-filled)
8. Hyperalimentation; nonfasting patient
9. Metastatic disease involving gallbladder
10. Pregnancy (last trimester)
11. Syndromes (eg, Dubin-Johnson S.; Kawasaki S.; Mirizzi S.)

[ ] This condition does not actually cause the gamuted imaging finding, but can produce imaging changes that simulate it.

References

1. Abbitt PL: Ultrasound: A Pattern Approach. New York: McGraw-Hill, 1995
2. Balthazar U, Dunn J, Gonzalez-Diaz S, et al: Agenesis of the gallbladder. South Med J 2000;93:914–915
3. Eisenberg RL: Gastrointestinal Radiology: A Pattern Approach. (ed 3) Philadelphia: Lippincott, 1996, pp 803–808
4. Gore RM: Gallbladder and biliary tract: Differential diagnosis. In: Gore RM, Levine MS: Textbook of Gastrointestinal Radiology. (ed 2) Philadelphia: WB Saunders, 2000, pp 1408–1414
5. Laing FC: Chapter 6. The gallbladder and bile ducts. The liver. In: Rumack CM, Wilson SR, Charboneau JW (eds): Diagnostic Ultrasound. St. Louis: Mosby, 1998, pp 175–223
6. Parulekar SG: Gallbladder and bile ducts. In: McGahan JP, Goldberg BB (eds): Diagnostic Ultrasound. Philadelphia: Lippincott-Raven, 1997, chapter 22
7. Shehadi WH: Radiologic examination of the biliary tract. Radiol Clin North Am 1966;4:463–482
8. Williamson, MR: Abdominal ultrasound. In: Essentials of Ultrasound. Philadelphia: WB Saunders, 1996, p 86

Gamut G-109

SMALL OR CONTRACTED GALLBLADDER (US, CT, MRI)

COMMON

1. Acute hepatitis
2. Chronic cholecystitis
3. Postprandial status

UNCOMMON

1. Adenomyomatosis of gallbladder
2. Congenital hypoplasia or multiseptate gallbladder
3. Cystic fibrosis (mucoviscidosis)

References

1. Eisenberg RL: Gastrointestinal Radiology: A Pattern Approach. (ed 3) Philadelphia: Lippincott, 1996, pp 809–812.
2. Gore RM: Gallbladder and biliary tract disease: Differential diagnosis. In: Gore RM, Levine MS (eds): Textbook of Gastrointestinal Radiology. ed 2 Philadelphia: WB Saunders, 2000, pp 1408–1415
3. Irie H, Honda H, Kuroiwa T, et al: Pitfalls in MR cholangiopancreatographic interpretation. RadioGraphics 2001; 21:23–38

Gamut G-110

ENLARGED GALLBLADDER (US, CT, MRI)

COMMON

1. Acute cholecystitis with cholelithiasis causing obstruction of cystic or common duct
2. Diabetes
3. Drugs (eg, anticholinergics; narcotics)
4. Hydrops; empyema
5. Hyperalimentation
6. Neoplasm arising in head of pancreas, ampulla of Vater, or lower common bile duct (Courvoisier gallbladder)

(continued)

7. Pancreatitis obstructing Vaterian segment
8. Postvagotomy; postsurgical
9. Pregnancy
10. Prolonged fasting

UNCOMMON

1. Acromegaly
2. AIDS-related cholangiopathy (cytomegalovirus; *Cryptosporidium*)
3. Alcoholism
4. Bedridden patient with chronic illness
5. Chagas' disease
6. Kawasaki S.
7. Leptospirosis
8. Mucocele
9. Normal variant

References
1. Eisenberg RL: Gastrointestinal Radiology: A Pattern Approach. (ed 3) Philadelphia: Lippincott, 1996, pp 809–811
2. Gore RM: Gallbladder and biliary tract: Differential diagnosis. In: Gore RM, Levine MS: Textbook of Gastrointestinal Radiology. (ed 2) Philadelphia: WB Saunders, 2000, pp 1408–1414
3. Kapicioglu S, Gurbuz S, Danalioglu A, et al: Measurement of gallbladder volume with ultrasonography in pregnant women. Can J Gastroenterol 2000;14:403–405
4. Parulekar SG: Gallbladder and bile ducts. In: McGahan JP, Goldberg BB (eds): Diagnostic Ultrasound. Philadelphia: Lippincott-Raven, 1997, chapter 22

Gamut G-111

DISTENDED GALLBLADDER IN A CHILD (US, CT)

COMMON

1. Kawasaki S.
2. Total parenteral nutrition

UNCOMMON

1. Gallstone in cystic duct
2. Gastroenteritis
3. Leptospirosis
4. Normal variant
5. Scarlet fever
6. Upper respiratory infection

References
1. Donaldson JS: Diseases of the pediatric gallbladder. In: Gore RM, Levine MS (eds): Textbook of Gastrointestinal Radiology. (ed 2) Philadelphia: WB Saunders, 2000, pp 2140–2148
2. Gilger MA: Diseases of the gallbladder. In: Wyllie R, Hyams JS: Pediatric Gastrointestinal Disease. Philadelphia: WB Saunders, 1999
3. Parulekar SG: Gallbladder and bile ducts. In: McGahan JP, Goldberg BB (eds): Diagnostic Ultrasound. Philadelphia: Lippincott-Raven, 1997, chapter 22
4. Siegel MJ: Pediatric Body CT. Philadelphia: Lippincott Williams & Wilkins, 1999

Gamut G-112

MULTISEPTATE GALLBLADDER (US, CT)

1. Adenomyomatosis
2. Cholesterolosis
3. Congenital malformation
4. Desquamated gallbladder mucosa
5. Normal folded gallbladder (incl. Phrygian cap)

References
1. Chapman S, Nakielny R: Aids to Radiological Differential Diagnosis. London: Bailliere Tindall, 1990
2. Rumack CM, Nilson SR, Charboneau JW (eds): Diagnostic Ultrasound. (ed 2) St. Louis: Mosby, 1998
3. Gore RM: Gallbladder and biliary tract disease: Differential diagnosis. In: Gore RM, Levine MS (eds): Textbook of Gastrointestinal Radiology. (ed 2) Philadelphia: WB Saunders, 2000, pp 1408–1415
4. Gore RM, Fulcher AS, Taylor AJ, et al: Anomalies and anatomic variants of the gallbladder and biliary tract. In Gore RM, Levine MS (eds): Textbook of Gastrointestinal Radiology. (ed 2) Philadelphia: WB Saunders, 2000, pp 1305–1320

Gamut G-113

GALLBLADDER DISEASE SECONDARY TO CYSTIC DUCT OR INFUNDIBULUM OBSTRUCTION

COMMON

1. Cholecystitis
2. Hydrops; empyema; mucocele of gallbladder
3. Milk of calcium bile
4. Porcelain gallbladder (calcified gallbladder wall)

UNCOMMON

1. Choledochoenteric fistula; gallstone ileus (eg, from gallstone perforation)
2. Emphysematous cholecystitis
3. Ruptured gallbladder

Reference

1. Zeman RK: Cholelithiasis and cholecystitis. In Gore RM, Levine MS (eds): Textbook of Gastrointestinal Radiology. (ed 2) Philadelphia: WB Saunders, 2000, pp 1321–1345

Gamut G-114

CALCIFICATION IN THE GALLBLADDER OR COMMON BILE DUCT

COMMON

1. Gallstone (eg, calcium bilirubinate or calcium carbonate)
2. [Other right upper quadrant density (eg, stone in kidney or retrocecal appendix; calcified aneurysm; barium in diverticulum)]

UNCOMMON

1. Milk of calcium bile
2. Mucinous adenocarcinoma of gallbladder

3. Porcelain gallbladder
4. Schistosomiasis
5. Stone in common duct or cystic duct remnant

[ ] This condition does not actually cause the gamuted imaging finding, but can produce similar imaging changes that simulate it.

References

1. Eisenberg RL: Gastrointestinal Radiology: A Pattern Approach. (ed 3) Philadelphia: Lippincott, 1996, pp 1002–1007
2. Fatoar S, Al Ansari AG, Bassiony H, et al: Calcified pancreas and bile ducts from schistosomiasis. Br J Radiol 1996;59:1064–1066

Gamut G-115-S1

ARTIFACTS THAT MIMIC GALLSTONES

1. Inspissated sludge
2. Intraluminal defect, any cause (See G-116)
3. Partial volume artifact with duodenal impression
4. Refraction from folds in gallbladder neck

References

1. Rumack CM, Nilson SR, Charboneau JW (eds): Diagnostic Ultrasound. (ed 2) St. Louis: Mosby, 1998
2. Gore RM: Gallbladder and biliary tract disease: Differential diagnosis. In: Gore RM Levine MS (eds): Textbook of Gastrointestinal Radiology. (ed 2) Philadelphia: WB Saunders, 2000, pp 1408–1415
3. Zeman RK: Cholelithiasis and cholecystitis. In Gore RM, Levine MS (eds): Textbook of Gastrointestinal Radiology. (ed 2) Philadelphia: WB Saunders, 2000, pp 1321–1345
4. Palanduz A, Yalcin I, Tonguc E, et al: Sonographic assessment of ceftriaxane-associated biliary pseudolithiasis in children. J Clin Ultrasound 2000;28:166–168

Gamut G-115-S2

STRUCTURES THAT SONOGRAPHICALLY MIMIC THE GALLBLADDER (US)

1. Abscess (esp. Near ligamentum teres)
2. Choledochal cyst
3. Dilated cystic duct remnant
4. Fluid-filled duodenal bulb
5. Hepatic cyst
6. Omental cyst
7. Renal cyst

Reference

1. Gore RM: Gallbladder and biliary tract disease: Differential diagnosis. In Gore RM, Levine MS (eds): Textbook of Gastrointestinal Radiology. (ed 2) Philadelphia: WB Saunders, 2000, pp 1408–1415

Gamut G-116

FIXED POLYPOID LESION(S) OR FILLING DEFECT(S) IN THE GALLBLADDER (US, CT, MRI)

COMMON

*1. Adenomyoma; adenomyomatosis; hyperplastic cholecystosis
*2. Cholesterol polyp
*3. Cholesterolosis ("strawberry" gallbladder)
*4. Gallstone, adherent
5. [Phrygian cap]

UNCOMMON

*1. Adenoma (incl. adenomatous polyp; villous adenoma; papilloma; fibroadenoma; cystadenoma)
*2. Cholecystitis glandularis proliferans
3. Congenital fold or septum
4. Cyst (epithelial; mucous retention)

5. Ectopic pancreatic or gastric tissue
*6. Hamartomas in Peutz-Jeghers S.
*7. Inflammatory polyp
8. Metachromatic leukodystrophy
*9. Metastasis (esp. melanoma)
10. Neoplasm, benign (eg, carcinoid; neurinoma; angioma)
11. Neoplasm, malignant (eg, adenocarcinoma; leiomyosarcoma)
*12. Parasitic granuloma (eg, *Ascaris*)
13. Postoperative defect
14. [Pseudodefect in neck of gallbladder; other pseudopolyps]
*15. Vascular lesion (eg, varix; aneurysm; tortuous artery)
16. Xanthogranulomatous cholecystitis

* May be multiple.

[ ] This condition does not actually cause the gamuted imaging finding, but can produce imaging changes that simulate it.

References

1. Berk RN, van der Vegt JH, Lichtenstein JE: The hyperplastic cholecystoses: Cholesterolosis and adenomyomatosis. Radiology 1983;146:593–601
2. Eisenberg RL: Gastrointestinal Radiology: A Pattern Approach. (ed 3) Philadelphia: Lippincott, 1996, pp 817–836
3. Lichtenstein JE: Adenomyomatosis and cholesterolosis: the "hyperplastic cholecystoses." In: Gore RM, Levine MS: Textbook of Gastrointestinal Radiology. (ed 2) Philadelphia: WB Saunders, 2000
4. Parra JA, Acinas O, Bueno J, et al: Xanthogranulomatous cholecystitis: clinical, sonographic, and CT findings in 26 patients. AJR 2000;174:979–983
5. Vogel T, Schumacher V, Saleh A, et al: Extraintestinal polyps in Peutz-Jeghers syndrome: presentation of four cases and review of the literature. Int J Colorectal Dis 2000;15:118–123

Gamut G-117

NONSHADOWING LESION IN THE GALLBLADDER (US)

COMMON

1. Gallstone, nonshadowing or not in the transducer focal zone
2. Polyp (adenomatous or cholesterol)
3. Sludge

UNCOMMON

1. Adenomyomatosis
2. Carcinoma of gallbladder
3. Desquamated mucosa
4. Fibrinous debris
5. Hematoma
6. Inspissated pus
7. Metastasis
8. Parasites (eg, *Ascaris; Clonorchis; Fasciola*)
9. Precipitated contrast medium from ERCP

References
1. Abbitt PL: Ultrasound: A Pattern Approach. New York: McGraw-Hill, 1995
2. Filly RA, Allen B, Minton MJ, et al: In vitro investigation of the origin of echoes within biliary sludge. J Clin Ultrasound 1980;8:193–200
3. Gore RM: Gallbladder and biliary tract: Differential diagnosis. In: Gore RM, Levine MS: Textbook of Gastrointestinal Radiology. (ed 2) Philadelphia: WB Saunders, 2000, pp 1408–1414
4. Rumack CM, Nilson SR, Charboneau JW (eds): Diagnostic Ultrasound. (ed 2) St. Louis: Mosby, 1998

Gamut G-118

ECHO(ES) WITHIN THE GALLBLADDER (US)

COMMON

1. Acute cholecystitis
2. Calculus
3. Fold in gallbladder wall
4. Polyp (adenomatous)
5. Sludge

UNCOMMON

1. AIDS-related cholangiopathy
2. Carcinoma of gallbladder
3. Clonorchiasis; fascioliasis
4. Ectopic pancreas or gastric mucosa
5. Emphysematous cholecystitis
6. Empyema of gallbladder
7. Feces (via fistula)
8. Food particles after cholecystojejunostomy
9. Gangrenous cholecystitis
10. Hemobilia
11. Hemorrhagic cholecystitis
12. Metastasis
13. Milk of calcium
14. Papilloma
15. Sarcoma of gallbladder

References
1. Gore RM: Gallbladder and biliary tract disease: Differential diagnosis. In: Gore RM, Levine MS (eds): Textbook of Gastrointestinal Radiology. (ed 2) Philadelphia: WB Saunders, 2000, pp 1408–1415
2. Kabaalio GB, Cubuk M, Senol U, et al: Fascioliasis: US, CT, and MRI findings with new observations. Abdom Imaging 2000;25:400–404
3. Williamson MR: Abdominal ultrasound. In: Essentials of Ultrasound. Philadelphia: WB Saunders, 1996, p 87

Gamut G-119-1

ECHOGENIC BILE/GALLBLADDER SLUDGE (US); HIGH DENSITY BILE (CT)

1. [Artifact (side lobe and slice thickness artifact on US; volume averaging of normal liver on CT)]
2. Cholelithiasis
3. Extrahepatic biliary obstruction
4. Hemolysis
5. Hemorrhage; hematobilia (esp. posttraumatic)
6. Inflammatory debris or pus
7. Milk of calcium
8. Prolonged fasting
9. Sickle cell disease; thalassemia
10. Vicarious excretion of contrast media (eg, renal failure; recent ERCP; occasionally normal)

[ ] This condition does not actually cause the gamuted imaging finding, but can produce imaging changes that simulate it.

References
1. Parulekar SG: Gallbladder and bile ducts. In: McGahan JP, Goldberg BB (eds): Diagnostic Ultrasound. Philadelphia: Lippincott-Raven, 1997, chapter 22
2. Rumack CM, Nilson SR, Charboneau JW (eds): Diagnostic Ultrasound. (ed 2) St. Louis: Mosby, 1998
3. Slone RM, Fisher AJ: Pocket Guide to Body CT Differential Diagnosis. New York: McGraw-Hill, 1999, p 230
4. Van Beers BE, Pringot JH: Imaging of cholelithiasis: helical CT. Abdom Imaging 2001;26:15–20
5. Zeman RK: Cholelithiasis and cholecystitis. In Gore RM, Levine MS (eds): Textbook of Gastrointestinal Radiology. (ed 2) Philadelphia: WB Saunders, 2000, pp 1321–1345

Gamut G-119-2

GALLSTONE OR SLUDGE IN FETAL OR NEONATAL GALLBLADDER (US)

1. Administration of parenteral nutrition and furosemide to premature infant
2. Biliary tree malformation
3. Cholestasis
4. Familial predisposition
5. Hemolysis (eg, Rh or ABO blood group alloimmunization; sickle cell disease; spherocytosis; thalassemia)
6. Hepatic dysfunction
7. Idiopathic
8. Methadone intake
9. Monochorionic twin after intrauterine death of its co-twin
10. Sepsis

References
1. Petrikoveky S, Klein V, Holsten N: Sludge in fetal gallbladder: natural history and neonatal outcome. Br J Radiol 1996; 69:1017–1018
2. Devonald KJ, Ellwood DA, Colditz PB: The variable appearance of fetal gallstones. J Ultrasound Med 1992; 11:579–585
3. Schweizer P, Lenz MP, Kirschner HJ: Pathogenesis and symptomatology of cholelithiasis in childhood. Dig Surg 2000;17:459–467

Gamut G-120

INCREASED ATTENUATION OF GALLBLADDER LUMEN (CT)

COMMON

1. Gallstones
2. Prior endoscopic retrograde cholangiopancreatography (ERCP) or oral cholecystography
3. Sludge; debris

UNCOMMON

1. Empyema of gallbladder with pus
2. Feces (via fistula)
3. Food particles after cholecystojejunostomy
4. Hemobilia
5. Hemorrhagic cholecystitis
6. Hydrops of gallbladder
7. Milk of calcium bile
8. Mucinous adenocarcinoma of the gallbladder
9. Polyp or papilloma projecting into lumen

10. Vicarious excretion of contrast medium
11. Volume averaging with adjacent structures

References
1. Gore RM: Gallbladder and biliary tract disease. In Gore RM, Levine MS (eds): Textbook of Gastrointestinal Radiology. (ed 2) Philadelphia: WB Saunders, 2000, pp 1408–1415
2. Van Beers BE, Pringot JH: Imaging of cholelithiasis: helical CT. Abdom Imaging 2001;26:15–20

Gamut G-121

HYPERECHOIC FOCUS IN THE GALLBLADDER WALL (US)

COMMON

1. Adenomyomatosis, cholesterolosis ("hyperplastic cholecystoses")
2. Gallstone (embedded)
3. Polyp, cholesterol or other

UNCOMMON

1. Cholecystitis glandularis proliferans
2. Emphysematous cholecystitis
3. Microabscess
4. Rokitansky-Aschoff sinuses

References
1. Graif M, Horovitz A, Itzchak Y, et al: Hyperechoic foci in the gallbladder wall as a sign of microabscess formation or diverticula. Radiology 1984;152:781–784
2. Lichtenstein JE: Adenomyomatosis and cholesterolosis: the "hyperplastic cholecystoses." In: Gore RM, Levine MS: Textbook of Gastrointestinal Radiology. (ed 2) Philadelphia: WB Saunders, 2000, pp 1353–1359

Gamut G-122

FOCAL THICKENING OF THE GALLBLADDER WALL (> 3MM) (US, CT)

COMMON

1. Adenomyomatosis
2. Adherent gallstone or sludge
3. Carcinoma of gallbladder
4. Polyp, inflammatory

UNCOMMON

1. Benign neoplasm (eg, adenoma; carcinoid; papilloma)
2. Ectopic mucosa
3. Gangrenous or hemorrhagic cholecystitis
4. Hematoma
5. Metastasis (esp. melanoma)
6. Varices

References
1. Abbitt PL: Ultrasound: A Pattern Approach. New York: McGraw-Hill, 1995
2. Pandey M, Sood BP, Shukla RC, et al: Carcinoma of the gallbladder: role of sonography in diagnosis and staging. J Clin Ultrasound 2000;28:227–232
3. Parulekar SG: Gallbladder and bile ducts. In: McGahan JP, Goldberg BB (eds): Diagnostic Ultrasound. Philadelphia: Lippincott-Raven, 1997, chapter 22
4. Slone RM, Fisher AJ: Pocket Guide to Body CT Differential Diagnosis. New York: McGraw-Hill, 1999, p 229
5. Ward LM, Fulcher AS, Pereles FS, et al: Neoplasms of the gallbladder and biliary tract. In Gore RM, Levine MS (eds): Textbook of Gastrointestinal Radiology. (ed 2) Philadelphia: WB Saunders, 2000, pp 1360–1374

Gamut G-123

DIFFUSE THICKENING OF THE GALLBLADDER WALL (US, CT, MRI)

COMMON

1. AIDS-related cholangiopathy (cytomegalovirus; *Cryptosporidium*)
2. Ascites with edema of gallbladder wall (eg, cirrhosis; renal failure; hypoalbuminemia; heart failure)
3. Carcinoma of gallbladder
4. Cholecystitis, acute or chronic, usually with cholelithiasis
5. Cirrhosis; schistosomiasis; liver failure
6. Hepatitis (viral or alcoholic)
7. Portal hypertension
8. Postprandial (physiolologic contraction); incomplete distension; inadequate fasting
9. Total parenteral nutrition

UNCOMMON

1. Adenomyomatosis; hyperplastic cholecystosis
2. Brucellosis
3. Extrahepatic portal vein obstruction (eg, pancreatitis; carcinoma of pancreas)
4. Folds in gallbladder wall
5. Gangrenous gallbladder
6. Graft-versus-host disease
7. Hemorrhagic cholecystitis
8. Infectious mononucleosis
9. Kaposi sarcoma (in AIDS)
10. Lymphatic obstruction at porta hepatis
11. Lymphoma_g
12. Multiple myeloma
13. Necrotizing enterocolitis in infants
14. Peptic ulcer adjacent to gallbladder
15. Pyelonephritis of right kidney
16. Sclerosing cholangitis
17. Torsion of gallbladder
18. Varices of gallbladder wall
19. Xanthogranulomatous cholecystitis

References

1. Abbitt PL: Ultrasound: A Pattern Approach. New York: McGraw-Hill, 1995
2. Cohen SM, Kurtz AB: Biliary sonography. Radiol Clin North Am 1991;29:1171–1192
3. Eisenberg RL: Gastrointestinal Radiology: A Pattern Approach. (ed 3) Philadelphia: Lippincott, 1996, pp 1067–1071
4. Fiske CE, Laing FC, Brown TW: Ultrasonographic evidence of gallbladder wall thickening in association with hypoalbuminemia. Radiology 1980;135:713–716
5. Gore RM: Gallbladder and biliary tract: Differential diagnosis. In: Gore RM, Levine MS: Textbook of Gastrointestinal Radiology. (ed 2) Philadelphia: WB Saunders, 2000, pp 1408–1414
6. Parulekar SG: Gallbladder and bile ducts. In: McGahan JP, Goldberg BB (eds): Diagnostic Ultrasound. Philadelphia: Lippincott-Raven, 1997, chapter 22
7. Ralls PW, Quinn MF, Juttner HU, et al: Gallbladder wall thickening: Patients without intrinsic gallbladder disease. AJR 1981;137:65–68
8. Sanders RC: The significance of sonographic gallbladder wall thickening. J Clin Ultrasound 1980;8:143–146
9. Shlaer WJ, Leopold GR, Scheible FW: Sonography of the thickened gallbladder wall: A nonspecific finding. AJR 1981;136:337–339
10. Williamson MR: Abdominal ultrasound. In: Essentials of Ultrasound. Philadelphia: WB Saunders, 1996, p 93

Gamut G-124

STRIATIONS IN A THICKENED GALLBLADDER WALL (US, CT)

COMMON

1. AIDS-related cholangiopathy (cytomegalovirus; *Cryptosporidium*)
2. Gangrenous cholecystitis
3. Non-biliary related edema or inflammation (eg, heart failure; renal failure; liver failure; hypoalbuminemia; ascites)

UNCOMMON

1. Adenomyomatosis
2. Blockage of lymphatic and venous drainage of gallbladder

3. Hepatitis
4. Pancreatitis
5. Varices of gallbladder wall
6. Xanthogranulomatous cholecystitis

References
1. MacCarty RL: Inflammatory disorders of the biliary tract. In: Gore RM, Levine MS: Textbook of Gastrointestinal Radiology. (ed 2) Philadelphia: WB Saunders, 2000, pp 1375–1395
2. Teefey SA, Baron RL, Bigler SA: Sonography of the gallbladder: significance of striated (layered) thickening of the gallbladder wall. AJR 1991;156:945–951
3. Williamson MR: Abdominal Ultrasound. In: Essentials of Ultrasound. Philadelphia: WB Saunders, 1996, p 90

Gamut G-125

EXTRINSIC DEFORMITY OR DISPLACEMENT OF THE GALLBLADDER (CAG, MRCP, CT)

COMMON

1. Liver mass (eg, hepatocellular carcinoma; hemangioma; metastases; regenerating nodule; abscess; hydatid cyst; polycystic disease)
2. Normal duodenum or colon

UNCOMMON

1. Choledochal cyst
2. Duodenal mass (eg, neoplasm; hematoma)
3. Lymphadenopathy (eg, lymphoma$_g$; metastases)
4. Pancreatic mass (eg, neoplasm; pseudocyst)
5. Retroperitoneal tumor or cyst (eg, renal, adrenal, soft tissue); polycystic kidney

Reference
1. Eisenberg RL: Gastrointestinal Radiology: A Pattern Approach. (ed 3) Philadelphia: Lippincott, 1996, pp 813–816

Gamut G-126

PERICHOLECYSTIC FLUID ON ULTRASOUND

COMMON

1. Acute cholecystitis (with or without perforation)
2. Ascites

UNCOMMON

1. AIDS-related cholangiopathy (cytomegalovirus; *Cryptosporidium*)
2. Hematoma
3. Pancreatitis
4. Peptic ulcer disease
5. Perforated appendix or diverticulum
6. Pericholecystic abscess
7. Peritonitis
8. Torsion of gallbladder

References
1. Rumack CM, Nilson SR, Charboneau JW (eds): Diagnostic Ultrasound. (ed 2) St. Louis: Mosby, 1998
2. Usui M, Matsuda S, Suzuki H, et al: Preoperative diagnosis of gallbladder torsion by magnetic resonance cholangiopancreatography. Scand J Gastroenterol 2000;35:218–222
3. Williamson MR: Abdominal ultrasound. In: Essentials of Ultrasound. Philadelphia: WB Saunders, 1996, p 90

Gamut G-127

DELAYED VISUALIZATION OF THE GALLBLADDER ON SCINTIGRAPHY

COMMON

1. Chronic cholecystitis

UNCOMMON

1. Acalculus cholecystitis
2. Carcinoma of gallbladder

(continued)

3. Dubin-Johnson syndrome
4. Hepatocellular disease (eg, cirrhosis; hepatitis)
5. Pancreatitis
6. Total parenteral nutrition

Reference
1. Gore RM: Gallbladder and biliary tract disease. In Gore RM, Levine MS (eds): Textbook of Gastrointestinal Radiology. (ed 2) Philadelphia: WB Saunders, 2000, pp 1408–1415

Gamut G-128

GAS IN THE GALLBLADDER OR BILIARY TRACT

COMMON

1. Biliary-enteric fistula to duodenum or colon (eg, perforated ulcer or adenocarcinoma of duodenum, ampulla, bile duct, gallbladder, stomach, pancreas, or colon; metastasis; lymphoma$_g$) (See G-139)
2. Cholecystitis with perforation
3. Emphysematous cholecystitis, cholangitis (esp. in diabetic)
4. [Gas in portal vein]
5. Postoperative (eg, sphincterotomy; biliary-intestinal anastomosis {cholecystoenterostomy; choledochoenterostomy; Whipple procedure}; internal or external biliary drainage)
6. Recent passage of gallstone from gallbladder or common duct (eg, gallstone ileus)

UNCOMMON

1. Common duct entry into duodenal diverticulum
2. Crohn's disease
3. [Gas in gallstone]
4. [Normal periductal fat]
5. Pancreatitis
6. Parasitic disease (clonorchiasis; ascariasis; ruptured amebic abscess of liver; strongyloidiasis of duodenum)
7. Peptic ulcer with perforation into common duct and fistula

8. Physiologic (incompetent, patulous sphincter, esp. in elderly)
9. Postbulbar duodenal ulcer adjacent to ampulla with spasm (acute) or fibrosis (healing)
10. Trauma, external penetrating or iatrogenic (eg, intubation; ERCP)

[ ] This condition does not actually cause the gamuted imaging finding, but can produce imaging changes that simulate it.

References
1. Eisenberg RL: Gastrointestinal Radiology: A Pattern Approach. (ed 3) Philadelphia: Lippincott, 1996, pp 888–893
2. Laing FC: The gallbladder and bile ducts. The liver. In: Rumack CM, Wilson SR, Charboneau JW (eds): Diagnostic Ultrasound. St. Louis: Mosby, 1998, pp 175–223
3. Martin DF, Tweedle DEF: The aetiology and significance of distal choledochoduodenal fistula. Br J Surg 1984;71: 632–634
4. Shimono T, Nishimura, Hayakawa K: CT imaging of biliary enteric fistula. Abdom Imaging 1998;23:172–176
5. Tamada K, Tomiyama T, Wada S, et al: Hyperechoic lines as a sonographic confirmatory sign during percutaneous transhepatic biliary drainage. Abdom Imaging 2001;26:39–42

Gamut G-129

CONGENITAL DISORDERS OR SYNDROMES WITH AN ABNORMAL BILIARY TRACT

COMMON

1. Asplenia S. (Ivemark S.); polysplenia S.
2. Biliary atresia
3. Caroli disease
4. Choledochal cyst
5. Cystic fibrosis (mucoviscidosis)

UNCOMMON

1. Bardet-Biedl S.
2. Bile duct hypoplasia (Alagille S. or arteriohepatic S.)
3. Bile plug S.
4. Hepatic fibrosis-renal cystic disease

---

5. Meckel S.
6. Spontaneous (idiopathic) perforation of common bile duct

References

1. Arcemont CM, Meza MP, Arumanla S, et al: MRCP in the evaluation of pancreaticobiliary disease in children. Pediatr Radiology 2001;31:92–97
2. Nicotra JJ, Kramer SS, Bellah RD, Redd DCB: Congenital and acquired biliary disorders in children. Semin Roentgenol 1997;32:215–227
3. Park KB, Auh YH, Kim JH, et al: Diagnostic pitfalls in the cholangiographic diagnosis of choledochoceles: cholangiographic quality and its effect on visualization. Abdom Imaging 2001;26:48–54
4. Rosenthal P: Biliary atresia and neonatal disorders of the bile ducts. In: Wyllie R, Hyams JS: Pediatric Gastrointestinal Disease. Philadelphia: WB Saunders, 1999, pp 568–578
5. Siegel MJ: Pediatric Body CT. Philadelphia: Lippincott Williams & Wilkins, 1999
6. Taybi H, Lachman RS: Radiology of Syndromes, Metabolic Disorders, and Skeletal Dysplasias. (ed 4) St. Louis: Mosby-Year Book, 1996, p 962

Gamut G-130

DILATATION OF BILE DUCTS (CAG, MRCP, US, CT, MRI)

COMMON

1. Advanced age
2. Calculus in biliary duct (choledocholithiasis)
3. Chronic pancreatitis
4. Lymphadenopathy with extrinsic compression
5. Neoplasm of pancreas, ampulla of Vater, common duct, or major bile duct (eg, papilloma; adenocarcinoma; mucin-producing cholangiocarcinoma)
6. Papillitis or fibrosis of ampulla of Vater
7. Parasitic disease (eg, ascariasis; clonorchiasis; opisthorchiasis; fascioliasis; hydatid disease)
8. Sclerosing cholangitis
9. Stricture of distal biliary duct (eg, postoperative; intubation; inflammatory; congenital)

UNCOMMON

1. Aneurysm of hepatic artery or aorta (compression)
2. Biliary atresia, extrahepatic
3. Biliary duct web or diaphragm
4. Caroli disease
5. Cholangitis, infectious (eg, AIDS-related; bacterial; parasitic)
6. Choledochal cyst
7. Choledochocele
8. Diverticulum of duodenum or biliary duct (compression)
9. Duodenal ulcer, penetrating
10. Hepatic fibrosis-renal cystic disease
11. Liver abscess (pyogenic, amebic, or fungal)
12. Liver infarcts following transcatheter embolization of hepatic artery branches
13. Lymphadenopathy in periportal area with ductal compression (eg, metastatic carcinoma of liver, stomach, or pancreas; lymphoma$_g$; sarcoidosis)
14. Metastasis
15. Mirizzi syndrome
16. Papillitis or fibrosis of ampulla
17. [Periportal edema]
18. Retroperitoneal fibrosis

[ ] This condition does not actually cause the gamuted imaging finding, but can produce imaging changes that simulate it.

References

1. Alexander ES, Mitchell SE: Dilatation of biliary ducts (extrahepatic, intrahepatic). Semin Roentgenol 1981;16:3–4
2. Berk RN, Clemett AR: Radiology of the Gallbladder and Bile Ducts. Philadelphia: WB Saunders, 1977
3. Eisenberg RL: Gastrointestinal Radiology: A Pattern Approach. (ed 3) Philadelphia: Lippincott, 1996, pp 872–881
4. Gore RM: Gallbladder and biliary tract: Differential diagnosis. In: Gore RM, Levine MS: Textbook of Gastrointestinal Radiology. (ed 2) Philadelphia: WB Saunders, 2000, pp 1408–1414
5. Lidofsky S, Scharschmidt BF: Jaundice. In: Feldman M, Scharschmidt BF, Sleisenger MH: Gastrointestinal and Liver Disease. (ed 6) Philadelphia: WB Saunders, 2000
6. Parulekar SG: Gallbladder and bile ducts. In: McGahan JP, Goldberg BB (eds): Diagnostic Ultrasound. Philadelphia: Lippincott-Raven, 1997, chapter 22
7. Slone RM, Fisher AJ: Pocket Guide to Body CT Differential Diagnosis. New York: McGraw-Hill, 1999, pp 226–227
8. Vitellas KM, Keogan MT, Spritzer CE, et al: MR cholangiopancreatography of bile and pancreatic duct abnormalities with emphasis on the single-shot fast spin-echo technique. RadioGraphics 2000;20:939–957

Gamut G-131

BILIARY DILATATION WITHOUT JAUNDICE OR OBSTRUCTION

1. Advanced age
2. Choledochal cyst (type I)
3. Common duct exploration sequela
4. Early ductal obstruction
5. Nonobstructive gallstone
6. Normal variant
7. Parasitic disease (eg, *Ascaris; Clonorchis; Fasciola; Opisthorchis;* ruptured hydatid cyst or amebic abscess into duct)
8. Postcholecystectomy
9. Post-ductal obstruction
10. Recent passage of stone with ampullary edema

Reference

1. Gore RM: Gallbladder and biliary tract disease. In Gore RM, Levine MS (eds): Textbook of Gastrointestinal Radiology. (ed 2) Philadelphia: WB Saunders, 2000, pp 1408–1415

Gamut G-132

BILIARY OBSTRUCTION WITHOUT DILATATION

1. Acute severe biliary obstruction (first 3 days)
2. Cholangiocarcinoma with tumor encasement
3. Cholangitis (eg, ascending; sclerosing; recurrent pyogenic)
4. Hemobilia
5. Pancreatitis
6. Parasitic disease (eg, solitary or few *Ascaris, Clonorchis, or Fasciola;* ruptured hydatid cyst or amebic abscess into duct with debris)

Reference

1. Gore RM: Gallbladder and biliary tract disease. In Gore RM, Levine MS (eds): Textbook of Gastrointestinal Radiology. (ed 2) Philadelphia: WB Saunders, 2000, pp 1408–1415

Gamut G-133-1

CYSTIC AND SACCULAR LESIONS OF THE BILE DUCTS— WITH NORMAL-SIZED INTRAHEPATIC BILE DUCTS (CAG, MRCP)

1. Choledochal cyst (common duct)
2. Choledochocele (intraduodenal)
3. Cystic duct remnant
4. Diverticulum of common duct or rarely, an intrahepatic duct
5. Simple central dilatation of common duct

References

1. Burgener FA, Kormano M: Differential Diagnosis in Conventional Radiology. (ed 2) New York: Thieme Medical Publ, 1991, pp 730–731
2. DeBacker AI, Van den Abbeele K, DeSchopper AM: Choledochocele: diagnosis by magnetic resonance imaging. Abdom Imaging 2000;25:508–510
3. Gore RM, Fulcher AS, Taylor AJ: Anomalies and anatomic variants of the gallbladder and biliary tract. In: Gore RM, Levine MS: Textbook of Gastrointestinal Radiology. (ed 2) Philadelphia: WB Saunders, 2000

Gamut G-133-2

CYSTIC AND SACCULAR LESIONS OF THE BILE DUCTS— WITH DILATATION OF INTRAHEPATIC BILE DUCTS (CAG, MRCP)

1. Bacterial cholangitis with tiny saccular abscesses (acute, suppurative, ascending cholangitis)
2. Caroli disease
3. Choledochal cyst
4. Hepatic fibrosis-renal cystic disease
5. Parasitic disease (esp. opisthorchiasis; also clonorchiasis; ascariasis)
6. Recurrent pyogenic cholangitis (Oriental cholangiohepatitis)

7. Reversible dilatation of intrahepatic bile ducts
8. Sclerosing cholangitis with prestenotic saccular out-pouchings

References

1. Burgener FA, Kormano M: Differential Diagnosis in Conventional Radiology. (ed 2) New York: Thieme Medical Publ, 1991, pp 730–731
2. Donaldson JS: Diseases of the pediatric gallbladder and biliary tract. In: Gore RM, Levine MS: Textbook of Gastrointestinal Radiology. (ed 2) Philadelphia: WB Saunders, 2000
3. Jequier S, Capusten B, Guttman F, et al: Childhood choledochal cyst with intrahepatic enlarged cyst-like bile ducts. J Can Assoc Radiol 1984;35:73–76
4. Turner MA, Fulcher AS: The cystic duct: normal anatomy and disease processes. RadioGraphics 2001;21:3–22

Gamut G-134

FILLING DEFECT OR SEGMENTAL LESION IN THE BILE DUCTS (CAG, MRCP, CT)

COMMON

1. Air bubble
2. Calculus
3. Contraction of choledochal sphincter (pseudo-calculus) in distal common duct
4. Edema of ampullary segment (eg, after passage of calculus; pancreatitis)
5. Extrinsic vascular impression (eg, right hepatic artery; bile duct varices)
6. Malignant neoplasm of bile duct (cholangiocarcinoma), gallbladder, ampulla, duodenum, or pancreas; hepatocellular carcinoma (hepatoma); Klatzkin tumor
7. Stricture (eg, cholangitis or Oriental cholangiohepatitis with dilated ducts and calculi)

UNCOMMON

1. Blood clot
2. Congenital membranous diaphragm (web) of common hepatic duct

3. Debris or mucus in ducts from obstructing tumor or parasites
4. Foreign body or food particle
5. Lymphadenopathy in porta hepatis
6. Metastasis (eg, lung; melanoma; lymphoma$_g$)
7. Mirizzi syndrome
8. Neoplasm, benign (eg, adenoma; papilloma; carcinoid; gastrointestinal stromal tumor$_g$; lipoma; hamartoma; polyp)
9. Normal variant (eg, cystic duct insertion; valves of Heister; redundant walls of tortuous duct)
10. Parasite (*Ascaris; Clonorchis; Fasciola;* hydatid cyst)
11. Pericholedochal adhesions
12. Postoperative defect (eg, plication defect at the site of duct-to-duct anastomosis)
13. Sarcoma botryoides (child)
14. Spasm of sphincter of Oddi

References

1. Eisenberg RL: Gastrointestinal Radiology: A Pattern Approach. (ed 3) Philadelphia: Lippincott, 1996, pp 837–871
2. Fulcher AS, Turner MA: Pitfalls of MR cholangiopancreatography. J Comput Assist Tomogr 1998;22:845–850
3. Gallix BP, Régent D, Bruel J-M: Use of magnetic resonance cholangiography in the diagnosis of choledocholithiasis. Abdom Imaging 2001;26:21–27
4. Pickuth D: Radiologic diagnosis of common bile duct stones. Abdom Imaging 2000;25:613–621
5. Vilgrain V, Palazzol L: Choledocholithiasis: role of US and endoscopic ultrasound. Abdom Imaging 2001:26:7-14

Gamut G-135

THICKENING OF BILE DUCT WALLS (US)

COMMON

1. AIDS-related cholangiopathy
2. Ascending (bacterial) cholangitis
3. Choledocholithiasis
4. Pancreatitis (common duct)
5. Recurrent pyogenic cholangitis (Oriental cholangio-hepatitis)
6. Sclerosing cholangitis

UNCOMMON

1. Cholangiocarcinoma
2. Parasitic disease (liver flukes {clonorchiasis; opisthorchiasis}; ascariasis; schistosomiasis; ruptured amebic hepatic abscess into bile ducts)

References
1. Berger J, Linsell DRM: Thickening of the walls of nondilated bile ducts. Clin Radiol 1997;52:474–476
2. Parulekar SG: Gallbladder and bile ducts. In: McGahan JP, Goldberg BB (eds): Diagnostic Ultrasound. Philadelphia: Lippincott-Raven, 1997, chapter 2
3. Vitellas KM, Keogan MT, Freed KS, et al: Radiologic manifestations of sclerosing cholangitis with emphasis on MR cholangiopancreatography. RadioGraphics 2000;20:959–975

Gamut G-136

ECHOES WITHIN THE BILE DUCTS (US)

COMMON

1. Calculus
2. Hemobilia
3. Pneumobilia
4. Pus
5. Sludge

UNCOMMON

1. Cholangiocarcinoma
2. Feces (via fistula)
3. Food particles (via reflux)
4. Hepatoma
5. Mesenchymal tumor, benign
6. Metastasis
7. Parasites (*Ascaris; Clonorchis; Fasciola;* hydatid debris)
8. Recurrent pyogenic cholangitis (Oriental cholangio-hepatitis)
9. Surgical clips

References
1. Kabaalio GB, Cubuk M, Senol U, et al: Fascioliasis: US, CT, and MRI findings with new observations. Abdom Imaging 2000;25:400–404
2. Williamson MR: Abdominal ultrasound. In: Essentials of Ultrasound. Philadelphia: WB Saunders, 1996, p 77

Gamut G-137

BILE DUCT NARROWING OR OBSTRUCTION (CAG, MRCP)

COMMON

1. Calculus in biliary duct (choledocholithiasis) (eg, impacted stone in Vaterian segment; papillary edema from recent passage of stone; Mirizzi syndrome)
2. Cholangitis
3. Contraction of choledochal sphincter (pseudo-calculus); papillary stenosis
4. Iatrogenic or posttraumatic (eg, surgical injury; trauma; radiation therapy; hepatic artery chemotherapy or embolization)
5. Neoplasm, malignant (eg, cholangiocarcinoma; ampullary, pancreatic, duodenal, or gallbladder carcinoma; hepatocellular carcinoma; Klatzkin tumor; villous tumor)
6. Pancreatitis, acute or chronic (incl. pseudocyst)
7. Sclerosing cholangitis

UNCOMMON

1. Abscess (pyogenic, amebic, or fungal)
2. AIDS-related cholangiopathy (eg, cytomegalovirus or *Cryptosporidium* infection)
3. Artifact from post-processing technique of MRCP
4. Biliary hypoplasia or atresia
5. Caroli disease (complicated)
6. Congenital membranous diaphragm (web)
7. Debris or mucus in ducts from obstructing tumor or parasites
8. Duodenal diverticulum
9. Hepatic fibrosis-renal cystic disease
10. Hepatocellular disease, advanced (eg, cirrhosis; cholangiolytic hepatitis)
11. Liver cyst, neoplasm, or abscess
12. Lymphadenopathy in porta hepatis (eg, metastasis; lymphoma$_g$; tuberculosis; sarcoidosis)
13. Metastasis (esp. from carcinoma of pancreas, gallbladder, stomach)
14. Neoplasm, benign (incl. adenoma; papilloma; gastrointestinal stromal tumor$_g$; myoblastoma; cystadenoma)
15. Papillitis of ampulla
16. Parasitic disease of bile ducts, liver, or duodenum (esp. ascariasis; clonorchiasis; fascioliasis; hydatid disease; amebic abscess; schistosomiasis; strongyloidiasis)
17. Postbulbar duodenal ulcer with scarring or perforation
18. Recurrent pyogenic cholangitis {Oriental cholangiohepatitis}
19. Stricture, traumatic or iatrogenic (eg, postoperative; intubation)
20. Vascular compression (eg, aneurysm of aorta or hepatic artery; calcified portal vein)

References
1. Dähnert W: Radiology Review Manual. Baltimore: Williams & Wilkins, 1999
2. Chapman S, Nakielny R: Aids to Radiological Differential Diagnosis. London: Bailliere Tindall, 1990
3. Eisenberg RL: Gastrointestinal Radiology: A Pattern Approach. (ed 3) Philadelphia: Lippincott, 1996, pp 851–871
4. Fulcher AS, Turner MA: Pitfalls of MR cholangiopancreatography. J Comput Assist Tomogr 1998;22:845–850
5. Gore RM: Gallbladder and biliary tract: Differential diagnosis. In: Gore RM, Levine MS: Textbook of Gastrointestinal Radiology. (ed 2) Philadelphia: WB Saunders, 2000, pp 1408–1414
6. Jacobson IM: ERCP and Its Applications. Philadelphia: Lippincott-Raven, 1998
7. Pavone P, Laghi A, Passariello R: MR cholangiopancreatography in malignant biliary obstruction. Semin Ultrasound CT MR 1999;20:317–323
8. Rajaram R, Ponsiden CY, Majoie CBLM, et al: Evaluation of a modified cholangiographic classification system for primary sclerosing cholangitis. Abdom Imaging 2001;26: 43–47
9. Semelka RC, Ascher SM, Reinhold C: MRI of the Abdomen and Pelvis. New York: Wiley-Liss, 1997

Gamut G-138

ENLARGED PAPILLA OF VATER

COMMON

1. Calculus impacted in distal common duct
2. Carcinoma of Vaterian segment
3. Idiopathic; normal variant
4. Mucinous (ductectatic) adenocarcinoma of pancreas
5. Pancreatitis
6. Papillitis

UNCOMMON

1. Edema secondary to active duodenal ulcer
2. Heterotopic pancreatic tissue
3. Neoplasm (eg, adenomatous polyp of papilla; carcinoid; gastrointestinal stromal tumor$_g$ of duodenum)
4. Pancreatic abscess
5. Parasitic disease (eg, strongyloidiasis; ascariasis)
6. Postoperative; instrumentation
7. Zollinger-Ellison syndrome

References
1. Eisenberg RL: Gastrointestinal Radiology: A Pattern Approach. (ed 3) Philadelphia: Lippincott, 1996, pp 882–887
2. Poppel MH, Jacobson HG, Smith RW: The Roentgen Aspects of the Papilla and Ampulla of Vater. Springfield, IL: CC Thomas, 1953

(continued)

3. Schutz SM: Papillary tumors. In: DiMarino AJ, Benjamin SB: Gastrointestinal Disease: An Endoscopic Approach. Malden, MA: Blackwell Science, 1997, pp 952–960

2. Zuckerman AM, Goldschmid S, Hunter JG, et al: Biliary fistulas. In: Pitt HA, Carr-Locke DL, Ferrucci JT, et al: Hepatobiliary and Pancreatic Disease. Boston: Little, Brown and Company, 1995

Gamut G-139

BILIARY-ENTERIC FISTULA
(See G-128)

COMMON

1. Cholecystitis (perforative, acute or chronic)
2. Gallstone fistula from gallbladder or bile duct (eg, choledochoduodenal fistula)
3. Malignant neoplasm of gallbladder, bile duct, pancreas, or intestine
4. Postoperative (eg, sphincterotomy; biliary-intestinal anastomosis—Whipple procedure)

UNCOMMON

1. Abscess (pancreatic; hepatic; pericolic; pericholecystic)
2. Common duct entry into duodenal diverticulum
3. Diverticulitis of duodenum or hepatic flexure of colon
4. Granulomatous disease of duodenum or colon (eg, Crohn's disease; tuberculosis; actinomycosis)
5. Lymphoma$_g$
6. Parasitic disease (esp. amebiasis; ascariasis; hydatid disease)
7. Passage of common duct stone
8. Peptic ulcer perforation into biliary tract
9. [Physiologic reflux at ampulla; incompetent sphincter]
10. Trauma, external or iatrogenic (eg, intubation; ERCP)

[ ] This condition does not actually cause the gamuted imaging finding, but can produce imaging changes that simulate it.

References
1. Martin DF, Tweedle DEF: The aetiology and significance of distal choledochoduodenal fistula. Br J Surg 1984;71:632–634

Gamut G-140

BILIARY-PLEURAL
(OR BRONCHIAL) FISTULA

1. Biliary obstruction
2. Congenital
3. Parasitic disease (eg, amebic abscess; hydatid disease)
4. Trauma, external or iatrogenic

References
1. Bamberger PK, Stojadinovic A, Shaked G, et al: Biliary-pleural fistula presenting as a massive pleural effusion after thoracoabdominal penetrating trauma. J Trauma 1997;43: 162–163
2. Böni RAH, Peter J, Marincek B: Amebic abscess of the liver manifested by "hemoptysis": US, CT, and MRI findings. Abdom Imag 1995;20:214–216
3. Feld R, Wechsler RJ, Bonn J: Biliary-pleural fistula without biliary obstruction. AJR 1997;169:381–383
4. Palmer PES, Reeder MM: The Imaging of Tropical Diseases. Heidelberg: Springer-Verlag, 2001

Gamut G-141-1

HEPATOMEGALY (See G-141-2)

COMMON

1. Abscess, solitary or multiple (pyogenic, amebic, or fungal)
2. Cirrhosis, early
3. Congenital hepatomegaly (See G-141-2)
4. Cyst (bile duct cyst; simple; posttraumatic; hydatid) (See G-157)

5. Elevated venous pressure (eg, heart failure; constrictive pericarditis; tricuspid stenosis or insufficiency)
6. Fatty change (steatosis) (See G-144)
7. Hemochromatosis
8. Hepatitis (viral, infectious, or serum)
9. Infectious disease, other (eg, infectious mononucleosis; candidiasis; brucellosis; miliary tuberculosis or histoplasmosis; malaria)
10. Metastases
11. Neoplasm (esp. hepatocellular carcinoma {hepatoma}; cholangiocarcinoma; hepatoblastoma; giant hemangioma; hemangioendothelioma; angiosarcoma)
12. Obstruction of common bile duct (biliary cirrhosis) (See G-137)

UNCOMMON

1. Amyloidosis
2. Anemia, primary (eg, thalassemia major)
3. Chronic granulomatous disease of childhood
4. Extramedullary hematopoiesis
5. Gaucher disease; Niemann-Pick disease
6. Glycogen storage disease (eg, type I—von Gierke)
7. Hematoma
8. Hydatid disease (*Echinococcus granulosus* and *E. multilocularis*)
9. Kala-azar
10. Langerhans cell histiocytosis$_g$
11. Lymphoma$_g$
12. Myeloid metaplasia; myelofibrosis
13. Polycystic disease of liver
14. Polycythemia vera
15. Reye S.
16. Sarcoidosis
17. Schistosomiasis
18. Thrombosis of hepatic vein or upper inferior cava (Budd-Chiari S.); veno-occlusive disease (See G-189)
19. Wilson disease

Reference
1. Lefkowitch JH: Pathologic diagnosis of liver disease. In: Zakim D, Boyer TD: Hepatology. (ed 3) Philadelphia: WB Saunders, 1996, pp 844–874

Gamut G-141-2

CONGENITAL HEPATOMEGALY

COMMON

1. Anemia$_g$, primary (esp. thalassemia; sickle cell disease)
2. Cystic fibrosis (mucoviscidosis)
3. Gaucher disease; Niemann-Pick disease
4. Glycogen storage disease, types I (von Gierke), III and IV
5. Infant of diabetic mother
6. Langerhans cell histiocytosis$_g$
7. Mucopolysaccharidoses (esp. Hurler S., Hunter S.); mucolipidosis II (I-cell disease) (See J-4)
8. Polycystic disease of liver

UNCOMMON

1. Aase S.
2. Alagille S. (arteriohepatic S.)
3. Alpha-1-antitrypsin deficiency
4. Beckwith-Wiedemann S.
5. Budd-Chiari S.
6. Chédiak-Higashi S.
7. Cholesterol ester storage disease
8. Chronic granulomatous disease of childhood
9. Congenital transplacental infection (eg, toxoplasmosis; rubella; cytomegalovirus; herpes simplex)
10. Cystinosis
11. Ethanolaminosis
12. Farber disease (lipogranulomatosis)
13. Felty S.
14. Galactosemia
15. Galactosialidosis
16. GM$_1$ gangliosidosis; fucosidosis; mannosidosis
17. Hepatic fibrosis-renal cystic disease
18. Homocystinuria
19. Hyperlipoproteinemia
20. Infantile multisystem inflammatory disease (NOMID)
21. Lipoatrophic diabetes
22. Mauriac S.
23. Osteopetrosis

(continued)

24. POEMS S.
25. Pyruvate kinase deficiency
26. Sea-blue histiocyte S.
27. Tyrosinemia (type I)
28. Weber-Christian S.
29. Wilson disease
30. Wolman disease (familial xanthomatosis)
31. Zellweger S. (cerebrohepatorenal S.)

References
1. Siafakis CG, Jonas MM: Neonatal hepatitis. In: Wyllie R, Hyams JS: Pediatric Gastrointestinal Disease. Philadelphia: WB Saunders, 1999, pp 563–567
2. Siegel MJ: Pediatric Body CT. Philadelphia: Lippincott, Williams & Wilkins, 1999
3. Taybi H, Lachman RS: Radiology of Syndromes, Metabolic Disorders, and Skeletal Dysplasias. (ed 4) St. Louis: Mosby-Year Book, 1996, p 959

Gamut G-142

DIFFUSE HEPATIC CALCIFICATIONS (PF, US, CT)

COMMON

1. Hyperparathyroidism, secondary (incl. chronic renal failure; uremia; hemodialysis)
2. Ischemia, with or without shock; infarction (chronic)
3. Metastatic disease (eg, mucinous adenocarcinoma of colon, stomach, breast, or thyroid; carcinoma of ovary, pancreas, or lung; islet cell carcinoma; melanoma; neuroblastoma; osteosarcoma; chondrosarcoma; teratoma; also postradiation and post-chemotherapy)
4. [Neoplasm of liver, large, advanced, often necrotic (eg, hepatocellular carcinoma; cholangiocarcinoma; hemangioma; infantile hemangioendothelioma; hepatoblastoma; fibrolamellar carcinoma; mesenchymal hamartoma)—calcifications may be extensive in a localized area or even multifocal, but not truly diffuse]

UNCOMMON

1. Amyloidosis
2. Chronic granulomatous disease of childhood
3. Congenital transplacental infection (eg, toxopolasmosis; rubella; cytomegalovirus; herpes simplex; varicella)
4. Granulomas, multiple healed (eg, tuberculosis; histoplasmosis; coccidioidomycosis; brucellosis)
5. Hemochromatosis
6. Hydatid disease (*Echinococcus multilocularis* or multiple calcified *E. granulosus* cysts)
7. Infection, severe (eg, multiple healed abscesses)
8. Pentastomiasis (*Armillifer* infection)
9. [Peritoneal calcifications overlying liver capsule in infancy (eg, meconium peritonitis; ruptured hydrometrocolpos)]
10. Schistosomiasis (esp. *S. japonica*)
11. [Thorotrast residual]

[ ] This condition does not actually cause the gamuted imaging finding, but can produce imaging changes that simulate it.

References
1. Gore RM: Liver: Differential diagnosis. In: Gore RM, Levine MS: Textbook of Gastrointestinal Radiology. (ed 2) Philadelphia: WB Saunders, 2000, pp 1712–1727
2. Kennan NM, Evans C: Hepatic and splenic calcification due to amyloid. Clin Radiol 1991;44:60–61
3. Milstein MJ, Moulton JS: Diffuse hepatic calcification after ischemic liver injury in a patient with chronic renal failure. AJR 1993;161:75–76
4. Parulekar SG, Bree RL: Liver. In: McGahan JP, Goldberg BB (eds): Diagnostic Ultrasound. Philadelphia: Lippincott-Raven, 1997, chapter 21

FETAL OR NEONATAL LIVER CALCIFICATION

COMMON

1. Congenital transplacental infection (eg, toxopolasmosis; rubella; cytomegalovirus; herpes simplex; varicella)
2. Metastatic neuroblastoma
3. [Peritoneal calcifications overlying liver capsule (eg, meconium peritonitis; ruptured hydrometrocolpos)]

UNCOMMON

1. Infarcts
2. Primary liver tumor (eg, hemangioma; hepatoblastoma; infantile hemangioendothelioma; hamartoma; teratoma)
3. Thromboemboli in portal vein [or IVC]

[ ] This condition does not actually cause the gamuted imaging finding, but can produce imaging changes that simulate it.

References

1. Brugman SM. Bjelland JJ, Thomason JE, et al: Sonographic findings with radiologic correlation in meconium peritonitis. J Clin Ultrasound 1979;7:305–306
2. Chapman S, Nakielny R: Aids to Radiological Differential Diagnosis. (ed 3) London: WB Saunders, 1995, p 267
3. Friedman AP, Haller JO, Boyer B, Cooper R: Calcified portal vein thromboemboli in infants: radiography and ultrasonography. Radiology 1981;140:381–382
4. Nguyen DL, Leonard JC: Ischaemic hepatic necrosis: a cause of fetal liver calcification. AJR 1986:147:596–597
5. Schackelford GD, Kirks DR: Neonatal hepatic calcification secondary to transplacental infection. Radiology 1977;122:753–757
6. Siegel MJ: Pediatric Body CT. Philadelphia: Lippincott, Williams & Wilkins, 1999

FATTY CHANGE IN THE LIVER (STEATOSIS) (US, CT, MRI)

COMMON

*1. AIDS
2. Alcoholism; cirrhosis
*3. Cystic fibrosis (mucoviscidosis)
4. Diabetes mellitus
*5. Drug therapy (esp. tetracycline; steroids; chemotherapy with cytotoxic agents)
*6. Idiopathic
*7. Obesity

UNCOMMON

1. Carbon tetrachloride exposure
*2. Cushing S.
*3. Fever, prolonged
*4. Hepatitis, acute or viral
*5. Hepatotoxins
6. Hyperalimentation
7. Hyperlipidemia, familial
8. Jejunoileal bypass
*9. Lipoatrophic diabetes (congenital total lipodystrophy)
*10. Malabsorption syndrome (See G-57)
11. Peritoneal dialysis
12. Pregnancy
*13. Reye S.
*14. Starvation, acute or chronic (incl. malnutrition; kwashiorkor)
*15. Storage diseases (eg, Gaucher disease; Niemann-Pick disease; glycogen storage disease, type I—von Gierke)

* Children affected.

References

1. Baron RL, Gore RM: Diffuse liver disease. In: Gore RM, Levine MS: Textbook of Gastrointestinal Radiology. (ed 2) Philadelphia: WB Saunders, 2000, pp 1590–1638

(continued)

2. Bashist B, Hecht HL, Harley WD: Computed tomographic demonstration of rapid changes in fatty infiltration of the liver. Radiology 1982;142:691–692

3. Taybi H, Lachman RS: Radiology of Syndromes, Metabolic Disorders, and Skeletal Dysplasias. (ed 4) St. Louis: Mosby-Year Book, 1996

4. Wilson SR, Rosen IE, Chin-Sang HB, et al: Fatty infiltration of the liver: an imaging challenge. J Can Assoc Radiol 1982; 33:227–232

Gamut G-145

PERFUSION ABNORMALITIES OF THE LIVER

LOBAR OR SEGMENTAL

1. Cirrhosis with arterial-portal shunt
2. Hypervascular gallbladder disease
3. Mass effect due to tumor, cyst, abscess within liver
4. Portal vein ligation, obstruction or thrombosis

SUBSEGMENTAL

1. Acute cholecystitis
2. Ethanol ablation
3. Obstruction of peripheral portal branches
4. Percutaneous needle biopsy

References

1. Gore RM: Liver: Differential diagnosis. In: Gore RM, Levine MS (eds): Textbook of Gastrointestinal Radiology. (ed 2) Philadelphia: WB Saunders, 2000, pp 1712–1727
2. Gore RM, Marn CS, Baron RL: Vascular disorders of the liver and splanchnic circulation. In: Gore RM, Levine MS (eds): Textbook of Gastrointestinal Radiology. (ed 2) Philadelphia: WB Saunders, 2000, pp 1639–1668
3. Gabata T, Kadoya M, Matsui O, et al: Dynamic CT of hepatic abscess: significance of transient segmental enhancement. AJR 2001;176:675–680
4. Rozeik PE, Huppert PE, Münch H: Angiographic pseudolesion in the liver in asymptomatic subacute cholecystitis. Eur Radiol 2001;11:346–347
5. Semelka RC, Chung J-J, Hussain SM, et al: Chronic hepatitis: correlation of early patchy and late enhancement patterns on gadolinium-enhanced MR images with histopathology. JMRI 2001;385–391

Gamut G-146

PATCHY HEPATOGRAM (AREAS OF LOW DENSITY ON ANGIOGRAPHY OR POSTCONTRAST CT)

COMMON

1. Budd-Chiari syndrome
2. Cirrhosis
3. Heart failure
4. Hepatitis
5. Portal vein thrombosis

UNCOMMON

1. Lymphomatous infiltration
2. Sarcoidosis
3. Schistosomiasis
4. Thyrotoxicosis
5. Tricuspid atresia

References

1. Gore RM: Liver: Differential diagnosis. In: Gore RM, Levine MS (eds): Textbook of Gastrointestinal Radiology. (ed 2) Philadelphia: WB Saunders, 2000, pp 1712–1727
2. Gore RM, Marn CS, Baron RL: Vascular disorders of the liver and splanchnic circulation. In: Gore RM, Levine MS (eds): Textbook of Gastrointestinal Radiology. (ed 2) Philadelphia: WB Saunders, 2000, pp 1639–1668
3. Gabata T, Kadoya M, Matsui O, et al: Dynamic CT of hepatic abscess: significance of transient segmental enhancement. AJR 2001;176:675–680
4. Rozeik PE, Huppert PE, Münch H: Angiographic pseudolesion in the liver in asymptomatic subacute cholecystitis. Eur Radiol 2001;11:346–347
5. Semelka RC, Chung J-J, Hussain SM, et al: Chronic hepatitis: correlation of early patchy and late enhancement patterns on gadolinium-enhanced MR images with histopathology. JMRI 2001;385–391

Gamut G-147

GENERALIZED OR MULTIFOCAL DECREASED ECHOGENICITY OF THE LIVER ON ULTRASOUND (HYPOECHOIC)

COMMON

1. Hepatitis, acute viral
2. Malignant infiltration of liver by primary or metastatic neoplasm
3. Schistosomiasis, early

UNCOMMON

1. Amyloidosis
2. Leukemia; lymphoma$_g$; Burkitt lymphoma
3. [Renal disease, end stage; nephrocalcinosis]

[ ] This condition does not actually cause the gamuted imaging finding, but can produce imaging changes that simulate it.

References

1. Baron RL, Gore RM: Diffuse liver disease. In: Gore RM, Levine MS: Textbook of Gastrointestinal Radiology. (ed 2) Philadelphia: WB Saunders, 2000, pp 1590–1638
2. Cosgrove DO: Liver and biliary tree. In: Barnett E, Morley P (eds): Clinical Diagnostic Ultrasound. Oxford: Blackwell Scientific Publ, 1985, pp 365–386
3. Gore RM: Liver: Differential diagnosis. In: Gore RM, Levine MS: Textbook of Gastrointestinal Radiology. (ed 2) Philadelphia: WB Saunders, 2000, pp 1712–1726
4. Konno K, Ishida H, Sato M, et al: Macronodular hepatic deformity on normal liver. Abdom Imaging 2000;25:592–595
5. Skolnick ML: Guide to the Ultrasound Examination of the Abdomen. New York: Springer-Verlag, 1986, pp 87–88
6. Weill FS: Ultrasound Diagnosis of Digestive Diseases. (ed 3 revised) Berlin: Springer-Verlag, 1990, pp 239–246

Gamut G-148

GENERALIZED OR MULTIFOCAL INCREASED ECHOGENICITY OF THE LIVER ON ULTRASOUND (HYPERECHOIC)

COMMON

1. AIDS
2. Fatty infiltration (eg, alcoholism; various toxins; diabetes; malabsorption S.; jejunoileal bypass; protein deficiency; starvation—malnutrition, kwashiorkor; familial hyperlipidemia) (See G-144)
3. Fibrosis of liver parenchyma (eg, alcoholism; cirrhosis; schistosomiasis; chronic hepatitis; glycogen storage disease)
4. Hepatocellular carcinoma (hepatoma), diffuse
5. Hydatid disease (*Echinococcosis multilocularis* or multiple healed, calcified *E. granulosus* cysts)
6. Idiopathic
7. Lipoatrophic diabetes
8. Obesity
9. Technical—excessive gain

UNCOMMON

1. Budd-Chiari S. (focal)
2. Carbon tetrachloride exposure
3. Cystic fibrosis (mucoviscidosis)
4. Drug therapy (esp. tetracycline; steroids; chemotherapy)
5. Gaucher disease
6. Hyperalimentation
7. Lipoatrophic diabetes (congenital total lipodystrophy)
8. Lymphoma$_g$; leukemia
9. Miliary tuberculosis
10. Pregnancy
11. Reye S.
12. Tyrosinemia
13. Wilson disease

References

1. Baron RL, Gore RM: Diffuse Liver Disease. In: Gore RM, Levine MS: Textbook of Gastrointestinal Radiology. (ed 2) Philadelphia: WB Saunders, 2000, pp 1590–1638

(continued)

2. Cosgrove DO: Liver and biliary tree. In: Barnett E, Morley P (eds): Clinical Diagnostic Ultrasound. Oxford: Blackwell Scientific Publ, 1985, pp 365–386
3. Skolnick ML: Guide to the Ultrasound Examination of the Abdomen. New York: Springer-Verlag, 1986, pp 87–88
4. Taybi H, Lachman RS: Radiology of Syndromes, Metabolic Disorders, and Skeletal Dysplasias. (ed 4) St. Louis: Mosby-Year Book, 1996, pp 959–960
5. Weill FS: Ultrasound Diagnosis of Digestive Diseases. (ed 3 revised) Berlin: Springer-Verlag, 1990, pp 239–246
6. Williamson, MR: Abdominal ultrasound. In: Essentials of Ultrasound. Philadelphia: WB Saunders, 1996, p 79
7. Wilson SR, Rosen IE, Chin-Sang HB, et al: Fatty infiltration of the liver: an imaging challenge. J Can Assoc Radiol 1982;33:227–232
8. Zweibel WJ: Sonographic diagnosis of diffuse liver disease. Semin Ultrasound CT and MRI 1995;16:8–15

Gamut G-149

GENERALIZED HIGH DENSITY LIVER (NONENHANCED CT)

COMMON

1. Hemochromatosis
2. Hemosiderosis

UNCOMMON

1. Chronic arsenic poisoning
2. Drug therapy (eg, amiodarone; gold; cisplatin)
3. Glycogen storage disease, type I—von Gierke (may be low density liver)
4. Iron overload of liver (eg, multiple transfusions)
5. Storage diseases (usually low density)
6. Thorotrast
7. Wilson disease

References
1. Bacon BR: Hemochromatosis: diagnosis and management. Gastroenterology 2001;120:718–725
2. Butler S, Smathers RL: Computed tomography of amiodarone pulmonary toxicity. J Comput Assist Tomogr 1985; 9:375–376

3. Foley WD, Jochem RJ: Computed tomography: focal and diffuse liver masses. Radiol Clin North Am 1991;20:1213
4. Gore RM: Liver: Differential diagnosis. In: Gore RM, Levine MS: Textbook of Gastrointestinal Radiology. (ed 2) Philadelphia: WB Saunders, 2000, pp 1712–1727
5. Rofsky NM, Fleishaker H: CT and MRI of diffuse liver disease. Semin Ultrasound CT and MRI 1995;16:33

Gamut G-150

GENERALIZED OR MULTIFOCAL LOW DENSITY LIVER (NONENHANCED CT)

COMMON

1. Diffuse malignancy, primary or metastatic (incl. lymphoma)
2. Fatty infiltration (steatosis) (See G-144)
3. Hepatic congestion (eg, heart failure; constrictive pericarditis; tricuspid stenosis or insufficiency)

UNCOMMON

1. Amyloidosis
2. Budd-Chiari syndrome, acute or chronic
3. Cysts, numerous (eg, hydatid disease; Caroli disease; polycystic liver disease; Von Hippel-Lindau disease)
4. Storage diseases (eg, Gaucher disease; Niemann-Pick disease; glycogen storage disease, type I—von Gierke)

References
1. Baron RL, Gore RM: Diffuse Liver Disease. In: Gore RM, Levine MS: Textbook of Gastrointestinal Radiology. (ed 2) Philadelphia: WB Saunders, 2000, pp 1590–1638
2. Foley WD, Jochem RJ: Computed tomography: focal and diffuse liver masses. Radiol Clin North Am 1991;20:1213
3. Gore RM: Liver: Differential diagnosis. In: Gore RM, Levine MS: Textbook of Gastrointestinal Radiology. (ed 2) Philadelphia: WB Saunders, 2000, pp 1712–1727
4. Halvorsen RA, Korobkin M, Ram PC, Thompson WM: CT appearance of focal fatty infiltration of the liver. AJR 1982;139:277–281
5. Mergo PJ, Ros PR: Benign lesions of the liver. Radiol Clin North Am 36:319–332, 1998

6. Siegel MJ: Pediatric Body CT. Philadelphia: Lippincott Williams & Wilkins, 1999
7. Slone RM, Fisher AJ: Pocket Guide to Body CT Differential Diagnosis. New York: McGraw-Hill, 1999, pp 203–204
8. Suzuki S, et al: CT findings in hepatic and splenic amyloidosis. J Comput Assist Tomog 1986;10:332–334
9. Vogelzang RL, Anscheutz SL, Gore RM: Budd Chiari syndrome: CT observations. Radiology 1987;163:329–333
10. Yates CK, Streight RA: Focal fatty infiltration of the liver simulating metastatic disease. Radiology 1986;159:83–84

Gamut G-151

MULTIPLE HYPOINTENSE LIVER LESIONS ON T2-WEIGHTED MR IMAGES

COMMON

1. Calcified granulomas
2. Regenerating nodules in cirrhosis

UNCOMMON

1. Gamna-Gandy bodies
2. Gas in biliary ducts or portal vein
3. Hydatid disease (*Echinococcus granulosus* or *E. multilocularis* with multiple calcified cysts)
4. Multifocal acute intrahepatic hemorrhages
5. Osler-Weber-Rendu disease
6. Periportal vascular collaterals

Reference
1. Gore RM: Liver: Differential diagnosis. In: Gore RM, Levine MS (eds): Textbook of Gastrointestinal Radiology. (ed 2) Philadelphia: WB Saunders, 2000, pp 1712–1727
2. Gore RM, Marn CS, Baron RL: Vascular disorders of the liver and splanchnic circulation. In: Gore RM, Levine MS (eds): Textbook of Gastrointestinal Radiology (ed 2) Philadelphia: WB Saunders, 2000, pp 1639–1668
3. Semelka RC, Kelekis NL: Liver. In: Semelka RC, Ascher SM, Reinhold C (eds): MRI of the Abdomen and Pelvis: A Text-Atlas. New York: Wiley-Liss, 1997, pp 19–136

Gamut G-152

DIFFUSELY DECREASED LIVER INTENSITY ON MRI

1. Hemochromatosis
2. Hemosiderosis
3. Superparamagnetic contrast medium
4. Wilson disease

References
1. Baron RL, Gore RM: Diffuse Liver Disease. In: Gore RM, Levine MS: Textbook of Gastrointestinal Radiology. (ed 2) Philadelphia: WB Saunders, 2000, pp 1590–1638
2. Gore RM: Liver: Differential diagnosis. In Gore RM, Levine MS (eds): Textbook of Gastrointestinal Radiology. (ed 2) Philadelphia: WB Saunders, 2000, pp 1712–1727
3. Mergo PJ, Ros PR: Benign lesions of the liver. Radiol Clin North Am 36:319–332, 1998

Gamut G-153

SPONTANEOUS LIVER RUPTURE

1. Hepatic tumor (eg, hepatocellular adenoma; hemangioma; hepatocellular carcinoma {hepatoma}
2. Oral contraceptive use
3. Oral estrogen therapy, long-term
4. Peliosis hepatis
5. Toxemia of pregnancy

Reference
1. Lundell CJ: Spontaneous hepatic rupture in postmenopausal women receiving oral estrogen replacement. JVIR 1993;4: 245–249

Gamut G-154

NEOPLASM OF THE LIVER (CHILD OR ADULT)

COMMON

1. Hepatocellular adenoma
2. Cholangiocarcinoma, intrahepatic
3. [Cyst (eg, simple; posttraumatic; hydatid)]
4. Hemangioma (cavernous; capillary)
5. Hepatocellular carcinoma (hepatoma)
6. Metastasis
7. Multiple bile duct hamartoma (von Meyenburg complex) (microbiliary hamartoma)
8. [Nodular regenerative hyperplasia; focal nodular hyperplasia]

UNCOMMON

1. [Adrenal rest]
2. Biliary cystadenoma
3. Carcinoid of liver, primary or metastatic
4. Cholangioma
5. Epithelioid hemangioendothelioma
6. Fibrolamellar carcinoma
7. Gastrointestinal stromal tumor$_g$ (eg, leiomyoma; fibroma)
8. Mesenchymal hamartoma (child)
9. Infantile hemangioendothelioma of liver (child)
10. Hepatoblastoma
11. Lymphangioma
12. Lymphoma$_g$
13. [Pancreatic rest]
14. Sarcoma (esp. angiosarcoma; also nonvascular sarcomas; Kaposi sarcoma)
15. [Splenosis]
16. Teratoma

[ ] This condition does not actually cause the gamuted imaging finding, but can produce imaging changes that simulate it.

References

1. Anthony CR: Tumors of the liver. Semin Roentgenol 1983;18:67–68
2. Buetow PC, Buck JL, Ros PR, et al: Malignant vascular tumors of the liver: radiologic-pathologic correlation. Radio-Graphics 1994;14:153
3. Del Pilar Fernandez M, Reduanly RD: Primary hepatic malignant neoplasms. Radiol Clin North Am 1998;36:333–348
4. Kew MC: Hepatic tumors and cysts. In: Feldman M, Scharschmidt BF, Sleisenger MH: Gastrointestinal and Liver Disease. (ed 6) Philadelphia: WB Saunders, 2000
5. Paley MR, Ros PR; Hepatic metastases. Radiol Clin North Am 1998;36:349–364
6. Ros PR, Taylor HM: Malignant tumors of the liver. In: Gore RM, Levine MS (eds): Textbook of Gastrointestinal Radiology. (ed 2) Philadelphia: WB Saunders, 2000, pp 1523–1568
7. Sato M, Ishida H, Konno K, et al: Liver tumors in children and young patients: sonographic and color Doppler findings. Abdom Imaging 2000;25:596–601
8. Siegel MJ: Pediatric Body CT. Philadelphia: Lippincott Williams & Wilkins, 1999
9. Stephens DH, Sheedy PF, Hattery RR, et al: Computed tomography of the liver. AJR 1977;128:579–590
10. Taybi H, Lachman RS: Radiology of Syndromes, Metabolic Disorders, and Skeletal Dysplasias. (ed 4) St. Louis: Mosby-Year Book, 1996
11. Welch TJ, Sheedy PF, Johnson CM, et al: Radiographic characteristics of benign liver tumors: focal nodular hyperplasia and hepatic adenoma. RadioGraphics 1985;5:673

Gamut G-155-1

SOLID LIVER LESION—ADULT (US, CT, MRI)

COMMON

1. Abscess (pyogenic, amebic, or fungal)
2. Focal fatty change (focal steatosis)
3. Focal nodular hyperplasia; adenomatous hyperplastic nodule
4. Hemangioma, cavernous or capillary
5. Hematoma
6. Hepatocellular adenoma
7. Hepatocellular carcinoma (hepatoma)—usually in cirrhotic or other damaged liver (eg, postradiation)
8. Metastasis (esp. from carcinoma of lung, breast, colon, kidney)

9. Multiple bile duct hamartoma (von Meyenburg complex) (microbiliary hamartoma)
10. Regenerating or dysplastic nodule (cirrhosis)

UNCOMMON

1. Aneurysm of hepatic artery
2. Angiomyolipoma of liver
3. Angiosarcoma of liver
4. Bacillary angiomatosis (in AIDS)
5. Biliary cystadenoma, cystadenocarcinoma
6. Cholangiocarcinoma
7. Extramedullary hematopoiesis
8. Fibrolamellar carcinoma
9. Fungus disease (esp. histoplasmosis; candidiasis)
10. Hydatid disease (*Echinococcus multilocularis* or healed *E. granulosus* cyst)
11. Infarct
12. Kaposi sarcoma
13. Lipoma
14. Lymphoma$_g$
15. Tuberculosis; other granulomatous disease
16. Visceral larval migrans granuloma

References

1. Kehagias D, Moulopoulos L, Antoniou A, et al: Focal nodular hyperplasia. Eur Radiol 2001;11:202–212
2. Kim CK, Lim JH, Lee WJ: Detection of hepatocellular carcinomas and dysplastic nodules in cirrhotic liver. J Ultrasound Med 2001;20:99–104
3. Ros PR, Taylor HM: Benign and malignant tumors of the liver. In: Gore RM, Levine MS: Textbook of Gastrointestinal Radiology. (ed 2) Philadelphia: WB Saunders, 2000, pp 1487–1568
4. Ros PR, Taylor HM, Barreda R, et al: Focal hepatic infections. In: Gore RM, Levine MS: Textbook of Gastrointestinal Radiology. (ed 2) Philadelphia: WB Saunders, 2000, pp 1569–1589
5. Semelka RC, Kelekis NL: Liver. In: Semelka RC, Ascher SM, Reinhold C (eds): MRI of the Abdomen and Pelvis: A Text-Atlas. New York: Wiley-Liss, 1997, pp 19–136
6. Taylor HM, Ros PR: Hepatic imaging: an overview. Radiol Clin North Am 1998;36:237–245
7. Williamson MR: Abdominal ultrasound. In: Essentials of Ultrasound. Philadelphia: WB Saunders, 1996, p 86

Gamut G-155-2

SOLID LIVER LESION—OLDER CHILD OR ADOLESCENT

COMMON

1. Abscess (pyogenic, amebic, or fungal)
2. Hepatocellular carcinoma (hepatoma)
3. Metastasis (esp. neuroblastoma; sarcoma)

UNCOMMON

1. Angiomyolipoma
2. Fibrolamellar carcinoma
3. Focal nodular hyperplasia
4. Hemangioma
5. Hematoma
6. Hepatocellular adenoma (usually associated with glycogen storage disease, type I or Fanconi anemia)
7. Hydatid disease (*Echinococcus multilocularis* or healed *E. granulosus* cyst)
8. Infarct
9. Lipoma
10. Lymphoma$_g$; leukemia; Burkitt lymphoma
11. Mesenchymal hamartoma
12. Multiple bile duct hamartoma
13. Peliosis hepatis
14. Sarcoma of liver (eg, undifferentiated (embryonal); mixed mesenchymal); rhabdomyosarcoma of bile ducts
15. Teratocarcinoma
16. Tuberculosis; other granulomatous disease

References

1. Ros PR, Taylor HM: Benign and malignant tumors of the liver. In: Gore RM, Levine MS: Textbook of Gastrointestinal Radiology. (ed 2) Philadelphia: WB Saunders, 2000, pp 1487–1568
2. Ros PR, Taylor HM, Barreda R, et al: Focal hepatic infections. In: Gore RM, Levine MS: Textbook of Gastrointestinal Radiology. (ed 2) Philadelphia: WB Saunders, 2000, pp 1569–1589
3. Sato M, Ishida H, Konno K, et al: Liver tumors in children and young patients: sonographic and color Doppler findings. Abdom Imaging 2000;25:596–601

(continued)

4. Siegel MJ: Pediatric Body CT. Philadelphia: Lippincott Williams & Wilkins, 1999
5. Taylor HM, Ros PR: Hepatic imaging: an overview. Radiol Clin North Am 1998;36:237–245

Gamut G-155-3

SOLID LIVER LESION—INFANT OR YOUNG CHILD (Under Age 5)

COMMON
*1. Hemangioma
2. Hepatoblastoma
*3. Infantile hemangioendothelioma

UNCOMMON
1. Abscess
2. Hematoma
3. Mesenchymal hamartoma
4. Metastasis (esp. neuroblastoma; sarcoma)

* Especially newborn to 6 months.

References
1. Cohen MD: Imaging of Children with Cancer. St. Louis: Mosby-Year Book, 1992, pp 20–42
2. Ros PR, Taylor HM: Benign and malignant tumors of the liver. In: Gore RM, Levine MS: Textbook of Gastrointestinal Radiology. (ed 2) Philadelphia: WB Saunders, 2000, pp 1487–1568
3. Sato M, Ishida H, Konno K, et al: Liver tumors in children and young patients: sonographic and color Doppler findings. Abdom Imaging 2000;25:596–601
4. Siegel MJ: Pediatric Body CT. Philadelphia: Lippincott Williams & Wilkins, 1999

Gamut G-156

SOLID LIVER MASSES—MULTIPLE

COMMON
1. Abscess (pyogenic, amebic, or fungal)
2. Fatty change in liver (steatosis)
3. Focal nodular hyperplasia
4. Fungus disease (eg, candidiasis; histoplasmosis)
5. Granulomatous disease (eg, sarcoidosis; tuberculosis)
6. Hemangioma
7. Hematoma (intrahepatic or subcapsular)
8. Lymphoma$_g$; Burkitt lymphoma
9. Metastases (esp. from carcinoma of lung, breast, colon, kidney)
10. Regenerating or dysplastic nodules (cirrhosis)

UNCOMMON
1. Angiosarcoma of liver
2. Bacillary angiomatosis (in AIDS)
3. Cholangiocarcinoma
4. Cytomegalovirus infection, multifocal
5. Drug-induced toxicity (eg, erythromycin; diphenyl-hydantoin)
6. Extramedullary hematopoiesis
7. Hepatic cystadenoma
8. Hepatocellular adenoma; adenomatosis
9. Hepatocellular carcinoma (hepatoma)
10. Hydatid disease (Echinococcus multilocularis or healed, calcified E. granulosus cysts)
11. Kaposi sarcoma
12. Mesenchymal hamartoma

References
1. Gore RM: Liver: Differential diagnosis. In: Gore RM, Levine MS: Textbook of Gastrointestinal Radiology. (ed 2) Philadelphia: WB Saunders, 2000, pp 1712–1727
2. Ros PR, Taylor HM: Benign and malignant tumors of the liver. In: Gore RM, Levine MS: Textbook of Gastrointestinal Radiology. (ed 2) Philadelphia: WB Saunders, 2000, pp 1487–1568
3. Ros PR, Taylor HM, Barreda R, et al: Focal hepatic infections. In: Gore RM, Levine MS: Textbook of Gastrointesti-

nal Radiology. (ed 2) Philadelphia: WB Saunders, 2000, pp 1569–1589

4. Sato M, Ishida H, Konno K, et al: Liver tumors in children and young patients: sonographic and color Doppler findings. Abdom Imaging 2000;25:596–601

5. Semelka RC, Kelekis NL: Liver. In: Semelka RC, Ascher SM, Reinhold C (eds): MRI of the Abdomen and Pelvis: A Text-Atlas. New York: Wiley-Liss, 1997, pp 19–136

6. Williamson MR: Abdominal ultrasound. In: Essentials of Ultrasound. Philadelphia: WB Saunders, 1996, p 86

7. Withers CE, Wilson SR: The liver. In: Rumack CM, Wilson SR, Charboneau JW (eds): Diagnostic Ultrasound. (ed 2) St. Louis: Mosby, 1998, pp 87–154

Gamut G-157

CYSTIC LIVER LESION(S) (US, CT, MRI) (Usually Anechoic or Hypoechoic on US and Low Density on CT)

COMMON

1. Abscess (pyogenic, amebic, or fungal)
2. Cyst, congenital or acquired (eg, epithelial; post-traumatic; hydatid)
3. Cystic metastasis (eg, mucinous adenocarcinoma of colon, stomach; cystadenocarcinoma of pancreas, ovary, or uterus; melanoma, carcinoid, or sarcoma with necrosis)
4. [Chilaiditi disease (interposition of colon between liver and diaphragm]
5. Hematoma, acute
6. Hydatid disease (*Echinococcus granulosus* and *E. multilocularis*)

UNCOMMON

1. Aneurysm of hepatic artery or portal vein
2. Biliary cystadenoma, cystadenocarcinoma
3. Biloma
4. Caroli disease
5. Cat-scratch disease
6. Cholangiocarcinoma

7. Choledochal cyst
8. Cystic duct remnant with mucocele
9. Cystic hepatocellular carcinoma (hepatoma)
10. Cystic lymphangioma, mesenchymal hamartoma, or other unusual cystic or necrotic tumor
11. Intrahepatic gallbladder
12. Mesenchmal hamartoma
13. Multiple bile duct hamartoma (Von Meyenburg complex)
14. Polycystic liver disease
15. Undifferentiated (embryonal) sarcoma
16. Von Hippel-Lindau disease

[ ] This condition does not actually cause the gamuted imaging finding, but can produce imaging changes that simulate it.

References

1. Eisenberg RL: Clinical Imaging: An Atlas of Differential Diagnosis. (ed 3) Philadelphia: Lippincott-Raven, 1997, pp 484–487

2. Ferrozzi F, Bova D, Campodonico F: Cystic primary neoplasms of the liver of the adult: CT features. Clin Imag 1993;17:292–296

3. Luo T, Itai Y, Eguchi N, et al: Von Meyenburg complexes of the liver: imaging findings. J Comput Assist Tomogr 1998; 22:372–378

4. Mergo PJ, Ros PR: Benign lesions of the liver. Radiol Clin North Am 1998;36:365–376

5. Parulekar SG, Bree RL: Liver. In: McGahan JP, Goldberg BB (eds): Diagnostic Ultrasound. Philadelphia: Lippincott-Raven, 1997, chapter 21

6. Semelka RC, Kelekis NL: Liver. In: Semelka RC, Ascher SM, Reinhold C (eds): MRI of the Abdomen and Pelvis: A Text-Atlas. New York: Wiley-Liss, 1997, pp 19–136

7. Singh Y, Winick AB, Tabbara SO: Multiloculated cystic liver lesions: radiologic-pathologic differential diagnosis. RadioGraphics 1997;17:219–224

8. Skolnick ML: Guide to the Ultrasound Examination of the Abdomen. New York: Springer-Verlag, 1986, pp 89–90

9. Withers CE, Wilson SR: The liver. In: Rumack CM, Wilson SR, Charboneau JW (eds): Diagnostic Ultrasound. (ed 2) St. Louis: Mosby, 1998, pp 87–154

Gamut G-158-1

LIVER LESION CHARACTERIZED BY LINEAR OR STELLATE CENTRAL SCAR (CT, US, ANGIO)

1. Cholangiocarcinoma
2. Fibrolamellar carcinoma
*3. Focal nodular hyperplasia
4. Hemangioma, giant cavernous
5. Hepatocellular adenoma
*6. Hepatocellular carcinoma (hepatoma)
7. Metastasis, hypervascular

* Usually isoechoic mass with hyperechoic linear or stellate central scar on ultrasound.

References
1. Gore RM: Liver: Differential diagnosis. In: Gore RM, Levine MS: Textbook of Gastrointestinal Radiology. (ed 2) Philadelphia: WB Saunders, 2000, pp 1712–1727
2. Parulekar SG, Bree RL: Liver. In: McGahan JP, Goldberg BB (eds): Diagnostic Ultrasound. Philadelphia: Lippincott-Raven, 1997, chapter 21
3. Ros PR, Taylor HM: Benign and malignant tumors of the liver. In: Gore RM, Levine MS: Textbook of Gastrointestinal Radiology. (ed 2) Philadelphia: WB Saunders, 2000, pp 1487–1568
4. Withers CW, Wilson SR: The liver. In: Rumack CM, Wilson SR, Charboneau JW (eds): Diagnostic Ultrasound. St. Louis: Mosby, 1998, pp 87–154

Gamut G-158-2

LIVER LESION WITH CENTRAL SCAR ON MRI

1. Cavernous hemangioma: hypo- or hyperintense T2-weighted image (either inflammatory or fibrous scar)
2. Fibrolamellar hepatocellular carcinoma: hypointense T1-WI, hyperintense T2-WI (fibrotic-repair of scar)
3. Focal nodular hyperplasia: hypointense T1-WI, hyperintense T2-WI (inflammatory scar)
4. Hepatocellular adenoma: variable signal

References
1. Pomeranz SJ; Gamuts and Pearls in MRI. (ed 2) Cincinnati: MRI-EFI Publications, 1993
2. Ros PR, Taylor HM: Benign and malignant tumors of the liver. In: Gore RM, Levine MS: Textbook of Gastrointestinal Radiology. (ed 2) Philadelphia: WB Saunders, 2000, pp 1487–1568
3. Semelka RC, Kelekis NL: Liver. In: Semelka RC, Ascher SM, Reinhold C (eds): MRI of the Abdomen and Pelvis: A Text-Atlas. New York: Wiley-Liss, 1997, pp 19–136

Gamut G-159

LIVER LESION CHARACTERIZED BY BLOOD OR HEMORRHAGE

COMMON

1. Hemangioma
2. Hematoma
3. Hepatocellular adenoma
4. Hepatocellular carcinoma (hepatoma)

UNCOMMMON

1. Angiosarcoma of liver
2. Bacillary angiomatosis (in AIDS)
3. Kaposi sarcoma
4. Peliosis hepatis

References
1. Mergo PJ, Ros PR: Benign lesions of the liver. Radiol Clin North Am 1998;36:365–376
2. Ros PR, Taylor HM: Benign and malignant tumors of the liver. In: Gore RM, Levine MS: Textbook of Gastrointestinal Radiology. (ed 2) Philadelphia: WB Saunders, 2000, pp 1487–1568

LIVER LESION CHARACTERIZED BY CALCIFICATION

COMMON

1. Abscess, healed (pyogenic, amebic, or fungal)
2. Calculus(i) in biliary tract
3. Granuloma (eg, tuberculosis; histoplasmosis; coccidioidomycosis; brucellosis)
4. Hemangioma, cavernous
5. Hematoma, old
6. Hepatocellular carcinoma (hepatoma), esp. treated
7. Hydatid disease (*Echinococcus granulosus* or *E. multilocularis)*
8. Metastases (eg, from osteosarcoma; chondrosarcoma; mucinous or colloid adenocarcinoma of colon, rectum, ovary, breast, pancreas, stomach, or thyroid; islet cell carcinoma; carcinoid; teratocarcinoma; leiomyosarcoma; neuroblastoma; pheochromocytoma; treated melanoma or lymphoma)

UNCOMMON

1. Biliary cystadenocarcinoma
2. Calcified gallbladder (porcelain gallbladder)
3. Calcified hepatic artery (incl. aneurysm)
4. Cholangiocarcinoma
5. Cyst, nonparasitic, congenital or acquired
6. Fibrolamellar carcinoma
7. Gumma (hepar lobatum)
8. Hemangioendothelioma (epithelioid or infantile)
9. Hepatoblastoma
10. Hepatocellular adenoma
11. Mesenchymal hamartoma
12. Regenerating nodules in cirrhosis (rarely)

13. Schistosomiasis (turtleshell appearance, esp. *S. japonica*)
14. Thromboembolus of portal vein, calcified

References
1. Darlak JJ, Moskowitz M, Katten KR: Calcifications in the liver. Radiol Clin North Am 1980;18:209–219
2. Paley MR, Ros PR: Hepatic calcification. Radiol Clin North Am 1998;36:391–398
3. Parulekar SG, Bree RL: Liver. In: McGahan JP, Goldberg BB: Diagnostic Ultrasound. Philadelphia: Lippincott-Raven, 1997, chapter 21
4. Stoupis C, Taylor HM, Paley MR, et al: The rocky liver: radiologic-pathologic correlation of calcified hepatic masses. Radiographics 1998;18:675–685

LIVER LESION CHARACTERIZED BY FAT (CT, MRI)

1. Angiomyolipoma of liver
2. Focal fatty change
3. Focal nodular hyperplasia
4. Hepatocellular adenoma
5. Hepatocellular carcinoma (hepatoma)
6. Langerhans cell histiocytosis$_g$
7. Lipoma
8. Metastasis (eg, liposarcoma; teratoid tumor)
9. Myelolipoma

References
1. Roberts JL, Fishman EK, Hartman DS, et al.: Lipomatous tumors of the liver: evaluation with CT and US. Radiology 1986;158:613–617
2. Ros PR: Hepatic angiomyolipoma: is fat in the liver friend or foe? Abdom Imaging 1994;19:552–553

Gamut G-162

LIVER LESION CHARACTERIZED BY BULL'S-EYE APPEARANCE

1. Fungus disease (eg, candidiasis, usually in immuno-compromised individual); other opportunistic infections
2. Kaposi sarcoma
3. Lymphoma$_g$; leukemia
4. Metastasis
5. Sarcoidosis
6. Septic emboli

References

1. Dähnert W: Radiology Review Manual. (ed 4) Baltimore, Williams & Wilkins, 1999
2. Paley MR, Ros PR: Hepatic metastases. Radiol Clin North Am 1998;36:349–364

Gamut G-163

LIVER LESION CHARACTERIZED BY FLUID-FLUID LEVEL

1. Biliary cystadenoma
2. Hemangioma
3. Hematoma
4. Hepatic cyst (with hemorrhage or infection)
5. Hepatocellular adenoma (hemorrhagic)
6. Hepatocellular carcinoma (hepatoma), cystic
7. Metastasis (eg, leiomyosarcoma; adenocarcinoma of lung or ovary; carcinoid)

Reference

1. Soyer P, Bluemke DA, Fishman EK, Rymer R: Fluid-fluid levels within focal hepatic lesions: imaging appearance and etiology. Abd Imag 1998;23:161–165

Gamut G-164

LIVER LESION CHARACTERIZED BY "FILL-IN" (ANGIO, POSTCONTRAST CT OR MRI)

1. Cholangiocarcinoma
2. Focal nodular hyperplasia
3. Hemangioendothelioma (epithelioid or infantile)
4. Hemangioma
5. Hepatocellular carcinoma (hepatoma)
6. Kaposi sarcoma
7. Leiomyosarcoma
8. Lymphoma$_g$
9. Metastasis
10. Vascular malformation

References

1. Ito K, Honjo K, Fujita T, et al: Liver neoplasms: diagnostic pitfalls in cross sectional imaging. RadioGraphics 1996; 16:273–283
2. Shirkhoda A, Salmanzadeh A: Hepatic lesions which "fill-in" on contrast-enhanced CT and MR imaging: patterns and diagnostic pitfalls

Gamut G-165-S

LIVER LESIONS—CLINICAL CONSIDERATIONS

Nonsurgical Liver Lesions

1. Abscess (except for possible drainage)
2. Cyst (eg, simple; posttraumatic; hydatid)
3. Fatty liver
4. Focal nodular hyperplasia
5. Hemangioma

Painless Liver Lesions

1. Cyst (eg, simple; hydatid)
2. Focal nodular hyperplasia
3. Hemangioma
4. Hepatocellular adenoma (small)

Liver Lesions Related to Excessive Steroids

1. Focal nodular hyperplasia
2. Hemangioma
3. Hepatocellular adenoma
4. Hepatocellular carcinoma (hepatoma)
5. Nodular regenerative hyperplasia

Liver Neoplasms With Elevated Alpha Fetal Protein (AFP)

1. Hepatoblastoma
2. Hepatocellular carcinoma (hepatoma)

Sex Predilection for Liver Neoplasms

1. Hepatic neoplasm is usually benign in women
2. Hepatic neoplasm is usually malignant in men

Reference

1. Ros PR, Taylor HM: Benign and malignant tumors of the liver. In: Gore RM, Levine MS: Textbook of Gastrointestinal Radiology. (ed 2) Philadelphia: WB Saunders, 2000, pp 1487–1568

Gamut G-166

LIVER METASTASES—CALCIFIED

COMMON

1. Endocrine carcinoma of pancreas (esp. islet cell tumor)
2. Malignant melanoma
3. Medullary or colloid carcinoma of breast or thyroid
4. Mucinous adenocarcinoma of colon or stomach
5. Neuroblastoma
6. Papillary serous cystadenocarcinoma of ovary
7. Sarcoma (esp. osteosarcoma; chondrosarcoma; leiomyosarcoma)

UNCOMMON

1. Carcinoma of lung or testis
2. Lymphoma$_g$, treated

3. Mesothelioma
4. Renal cell carcinoma

References

1. Burgener FA, Kormano M: Differential Diagnosis in Computed Tomography. New York: Thieme, 1996
2. Dähnert W: Radiology Review Manual. (ed 4) Baltimore: Williams & Wilkins, 1999, p 596
3. Paley MR, Ros PR: Hepatic metastases. Radiol Clin North Am 1998;36:349–364
4. Ros PR, Taylor HM: Malignant tumors of the liver. In: Gore RM, Levine MS (eds): Textbook of Gastrointestinal Radiology. (ed 2) Philadelphia: WB Saunders, 2000, pp 1523–1568

Gamut G-167

LIVER METASTASES— HYPERVASCULAR

COMMON

1. Carcinoid
2. Carcinoma of breast
3. Carcinoma of colon
4. Choriocarcinoma
5. Endocrine carcinoma of pancreas (esp. islet cell tumor)
6. Malignant melanoma
7. Renal cell carcinoma (hypernephroma)

UNCOMMON

1. Cystadenocarcinoma of ovary
2. Pheochromocytoma
3. Sarcoma (esp. osteosarcoma; chondrosarcoma; leiomyosarcoma)

References

1. Dähnert W: Radiology Review Manual. (ed 4) Baltimore: Williams & Wilkins, 1999, p 596
2. Paley MR, Ros PR: Hepatic metastases. Radiol Clin North Am 1998;36:349–364
3. Ros PR, Taylor HM: Malignant tumors of the liver. In: Gore RM, Levine MS (eds): Textbook of Gastrointestinal Radiology. (ed 2) Philadelphia: WB Saunders, 2000, pp 1523–1568

Gamut G-168

LIVER METASTASES—HEMORRHAGIC

COMMON

1. Carcinoma of breast
2. Carcinoma of colon
3. Carcinoma of thyroid
4. Choriocarcinoma
5. Malignant melanoma
6. Renal cell carcinoma (hypernephroma)

References
1. Dähnert W: Radiology Review Manual. (ed 4) Baltimore: Williams & Wilkins, 1999, p 597
2. Paley MR, Ros PR: Hepatic metastases. Radiol Clin North Am 1998;36:349–364
3. Ros PR, Taylor HM: Malignant tumors of the liver. In: Gore RM, Levine MS (eds): Textbook of Gastrointestinal Radiology. (ed 2) Philadelphia: WB Saunders, 2000, pp 1523–1568

Gamut G-169

LIVER METASTASES—CYSTIC

COMMON

1. Carcinoma of colon
2. Choriocarcinoma
3. Malignant melanoma
4. Mucinous carcinoma of ovary
5. Sarcoma (eg, osteosarcoma; chondrosarcoma; leiomyosarcoma)

UNCOMMON

1. Carcinoid
2. Carcinoma of lung (esp. small cell)
3. Carcinoma of stomach
4. Endometrial carcinoma of uterus

Reference
1. Dähnert W: Radiology Review Manual. (ed 4) Baltimore: Williams & Wilkins, 1999, p 597

Gamut G-170

LIVER METASTASES— ULTRASOUND CHARACTERISTICS

HYPOECHOIC LESIONS (37.5%)

COMMON

1. Carcinoma of breast
2. Carcinoma of pancreas (36%)
3. Carcinoma of cervix (20%)
4. Lymphoma$_g$

UNCOMMON

1. Adenocarcinoma of lung
2. Carcinoma of nasopharynx

MIXED ECHOGENICITY (37.5%)

COMMON

1. Carcinoma of breast
2. Carcinoma of rectum
3. Carcinoma of lung
4. Carcinoma of stomach
5. Hepatocellular carcinoma (hepatoma)

UNCOMMON

1. Anaplastic carcinoma
2. Carcinoma of cervix
3. Vascular primaries (carcinoid; islet cell carcinoma of pancreas; choriocarcinoma; renal cell carcinoma)

HYPERECHOIC LESIONS WITH SHADOWING (25%)

COMMON

1. Adenocarcinoma of stomach
2. Cystadenocarcinoma of pancreas
3. Melanoma
4. Mucinous or colloid carcinoma of colon or breast
5. Pseudomucinous cystadenocarcinoma of ovary

UNCOMMON

1. Chondrosarcoma
2. Neuroblastoma
3. Osteosarcoma
4. Teratocarcinoma

CYSTIC METASTASES (See G-169)

1. Central necrosis of any malignant lesion, esp. sarcomas
2. Mucin-secreting metastases from carcinoma of the ovary, colon, pancreas, or stomach

BULL'S-EYE OR TARGET PATTERN

1. Carcinoma of lung
2. Other carcinomas (occasionally)

INFILTRATIVE PATTERN

1. Carcinoma of breast
2. Carcinoma of lung
3. Melanoma

References

1. Dähnert W: Radiology Review Manual. (ed 4) Baltimore: Williams & Wilkins, 1999, p 597
2. Gore RM: Liver: Differential diagnosis. In Gore RM, Levine MS (eds): Textbook of Gastrointestinal Radiology. (ed 2) Philadelphia: WB Saunders, 2000, pp 1712–1727
3. Paley MR, Ros PR: Hepatic metastases. Radiol Clin North Am 1998;36:349–364

AVASCULAR OR HYPOVASCULAR LIVER LESION (ANGIO, POSTCONTRAST CT OR MRI)

COMMON

*1. Abscess (eg, pyogenic, amebic, or fungal)
2. Cholangiocarcinoma
*3. Cyst (congenital; inflammatory; hydatid; traumatic)
4. [Extrinsic mass (eg, gallbladder; adrenal neoplasm; subphrenic abscess)]
*5. Focal fatty change
*6. Metastasis

UNCOMMON

1. Adrenal rest
2. [Biloma, traumatic or iatrogenic (eg, needle biopsy)]
3. Hematoma
*4. Lymphoma$_g$
5. Mesenchymal hamartoma
6. Neoplasm, benign or malignant, other (eg, gastrointestinal stromal tumor$_g$; teratoma; lipoma)
*7. Polycystic disease of liver

* May be multiple.
[ ] This condition does not actually cause the gamuted imaging finding, but can produce imaging changes that simulate it.

References

1. Guermazi A, Brice P, de Kerviler E, et al: Extranodal Hodgkin disease: spectrum of disease. RadioGraphics 2001; 21:161–179
2. Ros PR, Taylor HM: Benign and malignant tumors of the liver. In: Gore RM, Levine MS: Textbook of Gastrointestinal Radiology. (ed 2) Philadelphia: WB Saunders, 2000, pp 1487–1568

HYPERVASCULAR OR HYPERDENSE LIVER LESION (ANGIO, POSTCONTRAST CT OR MRI)

COMMON

*1. Focal fatty sparing (simulates enhancing mass)
*2. Focal nodular hyperplasia
*3. Hemangioma, cavernous or capillary
 4. Hepatoblastoma
 5. Hepatocellular adenoma
 6. Hepatocellular carcinoma (hepatoma)
*7. Metastasis, hypervascular (eg, carcinoid; islet cell tumor of pancreas; pheochromocytoma; leiomyosarcoma; other sarcomas; choriocarcinoma; carcinoma of breast, colon, kidney, or thyroid; malignant melanoma)

UNCOMMON

 1. Aneurysm of hepatic artery, true or false (incl. arteriobiliary fistula) or portal vein
 2. Angiosarcoma of liver
*3. Arteriovenous fistula (eg, congenital; traumatic; iatrogenic); arterio-portal shunt in some hepatomas
 4. Fibrolamellar carcinoma
 5. Hemangioendothelioma, epithelioid
 6. Vascular phenomena (eg, SVC obstruction; Budd-Chiari S.; transient hepatic attenuation difference {THAD})

* May be multiple.

References

1. Adler J, Goodgold M, Mitty H, et al: Arteriovenous shunts involving the liver. Radiology 1978;129:315–322
2. Bressler EL, Alpern MB, Glazer GM, et al: Hypervascular hepatic metastases: CT evaluation. Radiology 1987;162;49–51
3. Kehagias D, Moulopoulos L, Antoniou A, et al: Focal nodular hyperplasia: imaging findings. Eur Radiol 2001;11:202–212
4. Murakami T, Kim T, Takamura M, et al: Hypervascular hepatocellular carcinoma: detection with double arterial phase multi-detector helical CT. Radiology 2001;218:763–767
5. Oliver JH, Baron RL, Federle MP, et al: Hypervascular liver metastasis: do unenhanced and hepatic arterial phase CT images affect tumor detection? Radiology 1997;205:709–715
6. Quiroga S, Sebastia C, Pallisa E, et al: Improved diagnosis of hepatic perfusion disorders: Value of hepatic arterial phase imaging during helical CT. RadioGraphics 2001;21:65–81
7. Slone RM, Fisher AJ: Pocket Guide to Body CT Differential Diagnosis. New York: McGraw-Hill, 1999, pp 219–220

ANECHOIC LIVER LESION (USUALLY CYSTIC ON US)

COMMON

*1. Caroli disease
*2. Congenital simple cyst
 3. Metastasis, cystic (eg, from mucinous carcinoma of colon; carcinoma of stomach or uterus; cystadenocarcinoma of ovary or pancreas; squamous cell carcinoma, esp. bronchogenic; carcinoid; malignant melanoma; sarcoma, esp. leiomyosarcoma)
*4. Polycystic liver disease

UNCOMMON

 1. Abscess (pyogenic, amebic, or fungal)
*2. Acquired cyst (eg, posttraumatic; inflammatory)
*3. Aneurysm of hepatic artery or portal vein
 4. Biliary cystadenoma, cystadenocarcinoma
*5. Biloma
*6. [Chilaiditi disease (interposition of colon between liver and diaphragm)]
*7. Choledochal cyst
 8. Cystic or necrotic neoplasm
*9. Cystic duct remnant with mucocele
10. Hematoma, acute
11. Hydatid cyst
*12. Intrahepatic gallbladder
13. Lymphoma$_g$

* Usually unilocular with smooth walls and distal acoustic enhancement.
[ ] This condition does not actually cause the gamuted imaging finding, but can produce imaging changes that simulate it.

References
1. Eisenberg RL: Clinical Imaging: An Atlas of Differential Diagnosis. (ed 3) Philadelphia: Lippincott-Raven, 1997, pp 484–487
2. Parulekar SG, Bree RL: Liver. In: McGahan JP, Goldberg BB (eds): Diagnostic Ultrasound. Philadelphia: Lippincott-Raven, 1997, chapter 21
3. Skolnick ML: Guide to the Ultrasound Examination of the Abdomen. New York: Springer-Verlag, 1986, pp 89–90
4. Williamson MR: Abdominal ultrasound. In: Essentials of Ultrasound. Philadelphia: WB Saunders, 1996, p 81
5. Withers CE, Wilson SR: The liver. In: Rumack CM, Wilson SR, Charboneau JW (eds): Diagnostic Ultrasound. (ed 2) St. Louis: Mosby, 1998, pp 87–154

Gamut G-174

HYPOECHOIC LIVER LESION (US)

COMMON

  1. Abscess (pyogenic, amebic, or fungal)
  2. Cyst, complicated (eg, with cholesterol crystals)
*3. Cystic liver tumor (eg, cholangiocarcinoma; biliary cystadenoma or cystadenocarcinoma; lymphangioma; mesenchymal hamartoma)
+4. Focal nodular hyperplasia
  5. Hematoma, acute
+6. Hepatocellular carcinoma (hepatoma)
  7. Infarct
  8. Lymphoma$_g$; Burkitt lymphoma
+9. Metastasis, incl. cystic metastasis (eg, from carcinoma of breast, lung, colon, stomach, ovary, pancreas)

UNCOMMON

  1. Biloma
+2. Candidiasis (wheel within a wheel)
  3. Extramedullary hematopoiesis
  4. Focal hepatic necrosis
  5. Focal sparing in fatty liver (steatosis)
  6. Granuloma (eg, tuberculosis)
  7. Hemangioendothelioma of liver
  8. Hemangioma, cavernous (more often hyperechoic)

+9. Hepatocellular adenoma
*10. Hydatid disease (*Echinococcus granulosus or E. multilocularis*)

* Usually a multicystic image on ultrasound.
+ Hepatic mass with hypoechoic halo.

References
1. Gore RM: Liver: differential diagnosis. In: Gore RM, Levine MS: Textbook of Gastrointestinal Radiology. (ed 2) Philadelphia: WB Saunders, 2000, pp 1712–1726
2. Parulekar SG, Bree RL: Liver. In: McGahan JP, Goldberg BB (eds): Diagnostic Ultrasound. Philadelphia: Lippincott-Raven, 1997, chapter 21
3. Skolnick ML: Guide to the Ultrasound Examination of the Abdomen. New York: Springer-Verlag, 1986, pp 91–92
4. Weill FS: Ultrasound Diagnosis of Digestive Diseases. (ed 3 revised) Berlin: Springer-Verlag, 1990, pp 239–246
5. Withers CE, Wilson SR: The liver. In: Rumack CM, Wilson SR, Charboneau JW (eds): Diagnostic Ultrasound. St. Louis: Mosby-Year Book, 1998, pp 87–154

Gamut G-175

HYPERECHOIC LIVER LESION (US)

COMMON

  1. Cirrhosis (multifocal regenerating nodules)
  2. Focal fatty infiltration (focal steatosis)
*3. Hemangioma
  4. Hepatocellular adenoma
*5. Hepatocellular carcinoma (hepatoma)
  6. Lipoma
  7. Metastasis {esp. from carcinoma of colon, stomach, ovary, kidney or pancreas {incl. islet cell carcinoma}; carcinoid*; choriocarcinoma)

UNCOMMON

  1. Angiomyolipoma
  2. Debris inside abscess or hematoma
  3. Dysplastic nodule
  4. Focal nodular hyperplasia
*5. Hemangioendothelioma
  6. Hepatic fissure

(continued)

7. Hydatid disease (old healed, calcified *E. granulosus* cyst; *Echinococcus multilocularis*—multifocal)
8. Infection (eg, cytomegalovirus or *Candida)*
9. Lymphoma$_g$
10. Omentum inserted into bed of hepatic resection
*11. Peliosis hepatis
12. Postradiation therapy
13. Solitary fibrous tumor of the liver

* Hyperechoic hepatic mass(es) with punctate calcifications and/or acoustic enhancement on ultrasound.

References

1. Fuksbrumer MS, Klimstra D, Panicek DM: Solitary fibrous tumor of the liver: Imaging findings. AJR 2000;175:1683–1687
2. Numata K, Tanaka K, Kiba T, et al: Contrast-enhanced, wide-band harmonic gray scale imaging of hepatocellular carcinoma. J Ultrasound Med 2001;20:89–98
3. Parulekar SG, Bree RL: Liver. In: McGahan JP, Goldberg BB (eds): Diagnostic Ultrasound. Philadelphia: Lippincott-Raven, 1997, chapter 21
4. Ros PR, Taylor HM: Benign and malignant tumors of the liver. In: Gore RM, Levine MS: Textbook of Gastrointestinal Radiology. (ed 2) Philadelphia: WB Saunders, 2000, pp 1487–1568
5. Rumack CM, Wilson SR, Charboneau JW (eds): Diagnostic Ultrasound. St. Louis: Mosby, 1998
6. Weill FS: Ultrasound Diagnosis of Digestive Diseases. (ed 3 revised) Berlin: Springer-Verlag, 1990, pp 239–246
7. Withers CW, Wilson SR: The liver. In: Rumack CM, Wilson SR, Charboneau JW (eds): Diagnostic Ultrasound. St. Louis: Mosby-Year Book, 1998, pp 87–154

Gamut G-176

ISOECHOIC LIVER LESION (US)

1. Focal nodular hyperplasia
2. Hepatocellular adenoma
3. Hepatocellular carcinoma (hepatoma)

Reference

1. Withers CW, Wilson SR: The liver. In: Rumack CM, Wilson SR, Charboneau JW (eds): Diagnostic Ultrasound. St. Louis: Mosby-Year Book, 1998, pp 87–154

Gamut G-177

HETEROGENEOUS HEPATIC ECHOGENICITY ON ULTRASOUND (COMPLEX HEPATIC MASS OR DIFFUSE PARENCHYMAL INVOLVEMENT)

COMMON

1. Abscess
2. Cavernous hemangioma
*3. Cirrhosis
*4. Fatty change in liver
5. Focal nodular hyperplasia
6. Hepatocellular carcinoma (hepatoma)
7. Hydatid cyst (with collapsed daughter cysts)
*8. Metastasis with mixed echogenicity or diffuse infiltration (eg, from carcinoma of breast, lung, or ovary; melanoma)
9. Neoplasm with liquefaction necrosis (hypoechoic) and infarcted nonliquefied areas (hyperechoic)

UNCOMMON

1. Biliary cystadenoma
2. Cholangiocarcinoma
3. Hemangioendothelioma; angiosarcoma
4. Hepatic adenoma, esp. after oral contraceptive use, or in glycogen storage disease, type I (von Gierke disease)
5. Hepatoblastoma
*6. Peliosis hepatitis

* Usually generalized or multifocal.

References

1. Eisenberg RL: Clinical Imaging: An Atlas of Differential Diagnosis. Gaithersburg, MD: Aspen Publ, 1992
2. Parulekar SG, Bree RL: Liver. In: McGahan JP, Goldberg BB (eds): Diagnostic Ultrasound. Philadelphia: Lippincott-Raven, 1997, chapter 21
3. Skolnick ML: Guide to the Ultrasound Examination of the Abdomen. New York: Springer-Verlag, 1986, p 93
4. Withers CW, Wilson SR: The liver. In: Rumack CM, Wilson SR, Charboneau JW (eds): Diagnostic Ultrasound. St. Louis: Mosby, 1998, pp 87–154

Gamut G178-S

HEPATIC PSEUDOLESION (US)

1. Diaphragmatic leaflets: peripheral echogenic pseudolesion may simulate hemangiomas
2. Falciform ligament: echogenic "mass" (pseudo-lesion) in left lobe
3. Focal fatty infiltration: echogenic pseudolesion may simulate metastases
4. Focal hepatic sparing in steatosis: hypoechoic pseudolesion often seen in porta hepatis
5. Gallbladder inflammation: hypoechoic hepatic pseudolesion in adjacent parenchyma
6. Ligamentum venosum: fibrous tissue attenuates sound, causing hypoechoic pseudolesion in caudate lobe
7. Perihepatic fat may invaginate liver causing hyper-echoic masses

Reference
1. Gore RM: Liver: Differential diagnosis. In Gore RM, Levine MS (eds): Textbook of Gastrointestinal Radiology. (ed 2) Philadelphia: WB Saunders, 2000, pp 1712–1727

Gamut G-179

INTRAHEPATIC ACOUSTIC SHADOWING (LINEAR VERSUS FOCAL) ON US

LINEAR OR BRANCHING SHADOWING
1. Air in biliary tract
2. Air in portal vein
3. Calculi in biliary ducts

FOCAL SHADOWING
1. Calcification (eg, primary or metastatic tumor; granuloma; healed abscess; aneurysm)
2. Foreign material (eg, surgical clips, drains, catheters, stents, sponges)

3. Gas (eg, in abscess; necrotic tumor; sequela of tumor embolization or biopsy)
4. Parasites in bile ducts (eg, *Clonorchis; Ascaris; Fasciola*) (may also show linear shadowing)
5. Parasitic disease in liver parenchyma (eg, hydatid disease; amebic abscess; pentastomiasis (*Armillifer* infection)
6. Refractile artifacts (eg, junction of vessels; gall-bladder neck)

References
1. Gore RM: Liver: Differential diagnosis. In Gore RM, Levine MS (eds): Textbook of Gastrointestinal Radiology. (ed 2) Philadelphia: WB Saunders, 2000, pp 1712–1727
2. Parulekar SG, Bree RL: Liver. In: McGahan JP, Goldberg BB (eds): Diagnostic Ultrasound. Philadelphia: Lippincott-Raven, 1997, chapter 21
3. Withers CW, Wilson SR: The liver. In: Rumack CM, Wilson SR, Charboneau JW (eds): Diagnostic Ultrasound. St. Louis: Mosby, 1998, pp 87–154

Gamut G-180

FOCAL LOW DENSITY (DECREASED ATTENUATION) LIVER LESION (NONENHANCED CT)

COMMON
1. Abscess (pyogenic, amebic, or fungal)
2. Cyst (eg, congenital; epithelial; posttraumatic; hydatid)
3. Focal fatty infiltration (focal steatosis)
4. Focal nodular hyperplasia
5. Hemangioma
6. Hematoma; laceration (posttraumatic)
7. Hepatocellular adenoma
8. Hepatocellular carcinoma (hepatoma)
9. Hydatid disease (*Echinococcus granulosis* and *E. multilocularis*)
10. Lymphoma$_g$
11. Metastasis (esp. from carcinoma of lung, breast, colon, kidney)

(continued)

UNCOMMON

1. Angiosarcoma of liver (may have high density regions with hemorrhage)
2. Biliary cystadenoma, cystadenoarcinoma (near water density on CT)
3. Biloma
4. Caroli disease
5. Cholangiocarcinoma
6. Choledochal cyst
7. Fibrolamellar carcinoma
8. Fungus disease with multiple microabscesses (eg, *Candida; Cryptococcus*)
9. Hemangioendothelioma
10. Hepatoblastoma
11. Infarct
12. Mesenchymal hamartoma
13. Multiple bile duct hamartoma
14. Polycystic liver disease
15. Radiation therapy (fatty replacement)
16. Schistosomiasis
17. Von Hippel-Lindau disease

References
1. Mathieu D, Bruneton JN, Drouillard J, et al: Hepatic adenomas and focal nodular hyperplasia: dynamic CT study. Radiology 1986;160:53–58
2. Slone RM, Fisher AJ: Pocket Guide to Body CT Differential Diagnosis. New York: McGraw-Hill, 1999, pp 212–214

Gamut G-181

FOCAL LOW DENSITY LIVER LESION (POSTCONTRAST CT)

COMMON

1. Abscess (pyogenic, amebic, or fungal)
2. Cyst (eg, congenital; epithelial; posttraumatic; hydatid)
3. Focal fatty infiltration (focal steatosis)
4. Hemangioma, giant
5. Hematoma
6. Hydatid disease (*Echinococcus granulosis* and *E. multilocularis*)

7. Metastasis (esp. from carcinoma of lung, breast, colon, kidney)
8. Regenerating nodules

UNCOMMON

1. Biloma
2. Caroli disease
3. Cholangiocarcinoma (late enhancement)
4. Fungus disease with multiple microabscesses (eg, *Candida; Cryptococcus*)
5. Lymphangioma
6. Polycystic liver disease
7. Radiation therapy (fatty replacement)
8. Schistosomiasis
9. Von Hipple-Lindau disease

Reference
1. Slone RM, Fisher AJ: Pocket Guide to Body CT Differential Diagnosis. New York: McGraw-Hill, 1999, pp 215–216

Gamut G-182

FOCAL HIGH DENSITY LIVER LESION (NONENHANCED CT)

1. Granuloma (esp. tuberculoma)
2. Hematoma, subcapsular or intrahepatic (first few days)
3. Hepatic tumor (eg, hepatocellular carcinoma {hepatoma}; hepatoblastoma; hemangioendothelioma)
4. Hepatocellular adenoma with acute hemorrhage
5. Hydatid disease (old healed, calcified *E. granulosus* cyst; *Echinococcus multilocularis*—with calcification)
6. Metastasis with calcification (eg, from colon, rectum, stomach, ovary)

References
1. Bressler EL, et al: Hypervascular hepatic metastases: CT evaluation. Radiology 1987; 162:49–51
2. Chapman S, Nakielny R: Aids to Radiological Differential Diagnosis. (ed 2) London, Bailliere Tindall, 1990, p 235.

---

3. Ros PR, Rosado de Christenson ML, Buetow PC, et al: Image interpretation session: 1997. Radiographics 1998;18: 199–202

4. Scatarige JC, Fishman EK, Saksouk FA, Siegelman SS: Computed tomography of calcified liver masses. J Comput Assist Tomogr 1983; 7:83–89

Gamut G-184-S

MRI CHARACTERISTICS OF VARIOUS LIVER LESIONS

	T1W	T2W	Gadolinium
1. Adenoma	Hyperintense	Hypointense	
2. Focal nodular hyperplasia			
central scar	Hypointense	Hyperintense+	+
margins	Isointense	Hyperintense	+/-
3. Hemangioma	Hypointense	Hyperintense ++	+ (like CT)
4. Hemochromatosis/ Iron deposition	Hypointense	Hypointense++	
5. Hepatocellular carcinoma	Hypo-, iso-, or hyperintense (due to fat degeneration)	Hyperintense	+
6. Metastasis	Hypointense	Hyperintense	+
7. Regenerating nodule	Hypo- or insointense	Hypointense	

References
1. Chapman S, Nakielny R: Aids to Radiological Differential Diagnosis. (ed 3) London: Saunders, 1995, p 279
2. Choi BI, Takayasu K, Han MC: Small hepatocellular carcinomas and associated nodular lesions of the liver: pathology, pathogenesis and imaging findings. AJR 1993;160:1177–1187
3. Vilgrain V, Flejou J-F, Arrive L: Focal nodular hyperplasia of the liver: MR imaging and pathologic correlation in 37 patients. Radiology 1992;184:699–703

Gamut G-185

LIVER LESIONS WITH CIRCUMFERENTIAL RIM ON MRI

HYPOINTENSE RIM ON T1-WEIGHTED IMAGE
1. Abscess, pyogenic or amebic (concentric rims; rim of collagen)
2. Hematoma, chronic (hemosiderin)
3. Hepatocellular carcinoma (hepatoma) (pseudocapsular rim is thin)
4. Hydatid cyst (thick, homogeneous rim; no perilesional edema)

HYPOINTENSE RIM ON T2-WEIGHTED IMAGE
1. Abscess, pyogenic or amebic (one or two concentric rings of mixed signal intensity)
2. Hematoma, subacute to chronic (white rim also seen on T1-weighted images)
3. Hydatid cyst (thick, homogeneous rim; no perilesional edema; high signal cyst contents on T2)
4. Metastasis (peritumoral edema with double ring pattern)

NO RIM
1. Cavernous hemangioma
2. Cyst, simple

(continued)

3. Focal nodular hyperplasia
4. Hepatocellular adenoma

References
1. Elizondo G, Weissleder R, Stark DD, et al: Amebic liver abscess—diagnosis and treatment evaluation with MR imaging. Radiology 1987;165:795–800
2. Gore RM: Liver: Differential diagnosis. In Gore RM, Levine MS (eds): Textbook of Gastrointestinal Radiology. (ed 2) Philadelphia: WB Saunders, 2000, pp 1712–1727
3. Hahn PF, Stark DD, Saini S, et al: The differential diagnosis of ringed hepatic lesions in MR imaging. AJR 1990;154:287–290
4. Hoff FL, Aisen AM, Walden ME, Glazer GM: MR imaging in hydatid disease of the liver. Gastrointest Radiol 1987;12:39–42
5. Rummeny E, Weissleder R, Stark DD, et al: Primary liver tumors: diagnosis by MR imaging. AJR 1989;152:63–72
6. Wittenberg J, Stark DD, Forman BH, et al: Differentiation of hepatic metastases from hepatic hemangiomas and cysts by using MR imaging. AJR 1988;151:79–84

10. Proteinaceous material in dependent portion of abscess or hematoma
11. [Pulsation artifact from aorta]

[ ] This condition does not actually cause the gamuted imaging finding, but can produce imaging changes that simulate it.

References
1. Chapman S, Nakielny R: Aids to Radiological Differential Diagnosis. (ed 3) London:WB Saunders, 1995, p 280
2. Gore RM: Liver: Differential diagnosis. In Gore RM, Levine MS (eds): Textbook of Gastrointestinal Radiology. (ed 2) Philadelphia: WB Saunders, 2000, pp 1712–1727
3. Lee MJ, Hahn PF, Saini S, Mueller PR: Differential diagnosis of hyperintense liver lesions on T1W MR images. AJR 1992;159:1017–1020
4. Mathieu D, Paret M, Mahfouz AE, et al.: Hyperintense benign liver lesions on spin-echo T1-weighted MR images: pathologic correlations. Abdom Imaging 1997;22:410–417
5. Mergo PJ, Ros PR: Benign lesions of the liver. Radiol Clin North Am 1998;36:319–332

Gamut G-186

FOCAL HIGH SIGNAL INTENSITY LIVER LESION ON T1-WEIGHTED MR IMAGES

1. [Contrast agent (eg, gadolinium; lipiodol)]
2. Dysplastic nodule(s)
3. Fatty lesion (eg, lipoma; angiomyolipoma; focal fatty deposit; surgical defect packed with omental fat; occasional hepatoma with fatty degeneration)
4. Focal nodular hyperplasia
5. Hematoma or hemorrhage, acute (eg, trauma; blood dyscrasia; anticoagulants)
6. Hepatocellular adenoma
7. Hepatocellular carcinoma (hepatoma)
8. Metastasis (esp. melanoma)
9. Normal signal intensity liver surrounded by low signal intensity liver (eg, hemochromatosis; hemosiderosis; cirrhosis with regenerating nodules; edema)

Gamut G-187

DAMPING OF HEPATIC VEIN DOPPLER WAVEFORM (US)

1. Budd-Chiari syndrome
2. Cirrhosis
3. Extrinsic compression of hepatic veins
4. Passive hepatic congestion
5. Various parenchymal abnormalities of liver

Reference
1. Gore RM, Marn CS, Baron RL: Vascular disorders of the liver and splanchnic circulation. In: Gore RM, Levine MS (eds): Textbook of Gastrointestinal Radiology. (ed 2) Philadelphia: WB Saunders, 2000, pp 1639–1668

Gamut G-188

HEPATIC VEIN DILATATION

COMMON

1. Constrictive pericarditis
2. Inferior vena cava obstruction or thrombus
3. Normal with Valsalva maneuver in young patient
4. Right-sided congestive heart failure
5. Thrombus in hepatic vein
6. Tricuspid atresia or stenosis

UNCOMMON

1. Right atrial tumor

Reference

1. Gore RM, Marn CS, Baron RL: Vascular disorders of the liver and splanchnic circulation. In: Gore RM, Levine MS (eds): Textbook of Gastrointestinal Radiology. (ed 2) Philadelphia: WB Saunders, 2000, pp 1639–1668

Gamut G-189

HEPATIC VEIN THROMBOEMBOLISM OR OBSTRUCTION (BUDD-CHIARI S.) (INCL. OBSTRUCTION OF UPPER INFERIOR VENA CAVA)

COMMON

1. Cirrhosis
2. Heart failure
3. Idiopathic
4. Neoplasm invading inferior vena cava (esp. renal cell carcinoma; hepatocellular carcinoma)
5. Thrombophlebitis

UNCOMMON

1. Alkaloid ingestion (bush tea disease)
2. Behçet syndrome

3. Coagulopathy (incl. polycythemia vera; sickle cell disease)
4. Iatrogenic (eg, catheterization; vena cavography)
5. Infection of liver (eg, aspergillosis)
6. Intravenous web
7. Metastasis, hepatic
8. Neoplastic compression (eg, carcinoma of pancreas; retroperitoneal sarcoma; lymphoma$_g$)
9. Oral contraceptive use
10. Parasitic disease (eg, amebic liver abscess; schistosomiasis; hydatid disease)
11. Postoperative (eg, splenectomy)
12. Pregnancy; postpartum
13. Trauma

References

1. Deutsch V, Rosenthal T, Adar R, et al: Budd-Chiari syndrome. AJR 1972;116:430–439
2. Gore RM, Marn CS, Baron RL: Vascular disorders of the liver and splanchnic circulation. In: Gore RM, Levine MS: Textbook of Gastrointestinal Radiology. (ed 2) Philadelphia: WB Saunders, 2000, pp 1639–1668
3. Henderson JM, Boyer TD: Budd-Chiari syndrome. In: Zakim D, Boyer TD: Hepatology. (ed 3) Philadelphia: WB Saunders, 1996
4. Young RC: The Budd-Chiari syndrome caused by aspergillus. Arch Intern Med 1969;124:754–757

Gamut G-190

PORTAL VEIN THROMBOSIS OR OBSTRUCTION*

COMMON

1. Cirrhosis plus portal hypertension
2. Extrinsic compression or invasion by carcinoma of pancreas or stomach; lymphadenopathy of porta hepatis
3. Hepatocellular carcinoma (hepatoma) or cholangiocarcinoma (tumor thrombus or invasion)
4. Hypercoagulable state (eg, blood dyscrasia; clotting disorder; polycythemia vera; protein c or s deficiency; paroxysmal nocturnal hemoglobinuria)

(continued)

5. Iatrogenic (eg, TIPS; umbilical venous catheterization; estrogen therapy; oral contraceptive use)
6. Idiopathic
7. Neonatal sepsis; perinatal omphalitis
8. Pancreatitis
9. Postoperative (esp. postsplenectomy)
10. Schistosomiasis (periportal fibrosis causing presinusoidal intrahepatic obstruction)
11. Sclerosing cholangitis

UNCOMMON
1. Behçet S.
2. [Budd-Chiari S. causing reversal of portal venous blood return]
3. Dehydration, severe
4. Liver transplantation
5. Portal phlebitis (from abdominal infection)
6. Postpartum
7. Trauma

* May result in cavernous transformation of portal vein.
[ ] This condition does not actually cause the gamuted imaging finding, but can produce imaging changes that simulate it.

References
1. Dähnert W; Radiology Review Manual. (ed 4) Baltimore: Williams & Wilkins, 1999, p 610
2. Gore RM, Marn CS, Baron RL: Vascular disorders of the liver and splanchnic circulation. In: Gore RM, Levine MS: Textbook of Gastrointestinal Radiology. (ed 2) Philadelphia: WB Saunders, 2000, pp 1639–1668
3. Mitchel DG, Nazarian LN: Hepatic vascular disease: CT and MRI. Semin US, CT, MR 1995;16:49–68

Gamut G-191

PORTAL HYPERTENSION

COMMON
1. Cardiac (eg, heart failure; constrictive pericarditis)
2. Cirrhosis (incl. hepatitis; liver atrophy)

3. Pancreatic disease with portal obstruction (eg, neoplasm; pancreatitis)
4. Portal vein thrombosis
5. Schistosomiasis (periportal fibrosis causing presinusoidal intrahepatic obstruction)
6. Splenic vein thrombosis

UNCOMMON
1. Alagille S. (arteriohepatic S.)
2. Alpha 1-antitrypsin deficiency
3. Banti S.
4. Budd-Chiari S.
5. Caroli disease
6. [Cavernous transformation of portal vein]
7. Cholesterol ester storage disease
8. Cruveilhier-Baumgarten S.
9. Cystic fibrosis (mucoviscidosis)
10. Fatty change in liver (steatosis) (See G-144)
11. Gaucher disease
12. Glycogen storage disease, types III and IV
13. Hemochromatosis; multiple transfusion effect
14. Hepatic fibrosis-renal cystic disease
15. Increased portal flow (eg, splenomegaly; splenic, mesenteric, or hepatic arteriovenous fistula)
16. Nodular regenerative hyperplasia
17. Osler-Weber-Rendu S.
18. Polycythemia vera
19. Retroperitoneal inflammatory disease
20. Tropical splenomegaly S.
21. Wilson disease

[ ] This condition does not actually cause the gamuted imaging finding, but can produce imaging changes that simulate it.

References
1. Baron RL, Gore RM: Diffuse liver disease. In: Gore RM, Levine MS: Textbook of Gastrointestinal Radiology. (ed 2) Philadelphia: WB Saunders, 2000, pp 1590–1638

2. Sutton D, Young JWR: A Short Textbook of Clinical Imaging. London: Springer-Verlag, 1990, p 252
3. Taybi H, Lachman RS: Radiology of Syndromes, Metabolic Disorders, and Skeletal Dysplasias. (ed 4) St. Louis: Mosby-Year Book, 1996, pp 973–974

Gamut G-192

GAS IN THE PORTAL VEINS

COMMON

1. Abscess, abdominal$_g$ or pelvic (eg, gas abscess of pancreas; diverticulitis)
2. [Gas in the biliary tract]
3. Iatrogenic (eg, catheterization of umbilical or mesenteric artery or vein; percutaneous abscess drainage; hydrogen peroxide enema or gastric lavage; post-hepatic artery embolization)
4. Mechanical bowel obstruction with ischemia (incl. closed loop obstruction)
5. Mesenteric ischemia or occlusion and bowel infarction (See G-69)
6. Necrotizing enterocolitis

UNCOMMON

1. Acute gastric dilatation
2. Carcinoma of colon, necrotic
3. Corrosive ingestion causing gastritis
4. Diabetic acidosis or coma
5. Emphysematous cholecystitis
6. Erythroblastosis fetalis
7. Gastric emphysema
8. Hemorrhagic pancreatitis

9. Neonatal gastroenteritis
10. Peptic ulcer eroding into mesenteric vein
11. Postcolonoscopy or post-air contrast barium enema in inflammatory bowel disease (eg, diverticulitis; Crohn's disease; ulcerative colitis;)
12. Postoperative (eg, bowel resection; operation for congenital bowel obstruction)
13. Pseudomembranous colitis
14. Sepsis
15. Toxic megacolon

[ ] This condition does not actually cause the gamuted imaging finding, but can produce imaging changes that simulate it.

References

1. Bach MC, Anderson LG, Martin TA: Gas in the hepatic portal venous system. A diagnostic clue to an occult intra-abdominal abscess. Arch Intern Med 1982; 142:1725–1726
2. Benson MB: Adult survival with intrahepatic portal venous gas secondary to acute gastric dilatation, with a review of portal venous gas. Clin Radiol 1985; 36:441–443
3. Eisenberg RL: Gastrointestinal Radiology: A Pattern Approach. (ed 3) Philadelphia: Lippincott, 1996, pp 894–899
4. Gore RM: Liver: differential diagnosis. In: Gore RM, Levine MS: Textbook of Gastrointestinal Radiology. (ed 2) Philadelphia: WB Saunders, 2000, pp 1712–1726
5. Kirks DR, O'Byrne SA: The value of the lateral abdominal roentgenogram in the diagnosis of neonatal hepatic portal venous gas (HPVG). AJR 1974;122:153–158
6. Merritt CRB, Goldsmith JP, Shary MJ: Sonographic detection of portal venous gas in infants with NEC. Am J Roentgenol 1984;143:1059
7. Mindelzun R, McCort JJ: Hepatic and perihepatic radiolucencies. Radiol Clin North Am 1980; 18:221–238
8. Sisk PB: Gas in the portal venous system. Radiology 1961;77:103–106
9. Wiot JF, Felson B: Gas in the portal venous system. AJR 1961;86:920–929

PERIPORTAL HYPOECHOGENICITY ON US/PERIPORTAL LOW DENSITY ON CT

1. AIDS-related cholangitis
2. Cholangitis
3. Congestive hepatomegaly
4. Liver transplant rejection (occasionally seen in non-rejecting liver transplant)
5. Malignant lymphatic obstruction
6. Schistosomiasis mansoni
7. Trauma, blunt abdominal
8. Viral hepatitis

References

1. Chapman S, Nakielny R: Aids to Radiological Differential Diagnosis. (ed 3) London: WB Saunders, 1995, p 272
2. Fataar S, Bassiony H, Satyanath S, et al: CT of hepatic Schistosomiasis mansoni. AJR 1985;145:63–66
3. Kaplan SB, Sumkin JH, Campbell WL, et al: Periportal low-attenuation areas on CT: value as evidence of liver transplant rejection. AJR 1989;152:285–287
4. Shanmuganathan K, Mirvis SE, Amorosa M: Periportal low density on CT in patients with blunt trauma: association with elevated venous pressure. AJR 1993;160:279–283
5. Siegel MJ, Herman TE: Periportal low attenuation at CT in childhood. Radiology 1992;183:685–688
6. Wechsler RJ, Munoz SJ, Needleman L, et al: The periportal collar: a CT sign of liver transplant rejection. Radiology 1987;165:57–60

PROMINENT PERIPORTAL ECHOES (STARRY SKY LIVER) IN ADULTS (US)

COMMON

1. Air in biliary tree (pneumobilia)
2. Cholangiocarcinoma
3. Cholangitis
4. Cholecystitis, acute or chronic

5. Hepatitis
6. Hepatocellular carcinoma (hepatoma)
7. Recurrent pyogenic cholangitis (Oriental cholangio-hepatitis)
8. Sclerosing cholangitis

UNCOMMON

1. Cystic fibrosis (mucoviscidosis)
2. Embolism of oily contrast medium after lymphangiogram
3. Infectious mononucleosis
4. Kaposi sarcoma of liver
5. Lymphoma$_g$; Burkitt lymphoma; leukemia
6. Periportal fibrosis (incl. schistosomiasis)
7. Right heart failure
8. Toxic shock syndrome

References

1. Gore RM: Liver: Differential diagnosis. In Gore RM, Levine MS (eds): Textbook of Gastrointestinal Radiology. (ed 2) Philadelphia: WB Saunders, 2000, pp 1712–1727
2. Williamson MR: Abdominal ultrasound. In: Essentials of Ultrasound. Philadelphia: WB Saunders, 1996, p 81

PROMINENT PERIPORTAL ECHOES IN NEONATES ON ULTRASOUND

COMMON

1. Acute hepatitis
2. Biliary atresia
3. [Idiopathic; transient (disappears within a year)]
4. Idiopathic neonatal jaundice

UNCOMMON

1. [Air in portal venous system]
2. Alpha-1-antitrypsin deficiency
3. Cytomegalovirus infection

[ ] This condition does not actually cause the gamuted imaging finding, but can produce imaging changes that simulate it.

Reference
1. Gore RM: Liver: Differential diagnosis. In Gore RM, Levine MS (eds): Textbook of Gastrointestinal Radiology. (ed 2) Philadelphia: WB Saunders, 2000, pp 1712–1727

Gamut G-196

INCREASED PERIPORTAL SIGNAL INTENSITY ON MRI

1. Acute hepatitis
2. AIDS-related cholangitis
3. Cholangiocarcinoma
4. Cholangitis
5. Cirrhosis
6. Obstructive jaundice

Reference
1. Gore RM: Liver: Differential diagnosis. In Gore RM, Levine MS (eds): Textbook of Gastrointestinal Radiology. (ed 2) Philadelphia: WB Saunders, 2000, pp 1712– 1727

Gamut G-197

SPLENOMEGALY: A CLASSIFICATION (See G-198)

BLOOD DYSCRASIA

1. Anemia$_g$ (esp. hemolytic, incl. sickle cell disease; thalassemia; hereditary spherocytosis; pyruvate kinase deficiency)
2. Dysgammaglobulinemia
3. Extramedullary hematopoiesis
4. Hemochromatosis
5. Leukemia (esp. chronic myelogenous)
6. Myelofibrosis (hypersplenism)
7. Osteopetrosis
8. Polycythemia vera
9. Thrombotic thrombocytopenic purpura
10. Waldenström macroglobulinemia

INFECTION

1. Bacterial (eg, miliary tuberculosis; tularemia; sub-acute bacterial endocarditis; septicemia; typhoid fever; brucellosis; syphilis; pyogenic abscess; tropical splenic abscess)
2. Chronic granulomatous disease of childhood
3. Fungal (esp. histoplasmosis; candidiasis)
4. Parasitic disease (eg, malaria; schistosomiasis; hydatid disease; kala-azar {leishmaniasis})
5. Rickettsial (eg, typhus)
6. Viral (eg, viral hepatitis; AIDS; infectious mononucleosis; cytomegalovirus infection; herpes simplex; rubella)

NEOPLASM

1. Benign neoplasm (eg, fibroma; hamartoma)
2. Cyst, epidermoid (simple, primary); dermoid; post-traumatic; hydatid
3. Hemangioma; cystic lymphangioma
4. Lymphoma$_g$
5. Metastases (esp. from carcinoma of breast, lung, colon, ovary; melanoma)
6. Sarcoma (esp. angiosarcoma)

PORTAL HYPERTENSION

1. Cirrhosis, nutritional or alcoholic
2. Congestive splenomegaly (Banti syndrome)
3. Schistosomiasis
4. Splenic or portal vein obstruction (eg, thrombosis; pancreatic neoplasm; lymphadenopathy)

STORAGE DISEASES

1. Gaucher disease
2. Glycogen storage disease
3. Langerhans cell histiocytosis$_g$
4. Mucopolysaccharidoses (incl. gargoylism); muco-lipidoses (See J-4)
5. Niemann-Pick disease

(continued)

TRAUMA

1. Hematoma (subcapsular; intrasplenic; perisplenic)
2. Hemorrhagic pseudocyst

OTHER

1. Alpha-1-antitrypsin deficiency
2. Amyloidosis
3. Congenital syndromes (See G-198)
4. Connective tissue diseases$_g$ (collagen vascular diseases) (esp. lupus erythematosus)
5. Cystic fibrosis (mucoviscidosis)
6. Diabetes
7. Heart failure
8. Hemodialysis
9. Infarction
10. Rheumatoid arthritis (Felty S.); juvenile rheumatoid arthritis; juvenile chronic arthritis (Still's disease)
11. Sarcoidosis
12. Tropical splenomegaly

References

1. Ayers AB: The spleen. In: Grainger RG, Allison DJ: Diagnostic Radiology. An Anglo-American Textbook of Imaging. (ed 2) Edinburgh: Churchill Livingstone, 1992, vol 3, p 2408
2. Dähnert W: Radiology Review Manual. (ed 4) Baltimore, Williams & Wilkins, 1999, p 556
3. Gore RM: Spleen: Differential diagnosis. In: Gore RM, Levine MS: Textbook of Gastrointestinal Radiology. (ed 2) Philadelphia: WB Saunders, 2000, pp 1925–1928
4. Siegel MJ: Pediatric Body CT. Philadelphia: Lippincott Williams & Wilkins, 1999
5. Teplick JG, Haskin ME: Roentgenographic Diagnosis. (ed 3) Philadelphia: WB Saunders, 1976

Gamut G-198

CONGENITAL SYNDROMES WITH SPLENOMEGALY

COMMON

1. Anemia$_g$ (eg, sickle cell disease; thalassemia; spherocytosis; pyruvate kinase deficiency)
2. Chronic granulomatous disease of childhood
3. Dysgammaglobulinemia
4. Fetal infection (eg, rubella; cytomegalovirus; herpes simplex)
5. Gaucher disease; Niemann-Pick disease
6. Glycogen storage disease, type I (von Gierke disease) and type III
7. Hemochromatosis
8. Langerhans cell histiocytosis$_g$
9. Mucopolysaccharidoses; mucolipidoses; GM$_1$ gangliosidosis (See J-4)

UNCOMMON

1. Aase S.
2. Alpha-1-antitrypsin deficiency
3. Aspartylglucosaminuria
4. Beckwith-Wiedemann S.
5. Chédiak-Higashi S.
6. Cholesterol ester storage disease
7. Cogan S.
8. Cruveilhier-Baumgarten S.
9. Cystinosis
10. Ethanolaminosis
11. Farber disease (lipogranulomatosis)
12. Felty S.
13. Fucosidosis; galactosialidosis; mannosidosis
14. Hepatic fibrosis-renal cystic disease
15. Hyperlipoproteinemia
16. Infantile multisystem inflammatory disease (NOMID)
17. Lipoatrophic diabetes
18. Osteopetrosis
19. POEMS S.
20. Sea-blue histiocyte S.

21. Tyrosinemia, type I
22. Vaquez-Osler S.
23. Wilson disease
24. Wolman disease

Reference
1. Taybi H, Lachman RS: Radiology of Syndromes, Metabolic Disorders, and Skeletal Dysplasias. (ed 4) St. Louis: Mosby-Year Book, 1996, p 961

Gamut G-199

SPLENOMEGALY WITH NORMAL ECHOGENICITY (US)

1. Congestion from portal hypertension
2. Felty syndrome
3. Hemolysis
4. Hereditary spherocytosis
5. Infection
6. Juvenile chronic arthritis (Still's disease) (eg, juvenile rheumatoid arthritis)
7. Myelofibrosis
8. Leukemia, myelogenous
9. Parasitic disease (eg, malaria; leishmaniasis {kala-azar}; schistosomiasis)
10. Polycythemia vera
11. Sickle cell disease (early)
12. Wilson disease

Reference
1. Gore RM: Spleen: Differential diagnosis. In: Gore RM, Levine MS: Textbook of Gastrointestinal Radiology. (ed 2) Philadelphia: WB Saunders, 2000, pp 1925–1928

Gamut G-200

SPLENOMEGALY WITH DIFFUSE HYPOECHOIC PATTERN (US)

1. Congestion from portal hypertension
2. Leukemia (esp. chronic lymphocytic)
3. Lymphoma$_g$
4. Multiple myeloma
5. Noncaseating granulomatous disease

Reference
1. Gore RM: Spleen: Differential diagnosis. In: Gore RM, Levine MS: Textbook of Gastrointestinal Radiology. (ed 2) Philadelphia: WB Saunders, 2000, pp 1925–1928

Gamut G-201

SPLENOMEGALY WITH DIFFUSE HYPERECHOIC PATTERN (US)

COMMON
1. Hematoma
2. Infection (eg, malaria; brucellosis; tuberculosis—esp. miliary)
3. Leukemia (acute lymphocytic, chronic lymphocytic, or myelogenous after chemotherapy or radiation therapy)
4. Lymphoma$_g$
5. Myelofibrosis (hypersplenism)

UNCOMMON
1. Dysgammaglobulinemia
2. Hereditary spherocytosis
3. Malignant neoplasm (esp. angiosarcoma)
4. Metastasis
5. Polycythemia
6. Portal vein thrombosis
7. Sarcoidosis

(continued)

References

1. Gore RM: Spleen: Differential diagnosis. In: Gore RM, Levine MS: Textbook of Gastrointestinal Radiology. (ed 2) Philadelphia: WB Saunders, 2000, pp 1925–1928
2. Mathieson JR, Cooperberg PL: The Spleen. In Rumack CM, Wilson SR, Charboneau JW (eds): Diagnostic Ultrasound. (ed 2) St. Louis: Mosby, 1998, pp 155–174
3. Siler J, Hunter TB, Weiss J, et al: Increased echogenicity of the spleen in benign and malignant disease. AJR 1980; 134:1011–1014

Gamut G-202

SMALL OR NONVISUALIZED SPLEEN

1. Asplenia S.; polysplenia S.
2. Atrophy
3. Hereditary hypoplasia
4. Inflammatory bowel disease
5. Postinfarction (esp. sickle cell disease)
6. Postradiation therapy
7. Sickle cell disease
8. Traumatic fragmentation
9. Wandering spleen

References

1. Dähnert W: Radiology Review Manual. (ed 4) Baltimore, Williams & Wilkins, 1999, p 556
2. Gore RM: Spleen: Differential diagnosis. In: Gore RM, Levine MS: Textbook of Gastrointestinal Radiology. (ed 2) Philadelphia: WB Saunders, 2000, pp 1925–1928

Gamut G-203

SPLENIC CALCIFICATION—SOLITARY

COMMON

1. Splenic artery aneurysm
2. Splenic artery atherosclerosis

UNCOMMON

1. Abscess, healed (eg, pyogenic; *Candida;* tuberculous)
2. Capsular ascites ("zuckerguss" spleen)
3. Cyst (eg, congenital; dermoid; epidermoid; hydatid; posttraumatic)
4. Granuloma (esp. tuberculosis)
5. Hamartoma
6. Hemangioma; phlebolith
7. Hematoma, healed
8. Infarct, healed
9. Metastasis

References

1. Eisenberg RL: Gastrointestinal Radiology: A Pattern Approach. (ed 3) Philadelphia: Lippincott, 1996, pp 991–997
2. Gore RM: Spleen: Differential diagnosis. In: Gore RM, Levine MS: Textbook of Gastrointestinal Radiology. (ed 2) Philadelphia: WB Saunders, 2000, pp 1925–1928

Gamut G-204

SPLENIC CALCIFICATIONS—MULTIPLE

COMMON

1. Granulomas, healed (eg, tuberculosis; histoplasmosis)
2. Phleboliths; hemangioma
3. Splenic artery

UNCOMMON

1. AIDS (healed *Pneumocystis carinii* infection)
2. Brucellosis

3. Hematomas
4. Hemochromatosis
5. Hemosiderosis
6. Infarcts
7. Metastases
8. Parasitic disease, esp. pentastomiasis (*Armillifer* infection); hydatid disease
9. Sarcoidosis
10. Sickle cell disease (stippled)
11. [Thorotrast residual]

[ ] This condition does not actually cause the gamuted imaging finding, but can produce imaging changes that simulate it.

References
1. Baker SR, Cho KC: The Abdominal Plain Film with Correlative Imaging. Norwalk, CT: Appleton & Lange, 1998
2. Eisenberg RL: Gastrointestinal Radiology: A Pattern Approach. (ed 3) Philadelphia: Lippincott, 1996, pp 991–997
3. Gore RM: Spleen: Differential diagnosis. In: Gore RM, Levine MS: Textbook of Gastrointestinal Radiology. (ed 2) Philadelphia: WB Saunders, 2000, pp 1925–1928

Gamut G-205

SOLITARY LESION OF THE SPLEEN (US, CT, MRI)

COMMON
1. Aneurysm of splenic artery
2. Cyst (congenital; epidermoid; dermoid or teratoma; hydatid; traumatic)
3. Hemangioma, cavernous or capillary
4. Hematoma (posttraumatic)
5. Infarct (esp. sickle cell disease)
6. Lymphoma$_g$; leukemia

UNCOMMON
1. Abscess (pyogenic; *Candida; Pneumocystis carinii*)
2. Arteriovenous malformation
3. Cystic lymphangioma
4. Hamartoma
5. Hemangiosarcoma

6. Metastasis (esp. from carcinoma of breast, lung, colon, ovary; melanoma)
7. Peliosis
8. Pseudocyst (secondary to pancreatitis)
9. Sarcoidosis
10. Splenic sequestration crisis

References
1. Dachman AH, Ros PR, Murari PJ, et al: Nonparasitic splenic cysts: A report of 52 cases with radiologic-pathologic correlation. AJR 1986;147:537–542
2. Guermazi A, Brice P, deKerviler E, et al: Extranodal Hodgkin disease: spectrum of disease. RadioGraphics 2001; 21:161–179
3. Mathieson JR, Cooperberg PL: Chapter 5. In: Rumack CM, Wilson SR, Charboneau JW (eds): Diagnostic Ultrasound. St. Louis: Mosby, 1998, pp 162–171
4. Reddy SC: Hemangiosarcoma of the spleen: Helical computed tomography features. South Med J 2000;93:825–827
5. Slone RM, Fisher AJ: Pocket Guide to Body CT Differential Diagnosis. New York: McGraw-Hill, 1999, pp 237–238
6. Solviati L, Bossi MC, Bellotti E, et al: Focal lesions in the spleen: Sonographic patterns and guided biopsy. AJR 1983; 140:59–65
7. Urrutia M, Mergo PJ, Ros LH, Torres GM, Ros PR: Cystic masses of the spleen: radiologic-pathologic correlation. RadioGraphics 1996;16:107–129

Gamut G-206

FOCAL CYSTIC OR LOW DENSITY SPLENIC LESION (CT, MRI—USUALLY HYPOECHOIC ON US)

COMMON
1. Abscess (pyogenic; *Candida; Pneumocystis carinii*)
2. Aneurysm of splenic artery
3. Cyst (congenital; epidermoid; dermoid or teratoma; hydatid; posttraumatic)
4. Hematoma
5. Infarction

UNCOMMON
1. Cystic lymphangioma
2. Hamartoma
3. Hemangioma, cavernous or capillary

(continued)

4. Hemangiosarcoma
5. Metastasis
6. Peliosis
7. Pseudocyst (secondary to pancreatitis)

References

1. Dachman AH, Ros PR, Murari PJ, et al: Nonparasitic splenic cysts: A report of 52 cases with radiologic-pathologic correlation. AJR 1986;147:537–542
2. Mathieson JR, Cooperberg PL: Chapter 5. In: Rumack CM, Wilson SR, Charboneau JW (eds): Diagnostic Ultrasound. St. Louis: Mosby, 1998, pp 162–171
3. Solviati L, Bossi MC, Bellotti E, et al: Focal lesions in the spleen: Sonographic patterns and guided biopsy. AJR 1983;140:59–65
4. Urrutia M, Mergo PJ, Ros LH, Torres GM, Ros PR: Cystic masses of the spleen: radiologic-pathologic correlation. RadioGraphics 1996;16:107–129

Gamut G-207

FOCAL HYPERECHOIC SPLENIC LESION (US)

COMMON

1. Hematoma
2. Infarct
3. Lymphoma$_g$

UNCOMMON

1. Abscess with gas bubbles
2. Hemangioma
3. Hemangiosarcoma
4. Hydatid cyst with "hydatid sand"
5. Metastasis
6. Plasmacytoma
7. Simple cyst with cholesterol crystals

References

1. Gore RM: Spleen: Differential diagnosis. In: Gore RM, Levine MS: Textbook of Gastrointestinal Radiology. (ed 2) Philadelphia: WB Saunders, 2000, pp 1925–1928

2. Mittelstaedt CA, Partain CL: Ultrasonic-pathologic classification of splenic abnormalities: Gray-scale patterns. Radiology 1980;134:697–705
3. Solviati L, Bossi MC, Bellotti E, et al: Focal lesions in the spleen: Sonographic patterns and guided biopsy. AJR 1983;140:59–65

Gamut G-208

DIFFUSE INCREASED SPLENIC DENSITY ON CT

1. Fanconi anemia
2. Hemochromatosis
3. Hemosiderosis
4. Lymphoma$_g$ (treated)
5. Sickle cell disease
6. Thorotrast residual

References

1. Kawashima A, Urban BA, Fishman EK: Benign lesions of the spleen. In: Gore RM, Levine MS (eds): Textbook of Gastrointestinal Radiology. (ed 2) Philadelphia: WB Saunders, 2000, pp. 1879–1904
2. Gore RM: Spleen: Differential diagnosis. In: Gore RM, Levine MS (eds): Textbook of Gastrointestinal Radiology. (ed 2) Philadelphia: WB Saunders, 2000, pp. 1925–1929

Gamut G-209

MULTIPLE SPLENIC HYPOINTENSITIES ON MRI*

COMMON

*1. Abscesses (pyogenic)
*2. Cysts (eg, congenital; hydatid; posttraumatic)
 3. Gamna-Gandy bodies
 4. Granulomas, calcified
*5. Hemangiomas
*6. Hematomas
*7. Infarcts

*8. Metastases (incl. hemorrhagic choriocarcinoma)

*9. Lymphoma$_g$

UNCOMMON

1. Amyloidosis
2. Flow void in arteriovenous malformation or Osler-Weber-Rendu S.
3. Fungemia with multifocal microabscess formation
*4. Peliosis
5. Sarcoidosis

* On T1-weighted images.

References

1. Gore RM: Spleen: Differential diagnosis. In: Gore RM, Levine MS: Textbook of Gastrointestinal Radiology. (ed 2) Philadelphia: WB Saunders, 2000, pp 1925–1928
2. Kelekis NL, Burdeny DA, Semelka RC: Spleen. In: Semelka RC, Ascher SM, Reinhold C (eds): MRI of the Abdomen and Pelvis. New York: Wiley-Liss, 1997, pp 239–256

Gamut G-210

MULTIPLE SPLENIC HYPERINTENSITIES ON T2-WEIGHTED MR IMAGES

COMMON

1. Abscesses (pyogenic)
2. Cysts (eg, congenital; hydatid; posttraumatic)
3. Hemangiomas
4. Hematomas
5. Infarcts
6. Metastases

UNCOMMON

1. Fungemia with multifocal microabscess formation
2. Lymphangioma (T1 and T2-WI)
3. Peliosis

References

1. Gore RM: Spleen: Differential diagnosis. In: Gore RM, Levine MS: Textbook of Gastrointestinal Radiology. (ed 2) Philadelphia: WB Saunders, 2000, pp 1925–1928
2. Kelekis NL, Burdeny DA, Semelka RC: Spleen. In: Semelka RC, Ascher SM, Reinhold C (eds): MRI of the Abdomen and Pelvis. New York: Wiley-Liss, 1997, pp 239–256

Gamut G-211

ABNORMALITY ON SPLENIC ARTERIOGRAPHY

COMMON

1. Accessory spleen
2. Anomalous origin of splenic or celiac artery
3. Splenic artery arteriosclerosis; aneurysm; fibromuscular hyperplasia (incl. stenosis; occlusion)
4. Splenic vein abnormality (See G-212)

UNCOMMON

1. Arteriovenous fistula; angiomatous malformation
2. Avascular mass
   a. Abscess
   b. Cyst (eg, dermoid; epidermoid; hydatid; posttraumatic)
   c. Infarction
   d. Lymphoma$_g$
   e. Metastasis
3. Displacement by extrinsic mass
4. Splenic artery encasement (eg, pancreatic carcinoma)
5. Splenic laceration; pericapsular hematoma
6. Thromboembolism
7. Vascular mass (eg, metastasis, esp. melanoma; hemangiosarcoma of spleen)

Gamut G-212

SPLENIC VEIN OBSTRUCTION (US, POSTCONTRAST CT, MRI, OR ANGIO)

COMMON

1. Lymphadenopathy (eg, lymphoma$_g$; metastases)
2. Neoplasm (eg, pancreatic; retroperitoneal sarcoma)
3. Pancreatitis (incl. pancreatic pseudocyst)
4. Thromboembolism of portal or splenic vein (esp. portal hypertension; polycythemia vera; heart failure)

UNCOMMON

1. Aneurysm of splenic artery or aorta
2. Postoperative
3. Retroperitoneal inflammation
4. Schistosomiasis
5. Trauma; hematoma

References

1. Gore RM, Marn CS, Baron RL: Vascular disorders of the liver and splanchnic circulation. In Gore RM, Levine MS (eds): Textbook of Gastrointestinal Radiology. (ed 2) Philadelphia: WB Saunders, 2000, pp 1639–1668
2. Rosch J, Dotter CT: Extrahepatic portal obstruction in childhood and its angiographic diagnosis. AJR 1971;112: 143–149
3. Yale CE, Crummy AB: Splenic vein thrombosis and bleeding esophageal varices. JAMA 1971; 217:317–320

Gamut G-213

SOLID PANCREATIC LESION (US, CT, MRI)

COMMON

1. Adenocarcinoma
2. Pancreatitis, focal

UNCOMMON

1. [Accessory spleen]
2. Aneurysm, thrombosed
3. Annular pancreas; pancreatic divisum
4. Hemangioma
5. Islet cell tumor (eg, insulinoma; gastrinoma; glucagonoma; somatostatinoma; VIPoma; non-functioning)
6. Lipoma
7. [Lymphadenopathy in celiac axis (eg, metastatic; tuberculous; Castleman disease)]
8. Lymphoma$_g$
9. Metastasis (esp. from carcinoma of breast, lung, stomach, gallbladder, kidney; melanoma)
10. Pancreaticoblastoma
11. Sarcoma
12. Serous cystadenoma (microcystic adenoma)
13. Solid and papillary epithelial neoplasm

[ ] This condition does not actually cause the gamuted imaging finding, but can produce imaging changes that simulate it.

References

1. Cheszmar JL: Pancreatic neoplasms. In: Gore RM, Levine MS (eds): Textbook of Gastrointestinal Radiology. (ed 2) Philadelphia: WB Saunders, 2000, pp 1796–1811
2. Clark LR, Jaffe MH, Choyke PL, et al: Pancreatic imaging. Radiol Clin North Am 1985;23:489–501
3. Helmberger TK, Ros LH, Baretton G, et al: Solid pancreatic lesions. Eur Radiol 1999;9(suppl 1):s195–s205
4. Sato M, Ishida H, Konno K, et al: Pancreatic metastasis: sonographic findings. Abdom Imaging 2001;26:72–75
5. Sato M, Ishida H, Konno K, et al: Pancreatic uncinate carcinoma: sonographic findings. Abdom Imaging 2001;26: 64–68
6. Scatarige JC, Horton KM, Sheth S, et al: Pancreatic parenchymal metastases: observations on helical CT. AJR 2001;176:695–701
7. Slone RM, Fisher AJ: Pocket Guide to Body CT Differential Diagnosis. New York: McGraw-Hill, 1999, pp 237–238

Gamut G-214

CYSTIC OR LOW DENSITY PANCREATIC LESION (CT, MRI—HYPOECHOIC ON US)

COMMON

1. Acute pancreatitis, focal
2. Chronic pancreatitis (inhomogeneous, often hyper-echoic)
3. Fluid collection, peripancreatic
4. Mucinous cystadenoma or cystadenocarcinoma (macrocystic adenoma)
5. Pancreatic duct dilatation, ectasia, or obstruction (from carcinoma; calculus; stricture)
6. Pancreatic ductal adenocarcinoma (eg, duct ectatic mucinous adenocarcinoma; papillary intraductal adenocarcinoma; anaplastic adenocarcinoma)
7. Pseudocyst of pancreas
8. Serous cystadenoma (microcystic adenoma)

UNCOMMON

1. Abscess$_g$
2. [Aneurysm or pseudoaneurysm of aorta, pancreati-coduodenal arcade, or splenic artery]
3. [Biloma]
4. [Cystic lymphangioma, retroperitoneal]
5. Cystic teratoma
6. Cysts, congenital (in adult polycystic kidney disease; Von Hippel-Lindau disease; or cystic fibrosis)
7. [Duodenal cyst or diverticulum]
8. Hemangioma
9. Hematoma
10. Hydatid cyst
11. Islet cell tumor or insulinoma, cystic
12. Liquefaction necrosis of pancreas
13. Lymphoma$_g$
14. Metastasis, cystic (eg, renal cell carcinoma; hepatoma; carcinoma of lung, breast, or ovary; melanoma)
15. Posttraumatic cyst
16. Solid and papillary epithelial neoplasm
17. [Varix of left renal vein]

[ ] This condition does not actually cause the gamuted imaging finding, but can produce imaging changes that simulate it.

References

1. Curry CA, Eng J, Horton KM, et al: CT of primary cystic pancreatic neoplasms: can CT be used for patient triage and treatment? AJR 2000;175:99–103
2. Kobayashi T, Kawabe A, Uenoyama S, et al: Macrocystic serous cystadenoma of the pancreas: case report. Abdom Imaging 2001;26:69–71
3. Ros PR, Hamrick-Turner JE, Chiechi MV, et al: Cystic pancreatic mass. Radiographics 1992;12:673–686
4. Ros LH, Helmberger T, Ros PR: Cystic pancreatic lesions. Eur Radiol 1999;9(suppl 1):s207–s215
5. Sato M, Ishida H, Konno K, et al: Pancreatic metastasis: sonographic findings. Abdom Imaging 2001:26:72–75
6. Scatarige JC, Horton KM, Sheth S, et al: Pancreatic parenchymal metastases: observations on helical CT. AJR 2001;176:695–701
7. Skolnick ML: Guide to the Ultrasound Examination of the Abdomen. New York: Springer-Verlag, 1986, pp 137–142
8. Williamson MR: Abdominal ultrasound. In: Essentials of Ultrasound. Philadelphia: WB Saunders, 1996, p 72

Gamut G-215

COMPLEX PANCREATIC LESION (US)

COMMON

1. Mucinous cystadenoma or cystadenocarcinoma (macrocystic adenoma)
2. Pseudocyst of pancreas

UNCOMMON

1. Hematoma, nonacute
2. Metastasis
3. Serous cystadenoma (microcystic adenoma)

References

1. Sato M, Ishida H, Konno K, et al: Pancreatic metastasis: sonographic findings. Abdom Imaging 2001:26:72–75
2. Skolnick ML: Guide to the Ultrasound Examination of the Abdomen. New York: Springer-Verlag, 1986, pp 137–142

Gamut G-216

INCREASED ECHOGENICITY OF PANCREAS (US)

COMMON

1. Advanced age
2. Chronic pancreatitis
3. Fatty infiltration
4. Hemorrhagic pancreatitis

UNCOMMON

1. Adenocarcinoma of pancreas
2. Cystic fibrosis
3. Diabetes
4. Hereditary pancreatitis
5. Malabsorption
6. Pancreatic insufficiency
7. Shwachman-Diamond S.
8. Steroid ingestion

References

1. Scafidi DE, Young LW: Diseases of the pediatric pancreas. In: Gore RM, Levine MS (eds): Textbook of Gastrointestinal Radiology. (ed 2) Philadelphia: WB Saunders, 2000, pp 2162–2173
2. Williamson MR: Abdominal ultrasound. In: Essentials of Ultrasound. Philadelphia: WB Saunders, 1996, p 70

Gamut G-217

FOCAL SHADOWING PANCREATIC LESION (US)

COMMON

1. Calcifications in chronic pancreatitis
2. Calculi in pancreatic duct

UNCOMMON

1. Arterial calcification
2. Gas in pancreatic abscess

3. Gas in pancreatic pseudocyst communicating with gut
4. Serous cystadenoma (microcystic adenoma) with calcifications
5. Solid and papillary epithelial neoplasm

References

1. Gore RM: Pancreas: Differential diagnosis. In: Gore RM, Levine MS: Textbook of Gastrointestinal Radiology. (ed 2) Philadelphia: WB Saunders, 2000, pp 1836–1843
2. Skolnick ML: Guide to the Ultrasound Examination of the Abdomen. New York: Springer-Verlag, 1986, pp 137–142

Gamut G-218

PANCREATIC CALCIFICATION WITHOUT MASS

COMMON

1. Chronic pancreatitis

UNCOMMON

1. Acute pancreatitis (saponification)
2. [Aneurysm or atherosclerosis of aorta or its branches]
3. Cystic fibrosis (mucoviscidosis)
4. Hemochromatosis
5. Hemorrhage (eg, trauma; infarction)
6. Hereditary pancreatitis (large clumps of calcium)
7. Hyperparathyroidism with pancreatitis
8. Idiopathic (pancreatic duct stenosis)
9. Kwashiorkor
10. Pancreatitis due to biliary disease (eg, gallstone in common duct)

[ ] This condition does not actually cause the gamuted imaging finding, but can produce imaging changes that simulate it.

References

1. Burgener FA, Kormano M: Differential Diagnosis in Conventional Radiology. (ed 2) New York: Thieme Medical Publ, 1991, pp 538–540

2. Eisenberg RL: Gastrointestinal Radiology: A Pattern Approach. (ed 3) Philadelphia: Lippincott, 1996, pp 997–1002
3. Ring EJ, Eaton SB, Ferrucci JT, Short WF: Differential diagnosis of pancreatic calcification. AJR 1973;177:446–452

Gamut G-219

PANCREATIC LESION CHARACTERIZED BY CALCIFICATION

COMMON

1. [Aneurysm of aorta, pancreaticoduodenal arcade, or splenic artery, thrombosed]
2. Chronic pancreatitis, focal
3. Hemorrhage, intraparenchymal (eg, old abscess; hematoma; infarction)

UNCOMMON

1. Adenocarcinoma of pancreas (rarely)
2. Hemangioma (plebolith)
3. Hydatid cyst
4. Islet cell tumor
5. Lymphangioma, cavernous
6. Lymphoma (treated)
7. Metastasis (esp. mucinous adenocarcinoma of colon)
8. Mucinous cystadenoma or cystadenocarcinoma (macrocystic adenoma) (peripheral calcium)
9. Pancreaticoblastoma
10. Pseudocyst of pancreas
11. Serous cystadenoma (microcystic adenoma) (central stellate calcium)
12. Solid and papillary epithelial neoplasm
13. Teratoma

[ ] This condition does not actually cause the gamuted imaging finding, but can produce imaging changes that simulate it.

References

1. Burgener FA, Kormano M: Differential Diagnosis in Conventional Radiology. (ed 2) New York: Thieme Medical Publ, 1991, pp 538–540
2. Eisenberg RL: Gastrointestinal Radiology: A Pattern Approach. (ed 3) Philadelphia: Lippincott, 1996, pp 997–1002
3. Ring EJ, Eaton SB, Ferrucci JT, Short WF: Differential diagnosis of pancreatic calcification. AJR 1973;177:446–452

Gamut G-220

PANCREATIC LESION CHARACTERIZED BY BLOOD OR HEMORRHAGE

1. [Aneurysm of aorta, pancreaticoduodenal arcade, or splenic artery]
2. Hemangioma
3. Hemorrhagic pancreatitis
4. Hemorrhagic pseudocyst
5. Islet cell tumor
6. Metastasis (esp. from carcinoma of colon)
7. Serous cystadenoma (microcystic adenoma)
8. Sarcoma
9. Solid and papillary epithelial neoplasm

[ ] This condition does not actually cause the gamuted imaging finding, but can produce imaging changes that simulate it.

Reference

1. Amano Y, Oishi, Takahashi M, et al: Nonenhanced magnetic resonance imaging of mild acute pancreatitis. Abdom Imaging 2001;26:59–63

Gamut G-221

PANCREATIC LESION CHARACTERIZED BY FAT

UNCOMMON

1. Focal fat deposit
2. Lipoma
3. Liposarcoma (possible in well-differentiated type)
4. Shwachman-Diamond S.
5. Teratoma

Reference

1. Itai Y, Saida Y, Kurosaki Y, et al: Focal fatty masses of the pancreas. Acta Radiol 1995;36:178–181

FATTY REPLACEMENT OR INFILTRATION OF PANCREAS

COMMON

1. Aging
2. Cystic fibrosis (mucoviscidosis)
3. Obesity
4. Steroid therapy

UNCOMMON

1. Chronic pancreatitis
2. Diabetes mellitus
3. Hemochromatosis
4. Hereditary pancreatitis
5. Johanson-Blizzard S.
6. Lipomatous pseudohypertrophy
7. Malnutrition
8. Shwachman-Diamond S.

References

1. Barzilai M, Lerner A, Branski D: Increased reflectivity of the pancreas in rare hereditary pancreatic insufficiency syndromes. Clin Radiol 1996;51:575–576
2. Gore RM: Pancreas: Differential diagnosis. In: Gore RM, Levine MS: Textbook of Gastrointestinal Radiology. (ed 2) Philadelphia: WB Saunders, 2000, pp 1836–1843
3. Matsumoto S, Mori H, Miyake H, et al: Uneven fatty replacement of the pancreas: evaluation with CT. Radiology 1995;194:453–458
4. Scafidi DE, Young LW: Diseases of the pediatric pancreas. In: Gore RM, Levine MS (eds): Textbook of Gastrointestinal Radiology. (ed 2) Philadelphia: WB Saunders, 2000, pp 2162–2173
5. Siegel MJ: Pediatric Body CT. Philadelphia: Lippincott Williams & Wilkins, 1999

HYPERVASCULAR PANCREATIC LESION (POSTCONTRAST CT, MRI, OR ANGIO)

COMMON

1. Acute pancreatitis
2. Adenocarcinoma, pancreatic ductal (hypovascular but with neovascularity)
3. Aneurysm or pseudoaneurysm of hepatic, gastroduodenal, pancreaticoduodenal or splenic arteries
4. Islet cell tumor, incl. insulinoma; gastrinoma (esp. with Zollinger-Ellison S. or MEN S. Type I (tumor blush); glucagonoma; nonfunctioning islet cell tumor; somatostatinoma)
5. Metastasis, hypervascular (eg, from angiosarcoma; leiomyosarcoma; carcinoid; melanoma; renal cell carcinoma; carcinoma of adrenal or thyroid)
6. Mucinous cystadenoma or cystadenocarcinoma (macrocystic adenoma)
7. Serous cystadenoma (microcystic adenoma)

UNCOMMON

1. Abscess of pancreas
2. Castleman disease
3. Hemangioma
4. Intraductal papillary mucinous tumor of pancreas
5. Solid and papillary epithelial neoplasm (hypovascular but with enhanced solid tissue toward center of mass)

References

1. Adsay NV, Longnecker DS, Klimstra DS: Pancreatic tumors with cystic dilatation of the ducts: intraductal papillary mucinous neoplasms and intraductal oncocytic papillary neoplasms. Semin Diagn Pathol 2000;17:16–30
2. Gore RM: Pancreas: Differential diagnosis. In: Gore RM, Levine MS: Textbook of Gastrointestinal Radiology. (ed 2) Philadelphia: WB Saunders, 2000, pp 1836–1843
3. Irie H, Honda H, Kuroiwa T, et al: Pitfalls in MR cholangiopancreatographic interpretation. RadioGraphics 2000; 24:229–234

4. Larena JA, Astigarraga E, Saralegui I, et al: Magnetic resonance cholangiopancreatography in the evaluation of pancreatic duct pathology. Br J Radiol 1998;71:1100–1106
5. Scatarige JC, Horton KM, Sheth S, et al: Pancreatic parenchymal metastases: observations on helical CT. AJR 2001;176:695–701

3. Pancreatic pseudocyst
4. Pancreatitis

OTHER

1. Microaneurysms (esp. pancreatitis; polyarteritis nodosa)
2. Occlusion or truncation, arterial or venous (eg, carcinoma; surgical ligation; vascular disease)

Gamut G-224

PANCREATIC ANGIOGRAPHIC ABNORMALITY (VIA CELIAC, SUPERIOR MESENTERIC, OR SUBSELECTIVE ARTERIOGRAPHY)

DISPLACEMENT OF VESSELS

1. Gallbladder enlargement
2. Lymphoma
3. Pancreatic mass (See G-213)

ENCASEMENT

1. Irregular (esp. carcinoma of pancreas)
2. Long segment with arterial cuffing (esp. carcinoma)
3. Smooth (eg, carcinoma; pancreatitis)

EXTRAVASATION

1. Pancreatic abscess
2. Pancreatitis

HYPERVASCULARITY (See G-223)

1. Carcinoma
2. Cystadenoma; cystadenocarcinoma (florid neovascularity)
3. Islet cell tumor, esp. Zollinger-Ellison S.; MEN S. Type I (tumor blush)
4. Pancreatic abscess
5. Pancreatitis

HYPOVASCULARITY

1. Lymphoma$_g$
2. Metastasis

Gamut G-225

DILATED PANCREATIC DUCT

1. Aging
2. Calculus in distal common duct
3. Chronic pancreatitis
4. Pancreatic or ampullary mass (esp. carcinoma of pancreas or ampulla; focal acute pancreatitis)

NOTE: NATURE OF DILATATION

Suggesting Pancreatitis

1. Calculi in duct
2. Irregular dilatation of duct

Suggesting Neoplasm

1. Duct occupies >50% of anteroposterior gland diameter
2. Smooth and beaded appearance of duct

References
1. Cheszmar JL: Pancreatic neoplasms. In: Gore RM, Levine MS (eds): Textbook of Gastrointestinal Radiology. (ed 2) Philadelphia: WB Saunders, 2000, pp 1796–1811
2. Gore RM: Pancreas: Differential Diagnosis. In Gore RM, Levine MS (eds): Textbook of Gastrointestinal Radiology. (ed 2) Philadelphia: WB Saunders, 2000, pp 1836–1843

Gamut G-226

PANCREATIC DUCT STRICTURE
(ERCP, MRCP)

WITH NORMAL PANCREATIC PARENCHYMA

1. Osteophyte of spine
2. Vascular compression (eg, aneurysm or pseudo-aneurysm of aorta, gastroduodenal, pancreatico-duodenal, or splenic arteries)

WITH ABNORMAL PARENCHYMA

1. Carcinoma of pancreas
2. Chronic pancreatitis
3. Duct hyperplasia

Reference

1. Gore RM: Pancreas: Differential Diagnosis. In Gore RM, Levine MS (eds): Textbook of Gastrointestinal Radiology. (ed 2) Philadelphia: WB Saunders, 2000, pp 1836–1843.

Gamut G-227

GAS IN PANCREATIC DUCT

COMMON

1. Abscess
2. Patulous Vaterian sphincter
3. Post-endoscopic retrograde cholangiopancrea-tography (ERCP)
4. Prior Vaterian papillotomy

UNCOMMON

1. Duodenal diverticulum communication
2. Enteropancreatic fistula (spontaneous; surgical)

Reference

1. Gore RM: Pancreas: Differential diagnosis. In: Gore RM, Levine MS: Textbook of Gastrointestinal Radiology. (ed 2) Philadelphia: WB Saunders, 2000, pp 1836–1843

Gamut G-228

CYSTIC MESENTERIC
OR INTRAPERITONEAL LESION
(US, CT, MRI)

COMMON

1. Abscess
2. Cystic lymphangioma
3. Hematoma
4. Mesenteric cyst

UNCOMMON

1. Ascites, complicated
2. Cystic mesothelioma
3. Cystic or necrotic stromal cell tumor$_g$ (eg, leio-myoma; leiomyosarcoma)
4. Duplication cyst (enteric)
5. Hydatid disease
6. Lymphadenopathy, cystic or necrotic (eg, bacillary angiomatosis in AIDS)
7. Papillary serous carcinoma of peritoneum
8. Pseudocyst of pancreas invading mesentery
9. Pseudomyxoma peritonei
10. Teratoma

References

1. Chopra S, Laurie LR, Chintapalli KN, et al: Primary papillary serous carcinoma of the peritoneum: CT-pathologic correlation. J Comput Assist Tomogr 2000;24:395–399
2. Inman DS, Lambert AW, Wilkins DC: Multicystic peritoneal inclusion cysts: the use of CT guided drainage for symptom control. Ann R Coll Surg Eng 2000; 82:196–197
3. Ros P, Olmsted W, Moser R, Dachman A, et al: Mesenteric and omental cysts: Histologic classification with imaging correlation. Radiology 1987;164:327–332
4. Ros PR: Bubbles and marbles of the belly: cystic and solid masses of the mesentery and omentum. In: Balfe DM, Levine MS: RSNA Categorical Course in Diagnostic Radiology: Gastrointestinal. 1997, pp 59–66
5. Silverman PM, Cooper C: Mesenteric and omental lesions. In Gore RM, Levine MS (eds): Textbook of Gastrointestinal Radiology. (ed 2) Philadelphia: WB Saunders, 2000, pp 1980–1992

Gamut G-229

SOLID LESION OF THE MESENTERY OR MESENTERIC ROOT (US, CT, MRI)

COMMON

1. Abscess$_g$
2. Hematoma (trauma; bleeding disorder)
3. Lymphadenopathy (eg, metastatic carcinoma; tuberculosis; Crohn's disease; Castleman disease; AIDS—bacillary angiomatosis)
4. Lymphoma$_g$
5. Metastasis (esp. from colon or ovary)
6. Omental "cakes" (eg, metastatic disease; carcinoid; lymphoma; tuberculosis)
7. Stromal cell tumor$_g$ (esp. leiomyosarcoma; leiomyoma; neurofibroma)

UNCOMMON

1. Desmoid tumor (mesenteric fibromatosis); desmoplastic small round cell tumor
2. Hemangioma
3. Hydatid disease
4. Lipoma; lipomatosis; liposarcoma
5. Lymphangioma
6. Malignant fibrous histiocytoma
7. Mesothelioma
8. Phlegmon (pancreatitis); pseudocyst of pancreas
9. Retractile mesenteritis (chronic fibrosing mesenteritis; mesenteric lipodystrophy; panniculitis; Weber-Christian disease)
10. Splenosis
11. Teratoma

References
1. Nicolas AI, Ros PR: Imaging of the mesentery and omentum. In: Grainger RG, Allison DJ: Grainger & Allison's Diagnostic Radiology. (ed 3) New York: Churchill Livingstone, 1997, pp 1059–1079
2. Silverman PM, Cooper C: Mesenteric and omental lesions. In Gore RM, Levine MS (eds): Textbook of Gastrointestinal Radiology. (ed 2) Philadelphia: WB Saunders, 2000, pp 1980–1992
3. Slone RM, Fisher AJ: Pocket Guide to Body CT Differential Diagnosis. New York: McGraw-Hill, 1999, pp 191–192

Gamut G-230

ALTERATION IN DENSITY OF THE MESENTERIC FAT ON CT ("Misty Mesentery")

1. Hemorrhage (eg, trauma)
2. Inflammation (eg, Crohn's disease)
3. Lymphedema
4. Mesenteric edema
5. Neoplasm, eg, carcinomatosis; mesothelioma (esp. after chemotherapy)
6. Retractile mesenteritis (chronic fibrosing mesenteritis; mesenteric lipodystrophy; panniculitis; Weber-Christian disease)

References
1. Mindelzun RE, Jeffrey RB Jr, Lane MJ, Silverman PM: The misty mesentery on CT: differential diagnosis. AJR 1996; 167:61–65
2. Silverman PM, Cooper C: Mesenteric and omental lesions. In Gore RM, Levine MS (eds): Textbook of Gastrointestinal Radiology. (ed 2) Philadelphia: WB Saunders, 2000, pp 1980–1992

Gamut G-231

PERITONEAL DISEASE

COMMON

1. Abscess$_g$, abdominal or pericolic (See G-89)
2. Adhesions (eg, inflammatory; postoperative); congenital peritoneal bands (Ladd's bands)
3. Crohn's disease
4. Endometriosis
5. Fluid, ascites (See G-233, 234)
6. Lymphoma$_g$
7. Metastasis, implantation, or invasion by malignant neoplasm
8. Obesity

(continued)

9. Pancreatitis (incl. saponification)
10. Peritonitis
11. Tuberculosis

UNCOMMON

1. Amyloidosis
2. Carcinoid
3. Cyst of mesentery
4. Desmoid tumor (mesenteric fibromatosis), isolated or with Gardner S.
5. Fungus disease$_g$ (eg, actinomycosis)
6. Medication (eg, practolol peritonitis; Sansert)
7. Mesothelioma
8. Parasitic disease (esp. hydatid disease; amebiasis; pentastomiasis-*Armillifer* infection)
9. Pseudomyxoma peritonei
10. Radiation peritonitis
11. Retractile mesenteritis (chronic fibrosing mesenteritis; mesenteric lipodystrophy; panniculitis; Weber-Christian disease)
12. Sarcoma
13. Typhoid fever

References

1. Banner MP, Gohel VK: Peritoneal mesothelioma. Radiology 1978; 129:637–640
2. Sacks B, Joffe N, Harris N: Isolated mesenteric desmoids (mesenteric fibromatosis). Clin Radiol 1978; 29:95–100
3. Silverman PM, Cooper C: Mesenteric and omental lesions. In Gore RM, Levine MS (eds): Textbook of Gastrointestinal Radiology. (ed 2) Philadelphia: WB Saunders, 2000, pp 1980–1992

DIFFUSE PERITONEAL THICKENING (US, CT, MRI)

COMMON

1. Carcinomatosis
2. Peritonitis
3. Postoperative state

UNCOMMON

1. Lymphoma$_g$
2. Mesothelioma
3. Pseudomyxoma peritonei
4. Sarcomatosis
5. Tuberculosis

Reference

1. Silverman PM, Cooper C: Mesenteric and omental lesions. In Gore RM, Levine MS (eds): Textbook of Gastrointestinal Radiology. (ed 2) Philadelphia: WB Saunders, 2000, pp 1980–1992

PERITONEAL FLUID COLLECTION (ASCITES) IN AN ADULT (ESP. ON US, CT, MRI)

INFECTION OR INFLAMMATION OF THE PERITONEAL CAVITY (PERITONITIS)

1. Abscess
2. Pancreatitis
3. Pelvic inflammatory disease (PID)
4. Rupture of a hollow viscus (eg, appendicitis; diverticulitis; empyema of gallbladder; peptic ulcer; typhoid fever)
5. Tuberculosis or other primary infection causing peritonitis

LYMPHATIC OBSTRUCTION WITH CHYLOUS OR LYMPH ASCITES (See G-235)

Congenital

1. Milroy disease
2. Tuberous sclerosis

Elevated lymphatic pressure

1. Cirrhosis
2. Constrictive pericarditis
3. Heart failure

Infection

1. Filariasis

Neoplastic disease

1. Lymphoma$_g$; leukemia
2. Metastatic disease in lymphatics

Radiation therapy

Trauma

1. Rupture of abdominal lymphatics

NEOPLASM

1. Benign (eg, Meigs S.— benign ovarian tumor)
2. Malignant (eg, carcinoma of gastrointestinal tract or ovary with mesenteric or peritoneal metastases; mesothelioma)

VENOUS OBSTRUCTION

Cardiac disease with chronic elevation of venous pressure

1. Chronic right heart failure due to other causes
2. Constrictive pericarditis
3. Mitral stenosis

External pressure on the portal vein

1. Inflammatory lymph nodes (eg, tuberculosis)
2. Lymphoma$_g$
3. Malignant tumor, primary or metastatic
4. Sarcoidosis

Obstruction of the inferior vena cava above the hepatic vein

1. Mediastinal mass
2. Thrombosis of IVC

Portal vein obstruction secondary to diffuse hepatic disease

1. Hepar lobatum
2. Portal cirrhosis
3. Schistosomiasis

Portal vein thrombosis

1. Chronically ill patients
2. Invasion by neoplastic disease

Veno-occlusive disease

Thrombosis or web in inferior vena cava

OTHER CAUSES

1. Bile peritonitis
2. Ectopic pregnancy
3. Hemoperitoneum (eg, trauma; surgery)
4. Hypoalbuminemia (eg, nephrotic S.; protein-losing gastroenteropathy)
5. Peritoneal lavage; dialysis

[CONDITIONS THAT MAY MIMIC ASCITES]

1. [Mesenteric cyst]
2. [Ovarian cyst]
3. [Pancreatic pseudocyst]
4. [Pregnancy]

References

1. Gore RM, Gore MD: Ascites and peritoneal fluid collections. In Gore RM, Levine MS (eds): Textbook of Gastrointestinal Radiology. (ed 2) Philadelphia: WB Saunders, 2000, pp 1969–1979
2. Williamson MR: Chapter 5. Abdominal Ultrasound. In: Essentials of Ultrasound. Philadelphia: WB Saunders, 1996, p 66

PERITONEAL FLUID (ASCITES) IN AN INFANT OR CHILD

COMMON

1. Appendiceal perforation
2. Cardiac disease (eg, anasarca; constrictive pericarditis)
3. Cirrhosis, portal or biliary (eg, biliary atresia; polycystic liver)
4. Hemorrhage
5. Hydrops fetalis; erythroblastosis fetalis
6. Hypoproteinemia (eg, malnutrition; kwashiorkor; intestinal lymphangiectasia)
7. Peritonitis (eg, meconium; sepsis; toxoplasmosis; rubella S.; cytomegalovirus infection; typhoid fever; amebiasis)
8. Portal vein or IVC obstruction, extrahepatic (eg, neoplasm; lymphadenopathy; thromboembolism)
9. Renal failure (eg, nephrotic S. with hypoproteinemia; glomerulonephritis; uremia)
10. Trauma; surgery
11. Urinary outlet obstruction with hydronephrosis (urine ascites)
12. Ventriculoperitoneal shunt

UNCOMMON

1. Antitrypsinase deficiency
2. Chylous or lymphatic ascites, neonatal (See G-235)
3. Galactosemia; tyrosinemia
4. Gaucher disease; lysosomal storage disease
5. Hemolytic anemia with ascites
6. Hydrometrocolpos with rupture and plastic peritonitis
7. Meckel diverticulum, perforated
8. Meigs S. (benign ovarian tumor)
9. Metastatic disease to peritoneum
10. Ovarian cyst, ruptured
11. Pancreatitis, acute
12. Preduodenal portal vein
13. Schistosomiasis
14. Thromboembolism of inferior vena cava, renal vein, or hepatic veins
15. Tuberculosis
16. Wilson disease

References

1. Meyer JI, Donaldson JS: Diseases of the pediatric abdominal wall, peritoneum, and mesentery. In Gore RM, Levine MS (eds): Textbook of Gastrointestinal Radiology. (ed 2) Philadelphia: WB Saunders, 2000, pp 2179–2185
2. Moncada R, Wang JJ, Love L, Bush I: Neonatal ascites associated with urinary outlet obstruction (urine ascites). Radiology 1968; 90:1165–1170
3. Siegel MJ: Pediatric Body CT. Philadelphia: Lippincott Williams & Wilkins, 1999
4. Silverman FN (ed): Caffey's Pediatric X-ray Diagnosis: An Integrated Imaging Approach. (ed 8) Chicago: Year Book Medical Publ, 1985
5. Swischuk LE: Radiology of the Newborn, Infant, and Young Child. (ed 3) Baltimore: Williams & Wilkins, 1989
6. Swischuk LE, John SD: Differential Diagnosis in Pediatric Radiology. (ed 2) Baltimore: Williams & Wilkins, 1995, pp 160–16

CHYLOUS OR LYMPHATIC ASCITES*

COMMON

1. Filariasis
2. Lymphoma$_g$
3. Metastatic disease (esp. to lymph nodes)
4. Neoplasm, benign (esp. lymphangioma)
5. Neoplasm, malignant, compressing or invading lymphatic system (eg, carcinoma of pancreas, lung, esopaghus; mediastinal tumor)
6. Postoperative
7. Trauma

UNCOMMON

1. Adhesive bands
2. Cirrhosis (hepatic lymphatics visible)
3. Congenital absence or hypoplasia of lymphatic system

4. Idiopathic
5. Lymphangioleiomyomatosis; tuberous sclerosis
6. Lymphangiomatosis, disseminated (benign metastasizing lymphangiomatosis)
7. Tuberculosis; histoplasmosis

* Obstruction of abdominal lymphatic vessels, cisterna chyli, or thoracic duct on lymphangiography.

References
1. Gore RM, Gore MD: Ascites and peritoneal fluid collections. In Gore RM, Levine MS (eds): Textbook of Gastrointestinal Radiology. (ed 2) Philadelphia: WB Saunders, 2000, pp 1969–1979
2. Griscom NT, Colodny AH, Rosenberg HK, et al: Diagnostic aspects of neonatal ascites: Report of 27 cases. AJR 1977;128:961–970

Gamut G-236

SPONTANEOUS PNEUMOPERITONEUM WITHOUT PERITONITIS

COMMON
1. Iatrogenic (incl. postoperative; anesthesia; respiratory therapy; peritoneal dialysis; Rubin test; bronchoscopy; endoscopy; diagnostic pneumoperitoneum)
2. Idiopathic
3. Perforation of GI tract, forme fruste type (eg, peptic ulcer; neoplasm; Crohn's disease; bowel infarction or obstruction)
4. Vaginal "aspiration" (eg, douching; sudden squatting; oral sex; postpartum exercises)

UNCOMMON
1. ARDS
2. Distention of stomach (eg, aerophagia; gastroscopy; sodium bicarbonate ingestion; misplaced oxygen tube)
3. Idiopathic dilatation of colon (eg, pseudo-obstruction)
4. Jejunal diverticulosis

5. Pneumatosis cystoides intestinalis (See G-70)
6. Pneumomediastinum (eg, pulmonary emphysema; ruptured bulla)
7. Pneumothorax (eg, via congenital pleuroperitoneal fistula)
8. Sclerotherapy of esophageal varices

References
1. Ashai S, Lipton D, Colon A, et al: Pneumoperitoneum secondary to cunnilingus. N Engl J Med 1976; 295:117
2. Baker SR, Cho KC: The Abdominal Plain Film with Correlative Imaging. Norwalk, CT: Appleton & Lange, 1998
3. Campbell RE, Boggs TR Jr, Kirkpatrick JA Jr: Early neonatal pneumoperitoneum from progressive massive tension pneumomediastinum. Radiology 1975;114:121–126
4. Eisenberg RL: Gastrointestinal Radiology: A Pattern Approach. (ed 3) Philadelphia: Lippincott, 1996, pp 939–949
5. Felson B, Wiot JF: Another look at pneumoperitoneum. Semin Roentgenol 1973; 8:437–443
6. Stringfield JT III, Graham JP, Watts CM, et al: Pneumoperitoneum: a complication of mechanical ventilation. JAMA 1976;235:744–746

Gamut G-237

PNEUMOPERITONEUM WITH PERITONITIS

COMMON
1. Perforated hollow viscus (eg, peptic ulcer; intestinal obstruction; diverticulitis; appendicitis; necrotic tumor; penetrating or blunt abdominal trauma; emphysematous cholecystitis) (See G-238)

UNCOMMON
1. Meconium peritonitis
2. Megacolon with rupture (eg, Chagas' disease; Hirschsprung disease)
3. Perforation of colon following immunosuppressive therapy in renal transplant patient
4. Septic peritonitis with gas forming organism

(continued)

5. Ulcerating bowel disease (eg, typhoid fever; amebiasis; toxic megacolon; ulcerative colitis; Crohn's disease; tuberculosis; pseudomembranous colitis; necrotizing enterocolitis; ischemic colitis; lymphogranuloma venereum)

References

1. Baker SR, Cho KC: The Abdominal Plain Film with Correlative Imaging. Norwalk, CT: Appleton & Lange, 1998
2. Eisenberg RL: Gastrointestinal Radiology: A Pattern Approach. (ed 3) Philadelphia: Lippincott, 1996, pp 939–946

Gamut G-238

PERFORATED HOLLOW VISCUS IN AN INFANT

COMMON

1. Iatrogenic (eg, intubation; rectal thermometer; enema; resuscitation; intrauterine transfusion)
2. Intestinal obstruction (eg, atresia; volvulus)
3. Meconium ileus (cystic fibrosis {mucoviscidosis})
4. Necrotizing enterocolitis
5. Respirator therapy
6. Trauma; battered child S.

UNCOMMON

1. Gastric rupture of newborn
2. Hirschsprung disease
3. Idiopathic
4. Ischemic enteritis (eg, umbilical artery thromboembolism; sepsis; malrotation with midgut volvulus)
5. Meconium plug S.
6. Perforated peptic or stress ulcer
7. [Pneumoperitoneum without peritonitis] (See G-236)
8. Small left colon S.

References

1. Fernbach SK: Neonatal gastrointestinal radiology. In: Gore RM, Levine MS (eds): Textbook of Gastrointestinal Radiology. (ed 2) Philadelphia: WB Saunders, 2000, pp 2042–2073
2. Leonidas JC, Hall RT, Rhodes PG, et al: Pneumoperitoneum in ventilated newborns. A medical or a surgical problem? Am J Dis Child 1974;128:677–6803.
3. Tucker AS, Soine L, Izant Jr RJ: Gastrointestinal perforations in infancy: Anatomic and etiologic gamuts. AJR 1975;123:755–763

Gamut G-239

ABNORMAL GAS COLLECTION IN THE RIGHT UPPER QUADRANT

COMMON

1. Abscess$_g$, abdominal (eg, subphrenic, hepatic, pericolic, renal, or perirenal) (See G-243)
2. Colon interposition (Chilaiditi S.); colon distention
3. Gas in the biliary tract; biliary fistula (See G-128, G-139)
4. Pneumoperitoneum, free or loculated (eg, perforation of hollow viscus; postoperative) (See G-236–238)
5. Subhepatic gas or abscess (eg, perforated duodenal ulcer or appendix)

UNCOMMON

1. Abdominal wall gas or abscess (postoperative; traumatic; drainage tube)
2. Emphysematous cholecystitis
3. Gastric rupture of newborn
4. Iatrogenic pneumoretroperitoneum (incl. interventional embolization of a viscus; needle or catheter drainage; postnephrectomy; endoscopy)
5. Pneumatosis intestinalis (See G-70)
6. Pneumomediastinum with retroperitoneal extension
7. Portal vein gas (See G-192)
8. Retroperitoneal rupture of gut (esp. duodenum or rectum)
9. Stomach (heterotaxy)

References

1. Anschuetz SL: Extraluminal gas in the upper abdomen. Semin Roentgenol 1984;19:255

2. Baker SR, Cho KC: The Abdominal Plain Film with Correlative Imaging. Norwalk, CT: Appleton & Lange, 1998
3. Eisenberg RL: Gastrointestinal Radiology: A Pattern Approach. (ed 3) Philadelphia: Lippincott, 1996, pp 950–964
4. Love L, Baker D, Ramey R: Gas producing perinephric abscess. AJR 1973;119:783–7925.
5. Rice RP, Thompson WM, Gedgaudas RK: The diagnosis and significance of extraluminal gas in the abdomen. Radiol Clin North Am 1982;20:819–837

3. Eisenberg RL: Gastrointestinal Radiology: A Pattern Approach. (ed 3) Philadelphia: Lippincott, 1996, pp 950–964.
4. Love L, Baker D, Ramey R: Gas producing perinephric abscess. AJR 1973;119:783–792

Gamut G-241

LARGE ABDOMINAL GAS POCKET

COMMON

1. Abscess$_g$, abdominal (eg, subphrenic, splenic, renal or perirenal, pericolic, pancreatic, lesser sac, abdominal wall)
2. Bladder distended with air (eg, iatrogenic; emphysematous cystitis)
3. Cecal distention (eg, nonobstructive "paralytic" ileus; pseudo-obstruction; colon obstruction)
4. Diabetic gastropathy; acute gastric dilatation (eg, cast S.)
5. Duodenal obstruction (See G-42, 43)
6. Gastric outlet obstruction (See G-30)
7. Hernia, obstructed (eg, hiatal; diaphragmatic; internal; external)
8. Pneumoperitoneum, free or loculated (subphrenic; lesser sac; greater sac)
9. Retroperitoneal or extraperitoneal gas (eg, duodenal or rectal perforation)
10. Sentinel loop (localized ileus) (See G-80)
11. Small bowel or colon obstruction, chronic (eg, Crohn's disease; adhesions; congenital stenosis)

UNCOMMON

1. Abdominal wall gas (postoperative)
2. Amnionitis; endometritis (physometra); infected fetus
3. Blind loop S. (esp. postoperative) (See G-58)
4. Diverticulum of colon or duodenum (giant size)
5. Duplication cyst, communicating
6. Emphysematous cholecystitis
7. Emphysematous peritonitis
8. Fibroid, infected

Gamut G-240

ABNORMAL GAS COLLECTION IN THE LEFT UPPER QUADRANT

COMMON

1. Abscess$_g$, other abdominal (eg, subphrenic, splenic, pericolic, renal or perirenal)
2. Pneumoperitoneum, free or loculated (eg, perforation of hollow viscus; postoperative) (See G-236–238)

UNCOMMON

1. Abdominal wall gas or abscess (postoperative; traumatic; drainage tube)
2. Emphysematous gastritis
3. Iatrogenic pneumoretroperitoneum (incl. interventional embolization of a viscus; needle or catheter drainage; postnephrectomy; endoscopy)
4. Lesser sac gas or abscess (eg, postsplenectomy; perforation of gut; pancreatic abscess or infected pseudocyst)
5. Pancreatic gas abscess (peritoneal fat necrosis)
6. Pneumatosis intestinalis
7. Pneumomediastinum with retroperitoneal extension
8. Retroperitoneal rupture of gut (esp. duodenum or rectum)

References
1. Anschuetz SL: Extraluminal gas in the upper abdomen. Semin Roentgenol 1984;19:255
2. Baker SR, Cho KC: The Abdominal Plain Film with Correlative Imaging. Norwalk, CT: Appleton & Lange, 1983.

(continued)

9. Gangrene of liver
10. Hydropneumometrocolpos; vaginitis emphysematosa
11. Meckel's diverticulum (giant size)
12. Ovarian cyst (eg, gas infection; intestinal fistula)

References

1. Altemeier WA, Culbertson WR, Fullen WD, et al: Intra-abdominal abscesses. Am J Surg 1973;125:70–79
2. Blatt ES, Schneider HJ, Wiot JF, et al: Roentgen findings in obstructed diaphragmatic hernia. Radiology 1962;79:648–6573.
3. Felson B, Wiot JF: Case of the Day. Springfield, IL: CC Thomas, 1967, p 764.
4. Gaillard S, Pascaud E, Chardac J, et al: An unusual cause of intra-abdominal gas pouches. Ann Radiol 1980;23:675–6785.
5. Messmer JM: Gas and soft tissue abnormalities. In Gore RM, Levine MS (eds): Textbook of Gastrointestinal Radiology. (ed 2) Philadelphia: WB Saunders, 2000, pp 157–177
6. Phillips JC: A spectrum of radiologic abnormalities due to tubo-ovarian abscess. Radiology 1974;110:307–311

Gamut G-242

ABDOMINAL OR PELVIC ABSCESS

COMMON

1. Appendicitis
2. Carcinoma or other malignancy with perforation
3. Crohn's disease
4. Diverticultis
5. Pancreatitis
6. Pelvic inflammatory disease (eg, endometritis)
7. Peptic ulcer perforation
8. Postoperative
9. Posttraumatic (eg, gunshot or knife wound)
10. Tubo-ovarian (eg, sexually transmitted diseases; ectopic pregnancy)

UNCOMMON

1. Intestinal perforation, other (eg, intestinal obstruction; meconium ileus)
2. Ischemic colitis
3. Lymphogranuloma venereum
4. Parasitic disease (eg, amebiasis; schistosomiasis; ascariasis)
5. Perinephric abscess; pyelonephritis
6. Tuberculosis
7. Typhoid fever

Gamut G-243

RIGHT ANTERIOR PARARENAL SPACE ABSCESS (ESPECIALLY ON US, CT, OR MRI)

1. Duodenal perforation secondary to
   a. Ulcer
   b. Foreign body
   c. Inflamed diverticulum of duodenum
2. Crohn's disease of small bowel or ascending colon
3. Colitis involving ascending colon
   a. Amebiasis
   b. Diverticulitis
   c. Tuberculosis
4. Ruptured retrocecal or retroperitoneal appendix
5. Pancreatic abscess or infected pseudocyst
6. Renal or perirenal abscess extending into pararenal space

Reference

1. Meyers MA: Dynamic Radiology of the Abdomen (ed 5) New York: Springer-Verlag, 2000

Gamut G-244-S

ABSCESS MIMICS ON ABDOMINAL US, CT, OR MRI

COMMON

1. Cyst (eg, ovarian; renal; splenic; dermoid; mesenteric; hepatic; hydatid)
2. Hematoma
3. Loop of bowel
4. Necrotic neoplasm (eg, hepatoma; metastasis)
5. Pseudocyst of pancreas

UNCOMMON

1. Biloma
2. Iatrogenic (eg, retained Foley catheter)
3. Herniation of bowel through diaphragm
4. Lymphocele
5. Seroma
6. Urinoma

Gamut G-245

DECREASED ABDOMINAL GAS IN A NEWBORN

COMMON

1. Congenital diaphragmatic hernia
2. Duodenal atresia or stenosis; annular pancreas
3. Endotracheal intubation
4. Esophageal obstruction (eg, atresia without T-E fistula; web) (See G-12, G-19)
5. Medication (esp. maternal)
6. Neonatal sepsis
7. Obstruction of pylorus (eg, hypertrophic pyloric stenosis at 2 to 8 weeks), duodenum, or proximal jejunum (esp. atresia or stenosis)
8. Suction, orogastric or nasogastric

UNCOMMON

1. Dehydration
2. Dysphagia; impaired swallowing physiology (eg, severe prematurity; depressed swallowing reflex; impending death)
3. Fluid-filled bowel
4. Large abdominal mass
5. Midgut volvulus
6. Normal
7. Peritoneal fluid (ascites)
8. Vomiting (eg, gastroenteritis; electrolyte imbalance)

References

1. Cohen MD, Jansen R, Lemons J, et al: Evaluation of the gasless abdomen in the newborn and young infant with metrizamide. AJR 1984;142:393–396
2. Fernbach SK: Neonatal gastrointestinal radiology. In Gore RM, Levine MS (eds): Textbook of Gastrointestinal Radiology. (ed 2) Philadelphia: WB Saunders, 2000, pp 2042–2073

Gamut G-246

DECREASED ABDOMINAL GAS IN AN ADULT

COMMON

1. Acute pancreatitis
2. Ascites
3. Normal

UNCOMMON

1. Dysphagia
2. Fluid-filled bowel (eg, closed loop obstruction)
3. Hernia (esp. hiatal)
4. Large abdominal mass displacing bowel laterally
5. Mesenteric infarction, early
6. Obstruction of esophagus (eg, cardiospasm; neoplasm), stomach (eg, volvulus; pyloric obstruction from ulcer or neoplasm), or duodenum (eg, neoplasm)
7. Vomiting; inanition

Gamut G-247-1

ABDOMINAL CALCIFICATION(S) IN AN INFANT OR CHILD
(See G-143, G-203, 204, G-247-2)

COMMON

1. Adrenal calcification (See H-123)
2. Appendiceal fecalith (calculus)
3. [Foreign material; pills; pica; medication; contrast medium; heavy metal]
4. Histoplasmosis or tuberculosis in liver, spleen, lymph node, peritoneum
5. Meconium in peritoneum (meconium peritonitis from intestinal perforation), intestinal lumen or wall
6. Neuroblastoma; other neurogenic neoplasm
7. Urinary tract calcification (See H-24)

UNCOMMON

1. Abscess$_g$, abdominal (esp. liver)
2. Arterial calcification (eg, metastatic calcinosis; primary or secondary hyperparathyroidism)
3. Calculus in Meckel's diverticulum or urachal cyst
4. Chronic granulomatous disease of childhood
5. Congenital syndromes (See G-247-2)
6. Cyst of spleen, kidney, pancreas, ovary, mesentery
7. Dermoid cyst; teratoma; fetus in fetu
8. Duplication, atresia, other obstruction of gut (mural or luminal calcification)
9. Enterolith; also enterolithiasis associated with anal atresia
10. Fetal infection (toxoplasmosis; rubella; cytomegalovirus; herpes simplex; varicella)
11. Gallstone (esp. thalassemia; sickle cell disease; other hemolytic anemia)
12. Hemangioma; lymphangioma (phlebolith; lympholith)
13. Hematoma, old (liver; spleen; retroperitoneal)
14. Hemochromatosis of liver
15. Hydrometrocolpos (ruptured) with plastic peritonitis
16. Ischemic infarct or necrosis of liver
17. Liver neoplasm (hemangioma; hamartoma; metastatic neuroblastoma; occasionally hepatoma; hepatoblastoma) (See G-154, 155)
18. Mucocele of appendix
19. Pancreatitis, chronic
20. Parasitic disease (eg, hydatid cysts or *Armillifer* infestation of peritoneum or mesentery; guinea worm infection or cysticercosis of abdominal wall or back)
21. Retroperitoneal neoplasm
22. Thromboembolism of inferior vena cava, portal vein, renal vein
23. Tuberculous psoas abscess

[ ] This condition does not actually cause the gamuted imaging finding, but can produce imaging changes that simulate it.

References

1. Baker SR, Cho KC: The Abdominal Plain Film with Correlative Imaging. Norwalk, CT: Appleton & Lange, 1998
2. Berdon WE, Baker DH, Wigger HJ, et al: Calcified intraluminal meconium in newborn males with imperforate anus: enterolithiasis in the newborn. AJR 1975;125:449–455
3. Friedman AP, Haller JO, Boyer B, Cooper R: Calcified portal vein thromboemboli in infants: Radiography and ultrasonography. Radiology 1981;140:381–382
4. Nguyen DL, Leonard JC: Ischemic hepatic necrosis: A cause of fetal liver calcification. AJR 1986;147:596–597
5. Schackelford GD, Kirks DR: Neonatal hepatic calcification secondary to transplacental infection. Radiology 1977;122: 753–757
6. Siegel MJ: Pediatric Body CT. Philadelphia: Lippincott Williams & Wilkins, 1999
7. Swischuk LE, John SD: Differential Diagnosis in Pediatric Radiology. (ed 2) Baltimore: Williams & Wilkins, 1995

Gamut G-247-2

CONGENITAL SYNDROMES WITH ABDOMINAL CALCIFICATIONS

1. Beckwith-Wiedemann S. (adrenal)
2. Cholesterol ester storage disease (adrenal)
3. Chondroectodermal dysplasia (Ellis-van Creveld S.) (gallstones; nephrocalcinosis)
4. Chronic granulomatous disease of childhood (liver; spleen; lymph nodes)

5. Cushing S. (adrenal)
6. Cystic fibrosis (mucoviscidosis) (pancreas; meconium peritonitis)
7. Cystinosis (urinary calculi)
8. Fetal cytomegalovirus infection (gonads)
9. Fetal herpes simplex infection (liver; adrenal)
10. Fetal toxoplasmosis infection (liver)
11. Fetal varicella infection (liver)
12. Gorlin S. (nevoid basal cell carcinoma S.) (ovarian)
13. Hirschsprung disease (enterolith)
14. Milk-alkali S. (nephrocalcinosis)
15. Multiple endocrine neoplasia (MEN) S., type IIA and IIB
   (eg, pheochromocytoma) (See J-5)
16. Oxalosis (nephrocalcinosis)
17. Prune-belly S. (Eagle-Barrett S.) (bladder wall; renal)
18. Renal tubular acidosis S. (nephrocalcinosis)
19. Wolman disease (familial xanthomatosis) (adrenal)

References
1. Kirks DR, Taybi H: Prune belly syndrome: an unusual cause of neonatal abdominal calcification. AJR 1975;123:778–7822.
2. Swischuk LE, John SD: Differential Diagnosis in Pediatric Radiology. (ed 2) Baltimore: Williams & Wilkins, 1995
3. Taybi H, Lachman RS: Radiology of Syndromes, Metabolic Disorders, and Skeletal Dysplasias. (ed 4) St. Louis: Mosby-Year Book, 1996, p 958

Gamut G-248

NONVISCERAL ABDOMINAL CALCIFICATION

COMMON
1. Aneurysm; arteriovenous malformation
*2. Appendiceal fecalith (calculus), extruded into peritoneal sac
3. Atherosclerosis
*4. Dermoid cyst; teratoma; fetus in fetu
*5. [Foreign material (eg, pill; pica; medication; contrast medium; heavy metal)]

*6. Gallstone extruded into peritoneal sac
*7. Lymph nodes (eg, tuberculosis; histoplasmosis)
*8. Meconium in peritoneum, intestinal wall or lumen
*9. Phlebolith; lympholith (incl. hemangioma; lymphangioma)
*10. [Rib cartilage]

UNCOMMON
*1. [Barium in peritoneum]
2. [Bone lesion with matrix or sclerosis]
*3. Epiploic appendage
4. Fluorosis (ligamentous)
5. Hydrometrocolpos
6. Lipoma
*7. Lithopedion; extrauterine pregnancy
*8. Mesenteric cyst
9. Mesothelioma of peritoneum
10. Metastasis (esp. from colloid carcinoma; papillary cystadenocarcinoma of ovary)
*11. Mineral oil granuloma (instilled in peritoneum)
12. Myositis (fibrodysplasia) ossificans progressiva
13. Neoplasm of soft tissues (eg, osteoma; osteosarcoma; chondrosarcoma; undifferentiated abdominal malignancy)
14. Neuroblastoma
15. Pancreatitis with saponification; fat necrosis; Weber-Christian disease
*16. Parasitic disease (eg, hydatid cysts or *Armillifer* infestation of peritoneum or mesentery; guinea worm infection or cysticercosis of abdominal wall or back)
17. Pheochromocytoma
18. Pseudomyxoma peritonei (eg, from pseudomucinous cystadenoma of ovary; mucocele of appendix)
19. Retroperitoneal hematoma
20. Retroperitoneal neoplasm
21. Scar or burn (abdominal wall)
22. Scleroderma; dermatomyositis
23. Thrombosis of portal vein, renal vein, or inferior vena cava
24. Tuberculous peritonitis, psoas abscess

* May be mobile.
[ ] This condition does not actually cause the gamuted imaging finding, but can produce imaging changes that simulate it.

(continued)

References
1. Baker SR, Cho KC: The Abdominal Plain Film with Correlative Imaging. Norwalk, CT: Appleton & Lange, 1998
2. Eisenberg RL: Gastrointestinal Radiology: A Pattern Approach. (ed 3) Philadelphia: Lippincott, 1996, pp 1043–1064

Gamut G-249

ABDOMINAL CALCIFICATIONS THAT LAYER IN THE UPRIGHT POSITION

COMMON
1. Bladder calculi
2. Gallstones

UNCOMMON
1. [Contrast medium; barium]
2. Dermoid cyst (eg, teeth)
3. Enteroliths in small bowel or Meckel's diverticulum
4. Milk of calcium (eg, in gallbladder or kidney, Pott's abscess, meconium, granulomatous lymph node, or chronic tubo-ovarian abscess)
5. Myxoglobulosis of appendix
6. Renal calculi (eg, in calyceal diverticulum or hydronephrosis)
7. Urachal cyst calculi

[ ] This condition does not actually cause the gamuted imaging finding, but can produce imaging changes that simulate it.

Reference
1. Baker SR, Cho KC: The Abdominal Plain Film with Correlative Imaging. Norwalk, CT: Appleton & Lange, 1998

Gamut G-250

ABDOMINAL CALCIFICATION(S) WITH A CONCRETION OR ANNULAR MORPHOLOGY

COMMON
1. Aneurysm; arteriovenous malformation; atherosclerosis
2. Appendiceal fecalith (calculus)
3. [Foreign body (eg, pill)]
4. Gallstone
5. Meconium
6. Pancreatic calculus
7. Phlebolith or lympholith (eg, normal pelvic veins; splenolith or hepatolith; hemangioma or lymphangioma; varicocele)
8. Prostatic calculus
9. Urinary tract calculus
10. Varix

UNCOMMON
1. Cyst (mesenteric; ovarian; renal; splenic)
2. Dermoid cyst
3. Diverticulum calculus (eg, colonic; duodenal; Meckel's)
4. Enterolith
5. Epiploic appendage
6. Lithopedion
7. Mineral oil granuloma
8. Mucocele or myxoglobulosis of appendix
9. Parasitic disease (esp. hydatid disease—*Echinococcus granulosus* or *E. multilocularis; Armillifer* infection; guinea worm infection or cysticercosis of abdominal wall or back)
10. Pseudomyxoma peritonei (eg, from pseudomucinous cystadenoma of ovary; mucocele of appendix)
11. Urachal calculus
12. Urethral calculus

[ ] This condition does not actually cause the gamuted imaging finding, but can produce imaging changes that simulate it.

Reference
1. Baker SR, Cho KC: The Abdominal Plain Film with Correlative Imaging. Norwalk, CT: Appleton & Lange, 1998

Gamut G-251

WIDESPREAD ABDOMINAL CALCIFICATIONS

COMMON

1. Atherosclerosis
2. Phleboliths (eg, normal; hemangioma)
3. Tuberculosis or histoplasmosis in liver, spleen, lymph nodes, or peritoneum

UNCOMMON

1. Fat necrosis (esp. pancreatitis; Weber-Christian disease)
2. [Hemochromatosis (liver and spleen)]
3. Meconium peritonitis
4. Metastases (eg, neuroblastoma; ovarian cystadenocarcinoma; colloid carcinoma of colon)
5. Mineral oil granulomas (peritoneal instillation)
6. Myositis (fibrodysplasia) ossificans progressiva (esp. abdominal wall)
7. Parasitic disease (esp. hydatid cysts or *Armillifer* infestation of peritoneum or mesentery; guinea worm infection or cysticercosis of abdominal wall or back)
8. Pseudomyxoma peritonei (eg, from pseudomucinous cystadenoma of ovary; mucocele of appendix)
9. Scleroderma; dermatomyositis (abdominal wall)
10. Undifferentiated abdominal malignancy

[ ] This condition does not actually cause the gamuted imaging finding, but can produce imaging changes that simulate it.

References
1. Baker SR, Cho KC: The Abdominal Plain Film with Correlative Imaging. Norwalk, CT: Appleton & Lange, 1998
2. Eisenberg RL: Gastrointestinal Radiology: A Pattern Approach. (ed 3) Philadelphia: Lippincott, 1996, pp 1044–1049
3. Swischuk LE, John SD: Differential Diagnosis in Pediatric Radiology. (ed 2) Baltimore: Williams & Wilkins, 1995

Gamut G-252

ABDOMINAL WALL CALCIFICATION

1. Fat necrosis
2. Hypercalcemic state; idiopathic calcinosis
3. Myositis (fibrodysplasia) ossificans progressiva; myositis ossificans
4. Neoplasm of abdominal wall (incl. osteoma; osteosarcoma; chondrosarcoma)
5. [Opaque medication]
6. Parasitic disease (esp. guinea worm infection or cysticercosis of abdominal wall or back; *Armillifer* infection of peritoneum)
7. Scar; burn
8. Scleroderma; dermatomyositis
9. [Skin nodule; tattoo; colostomy orifice]

[ ] This condition does not actually cause the gamuted imaging finding, but can produce imaging changes that simulate it.

References
1. Baker SR, Cho KC: Abdominal calcifications. In Gore RM, Levine MS (eds): Textbook of Gastrointestinal Radiology. (ed 2) Philadelphia: WB Saunders, 2000, pp 178–189
2. Eisenberg RL: Gastrointestinal Radiology: A Pattern Approach. (ed 3) Philadelphia: Lippincott, 1996, pp 1049–1051

Gamut G-253

ABDOMINAL WALL MASS (ESP. ON US, CT, OR MRI)

COMMON

1. Abscess$_g$
2. Hematoma
3. Umbilical or ventral hernia

UNCOMMON

1. Endometrioma in scar
2. Neoplasm (eg, desmoid tumor; lipoma; neurofibroma; malignant fibrous histiocytoma; metastasis)
3. Omphalomesenteric cyst
4. Seroma; cellulitis
5. Urachal cyst

References

1. Marn CS: Anterior abdominal wall. In: Gore RM, Levine MS (eds): Textbook of Gastrointestinal Radiology. (ed 2) Philadelphia: WB Saunders, 2000, pp 2010–2019
2. Siegel MJ: Pediatric Body CT. Philadelphia: Lippincott Williams & Wilkins, 1999
3. Williamson MR: Chapter 5. Abdominal ultrasound. In: Essentials of Ultrasound. Philadelphia: WB Saunders, 1996, p 68

Gamut G-254

CYSTIC ABDOMINAL MASS IN A FETUS OR NEWBORN (US)

COMMON

1. Dilated bladder
2. [Dilated bowel]
3. Hydronephrosis
4. Multicystic dysplastic kidney
5. Ovarian cyst

UNCOMMON

1. Choledochal cyst
2. Dilated ureter
3. Enteric duplication cyst
4. Hepatic cyst or cystic tumor (eg, mesenchymal hamartoma)
5. Hydrometrocolpos
6. Lymphangioma (incl. mesenteric cyst)
7. Persistent cloaca
8. Splenic cyst
9. Urachal cyst
10. Urinoma

[ ] This condition does not actually cause the gamuted imaging finding, but can produce imaging changes that simulate it.

References

1. Bryan, PJ: Lecture at Eastern Radiological Society Meeting, Dublin, Ireland, 1990.
2. Fernbach SK: Neonatal gastrointestinal radiology. In: Gore RM, Levine MS (eds): Textbook of Gastrointestinal Radiology. (ed 2) Philadelphia: WB Saunders, 2000, pp 2042–2073

Gamut G-255

UPPER ABDOMINAL MASS IN A NEONATE OR CHILD

COMMON

1. Abscess$_g$, abdominal (eg, retrocecal appendiceal)
2. Adrenal hemorrhage, cyst, or tumor (See H-124)
3. Fecal masses (esp. Hirschsprung disease)
4. Gastric dilatation (fluid filled stomach)
5. Hematoma (esp. splenic)
6. Hepatomegaly (See G-141-1 and -2)
7. Hydronephrosis
8. Intestinal obstruction (fluid-filled loop)
9. Intussusception
10. Lymphoma$_g$
11. Metastasis
12. Multicystic dysplastic kidney
13. Neuroblastoma; other neural tumor

14. Pyloric stenosis
15. Renal neoplasm (eg, Wilms' tumor; mesoblastic nephroma) (See H-42)
16. Splenomegaly (See G-197, 198)

UNCOMMON

1. Bezoar, gastric
2. Bone lesion (eg, aneurysmal bone cyst or sarcoma of spine)
3. Cyst (eg, mesenteric; omental; renal; splenic; pancreatic; hepatic; choledochal; duplication; dermoid; hydatid)
4. Hepatic mass (eg, abscess; cyst; hepatoblastoma; hemangioma; hemangioendothelioma; hepatoma) (See G-154–157)
5. Infantile polycystic kidneys
6. Lymphangioma of mesentery or omentum
7. Meconium (eg, in cystic fibrosis)
8. Meningocele (anterior; lateral)
9. Renal vein thrombosis
10. Retroperitoneal lesion (eg, teratoma; sarcoma; hematoma)
11. Urinoma; lymphocele

References

1. Chan CY, Chan SM, Liauw L: A large abdominal mass in a young girl. Br J Radiol 2000;7:913–914
2. Fernbach SK: Neonatal gastrointestinal radiology. In: Gore RM, Levine MS (eds): Textbook of Gastrointestinal Radiology. (ed 2) Philadelphia: WB Saunders, 2000, pp 2042–2073
3. Kirks DR, Merten DF, Grossman H, Bowie JD: Diagnostic imaging of pediatric abdominal masses: an overview. Radiol Clin North Am 1981;19:527–545
4. Koop CE: Abdominal mass in the newborn infant. N Engl J Med 1973;289:569–571
5. Melicow MM, Uson AC: Palpable abdominal masses in infants and children: A report based on a review of 653 cases. J Urol 1959;81:705–710
6. Siegel MJ: Pediatric Body CT. Philadelphia: Lippincott Williams & Wilkins, 1999
7. Swischuk LE, John SD: Differential Diagnosis in Pediatric Radiology. (ed 2) Baltimore: Williams & Wilkins, 1995
8. Tank ES, Poznanski AK, Holt JF: The radiologic discrimination of abdominal masses in infants. J Urol 1973;109:128–132
9. Wedge JJ, Grosfeld JL, Smith JP: Abdominal masses in the newborn: 63 cases. J Urol 1971;106:770–775

LOWER ABDOMINAL MASS IN A NEONATE OR CHILD

COMMON

1. Abscess$_g$, abdominal (eg, appendiceal)
2. Bladder, distended
3. Fecal impaction and masses (esp. Hirschsprung disease)
4. Intestinal obstruction (fluid-filled loop)
5. Intussusception
6. Lymphoma$_g$
7. Metastasis
8. Ovarian cyst
9. Pregnancy

UNCOMMON

1. Bone lesion (eg, aneurysmal bone cyst or sarcoma of pelvis or LS spine)
2. Cyst, other (eg, mesenteric; dermoid; urachal; duplication; hydatid)
3. Hydrometrocolpos
4. Meconium (eg, in cystic fibrosis)
5. Meningocele (anterior; lateral)
6. Retroperitoneal lesion (eg, teratoma; sarcoma; hematoma)
7. Urinoma; lymphocele

References

1. Chan CY, Chan SM, Liauw L: A large abdominal mass in a young girl. Br J Radiol 2000;7:913–914
2. Fernbach SK: Neonatal gastrointestinal radiology. In: Gore RM, Levine MS (eds): Textbook of Gastrointestinal Radiology. (ed 2) Philadelphia: WB Saunders, 2000, pp 2042–2073
3. Kirks DR, Merten DF, Grossman H, Bowie JD: Diagnostic imaging of pediatric abdominal masses: an overview. Radiol Clin North Am 1981;19:527–545
4. Koop CE: Abdominal mass in the newborn infant. N Engl J Med 1973;289:569–571
5. Melicow MM, Uson AC: Palpable abdominal masses in infants and children: A report based on a review of 653 cases. J Urol 1959;81:705–710

(continued)

6. Moss H, Wright DW, Weiss RG: Abdominal masses in pediatric patients. In: Wyllie R, Hyams JS: Pediatric Gastrointestinal Disease. (ed 2) Philadelphia: WB Saunders, 1999, pp 126–127
7. Siegel MJ: Pediatric Body CT. Philadelphia: Lippincott Williams & Wilkins, 1999
8. Swischuk LE, John SD: Differential Diagnosis in Pediatric Radiology. (ed 2) Baltimore: Williams & Wilkins, 1995
9. Tank ES, Poznanski AK, Holt JF: The radiologic discrimination of abdominal masses in infants. J Urol 1973;109:128–132
10. Wedge JJ, Grosfeld JL, Smith JP: Abdominal masses in the newborn: 63 cases. J Urol 1971;106:770–775

References
1. Chintapalli KN, Esola CC, Chopra S, et al: Pericolic mesenteric lymph nodes: an aid in distinguishing diverticulitis from cancer of the colon. AJR 1997;1253
2. Dodd GD, Baron RL, Oliver JH, et al: Enlarged abdominal lymph nodes in end-stage cirrhosis: CT—histopathologic correlation in 507 patients. Radiology 1997; 203:127–130
3. Dodd GD, Baron RL, Oliver JH, et al: Spectrum of imaging findings of the liver in endstage cirrhosis: part 1, gross morphology and diffuse abnormalities. AJR 1999;173:1185–1192
4. Okada Y, Yao YK, Yunoki M, et al: Lymph nodes in the hepatoduodenal ligament: US appearances with CT and MR correlation. Clin Radiol 1996;51:160–166
5. Warshauer DM, Dumbleton SA, Molina PL, et al: Abdominal CT findings in sarcoidosis: radiologic and clinical correlation. Radiology 1994;192:93–98

Gamut G-257

ABDOMINAL LYMPHADENOPATHY (US, CT, MRI)

BENIGN

+1. AIDS (eg, bacillary angiomatosis); AIDS related complex
2. Amyloidosis
3. Castleman disease
4. Cavitary mesenteric lymph node syndrome
5. Cirrhosis (alcohol induced); primary biliary cirrhosis
6. Crohn's disease
7. Diverticulitis
*8. Mycobacterial infection (eg, *Mycobacterium tuberculosis; M. avium intracellulare*)
9. Pyogenic infection
10. Sarcoidosis
11. Sclerosing cholangitis
12. Whipple's disease

MALIGNANT

+1. Kaposi sarcoma
2. Lymphoma$_g$; Hodgkin disease; leukemia
*3. Metastatic disease

* Lymph nodes may show low attenuation.
+ Lymph nodes may show very high attenuation.

Gamut G-258

FAT DENSITY IN THE ABDOMEN (CT, MRI)

COMMON

1. Dermoid cyst; teratoma
2. Fatty change in liver or pancreas
3. Lipoma; liposarcoma
4. Lipomatosis (pelvic; retroperitoneal; renal sinus)
5. Obesity

UNCOMMON

1. Angiomyolipoma of kidney or liver
2. Omental or mesenteric hernia
3. Steroid therapy; Cushing syndrome
4. Xanthogranulomatous pyelonephritis

Reference
1. Katz DL: Fatty densities on CT. Semin Roentgenol 1978; 13:187

Gamut G-259

"PSEUDOKIDNEY" OR "BULL'S-EYE" SIGN IN THE ABDOMEN (US)

COMMON

1. Gastroesophageal junction
2. Hypertrophic pyloric stenosis
3. Inflammatory bowel disease with wall thickening (eg, amebiasis; Crohn's disease; diverticulitis; Whipple's disease)
4. Intussusception (multiple concentric rings)
5. Malignant neoplasm with thickening of bowel wall (eg, carcinoma; lymphoma$_g$; leiomyosarcoma; metastasis to serosa)

UNCOMMON

1. Amyloidosis
2. Intramural hematoma (eg, trauma; anticoagulants; blood dyscrasia$_g$)

Reference

1. Eisenberg RL: Clinical Imaging: An Atlas of Differential Diagnosis. Gaithersburg, MD: Aspen Publ, 1992, pp 452–453

Gamut G-260

ABNORMAL ABDOMINAL VESSELS ON ANGIOGRAPHY

COMMON

1. Aneurysm$_g$
2. Anomalous origin or congenital absence of a vessel (eg, sequestration of lung)
3. Arterial occlusion, incl. collateral circulation (eg, via artery of Drummond; arc of Riolan; meandering mesenteric artery)
4. Arteritis, microaneurysms (eg, Behçet S.; Takayasu arteritis; necrotizing angiitis from drug abuse; my-

cotic aneurysms; polyarteritis nodosa; other connective tissue disease {collagen disease}$_g$)
5. Atherosclerosis
6. Fibromuscular dysplasia
7. Neoplasm, incl. neovascularity (eg, angiomyolipoma; pheochromocytoma; renal cell carcinoma) or vascular cuffing or displacement (esp. carcinoma)
8. Thromboembolism
9. Trauma (lacerated or transected vessel)
10. Varices (eg, portal venous hypertension or obstruction; inferior vena cava obstruction)

UNCOMMON

1. Anomalous pulmonary vein draining below the diaphragm (incl. venolobar S.)
2. Arteriovenous communication
3. Azygos continuation of inferior vena cava
4. Coarctation of abdominal aorta
5. Neurofibromatosis, arterial
6. Phlebitis (esp. pylephlebitis)
7. Portal vein occlusion ("cavernous transformation")
8. Pregnancy (eg, hypertrophied uterine vessels; compression of iliac vein)
9. Pseudoxanthoma elasticum
10. Telangiectasia (eg, Osler-Weber-Rendu S.)

References

1. Moskowitz M, Zimmerman H, Felson B: The meandering mesenteric artery of the colon. AJR 1964;92:1088–1099
2. Nemcek AA, Vogelzang RL: Angiography and interventional radiology of the alimentary tract. In: Gore RM, Levine MS (eds): Textbook of Gastrointestinal Radiology. (ed 2) Philadelphia: WB Saunders, 2000, pp 509–511

COMPLICATIONS OF AIDS IN THE GASTROINTESTINAL TRACT AND ABDOMEN

ESOPHAGITIS
1. Candidiasis (moniliasis)
2. Cytomegalovirus
3. Herpes
4. HIV

GASTRITIS
1. *Cryptosporidium* antritis
2. Cytomegalovirus infection (aphthoid ulcers; thick rugae, esp. at esophagogastric junction and antrum)

ENTERITIS WITH THICK IRREGULAR FOLDS, SPASM, AND OCCASIONAL DILATATION
1. Cryptosporidiosis
2. Cytomegalovirus infection
3. *Mycobacterium avium-intracellulare* infection
4. Parasitic disease (esp. giardiasis; strongyloidiasis)

COLITIS
1. Acute appendicitis
2. Cytomegalovirus infection of ileum and colon
3. Infectious colitis, esp. in rectum of homosexual men (eg, amebiasis; shigellosis; lymphogranuloma venereum {chlamydial proctitis}; gonorrhea)
4. Pseudomembranous colitis

NEOPLASM OF GI TRACT, OCCASIONALLY WITH INTUSSUSCEPTION OR OBSTRUCTION
1. Kaposi sarcoma
2. Lymphoma$_g$

LIVER AND BILE DUCT INVOLVEMENT
1. AIDS-related cholangitis (eg, cytomegalovirus; *Cryptosporidium*)
2. Liver abscess, infection (eg, *Mycobacterium avium-intracellulare; Pneumocystis carinii;* cytomegalovirus; histoplasmosis; cryptococcosis; bacillary angiomatosis)
3. Neoplasm (incl. lymphoma)
4. Peliosis hepatis

SPLENIC INVOLVEMENT
1. Lymphoma$_g$
2. Splenic abscess, infection (eg, *Mycobacterium avium-intracellulare;* istoplasmosis; cryptococcosis; cytomegalovirus; *Pneumocystis carinii*)
3. Splenic infarcts (septic emboli)
4. Splenomegaly

References
1. Gore RM, Miller FH, Yaghmai V: Acquired immunodeficiency syndrome (AIDS) of the abdominal organs; imaging features. Semin US, CT, and MR 1998;19:175–189
2. Janoff EN, Smith PD: Emerging concepts in gastrointestinal aspects of HIV-1 pathogenesis and management. Gastroenterology 2001;120:607–621

Genitourinary Tract, Retroperitoneum, Pelvis, GYN Ultrasound

H

H

H

H

H

H

H

Gamut H-1

CONGENITAL SYNDROMES WITH RENAL OR URETERAL MALFORMATION OR ANOMALY

COMMON

1. Adrenogenital S.
2. Asplenia S. (Ivemark S.); polysplenia S.
3. Ehlers-Danlos S.
4. Fetal alcohol S.
5. Fetal rubella infection
6. Glycogen storage disease
7. Hepatic fibrosis-renal cystic disease
8. Potter sequence (absent or multicystic dysplastic kidneys)
9. Prune-belly S. (Eagle-Barrett S.)
10. Turner S.

UNCOMMON

1. Acrorenal S.
2. Aminopterin fetopathy
3. Anorectal malformation
4. Antley-Bixler S.
5. Baller-Gerold S. (craniosynostosis-radial aplasia S.)
6. Bartter S.
7. Beckwith-Wiedemann S.
8. Brachmann de Lange S. (de Lange S.)
9. Branchio-oto-renal S.
10. Cat-eye S. (chromosome 22 trisomy/tetrasomy)
11. Cocaine abuse (maternal)
12. Craniosynostosis syndromes
13. Dietl S.
14. EEC syndrome
15. Fanconi anemia (pancytopenia-dysmelia S.)
16. Femoral hypoplasia-unusual facies S.
17. Fetal trimethadione S.
18. Fraser S. (cryptophthalmia S.)
19. Freeman-Sheldon S. (whistling face S.)
20. Frontometaphyseal dysplasia
21. Fryns S.
22. Hemihypertrophy
23. Johanson-Blizzard S.
24. Kallmann S.
25. Klippel-Feil S.
26. Lenz microphthalmia S.
27. Mayer-Rokitansky-Köster S.
28. Mesomelic dysplasia (multiple types)
29. MURCS association
30. Noonan S.
31. Perlman S.
32. Poland sequence
33. Renal-hepatic-pancreatic dysplasia
34. Roberts S.
35. Robinow S.
36. Ruvalcaba S. (trichorhinophalangeal dysplasia, type III)
37. Schinzel-Giedion S.
38. Sirenomelia
39. TAR S. (thrombocytopenia-absent radius S.)
40. Trisomy 13 S.
41. Trisomy 18 S.
42. VATER association
43. Zellweger S. (cerebrohepatorenal S.)

References
1. Felson B, ed: Dwarfs and other little people. Semin Roentgenol 1973;8:260
2. Taybi H, Lachman RS: Radiology of Syndromes, Metabolic Disorders, and Skeletal Dysplasias. (ed 4) St. Louis: Mosby-Year Book Inc., 1996, p 979

Gamut H-2

CONGENITAL SYNDROMES WITH RENAL INSUFFICIENCY OR NEPHROPATHY

COMMON

1. AIDS (congenital)
2. Alkaptonuria (ochronosis)
3. Fanconi S. (de Toni-Debré-Fanconi S.)
4. Glycogen storage disease (types I and V)

(continued)

5. Hemophilia
6. Polycystic kidneys and liver
   a. Autosomal recessive (infants and children with massive renomegaly, numerous cysts less than 2 cm, dilated collecting tubules, and progressive hepatic fibrosis and liver cysts)
   b. Autosomal dominant (adults and children with multiple cysts in kidneys and liver)
7. Potter sequence (absent or multicystic dysplastic kidneys)
8. Prune-belly S. (Eagle-Barrett S.)
9. Renal tubular acidosis
10. Sickle cell disease

UNCOMMON

1. Acrodysplasia with retinitis pigmentosa and nephropathy (Saldino-Mainzer S.)
2. Alagille S. (arteriohepatic S.)
3. Alport S. (hereditary nephritis)
4. Asphyxiating thoracic dysplasia
5. Bardet-Biedl S.
6. Bartter S.
7. Behcet S.
8. Chondroectodermal dysplasia (Ellis-van Creveld S.)
9. Cockayne S.
10. Cystinosis; cystinuria
11. Drash S.
12. Fabry disease
13. Familial hyperuricosuria
14. Familial Mediterranean fever
15. Gaucher disease
16. Hemolytic-uremic S.
17. Henoch-Schönlein purpura
18. Hepatic fibrosis-renal cystic disease
19. Laurence-Moon-Biedl S.
20. Lesch-Nyhan S.
21. Lowe S. (oculocerebrorenal S.)
22. Nail-patella S. (osteo-onychodysplasia)
23. Nephronophthisis
24. Osteolysis with nephropathy
25. Oxalosis
26. Paraneoplastic syndromes
27. Riley-Day S. (familial dysautonomia)

28. Senior-Loken S.
29. Tyrosinemia
30. Wilson disease
31. Wiskott-Aldrich S.
32. Zellweger S. (cerebrohepatorenal S.)

Reference
1. Taybi H, Lachman RS: Radiology of Syndromes, Metabolic Disorders, and Skeletal Dysplasias. (ed 4) St. Louis: Mosby-Year Book Inc., 1996, pp 981–982

Gamut H-3

MISPLACED OR DISPLACED KIDNEY

COMMON

1. [Absent kidney (congenital; nephrectomy)]
2. Ectopic kidney (pelvic, thoracic, crossed)
3. Hepatomegaly or splenomegaly displacing kidney
4. Horseshoe kidney
5. Malrotation
6. Mass displacing kidney (intra- or extrarenal) (See H-4)
7. Ptosis
8. Transplanted kidney

UNCOMMON

1. Colon distention
2. Hepatic atrophy; cirrhosis (elevated right kidney)
3. Hernia
4. Psoas muscle hypertrophy
5. Retroperitoneal lipomatosis or fibrosis

References
1. Rao AKR, Silver TM: Normal pancreas and splenic variants simulating suprarenal and renal tumors. AJR 1976;126: 530–537
2. Silverman PM, Kelvin FM, Korobkin M: Lateral displacement of the right kidney by the colon: An anatomic variation demonstrated by CT. AJR 1983;140:313–314

Gamut H-4

MASS DISPLACING A KIDNEY

COMMON

1. Abscess (retroperitoneal, peri- or pararenal, renal)
2. Hematoma (retroperitoneal)
3. Hepatomegaly; splenomegaly
4. Intrarenal neoplasm (eg, renal cell carcinoma; Wilms' tumor)

UNCOMMON

1. Aneurysm of aorta
2. Intracapsular extrarenal neoplasm (eg, lipoma)
3. Lymphadenopathy (eg, tuberculosis; sarcoidosis; metastases, esp. from testicular tumor)
4. Lymphoma$_g$
5. [Psoas muscle hypertrophy]
6. Retroperitoneal neoplasm (eg, sarcoma)
7. Suprarenal neoplasm (eg, neuroblastoma; adrenal adenoma or carcinoma; pheochromocytoma)

Gamut H-5

UNILATERAL ABSENCE OR BLURRING OF RENAL OUTLINE

COMMON

1. Abscess, perinephric or paranephric (See H-55-2)
2. Congenital absence or aplasia of kidney
3. Displaced kidney (See H-3)
4. Hemorrhage or hematoma (perirenal or retroperitoneal)
5. Nephrectomy
6. Normal (eg, technical factors; insufficient perirenal fat; overlying intestinal gas)

UNCOMMON

1. Atrophic kidney
2. Ectopic kidney (eg, presacral, thoracic)
3. Lymphocele
4. Thromboembolism of renal artery or vein, or inferior vena cava
5. Urinoma

References

1. Clark RE, Jacobson AC, Petty WE: Intrarenal mycotic (false) aneurysm secondary to staphylococcal septicemia. Radiology 1975;115:421–422
2. Pollack HM, Popky GL: Roentgenographic manifestations of spontaneous renal hemorrhage. Radiology 1974;110:1–6

Gamut H-6

DECREASED SIZE OF PART OF A KIDNEY

COMMON

1. Ischemia; infarction
2. Postobstructive atrophy (eg, from calculus)
3. Postoperative (eg, partial resection)
4. Reflux nephropathy (chronic atrophic pyelo-nephritis)
5. Traumatic atrophy

UNCOMMON

1. Abscess, healed
2. Interstitial nephritis
3. Papillary necrosis
4. Radiation therapy
5. Segmental hypoplasia (Ask-Upmark S.)
6. Thromboembolism of renal vein
7. Tuberculosis

Gamut H-7

UNILATERAL SMALL KIDNEY

Small Smooth Kidney

COMMON

1. Congenital hypoplasia (incl. Ask-Upmark kidney with focal hypoplasia)
2. Ischemia, renal artery stenosis (eg, arteriosclerosis; thromboembolism; fibromuscular hyperplasia; polyarteritis nodosa)
3. Postobstructive atrophy (eg, calculus)
4. Postoperative (partial nephrectomy)
5. Posttraumatic atrophy
6. Reflux nephropathy (chronic atrophic pyelonephritis)

UNCOMMON

1. Papillary necrosis (late after analgesic abuse)
2. Postinflammatory atrophy following acute bacterial nephritis (esp. in diabetic)
3. Radiation nephritis
4. Renal infarction, total, late (eg, embolus; thrombosis)
5. Thrombosis of renal vein (chronic with atrophy)

Small Scarred or Irregular Kidney

1. Multicystic dysplastic kidney (diminutive form)
2. Renal infarction (lobar)
3. Reflux nephropathy (chronic atrophic pyelonephritis)
4. Segmental hypoplasia (Ask-Upmark S.)
5. Tuberculosis (eg, autonephrectomy)

References

1. Davidson AJ: Radiologic Diagnosis of Renal Parenchymal Disease. Philadelphia: WB Saunders, 1977, p 39
2. Davidson AJ, Hartman DS: Radiology of the Kidney and Urinary Tract. Philadelphia: WB Saunders, 1994, Chapter 26, Angiography in diseases of the kidney, p 106
3. Eisenberg RL: Clinical Imaging: An Atlas of Differential Diagnosis. (ed 3) Philadelphia: Lippincott-Raven, 1997, pp 542–545
4. Friedland GW, Dale RL: Miniature kidneys due to obstructive atrophy. Radiology 1971;99:273–277
5. Hodson CJ, Carven JD: The radiology of obstructive atrophy of the kidney. Clin Radiol 1966;17:305–320
6. Morillo G: The differential diagnosis of the unilateral small kidney. CRC Crit Rev Diagn Imaging 1979;11:261–296
7. Swischuk LE, John SD: Differential Diagnosis in Pediatric Radiology. (ed 2) Baltimore: Williams & Wilkins, 1995, p 182

Gamut H-8

BILATERAL SMALL KIDNEYS

COMMON

1. Arteriolar nephrosclerosis (benign or malignant)
2. Glomerulonephritis, chronic
3. Ischemia, bilateral renal artery stenosis (eg, arteriosclerosis; fibromuscular hyperplasia; thromboembolism; polyarteritis nodosa; chronic arteritis)
4. Normal variant; idiopathic
5. Pyelonephritis, chronic atrophic
6. Reflux atrophy
7. Senile atrophy

UNCOMMON

1. Alport S. (hereditary chronic nephritis)
2. Amyloidosis (late)
3. Arterial hypotension, acute (eg, shock; reaction to contrast medium)
4. Bardet-Biedl S.
5. Collagen vascular disease$_g$ (eg, scleroderma)
6. Congenital hypoplasia
7. Cortical necrosis (late)
8. Diabetic nephropathy, late (eg, Kimmelstiel-Wilson S.)
9. Gouty nephropathy
10. Hyperparathyroidism, primary or secondary (renal osteodystrophy)
11. Hypertension, chronic (hypertensive nephropathy)
12. Infarction, bilateral
13. Interstitial nephritis, chronic
14. Juvenile nephronophthisis (medullary cystic disease)

15. Lead nephropathy
16. Multiple myeloma
17. Oxalosis (late)
18. Papillary necrosis, late
19. Postinflammatory atrophy
20. Postobstructive atrophy
21. Radiation nephritis
22. Segmental hypoplasia, bilateral (Ask-Upmark S.)
23. Thromboembolism of renal veins or inferior vena cava

References

1. Burgener FA, Kormano M: Differential Diagnosis in Conventional Radiology. (ed 2) New York: Thieme Medical Publ, 1991, pp 744–745
2. Cochlin DL: Chapter 24. Urinary tract. In: McGahan JP, Goldberg BB (eds): Diagnostic Ultrasound. Philadelphia: Lippincott-Raven, 1997
3. Davidson AJ, Hartman DS: Radiology of the Kidney and Urinary Tract. Philadelphia: WB Saunders, 1994, Chapter 26, Angiography in diseases of the kidney, p 106
4. Eisenberg RL: Clinical Imaging: An Atlas of Differential Diagnosis. (ed 3) Philadelphia: Lippincott-Raven, 1997, pp 550–553
5. Friedland GW, Dale RL: Miniature kidneys due to obstructive atrophy. Radiology 1971;99:273–277
6. Swischuk LE, John SD: Differential Diagnosis in Pediatric Radiology. (ed 2) Baltimore: Williams & Wilkins, 1995, p 182
7. Taybi H, Lachman RS: Radiology of Syndromes, Metabolic Disorders, and Skeletal Dysplasias. (ed 4) St. Louis: Mosby-Year Book Inc., 1996, p 980
8. Teplick JG, Haskin ME: Roentgenologic Diagnosis. (ed 3) Philadelphia: WB Saunders, 1976

Gamut H-9

UNILATERAL LARGE KIDNEY

COMMON

1. Abscess, renal (eg, carbuncle; nephronia) or perirenal
2. Compensatory hypertrophy due to disease or absence of opposite kidney
3. Cyst (simple; hydatid; parapelvic) (See H-30)
4. Double or triple collecting system
5. Hydronephrosis (See H-49); obstructive uropathy

6. Idiopathic; normal variant
7. [Malrotation]
8. Multicystic dysplastic kidney with numerous cysts in infants and children (they decrease in size by adulthood)
9. Neoplasm, malignant (eg, renal cell carcinoma; Wilms' tumor; sarcoma; metastasis)
10. Polycystic kidney disease with unilateral enlargement
11. Pyelonephritis, acute

UNCOMMON

1. Bartter S.
2. Congenital megacalyces
3. Crossed fused renal ectopy; horseshoe kidney
4. Hemihypertrophy, congenital
5. Hemorrhage (eg, hemophilia; anticoagulant therapy; trauma)
6. Infarction, acute arterial
7. Malakoplakia
8. Multilocular cystic nephroma
9. Neoplasm, benign, esp. angiomyolipoma (hamartoma)
10. Renal vein thrombosis
11. Transplant rejection, acute
12. Trauma (eg, contusion; hematoma; urinoma)
13. Xanthogranulomatous pyelonephritis

References

1. Ambos MA, Bosniak MA, Madayag MA, et al: Infiltrating neoplasms of the kidney. AJR 1977;129:859–864
2. Burgener FA, Kormano M: Differential Diagnosis in Conventional Radiology. (ed 2) New York: Thieme Medical Publ, 1991, pp 738–741
3. Cochlin DL: Chapter 24. Urinary tract. In: McGahan JP, Goldberg BB (eds): Diagnostic Ultrasound. Philadelphia: Lippincott-Raven, 1997
4. Davidson AJ: A systematic approach to the radiologic diagnosis of renal parenchymal disease. In: Pollack HM (ed): Clinical Urography. Philadelphia: WB Saunders, 1990
5. Davidson AJ, Hartman DS: Radiology of the Kidney and Urinary Tract. Philadelphia: WB Saunders, 1994, Chapter 26, Angiography in diseases of the kidney, p 106
6. Neuenschwander S, Cordier MD, Montagne JP: Unilateral "enlarged kidney" in the neonate: Ultrasonographic approach to the diagnosis. Ann Radiol 1981;24:141–146

(continued)

7. Parker M: Diagnostic skills. In: Friedland GW, Filly R, Goris ML, et al: Uroradiology: An Integrated Approach. New York: Churchill Livingstone, 1983, p 1654

Gamut H-10

BILATERAL LARGE KIDNEYS

COMMON

1. Diabetic nephropathy (eg, glomerulosclerosis; Kimmelstiel-Wilson S.)
2. Duplication of pelvocalyceal systems, bilateral
3. Glomerulonephritis (eg, acute {streptococcal infection}; lobular; hereditary; idiopathic; glomerulosclerosis)
4. Hydronephrosis (See H-49)
5. Multiple simple cysts
6. Nephrosis (eg, nephrotic S.; toxic nephrosis; lipoid nephrosis; bile nephrosis)
7. Normal variant; idiopathic
8. Polycystic kidney disease, adult autosomal dominant or infantile autosomal recessive; other cystic disease (See H-30)

UNCOMMON

1. Acquired cystic disease (eg, in hemodialysis for chronic renal failure)
2. Acromegaly
3. Acute cortical necrosis
4. Acute interstitial nephritis (allergic reaction to drugs—eg, methicillin)
5. Acute tubular necrosis
6. Agnogenic myeloid metaplasia
7. Allergic angiitis (necrotizing vasculitis)
8. Amyloidosis
9. Angiomyolipomas, multiple (esp. with tuberous sclerosis)
10. Bartter S.
11. Beckwith-Wiedemann S.
12. Bilateral renal neoplasms (eg, renal cell carcinoma {hypernephroma}; Wilms' tumor)
13. Bleeding disorder$_g$ (eg, hemophilia; Henoch-Schönlein purpura)
14. Collagen vascular disease$_g$ (esp. lupus nephritis; polyarteritis nodosa; thrombotic thrombocytopenic purpura)
15. Congenital megacalyces
16. Cyst in one kidney, hypernephroma in the other
17. Diuresis or vasodilatation secondary to diuretics or contrast media
18. Gaucher disease; Niemann-Pick disease
19. Glycogen storage disease, type I (von Gierke S.)
20. Goodpasture S.
21. Hemolytic-uremic S.
22. [Horseshoe kidney]
23. Infant of diabetic mother
24. Infarction (acute arterial)
25. Langerhans cell histiocytosis$_g$
26. Leukemia; lymphoma$_g$
27. Lipodystrophy (lipoatrophic diabetes)
28. Metastases (esp. from carcinoma of lung, breast, contralateral kidney)
29. Multiple myeloma; POEMS S.
30. Nephroblastomatosis
31. Nephromegaly with other conditions (eg, neonatal transient nephromegaly; hyperalimentation {total parenteral nutrition}; cirrhosis; Fabry's disease; paroxysmal nocturnal hemoglobinuria; AIDS nephropathy)
32. Pyelonephritis (acute)
33. Sarcoidosis
34. Sickle cell disease (homozygous)
35. Steroid therapy (prolonged)
36. Subacute infective endocarditis (glomerulonephritis)
37. Thromboembolism of renal veins or vena cava
38. Tuberous sclerosis
39. Tyrosinosis (hereditary)
40. Urate nephropathy (acute)
41. von Hippel-Lindau S.
42. Waldenström's macroglobulinemia
43. Wegener's granulomatosis
44. Wolman's disease
45. Work hypertrophy (eg, beer-drinker kidneys; diabetes insipidus)

References

1. Cochlin DL: Chapter 24. Urinary tract. In: McGahan JP, Goldberg BB (eds): Diagnostic Ultrasound. Philadelphia: Lippincott-Raven, 1997
2. Davidson AJ: Radiologic Diagnosis of Renal Parenchymal Disease. Philadelphia: WB Saunders, 1977
3. Davidson AJ, Hartman DS: Radiology of the Kidney and Urinary Tract. Philadelphia: WB Saunders, 1994, Chapter 26, Angiography in diseases of the kidney, p 106
4. Eisenberg RL: Clinical Imaging: An Atlas of Differential Diagnosis. (ed 3) Philadelphia: Lippincott-Raven, 1997, pp 554–561
5. Parker M: Diagnostic skills. In: Friedland GW, Filly R, Goris ML, et al: Uroradiology: An Integrated Approach. New York: Churchill Livingstone, 1983, p 1668
6. Segel MC, Lecky JW, Slasky BS: Diabetes mellitus. The predominant cause of bilateral renal enlargement. Radiology 1984;153:341–342
7. Swischuk LE, John SD: Differential Diagnosis in Pediatric Radiology. (ed 2) Baltimore: Williams & Wilkins, 1995, pp 179–183
8. Taybi H, Lachman RS: Radiology of Syndromes, Metabolic Disorders, and Skeletal Dysplasias. (ed 4) St. Louis: Mosby-Year Book Inc., 1996, p 980
9. Thurston W, Wilson SR: Chapter 9. The urinary tract. In: Rumack CM, Wilson SR, Charboneau JW (eds): Diagnostic Ultrasound. St. Louis: Mosby, 1998, pp 382–384

Gamut H-11

BILATERAL LARGE KIDNEYS WITH MULTIFOCAL MASSES

COMMON

1. Multiple cysts (simple or hydatid)
2. Polycystic kidney disease (adult—autosomal dominant)

UNCOMMON

1. Acquired cystic disease (eg, from dialysis)
2. Angiomyolipomas (eg, with tuberous sclerosis)
3. Bilateral renal neoplasms (eg, renal cell carcinoma; Wilms' tumor)
4. Cyst in one kidney, neoplasm in the other

5. Lymphoma$_g$ (incl. Burkitt's lymphoma)
6. Metastases
7. Nephroblastomatosis
8. von Hippel-Lindau disease

Reference

1. Davidson AJ: A systematic approach to the radiologic diagnosis of renal parenchymal disease. In: Pollack HM (ed): Clinical Urography. Philadelphia: WB Saunders, 1990, pp 2253–2263

Gamut H-12

DIMINISHED OR ABSENT NEPHROGRAM

UNILATERAL

COMMON

1. Ureteral obstruction

UNCOMMON

1. Renal artery occlusion
2. Renal vein occlusion
3. Trauma

BILATERAL

COMMON

1. Contrast administration error
2. Hypotension
3. Renal failure (acute or chronic)

Gamut H-13
FOCAL DEFECT(S) IN THE NEPHROGRAM

COMMON
1. Acute pyelonephritis
2. Cyst (simple; hydatid; parapelvic)
3. Infarction; arterial branch occlusion
4. Lipomatosis of renal sinus
5. Neoplasm, malignant (eg, renal cell carcinoma; transitional cell carcinoma of renal pelvis; Wilms' tumor; sarcoma)
6. Polycystic kidney disease, adult
7. Trauma (eg, contusion; laceration)

UNCOMMON
1. Abscess, acute or chronic
2. Aneurysm of renal artery (intrarenal); arteriovenous malformation
3. Angiomyolipoma (hamartoma), esp. with tuberous sclerosis
4. Hematoma, intrarenal
5. Localized hydronephrosis (due to congenital or tuberculous obstruction)
6. Lymphoma$_g$
7. Medullary cystic disease
8. Metastasis
9. Tuberculosis
10. Xanthogranulomatous pyelonephritis

References
1. Burgener FA, Kormano M: Differential Diagnosis in Conventional Radiology. (ed 2) New York: Thieme Medical Publ, 1991, pp 762–766
2. Davidson AJ: A systematic approach to the radiologic diagnosis of renal parenchymal disease. Chapter 23. The Nephrogram. In: Pollack HM (ed): Clinical Urography. Philadelphia: WB Saunders, 1990, pp 751–775

Gamut H-14
DENSE OR PROLONGED NEPHROGRAM ON IV UROGRAPHY

COMMON
1. Contrast reaction (acute contrast nephropathy)
2. Glomerulonephritis, acute or chronic
3. Hydronephrosis, severe (See H-49)
4. Hypotension; shock
5. Ischemia (reduced flow; acute renal arterial insufficiency) (See H-58)
6. Normal kidneys with rapid bolus contrast medium injection
7. Obstruction of bladder (See H-110)
8. Obstructive uropathy (eg, calculus or blood clot in ureter)
9. Pyelonephritis, acute severe (esp. in diabetic)
10. Renal failure (acute oliguric)
11. Traumatic reflex anuria

UNCOMMON
1. Collagen disease$_g$ (esp. polyarteritis nodosa)
2. Cortical necrosis
3. Iatrogenic (eg, ureteral catheter)
4. Idiopathic
5. Lymphoma$_g$ with urate nephropathy
6. Medullary cystic disease (early stage)
7. Nephrosis
8. Papillary necrosis (acute tubular obstruction by necrotic papillary tips)
9. Polycystic kidney disease, infantile type
10. Thromboembolism of renal vein or inferior vena cava
11. Trueta phenomenon
12. Tubular blockage (eg, sulfonamide therapy; multiple myeloma; amyloidosis; hemoglobinuria; myoglobinuria; hyperuricemia {urate nephropathy}; Tamm-Horsfall proteinuria)
13. Tubular necrosis, acute
14. Waldenström's macroglobulinemia

References

1. Burgener FA, Kormano M: Differential Diagnosis in Conventional Radiology. (ed 2) New York: Thieme Medical Publ, 1991, pp 760–761
2. Davidson AJ: A systematic approach to the radiologic diagnosis of renal parenchymal disease. Chapter 23. The Nephrogram. In: Pollack HM (ed): Clinical Urography. Philadelphia: WB Saunders, 1990, pp 751–775
3. Mandell GA, Swacus JR, Rosenstock J, et al: Danger of urography in hyperuricemic children with Burkitt's lymphoma. J Can Assoc Radiol 1983;34:273–277
4. Martin DJ, Jaffe N: Prolonged nephrogram due to hyperuricaemia. Br J Radiol 1971;44:806–809
5. Newhouse JH, Pfister RC: The nephrogram. Radiol Clin North Am 1979;17:213–225

Gamut H-15

STRIATED NEPHROGRAM

COMMON

*1. Acute obstruction
2. Acute renal failure
3. Medullary sponge kidney
4. Medullary tubular ectasia
*5. Pyelonephritis
*6. Trauma

UNCOMMON

*1. Arterial emboli
2. Arteritis (eg, polyarteritis nodosa; drug abuse; Wegener's granulomatosis)
3. Polycystic kidney disease (infantile—autosomal recessive)
*4. Renal vein thrombosis

* Usually unilateral. Others are usually or always bilateral.

Reference

1. Davidson AJ: A systematic approach to the radiologic diagnosis of renal parenchymal disease. Chapter 23. The Nephrogram. In: Pollack HM (ed): Clinical Urography. Philadelphia: WB Saunders, 1990, pp 751–775

Gamut H-16-1

NONVISUALIZATION OR NONFUNCTION OF ONE KIDNEY ON IV UROGRAPHY, CT, OR NUCLEAR SCAN (See H-16-2, H-17-1)

COMMON

1. [Ectopic kidney]
2. Hydronephrosis (See H-49)
3. Neoplasm (eg, renal cell carcinoma)
4. Obstruction of ureter (esp. calculus) (See H-93)
5. Postoperative (eg, nephrectomy)
6. Renal artery obstruction (eg, stenosis; thromboembolism; trauma)
7. Trauma (esp. fractured kidney)

UNCOMMON

1. Abscess; carbuncle; nephrosia; pyonephrosis
2. Absence or hypoplasia of kidney (congenital)
3. Acute bacterial nephritis (esp. diabetes)
4. Arteriovenous malformation of kidney
5. Lymphoma$_g$
6. Multicystic dysplastic kidney
7. Perinephric hematoma
8. Radiation injury
9. Renal vein obstruction (eg, thromboembolism; neoplasm)
10. Tuberculosis (autonephrectomy); other severe infection (eg, xanthogranulomatous pyelonephritis)

References

1. Karasick SR, Herring W: Computed tomography evaluation of the poorly or nonvisualized kidney. CT 1980;4:39–46
2. Parker M: Diagnostic skills. In: Friedland GW, Filly R, Goris ML, et al: Uroradiology: An Integrated Approach. New York: Churchill Livingstone, 1983, p 1632
3. Patasnick JP, Patel SK: Angiographic evaluation of the nonvisualizing kidney. AJR 1973;119:757–766
4. Zagoria RJ, Tung GA: Genitourinary Radiology: The Requisites. St. Louis: Mosby, 1997, p 55

Gamut H-16-2

NONVISUALIZATION OR NONFUNCTION OF A CALYX OR PART OF A KIDNEY ON IV UROGRAPHY, CT, OR NUCLEAR SCAN

1. Abscess; carbuncle; nephronia
2. Cyst (See H-30)
3. Duplication of collecting system with obstruction of one division (eg, ectopic ureterocele)
4. Metastasis
5. Neoplasm, benign or malignant (esp. transitional cell or renal cell carcinoma)
6. Obstruction (eg, calculus; crossing vessel)
7. Postoperative (eg, partial nephrectomy)
8. Trauma (esp. fractured kidney)
9. Tuberculosis or other infection

Gamut H-17-1

DIMINISHED CONCENTRATION OF CONTRAST MEDIUM IN PELVOCALICEAL SYSTEM ON IV UROGRAPHY—UNILATERAL

1. Compression of kidney by adjacent mass (eg, splenomegaly; neoplasm)
2. [Contralateral hyperconcentration (eg, renal artery stenosis involving opposite kidney)]
3. Cyst (esp. parapelvic)
4. Infection, acute (eg, bacterial pyelonephritis) or chronic (eg, tuberculosis)
5. Neoplasm
6. Radiation injury
7. Renal parenchymal disease, unilateral (eg, tuberculosis; abscess; carbuncle)
8. Renal vein thrombosis (See H-63)
9. Trauma with spasm of pelvocaliceal system
10. Urinary tract obstruction; hydronephrosis (See H-49)

Gamut H-17-2

DIMINISHED CONCENTRATION OF CONTRAST MEDIUM IN PELVOCALICEAL SYSTEM ON IV UROGRAPHY—BILATERAL

1. Arteriolar nephrosclerosis; hypertensive renal disease
2. Hydronephrosis (See H-49)
3. Idiopathic
4. Infection, acute (eg, bacterial pyelonephritis)
5. Lipomatosis of renal sinus
6. Myeloma kidney; amyloidosis
7. Overhydration or inadequate dehydration
8. Polyuria (eg, diuresis; diabetes insipidus or mellitus with renal disease)
9. Renal artery stenosis or thromboembolism
10. Renal failure; uremia
11. Tamm-Horsfall proteinuria
12. [Technical (eg, inadequate contrast dose)]
13. Thromboembolism of renal veins or inferior vena cava (See H-63)
14. Trauma

[ ] This condition does not actually cause the gamuted imaging finding, but can produce imaging changes that simulate it.

Gamut H-18

INTRARENAL CONTRAST COLLECTIONS (IVP, CT)

COMMON
1. Calyceal diverticulum
2. Dilated calyx

UNCOMMON
1. Communicating cyst (eg, ruptured hydatid)
2. Communicating urinoma
3. Medullary sponge kidney ("paint brush" effect)

4. Papillary necrosis
5. Trauma (eg, fractured kidney or calyces)

Reference
1. Ney C, Friedenberg R: Radiographic Atlas of the Genitourinary System. Philadelphia: Lippincott, 1966, pp 148, 189, 193, 199, 214, 216, 219

Gamut H-19

CLUBBING OR DESTRUCTION OF RENAL CALYCES

COMMON
1. Caliectasis, localized, from obstruction of infundibulum (eg, stone; neoplasm; stricture; clot; anomalous vessel)
2. Hydronephrosis
3. Papillary necrosis (See H-20)
4. Pyelonephritis (incl. xanthogranulomatous)
5. Tuberculosis
6. Vesicopelvic reflux

UNCOMMON
1. Abscess
2. [Congenital megacalyx]
3. Fungus disease_g
4. Neoplasm (esp. transitional cell carcinoma)
5. Postoperative scarring

Gamut H-20

RENAL PAPILLARY NECROSIS

COMMON
1. Analgesic abuse (eg, phenacetin; aspirin)
2. Diabetes mellitus

3. Obstruction of urinary tract
4. Pyelonephritis
5. Sickle cell disease

UNCOMMON
1. Abscess or carbuncle of kidney
2. Arteritis (eg, thromboembolism; polyarteritis nodosa; necrotizing)
3. Cirrhosis
4. Contrast medium reaction (intravenous; retrograde)
5. Disseminated intravascular coagulation (DIC); sepsis
6. Renal vein thrombosis
7. Shock; asphyxia; dehydration (esp. child)
8. Tuberculosis

References
1. Anand SK, Northway JD, Smith JA: Neonatal renal papillary and cortical necrosis. Am J Dis Child 1977:131: 773–777
2. Davidson AJ: A systematic approach to the radiologic diagnosis of renal parenchymal disease. Chapter 23. Chronic parenchymal disease. In: Pollack HM (ed): Clinical Urography. Philadelphia: WB Saunders, 1990, pp 2277–2288
3. Kozlowski K, Brown RW: Renal medullary necrosis in infants and children. Pediatr Radiol 1978;7:85–89
4. Mellins HZ: Chronic pyelonephritis and renal medullary necrosis. Semin Roentgenol 1971;6:292–309
5. Muhalwas KK, Shah GM, Winer RL: Renal papillary necrosis caused by long-term ingestion of pentazocine and aspirin. JAMA 1981;246:867–868

Gamut H-21

INFUNDIBULAR NARROWING OR AMPUTATION (FOCAL OR DIFFUSE)

COMMON
1. Carcinoma (eg, transitional cell; renal cell)
2. Normal variant (eg, crossing vessel)
3. Renal sinus lipomatosis or mass
4. Spasm or irritability (eg, acute pyelonephritis; trauma; hemorrhage)

(continued)

UNCOMMON

1. Abscess; carbuncle; nephronia
2. Congenital infundibular stenosis (Fraley S.)
3. Extrarenal pelvis
4. Extrinsic compression
5. Infarct (renal)
6. Neoplasm, other benign or malignant (eg, angiomyolipoma; lymphoma$_g$; squamous cell carcinoma)
7. Parapelvic cyst (simple; hydatid)
8. Postoperative (eg, partial resection)
9. Stricture, inflammatory
10. Tuberculosis; other infection (eg, brucellosis)

References

1. Dunnick NR, et al: Textbook of Uroradiology. Baltimore: Williams & Wilkins, 1997, p 288
2. Parker M: Diagnostic skills. In: Friedland GW, Filly R, Goris ML, et al: Uroradiology: An Integrated Approach. New York: Churchill Livingstone, 1983, p 1673

Gamut H-22

FILLING DEFECT OR MASS IN A RENAL PELVIS, INFUNDIBULUM, OR CALYX

COMMON

*1. Blood clot (eg, trauma; neoplasm)
*2. Calculus (See H-24– 26)
*3. Gas (eg, air from retrograde pyelogram; percutaneous or retrograde stone removal; sinus tract or fistula; gas infection; ureterointestinal anastomosis)
4. Metastasis
*5. Neoplasm (eg, hemangioma; hamartoma; angiomyolipoma; papilloma; oncocytoma; transitional cell carcinoma; hypernephroma; Wilms' tumor; lymphoma$_g$)
6. [Normal anatomic variation (eg, bifid pelvis; duplication; overlapping calyces; calyx on end)]

7. Normal renal artery or vein impression
8. Renal sinus lipomatosis
9. [Technical (incomplete filling with contrast medium; overlying intestinal gas)]

UNCOMMON

1. Amyloidosis
2. Cholesteatoma (squamous metaplasia of urothelium)
3. Cyst (eg, parapelvic, parenchymal, hydatid)
*4. Fungus ball (esp. *Candida*)
5. Inflammatory polyp
*6. Leukoplakia
7. Malakoplakia
*8. Multicystic kidney with pelvoinfundibular atresia (congenital)
9. Papilla, aberrant or sloughed (eg, papillary necrosis) (See H-20)
*10. Polycystic kidney
11. Pyelitis cystica
*12. Pyelonephritis with inspissated pus, necrotic debris (eg, suppurative; xanthogranulomatous; tuberculous)
13. Saccular aneurysm
14. Urinoma

* May fill entire renal pelvis.

References

1. Brown RC, Jones MC, Boldus R, et al: Lesions causing radiolucent defects in the renal pelvis. AJR 1973;119: 770–778
2. Goldman SM, Gatewood OMB: Neoplasms of the renal collecting system, pelvis, and ureters. In: Pollack HM (ed): Clinical Urography. Philadelphia: WB Saunders, 1990
3. Thurston W, Wilson SR: Chapter 9. The urinary tract. In: Rumack CM, Wilson SR, Charboneau JW (eds): Diagnostic Ultrasound. St. Louis: Mosby, 1998, pp 329–397

Gamut H-23

FOCAL OR ANNULAR CALCIFICATION IN THE KIDNEY

COMMON

1. Aneurysm of renal artery
2. Atherosclerosis of renal artery
3. Calculus (See H-24-26)
4. Neoplasm, malignant (eg, renal cell carcinoma; chondrosarcoma; neuroblastoma; osteosarcoma; transitional cell carcinoma; Wilms' tumor; metastasis)

UNCOMMON

1. Abscess (renal or perinephric)
2. [Adrenal cyst or neoplasm]
3. Arteriovenous communication; angioma
4. Caliceal diverticulum containing calculus or milk of calcium
5. [Cortical necrosis]
6. Cyst (eg, simple; hydatid)
7. [Glomerulonephritis, chronic (cortical)]
8. Hematoma
9. Hydronephrosis or pyonephrosis containing calculus or milk of calcium
10. Infarction
11. Leukoplakia
12. Multicystic kidney; polycystic kidney
13. Neoplasm, benign (eg, dermoid; teratoma; angiomyolipoma; hemangioendothelioma; medullary fibroma; hamartoma; spindle cell tumor $_g$; adenoma; multilocular cystic nephroma {Perlman tumor} oncocytoma)
14. Papillary necrosis
15. Thromboembolus
16. Tuberculosis

References

1. Cochlin DL: Chapter 24. Urinary tract. In: McGahan JP, Goldberg BB (eds): Diagnostic Ultrasound. Philadelphia: Lippincott-Raven, 1997
2. Margolin EG, Cohen LH: Genitourinary calcification: An overview. Semin Roentgenol 1982;17:95–100
3. Mencini RA: Gamut: Calcification in a renal mass. Semin Roentgenol 1982;17:90–91
4. Parker M: Diagnostic skills. In: Friedland GW, Filly R, Goris ML, et al: Uroradiology: An Integrated Approach. New York: Churchill Livingstone, 1983, p 1637
5. Weyman PJ, McClennan BL, Lee JKT: CT of calcified renal masses. AJR 1982;138:1095–1099

Gamut H-24

CAUSES OF RENAL AND OTHER URINARY TRACT CALCULI
(See also H-25-S)

COMMON

1. Hyperparathyroidism
2. Idiopathic
3. Infection
4. Osteoporosis (eg, senile; postmenopausal; immobilization) (See D-43-1)
5. Stasis (eg, urinary tract obstruction; neurogenic bladder; paralysis)

UNCOMMON

1. Bone destruction (eg, osteolytic bone metastases; multiple myeloma)
2. Cushing's disease; steroid therapy
3. Dehydration
4. Excessive calcium intake (eg, milk-alkali S.) or absorption
5. Hyperthyroidism
6. Hyperuricosuria
7. Hypervitaminosis D
8. Idiopathic hypercalciuria
9. Malabsorption S. (See G-57)
10. Medullary sponge kidney
11. Osteomalacia (See D-44)
12. Oxaluria
13. Paget's disease

(continued)

14. Papillary necrosis
15. Renal osteodystrophy
16. Renal tubular acidosis
17. Sarcoidosis
18. Schistosomiasis haematobium
19. Tuberculosis
20. Williams S. (idiopathic hypercalcemia)

References
1. Kirks DR: John Caffey Award: Lithiasis due to interruption of the enterohepatic circulation of bile salts. AJR 1979;133: 383–388
2. Malik, RS: Calculus disease of the genitourinary tract. In: Witten DM, Myers GH Jr, Utz DC: Emmett's Clinical Urography. (ed 4) Philadelphia: WB Saunders, 1977, p 1177
3. Margolin EG, Cohen LH: Genitourinary calcification: An overview. Semin Roentgenol 1982;17:95–100
4. Parker M: Diagnostic skills. In: Friedland GW, Filly R, Goris ML, et al: Uroradiology: An Integrated Approach. New York: Churchill Livingstone, 1983, p 1637

Gamut H-25-S

CLASSIFICATION OF CALCIUM STONES IN THE URINARY TRACT*

IDIOPATHIC

Hypercalciuria
1. Increased intestinal absorption of calcium
2. "Renal leak" of calcium

Hyperuricosuria

No Metabolic Abnormality Yet Defined
1. ? Decreased inhibitors of stone formation
2. ? Increased promoters of stone formation
3. ? Decreased urine volume

HYPERCALCEMIC HYPERCALCIURIA

Increased Bone Resorption
1. Hyperparathyroidism, primary
2. Hyperthyroidism

3. Immobilization
4. Neoplasm, widespread (eg, carcinomatosis; multiple myeloma)
5. Paget's disease

Increased Intestinal Absorption of Calcium
1. Milk-alkali S.
2. Sarcoidosis
3. Vitamin D intoxication

RENAL TUBULAR ACIDOSIS

Hyperoxaluria
1. Malabsorption S.
2. Primary hyperoxaluria

* Noncalcium stones are excluded: uric acid, struvite (magnesium ammonium phosphate), and cystine stones.

References
1. Kirks DR: John Caffey Award: Lithiasis due to interruption of the enterohepatic circulation of bile salts. AJR 1979; 133:383–388
2. Margolin EG, Cohen LH: Genitourinary calcification: An overview. Semin Roentgenol 1982;17:95–100
3. Parker M: Diagnostic skills. In: Friedland GW, Filly R, Goris ML, et al: Uroradiology: An Integrated Approach. New York: Churchill Livingstone, 1983, p 1637

Gamut H-26-S

DENSE VERSUS LUCENT CALCULI ON RADIOGRAPHY

RADIODENSE CALCULI

COMMON
1. Calcium oxalate

UNCOMMON
1. Calcium phosphate
2. Cystine (slightly radiopaque)
3. Struvite plus calcium phosphate

RADIOLUCENT CALCULI

COMMON

1. Uric acid (urates of ammonium, magnesium, potassium, or sodium)

UNCOMMON

1. Indinavir crystals
2. Matrix (mucoproteinaceous material)
3. Struvite (magnesium ammonium phosphate)
4. Xanthine

References

1. Brown RC, Loening SA, Ehrhardt JC, et al: Cystine calculi are radiopaque. AJR 1980;135:565–567
2. Spirnak JP, Resnick MI, Banner MP: Calculous disease of the urinary tract: General considerations. In: Pollack HM (ed): Clinical Urography. Philadelphia: WB Saunders, 1990

Gamut H-27

NEPHROCALCINOSIS (CORTICAL AND MEDULLARY)

CORTICAL

COMMON

1. Chronic glomerulonephritis
2. Renal cortical necrosis (eg, shock; abruptio placenta; hypotension; dehydration)

UNCOMMON

*1. AIDS-associated infection (eg, *Mycobacterium avium intracellulare; Pneumocysytis carinii;* cytomegalovirus)
2. Alport S. (hereditary nephritis)
3. Chronic hypercalcemia; paraneoplastic hypercalcemia
4. Drug therapy (eg, cyclamate)
5. Ethylene glycol (antifreeze) or mercury poisoning
6. Methoxyflurane anesthesia
*7. Oxalosis (primary or secondary hyperoxaluria)
8. Pyroxidine deficiency; xanthine oxidase deficiency

9. Renal transplant rejection
10. Renal vein thrombosis

* May show medullary as well as cortical nephrocalcinosis.

MEDULLARY

COMMON

1. Hyperparathyroidism, primary or secondary
2. Hypercalcemia (eg, widespread bone destruction or metastatic disease {carcinomatosis; myelomatosis}; Cushing S.; steroid therapy; milk-alkali S.; excessive calcium intake or absorption; Paget's disease; hypervitaminosis D; sarcoidosis)
3. Medullary sponge kidney
4. Osteoporosis (esp. immobilization; postmenopausal; senile)
5. Renal tubular acidosis (deToni-Fanconi S.; cystinuria)

UNCOMMON

*1. AIDS-associated infection (eg, *Mycobacterium avium intracellulare; Pneumocystis carinii;* cytomegalovirus)
2. Alkaptonuria (ochronosis)
3. Aminoaciduria
4. Barrter S.
5. Blue diaper S. (tryptophan malabsorption)
6. Chondroectodermal dysplasia (Ellis-van Creveld S.)
7. Dialysis therapy
8. Drug therapy (acetazolamide; amphotericin B; adrenocorticotrophic hormone; furosemide; triamterene; sulfonamide)
9. Ehlers-Danlos S.
10. Familial hypercholesterolemia
11. Glycogen storage disease (type I)
12. Hepatic fibrosis-renal cystic disease
13. Hyperthyroidism
14. Hyperuricemia (eg, gout; antimetabolite treatment of leukemia)
15. Hypochloremic acidosis
16. Hypophosphatasia
17. Hypothyroidism, juvenile; cretinism
18. Idiopathic renal hypercalciuria

(continued)

19. McCune-Albright S.
20. Metaphyseal chondrodysplasia (Jansen and Shwachman types)
21. Nail-patella S. (osteo-onychodysplasia)
*22. Oxalosis (hyperoxaluria)
23. Papillary necrosis (See H-20)
24. Pseudohypoparathyroidism
25. Pyelonephritis, chronic
26. Radiation therapy
27. Renal medullary necrosis
*28. Sickle cell disease
29. Sjögren S.
30. Tuberculosis (autonephrectomy)
31. Vesicoureteral reflux
32. Vitamin D-resistant rickets
33. Williams S. (idiopathic hypercalcemia)
34. Wilson's disease
35. Zollinger-Ellison S.

* May show cortical as well as medullary nephrocalcinosis.

References

1. Banner MP: Nephrocalcinosis. In: Pollack HM (ed): Clinical Urography. Philadelphia: WB Saunders, 1990, vol 2, pp 1768–1775
2. Lalli AF: Renal parenchyma calcifications. Semin Roentgenol 1982;17:101–112
3. Malik RS: Calculus disease of the genitourinary tract. In: Witten DM, Myers GH Jr, Utz DC: Emmett's Clinical Urography. (ed 4) Philadelphia: WB Saunders, 1977, p 1285
4. McAlister WH, Nedelman SH: The roentgen manifestations of bilateral renal cortical necrosis. AJR 1961;86:129–135
5. Ramchandani P: Radiological evaluation of renal calculous disease. In: Pollack HM, McClennan BL (eds): Clinical Urography. (ed 2) Philadelphia: WB Saunders, 2000, pp 2187–2196
6. Taybi H, Lachman RS: Radiology of Syndromes, Metabolic Disorders, and Skeletal Dysplasias. (ed 4) St. Louis: Mosby-Year Book Inc., 1996, p 981
7. Teplick JG, Haskin ME: Roentgenologic Diagnosis. (ed 3) Philadelphia: WB Saunders, 1976
8. Thurston W, Wilson SR: Chapter 9. The urinary tract. In: Rumack CM, Wilson SR, Charboneau JW (eds): Diagnostic Ultrasound. St. Louis: Mosby, 1998, pp 329–397
9. Wiggelinkhuizen J, Sinclaire-Smith C: Radiological case of the month: Nephroxalosis. Am J Dis Child 1978;132: 517–518

Gamut H-28-S

RENAL CORTICAL NECROSIS

Shock or Hypotension related to:

1. Aortic dissection
2. Burn
3. Dehydration
4. Diabetic ketoacidosis
5. Hemolytic-uremic S.
6. Hemorrhage
7. Myocardial failure
8. Obstetrical bleeding complications (eg, abruptio placentae)
9. Pancreatitis
10. Peritonitis
11. Renal transplantation
12. Scarlet fever
13. Sepsis
14. Sickle cell disease
15. Snakebite
16. Thrombotic thrombocytopenic purpura
17. Transfusion reaction
18. Tuberculosis

Reference

1. Ramchandani P: Radiological evaluation of renal calculous disease. In: Pollack HM, McClennan BL (eds): Clinical Urography. (ed 2) Philadelphia: WB Saunders, 2000, pp 2187–2188

CLASSIFICATION OF RENAL CYSTIC DISEASE

Simple renal cyst

Hydatid cyst

Cysts of the renal medulla
1. Medullary cystic disease
2. Medullary sponge kidney

Cysts of the renal sinus
1. Parapelvic cyst

Multicystic dysplastic kidney
1. Hydronephrotic multicystic kidney
2. Pyeloinfundibular atresia

Polycystic kidney disease
1. Adult—autosomal dominant polycystic kidney disease
2. Juvenile—autosomal recessive polycystic kidney disease

Miscellaneous cystic diseases
1. Congenital syndromes including renal cysts (see H-31)
2. Glomerulocystic kidney disease
3. Microcystic disease

Renal cystic disease associated with multiple renal neoplasms
1. Acquired renal cystic disease
2. Tuberous sclerosis
3. von Hippel-Lindau S.

Reference
1. Hartman DS: Overview of renal cystic disease. In: Pollack HM, McClennan BL (eds): Clinical Urography. (ed 2) Philadelphia: WB Saunders, 2000, pp 1245–1250

CYSTIC DISEASES OF THE KIDNEY

COMMON
*1. Acquired cystic disease (eg, from dialysis)
2. Caliceal diverticulum (pyelogenic cyst)
*3. Congenital syndromes (See H-31)
*4. [Cyst secondary to tuberculosis, pyelonephritis, medullary necrosis, or trauma)]
5. Hydronephrosis (focal)
*6. Medullary sponge kidney
*7. Multicystic dysplastic kidney
8. [Neoplasm with cystic degeneration (esp. necrotic renal cell carcinoma)
9. Parapelvic cyst
*10. Polycystic kidney disease (adult type—autosomal dominant)
*11. Simple cortical cyst (solitary or multiple)

UNCOMMON
*1. Cortical sponge kidney; congenital cortical cystic disease (trisomy syndromes; tuberous sclerosis; von Hippel-Lindau disease; Zellweger S.)
*2. Cystic dysplasia of cortex (esp. associated with urethral valves or other low obstruction)
3. Dermoid cyst; teratoma
4. Endometrial cyst
*5. Hepatic fibrosis—renal cystic disease
*6. Hydatid cyst
*7. Juvenile nephronopthosis (medullary cystic disease—incl. small fibrotic kidneys with uremia)
8. Multilocular cyst
9. Multilocular cystic renal tumor (cystic nephroma; cystic partially differentiated nephroblastoma)
10. Pericaliceal lymphangiectasis
*11. Polycystic kidney disease, infantile or juvenile type—autosomal recessive (incl. large sponge kidneys with cystic liver)
12. [Urinoma]

* May be multiple.

(continued)

References
1. Banner MP, Pollack HM, Chatten J, et al: Multilocular renal cysts: Radiologic-pathologic correlation. AJR 1981; 136:239–247
2. Cho KJ, Thornbury JR, Bernstein J, et al: Localized cystic disease of the kidney: Angiographic pathologic correlation. AJR 1979;132:891–895
3. Elkin M: Renal cystic disease: An overview. Semin Roentgenol 1975;10:99–102
4. Felson B (ed): Renal cystic disease. Semin Roentgenol 1975;10:93
5. Madewell JE, Hartman DS, Lichtenstein JE: Radiologic-pathologic correlations in cystic disease of the kidney. Radiol Clin North Am 1979;17:261–279
6. Mellins HZ: Cystic dilatations of the upper urinary tract: A radiologist developmental model. Radiology 1985;153: 291–301
7. Williamson MR: Renal ultrasound. In: Essentials of Ultrasound. Philadelphia: WB Saunders, 1996, p 111

Gamut H-31

CONGENITAL SYNDROMES ASSOCIATED WITH RENAL CYSTIC DISEASE

COMMON
1. Hepatic fibrosis-renal cystic disease
2. Polycystic kidney disease (adult—autosomal dominant)
3. Polycystic kidney disease (juvenile—autosomal recessive)
4. Potter S.
5. Tuberous sclerosis

UNCOMMON
1. Acrocephalosyndactyly (Apert type)
2. Aplasia cutis congenita
3. Asphyxiating thoracic dysplasia (Jeune S.)
4. Asplenia S. (Ivemark S.)
5. Axial osteomalacia
6. Bardet-Biedl S.
7. Beckwith-Wiedemann S.
8. Brachymesomelia-renal S.
9. Branchio-oto-renal S.
10. Caroli disease
11. Cerebro-costo-mandibular S.
12. Cutis laxa
13. Darier disease
14. DiGeorge sequence
15. Ehlers-Danlos S.
16. Eronen S. (digito-reno-cerebral S.)
17. Femoral hypoplasia-unusual facies S.
18. Fetal alcohol S.
19. Fetal hydantoin S.
20. Fryns S.
21. Glomerulocystic kidney disease
22. Goldston S.
23. Hemihypertrophy
24. Joubert S.
25. Kaufman-McKusick S.
26. Lissencephaly
27. Marden-Walker S.
28. Meckel S.
29. Nail-patella S. (osteo-onychodysplasia)
30. Nephronophthisis
31. Noonan S.
32. Oculoauriculovertebral spectrum (Goldenhar S.)
33. Opitz trigonocephaly S. (C syndrome)
34. Orofaciodigital S. I
35. Polysplenia S.
36. Renal-hepatic-pancreatic dysplasia
37. Roberts S. (pseudothalidomide S.)
38. Short-rib polydactyly S. (types I and II)
39. Trisomy 13-15 S. (Patau S.)
40. Trisomy 18 S. (Edwards S.; E syndrome)
41. Trisomy 21 (Down S.)
42. Turner S.
43. von Hippel-Lindau S.
44. Zellweger S. (cerebrohepatorenal S.)

References
1. Hartman DS: Overview of renal cystic disease. In: Pollack HM, McClennan BL (eds): Clinical Urography. (ed 2) Philadelphia: WB Saunders, 2000, pp1245–1250
2. Taybi H, Lachman RS: Radiology of Syndromes, Metabolic Disorders, and Skeletal Dysplasias. (ed 4) St. Louis: Mosby-Year Book Inc., 1996, pp 979–980

Gamut H-32

MULTILOCULATED RENAL LESIONS CONTAINING MULTIPLE INTERNAL CYSTIC AREAS

COMMON

1. Cystic or necrotic neoplasm (esp. renal cell carcinoma {hypernephroma})
2. Wilm's tumor

UNCOMMON

1. Abscess
2. Arteriovenous fistula
3. Hematoma (organizing)
4. Hydatid cyst
5. Localized renal cystic disease
6. Malakoplakia
7. Multicystic dysplastic kidney (segmental)
8. Multilocular cystic nephroma
9. Septated cyst
10. Xanthogranulomatous pyelonephritis (segmental)

Reference

1. Hartman DS: Overview of renal cystic disease. In: Pollack HM, McClennan BL (eds): Clinical Urography. (ed 2) Philadelphia: WB Saunders, 2000, pp 1245–1250

Gamut H-33

BILATERAL OR MULTIPLE CYSTIC RENAL MASSES ON CT OR ULTRASOUND (ESPECIALLY IN CHILDREN)

COMMON

1. Acquired cystic disease (from dialysis)
2. Multiple simple cysts
3. Polycystic kidney disease (infantile—autosomal recessive, or esp. adult—autosomal dominant)

UNCOMMON

1. Glomerulocystic disease
2. Hydatid cysts
3. Juvenile nephronophthisis (medullary cystic disease)
4. Multicystic dysplastic kidney (usually unilateral)
5. Multiple abscesses
6. Tuberous sclerosis
7. von Hippel-Lindau S.

References

1. Cochlin DL: Chapter 24. Urinary tract. In McGahan JP, Goldberg BB (eds): Diagnostic Ultrasound. Philadelphia: Lippincott-Raven, 1997
2. Dunnick NR, et al: Textbook of Uroradiology. Baltimore: Williams & Wilkins, 1997, Chapter 5, pp 116–135
3. Thurston W, Wilson SR: Chapter 4. The urinary tract. In: Rumack CM, Wilson SR, Charboneau JW (eds): Diagnostic Ultrasound. St. Louis: Mosby, 1998, pp 371–378

Gamut H-34

HIGH DENSITY RENAL CYST(S) ON CT (62–82 HU)

1. Cystic or necrotic neoplasm (eg, renal cell carcinoma)
2. Hemorrhagic cyst
3. Hydatid cyst
4. Multicystic dysplastic kidney
5. Polycystic kidney disease

Gamut H-35-1

FOCAL RENAL PARENCHYMAL SCAR(S)

COMMON
1. Calyceal calculi
2. Infarct (old)
3. Vesicoureteral reflux

UNCOMMON
1. Papillary necrosis
2. Postoperative
3. Pyelonephritis, acute
4. Radiation injury
5. Renal artery branch stenosis or emboli
6. Trauma (including lithotripsy)
7. Tuberculosis

References
1. Anderson BL, et al: Demonstration of radiation nephritis by computed tomography. CT 1982;6:187–191
2. Friedland GW, et al (eds): Uroradiology: An Integrated Approach. London: Churchill Livingstone, 1983, pp 363–364, 649
3. Lechevallier E, et al: J Endocrinol 1993;7:465–467
4. Meyrier A: Kidney International 1989;35:696–703
5. Surana R, Khan A, Fitzgerald RJ: Scarring following renal trauma in children. Br J Urol 1995;75:663–665

Gamut H-35-2

DEPRESSION OR SCAR IN RENAL MARGIN (SOLITARY OR MULTIPLE)

COMMON
1. Arterionephrosclerosis
2. Extrinsic pressure (eg, spleen)
3. Fetal lobulation
4. Infarct
5. Postoperative defect

6. Pyelonephritis (chronic atrophic)
7. Trauma (laceration of kidney)

UNCOMMON
1. Chronic interstitial nephritis
2. Glomerulonephritis
3. Papillary necrosis
4. Radiation therapy
5. Tuberculosis

Gamut H-36

LOCALIZED BULGE OF RENAL OUTLINE

COMMON
1. Cyst (eg, simple; hydatid) (See H-30)
2. Localized hypertrophy with atrophy of remaining portion of kidney (eg, chronic atrophic pyelonephritis; infarction; trauma)
3. Metastasis
4. Neoplasm, benign (esp. angiomyolipoma) or malignant (eg, hypernephroma; sarcoma; lymphoma$_g$; Wilms' tumor)
5. Renal pseudotumor (eg, dromedary hump; fetal lobulation) (See H-37)

UNCOMMON
1. Abscess; carbuncle; nephronia; inflammatory mass (eg, tuberculosis; fungus disease$_g$)
2. Acute lobar pyelonephritis
3. Amyloidosis
4. Hematoma (subcapsular)
5. Localized hydronephrosis
6. Xanthogranulomatous pyelonephritis

References
1. Burgener FA, Kormano M: Differential Diagnosis in Conventional Radiology. (ed 2) New York: Thieme Medical Publ, 1991, pp 752–753

2. Felson B, Moskowitz M: Renal pseudotumors: The regenerated nodule and other lumps, bumps, and dromedary humps. AJR 1969;107:720–729
3. Rosenfield AT, Glickman MG, Taylor KJW, et al: Acute focal bacterial nephritis (acute lobar nephronia). Radiology 1979;132:553–561

Gamut H-37

RENAL PSEUDOTUMOR (NORMAL STRUCTURE)

COMMON

1. Dromedary hump
2. Duplicated collecting system
3. Fetal lobulation
4. Hypertrophy, localized (regenerated nodule)
5. Lipomatosis of renal pelvis
6. Malrotation
7. Prominent column of Bertin (lobar dysmorphism)
8. Prominent hilar lip; hilum profile
9. Splenic imprint
10. Superimposed abdominal shadow (eg, gallbladder; duodenal bulb; gastric fundus; accessory spleen)
11. Vascular impression

UNCOMMON

1. Aberrant papilla
2. Renunculus

References
1. Depner TA, Ryan KG, Yamauchi H: Pseudotumor of the kidney: A sequel to regional glomerulonephritis. AJR 1976; 126:1197–1202
2. Feldman AE, Pollack HM, Perri AJ Jr, et al: Renal pseudotumors: An anatomic-radiologic classification. J Urol 1978; 120:133–139
3. Felson B, Moskowitz M: Renal pseudotumors: The regenerated nodule and other lumps, bumps, and dromedary humps. AJR 1969;107:720–729
4. Friedenberg RM, Dunbar JS: Excretory urography. In: Pollack HM (ed): Clinical Urography. Philadelphia: WB Saunders, 1990, pp 101–255
5. Lopez FA: Renal pseudotumors. AJR 1970;109:172–184

Gamut H-38-S

TUMORS OF THE RENAL COLLECTING SYSTEM, PELVIS, AND URETERS

Epithelial Neoplasms
1. Inverted papilloma
2. Papilloma and transitional cell carcinoma
3. Transitional cell carcinoma with squamous, glandular, or mixed differentiation
4. Squamous cell carcinoma (pure or predominantly squamous)
5. Adenocarcinoma (pure or predominantly adenocarcinoma)
6. Carcinosarcoma
7. Small cell (undifferentiated) carcinoma

Mesodermal Neoplasms
1. Smooth Muscle
   a. Leiomyoma
   b. Leiomyoblastoma
   c. Leiomyosarcoma
2. Neural Neoplasms
   a. Neurilemmoma
   b. Neurofibroma
3. Vascular Neoplasms
   a. Hemangioma
   b. Lymphangioma
   c. Hemangiosarcoma
4. Fibrous Tissue
   a. Fibroepithelial polyp
   b. Renal medullary fibroma
5. Mixed Neoplasms
   a. Fibromyoma
   b. Fibromyxoma
   c. Fibrolipoma
6. Lymphoma; Burkitt lymphoma
7. Other Sarcomas
   a. Spindle cell sarcoma
   b. Osteosarcoma Secondary Neoplasms (Metastases)

(continued)

Secondary Neoplasms (Metastases)

1. Direct invasion from renal medullary tumor (esp. renal cell carcinoma) or adjacent extrinsic neoplasm (eg, gastrointestinal or pancreatic carcinoma or retroperitoneal sarcoma)
2. Seeding (eg, transitional cell carcinoma)
3. Lymphohematogenous spread

Gamut H-39

TUMORS OF THE RENAL PARENCHYMA (BENIGN AND MALIGNANT)

BENIGN

COMMON

1. Adenoma (usually too small to be seen by imaging)
2. Angiomyolipoma (eg, with tuberous sclerosis)

UNCOMMON

1. Benign mesenchymal tumor (eg, leiomyoma; lipoma; myolipoma; hemangioma; benign hemangiopericytoma; lymphangioma)
2. Juxtaglomerular cell tumor (reninoma)
3. Multilocular cystic renal tumor (multilocular cystic nephroma)
4. Oncocytoma
5. Renomedullary interstitial cell tumor (fibroma)

MALIGNANT

COMMON

1. Renal cell carcinoma (hypernephroma)
2. Wilm's tumor

UNCOMMON

1. Carcinoid tumor
2. Carcinoma, other (eg, small cell {undifferentiated}; renal medullary; invasive renal pelvic)
3. Lymphoma$_g$; Burkitt lymphoma; leukemia
4. Malignant mesenchymal tumors (eg, leiomyosarcoma; liposarcoma; rhabdomyosarcoma; angiosarcoma; osteosarcoma; malignant fibrous histiocytoma and fibrosarcoma; hemangiopericytoma)
5. Metastasis (eg, carcinoma; sarcoma; melanoma)
6. Neoplasm invading from an adjacent organ (eg, gastrointestinal or pancreatic carcinoma; retroperitoneal sarcoma)
7. Plasmacytoma; myeloma

References
1. Dunnick NR, et al: Textbook of Uroradiology. Baltimore: Williams & Wilkins, 1997, Chapter 6, pp 136–162
2. Levine E, King BF Jr: Adult malignant renal parenchymal neoplasms. In: Pollack HM, McClennan BL (eds): Clinical Urography. (ed 2) Philadelphia: WB Saunders, 2000, pp 1440–1559
3. Williamson B Jr, King BF Jr: Benign neoplasms of the renal parenchyma. In: Pollack HM, McClennan BL (eds): Clinical Urography. (ed 2) Philadelphia: WB Saunders, 2000, pp 1414–1439

Gamut H-40

PEDIATRIC RENAL MASSES (BENIGN AND MALIGNANT)

BENIGN

*1. Abscess
*2. Angiomyolipoma (esp. with tuberous sclerosis)
3. Benign adenomatous neoplasm (eg, embryonal adenoma; nephrogenic adenofibroma)
*4. Cyst (simple; hydatid; parapelvic; traumatic)
5. Fibroepithelial polyp of renal pelvis or ureter
6. Hydronephrosis (focal)
7. Mesoblastic nephroma (mesenchymal hamartoma)
8. Multilocular cystic renal tumor
   a. Multilocular cystic nephroma (multilocular renal cyst or cystic adenoma)

b. Cystic partially differentiated nephroblastoma (CPDN)

*9. Nephroblastomatosis

   a. Multifocal (juvenile)

   b. Superficial diffuse (late infantile)—high association with Wilms' tumor

   c. Universal/panlobar (infantile)

10. Ossifying renal tumor of infancy

*11. Polycystic kidney disease

MALIGNANT

1. Clear cell sarcoma

*2. Leukemia; lymphoma$_g$; Burkitt lymphoma

*3. Metastasis (eg, neuroblastoma with direct invasion)

4. Renal cell carcinoma

5. Rhabdoid tumor; rhabdomyosarcoma

*6. Wilms' tumor

* May be multiple.

References

1. Carpenter BLM, Day DL: Pediatric Renal Tumors: Nonspecificity of radiographic findings. Scientific Exhibit at the Radiological Society of North America Meeting, Chicago, 1991
2. Paltiel HJ, Kirks DR: Pediatric urological neoplasms. In: Pollack HM, McClennan BL (eds): Clinical Urography. (ed 2) Philadelphia: WB Saunders, 2000, pp 1743–1765

Gamut H-41

CONGENITAL SYNDROMES OR ANOMALIES ASSOCIATED WITH WILMS' TUMOR

1. Aniridia-Wilms' tumor association
2. Beckwith-Wiedemann S.
3. Drash S. (male pseudohermaphroditism)
4. Hemihypertrophy
5. Horseshoe kidney
6. Klippel-Trenaunay-S.; Parkes Weber S.
7. Perlman S.
8. Trisomy 13 S.
9. Trisomy 18 S.

Reference

1. Taybi H, Lachman RS: Radiology of Syndromes, Metabolic Disorders, and Skeletal Dysplasias. (ed 4) St. Louis: Mosby-Year Book Inc., 1996, p 1066

Gamut H-42

NEONATAL RENAL MASS

COMMON

1. Hydronephrosis (esp. UPJ obstruction; duplication of collecting system) (See H-49)
2. Multicystic dysplastic kidney (pelvoinfundibular or hydronephrotic types)

UNCOMMON

1. Mesoblastic nephroma
2. Metastasis (eg, neuroblastoma with direct invasion)
3. Multilocular cystic renal tumor

   a. Multilocular cystic nephroma (multilocular renal cyst or cystic adenoma)

   b. Cystic partially differentiated nephroblastoma (CPDN)

4. Neoplasm, other (eg, teratoma; ossifying renal tumor of infancy)
5. Nephroblastomatosis

   a. Multifocal (juvenile)

   b. Superficial diffuse (late infantile)—high association with Wilms' tumor

   c. Universal/panlobar (infantile)

6. Polycystic kidney disease
7. Wilms' tumor

References

1. Felson B, Cussen LJ: The hydronephrotic type of unilateral congenital multicystic disease of the kidney. Semin Roentgenol 1975;10:113–123
2. Paltiel HJ, Kirks DR: Pediatric urological neoplasms. In: Pollack HM, McClennan BL (eds): Clinical Urography. (ed 2) Philadelphia: WB Saunders, 2000, pp 1743–1765
3. Swischuk LE: Imaging of the Newborn, Infant, and Young Child. (ed 3) Baltimore: Williams & Wilkins, 1989

Gamut H-43

SOLID RENAL MASS (US, CT)

COMMON

1. Abscess; carbuncle
2. Angiomyolipoma (hamartoma), esp. in tuberous sclerosis
3. Calculus
4. Cyst (calcified; hemorrhagic; infected; multilocular; hydatid)
5. Hematoma or contusion (intrarenal or subcapsular)
6. Infarct
7. Metastasis (esp. from carcinoma of lung, breast, stomach, colon, cervix, pancreas, contralateral kidney, or choriocarcinoma)
8. Normal parenchyma; pseudotumor (eg, hypertrophied column of Bertin; regenerated nodule; dromedary hump; lobar dysmorphism)
9. Renal cell carcinoma (hypernephroma)
10. Wilms' tumor

UNCOMMON

1. Arteriovenous malformation; hemangioma (cavernous)
2. Benign neoplasm, other (eg, adenoma; oncocytoma; lipoma; fibroma; mesoblastic nephroma)
3. Calcified renal mass (eg, hydatid cyst; abscess; hematoma)
4. Granuloma (eg, tuberculosis)
5. Leukoplakia; cholesteatoma
6. Lipomatosis of renal sinus
7. Lymphoma$_g$; leukemia; Burkitt lymphoma
8. Malakoplakia
9. Polycystic kidney disease (infantile—autosomal recessive)
10. Pyelonephritis, acute focal bacterial (nephronia) (on postcontrast scan)
11. Sarcoma (eg, osteosarcoma)
12. Transitional cell carcinoma
13. Xanthogranulomatous pyelonephritis (focal)

References

1. Amis ES Jr, Hartman DS: Renal ultrasonography 1984: A practical overview. Radiol Clin North Am 1984;22:315–332
2. Eisenberg RL: Clinical Imaging: An Atlas of Differential Diagnosis. (ed 3) Philadelphia: Lippincott-Raven, 1997, pp 644–653
3. Elyaderani MK, Gabriele OF: Ultrasound of renal masses. Semin Ultrasound 1981;11:21–43
4. Fleischer AC, James AE: Introduction to Diagnostic Sonography. New York: John Wiley & Sons, 1980
5. Williamson MR: Chapter 6. Renal ultrasound. In: Essentials of Ultrasound. Philadelphia: WB Saunders, 1996, p 115

Gamut H-44

CYSTIC RENAL MASS (US, CT)

COMMON

1. Abscess; carbuncle; nephronia
2. Cyst (simple; hydatid; parapelvic)
3. Hydronephrosis (focal)
4. Necrotic neoplasm (esp. cystic renal cell carcinoma)
5. Polycystic kidney disease (adult—autosomal dominant)

UNCOMMON

1. Acquired cystic disease (dialysis)
2. Calyceal diverticulum
3. Cystic hematoma
4. Infection with necrosis (eg, tuberculosis)
5. Multicystic dysplastic kidney
6. Multilocular cystic renal tumor (multilocular cystic nephroma, multilocular renal cyst)
7. Urinoma
8. Vascular anomaly (aneurysm; pseudoaneurysm; arteriovenous fistula)

References

1. Eisenberg RL: Clinical Imaging: An Atlas of Differential Diagnosis. (ed 3) Philadelphia: Lippincott-Raven, 1997, pp 644–653
2. Williamson MR: Chapter 6. Renal ultrasound. In: Essentials of Ultrasound. Philadelphia: WB Saunders, 1996, p 111

Gamut H-45

CYSTIC RENAL MASS WITH INTERNAL DEBRIS (US, CT)

1. Abscess, renal or perinephric (thick wall)
2. Cystic or necrotic neoplasm (eg, renal cell carcinoma {hypernephroma})
3. Hemorrhagic cyst
4. Hydatid cyst
5. Infected cyst
6. Multilocular cystic nephroma (multilocular renal cyst)

Reference
1. Thurston W, Wilson SR: Chapter 9. The urinary tract. In: Rumack CM, Wilson SR, Charboneau JW (eds): Diagnostic Ultrasound. St. Louis: Mosby, 1998, pp 329–397

Gamut H-46

CYSTIC RENAL MASS WITH WALL CALCIFICATION

1. Aneurysm; arteriovenous malformation
2. Hydatid cyst
3. Polycystic kidney disease
4. [Renal artery or its branches]
5. Renal cell carcinoma (hypernephroma), necrotic
6. Simple cortical cyst

Reference
1. Thurston W, Wilson SR: Chapter 9. The urinary tract. In: Rumack CM, Wilson SR, Charboneau JW (eds): Diagnostic Ultrasound. St. Louis: Mosby, 1998, pp 371–378

Gamut H-47

RENAL MASS WITH CALCIFICATION

COMMON
1. Calcified stone with hydronephrosis
2. Hemorrhagic cyst; complicated simple cyst
3. Renal cell carcinoma (hypernephroma)

UNCOMMON
1. Acquired polycystic kidney disease (from dialysis)
2. Brucellosis
3. Hematoma
4. Hydatid cyst
5. Multilocular cystic kidney, segmental
6. Multilocular cystic nephroma
7. Polycystic kidney disease (adult—autosomal dominant)
8. Sarcoma (eg, leiomyosarcoma; osteosarcoma)
9. Transitional cell carcinoma
10. Tuberculosis
11. Wilms' tumor
12. Xanthogranulomatous pyelonephritis

References
1. Cochlin DL: Chapter 24. Urinary tract. In: McGahan JP, Goldberg BB (eds): Diagnostic Ultrasound. Philadelphia: Lippincott-Raven, 1997
2. Pollack HM (ed): Clinical Urography. Philadelphia: WB Saunders, 1990, pp 791, 1012, 1024, 1026, 1056, 1072, 1094, 1127, 1160, 1209, 1227, 1279, 1280, 1294

Gamut H-48

RENAL MASS WITH FAT ON CT

COMMON

1. Angiomyolipoma (eg, with tuberous sclerosis)

UNCOMMON

1. Lipoma; liposarcoma
2. Renal cell carcinoma (entrapping perinephric or sinus fat, or intratumoral metaplasia)
3. Teratoma
4. Wilms' tumor
5. Xanthogranulomatous pyelonephritis

Reference

1. Slone RM, Fisher AJ: Pocket Guide to Body CT Differential Diagnosis. New York: McGraw-Hill, 1999, p 273

Gamut H-49

HYDRONEPHROSIS

COMMON

1. Neurogenic bladder (See H-98)
2. Pregnancy
3. Ureteral or ureteropelvic obstruction (eg, calculus; stricture; neoplasm {esp. transitional cell carcinoma}) (See H-93)
4. Ureterectasis (See H-91)
5. Urethral or bladder outlet obstruction (eg, urethral valves; stricture) (See H-110, 111)
6. Urinary tract infection with stricture (incl. tuberculosis; schistosomiasis haematobium)
7. Vesicoureteral reflux (See H-92)

UNCOMMON

1. Bardet-Biedl S.
2. Bartter S.
3. Beckwith-Wiedeman S.

4. Bladder distention (See H-96)
5. Constipation; fecal impaction; colon distention
6. Diuresis
7. Extrarenal pelvis
8. Megaureter (congenital)
9. Papillary necrosis (obstruction by sloughed papilla)
10. Prune-belly S. (Eagle-Barrett S.)
11. Pyonephrosis (debris or fluid-fluid level in collecting system)
12. Urinary flow increase, overhydration (eg, diabetes insipidus; beer-drinker kidneys)

References

1. Friedland GW: Hydronephrosis in infants and children, Part I. Curr Probl Diagn Radiol 1978;7:3–52
2. Talner LB: Urinary obstruction. In: Pollack HM (ed): Clinical Urography. Philadelphia: WB Saunders, 1990, pp 1535–1628
3. Thurston W, Wilson SR: Chapter 9. The urinary tract. In: Rumack CM, Wilson SR, Charboneau JW (eds): Diagnostic Ultrasound. St. Louis: Mosby, 1998, pp 329–397

Gamut H-50

RENAL HEMORRHAGE

COMMON

1. Anticoagulant therapy
2. Biopsy and other invasive procedure
3. Bleeding disorder$_g$ (eg, hemophilia)
4. Coagulopathy
5. Neoplasm (eg, angiomyolipoma; hemangioma; renal cell carcinoma; other primary malignancy; metastasis)
6. Trauma

UNCOMMON

1. Aneurysm
2. Arteritis (eg, polyarteritis nodosa; drug abuse; Wegener's granulomatosis)
3. Arteriovenous malformation
4. Glomerulonephritis

5. Hydronephrosis, severe
6. Postoperative
7. Pyelonephritis, severe

Reference

1. Spataro R, Thornbury JR: Renal hemorrhage and renal complications of hemorrhagic hypotension. In: Pollack HM (ed): Clinical Urography. Philadelphia: WB Saunders, 1990, pp 2188–2209

Gamut H-51

RENAL PARENCHYMAL GAS

1. Abscess
2. Acute pyelonephritis
3. Emphysematous pyelonephritis
4. Infected or ruptured cyst (eg, hydatid)
5. Nephrointestinal fistula (See H-52)
6. Post-instrumentation

Reference

1. Thurston W, Wilson SR: Chapter 9. The urinary tract. In: Rumack CM, Wilson SR, Charboneau JW (eds): Diagnostic Ultrasound. St. Louis: Mosby, 1998, pp 329–397

Gamut H-52

NEPHROINTESTINAL FISTULA

1. Chronic renal infection
2. Carcinoma or other malignancy of colon or duodenum
3. Foreign body
4. Peptic ulcer disease (perforating from duodenum)
5. Renal calculus (perforating)
6. Trauma

Reference

1. Balfe DM, Bova JG: Genitourinary manifestations of gastrointestinal disease. In: Pollack HM (ed): Clinical Urography. Philadelphia: WB Saunders, 1990, pp 961–979

Gamut H-53

DARK KIDNEY ON T2-WEIGHTED MRI

COMMON

1. Hemolytic anemia$_g$
2. Multiple blood transfusions

UNCOMMON

1. Hemochromatosis
2. Nephrocalcinosis
3. Paroxysmal nocturnal hemoglobinuria

Reference

1. Roubidoux MA: MR imaging of hemorrhage and iron deposition in the kidney. RadioGraphics 1994;14:1033–1044

Gamut H-54

LESIONS INVOLVING THE PERIRENAL SPACE (See G-243)

COMMON

1. Hemorrhage (See H-55-3)
2. Neoplasm, metastatic or invasive (eg, carcinoma of kidney or colon)
3. Neoplasm, primary renal (eg, hypernephroma; Wilms' tumor; lymphoma$_g$)
4. Pancreatitis
5. Perinephric abscess originating from infection in kidney, colon, duodenum, or retrocecal appendix (See H-55-2)
6. Urinoma (traumatic or postoperative)

UNCOMMON

1. Lipomatosis
2. Lymphocele (traumatic; postoperative; lymphangioma; obstruction to thoracic duct)
3. Lymphoma$_g$ of retroperitoneum

(continued)

4. Retroperitoneal fibrosis (See H-128)
5. Spindle cell neoplasm$_g$ of retroperitoneum (esp. sarcoma)
6. Suprarenal lesion (eg, adrenal cyst, adenoma, or carcinoma; neuroblastoma; pheochromocytoma)

References
1. Meyers MA: Uriniferous perirenal pseudocyst: New observations. Radiology 1975;117:539–545
2. Pummill CL: Gamut: Lesions involving the perirenal space. Semin Roentgenol 1981;16:237–238

Gamut H-55-1

PERIRENAL FLUID COLLECTION

COMMON
1. Cyst
2. Loculated ascites

UNCOMMON
1. Abscess (See H-55-2)
2. Adrenal cyst
3. Hemorrhage or hematoma (See H-55-3)
4. Hepatic cyst
5. Lymphocele (common after renal transplant)
6. Pancreatic pseudocyst
7. Urinoma (common after renal transplant)

References
1. Blandino A, et al: Subcapsular renal spread of a pancreatic pseudocyst. Abdominal Imaging 1996;21:73–74
2. Morley P, et al: Ultrasound in the diagnosis of fluid collections following renal transplantation. Clinical Radiology 1975;26:199–207

Gamut H-55-2

PERINEPHRIC ABSCESS

1. Extraurinary infection with direct or hematogenous spread
   a. Deep infection (eg, osteomyelitis; pharyngitis; tonsillitis; perforated ulcer; diverticulitis; pancreatitis)
   b. Superficial infection (eg, furuncle; carbuncle; wound infection)
2. Gas abscess
3. Iatrogenic (eg, removal of ureteral calculus; ureteral catheterization)
4. Obstructive uropathy
5. Trauma to kidney or ureter
6. Tuberculosis; fungus infection$_g$
7. Urinary tract infection (esp. in diabetic)
8. Urinoma or hematoma (infected)

Reference
1. Love L, Baker D, Ramsey R: Gas producing perinephric abscess. AJR 1973;119:783–792

Gamut H-55-3

PERINEPHRIC HEMORRHAGE OR HEMATOMA

COMMON
1. Aneurysm, aortic, renal artery, or other (incl. atherosclerotic; mycotic; dissecting)
2. Iatrogenic (eg, needle biopsy; catheter; surgery)
3. Neoplasm, adrenal or renal (eg, carcinoma; angioma; angiomyolipoma)
4. Thromboembolism of inferior vena cava or renal vein
5. Trauma, external

UNCOMMON

1. Arterial disease (fibromuscular disease; polyarteritis nodosa)
2. Arteriovenous fistula (congenital or traumatic)
3. Bleeding disorder$_g$ (incl. anticoagulant therapy)
4. Calculus, perforated
5. Hypertension
6. Idiopathic
7. Infarction of kidney
8. Infection (eg, abscess; tuberculosis)
9. Rupture of kidney (eg, spontaneous; infarct; hydronephrosis; cyst)
10. Sickle cell disease
11. Stress (adrenal bleeding)

References

1. Burgener FA, Kormano M: Differential Diagnosis in Conventional Radiology. (ed 2) New York: Thieme Medical Publ, 1991, p 754
2. Pollack HM, Popky GL: Roentgenographic manifestations of spontaneous renal hemorrhage. Radiology 1974;110:1–6

Gamut H-56

PERIPELVIC EXTRAVASATION (SINUS LEAKAGE) (See H-95)

COMMON

1. Abdominal compression (binder)
2. Iatrogenic (instrumentation; retrograde pyelography; accidental ureteral ligation; postoperative)
3. Trauma
4. Ureteral calculus

UNCOMMON

1. [Communicating renal cyst or hydatid]
2. Hydronephrosis (eg, ureteral tumor or stricture)
3. Neoplasm of renal pelvis (esp. with rupture or hemorrhage)
4. Parturition
5. Polycystic kidney

References

1. Bramwit DN, Rosen LS, Cukier DS: Peripelvic extravasation in chronic ureteral obstruction by reticulum-cell sarcoma. Radiology 1970;96:421–422
2. Braun WT: Peripelvic extravasation during intravenous urography. AJR 1966;98:41–46
3. Meyers MA: Uriniferous perirenal pseudocyst: New observations. Radiology 1975;117:539–545
4. Parker M: Diagnostic skills. In: Friedland GW, Filly R, Goris ML, et al: Uroradiology: An Integrated Approach. New York: Churchill Livingstone, 1983, pp 1675, 1678
5. Pummill CL: Gamut: Lesions involving the perirenal space. Semin Roentgenol 1981;16:237–238

Gamut H-57

PERIPHERAL RIM ENHANCEMENT (ANGIO, IVP)

COMMON

1. Abscess
2. Neoplasm (eg, necrotic or cystic, esp. at periphery of cortex)
3. Severe hydronephrosis

UNCOMMON

1. Acute renal artery occlusion
2. Acute renal vein thrombosis

Reference

1. Davidson AJ: A systematic approach to the radiologic diagnosis of renal parenchymal disease. Chapter 23. The Nephrogram. In: Pollack HM (ed): Clinical Urography. Philadelphia: WB Saunders, 1990, pp 751–775

Gamut H-58

RENAL ANGIOGRAPHY: RENAL ISCHEMIA

COMMON

1. Arteriolar nephrosclerosis
2. Atherosclerosis
3. Chronic pyelonephritis
4. Thromboembolism, spasm, or stenosis of renal artery
5. Trauma (eg, fractured kidney; avulsion of renal artery)

UNCOMMON

1. Arteritis (eg, polyarteritis nodosa; Takayasu S.)
2. Arteriovenous communication
   a. Congenital
   b. Iatrogenic (eg, stump fistula following partial nephrectomy; needle biopsy)
   c. Renal carcinoma eroding renal vein
   d. Ruptured aneurysm
   e. Traumatic
3. Extrinsic pressure on the renal artery (eg, neoplasm; cyst; aortic aneurysm$_g$; lymphadenopathy; fibrous band)
4. Fibromuscular hyperplasia (intimal, medial, subadventitial)
5. [Lipomatosis of renal sinus]
6. Renal artery aneurysm
7. Renal compression (eg, perirenal or subcapsular hematoma; splenomegaly)
8. Thrombosis of renal vein (See H-63)

References

1. Baum S: Renal ischemic lesions. Radiol Clin North Am 1967;5:543–558
2. Newhouse JH, Pfister RC: The nephrogram. Radiol Clin North Am 1979;17:213–225

Gamut H-59-1

RENAL ANGIOGRAPHY: UNILATERAL RENAL LESION THAT MAY CAUSE HYPERTENSION (NARROWING OR OTHER LESION OF RENAL ARTERY OR ITS BRANCHES)

1. [Acute glomerulonephritis (bilateral)]
2. Aneurysm (See H-60)
3. [Arteriolar nephrosclerosis (bilateral)]
4. Arteriovenous malformation
5. Arteritis (eg, Takayasu S.; thromboangiitis obliterans; congenital rubella S.; syphilis; idiopathic)
6. Atherosclerosis
7. [Collagen vascular disease$_g$ (eg, polyarteritis nodosa; scleroderma; lupus erythematosus) (bilateral)]
8. Congenital narrowing
9. Dissection
10. Drug abuse
11. Extrinsic pressure from adjacent mass
12. Fibromuscular hyperplasia
13. Neurofibromatosis
14. Perivascular fibrosis
15. Radiation injury
16. Thrombosis or embolism
17. Transplant rejection
18. Trauma

References

1. Bookstein JJ: Cooperative study of radiologic aspects of renovascular hypertension. JAMA 1977;237:1706–1709
2. Davidson AJ, Hartman DS: Radiology of the Kidney and Urinary Tract. Chapter 26, Angiography in diseases of the kidney. Philadelphia: WB Saunders, 1994, pp 789–800
3. Hanenson IB, Gaffney TE: Clinical recognition of renal hypertension. Semin Roentgenol 1967;2:115–125
4. Johnsrude IS, Jackson DC: A Practical Approach to Angiography. Boston: Little, Brown, 1979, pp 167–185

RENAL ANGIOGRAPHY: UNILATERAL RENAL LESION THAT MAY CAUSE HYPERTENSION (RENAL PARENCHYMAL DISEASE AND OTHER CAUSES)

RENAL PARENCHYMAL DISEASE

1. Neoplasm, malignant (eg, carcinoma; sarcoma; Wilms' tumor; metastasis)
2. Obstructive uropathy
3. Ptosis of kidney
4. Pyelonephritis
5. Radiation nephritis

RENAL VEIN THROMBOEMBOLISM

RENAL COMPRESSION (PAGE KIDNEY)

1. Extrarenal mass (eg, aortic aneurysm$_g$; retroperitoneal hematoma or neoplasm; peripelvic cyst)
2. Subcapsular hemorrhage

References
1. Bookstein JJ: Cooperative study of radiologic aspects of renovascular hypertension. JAMA 1977;237:1706–1709
2. Davidson AJ, Hartman DS: Radiology of the Kidney and Urinary Tract. Chapter 26, Angiography in diseases of the kidney. Philadelphia: WB Saunders, 1994, pp 789–800
3. Hanenson IB, Gaffney TE: Clinical recognition of renal hypertension. Semin Roentgenol 1967;2:115–125
4. Johnsrude IS, Jackson DC: A Practical Approach to Angiography. Boston: Little, Brown, 1979, pp 167–185

RENAL ANGIOGRAPHY: RENAL ARTERY ANEURYSMS OR MICROANEURYSMS

COMMON
*1. Atherosclerosis
*2. Iatrogenic (eg, post-needle biopsy; postsurgical)
 3. Polyarteritis nodosa

UNCOMMON
 1. Angiomyolipoma (esp. with tuberous sclerosis)
 2. Arteriolar nephrosclerosis, malignant
 3. Atrial myxoma (metastatic)
*4. Arteriovenous communication (congenital; acquired)
 5. Bacterial endocarditis
 6. Collagen disease$_g$, other (eg, lupus erythematosus)
*7. Dissecting aneurysm
 8. Drug abuse angiitis
*9. Fibromuscular hyperplasia
 10. Homocystinuria
*11. Mycotic aneurysm
 12. Neurofibromatosis
 13. Renal cell carcinoma (hypernephroma)
 14. Renal transplant rejection
 15. Rheumatic or rheumatoid arteritis
*16. Takayasu's arteritis
 17. Thrombocytopenic purpura
*18. Traumatic aneurysm
 19. Wegener's granulomatosis; hypersensitivity angiitis

* May be solitary.

References
1. Clark RE, Jacobson AC, Petty WE: Intrarenal mycotic (false) aneurysm secondary to staphylococcal septicemia. Radiology 1975;115:421–422
2. Davidson AJ, Hartman DS: Radiology of the Kidney and Urinary Tract. Philadelphia: WB Saunders, 1994, Chapter 26, Angiography in diseases of the kidney, pp 789–800

(continued)

3. Easterbrook JS: Renal and hepatic microaneurysms: Report of a new entity simulating polyarteritis nodosa. Radiology 1980;137:629–630
4. Pope TL Jr, Buschi AJ, Moore TS, et al: CT features of renal polyarteritis nodosa. AJR 1981;136:986–989

Gamut H-61

RENAL ANGIOGRAPHY: AVASCULAR RENAL MASS

COMMON

1. Abscess
2. [Arterial occlusion; infarction]
3. Cyst (eg, simple; hydatid) (See H-30)
4. Hematoma
5. Polycystic kidney disease

UNCOMMON

1. [Dilated calyx]
2. Lymphoma$_g$
3. Metastasis
4. Multilocular cystic nephroma (multilocular renal cyst)
5. Neoplasm, benign (eg, adenoma; spindle cell tumor$_g$; lipoma)
6. Neoplasm, malignant, necrotic (eg, renal cell carcinoma; Wilms' tumor)
7. Xanthogranulomatous pyelonephritis

Gamut H-62

RENAL ANGIOGRAPHY: EARLY VENOUS OPACIFICATION (LESS THAN 5 SEC)

COMMON

1. Arteriovenous communication, congenital or acquired (eg, traumatic; needle biopsy; postoperative)
2. Renal neoplasm (eg, hemangioma; angiomyolipoma; renal cell carcinoma)

UNCOMMON

1. Inflammatory disease, diffuse
2. Inflammatory lesion, localized (renal abscess; carbuncle; nephronia; perinephric abscess)
3. Renal artery obstruction, acute (eg, catheter in wedge position)
4. Trueta phenomenon

Reference

1. Becker JA, Kanter IE, Perl S: Rapid intrarenal circulation. AJR 1970;109:167–171

Gamut H-63

RENAL ANGIOGRAPHY: RENAL VEIN THROMBOSIS

COMMON

1. Dehydration; diarrhea (in a child)
2. Idiopathic (primary)
3. Neoplasm with renal vein invasion or obstruction (esp. renal cell carcinoma; sarcoma, esp. of inferior vena cava)
4. Thromboembolism of inferior vena cava with retrograde extension

UNCOMMON

1. Amyloidosis; multiple myeloma
2. Ascending phlebitis
3. Clotting disorder; polycythemia vera; sickle cell disease
4. Congenital heart disease
5. Diabetic glomerulosclerosis
6. Glomerulonephritis (membranous or proliferative)
7. Nephrotic S.
8. Postoperative
9. Postpartum
10. Pyelonephritis
11. Renal hypertension
12. Trauma

References
1. Clark RA, Wyatt GM, Colley DP: Renal vein thrombosis: An underdiagnosed complication of multiple renal abnormalities. Radiology 1979;132:43–50
2. Coel MN, Talner LB: Obstructive nephrogram due to renal vein thrombosis. Radiology 1971;101:573–574
3. Mulhern CB, Arger PH, Miller WT, et al: The specificity of renal vein thrombosis. AJR 1975;125:291–299

3. Elyaderani MK, Gabriele OF: Ultrasound of renal masses. Semin Ultrasound 1981;11:21–43
4. Hayes WS, Hartman DS, Sesterhenn IA: From the Archives of the AFIP. Xanthogranulomatous pyelonephritis. RadioGraphics 1991;11:485–498
5. Itoh S, et al. Ultrasonographic diagnosis of uriniferous perirenal pseudocyst. Pediat Rad 1982;12:156–158
6. Morley P, et al: Ultrasound in the diagnosis of fluid collections following renal transplantation. Clin Radiol 1975;26:199–207
7. Ralls PW, Halls J: Hydronephrosis, renal cystic disease, and renal parenchymal disease. Semin Ultrasound 1981;11:49–60
8. Schnabel SI, et al: Ultrasound detection of milk of calcium within a calyceal diverticulum. J Clin Ultrasound 1980;8:154–155
9. Thurston W, Wilson SR: Chapter 9. The urinary tract. In: Rumack CM, Wilson SR, Charboneau JW (eds): Diagnostic Ultrasound. St. Louis: Mosby, 1998, pp 329–397
10. Townsend RR, et al: Abdominal lymphoma in AIDS: evaluation with US. Radiology 1989;171:719–724

Gamut H-64

SONOGRAPHY: ECHO-FREE (ANECHOIC) RENAL MASS

COMMON
1. Abscess, renal or perirenal
2. Cyst (eg, simple; hydatid; parapelvic) (See H-30)
3. Hydronephrosis, focal (See H-49)
4. Neoplasm (esp. lymphoma$_g$; necrotic renal cell carcinoma; cyst with small mural tumor)
5. Polycystic kidney disease (autosomal dominant—adult)

UNCOMMON
1. Aneurysm (noncalcified) of renal artery
2. Arteriovenous malformation
3. Calyceal diverticulum
4. Caliectasis (esp. duplication with ectopic ureterocele)
5. Fluid collection, renal or perirenal (eg, hemorrhage; seroma; urinoma; lymphocele)
6. Medullary cystic disease
7. Multicystic dysplastic kidney
8. Pyonephrosis
9. Tuberculous cavity

References
1. Amis ES Jr, Hartman DS: Renal ultrasonography 1984: A practical overview. Radiol Clin North Am 1984;22:315–332
2. Brondum V, Fiirgaard B: Renal artery aneurysm detected by pulsed Doppler ultrasound. Röntgen-Blatter 1990;43:510–511

Gamut H-65

SONOGRAPHY: HYPOECHOIC RENAL MASS

COMMON
1. Abscess with debris
2. Cyst with debris (eg, simple; hydatid; parapelvic; hemorrhagic)
3. Pyelonephritis, acute
4. Renal cell carcinoma (hypernephroma)

UNCOMMON
1. Calyceal diverticulum with debris
2. Duplication of collecting system (obstructed with debris)
3. Hematoma
4. Infarction (focal)
5. Localized hydronephrosis with debris
6. Lymphoma$_g$; leukemia
7. Metastasis
8. Oncocytoma

(continued)

9. Transitional cell carcinoma
10. Xanthogranulomatous pyelonephritis

References

1. Cochlin DL: Chapter 24. Urinary tract. In: McGahan JP, Goldberg BB (eds): Diagnostic Ultrasound. Philadelphia: Lippincott-Raven, 1997
2. Pollack HM (ed): Clinical Urography. Philadelphia: WB Saunders, 1990, pp 806, 1077, 1251, 1273, 1283, 1482, 1561

Gamut H-66

SONOGRAPHY: ISOECHOIC RENAL MASS

1. Hypertrophied column of Bertin
2. Lymphoma$_g$
3. Pyelonephritis (focal)
4. Renal cell carcinoma (hypernephroma)
5. Renal pseudotumor (eg, dromedary hump; focal compensatory hypertrophy)
6. Transitional cell carcinoma

Gamut H-67

SONOGRAPHY: HYPERECHOIC RENAL MASS

COMMON

1. Angiomyolipoma (incl. tuberous sclerosis)
2. Nephrocalcinosis (focal)
3. Renal cell carcinoma (hypernephroma)
4. Renal sinus lipomatosis or duplication

UNCOMMON

1. Abscess with microbubble gas formation
2. Benign renal neoplasm (eg, cavernous hemangioma; oncocytoma; hamartoma; lipoma; juxtaglomerular cell tumor)

3. Calcified or complicated renal cyst (esp. hydatid)
4. Calcified or thrombosed renal artery aneurysm
5. Focal renal dysplasia
6. Hematoma; hemorrhage; hemorrhagic pyelonephritis
7. Hypertrophied column of Bertin (viewed en face)
8. Infarct with focal scar
9. Malakoplakia
10. Multilocular cystic nephroma
11. Sarcoma (eg, angiosarcoma; liposarcoma; undifferentiated sarcoma)
12. Tuberculosis (early)
13. Wilms' tumor

References

1. Bisset RAL, Khan AN: Differential Diagnosis in Abdominal Ultrasound. London: Baillière Tindall, 1990, p 220
2. Pollack HM (ed): Clinical Urography. Philadelphia: WB Saunders, 1990, pp 349–355, 838, 1212, 1214
3. Thurston W, Wilson SR: Chapter 9. The urinary tract. In: Rumack CM, Wilson SR, Charboneau JW (eds): Diagnostic Ultrasound. St. Louis: Mosby, 1998, pp 329–397

Gamut H-68-1

SONOGRAPHY: MULTILOCULAR OR COMPLEX RENAL MASS

NEOPLASM

1. Angiomyolipoma (esp. with tuberous sclerosis)
2. Cystic Wilms' tumor
3. Mesoblastic nephroma
4. Metastasis
5. Multilocular cystic nephroma (multilocular renal cyst)
6. Necrotic tumor with debris
7. Renal cell carcinoma (hypernephroma) (incl. von Hippel-Lindau S.)

RENAL CYSTIC DISEASE

1. Cyst containing debris (eg, infected cyst; ruptured hydatid cyst) or clot (hemorrhagic cyst)
2. Multicystic dysplastic kidney (segmental)
3. Polycystic kidney
4. Segmental cystic disease
5. "Septated" cyst

INFLAMMATION/INFECTION

1. Abscess with debris
2. Fungus ball (renal candidasis)
3. Hydatid cyst
4. Pyonephrosis (infected hydronephrosis)
5. Malakoplakia of renal parenchyma
6. Tuberculosis (late)
7. Xanthogranulomatous pyelonephritis (segmental)

MISCELLANEOUS

1. Arteriovenous malformation
2. Hemorrhage
3. Hemorrhagic infarct (as in renal vein thrombosis)
4. Posttraumatic (organizing hematoma)

References

1. Amis ES Jr, Hartman DS: Renal ultrasonography 1984: A practical overview. Radiol Clin North Am 1984;22:315–332
2. Eisenberg RL: Clinical Imaging: An Atlas of Differential Diagnosis. (ed 3) Philadelphia: Lippincott-Raven, 1997, pp 636–639
3. Elyaderani MK, Gabriele OF: Ultrasound of renal masses. Semin Ultrasound 1981;11:21–43
4. Thurston W, Wilson SR: Chapter 9. The urinary tract. In: Rumack CM, Wilson SR, Charboneau JW (eds): Diagnostic Ultrasound. St. Louis: Mosby, 1998, pp 329–397

Gamut H-68-2

SONOGRAPHY: ILL-DEFINED RENAL PARENCHYMAL MASS

COMMON

1. Acute pyelonephritis
2. Normal variant (eg, hypertrophied column of Bertin; focal compensatory hypertrophy)
3. Renal cell carcinoma (hypernephroma)

UNCOMMON

1. Contusion; hematoma
2. Oncocytoma
3. Lymphoma$_g$; leukemia
4. Metastasis
5. Renal vein thrombosis
6. Transitional cell carcinoma
7. Tuberculosis (early)

Reference

1. Thurston W, Wilson SR: Chapter 9. The urinary tract. In: Rumack CM, Wilson SR, Charboneau JW (eds): Diagnostic Ultrasound. St. Louis: Mosby, 1998, pp 329–397

Gamut H-69

SONOGRAPHY: MASS IN RENAL COLLECTING SYSTEM OR PELVIS WITH ACOUSTICAL SHADOWING

COMMON

1. Calculus (uric acid or calcium)
2. Renal artery calcification (eg, aneurysm, atherosclerosis)
3. Renal gas or air

(continued)

UNCOMMON

1. Calcification in cyst wall (esp. hydatid)
2. Transitional cell carcinoma with calcification

References

1. Amis ES Jr, Hartman DS: Renal ultrasonography 1984: A practical overview. Radiol Clin North Am 1984;22:315–332
2. Cochlin DL: Chapter 24. Urinary tract. In McGahan JP, Goldberg BB (eds): Diagnostic Ultrasound. Philadelphia: Lippincott-Raven, 1997

Gamut H-70

SONOGRAPHY: DECREASED RENAL CORTICAL ECHOGENICITY

COMMON

1. Acute glomerulonephritis
2. Acute pyelonephritis
3. Renal vein thrombosis
4. Transplant rejection

UNCOMMON

1. Multicentric renal cell carcinoma
2. Lupus nephritis
3. Lymphoma$_g$
4. Xanthogranulomatous pyelonephritis

References

1. Cochlin DL: Chapter 24. Urinary tract. In McGahan JP, Goldberg BB (eds): Diagnostic Ultrasound. Philadelphia: Lippincott-Raven, 1997
2. Williamson MR: Chapter 6. Renal ultrasound. In: Essentials of Ultrasound. Philadelphia: WB Saunders, 1996, p 106

Gamut H-71

SONOGRAPHY: HYPERECHOIC RENAL CORTEX (WITH NORMAL MEDULLA)

COMMON

1. Acute interstitial nephritis
2. Acute pyelonephritis (hemorrhagic)
3. Acute tubular necrosis
4. AIDS nephropathy
5. Diabetic nephropathy
6. Glomerulonephritis (acute or chronic)
7. Nephrosclerosis
8. Renal vein thrombosis
9. Transplant rejection

UNCOMMON

1. Acute cortical necrosis
2. Alport S. (hereditary nephritis)
3. Amyloidosis
4. Beckwith-Wiedemann S.
5. Hypercalcemia (eg, Williams S.)
6. Leukemia
7. Lupus nephritis; scleroderma
8. Myoglobinuria
9. Nephrocalcinosis (cortical)
10. Oxalosis
11. Papillary necrosis (eg, sickle cell disease; phenacetin abuse)
12. Pre-eclampsia

References

1. Anderson G, Fiskes RV, Lauridsen KN: Renal vein thrombosis in the neonatal period. Ugeskrift for Laeger 1993;155: 3301–3302
2. Cochlin DL: Chapter 24. Urinary tract. In McGahan JP, Goldberg BB (eds): Diagnostic Ultrasound. Philadelphia: Lippincott-Raven, 1997, pp 357; 371–378
3. Williamson MR: Chapter 6. Renal ultrasound. In: Essentials of Ultrasound. Philadelphia: WB Saunders, 1996, p 105

Gamut H-72

SONOGRAPHY: HYPERECHOIC RENAL MEDULLA

COMMON
1. Dehydration
2. Medullary sponge kidney
3. Nephrocalcinosis (medullary)
4. Renal pyramidal fibrosis
5. Sepsis

UNCOMMON
1. Aldosteronism (primary)
2. Glycogen storage disease (type 1)
3. Gout
4. Hypokalemia
5. Lesch-Nyhan S.
6. Pseudo-Bartter S.
7. Pyelonephritis
8. Renal candidiasis
9. Renal tubular necrosis
10. Sjögren S.
11. Tamm-Horsfall proteinuria
12. Williams S. (idiopathic hypercalcemia)
13. Wilson's disease

References
1. Shultz PK, et al: Hyperechoic Renal Medullary Pyramids in Infants and Children. Radiology 181:163–167; 1991
2. Williamson MR: Chapter 6. Renal ultrasound. In: Essentials of Ultrasound. Philadelphia: WB Saunders, 1996, p 106

Gamut H-73

SONOGRAPHY: HYPERECHOIC RENAL PARENCHYMA (CORTEX AND MEDULLA)

COMMON
1. Chronic glomerulonephritis
2. Chronic pyelonephritis
3. Chronic renal failure

UNCOMMON
1. Acquired cystic disease (eg, from dialysis)
2. AIDS nephropathy
3. Infarction (healing)
4. Medullary cystic disease
5. Nephronia (focal bacterial pyelonephritis)
6. Nephrotic S.
7. Polycystic renal disease (infantile type—autosomal recessive, or adult type—autosomal dominant)
8. Renal tubular ectasia

References
1. Gray-Woodford LM, et al: Diffuse renal cystic disease in children. Pediatr Nephrol 1998;12:173–182
2. Hricak H, et al: Renal parenchymal disease: sonographic-histologic correlation. Radiology 1982;144:141–147
3. Kraus AK, Gaisie G, Young LW: Increased renal parenchymal echogenesity. RadioGraphics 1990;10:1009–1018
4. Williamson MR: Chapter 6. Renal ultrasound. In: Essentials of Ultrasound. Philadelphia: WB Saunders, 1996, p 105

Gamut H-74

SONOGRAPHY: RENAL COLLECTING SYSTEM ECHOES

COMMON

1. Blood clot
2. Calculus
3. Emphysematous pyelonephritis
4. Nephrostomy tube or stent
5. Pyonephrosis

UNCOMMON

1. Fungus ball (renal candidasis)
2. Sloughed papilla (papillary necrosis)
3. Transitional cell carcinoma

References

1. Thurston W, Wilson SR: Chapter 9. The urinary tract. In: Rumack CM, Wilson SR, Charboneau JW (eds): Diagnostic Ultrasound. St. Louis: Mosby, 1998, pp 329–397
2. Williamson MR: Chapter 6. Renal ultrasound. In: Essentials of Ultrasound. Philadelphia: WB Saunders, 1996, p 112

Gamut H-75

DOPPLER SONOGRAPHY: INCREASED RENAL ARTERY DIASTOLIC FLOW
(Low Resistive Index)

1. Arteriovenous fistula
2. Inflammation (eg, acute pyelonephritis; renal abscess)
3. Renal malignancy (esp. renal cell carcinoma)

Reference

1. Scoutt LM, Burns P, Brown JL, et al: Ultrasound evaluation of the urinary tract. In: Pollack HM, McClennan BL: Clinical Urography. (ed 2) Philadelphia: WB Saunders Co., 2000, pp 459–469

Gamut H-76

DOPPLER SONOGRAPHY: DECREASED RENAL ARTERY DIASTOLIC FLOW
(Increased Resistance Index > 0.70)

1. Compression of kidney from perinephric abscess or hematoma (Page kidney; lymphocele)
2. Edema of kidney (severe pyelonephritis or trauma)
3. Hemolytic-uremic S.
4. Hepatorenal S.
5. Medical renal disease (eg, acute tubular necrosis— flow may be reversed; diabetes mellitus; vasculitis)
6. Obstructive uropathy (eg, ureteral obstruction)
7. Renal transplant rejection
8. Renal vein thrombosis or occlusion (flow may be reversed)

Reference

1. Scoutt LM, Burns P, Brown JL, et al: Ultrasound evaluation of the urinary tract. In: Pollack HM, McClennan BL: Clinical Urography. (ed 2) Philadelphia: WB Saunders Co., 2000, pp 459–469

Gamut H-77

DOPPLER SONOGRAPHY: RENAL TRANSPLANT— INCREASED RENAL ARTERIAL RESISTANCE INDEX (> 0.70)

COMMON

1. Arterial obstruction, severe acute (eg, renal artery stenosis)
2. Cyclosporine nephrotoxicity (acute)
3. Pyelonephritis (acute)
4. Transplant rejection (acute)
5. Tubular necrosis (acute)

UNCOMMON

1. Hydronephrosis (high grade obstruction)
2. Page kidney (eg, renal compression by perirenal collection {urinoma; hematoma; lymphocele; abscess})
3. [Renal compression by transducer]
4. Renal vein thrombosis

References
1. Cochlin DL: Chapter 24. Urinary tract. In McGahan JP, Goldberg BB (eds): Diagnostic Ultrasound. Philadelphia: Lippincott-Raven, 1997
2. Dunnick NR, et al: Textbook of Uroradiology. Baltimore: Williams & Wilkins, 1997, p 234
3. Thurston W, Wilson SR: Chapter 9. The urinary tract. In: Rumack CM, Wilson SR, Charboneau JW (eds): Diagnostic Ultrasound. St. Louis: Mosby, 1998, pp 382–384

Gamut H-78

SONOGRAPHY: ENLARGEMENT OF RENAL TRANSPLANT

1. Hypertrophy of transplanted kidney
2. Rejection of transplanted kidney (acute)
3. Renal infection
4. Renal vein thrombosis
5. Ureteral obstruction

Reference
1. Cochlin DL: Chapter 24. Urinary tract. In McGahan JP, Goldberg BB (eds): Diagnostic Ultrasound. Philadelphia: Lippincott-Raven, 1997

Gamut H-79

SONOGRAPHY: DIMINISHED SIZE OF RENAL TRANSPLANT

1. Chronic rejection
2. Renal ischemia

Reference
1. Cochlin DL: Chapter 24. Urinary tract. In McGahan JP, Goldberg BB (eds): Diagnostic Ultrasound. Philadelphia: Lippincott-Raven, 1997

Gamut H-80

DIMINISHED FUNCTION OF TRANSPLANTED KIDNEY

COMMON

1. Chronic rejection
2. Cyclosporine toxicity

UNCOMMON

1. Acute or hyperacute rejection
2. Renal arterial insufficiency
3. Renal vein thrombosis
4. Ureteral obstruction

Reference
1. Dunnick NR, et al: Textbook of Uroradiology. Baltimore: Williams & Wilkins, 1997, pp 236–253

Gamut H-81-S

COMPLICATIONS OF RENAL TRANSPLANTATION

CARDIOPULMONARY

1. Mediastinal widening due to steroid-induced fat deposition
2. Metastatic pulmonary calcinosis
3. Opportunistic infection
4. Pleural effusion
5. Pulmonary edema or hemorrhage

GASTROINTESTINAL

1. Appendicitis
2. Cholecystitis
3. Esophagitis
4. Fecal impaction
5. Hemorrhage
6. Hepatitis
7. Ileus (nonobstructive)
8. Infarction
9. Inflammation (diffuse)
10. Pancreatitis
11. Perforation
12. Peritonitis
13. Pneumatosis intestinalis
14. Ulceration

BONE AND SOFT TISSUE

1. Hyperparathyroidism, secondary
2. Osteomalacia
3. Osteomyelitis
4. Osteonecrosis
5. Osteoporosis
6. Periostitis
7. Slipped epiphysis
8. Soft tissue calcifications
9. Tendon rupture
10. Vascular calcification

UROLOGIC

1. Acute tubular necrosis
2. Bladder neck contraction
3. Calculus formation
4. Extraurinary fluid collections
   a. Abscess
   b. Hematoma
   c. Lymphocele (most common)
   d. Urinoma
5. Fistula
6. Malignant neoplasm
7. Obstruction
8. Papillary necrosis
9. Rejection
10. Vascular (arterial or venous obstruction; hemorrhage; arteriovenous fistula)
11. Vesicoureteral reflux

Reference
1. Colley DP: Complications of renal transplants. Semin Roentgenol 1978;13:299–300

Gamut H-82

MEDIAL DEVIATION OF THE UPPER URETER

COMMON

1. Horseshoe kidney; crossed renal ectopia
2. Normal (eg, prominent psoas muscle)
3. Postoperative (eg, renal or ureteral surgery)

UNCOMMON

1. Hydronephrosis
2. Lymph node enlargement (eg, lymphoma$_g$; metastasis)
3. Neoplasm, extrinsic, benign or malignant (eg, renal; adrenal; colonic; retroperitoneal)
4. Ptosis of kidney; displacement (eg, large liver or spleen)

5. Renal cyst (eg, parapelvic or lower pole)
6. Retrocaval ureter
7. Retroperitoneal fibrosis, lipomatosis, or hemorrhage
8. Tortuous aorta
9. Urinoma; lymphocele

References
1. Dunnick NR, et al: Textbook of Uroradiology. Baltimore: Williams & Wilkins, 1997, pp 371–372
2. Flatman JG: Displacement of the kidneys and ureters by retroperitoneal fat. J Can Assoc Radiol 1978;29:195–196
3. Ziter FMH Jr: Unilateral ureteral deviation due to unilateral iliopsoas muscle hypertrophy. J Can Assoc Radiol 1974; 25:327–328

2. Effusion (extraperitoneal)
3. Hydronephrosis
4. Retroperitoneal fibrosis or lipomatosis
5. Venous anomaly (eg, ovarian vein S.)

References
1. Dunnick NR, et al: Textbook of Uroradiology. Baltimore: Williams & Wilkins, 1997, pp 371–372
2. Flatman JG: Displacement of the kidneys and ureters by retroperitoneal fat. J Can Assoc Radiol 1978;29:195–196
3. Ziter FMH Jr: Unilateral ureteral deviation due to unilateral iliopsoas muscle hypertrophy. J Can Assoc Radiol 1974; 25:327–328

Gamut H-83

LATERAL DEVIATION OF THE UPPER URETER

COMMON

1. Aneurysm$_g$ (esp. aortic) (See H-127)
2. Fat deposition (retroperitoneal)
3. Hemorrhage or hematoma in retroperitoneum (traumatic or bleeding disorder$_g$)
4. Horseshoe kidney; crossed renal ectopia
5. Lymph node enlargement, para-aortic (eg, lymphoma$_g$; sarcoidosis; metastasis)
6. Neoplasm, extrinsic, benign or malignant (eg, renal; adrenal; colonic; retroperitoneal)
7. Normal (eg, prominent psoas muscle)
8. Postoperative (eg, ureteroileal diversion; renal transplant)
9. Psoas abscess
10. Ptosis or displacement of kidney (eg, enlarged liver or spleen)
11. Spinal lesion (eg, tuberculosis; metastasis)
12. Urinoma; lymphocele

UNCOMMON

1. Duplication of kidney with dilated ectopic ureterocele

Gamut H-84

DISPLACEMENT OF THE PELVIC URETER

COMMON

1. Abscess, pelvic (eg, appendiceal; retroperitoneal; tuboovarian; pericolic)
2. Bone lesion of spine, sacrum, or pelvis
3. Diverticulitis of colon
4. Diverticulum of bladder (esp. Hutch type)
5. Hematoma, traumatic or other
6. Lymph node enlargement (eg, lymphoma$_g$; metastasis)
7. Neoplasm, extrinsic or malignant (eg, carcinoma of uterus, adnexa, bladder, rectum, prostate; retroperitoneal sarcoma or lymphoma$_g$)
8. Postoperative (eg, abdominoperineal resection; renal transplantation; ureteral reimplantation)

UNCOMMON

1. Aneurysm$_g$, iliac artery or other (See H-127)
2. Ectopic kidney
3. Endometriosis
4. Hernia (eg, obturator; sciatic; inguinal; femoral)
5. Pelvic lipomatosis
6. Radiation fibrosis

(continued)

7. Retroperitoneal fibrosis
8. Venous anomaly (eg, ovarian vein S.)

References
1. Dunnick NR, et al: Textbook of Uroradiology. Baltimore: Williams & Wilkins, 1997, pp 371–372
2. Goldin RR, Rosen RA: Effects of inguinal hernia upon the bladder and ureters. Radiology 1975;115:55–58
3. Lebowitz RL: Ureteral sciatic hernia. Pediatr Radiol 1973; 1:178–182

Gamut H-85

URETERAL AND RENAL PELVIC CALCIFICATION

COMMON
1. Calculus (See H-24)

UNCOMMON
*1. Amyloidosis
*2. [Argyrosis (etched ureter)]
*3. Brucellosis
 4. [Foreign body]
 5. Milk of calcium ureter
*6. Neoplasm, benign (eg, hemangioma; papilloma; lipoma)
*7. Neoplasm, malignant (eg, primary transitional cell carcinoma; metastatic or invasive from ovarian cystadenocarcinoma or colloid colon carcinoma)
 8. Papillary necrosis (sloughed calcified renal papilla)
*9. Postoperative (eg, osteocartilaginous metaplasia after ureterotomy)
*10. Radiation effect
*11. Schistosomiasis haematobium
*12. Tuberculosis

* Mural calcification. Others are intraluminal.
[ ] This condition does not actually cause the gamuted imaging finding, but can produce imaging changes that simulate it.

References
1. Dunnick NR, et al: Textbook of Uroradiology. Baltimore: Williams & Wilkins, 1997, pp 382–384

2. Gross BH: Gamut: Bladder and ureteral calcifications. Semin Roentgenol 1979;14:261–262
3. Moul JW, McLeod DG: Bilateral organ-limited amyloidosis of the distal ureter associated with osseous metaplasia radiographic calcification. J Urology 1988;139:807–809
4. Thomas SD, Sanders PW III, Pollack HM: Primary amyloidosis of urinary bladder and ureter: cause of mural calcification. Urology 1977;9:586–589

Gamut H-86

URETERAL INTRALUMINAL FILLING DEFECT(S) (See also H-87)

COMMON
1. Air bubble from catheter
2. Blood clot; hemorrhage; inspissated pus; necrotic debris
3. Calculus
4. [Malacoplakia]
5. Neoplasm (eg, papilloma; polyp; transitional cell carcinoma, primary or seeding from kidney)
6. [Technical (incomplete filling with contrast medium; artifact)]

UNCOMMON
1. Eosinophilic ureteritis
2. Fungus ball
3. Leukoplakia (squamous metaplasia; cholesteatoma)
4. Sloughed papilla from papillary necrosis
5. Ureteritis cystica

[ ] This condition does not actually cause the gamuted imaging finding, but can produce imaging changes that simulate it.

References
1. Banner MP, Pollack HM: Fibrous ureteral polyps. Radiology 1979;130:73–76
2. Dunnick NR, et. al: Textbook of Uroradiology. Baltimore: Williams & Wilkins, 1997, pp 375–385
3. Witten DM, Myers GH Jr, Utz DC: Emmett's Clinical Urography. (ed 4) Philadelphia: WB Saunders, 1977

Gamut H-87

URETERAL MURAL FILLING DEFECT(S) (See also H-86)

COMMON

1. Neoplasm, benign (eg, papilloma; polyp; spindle cell tumor$_g$; lipoma; hamartoma; hemangioma)
2. Neoplasm, malignant (esp. transitional cell carcinoma, primary or seeding from kidney)
3. [Peristaltic wave; transverse folds (kinks)]
4. Ureteritis cystica

UNCOMMON

1. Endometriosis
2. Eosinophilic ureteritis
3. Granuloma or stricture (eg, tuberculosis; schistosomiasis haematobium)
4. Hematoma
5. [Leukoplakia (squamous metaplasia; cholesteatoma)]
6. Malakoplakia
7. Metastasis (eg, ureteral; lymph node)
8. [Neoplasm, extrinsic, compression or invasion (eg, retroperitoneal lymphoma$_g$ or sarcoma; carcinoma of cervix; ovarian cyst; uterine fibroid)]
9. Postoperative
10. Renal vein thrombosis; varicosities
11. Striations (from reflux or relieved obstruction)

Reference

1. Dunnick NR, et. al: Textbook of Uroradiology. Baltimore: Williams & Wilkins, 1997, pp 375–388

Gamut H-88

URETERAL TUMORS

COMMON

1. Direct invasion by extrinsic malignancy (eg, carcinoma of colon, cervix, bladder, or prostate)
2. Transitional cell carcinoma

UNCOMMON

1. Carcinoma, other (adenocarcinoma; squamous cell carcinoma)
2. Fibroepithelial polyp
3. Lymphoma$_g$
4. Mesenchymal tumors
5. Metastasis
6. Papilloma; inverted papilloma

Reference

1. Dunnick NR, et. al: Textbook of Uroradiology. Baltimore: Williams & Wilkins, 1997, p 377

Gamut H-89

MULTIPLE URETERAL FILLING DEFECTS

COMMON

1. Air bubbles
2. Blood clots
3. Multiple calculi
4. [Ureteral peristalsis; kinks]
5. Vascular indentations (eg, arterial or venous collaterals; varicosities) (See H-90)

UNCOMMON

1. Endometriosis
2. Eosinophilic ureteritis
3. Granulomas or strictures (eg, tuberculosis; schistosomiasis haematobium)

(continued)

4. Hemorrhage, submucosal (esp. anticoagulant therapy)
5. Leukoplakia (squamous metaplasia; cholesteatoma)
6. Malacoplakia
7. Neoplasms, multiple (eg, papillomatosis; polyps; seeding from transitional cell carcinoma of kidney)
8. Striations (from reflux or relieved obstruction)
9. Ureteritis cystica

References
1. Campbell JE, Aldis HW: Lymphangitic ureteral metastases from prostatic carcinoma. J Can Assoc Radiol 1980;31: 158–162
2. Chait A, Matasar KW, Fabian CE, et al: Vascular impressions on the ureters. AJR 1971;111:729–749
3. Hughes FA III, Davis CS Jr: Multiple benign ureteral fibrous polyps. AJR 1976;126:723–727
4. Padovani J , Grangier ML, Faure F, et al: Idiopathic ureteral varicose veins in children: Review of four cases. Ann Radiol 1984;27:482–486
5. Parker M: Diagnostic skills. In: Friedland GW, Filly R, Goris ML, et al: Uroradiology: An Integrated Approach. New York: Churchill Livingstone, 1983, p 1690
6. Smith WL, Weinstein AS, Wiot JF: Defects of the renal collecting systems in patients receiving anticoagulants. Radiology 1974;113:649–651

Gamut H-90

VASCULAR INDENTATIONS ON THE URETER OR RENAL PELVIS (NOTCHING)

COMMON
1. Collateral arterial circulation (eg, aortic, renal artery, or iliac artery stenosis or occlusion)
2. Collateral venous circulation (eg, obstruction of inferior or superior vena cava, renal, gonadal, azygos, splenic, or portal vein)
3. Normal accessory renal artery
4. Normal iliac artery

UNCOMMON
1. Aneurysm of aorta or iliac artery$_g$ (See H-127)
2. Arteriovenous communication of renal or juxtarenal vessels
3. Azygos continuation of inferior vena cava
4. Cirsoid aneurysm of renal artery
5. Lymphangiectasis; lymphangioma
6. Normal gonadal vein
7. Varices of ureter, gonad, or broad ligament (idiopathic or from portal hypertension)

References
1. Beckmann CF, Abrams HL: Idiopathic renal vein varices: Incidence and significance. Radiology 1982;143:649–652
2. Chait A, Matasar KW, Fabian CE, et al: Vascular impressions on the ureters. AJR 1971;111:729–749
3. Cleveland RH, Fellows KE, Lebowitz RL: Notching of the ureter and renal pelvis in children. AJR 1977;129:837–844

Gamut H-91

DILATATION OF URETER (SEGMENTAL OR DIFFUSE URETERECTASIS)

COMMON
*1. Congenital or idiopathic (fusiform terminal ureterectasis; primary megaureter)
2. Infection
*3. Mid-ureteral "spindle" proximal to iliac artery crossing
4. Neurogenic bladder (See H-98)
*5. Obstruction of ureter, intrinsic or extrinsic, esp. at ureterovesical junction (eg, stone, stricture or stenosis, neoplasm, clot, sloughed papilla, postoperative, radiation, pelvic lipomatosis, endometriosis, bladder prolapse) (See H-93)
6. Obstruction of urethra (eg, valve; stricture; diverticulum) or bladder outlet (eg, prostatic enlargement)
7. Ureteral duplication with obstruction
*8. Ureterocele
9. Vesicoureteral reflux (See H-92)

UNCOMMON

1. Aganglionosis; Chagas' disease
2. Bartter S.
3. Fluid overload (eg, polydypsia; diabetes insipidus; beer-drinker's kidneys)
4. Prune-belly S. (Eagle-Barrett S.)

* Segmental ureterectasis (focal ureteral dilatation).

References

1. Dunnick NR, et. al: Textbook of Uroradiology. Baltimore: Williams & Wilkins, 1997, pp 369–370
2. Francis DA, Martinez LO: Primary megaloureter. Rev Interamer Radiol 1983;8:9–14
3. Garel L, Frija J, Lortat-Jacob S: Segmental dilatation of the ureter. Ann Radiol 1980;23:124–126
4. Pollack HM (ed): Clinical Urography. Philadelphia: WB Saunders, 1990, pp 1651–1692
5. Swischuk LE, John SD: Differential Diagnosis in Pediatric Radiology. (ed 2) Baltimore: Williams & Wilkins, 1995
6. Witten DM, Myers GH Jr, Utz DC: Emmett's Clinical Urography. (ed 4) Philadelphia: WB Saunders, 1977

Gamut H-92

VESICOURETERAL REFLUX

COMMON

1. Idiopathic
2. Infection (severe cystisis—eg, tuberculosis; schistosomiasis haematobium; chemotherapy-induced; interstitial))
3. Neurogenic bladder (See H-98)
4. Postoperative (prior ureterovesical surgery)

UNCOMMON

1. Anomaly of ureterovesical junction
2. Diverticulum of bladder
3. Duplication of ureters
4. Ectopic ureter emptying into bladder neck or urethra
5. Exstrophy of bladder
6. Iatrogenic; irritative contrast medium
7. Megacolon

8. Megaureter-megacystis S.
9. Nonfuncioning or absent kidney
10. Pelvic mass
11. Postradiation
12. Prune-belly S. (Eagle-Barrett S.)
13. Urethral obstruction (eg, valve or stenosis)

References

1. Burgener FA, Kormano M: Differential Diagnosis in Conventional Radiology. (ed 2) New York: Thieme Medical Publ, 1991, pp 800–801
2. Spartaro RF: Inflammatory conditions of the renal pelvis and ureter. In: Pollack HM (ed): Clinical Urography. Philadelphia: WB Saunders, 1990, pp 884–903

Gamut H-93

OBSTRUCTION OF THE URETER (WITH OR WITHOUT HYDRONEPHROSIS)

COMMON

1. Blood clot; inspissated pus
2. Calculus
3. Congenital ureteropelvic junction obstruction (eg, band; valve; vessel)
4. Cystitis or carcinoma of bladder (obstruction of intramural ureter)
5. Inflammation, edema (eg, pelvic inflammatory disease)
6. Metastasis to ureter or retroperitoneal lymph nodes
7. Neoplasm, extrinsic, compression or invasion (eg, retroperitoneal lymphoma$_g$ or sarcoma; carcinoma of cervix; ovarian cyst; uterine fibroid)
8. Postoperative (eg, ligature; edema)
9. Pregnancy
10. Stricture (eg, congenital; traumatic; postoperative; postradiation; inflammatory—tuberculosis; schistosomiasis)
11. Ureterocele
12. Vascular compression (eg, normal or abnormal vessel; aneurysm$_g$)

(continued)

UNCOMMON

1. Bladder diverticulum (Hutch type)
2. Carcinoma of ureter (esp. transitional cell)
3. Endometriosis
4. Megacolon
5. Neoplasm of ureter, benign (eg, polyp; papilloma; spindle cell tumor$_g$)
6. Papillary necrosis with sloughed papilla
7. Pelvic lipomatosis
8. Radiation fibrosis
9. Retrocaval ureter
10. Retroperitoneal fibrosis (periureteric)

14. Retroperitoneal fibrosis
15. Retroperitoneal hematoma
16. Ureteritis cystica
17. Xanthogranulomatous stricture

[ ] This condition does not actually cause the gamuted imaging finding, but can produce imaging changes that simulate it.

References

1. Kruglik GD, et al: Urologic complications of regional enteritis. Gastrointest Radiol, 1977;1:375–378
2. Ney C, Friedenberg R: Radiographic Atlas of the Genitourinary System. Philadelphia: JP Lippincott, 1966, pp 384, 402–450
3. Spark RP, et al: Is eosinophilic ureteritis an entity? J Urology 1991;145:1256–1260

Gamut H-94

URETERAL STRICTURE

COMMON

1. Neoplasm (primary, esp. transitional cell carcinoma; invasive or metastatic)
2. [Pseudostricture (vascular indentation; crossing vessels {eg, ovarian vein}; peristaltic wave)]
3. Schistosomiasis haematobium
4. Tuberculosis

UNCOMMON

1. Amyloidosis
2. Congenital
3. Endometriosis
4. Eosinophilic ureteritis
5. Inflammatory bowel disease (eg, Crohn's disease; amebiasis)
6. Leukoplakia
7. Lymphoma$_g$
8. Pelvic inflammatory disease
9. Polyarteritis nodosa
10. Postoperative
11. Postradiation therapy
12. Posttraumatic
13. Pseudodiverticulosis

Gamut H-95

URETERAL EXTRAVASATION OR FISTULA (See H-56)

COMMON

1. Instrumentation (eg, retrograde pyelography)
2. Postoperative (eg, ureteral injury)
3. Trauma

UNCOMMON

1. Actinomycosis
2. Calculus in ureter
3. Crohn's disease
4. Diverticulitis (colonic)
5. Endometriosis
6. Neoplasm, malignant (eg, transitional cell carcinoma of ureter; carcinoma of cervix or intestinal tract)
7. Tuberculosis

Reference

1. Lang EK, Fritzsche P: Fistulas of the genitourinary tract. In: Pollack HM (ed) Clinical Urography. Philadelphia: WB Saunders, 1990, pp 2579–2593

Gamut H-96

DISTENDED BLADDER

COMMON

1. Calculus in bladder neck
2. Fluid overload (eg, polydypsia; diabetes mellitus or insipidus)
3. Infrequent voiding
4. Malignant neoplasm with bladder outlet obstruction (carcinoma of bladder neck, urethra, or prostate; metastasis)
5. Neurogenic bladder (eg, cerebral palsy; multiple sclerosis; paralysis) (See H-98)
6. Postoperative
7. Prostatic hypertrophy
8. Urethral obstruction (See H-111–115)

UNCOMMON

1. Bartter S.
2. Drug therapy (eg, ephedrine; levodopa; diuretic)
3. Foreign body obstruction
4. Hydrometrocolpos
5. Idiopathic
6. Intraluminal mass (eg, large clots; calculi; fungus ball)
7. Megacystis-microcolon-intestinal hypoperistalsis S. (Berdon S.)
8. Prune-belly S. (Eagle-Barrett S.)
9. Psychogenic
10. Ureterocele (ectopic)

References
1. Lalli AF, Thornbury JR, Lapides J: Large capacity smooth-walled bladders as an indication of the infrequent voiding syndrome. J Urol 1971;105:662–663
2. Rubin A: Colonic obstruction: A pelvic mass in a 46-year-old man. JAMA 1983;249:1195–1196
3. Swischuk LE, John SD: Differential Diagnosis in Pediatric Radiology. (ed 2) Baltimore: Williams & Wilkins, 1995

Gamut H-97

SMALL OR CONTRACTED BLADDER

COMMON

1. Carcinoma of bladder, infiltrating
2. Cystitis, severe (eg, aseptic, eosinophilic, interstitial, or hemorrhagic cystitis)
3. Drug reaction (eg, cyclophosphamide {Cytoxan} cystitis)
4. Hypertrophy from bladder outlet obstruction (eg, chronic urethral obstruction by stricture or prostatic hypertrophy)
5. Neurogenic bladder (See H-98)
6. Pelvic hematoma or hemorrhage
7. Pelvic inflammatory disease
8. Pelvic lipomatosis
9. Postoperative (eg, ileal conduit, bladder diversion; partial resection)
10. Radiation therapy
11. Recent voiding
12. Retroperitoneal fibrosis
13. Total incontinence (eg, postprostatectomy)

UNCOMMON

1. Bladder hernia (eg, inguinal; femoral)
2. [Congenital small bladder]
3. Cystitis glandularis
4. Lymphoma$_g$
5. Schistosomiasis haematobium
6. Tuberculosis

[ ] This condition does not actually cause the gamuted imaging finding, but can produce imaging changes that simulate it.

References
1. Burgener FA, Kormano M: Differential Diagnosis in Conventional Radiology. (ed 2) New York: Thieme Medical Publ, 1991, pp 815–817
2. Dunnick NR, et al: Textbook of Uroradiology. Baltimore: Williams & Wilkins, 1997, pp 396–439
3. Swischuk LE, John SD: Differential Diagnosis in Pediatric Radiology. (ed 2) Baltimore: Williams & Wilkins, 1995

Gamut H-98

NEUROGENIC BLADDER

COMMON

1. Cerebral palsy
2. Detrusor areflexia
   a. Cord neoplasm
   b. Disk disease
   c. Neuropathy
   d. Sacral anomaly; caudal regression S. (eg, sacral agenesis or hypoplasia; scoliosis; hemisacrum)
   e. Tethered cord
3. Detrusor hyperreflexia/detrusor-external sphincter dyssynergia
   a. Cord arteriovenous malformation
   b. Cord neoplasm
   c. Cord trauma
   d. Disk disease
   e. Multiple sclerosis
   f. Myelodysplasia
4. Idiopathic uninhibited bladder
5. Neoplasm of spine, spinal cord, or brain
6. Paralytic disorder$_g$
7. Parkinson's disease
8. Spina bifida vera with meningomyelocele
9. Stroke

UNCOMMON

1. Arachnoiditis
2. Block vertebrae
3. Diabetes mellitus
4. Diastematomyelia
5. Neurofibromatosis
6. Neurosyphilis
7. Normal pressure hydrocephalus
8. Syringomyelia
9. Transverse myelitis
10. Tuberculosis of spine (Pott's disease) or meninges

References

1. Dunnick NR, et al: Textbook of Uroradiology. Baltimore: Williams & Wilkins, 1997, p 432

2. Grossman H, Winchester PH, Colston WC: Neurogenic bladder in childhood. Radiol Clin North Am 1968;6: 155–163

Gamut H-99

EXTRINSIC PRESSURE DEFORMITY OF THE BLADDER
(Incl. Teardrop or Pear-Shaped Bladder)

COMMON

*1. Abscess (eg, tubo-ovarian; appendiceal; pericolic)
2. Bone lesion of sacrum or pelvis (eg, osteophyte of pubic symphysis; bone sarcoma)
3. Colon distention
4. [Diverticulum of bladder or female urethra]
*5. Hematoma; hemorrhage (traumatic; bleeding disorder$_g$)
*6. Lymph node enlargement (eg, metastasis; lymphoma$_g$)
7. [Neoplasm of bladder, intrinsic]
*8. Pelvic lipomatosis
9. Pelvic mass (eg, carcinoma of cervix, uterus, or ovary; uterine fibroid; gastrointestinal neoplasm; mesenchymal neoplasm)
10. Pregnancy
11. Prostatic enlargement (hypertrophy; carcinoma)

UNCOMMON

1. Aneurysm$_g$ of iliac artery (See H-127)
2. Anterior myelomeningocele
3. [Carcinoma in a bladder diverticulum]
4. Cyst (eg, ovarian; hydatid; Müllerian duct cyst; seminal vesicle cyst)
*5. Inferior vena cava obstruction (eg, thromboembolism) with venous collaterals
6. [Inguinal hernia]
*7. Lymphocele; urinoma; extravasated urine or lymph
*8. Normal or prominent soft tissue structure (eg, levator ani muscle; iliopsoas muscle; sacrospinous ligament)

9. Postoperative (eg, hip replacement)
*10. Retroperitoneal fibrosis
*11. Retroperitoneal sarcoma
12. Rheumatoid synovial cyst of hip joint
13. Urachal remnant
14. Ureterocele (ectopic)
15. Urethral neoplasm
16. Vaginal neoplasm
17. Varices

* May be teardrop or pear-shaped bladder.
[ ] This condition does not actually cause the gamuted imaging finding, but can produce imaging changes that simulate it.

References
1. Ambos MA, Bosniak MA, Lefleur RS: The pear-shaped bladder. Radiology 1977;122:85–88
2. Chang SF: Pear-shaped bladder caused by large iliopsoas muscles. Radiology 1978;128:349–350
3. Dunnick NR, et al: Textbook of Uroradiology. Baltimore: Williams & Wilkins, 1997, pp 410–412
4. Korobkin M, Minagi H, Palubinskas AJ: Lateral displacement of the bladder. AJR 1975;125:337–347
5. Pope TL Jr, Harrison RB, Clark RL, et al: Bladder base impressions in women: "Female prostate." AJR 1981;136:1105–1109

Gamut H-100

FOCAL THICKENING OF THE BLADDER WALL

COMMON

1. Cystitis which may at times be localized (eg, cyclophosphamide {Cytoxan} cystitis; cystitis cystica {glandularis})
2. Indwelling catheter
3. Invasion by adjacent tumor
4. Transitional cell carcinoma
5. Ureterocele
6. Ureterovesicle junction edema (eg, from calculus at UVJ)

UNCOMMON

1. Adjacent abscess

2. Amyloidosis
3. Endometriosis
4. Fistula (eg, colovesical; vaginovesical)
5. Gastrointestinal inflammatory disease (esp. Crohn's disease; diverticulitis)
6. Hematoma
7. Leukoplakia
8. Malacoplakia
9. Neoplasm of bladder, benign (eg, leiomyoma; pheochromocytoma; neurofibroma; hemangioma; nephrogenic adenoma)
10. Pelvic inflammatory disease
11. Postoperative
12. Schistosomiasis haematobium
13. Tuberculosis

References
1. Dunnick NR, et al: Textbook of Uroradiology. Baltimore: Williams & Wilkins, 1997, pp 396–439
2. Williamson MR: Chapter 6. Renal ultrasound. In: Essentials of Ultrasound. Philadelphia: WB Saunders, 1996, p 124

Gamut H-101

GENERALIZED BLADDER WALL THICKENING

COMMON

1. Cystitis (eg, bacterial, eosinophilic, hemorrhagic or acute radiation cystitis; cyclophosphamide {Cytoxan) cystitis; cystitis cystica {glandularis})
2. Muscular hypertrophy and trabeculation (eg, chronic bladder outlet obstruction; neurogenic bladder)

UNCOMMON

*1. Amyloidosis
*2. Carcinoma, extensive (transitional cell; squamous cell; adenocarcinoma)
*3. Endometriosis
*4. Lymphoma
5. Schistosomiasis haematobium

(continued)

6. Radiation therapy (late fibrosis)
7. Tuberculosis

* Infiltrative and proliferative diseases of the bladder.

Reference
1. Dunnick NR, et al: Textbook of Uroradiology. Baltimore: Williams & Wilkins, 1997, pp 396–439

Gamut H-102

CYSTITIS

COMMON
1. Bacterial (gram negative) cystitis

UNCOMMON
1. Cyclophosphamide (Cytoxan) cystitis
2. Cystitis cystica (cystitis glandularis)
3. Emphysematous cystitis
4. Eosinophilic cystitis
5. Interstitial cystitis
6. Malakoplakia
7. Postradiation therapy
8. Schistosomiasis haematobium
9. Tuberculosis

Reference
1. Davidson AJ, Hartman DS: Radiology of the Kidney and Urinary Tract. Chapter 19, The urinary bladder. Philadelphia: WB Saunders, 1994, pp 607–648

Gamut H-103

BLADDER TUMORS

COMMON
1. Direct invasion by carcinoma of colon, cervix, vagina, or prostate
2. Transitional cell carcinoma

UNCOMMON
1. Carcinoma, other (eg, adenocarcinoma; squamous cell carcinoma; carcinosarcoma; urachal)
2. [Cyst (eg, hydatid)]
3. Fibroepithelial polyp
4. [Hematoma]
5. Lymphoma$_g$
6. Metastasis
7. Mesenchymal neoplasm
8. Papilloma
9. Pheochromocytoma
10. Schistosomiasis haematobium (eg, granulomatous polyp, urticarial edema, or complicating carcinoma)

Reference
1. Hahn D: Neoplasms of the urinary bladder. In: Pollack HM (ed): Clinical Urography. Philadelphia: WB Saunders, 1990, pp 1353–1380

Gamut H-104

FILLING DEFECT(S) IN THE BLADDER WALL OR LUMEN

COMMON
1. Air bubbles
2. Blood clot
3. Calculus
4. Carcinoma (esp. transitional cell; also squamous cell; adenocarcinoma; carcinosarcoma)
5. Instrument (eg, Foley or other catheter)
6. Polyp (fibrous or inflammatory); papilloma
7. Prostatic enlargement (hypertrophy of median lobe; carcinoma)
8. Ureterocele, simple or ectopic

UNCOMMON
1. Amyloidosis
2. Brunn's nests
3. Condyloma acuminata

4. Cystitis (eg, bullous; eosinophilic; cystitis cystica {cystitis glandularis})
5. Endometriosis
6. Foreign body
7. Fungus ball (eg, *Candida,* esp. in diabetic)
8. Hematoma (intramural)
9. Hydatid cyst
10. Infection; granuloma; fistula; abscess (eg, Crohn's disease; diverticulitis; tuberculosis; lymphogranuloma venereum)
11. Leukoplakia
12. Malakoplakia
13. Metastasis
14. Mural edema or hemorrhage (eg, impacted ureteral calculus; hemorrhagic cystitis)
15. Nephrogenic adenoma
16. Non-epithelial neoplasm (eg, mesenchymal tumor; pheochromocytoma; neurofibroma; sarcoma; lymphoma$_g$; mixed mesodermal neoplasm)
17. Postoperative (eg, suture granuloma; ureteral anastomosis)
18. Prolapsing urethral polyp
19. Schistosomiasis haematobium (granuloma; inflammatory polyp; urticarial edema)
20. Squamous metaplasia

References

1. Bernstein RG, Siegelman SS, Tein AB, et al: Huge filling defect in the bladder caused by intravesical enlargement of the prostate. Radiology 1969;92:1447–1452
2. Parker M: Diagnostic skills. In: Friedland GW, Filly R, Goris ML, et al: Uroradiology: An Integrated Approach. New York: Churchill Livingstone, 1983, p 1698

CALCIFICATION IN THE BLADDER WALL OR LUMEN (See H-85)

COMMON

1. Calculus (See H-24, 106)

UNCOMMON

1. Alkaptonuria (ochronosis)
2. Amyloidosis
3. [Calculus in urachal cyst or in bladder diverticulum]
4. Carcinoma, esp. transitional cell (encrusted)
5. Cystinuria
6. Cystitis (alkaline encrusted)
7. Drug reaction (esp. cyclophosphamide {Cytoxan} cystitis; Mitomycin C instillation)
8. [Fetal head]
9. Foreign body or blood clot (encrusted)
10. Hematoma
11. Hyperparathyroidism, primary or secondary
12. Neoplasm, benign (eg, hemangioma)
13. Neoplasm, invasive (esp. ovarian cystadenocarcinoma; rectal colloid carcinoma)
14. Neuroblastoma; pheochromocytoma
15. Oxalosis
16. Prune-belly S. (Eagle-Barrett S.)
17. Radiation reaction
18. Renal tubular acidosis
19. Schistosomiasis haematobium
20. Stevens-Johnson S.
21. Tuberculosis
22. Wilson's disease

[ ] This condition does not actually cause the gamuted imaging finding, but can produce imaging changes that simulate it.

References

1. Dunnick NR, et al: Textbook of Uroradiology. Baltimore: Williams & Wilkins, 1997, p 401
2. Ferris EJ, O'Connor SJ: Calcification in urinary bladder tumors. AJR 1965;95:447–449
3. Harrison RB, Stier FM, Cochran EJA: Alkaline encrusting cystitis. AJR 1978;130:575–577

(continued)

4. Irwin GA, Craig R, Novotny P: CT of calcified bladder masses. Comput Radiol 1985;9:181–184
5. Pollack HM, Banner MP, Martinez LO, et al: Review: Diagnostic considerations in urinary bladder wall calcification. AJR 1981;136:791–797

Gamut H-106

CAUSES FOR BLADDER STONES

COMMON
1. Bladder outlet obstruction
2. Chronic catheterization
3. Chronic infection (incl. *Schistosoma haematobium*)
4. Diverticulum of bladder
5. Neurogenic bladder (See H-98)
6. Urea-splitting microorganisms

UNCOMMON
1. Bladder wall sutures
2. Cystinuria
3. Foreign body
4. Hypercalcuria
5. Hyperuricosuria

Reference
1. Dunnick NR, et al: Textbook of Uroradiology. Baltimore: Williams & Wilkins, 1997, pp 420–424

Gamut H-107

GAS IN THE BLADDER WALL OR LUMEN

COMMON
1. Bladder fistula (See H-108)
2. Emphysematous cystitis (gas-forming organism, esp. in a diabetic)
3. Iatrogenic (eg, air cystogram; instrumentation)
4. Postoperative (eg, ureteral transposition; ileal bladder)
5. Trauma

UNCOMMON
1. Abscess (incl. appendiceal, pericolic)
2. Fungus ball in bladder

References
1. Dunnick NR, et al: Textbook of Uroradiology. Baltimore: Williams & Wilkins, 1997, pp 396–439
2. Witten DM, Myers GH Jr, Utz DC: Emmett's Clinical Urography. (ed 4) Philadelphia: WB Saunders, 1977

Gamut H-108

BLADDER FISTULA

COMMON
1. Congenital anal atresia
2. Crohn's disease
3. Diverticulitis of colon
4. Iatrogenic (eg, instrumentation)
5. Neoplasm, malignant (eg, carcinoma of colon, bladder, cervix, ovary, genital system)
6. Pelvic inflammatory disease; endometritis
7. Postoperative
8. Postpartum
9. Radiation therapy
10. Trauma

UNCOMMON
1. Appendiceal perforation
2. Calculus eroding through bladder wall
3. Foreign body
4. Lymphogranuloma venereum
5. Schistosomiasis
6. Tuberculous enterocolitis
7. Ulcerative colitis

References
1. Amendola MA, Agaha FP, Dent TL, et al: Detection of occult colovesical fistula by the Bourne test. AJR 1984;142:715–718
2. Joffe N: Roentgenologic abnormalities of the urinary bladder secondary to Crohn's disease. AJR 1976;127:297–302

3. Lang EK, Fritzsche P: Fistulas of the genitourinary tract. In: Pollack HM (ed): Clinical Urography. Philadelphia: WB Saunders, 1990, pp 2579–2593

BLADDER OUTLET OBSTRUCTION

COMMON

1. Bladder neck obstruction (anatomical versus functional)
2. Bladder sphincter dyssynergia
3. Prostatic enlargement (hypertrophy; carcinoma)
4. Urethral obstruction (eg, neoplasm; stricture; valve)

UNCOMMON

1. Acquired bladder neck stricture (postsurgical; post-traumatic)
2. Hydrocolpos; hydrometrocolpos; hematometro-colpos
3. Leiomyoma of cervix or lower uterine segment
4. Miscellaneous (eg, calculus; Brunn's cyst; epider-molysis bullosa; gelatinous plug; trigonal polyp; prolapsing ectopic ureterocele)
5. Pelvic neoplasm, large (eg, malignant schwannoma; fibrous mesothelioma)
6. Prostatic lesions, other (Wegener's granulomatosis; lymphomatosis; lymphoma$_g$; hemangiopericytoma; rhabdomyosarcoma)
7. Vaginal neoplasm (eg, carcinoma; leiomyoma; fibroma; rhabdomyosarcoma)

Reference

1. Pollack HM (ed): Clinical Urography. Philadelphia: WB Saunders, 1990, p l692

BLADDER DIVERTICULA

PRIMARY (CONGENITAL, IDIOPATHIC)

1. Hutch (in paraureteral region)

SECONDARY

1. Bladder outlet obstruction
   a. Bladder neck stenosis
   b. Neurogenic bladder
   c. Posterior urethral valve
   d. Prostatic enlargement (hypertrophy; carcinoma)
   e. Ureterocele (large)
   f. Urethral stricture
2. Congenital syndromes
   a. Diamond-Blackfan S.
   b. Ehlers-Danlos S.
   c. Menkes S. (kinky-hair S.)
   d. Prune-belly S. (Eagle-Barrett S.)
   e. Williams S. (idiopathic hypercalcemia)
3. Postoperative

References

1. Dähnert W: Radiology Review Manual. (ed 4) Baltimore: Williams & Wilkins, 1999, p 762
2. Dunnick NR, et al: Textbook of Uroradiology. Baltimore: Williams & Wilkins, 1997, p 405

URINARY TRACT OBSTRUCTION BELOW THE BLADDER IN A CHILD

COMMON

1. Foreign body
2. Meatal stenosis
3. [Neurogenic bladder]
4. Trauma
5. Ureterocele (ectopic)
6. Urethral stricture
7. Urethral valve

UNCOMMON

1. Hydrometrocolpos
2. Neoplasm (esp. urethral)
3. Normal folds
4. Prostatic enlargement (fibroelastosis)
5. Prune-belly S. (Eagle-Barrett S.)
6. Urethral calculus
7. Urethral diverticulum
8. Urethral polyp
9. Urethritis
10. Verumontanum hypertrophy

References

1. Currarino G: Narrowing of the male urethra caused by contractions or spasm of the bulbocavernosus muscle: Cystourethrographic observations. AJR 1970;108:641–647
2. Friedland GW, Fair WR, Govan DE, et al: Posterior urethral valves. Clin Radiol 1977;23:367–380
3. Gaisie G, Mandell J, Scatliff JH: Review: Congenital stenosis of the male urethra. AJR 1984;142:1269–1271

STRICTURE OF ANTERIOR URETHRA

COMMON

1. Iatrogenic (eg, post-instrumentation or catheterization)
2. Postoperative
3. Posttraumatic
4. Urethritis (eg, gonococcal; non-gonococcal; chlamydia)
5. [Urinal defect]

UNCOMMON

1. Amyloidosis
2. Balanitis xerotica obliterans
3. Carcinoma (eg, transitional cell; squamous cell)
4. Congenital
5. Reiter S.; Reiter/reactive arthritis
6. *Schistosoma haematobium* infection
7. Tuberculosis
8. Wegener's granulomatosis

[ ] This condition does not actually cause the gamuted imaging finding, but can produce imaging changes that simulate it.

Reference

1. DiSantis DJ: Urethral inflammation. In: Pollack HM (ed): Clinical Urography. Philadelphia: WB Saunders, 1990, pp 925–939, 1692

Gamut H-113

DILATED POSTERIOR URETHRA

COMMON
1. Neurogenic voiding dysfunction (esp. detrusor/external sphincter dyssynergy)
2. Posterior urethral valve
3. Previous prostatectomy
4. Stricture of anterior urethra (See H-112)

UNCOMMON
1. Prune-belly S. (Eagle-Barrett S.)

Reference
1. Dunnick NR, et al: Textbook of Uroradiology. Baltimore: Williams & Wilkins, 1997, pp 34–35, 38–39, 432–433, 484–485

Gamut H-114

URETHRAL TUMORS

BENIGN
1. Adenomatous polyp
2. Condyloma acuminata/penile squamous papilloma
3. Fibroepithelial polyp
4. [Inflammatory polyp]
5. Papillary adenoma
6. Transitional cell papilloma

MALIGNANT
COMMON
1. Squamous cell carcinoma

UNCOMMON
1. Adenocarcinoma
2. Melanoma
3. Metastasis (from carcinoma of bladder or prostate)

4. Sarcoma (eg, rhabdomyosarcoma; fibrosarcoma)
5. Transitional cell carcinoma

[ ] This condition does not actually cause the gamuted imaging finding, but can produce imaging changes that simulate it.

References
1. Dähnert W: Radiology Review Manual. (ed 4) Baltimore: Williams & Wilkins, 1999, pp747–748
2. McCallum R: Urethral neoplasms. In: Pollack HM (ed): Clinical Urography. Philadelphia: WB Saunders, 1990, pp 1404–1414, 1692

Gamut H-115

URETHRAL FILLING DEFECT(S), INTRINSIC OR EXTRINSIC

COMMON
1. Abscess (periurethral)
2. Carcinoma (esp. squamous cell; also transitional cell carcinoma; adenocarcinoma)
3. Foreign body
4. Hematoma (traumatic; iatrogenic)
5. Postoperative (eg, scar; granulation tissue; blood clot; sinus tract)
6. Stricture (gonorrheal, iatrogenic, or other)
7. Valve, anterior or posterior

UNCOMMON
1. Calculus
2. Condyloma acuminata
3. Diverticulum, congenital or acquired
4. Hemangioma; lymphangioma
5. Melanoma, primary or metastatic
6. Metastasis, implantation or invasion by neoplasm of prostate, testis, or urinary tract
7. Müllerian duct cyst
8. Neoplasm, other (spindle cell$_g$; rhabdomyosarcoma)
9. Nephrogenic adenoma
10. Papilloma
11. Polyp (eg, fibroepithelial; adenomatous; inflammatory)

(continued)

12. Ureterocele (ectopic)
13. Urethritis (incl. urethritis cystica)
14. Verumontanum hypertrophy

References

1. Dunnick NR, et al: Textbook of Uroradiology. Baltimore: Williams & Wilkins, 1997, pp 473–480
2. Hanslits ML: Urethral filling defect (solitary or multiple). Semin Roentgenol 1983;18:245
3. Pollack HM, DeBenedictus TJ, Marmar JL, et al: Urethrographic manifestations of venereal warts (condyloma acuminata). Radiology 1978;126:643–646

Gamut H-116

URETHRAL OUTPOUCHING

COMMON

1. Diverticulum
2. False passage (eg, iatrogenic or gonorrheal)
3. Fistula, gonorrheal or other
4. Postoperative (esp. prostatectomy; urethroplasty)

UNCOMMON

1. Ambiguous genitalia
2. Cowper's glands, normal or enlarged
3. Glands of Littré, enlarged
4. Prolapse
5. Utriculus masculinus
6. Valve

Gamut H-117

URETHRAL FISTULA

COMMON

1. Postoperative; post-instrumentation

UNCOMMON

1. Gonorrhea
2. Schistosomiasis haematobium
3. Tuberculosis

Reference

1. Dunnick NR, et al: Textbook of Uroradiology. Baltimore: Williams & Wilkins, 1997, p 471

Gamut H-118

UNILATERAL ADRENAL MASS OR ENLARGEMENT

SMALL (LESS THAN 4 CM)

1. Adenoma
2. Ganglioneuroma
3. Hyperplasia
4. Metastasis (esp. lung, breast)
5. Pheochromocytoma

LARGE (GREATER THAN 4 CM)

1. Carcinoma of adrenal cortex
2. Cyst
3. Hemorrhage; hematoma
4. Infection (eg, abscess; tuberculosis; histoplasmosis)
5. Metastasis (esp. from carcinoma of lung or breast)
6. Myelolipoma
7. Neuroblastoma; ganglioneuroblastoma; ganglioneuroma
8. Pheochromocytoma associated with multiple endocrine neoplasia S., type IIA (MEN IIA) and type IIB (MEN IIB)

References
1. Costello P, Clouse ME, Kane RA, et al: Problems in the diagnosis of adrenal tumors. Radiology 1977;125:335–341
2. Prinz RA, Brooks MH, Churchill R, et al: Incidental asymptomatic adrenal masses detected by computed tomographic scanning. JAMA 1982;248:701–704

Gamut H-119

BILATERAL ADRENAL ENLARGEMENT

COMMON
1. Hemorrhage (spontaneous, esp. in infants; traumatic; bleeding disorder$_g$)
2. Histoplasmosis
3. Hyperplasia
4. Metastases (esp. from carcinoma of lung or breast)
5. Neuroblastomas
6. Tuberculosis

UNCOMMON
1. Addison's disease (See H-125)
2. Adenomas
3. Amyloidosis
4. Carcinomas, multiple primary
5. Infection, other
6. Lymphoma$_g$
7. Pheochromocytomas associated with multiple endocrine neoplasia S., type IIA (MEN IIA) and type IIB (MEN IIB)
8. Wolman's disease (familial xanthomatosis)

References
1. Bosniak MA: Introduction. In: Pollack HM (ed): Clinical Urography. Philadelphia: WB Saunders, 1990, pp 2289–2290
2. Morgan HE, Austin JHM, Follett DA: Bilateral adrenal enlargement in Addison's disease caused by tuberculosis: nephrotomographic demonstration. Radiology 1975;115:357–358

Gamut H-120

CYSTIC ADRENAL LESION

1. Abscess
2. Cystic or necrotic neoplasm (eg, pheochromocytoma)
3. Endothelial cyst
4. Epithelial cyst
5. Hemorrhage
6. Hydatid cyst
7. Lymphatic cyst
8. Pseudocyst

Reference
1. Dunnick NR, et al: Textbook of Uroradiology. Baltimore: Williams & Wilkins, 1997, pp 325–357

Gamut H-121

ADRENAL TUMORS

COMMON
1. Adenomas (functioning and non-functioning)
2. Metastasis (esp. from carcinoma of lung, breast, or kidney)
3. Neuroblastoma
4. Pheochromocytoma

UNCOMMON
1. Adrenocortical carcinoma
2. Fibroma
3. Hemangioma
4. Lipoma
5. Lymphangioma
6. Lymphoma$_g$
7. Myelolipoma
8. Neurogenic tumors, other (eg, neurofibroma; neurilemoma; schwannoma; ganglioneuroma; ganglioneuroblastoma)

(continued)

Reference
1. Bosniak MA: Introduction. In Pollack HM (ed): Clinical Urography. Philadelphia: WB Saunders, 1990, pp 2289–2290

Gamut H-122

ADRENAL PSEUDOTUMORS*

COMMON

1. Fluid-filled bowel
2. Pancreatic tail
3. Pseudomyelolipoma
4. Splenule; accessory spleen
5. Stomach fundus
6. Upper pole renal neoplasms
7. Varices

UNCOMMON

1. Diverticulum of stomach
2. Duplication of stomach
3. Hepatic mass
4. Pancreatic pseudocyst
5. Splenic artery aneurysm

* Entities that can be mistaken for an adrenal lesion.

Reference
1. Dunnick NR, et al: Textbook of Uroradiology. Baltimore: Williams & Wilkins, 1997, pp 354–355

Gamut H-123

ADRENAL CALCIFICATION

COMMON

1. Hemorrhage (neonatal or other) (See H-124)
2. Histoplasmosis
3. Idiopathic
4. Neuroblastoma
5. Tuberculosis

UNCOMMON

1. Addison's disease (See H-125)
2. Amyloidosis
3. Beckwith-Wiedeman S.
4. Cushing S.
5. Cyst
6. Metastasis (mucinous primary or post hemorrhagic)
7. Neoplasm of adrenal, other (eg, adenoma; adreno-cortical carcinoma; dermoid; aldosteronoma; hemangioma; ganglioneuroma; myelolipoma)
8. Pheochromocytoma
9. Waterhouse-Friderichsen S.
10. Wolman's disease (familial xanthomatosis)

References
1. Cohen KL, Harris S, Keohane M: Upper abdominal calcification in a young man. JAMA 1978;240:1639–1640
2. Kenney PJ, Stanley RJ: Calcified adrenal masses. Urologic Radiol 1987;9:9–15
3. Moss A: Milk of calcium of the adrenal gland. Br J Radiol 1976;49:186–187
4. Queloz JM, Capitanio MA, Kirkpatrick JA: Wolman's disease. Radiology 1972;104:357–359
5. Taybi H, Lachman RS: Radiology of Syndromes, Metabolic Disorders, and Skeletal Dysplasias. (ed 4) St. Louis: Mosby-Year Book, Inc., 1996

Gamut H-124

ADRENAL HEMORRHAGE

COMMON

1. Post-biopsy

UNCOMMON

1. Bleeding disorder (eg, hemophilia)
2. Coagulopathy
3. Neonatal
4. Neoplasm
5. Primary antiphospholipid S.
6. Sepsis (Waterhouse-Friderichsen S.)

7. Shock
8. Trauma

Reference

1. Dunnick NR, et al: Textbook of Uroradiology. Baltimore: Williams & Wilkins, 1997, pp 347–348

Gamut H-125

ADRENAL INSUFFICIENCY (ADDISON'S DISEASE)

COMMON

1. Histoplasmosis
2. Idiopathic
3. Metastases (esp. from carcinoma of lung or breast)
4. Post-adrenalectomy
5. Post-withdrawal of exogenous steroids
6. Tuberculosis

UNCOMMON

1. Amyloidosis
2. Hemochromatosis
3. Hemorrhage (spontaneous; traumatic; bleeding diathesis$_g$)
4. Infarction
5. Lymphoma$_g$
6. Neoplasm, primary (adenoma; carcinoma; neuroblastoma)
7. Postoperative
8. Wolman's disease (familial xanthomatosis)

Reference

1. Dunnick NR, et al: Textbook of Uroradiology. Baltimore: Williams & Wilkins, 1997, p 328

Gamut H-126-S1

CUSHING SYNDROME

COMMON

1. Exogenous steroids
2. Hyperplasia from pituitary or ectopic ACTH

UNCOMMON

1. Adrenal adenoma
2. Adrenocortical carcinoma

Reference

1. Dunnick NR, et al: Textbook of Uroradiology. Baltimore: Williams & Wilkins, 1997, p 326

Gamut H-126-S2

PHEOCHROMOCYTOMA SYNDROMES

1. Carney's triad
2. Multiple endocrine neoplasia S. (IIA and IIB)
3. Neurofibromatosis
4. von Hippel-Lindau S.

Reference

1. Dunnick NR, et al: Textbook of Uroradiology. Baltimore: Williams & Wilkins, 1997, p 335

Gamut H-127

ANEURYSM OF THE ABDOMINAL AORTA OR ITS BRANCHES (See H-60)

COMMON
1. Atherosclerosis
2. Dissecting aneurysm
3. Drug abuse (necrotizing angiitis)

UNCOMMON
1. Angiomyolipoma
2. Arteritis (eg, polyarteritis nodosa; other collagen disease$_g$; syphilis; Takayasu S.)
3. Fibromuscular dysplasia
4. Mycotic aneurysm (sepsis, usually *Salmonella* or *Streptococcus;* bacterial endocarditis; tuberculosis)
5. Neurofibromatosis
6. Pseudoxanthoma elasticum
7. Osler-Weber-Rendu S.; arteriovenous malformation
8. Trauma (false aneurysm)

Gamut H-128

RETROPERITONEAL FIBROSIS

COMMON
1. Drug reaction (eg, methysergide; ergotamine; hydralazine)
2. Idiopathic

UNCOMMON
1. Amyloidosis
2. Appendicitis, perforated
3. Carcinoid tumor
4. Collagen disease$_g$
5. Crohn's disease (fistula)
6. Diverticulitis of colon
7. Extravasated contrast medium (esp. Thorotrast)
8. Fungus disease$_g$ (esp. histoplasmosis)

9. Hemorrhage, traumatic or bleeding disorder$_g$
10. Lymphogranuloma venereum
11. Lymphoma$_g$ (esp. nodular sclerosing Hodgkin's disease)
12. Mediastinitis (extension)
13. Mesenteritis, retractile; Weber-Christian S.
14. Pancreatitis
15. [Pelvic lipomatosis]
16. Postoperative
17. [Psoas muscle hypertrophy]
18. Radiation fibrosis
19. Retroperitoneal extension of scirrhous or desmoplastic carcinoma of stomach, colon, or prostate
20. Riedel struma
21. Sclerosing agent (for hemorrhoids)
22. Tuberculosis
23. Urinary extravasation (eg, trauma)

[ ] This condition does not actually cause the gamuted imaging finding, but can produce changes that simulate it.

References
1. Arger PH, Stolz JL, Miller WT: Retroperitoneal fibrosis: an analysis of the clinical spectrum and roentgenographic signs. AJR 1973;119:812–821
2. Krane RJ, Cho SI, Olsson CA: Renal-transplant ureteral obstruction simulating retroperitoneal fibrosis. JAMA 1973; 225:607–609
3. Larrieu AJ, Weiner I, Abston S, et al: Retroperitoneal fibrosis. Surg Gynecol Obstet 1980;150:699–702
4. Lepor H, Walsh PC: Review article. Idiopathic retroperitoneal fibrosis. J Urol 1979;122:1–6
5. Williams RG, Nelson JA: Retractile mesenteritis: Initial presentation as colonic obstruction. Radiology 1978;126: 35–37

Gamut H-129

RETROPERITONEAL LYMPHADENOPATHY

COMMON
1. Lymphoma$_g$; leukemia
2. Metastatic disease (from carcinoma of breast, lung, colon, pancreas, kidney, bladder, cervix, or testis)

UNCOMMON

1. AIDS
2. Chronic granulomatous disease (eg, tuberculosis; *Mycobacterium avium-intracellulare* infection; sarcoidosis; histoplasmosis)
3. Inflammatory bowel disease (eg, Crohn's disease)
4. Lymphangioleiomyomatosis
5. Mesenteritis
6. Whipple's disease

References

1. Apter S, et. al: CT of the urinary tract after abdominal-perineal resection for rectal carcinoma. Urol Rad 1992;14: 177–182
2. Balthazar EJ, et al: CT of small-bowel lymphoma in immunocompetent patients and patients with AIDS. AJR 1997;168:675–680
3. Chou CK, et al: MRI manifestations of gastrointestinal lymphoma. Abdom Imaging 1994;19:495–500
4. Ellis JH, et al: Transitional cell carcinoma of the bladder. AJR 1991;157:999–1002
5. Gilks CD, Clemet PB: Papillary serous adenocarcinoma of the uterine cervix. Modern Path 1992;5:426–431
6. Hung CC, et al: Intestinal obstruction and peritonitis resulting from gastrointestinal histoplasmosis in an AIDS patient. J Formosa Med Assoc 1998;97:577–580
7. Liel Y, et al: Carcinoma of the prostate clinically and radiologically simulating malignant lymphoma. J Surg Oncol 1987;35:1113–1116
8. Lucey B, et al: Small cell carcinoma of the lung presenting as chylous ascites. Italian J Gastroenterol 1998;29:1845
9. Pescowitz MD, et al: Diffuse retroperitoneal lymphadenopathy following liver transplantation. Transplantation 1995;60:393–396
10. Sherazi ZA, et al: Neuroblastoma and diagnostic imaging. Annals Academic Med Singapore 1993;22:7801–7806
11. Spencer J, Golding S: CT evaluation of lymph nodes status at presentation of prostate carcinoma. Brit J Radiol 1992; 65:99–201
12. Stein BS, Shea FJ: Metastatic carcinoma of the prostate presenting radiologically as lymphoma. J Urol 1983;130: 362–364
13. Woodring SH, Howard RS, Johnson MV: Massive low-attenuation mediastinal, retroperitoneal and pelvic lymphadenopathy on CT from lymphangioleiomyomatosis. Clinical Imaging 1994;18:7–11
14. Tesoro-Tess JD, et al: Reliability of diagnostic imaging after orchiectomy alone in follow-up of clinical stage I testicular carcinoma. Lymphology 1987;20:161–165
15. Zalev AH, Sacks JH, Warren RE: Pancreaticoduodenal tuberculosis simulating metastatic ovarian carcinoma. Can J Gastroenterol 1997;11:41–43

Gamut H-130

ENLARGED ILIOPSOAS MUSCLE OR COMPARTMENT

INFECTION or ABSCESS (BACTERIAL or TUBERCULOUS)

1. From retroperitoneal organs
   a. Complicated pancreatitis
   b. Kidney infection
   c. Postoperative aortic graft infection
2. From spine
   a. Hydatid disease
   b. Osteomyelitis or discitis (postoperative complication of bone or disc surgery)
3. From gastrointestinal tract
   a. Amebiasis
   b. Appendicitis
   c. Crohn's disease
4. Others
   a. Pelvic inflammatory disease (PID)
   b. Postpartum infection
   c. Sepsis
   d. Tuberculosis

HEMORRHAGE

1. Bleeding or coagulation disorder$_g$ (eg, hemophilia; anticoagulant therapy)
2. Postoperative aneurysm repair; other surgery
3. Ruptured aortic aneurysm
4. Trauma (blunt or penetrating)

NEOPLASM

1. Bone metastases or primary spinal tumor with soft tissue extension
2. Lipoma; liposarcoma
3. Lymphoma$_g$

(continued)

4. Metastatic lymphadenopathy
5. Muscle tumor (eg, rhabdomyosarcoma; fibrosarcoma)
6. Neurogenic tumor (eg, neuroblastoma; neuro-fibroma; ganglioneuroma)
7. Retroperitoneal sarcoma

Miscellaneous

1. Fluid collections (eg, urinoma; lymphocele; pancreatic pseudocyst; fluid in iliopsoas bursa)
2. Pseudoenlargement of psoas muscle (compared to atrophy of contralateral muscle)
3. Thrombosis of pelvic veins with diffuse swelling (edema) of muscles

Reference
1. Dähnert W: Radiology Review Manual. (ed 4) Baltimore: Williams & Wilkins, 1999, p 728

Gamut H-131

CYSTIC RETROPERITONEAL MASS (US, CT, MRI)

COMMON

1. Abscess$_g$
2. Hematoma (late)
3. Hydronephrosis
4. Pseudocyst of pancreas
5. Renal cystic disease (eg, simple cyst; polycystic kidney; multicystic dysplastic kidney; cystic renal cell carcinoma)

UNCOMMON

1. Cystadenoma or cystadenocarcinoma of pancreas
2. Cystic para-aortic lymphadenopathy (eg, carcinoma of cervix; teratoma of testis)
3. Hemangiopericytoma
4. Hydatid cyst
5. Leiomyosarcoma

6. Lymphangioma
7. Lymphocele
8. Meningocele
9. von Hippel-Lindau S.

References
1. Chapman S, Nakielny R: Aids to Radiological Differential Diagnosis. London: Baillière Tindall, 1990, p 218
2. Munechika H, et al: Computed tomography of retroperitoneal cystic lymphangiomas. J Comput Assist Tomogr 1986;11:116–119

Gamut H-132

EXTRAPERITONEAL GAS (See H-139)

COMMON

1. Abscess$_g$
2. Iatrogenic (eg, postoperative; rectal biopsy; enema; needle aspiration; gas insufflation)
3. [Interposition of colon (Chilaiditi S.)]
4. Perforation of gastrointestinal tract (eg, peptic ulcer; diverticulum; carcinoma; Crohn's disease)
5. Trauma (eg, gunshot wound; duodenal or colonic rupture)

UNCOMMON

1. Emphysematous cholecystitis (perforated)
2. Pneumatosis intestinalis with leakage
3. Pneumomediastinum with caudal tracking (eg, spontaneous; traumatic; tracheotomy)
4. [Portal vein gas]

[ ] This condition does not actually cause the gamuted imaging finding, but can produce imaging changes that simulate it.

References
1. Calenoff L, Poticha SM: Combined occurrence of retro-pneumoperitoneum and pneumoperitoneum. AJR 1973; 117:366–372
2. Love L, Baker D, Ramsey R: Gas producing perinephric abscess. AJR 1973;119:783–792

Gamut H-133

LARGE SOFT TISSUE MASS IN THE PELVIS (See also H-134–137)

COMMON
1. Abscess$_g$
2. Bladder enlargement (See H-96)
3. Feces in colon
4. Fluid-filled loop of bowel
5. Hematoma
6. Hydrosalpinx
7. Ovarian cyst or neoplasm (eg, dermoid; carcinoma) (See H-182, H-183)
8. Pregnancy (incl. ectopic pregnancy)
9. Uterine neoplasm (eg, fibroid; mole; carcinoma)

UNCOMMON
1. Bone tumor (eg, chordoma; Ewing sarcoma; osteosarcoma; chondrosarcoma)
2. Extraperitoneal neoplasm, other (lymphoma$_g$; Burkitt lymphoma; spindle cell tumor$_g$; neurogenic tumor)
3. Hemato- or hydrometrocolpos
4. Hydatid cyst
5. Meningocele, anterior sacral
6. Pelvic kidney
7. Pelvic lipomatosis
8. Soft tissue sarcoma (eg, rhabdomyosarcoma; liposarcoma; leiomyosarcoma)
9. Teratoma (eg, retroperitoneal; presacral; ovarian)

5. Lymph node enlargement
6. Lymphoma$_g$
7. Metastasis
8. Neoplasm of ovary (eg, carcinoma; dysgerminoma; yolk sac tumor; granulosa and theca cell tumors; fibroma)
9. Neoplasm of uterus, malignant (eg, carcinoma of cervix or endometrium; leiomyosarcoma)
10. Prostatic enlargement (eg, benign prostatic hypertrophy; carcinoma; prostatitis; abscess) (See H-140)
11. Torsion of ovary
12. Trophoblastic tumor (eg, hydatidiform mole; choriocarcinoma)

UNCOMMON
1. Hemangiopericytoma
2. Lipoma; liposarcoma
3. Neoplasm, extraperitoneal
4. Neurogenic tumor (eg, neurofibroma; ganglioneuroma; neuroblastoma); pheochromocytoma
5. Spindle cell tumor$_g$
6. Teratoma

[ ] This condition does not actually cause the gamuted imaging finding, but can produce imaging changes that simulate it.

References
1. Bree RL, Silver TM: Sonography of bladder and perivesical abnormalities. AJR 1981;136:1101–1104
2. Eisenberg RL: Clinical Imaging: An Atlas of Differential Diagnosis. (ed 3) Philadelphia: Lippincott-Raven, 1997, pp 676–679
3. Fleischer AC, James AE Jr: Introduction to Diagnostic Sonography. New York: John Wiley & Sons, 1980, p 107

Gamut H-134

SOLID PELVIC MASS (US, CT)

COMMON
1. [Bowel, fluid-filled]
2. Ectopic kidney
3. Fat, intraperitoneal
4. Leiomyoma (fibroid) of uterus

Gamut H-135

CYSTIC PELVIC MASS (US, CT)*

COMMON
1. Dermoid cyst
2. Ectopic pregnancy
3. Endometrioma
4. Hydrosalpinx

(continued)

5. Ovarian cyst, physiologic (follicular; corpus luteum; theca lutein; retention)
6. Ovarian serous or mucinous cystic lesion (cystadenoma or cystadenocarcinoma)
7. Paraovarian cyst
8. Urinary tract mass (eg, bladder enlargement; diverticulum; urinoma; ureterocele; hydroureter; urachal cyst)

UNCOMMON

1. Abscess$_g$ (incl. appendiceal; tubo-ovarian)
2. Ascites (loculated)
3. Hemato- or hydrometrocolpos
4. Hematoma
5. Hydatid cyst
6. Lymphocele
7. Mesenteric cyst
8. Peritoneal inclusion cyst
9. Polycystic ovary

* Cystic (homogeneous, septated, or with few solid foci).

References

1. Bree RL, Silver TM: Sonography of bladder and perivesical abnormalities. AJR 1981;136:1101–1104
2. Eisenberg RL: Clinical Imaging: An Atlas of Differential Diagnosis. (ed 3) Philadelphia: Lippincott-Raven, 1997, pp 668–671
3. Fleischer AC, James AE Jr: Introduction to Diagnostic Sonography. New York: John Wiley & Sons, 1980, p 107

Gamut H-136

COMPLEX PELVIC MASS (US, CT)*

COMMON

1. Abscess (tubo-ovarian or other)
2. Ectopic pregnancy
3. Endometrioma
4. Hemorrhagic corpus luteum cyst
5. Leiomyoma (fibroid) of uterus
6. Ovarian neoplasm (incl. dermoid cyst; mucinous cystadenoma, cystadenocarcinoma)
7. Pregnancy (fetus)

UNCOMMON

1. Adenomyosis of uterus
2. [Bowel, fluid- and air-filled]
3. Hydatid cyst
4. [Meningomyelocele]
5. Neoplasm of uterus, malignant (eg, carcinoma of endometrium; leiomyosarcoma)
6. Polycystic ovary
7. Pyometrium
8. Torsion of ovary
9. Trophoblastic tumor (eg, hydatidiform mole; choriocarcinoma)

* Complex (partly cystic, partly solid).
[ ] This condition does not actually cause the gamuted imaging finding, but can produce imaging chanes that can simulate it.

References

1. Bree RL, Silver TM: Sonography of bladder and perivesical abnormalities. AJR 1981;136:1101–1104
2. Eisenberg RL: Clinical Imaging: An Atlas of Differential Diagnosis. (ed 3) Philadelphia: Lippincott-Raven, 1997, pp 672–675
3. Fleischer AC, James AE Jr: Introduction to Diagnostic Sonography. New York: John Wiley & Sons, 1980, p 107

Gamut H-137

LOWER ABDOMINAL OR PELVIC MASS IN AN INFANT OR CHILD (See H-133–136)

COMMON

1. Appendiceal abscess
2. Bladder enlargement (See H-96)
3. Bone lesion of spine or pelvis
4. Hematoma (trauma; bleeding or coagulation disorder$_g$)
5. Ovarian cyst or neoplasm (See H-182–183)

UNCOMMON

1. Anterior sacral meningocele
2. Duplication cyst of gut or genital tract

3. Ectopic kidney
4. Fecal impaction (eg, Hirschsprung's disease)
5. Foreign body, vaginal or rectal
6. Hemato- or hydrometrocolpos
7. Hydatid cyst
8. Hydroureter
9. Intestinal obstruction
10. Intussusception
11. Lymphoma$_g$; Burkitt lymphoma
12. Meconium (eg, imperforate anus; meconium ileus; meconium plug S.)
13. Mesenteric or omental cyst
14. Metastasis
15. Neurogenic neoplasm (eg, neuroblastoma)
16. Perirectal abscess
17. Retroperitoneal neoplasm (eg, teratoma; sarcoma)
18. Rhabdomyosarcoma (botryoides) of bladder or vagina
19. Tubo-ovarian abscess; hydrosalpinx; pyosalpinx
20. Urachal cyst

References

1. Koop CE: Abdominal mass in the newborn infant. N Engl J Med 1973;289:569–571
2. Melicow MM, Uson AC: Palpable abdominal masses in infants and children: a report based on a review of 653 cases. J Urol 1959;81:705–710
3. Tank ES, Poznanski AK, Holt JF: The radiologic discrimination of abdominal masses in infants. J Urol 1973;109:128–132
4. Wedge JJ, Grosfeld JL, Smith JP: Abdominal masses in the newborn: 63 cases. J Urol 1971;106:770–775

Gamut H-138

PELVIC OR LOWER QUADRANT CALCIFICATION (See also G-247-1 to G-251)

COMMON

1. Appendiceal calculus (fecalith)
2. Dermoid cyst

3. [Foreign material: eg, pica; foreign body; intrauterine device; vaginal pessary; medicinal injections (eg, bismuth); residual barium (eg, in appendix or diverticula); pills; contrast medium (eg, Pantopaque, Ethiodol); radon seeds; metallic clips and sutures; catheter; gauze sponge]
4. Leiomyoma or leiomyosarcoma of uterus
5. Lithopedion
6. Lymph node (eg, tuberculosis; histoplasmosis)
7. Pregnancy (fetus; placenta)
8. Prostatic calculi
9. [Soft tissue or skin lesion]
10. Urinary tract calculus (in ureter, bladder, bladder diverticulum, urethra, pelvic kidney) (See H-24, 106)
11. Vas deferens, seminal vesicle, fallopian tube (eg, diabetes; tuberculosis; schistosomiasis)
12. Vascular (eg, arteries; phleboliths)

UNCOMMON

1. Bladder neoplasm
2. Bladder or ureteral wall calcification (eg, schistosomiasis; tuberculosis) (See H-85, 105)
3. Bone neoplasm (eg, osteochondroma; chondrosarcoma; osteosarcoma)
4. Calcified epiploic appendage; omental fat
5. Calculus in Meckel's diverticulum or colon diverticulum
6. Colloid carcinoma of colon or appendix
7. Cystadenoma or cystadenocarcinoma of ovary with psammomatous calcifications
8. Enterolith (esp. with small bowel tuberculosis)
9. Fluorosis (ligament calcification)
10. Gallstone in ileum (gallstone ileus)
11. Hemangioma (phleboliths)
12. Hydatid cyst
13. Lymphoma$_g$ (radiation treated)
14. Myxoglobulosis or mucocele of appendix
15. Neuroblastoma
16. Ovarian neoplasm; other (eg, fibroma; gonadoblastoma; teratoma; dysgerminoma; sclerosing stromal neoplasm, corpus albicans; nevoid basal cell carcinoma S. {Gorlin S.})

(continued)

17. Parasites (*Cysticercus; Armillifer;* guinea worm)
18. Pseudomyxoma peritonei

[ ] This condition does not actually cause the gamuted imaging finding, but can produce imaging changes that simulate it.

Gamut H-139

ABNORMAL GAS COLLECTION IN THE PELVIS AND FEMALE GENITAL TRACT (See H-132)

COMMON

1. Abscess$_g$
2. Bladder (eg, emphysematous cystitis; colovesical fistula) (See H-107)
3. Endometritis
4. Perforated appendix or colon (eg, diverticulum)
5. Pneumatosis cystoides of pelvic colon
6. Recent instrumentation
7. Rectal laceration or fistula

UNCOMMON

1. Carcinoma of cervix or endometrium with fistula to intestinal tract
2. *Clostridium* infection (gas gangrene of abdominal wall or uterus, esp. after septic abortion)
3. Emphysematous vaginitis
4. Gas in dead fetus
5. Giant colon diverticulum
6. Hydrogen peroxide enema (mural gas)
7. Infected uterine leiomyoma (fibroid)
8. Intestinal necrosis
9. Ovarian gas abscess (esp. in neoplasm)
10. Pyometra from obstruction by carcinoma of cervix

Reference
1. Seaman WB, Fleming RJ: Pneumatosis of pelvic viscera. Semin Roentgenol 1969;4:202–211

Gamut H-140

ENLARGED PROSTATE

COMMON

1. Benign prostatic hypertrophy (BPH)
2. Carcinoma of prostate
3. Prostatitis

UNCOMMON

1. Abscess
2. Amyloidosis
3. Sarcoma

Reference
1. Dunnick NR, et al: Textbook of Uroradiology. Baltimore: Williams & Wilkins, 1997, pp 440–457

Gamut H-141

SONOGRAPHY: ANECHOIC (USUALLY CYSTIC) LESION IN OR NEAR PROSTATE

COMMON

1. Cystic degeneration in benign prostatic hypertrophy (BPH)
2. Ejaculatory duct cyst
3. Müllerian duct cyst
4. Seminal vesicle cyst
5. Surgical defect (eg, transurethral prostatectomy—TURP)

UNCOMMON

1. Abscess
2. Cavitary/diverticular prostatitis (from fibrosis of chronic prostatitis—"Swiss cheese" prostate)
3. Cystic carcinoma of prostate
4. Cystocele

5. Ureterocele (ectopic)
6. Utricle cyst

References

1. Dähnert W: Radiology Review Manual. (ed 4) Baltimore: Williams & Wilkins, 1999, pp 746–747
2. Zagoria RJ, Tung GA: Genitourinary Radiology: The Requisites. St. Louis: Mosby, 1997, p 327
3. Williamson MR: Chapter 4. Renal ultrasound. In: Essentials of Ultrasound. Philadelphia: WB Saunders, 1996, p 128

Gamut H-142

SONOGRAPHY:
HYPOECHOIC PROSTATE LESION

COMMON

1. Acute prostatitis / abscess
2. Atypical prostatic hyperplasia
3. Carcinoma of prostate
4. Normal prostatic tissue (eg, prostate retention cysts in a cluster; prominent ejaculatory ducts; vessel)

UNCOMMON

1. Atrophy or dysplasia of prostate
2. Complex cyst
3. Fibrosis
4. Granulomatous prostatitis (eg, tuberculosis; BCG bacillus)
5. Hematoma
6. Infarct

References

1. Dähnert W: Radiology Review Manual. (ed 4) Baltimore: Williams & Wilkins, 1999, p 747
2. Kuligowska E, Pomeroy OH: Chapter 25. Prostate. In: McGahan JP, Goldberg BB (eds): Diagnostic Ultrasound. Philadelphia: Lippincott-Raven, 1997

Gamut H-143

SONOGRAPHY:
ISOECHOIC PROSTATE LESION

1. Atypical hyperplasia
2. Carcinoma of prostate
3. Fibrosis
4. Granulomatous prostatitis
5. Hematoma
6. Infarct

Reference

1. Kuligowska E, Pomeroy OH: Chapter 25. Prostate. In: McGahan JP, Goldberg BB (eds): Diagnostic Ultrasound. Philadelphia: Lippincott-Raven, 1997

Gamut H-144

SONOGRAPHY:
HYPERECHOIC PROSTATE LESION

1. Calcification
2. Carcinoma of prostate (esp. comedocarcinoma)
3. Chronic prostatitis

Reference

1. Kuligowska E, Pomeroy OH: Chapter 25. Prostate. In: McGahan JP, Goldberg BB (eds): Diagnostic Ultrasound. Philadelphia: Lippincott-Raven, 1997

Gamut H-145

HYPERVASCULAR PROSTATE LESION ON COLOR DOPPLER ULTRASOUND

1. Arteriovenous fistula (post biopsy); other vascular malformation
2. Carcinoma of prostate
3. Infection (prostatitis)

Reference
1. Kuligowska E, Pomeroy OH: Chapter 25. Prostate. In: Mc-Gahan JP, Goldberg BB (eds): Diagnostic Ultrasound. Philadelphia: Lippincott-Raven, 1997

Gamut H-146

LOW-INTENSITY PERIPHERAL ZONE OF PROSTATE ON T2-WEIGHTED MR IMAGES

COMMON
1. Carcinoma of prostate
2. Hematoma
3. Prostatitis (chronic and granulomatous)

UNCOMMON
1. Amyloidosis
2. Benign prostatic hypertrophy (atypical)
3. Infarct
4. Intraepithelial neoplasia of prostate
5. Post-hormonal therapy
6. Post-radiation therapy

Gamut H-147

LOW-INTENSITY SEMINAL VESICLE ON T2-WEIGHTED MR IMAGES

COMMON
1. Blood
2. Carcinoma
3. [Vasa deferentia]

UNCOMMON
1. Amyloidosis
2. Post-hormonal therapy
3. Post-radiation therapy
4. Seminal vesiculitis

[ ] This condition does not actually cause the gamuted imaging finding, but can produce imaging changes that simulate it.

Reference
1. Ramchandani P, Banner MP, Pollack HM: Imaging of the seminal vesicles. Semin Roentgenol 1993;28:83–91

Gamut H-148

CYSTIC STRUCTURE NEAR SEMINAL VESICLE

1. Müllerian remnant cyst
2. Seminal vesicle cyst
3. Ureterocele (ectopic)
4. Utricle

Reference
1. Nghiem HT, et. al: RadioGraphics 1990;10:635–650

Gamut H-149

CALCIFICATION IN THE SEMINAL VESICLE, VAS DEFERENS, OR FALLOPIAN TUBE

COMMON

1. Aging; degenerative
2. [Atherosclerosis]
3. Diabetes
4. Idiopathic
5. Tuberculosis

UNCOMMON

1. Calculus
2. Chronic nonspecific infection
3. Hemorrhage (traumatic or other)
4. Paraplegia
5. Schistosomiasis haematobium
6. Syphilis

[ ] This condition does not actually cause the gamuted imaging finding, but can produce imaging changes that simulate it.

References

1. Dunnick NR, et al: Textbook of Uroradiology. Baltimore: Williams & Wilkins, 1997, pp 45, 460–463
2. Grunebaum M: The calcified vas deferens. Isr J Med Sci 1971;7:311–314
3. King JC Jr, Rosenbaum HD: Calcification of the vasa deferentia in nondiabetics. Radiology 1971;100:603–606
4. Pollack HM (ed): Clinical Urography. Philadelphia: Saunders, 1990
5. Rodriguez de Velasquez A, Yoder IC, Velasquez PA, Papanicolaou N: Imaging the effects of diabetes on the genitourinary system. RadioGraphics 1995;15:1051–1068

Gamut H-150

ABNORMALITLES INVOLVING THE ENTIRE TESTIS

COMMON

1. Orchitis
2. Torsion

UNCOMMON

1. Testicular neoplasms (rarely)
2. Trauma (hemorrhage; hematoma)

Gamut H-151

SOLID TESTICULAR MASS (US, MRI)

COMMON

1. Hematoma
2. Infarct
3. Infection
4. Lymphoma$_g$; leukemia
5. Neoplasm, benign or malignant (See H-155–157)

UNCOMMON

1. Adrenal rest
2. Metastasis

Gamut H-152

CYSTIC TESTICULAR MASS (US, MRI)

1. Abscess
2. Cystic dysplasia
3. Cystic or necrotic neoplasm, benign or malignant (See H-155–157)
4. Hematoma
5. Intratesticular tubular ectasia (dilatation of rete testis)
6. Simple testicular cyst (often with spermatocele)
7. Tunica albuginea cyst

Gamut H-153

UNILATERAL TESTICULAR MASS (US, MRI)

COMMON

1. Choriocarcinoma
2. Embryonal cell carcinoma
3. Seminoma
4. Teratoma
5. Yolk sac tumor (endodermal sinus tumor)

UNCOMMON

1. Leydig cell tumor
2. Metastasis
3. Sertoli cell tumor

Gamut H-154

BILATERAL TESTICULAR MASSES (US, MRI)

COMMON

1. Lymphoblastic leukemia (acute or chronic)
2. Lymphoma (non-Hodgkins)
3. Metastases

UNCOMMON

1. Adrenal rest hyperplasia

Gamut H-155-S

GERM CELL TUMORS OF THE TESTES

COMMON

1. Mixed germ cell tumor
   a. Embryonal cell carcinoma plus seminoma
   b. Seminoma plus teratoma
   c. Teratocarcinoma (teratoma plus embryonal cell carcinoma)
2. Seminoma

UNCOMMON

1. Choriocarcinoma
2. Embryonal cell carcinoma
3. Polyembryoma
4. Spermatocytic seminoma
5. Teratoma
6. Yolk sac tumor (endodermal sinus tumor)

Reference

1. Heiken JP: Tumors of the testis and testicular adnexa. World Health Organization Classification of Testicular Germ Cell Tumors. In: Pollack HM, McClennan BL (eds): Clinical Urography. (ed 2) Philadelphia: WB Saunders, 2000, pp 1716–1741

Gamut H-156-S

NON-GERM CELL TUMORS OF THE TESTES

COMMON

1. Lymphoma$_g$; leukemia

UNCOMMON

1. Adrenal rest tumor
2. Adenocarcinoma of rete testis
3. Carcinoid tumor
4. Epidermoid cyst
5. Extramedullary plasmacytoma
6. Fibroma
7. Gonadoblastoma
8. Granulosa cell tumor
9. Leydig cell tumor
10. Metastasis
11. Papillary adenocarcinoma of rete testis
12. Sertoli cell tumor

Reference

1. Heiken JP: Tumors of the testis and testicular adnexa. In: Pollack HM, McClennan BL (eds): Clinical Urography. (ed 2) Philadelphia: WB Saunders, 2000, pp 1716–1741

Gamut H-157

TESTICULAR TUMOR IN A CHILD (US)

COMMON

1. Teratoma
2. Yolk sac tumor

UNCOMMON

1. Gonadoblastoma
2. Granulosa cell tumor
3. Leydig cell tumor
4. Sertoli cell tumor

Gamut H-158

TESTICULAR CALCIFICATION (PF, US)

COMMON

1. Embryonal cell carcinoma
2. Hematoma (old)
3. Metastatic neuroblastoma
4. Microlithiasis of testis (may occur with pulmonary alveolar microlithiasis)
5. Scar
6. Spermatic granuloma
7. Tumor (posttreatment)

UNCOMMON

1. Cryptorchidism
2. Epidermoid cyst
3. Germ cell tumor ("burned-out")
4. Granulomatous orchitis (eg, tuberculosis)
5. Kleinfelter S. (XXY S.)
6. Leydig cell tumor
7. Phlebolith
8. Sertoli cell tumor

Reference

1. Williamson MR: In: Essentials of Ultrasound. Philadelphia: WB Saunders, 1996, p 134

Gamut H-159

EPIDIDYMAL LESION (US, MRI)

COMMON

1. Adenomatoid tumor
2. Epididymitis
3. Spermatocele
4. Torsion

UNCOMMON

1. Abscess
2. Cyst

(continued)

3. Cystadenoma
4. Mesenchymal tumor (eg, leiomyoma)

References
1. Choyke PL, et al: Epididymal cystadenomas in von Hippel-Lindau disease. Urology 1997;49:926–931
2. Dunnick NR, et al: Textbook of Uroradiology. Baltimore: Williams & Wilkins, 1997, pp 500–503
3. Heiken JP: Tumors of the testis and testicular adnexa. In: Pollack HM, McClennan BL (eds): Clinical Urography. (ed 2) Philadelphia: WB Saunders, 2000, pp 1716–1741
4. Makarainen HP, et al: Intrascrotal adenomatoid tumors and their ultrasound findings. J Clin Ultrasound 1993;21:33–37

Gamut H-160

MASS IN THE SCROTUM

COMMON

1. Cyst of testis, epididymis, vas deferens, or seminal vesicle
2. Hematoma
3. Hydrocele
4. Infection, chronic (eg, epididymitis; seminal vesiculitis)
5. Malignant neoplasm of testis or testicular adnexa (eg, seminoma; choriocarcinoma; embryonal cell carcinoma; teratoma; lymphoma$_g$; rhabdomyo-sarcoma of spermatic cord)
6. Orchitis (traumatic or other)
7. Varicocele

UNCOMMON

1. Abscess
2. Benign hypertrophy of testis
3. Benign neoplasm of testis or testicular adnexa (eg, adenomatoid tumor; fibroma)
4. Hernia
5. Hydatid of Morgagni (appendix testis)
6. Metastasis
7. Torsion of testicle

8. Tuberculosis (esp. epididymis)
9. Ureterocele (ectopic)

References
1. Heiken JP: Tumors of the testis and testicular adnexa. In: Pollack HM, McClennan BL (eds): Clinical Urography. (ed 2) Philadelphia: WB Saunders, 2000, pp 1716–1741
2. Loveday BJ, Price JL: Soft tissue radiography of the testes. Clin Radiol 1978;29:685–689

Gamut H-161

EXTRATESTICULAR TUMORS IN THE SCROTUM

COMMON

1. Adenomatoid tumor
2. Fibrous pseudotumor (fibroma)
3. Rhabdomyosarcoma of spermatic cord

UNCOMMON

1. Cystadenoma
2. Dermoid cyst; teratoma
3. Fibrosarcoma; malignant fibrous histiocytoma
4. Leiomyoma; leiomyosarcoma
5. Lipoma (esp. of spermatic cord); liposarcoma
6. Mesothelioma
7. Metastases
8. Myxochondrosarcoma

Reference
1. Heiken JP: Tumors of the testis and testicular adnexa. In: Pollack HM, McClennan BL (eds): Clinical Urography. (ed 2) Philadelphia: WB Saunders, 2000, pp 1716–1741

Gamut H-162

SOLID EXTRATESTICULAR MASS IN THE SCROTUM (US, MRI)

COMMON
1. Hematoma
2. Hernia
3. Infection; phlegmon
4. Neoplasm, benign or malignant (esp. adenomatoid tumor; rhabdomyosarcoma; fibroma) (See H-161)

UNCOMMON
1. Adrenal rest
2. Metastasis

Gamut H-163

CYSTIC EXTRATESTICULAR MASS IN THE SCROTUM (US, MRI)

1. Abscess
2. Epididymal cyst
3. Hematoma
4. Hernia
5. Hydrocele
6. Post-vasectomy
7. Spermatocele
8. Varicocele

Gamut H-164

CALCIFICATIONS IN THE SCROTUM (PF, US)

COMMON
1. Aging; degenerative
2. Atherosclerosis (esp. diabetic)
3. Hemorrhage, old; hematoma (traumatic or other)
4. Testicular calcification (eg, microlithiasis) (See H-158)
5. Varicocele, hemangioma (phleboliths)

UNCOMMON
1. Hydrocele
2. Idiopathic scrotal calcinosis
3. Infarction of testis
4. Meconium peritonitis (in hydrocele)
5. Neoplasm (eg, teratoma)
6. Parasites (esp. guinea worm; *Armillifer;* filariasis)
7. Sebaceous cyst
8. Spermatocele
9. Syphilis
10. Testicular atrophy
11. Tuberculosis
12. Vas deferens calcification (See H-149)

References
1. Backus MC, et al: Testicular microlithiasis. Radiology 1994;192:781
2. Dare AJ, Axelsen RA: Scrotal calcinosis. J Cutaneous Path 1988;15:142–149
3. Koh E, et al: The case of chronic huge hematocele. Acta Urologica Japanica 1989;35:1421–1424
4. Martin B, Tubiana JM: Significance of scrotal calcifications detected by sonography. J Clin Ultrasound 1988;16:545–552
5. Plata C, et al: Large cell calcifying sertoli-cell tumor of the testis. Histopathology 1995;26:255–259
6. Rhaghavaiah NV: Epididymal calcification in genital filariasis. Urology 1981;18:78–79
7. Ring KS, et al: Meconium hydrocele. J Urology 1989;141:1172–1173

Gamut H-165

FLUID COLLECTION IN THE SCROTUM (US)

1. Abscess
2. Cyst of testis or epididymis
3. Hematoma
4. Hernia
5. Hydrocele
6. Spermatocele
7. Varicocele

Reference
1. Dunnick NR, et al: Textbook of Uroradiology. Baltimore: Williams & Wilkins, 1997, pp 493–506

Gamut H-166

CONGENITAL SYNDROMES WITH HYPOSPADIAS OR OTHER AMBIGUOUS EXTERNAL GENITALIA

1. Bardet-Biedl S. (Laurence-Moon-Biedl S.)
2. Chondroectodermal dysplasia (Ellis-van Creveld S.)
3. Chromosomal syndromes (eg, 4 p - S.; trisomy 3, 13, and 18 S.; XXXXY S.)
4. Dubowitz S.
5. Familial hypospadias
6. Fanconi anemia (pancytopenia-dysmelia S.)
7. Fetal primidone S.
8. Fraser S. (cryptophthalmia S.)
9. Hand-foot-genital S.
10. Hypertelorism-hypospadias S.
11. Lenz microphthalmia S.
12. LEOPARD S. (multiple lentigenes S.)
13. Male pseudohermaphroditism
14. Opitz BBBG S. (hypertelorism-hypospadias S. or GS.)
15. Popliteal pterygium S.
16. Reifenstein S. (hereditary familial hypogonadism)
17. Rieger S.
18. Schinzel-Giedion S.
19. Silver-Russell S.
20. Smith-Lemli-Opitz S.
21. VATER association
22. Zellweger S. (cerebrohepatorenal S.)

Reference
1. Taybi H, Lachman RS: Radiology of Syndromes, Metabolic Disorders, and Skeletal Dysplasias. (ed 4) St. Louis: Mosby-Yearbook Inc., 1996, pp 978–979

Gamut H-167

CALCIFICATIONS IN THE FEMALE GENITAL TRACT

OVARIES

1. Cystadenocarcinoma
2. Dermoid cyst
3. Gonadoblastoma
4. Papillary cystadenoma (psammomatous bodies)
5. Pseudomyxoma peritonei
6. Torsion of ovary (chronic)

UTERUS

1. Arcuate arteries
2. Leiomyoma (fibroid)
3. Lithopedion
4. Placenta

FALLOPIAN TUBES

1. Aging
2. Diabetes
3. Schistosomiasis haematobium
4. Tuberculous salpingitis

Gamut H-168

VAGINAL FISTULA

COMMON

1. Abscess$_g$ (esp. pelvic; appendiceal; colon diverticulitis)
2. Crohn's disease
3. Endometriosis
4. Lymphogranuloma venereum
5. Metastatic disease
6. Neoplasm, malignant (eg, carcinoma of rectum, sigmoid, vagina, uterus, or bladder)
7. Parturition (eg, arrested fetal passage; dystocia)
8. Pelvic inflammatory disease; endometritis
9. Postoperative (eg, pelvic surgery)
10. Radiation therapy (esp. radium)
11. Trauma (external; iatrogenic; sexual)

UNCOMMON

1. Amebiasis
2. Congenital
3. Ectopic pregnancy
4. Foreign body perforation
5. Fungus infection$_g$ (esp. actinomycosis)
6. Hemato- or hydrometrocolpos
7. Osteomyelitis of pelvic bones
8. Polyarteritis nodosa
9. Tuberculosis
10. Vaginitis

References
1. Cooper RA: Vaginography: A presentation of new cases and subject review. Radiology 1982;143:421–425
2. Shieh CJ, Gennaro AR: Rectovaginal fistula: a review of 11 years' experience. Int Surg 1984;69:69–72

Gamut H-169-S

COMMON INDICATIONS FOR GYNECOLOGICAL ULTRASOUND

1. Evaluation of location, size, and consistency of a pelvic mass (eg, ovarian, tubal, uterine)
2. Evaluation of pelvic pain
3. Evaluation of vaginal bleeding (eg, endometrial hyperplasia, polyp, or carcinoma)
4. Follicular monitoring and guided aspiration
   a. Gamete intrafallopian transfer (GIFT)
   b. In vitro fertilization; embryo transfer
   c. Ovulation induction
5. IUD complications

Reference
1. Fleischer AC, Boehm FH, James AE Jr: Ultrasonography in obstetrics and gynaecology: obstetric radiology. In: Grainger RG, Allison DJ: Diagnostic Radiology. (ed 2) Edinburgh: Churchill Livingstone, 1992, pp 1809–1819

Gamut H-170

SONOGRAPHY: HYPERECHOIC FOCAL UTERINE LESIONS

1. Calcified arcuate artery
2. Calcified leiomyoma (fibroid)
3. Endometrial calcification (post D&C or infection)
4. Gas (from recent instrumentation)
5. Intrauterine contraceptive device (IUD)
6. Retained products of conception

Reference
1. Williamson MR: Chapter 7. Ultrasound of the female pelvis. In: Essentials of Ultrasound. Philadelphia: WB Saunders, 1996, p 149

Gamut H-171

SONOGRAPHY:
DIFFUSE UTERINE ENLARGEMENT

COMMON

*1. Carcinoma of endometrium
*2. Leiomyomas (fibroids)
 3. Multiparity
 4. Normal parous uterus
 5. Postpartum uterus
 6. Pregnancy
 7. Recent abortion

UNCOMMON

*1. Adenomyosis (endometriosis) of uterus
 2. Arteriovenous malformation involving uterus
 3. Congenital anomaly
 4. Hemato-, hydro-, or pyometrocolpos
*5. Obstruction of uterus (eg, extensive carcinoma of cervix; fibroids)
 6. Precocious puberty
 7. Pseudocyesis (false pregnancy)
*8. Sarcoma of uterus
 9. Trophoblastic disease (eg, hydatidiform mole; chориocarcinoma)

* Seen especially in postmenopausal women.

References

1. Lawson TL, Albarelli JN: Diagnosis of gynecologic pelvic masses by gray scale ultrasonography: (A) Analysis of specificity and accuracy. AJR 1977;128:1003–1006
2. Levine D: Chapter 29. Postmenopausal pelvis. In: McGahan JP, Goldberg BB (eds): Diagnostic Ultrasound. Philadelphia: Lippincott-Raven, 1997
3. Williamson MR: Chapter 7. Ultrasound of the female pelvis. In: Essentials of Ultrasound. Philadelphia: WB Saunders, 1996, p 145

Gamut H-172

SONOGRAPHY:
ENDOMETRIAL THICKENING

*1. Adenomyosis (endometriosis) of uterus
*2. Carcinoma of endometrium
 3. Early pregnancy
 4. Ectopic pregnancy
 5. Endometritis
 6. Gestational trophoblastic disease
 7. Hematometria
*8. Hormone therapy
*9. Hyperplasia of endometrium
 10. Intrauterine contraceptive device (IUD)
*11. Leiomyoma (fibroid)
 12. Missed abortion
 13. Normal secretory phase
*14. Polyp of endometrium
 15. Pyometria
 16. Retained products of conception
*17. Tamoxifen therapy

* Seen especially in postmenopausal women.

References

1. Levine D: Chapter 29. Postmenopausal pelvis. In: McGahan JP, Goldberg BB (eds): Diagnostic Ultrasound. Philadelphia: Lippincott-Raven, 1997
2. Williamson MR: Chapter 7. Ultrasound of the female pelvis. In: Essentials of Ultrasound. Philadelphia: WB Saunders, 1996, p 144

Gamut H-173

SONOGRAPHY:
ENDOMETRIAL FLUID

COMMON

*1. Carcinoma of cervix
*2. Carcinoma of endometrium
*3. Cervical stenosis

*4. Degenerating leiomyomas (fibroids)
*5. Dilatation and curettage (D&C), recent
*6. Hyperplasia of endometrium
7. Imperforate hymen
*8. Infection (endometritis)
9. Normal (menstrual phase)
*10. Polyps of endometrium
11. Pregnancy-related (incomplete abortion; ectopic pregnancy)

UNCOMMON

1. Duplication anomaly with obstruction
2. Vaginal or cervical atresia

* Seen especially in postmenopausal women.

Reference

1. Levine D: Chapter 28. Female pelvis, and Chapter 29. Postmenopausal pelvis. In: McGahan JP, Goldberg BB (eds): Diagnostic Ultrasound. Philadelphia: Lippincott-Raven, 1997

Gamut H-174

SONOGRAPHY: INDEFINITE UTERUS SIGN ("SILHOUETTE SIGN")

1. Endometriosis
2. Hemorrhage (trauma; bleeding or coagulation disorder$_g$)
3. Leiomyoma (fibroid) of uterus
4. Malignant neoplasm
5. Pelvic inflammatory disease (acute)
6. Ruptured ectopic pregnancy

References

1. Berland LL, Lawson TL, Foley WD, et al: Ultrasound evaluation of pelvic infections. Radiol Clin North Am 1982; 20:367–382
2. Lawson TL, Albarelli JN: Diagnosis of gynecologic pelvic masses by gray scale ultrasonography: (A) Analysis of specificity and accuracy. AJR 1977;128:1003–1006

Gamut H-175

SONOGRAPHY: PROMINENCE OF CENTRAL UTERINE ECHO

COMMON

1. Endometrial hyperplasia
2. Endometritis (incl. tuberculous)
3. Hydatidiform mole
4. Intrauterine device
5. Neoplasm, malignant (eg, carcinoma of endometrium; leiomyosarcoma; choriocarcinoma; invasive ovarian carcinoma)
6. Normal menstrual endometrium
7. Placenta (tangential scan)
8. Polyp of endometrium
9. Pregnancy (early intrauterine or ectopic)
10. Retained products of conception; missed abortion

UNCOMMON

1. Atrophic endometrium
2. Foreign body
3. Gas; physometra
4. Leiomyoma (degenerating)
5. Multiple gestation (early)

References

1. Grossman M: Gamut: Diffuse formless intrauterine echoes. Semin Roentgenol 1975;10:251
2. Slezak P, Tillinger KG: Hysterographic evidence of polypoid filling defects in the uterine cavity. Radiology 1975; 115:79–83

Gamut H-176

SONOGRAPHY: CERVICAL MASS

1. Carcinoma of cervix
2. Ectopic pregnancy
3. Leiomyoma (fibroid) of cervix
4. Nabothian cyst
5. Polyp

Reference
1. Levine D: Chapter 28. Female pelvis. In: McGahan JP, Goldberg BB (eds): Diagnostic Ultrasound. Philadelphia: Lippincott-Raven, 1997

Gamut H-177

SONOGRAPHY: FREE FLUID IN CUL-DE-SAC

1. Ascites
2. Ectopic pregnancy
3. Follicular rupture
4. Neoplasm (esp. of ovary)
5. Ovulation
6. Pelvic inflammatory disease
7. Postculdocentesis

Reference
1. Dähnert W: Radiology Review Manual. (ed 4) Baltimore: Williams & Wilkins, 1999, p 836

Gamut H-178

SONOGRAPHY: FALLOPIAN TUBE MASS

1. Carcinoma
2. Ectopic pregnancy
3. Hydrosalpinx
4. Paratubal cyst
5. Pyosalpinx
6. Tubo-ovarian abscess

Reference
1. Levine D: Chapter 28. Female pelvis. In: McGahan JP, Goldberg BB (eds): Diagnostic Ultrasound. Philadelphia: Lippincott-Raven, 1997

Gamut H-179

SONOGRAPHY: SIMPLE ANECHOIC OR HYPOECHOIC CYSTIC ADNEXAL LESION

1. [Bladder diverticulum]
2. [Bowel loop]
3. Corpus luteum cyst
4. Follicular cyst
5. Functional/retention cyst
6. Hydrosalpinx
7. Hydroureter
8. Loculated ascites
9. Lymphocele
10. Mesenteric cyst
11. Paraovarian or paratubal cyst
12. Peritoneal inclusion cyst
13. Theca lutein cyst
14. Varices

[ ] This condition does not actually cause the gamuted imaging finding, but can produce imaging changes that simulate it.

References

1. Bisset RAL, Khan AN: Differential Diagnosis in Abdominal Ultrasound. London: Bailliere Tindall, 1990, pp 273–275
2. Levine D: Chapter 28. Female pelvis. In: McGahan JP, Goldberg BB (eds): Diagnostic Ultrasound. Philadelphia: Lippincott-Raven, 1997

Gamut H-180

SONOGRAPHY: COMPLEX (USUALLY CYSTIC) ADNEXAL MASS

1. Abscess (tubo-ovarian; appendiceal; diverticular; postoperative)
2. Cystic ovarian tumor (eg, dermoid; mucinous or serous cystadenoma or cystadenocarcinoma)
3. Degenerated pedunculated uterine leiomyoma (fibroid)
4. Ectopic pregnancy
5. Endometrioma
6. Fallopian tube carcinoma
7. Hematoma
8. Hemorrhagic cyst of ovary
9. Hydatid cyst
10. Hydrosalpinx
11. Peritoneal inclusion cyst
12. Polycystic ovary S.
13. Theca lutein cyst
14. Torsion of adnexa

References

1. Bisset RAL, Khan AN: Differential Diagnosis in Abdominal Ultrasound. London: Bailliere Tindall, 1990, pp 273–275
2. Levine D: Chapter 28. Female pelvis. In: McGahan JP, Goldberg BB (eds): Diagnostic Ultrasound. Philadelphia: Lippincott-Raven, 1997

Gamut H-181

ADNEXAL LESIONS WITH LOW RESISTIVE INDEX (< 0.4) ON DOPPLER ULTRASOUND

1. Adenofibroma
2. Dermoid cyst of ovary
3. Ectopic pregnancy
4. Endometrioma
5. Luteal cyst
6. Luteal phase of functioning ovary
7. Malignant neoplasm (eg, carcinoma of ovary)
8. Pedunculated leiomyoma (fibroid) of uterus
9. Tubo-ovarian abscess

Reference

1. Levine D: Chapter 28. Female pelvis. In: McGahan JP, Goldberg BB (eds): Diagnostic Ultrasound. Philadelphia: Lippincott-Raven, 1997

Gamut H-182

SONOGRAPHY: SOLID OVARIAN TUMOR

1. Adenocarcinoma of ovary
2. Brenner tumor
3. Burkitt lymphoma
4. Dysgerminoma
5. Endometrioma
6. Fibroma
7. Germ cell tumor (non-teratomatous)
8. Granulosa cell tumor
9. Metastasis
10. Sarcoma of ovary
11. Sertoli-Leydig cell tumor
12. Teratoma
13. Thecoma
14. Yolk sac tumor (endodermal sinus tumor)

(continued)

References
1. Dähnert W: Radiology Review Manual. (ed 4) Baltimore: Williams & Wilkins, 1999, p 837
2. Levine D: Chapter 28. Female pelvis. In: McGahan JP, Goldberg BB (eds): Diagnostic Ultrasound. Philadelphia: Lippincott-Raven, 1997

Gamut H-183

OVARIAN NEOPLASM OR CYST IN A CHILD

SIMPLE EPITHELIAL CYST
1. Cystadenoma, serous or mucinous
2. Paraovarian cyst (mesonephric origin)

CYST OF GRAAFIAN FOLLICLE ORIGIN
1. Follicular cyst
2. Theca lutein cyst

TUMOR OF OVARIAN STROMAL ORIGIN
1. Granulosa-thecal cell tumor
2. Pure granulosa cell tumor (benign or malignant)
3. Thecoma

GERM CELL TUMOR
1. Dysgerminoma
2. Endodermal sinus tumor (yolk sac tumor)
3. Gonadoblastoma (dysgenetic ovary)
4. Teratoma, cystic
5. Teratoma, immature (embryonal)
6. Teratoma with malignant elements

BURKITT LYMPHOMA

Reference
1. Kevin E Bove, Department of Pathology, Cincinnati Children's Hospital: Personal communication

I

Mammography

I

I

Gamut I-1-1

CIRCUMSCRIBED BREAST LESION EVALUATED BY SIZE OF LESION— SMALL TO INTERMEDIATE (LESS THAN 4 CM)

COMMON

1. Axillary lymph node (eg, lymphoma$_g$; leukemia; metastasis; tuberculosis) (See I-17)
2. Carcinoma (esp. mucinous or papillary)
3. Cyst
4. Fibroadenoma
5. Fibrocystic change (esp. sclerosing adenosis)
*6. Intramammary lymph node
*7. Oil or lipid cyst (posttraumatic or postsurgical fat necrosis)
8. Papilloma, papillomatosis
9. Skin lesion (eg, wart; mole; neurofibroma; sebaceous cyst; nipple out of profile)

UNCOMMON

*1. Galactocele
2. Hemangioma (cavernous)
*3. Hematoma or seroma
*4. Lipoma
5. Metastasis
6. Phyllodes tumor (formerly cystosarcoma phyllodes)

*Radiolucent or partially lucent lesions containing fat.

References

1. DeParedes ES: Atlas of Film Screen Mammography. (ed 2) Baltimore: Williams & Wilkins, 1992, p 134
2. Dershaw DD (ed): Interventional Breast Procedures. Edinburgh: Churchill Livingstone, 1996
3. Friedrich M, Sickles EA: Radiologic Diagnosis of Breast Diseases. New York: Springer, 2000
4. Hall FM: Probably benign breast nodules: follow-up of selected cases without initial full problem-solving imaging. Radiology 1995;194:305
5. Jackson VP: Management of solid breast nodules: what is the role of sonography? Radiology 1995;196:14–15
6. Kopans DB: Breast Imaging. (ed 2) Philadelphia: Lippincott-Raven, 1998
7. Powell DE, Stelling CB: The Diagnosis and Detection of Breast Disease. Stromal, vascular, hematolymphoid, and metastatic breast lesions. St. Louis: Mosby-Year Book, Inc., 1994, pp 344–353
8. Sickles EA: Periodic mammographic following of probably benign lesions: results in 3,184 consecutive cases. Radiology 1991;179:463–468
9. Sickles EA: Non-palpable, circumscribed non-calcified solid breast masses: likelihood of malignancy based on lesion size and age of patient. Radiology 1994;192:439–432
10. Stavros AT, Thickman D, Rapp CL, et al: Solid breast nodules: use of sonography to distinguish between benign and malignant lesions. Radiology 1995;196:123–124
11. Stavros A: Breast Ultrasound. Philadelphia: Lippincott-Williams & Wilkins, 2002
12. Tabar L, Dean PB: Teaching Atlas of Mammography. (ed 3) New York: Thieme, 2000
13. Tavassoli FA: Pathology of the Breast. (ed 2) New York: McGraw-Hill, 1999

Gamut I-1-2

CIRCUMSCRIBED BREAST LESION — LARGE (OVER 4 CM)

COMMON

1. Carcinoma (unusual to be circumscribed at this size)
2. Cyst (simple or complicated)

UNCOMMON

1. Abscess
2. Axillary or unusual intramammary lymphadenopathy (eg, lymphoma$_g$, metastasis) (See I-17)
*3. Fibroadenolipoma (hamartoma)
4. Hematoma
*5. Lipoma
6. Metastasis to breast
*7. Oil or lipid cyst, large (posttraumatic or postsurgical fat necrosis)
8. Phyllodes tumor (formerly cystosarcoma phyllodes; giant fibroadenoma)
9. Postoperative seroma (eg, after implant removal— usually not well circumscribed)

10. Sarcoma
11. [Sebaceous cyst]

*Radiolucent or partially lucent lesions containing fat.
[ ] This condition does not actually cause the gamuted imaging finding,
but can produce imaging changes that simulate it.

References
1. DeParedes ES: Atlas of Film Screen Mammography. (ed 2) Baltimore: Williams & Wilkins, 1992, p 134
2. Dershaw DD (ed): Interventional Breast Procedures. Edinburgh: Churchill Livingstone, 1996
3. Friedrich M, Sickles EA: Radiologic Diagnosis of Breast Diseases. New York: Springer, 2000
4. Hall FM: Probably benign breast nodules: follow-up of selected cases without initial full problem-solving imaging. Radiology 1995;194:305
5. Jackson VP: Management of solid breast nodules: what is the role of sonography? Radiology 1995;196:14–15
6. Kopans DB: Breast Imaging. (ed 2) Philadelphia: Lippincott-Raven, 1998
7. Powell DE, Stelling CB: The Diagnosis and Detection of Breast Disease. Stromal, vascular, hematolymphoid, and metastatic breast lesions. St. Louis: Mosby-Year Book, Inc., 1994, pp 344–353
8. Sickles EA: Periodic mammographic following of probably benign lesions: results in 3,184 consecutive cases. Radiology 1991;179:463–468
9. Sickles EA: Non-palpable, circumscribed non-calcified solid breast masses: likelihood of malignancy based on lesion size and age of patient. Radiology 1994;192:439–432
10. Stavros AT, Thickman D, Rapp CL, et al: Solid breast nodules: use of sonography to distinguish between benign and malignant lesions. Radiology 1995;196:123–124
11. Stavros A: Breast Ultrasound. Philadelphia: Lippincott-Williams & Wilkins, 2002
12. Tabar L, Dean PB: Teaching Atlas of Mammography. (ed 3) New York: Thieme, 2000
13. Tavassoli FA: Pathology of the Breast. (ed 2) New York: McGraw-Hill, 1999

Gamut I-2

WELL-DEFINED CIRCUMSCRIBED LESION OF THE BREAST

COMMON

1. Carcinoma, usually not "well" circumscribed on magnification views (eg, ductal in situ; invasive ductal; medullary; colloid or mucinous; papillary; intracystic papillary)

*2. Cyst
*3. Fibroadenoma
*4. Fibrocystic change (esp. sclerosing adenosis)
5. Intramammary (or axillary) lymph node
6. [Normal variant (circumscribed parenchyma of puberty; retracted or normal nipple out of profile; end-on vein)]
7. Oil or lipid cyst (posttraumatic or postsurgical fat necrosis)
*8. Papilloma (intraductal)
*9. [Skin lesion (eg, mole; wart; neurofibroma; epidermal inclusion or sebaceous cyst)]

UNCOMMON

1. Abscess
*2. Fibroadenolipoma (hamartoma)
3. Galactocele
4. Granular cell myoblastoma
5. Hemangioma (cavernous)
6. Hematoma
7. Lipoma
8. Lymphoma, primary
*9. Metastasis to breast (eg, from melanoma; carcinoma of lung, ovary, GI or GU tract; lymphoma$_g$; sarcoma)
10. Phyllodes tumor (formerly cystosarcoma phyllodes; giant fibroadenoma)
11. Pseudoangiomatous stromal hyperplasia (PASH)
12. Sarcoma of breast (eg, angiosarcoma)
*13. [Silicone globule or implant artifact]

* May be multiple.
[ ] This condition does not actually cause the gamuted imaging finding,
but can produce imaging changes that simulate it.

References
1. Burgener FA, Kormano M: Differential Diagnosis in Conventional Radiology. (ed 2) New York: Thieme Medical Publ, 1991, pp 492–494
2. DeParedes ES: Atlas of Film Screen Mammography. (ed 2) Baltimore: Williams & Wilkins, 1992, pp 131–134
3. Dershaw DD (ed): Interventional Breast Procedures. Edinburgh: Churchill Livingstone, 1996
4. Eisenberg RL: Clinical Imaging. An Atlas of Differential Diagnosis. (ed 3) Philadelphia: Lippincott-Raven, 1997, pp 1172–1177

5. Feig SA: Breast masses: Mammographic and sonographic evaluation. Radiol Clin North Am 1992;30:67–92
6. Friedrich M, Sickles EA: Radiologic Diagnosis of Breast Diseases. New York: Springer, 2000
7. Hall FM: Probably benign breast nodules: follow-up of selected cases without initial full problem-solving imaging. Radiology 1995;194:305
8. Jackson VP: Management of solid breast nodules: what is the role of sonography? Radiology 1995;196:14–15
9. Kopans DB: Breast Imaging. (ed 2) Philadelphia: Lippincott-Raven, 1998
10. Powell DE, Stelling CB: The Diagnosis and Detection of Breast Disease. Stromal, vascular, hematolymphoid, and metastatic breast lesions. St. Louis: Mosby-Year Book, Inc., 1994, pp 344–353
11. Sickles EA: Periodic mammographic following of probably benign lesions: results in 3,184 consecutive cases. Radiology 1991;179:463–468
12. Sickles EA: Non-palpable, circumscribed non-calcified solid breast masses: likelihood of malignancy based on lesion size and age of patient. Radiology 1994;192:439–432
13. Stavros AT, Thickman D, Rapp CL, et al: Solid breast nodules: use of sonography to distinguish between benign and malignant lesions. Radiology 1995;196:123–124
14. Stavros A: Breast Ultrasound. Philadelphia: Lippincott-Williams & Wilkins, 2002
15. Tabar L, Dean PB: Teaching Atlas of Mammography. (ed 3) New York: Thieme, 2000
16. Tavassoli FA: Pathology of the Breast. (ed 2) New York: McGraw-Hill, 1999

Gamut I-3

HALO SIGN OR CAPSULE AROUND THE PERIPHERY OF A BREAST LESION

COMMON

1. Benign well-circumscribed mass esp. cyst; fibroadenoma; fibrocystic change (solid nodule); sebaceous cyst (contiguous with skin); nipple out of profile

RARE

1. Carcinoma (intracystic, papillary, or arising in or near a fibroadenoma) (rarely holds up on magnification views)

References
1. Kopans, DB: Analyzing the Mammogram: Breast Imaging (ed 2). Philadelphia: Lippincott, 1988, pp 279–330
2. Lane EJ, Proto AV, Phillips TW: Mach bands and density perception. Radiology 1976;121:9–17

Gamut I-4

POORLY DEFINED OR IRREGULARLY MARGINATED LESION OF THE BREAST

COMMON

*1. Carcinoma (esp. scirrhous; invasive ductal; invasive lobular; medullary; mucinous; papillary)
*2. Fat necrosis (traumatic; postsurgical; postbiopsy scar; idiopathic)
*3. Fibrocystic change (esp. sclerosing adenosis)
 4. [Superimposed densities or summation shadows creating a "pseudomass"]

UNCOMMON

*1. Abscess, acute or chronic
 2. Complicated cyst (hemorrhagic, inspissated, or infected)
*3. Fibroadenoma (hyalinized)
*4. Fibromatosis (extra-abdominal desmoid)
 5. Foreign body granuloma (eg, suture)
*6. Granular cell myoblastoma
 7. Hematoma
 8. Lymphoma$_g$
 9. Plasma cell mastitis
*10. Radial scar (complex sclerosing lesion)
 11. Sarcoma
 12. Tuberculosis; fungus disease; nocardiosis

*May present as a spiculated lesion.
[ ] This condition does not actually cause the gamuted imaging finding, but can produce imaging changes that simulate it.

References
1. Bassett LW, Cove HC: Myoblastoma of the breast. Am J Roentgenol 1979;132:122
2. DeParedes ES: Atlas of Film-Screen Mammography. (ed 2) Baltimore: Williams & Wilkins, 1992, pp 233–236

3. Dershaw DD (ed): Interventional Breast Procedures. Edinburgh: Churchill Livingstone, 1996
4. Eisenberg RL: Clinical Imaging. An Atlas of Differential Diagnosis. (ed 3) Philadelphia: Lippincott-Raven, 1997, pp 1178–1181
5. Feig SA: Breast masses: Mammographic and sonographic evaluation. Radiol Clin North Am 1992;30:67–92
6. Friedrich M, Sickles EA: Radiologic Diagnosis of Breast Diseases. New York: Springer, 2000
7. Jackson VP: Management of solid breast nodules: what is the role of sonography? Radiology 1995;196:14–15
8. Kopans DB: Breast Imaging. (ed 2) Philadelphia: Lippincott-Raven, 1998
9. Powell DE, Stelling CB: The Diagnosis and Detection of Breast Disease. Stromal, vascular, hematolymphoid, and metastatic breast lesions. St. Louis: Mosby-Year Book, Inc., 1994, pp 344–353
10. Stavros AT, Thickman D, Rapp CL, et al: Solid breast nodules: use of sonography to distinguish between benign and malignant lesions. Radiology 1995;196:123–124
11. Stavros A: Breast Ultrasound. Philadelphia: Lippincott-Williams & Wilkins, 2002
12. Tabar L, Dean PB: Teaching Atlas of Mammography. (ed 3) New York: Thieme, 2000
13. Tavassoli FA: Pathology of the Breast. (ed 2) New York: McGraw-Hill, 1999
14. Wolverton DE, Sickles EA: Clinical outcome of doubtful mammographic findings. AJR 1996;167:1041–1045

Gamut I-5

SPICULATED LESION OF THE BREAST (INCLUDING STELLATE LESION)

COMMON

1. Carcinoma (esp. scirrhous infiltrating ductal; also tubular, invasive lobular, intraductal)
2. Fat necrosis (traumatic; postsurgical; postbiopsy scar; idiopathic)
*3. Radial scar (sclerosing duct hyperplasia; complex sclerosing lesion; indurative mastopathy)
4. Scarring (posttraumatic; postoperative)
5. [Summation shadows]

UNCOMMON

1. Abscess (occasionally)
2. Fibroadenoma, hyalinized with fibrosis and myxoid degeneration

3. Fibrocystic change (esp. sclerosing adenosis)
4. Fibromatosis (extra-abdominal desmoid)
5. Granular cell myoblastoma

*Associated carcinoma of breast is present in about 25% of radial scars (20% in situ, 5% invasive carcinoma).

[ ] This condition does not actually cause the gamuted imaging finding, but can produce imaging changes that simulate it.

References

1. Bassett LW, Cove HC: Myoblastoma of the breast. Am J Roentgenol 1979;132:122
2. DeParedes ES: Atlas of Film-Screen Mammography. (ed 2) Baltimore, Williams & Wilkins, 1992, pp 233–236
3. Dershaw DD (ed): Interventional Breast Procedures. Edinburgh: Churchill Livingstone, 1996
4. Eisenberg RL: Clinical Imaging. An Atlas of Differential Diagnosis. (ed 3) Philadelphia: Lippincott-Raven, 1997, pp 1178–1181
5. Feig SA: Breast masses: Mammographic and sonographic evaluation. Radiol Clin North Am 1992;30:67–92
6. Friedrich M, Sickles EA: Radiologic Diagnosis of Breast Diseases. New York: Springer, 2000
7. Kopans DB: Breast Imaging, ed 2. Philadelphia: Lippincott-Raven, 1998
8. Powell DE, Stelling CB: The Diagnosis and Detection of Breast Disease. Stromal, vascular, hematolymphoid, and metastatic breast lesions. St. Louis: Mosby-Year Book, Inc., 1994, pp 344–353
9. Stavros A: Breast Ultrasound. Philadelphia: Lippincott-Williams & Wilkins, 2002
10. Tabar L, Dean PB: Teaching Atlas of Mammography. (ed 3) New York: Thieme, 2000
11. Tavassoli FA: Pathology of the Breast. (ed 2) New York: McGraw-Hill, 1999
12. Wolverton DE, Sickles EA: Clinical outcome of doubtful mammographic findings. AJR 1996;167:1041–1045
13. Bassett LW, Jackson VP, Jahan R, Fu YS, Gold RH: Diagnosis of Diseases of the Breast. Invasive Malignancies in Breast Disease. Philadelphia: Saunders, 1997, pp 461–500

Gamut I-6

BREAST LESION CONTAINING FAT

COMMON

1. Intramammary lymph node
2. Lipoma

3. Normal fat lobule
4. Oil or lipid cyst (posttraumatic or postsurgical fat necrosis)
5. Radial scar (central lucency)

UNCOMMON

1. Fibroadenolipoma (hamartoma)
2. Galactocele
3. Hematoma, acute (fat-fluid level)
4. Liposarcoma
5. Steatocystoma (simple or complex)

References
1. Bassett LW, Cove HC: Myoblastoma of the breast. Am J Roentgenol 1979;132:122
2. DeParedes ES: Atlas of Film-Screen Mammography. (ed 2) Baltimore: Williams & Wilkins, 1992, pp 233–236
3. Dershaw DD (ed): Interventional Breast Procedures. Edinburgh: Churchill Livingstone, 1996
4. Eisenberg RL: Clinical Imaging. An Atlas of Differential Diagnosis. (ed 3) Philadelphia: Lippincott-Raven, 1997, pp 1178–1181
5. Feig SA: Breast masses: Mammographic and sonographic evaluation. Radiol Clin North Am 1992;30:67–92
6. Friedrich M, Sickles EA: Radiologic Diagnosis of Breast Diseases. New York: Springer, 2000
7. Hoeffken W, Lanyi M: Mammography. Transl by Rigler LG, et al. Philadelphia: WB Saunders, 1977
8. Jackson VP: Management of solid breast nodules: what is the role of sonography? Radiology 1995;196:14–15
9. Kopans DB: Breast Imaging: Analyzing the Mammogram, Calcified fat necrosis and cysts. New York: JB Lippincott Co., 1989, p 81
10. Kopans DB: Breast Imaging. (ed 2) Philadelphia: Lippincott-Raven, 1998
11. Magid ML, Wentzell JM, Roenigk HM: Multiple cystic lesions: Steatocystoma multiplex. Arch Dermatol 1990;26: 101–102
12. Powell DE, Stelling CB: The Diagnosis and Detection of Breast Disease. Stromal, vascular, hematolymphoid, and metastatic breast lesions. St. Louis: Mosby-Year Book, Inc., 1994, pp 344–353
13. Stavros AT, Thickman D, Rapp CL, et al: Solid breast nodules: use of sonography to distinguish between benign and malignant lesions. Radiology 1995;196:123–124
14. Stavros A: Breast Ultrasound. Philadelphia: Lippincott-Williams & Wilkins, 2002
15. Tabar L, Dean PB: Teaching Atlas of Mammography. (ed 3) New York: Thieme, 2000
16. Tavassoli FA: Pathology of the Breast. (ed 2) New York: McGraw-Hill, 1999

Gamut I-7-1

BREAST CALCIFICATIONS—COARSE

COMMON

1. Carcinoma with central necrosis
2. Fat necrosis (traumatic; postsurgical; postbiopsy scar; idiopathic)
3. Fibroadenoma (bizarre or popcorn-like calcifications)

UNCOMMON

1. Granulomatous disease (tuberculosis and fungus disease, usually in axillary lymph nodes)
2. Renal osteodystrophy (secondary hyperparathyroidism); hypercalcemia

Reference
1. See References listed under I-7-6

Gamut I-7-2

BREAST CALCIFICATIONS— SEMICIRCULAR, CIRCULAR, OR EGGSHELL

COMMON

1. Calcified sebaceous gland cysts; other skin lesions
2. Fibroadenoma
3. Oil or lipid cyst (posttraumatic or postsurgical fat necrosis)

UNCOMMON

1. Galactocele (in capsule)
2. Lipoma with fat necrosis
3. Liponecrosis microcystica calcificans (subcutaneous fat necrosis)
4. Panniculitis nodularis, nonsuppurative (Weber-Christian disease)
5. Papilloma

6. Plasma cell mastitis* (periductal mastitis; also known as secretory disease)
7. Postradiation therapy (dystrophic round or ring-like calcifications)
8. Silicone globules

* May occasionally show dense, regular, elongated, linear or branching intraductal calcifications as well as more common large, smooth, dense, round, or oval calcifications.

Reference
1. See References listed under I-7-6

Gamut I-7-3

BREAST CALCIFICATIONS— LOBULAR (HOMOGENEOUS, SOLID, WELL-DEFINED, SPHERULES OR PEARLS IN DILATED DUCTULES AND LOBULES)

1. Atypical lobular hyperplasia
2. Blunt duct adenosis
3. Fibrocystic change (esp. sclerosing adenosis) with "milk of calcium" crystals in cyst fluid

Reference
1. See References listed under I-7-6

Gamut I-7-4

BREAST CALCIFICATIONS—LINEAR

COMMON
1. Arterial (Mönckeberg's medial sclerosis and athero-sclerosis)
2. Carcinoma (intraductal)
3. Fibrocystic change with "milk of calcium" crystals in cyst fluid

*4. Plasma cell mastitis (periductal mastitis; secretory disease)

UNCOMMON
1. Parasites (*Loa Loa; Dracunculus medinensis* (guinea worm) (serpiginous outline in subcutaneous tissues of breast)

* May occasionally show dense, regular, elongated, linear or branching intraductal calcifications as well as more common large, smooth, dense, round, or oval calcifications.

Reference
1. See References listed under I-7-6

Gamut I-7-5

BREAST CALCIFICATIONS— MICROCALCIFICATIONS LOCALIZED INTO GROUPS

1. Carcinoma, intraductal (may present as (a) casts of the ductal lumen, or as (b) tiny granular, dot-like or elongated, multiple, irregularly grouped microcalcifications very close together)
2. Carcinoma (lobular in situ)
3. Early calcification within a fibroadenoma or artery
4. Fibrocystic change (sclerosing adenosis)
5. Papilloma; papillomatosis (intraductal)
6. Scar calcification

Reference
1. See References listed under I-7-6

Gamut I-7-6

BREAST CALCIFICATIONS—DIFFUSE SCATTERED MICROCALCIFICATIONS

1. [Artifacts or pseudocalcifications from powders, creams, ointments, or deodorants on skin surface of breast or axilla]
2. Atrophic
3. Carcinoma (intraductal or multicentric lobular)
4. Fibrocystic change (esp. sclerosing adenosis)
5. Involutional glandular
6. Plasma cell mastitis* (secretory disease; periductal mastitis; ductal ectasia)

*May occasionally show dense, regular, elongated, linear or branching intraductal calcifications as well as more common large, smooth, dense, round or oval calcifications.

[ ] This condition does not actually cause the gamuted imaging finding, but can produce imaging changes that simulate it.

References

1. Bassett, LW: Mammographic analysis of calcifications. Radiol Clin North Am 1992;30:93–105
2. Burgener FA, Kormano M: Differential Diagnosis in Conventional Radiology. (ed 2) New York: Thieme Medical Publ, 1991, pp 498–499
3. DeParedes ES: Atlas of Film-Screen Mammography. (ed 2) Baltimore: Williams & Wilkins, 1992, pp 299–303
4. Dershaw DD (ed): Interventional Breast Procedures. Edinburgh: Churchill Livingstone, 1996
5. Eisenberg RL: Clinical Imaging. An Atlas of Differential Diagnosis. (ed 3) Philadelphia: Lippincott-Raven, 1997, pp 1182–1187, 1996
6. Friedrich M, Sickles EA: Radiologic Diagnosis of Breast Diseases. New York: Springer, 2000
7. Kopans DB: Breast Imaging. (ed 2) Philadelphia: Lippincott-Raven, 1998
8. Lanyi M: Differential Diagnosis of Microcalcifications. In: Friedrich M, Sickles EA (eds): Radiological Diagnosis of Breast Diseases. New York: Springer, 2000
9. Sickles EA: Breast calcification: Mammographic evaluation. Radiology 1986;160:289–293
10. Stomper PC, Connolly JL: Ductal carcinoma of the breast: correlation between mammographic calcification & tumor subtype. AJR 1992;159:483–485
11. Tabar L, Dean PB: Teaching Atlas of Mammography. (ed 3) New York: Thieme, 2000
12. Tavassoli FA: Pathology of the Breast. (ed 2) New York: McGraw-Hill, 1999

Gamut I-8

PROMINENT (DENSE) DUCTAL PATTERN ON MAMMOGRAPHY

COMMON

1. Carcinoma (intraductal)
2. [Dense breast]
3. Ductal ectasia; periductal inflammation and fibrosis
4. Lactation
5. Papilloma (solitary or multiple, intraductal)
6. Papillomatosis (intraductal)

UNCOMMON

1. Ductal adenoma
2. Ductal hyperplasia

[ ] This condition does not actually cause the gamuted imaging finding, but can produce imaging changes that simulate it.

References

1. DeParedes ES: Atlas of Film-Screen Mammography (ed 2). Baltimore: Williams & Wilkins, 1992, pp 417–418
2. Friedrich M, Sickles EA: Radiologic Diagnosis of Breast Diseases. New York: Springer, 2000
3. Kopans DB: Breast Imaging. (ed 2) Philadelphia: Lippincott-Raven, 1998
4. Tabar L, Dean PB: Teaching Atlas of Mammography. (ed 3) New York: Thieme, 2000
5. Tavassoli FA: Pathology of the Breast. (ed 2) New York: McGraw-Hill, 1999

Gamut I-9

DIFFUSE BREAST CHANGES

COMMON

1. Carcinoma, "inflammatory" or diffuse spread within breast
2. Fibrocystic change
3. Hormone replacement therapy
4. Lymphatic obstruction (eg, postsurgical or secondary to infiltrating neoplasm or lymph node metastases)
5. Mastitis, extensive acute

6. Postoperative; multiple biopsies
7. Radiation therapy
8. Silicone injection (direct); prosthesis or implant surgery

UNCOMMON
1. Edema (eg, heart, liver, or kidney failure)
2. Fibroliposarcoma
3. Filariasis (with lymphedema)
4. Hemorrhage
5. Lymphoma$_g$
6. Tuberculosis, fungus disease, or nocardiosis (diffuse)

References
1. DeParedes ES: Atlas of Film-Screen Mammography (ed 2). Baltimore: Williams & Wilkins, 1992
2. Friedrich M, Sickles EA: Radiologic Diagnosis of Breast Diseases. New York: Springer, 2000
3. Hoeffken W, Lanyi M: Mammography. Transl by Rigler LG, et al. Philadelphia: WB Saunders, 1977, p 275
4. Kopans DB: Breast Imaging. (ed 2) Philadelphia: Lippincott-Raven, 1998
5. Stavros A: Breast Ultrasound. Philadelphia: Lippincott-Williams & Wilkins, 2002
6. Tabar L, Dean PB: Teaching Atlas of Mammography. (ed 3) New York: Thieme, 2000
7. Tavassoli FA: Pathology of the Breast. (ed 2) New York: Mc-Graw-Hill, 1999

6. Postoperative (recent); postbiopsy; reduction mammoplasty
7. Radiation therapy

UNCOMMON
1. Abscess (esp. retromammillary)
2. Burn
3. Fat necrosis and interstitial hematoma (incl. Coumadin therapy)
4. Insect bite (usually spider)
5. Lymphoma$_g$
6. Metastatic disease to breast (esp. from opposite breast)
7. Pachydermoperiostosis

References
1. DeParedes ES: Atlas of Film-Screen Mammography (ed 2). Baltimore: Williams & Wilkins, 1992, p 451
2. Friedrich M, Sickles EA: Radiologic Diagnosis of Breast Diseases. New York: Springer, 2000
3. Hoeffken W, Lanyi M: Mammography. Transl by Rigler LG, et al. Philadelphia: WB Saunders, 1977
4. Kopans DB: Breast Imaging. (ed 2) Philadelphia: Lippincott-Raven, 1998
5. Tabar L, Dean PB: Teaching Atlas of Mammography. (ed 3) New York: Thieme, 2000
6. Tavassoli FA: Pathology of the Breast. (ed 2) New York: Mc-Graw-Hill, 1999

Gamut I-10

SKIN THICKENING OVER THE BREAST

COMMON
1. Carcinoma, esp. scirrhous (locally advanced with focal skin thickening, or recurrent after lumpectomy and radiation therapy)
2. Fluid overload, systemic (eg, heart failure; renal failure; anasarca hypoalbuminemia; cirrhosis)
3. "Inflammatory" carcinoma (neoplastic lymphatic obstruction)
4. Lymphatic obstruction (eg, following axillary node dissection or secondary to axillary or mediastinal nodal metastases from breast or other primary malignancy)
5. Mastitis (incl. bacterial, fungal, tuberculous, filarial infection)

Gamut I-11-S

LESIONS OR ARTIFACTS THAT CAN MIMIC A TRUE BREAST LESION

1. Fat necrosis (oil or lipid cyst, posttraumatic or post-surgical)
2. Film or screen artifacts (scratches; fingerprints)
3. Foreign substance on skin surface (eg, medicinal ointment; bandage; axillary deodorant)
4. Lymph nodes (in axilla, axillary tail of breast, or intramammary)
5. Lymphedema (eg, obstruction of lymph drainage from metastases or surgery; heart failure)
6. Nipple out of profile; retracted nipple

7. Postbiopsy scar
8. Silicone injection
9. Skin calcifications
10. Skin lesion (eg, wart; mole; neurofibroma; sebaceous or epidermal inclusion cyst)
11. Superimposition of fibroglandular breast tissue

Gamut I-12

GYNECOMASTIA

PHYSIOLOGICAL

*1. Idiopathic
2. Neonatal (high placental estrogens)
3. Pubertal (excess of estradiol over testosterone)
*4. Senile (falling androgen and rising estrogen levels with age)

PHARMACOLOGICAL

1. Anti-androgens (eg, spironolactone)
2. Antidepressants, tricyclic
*3. Chemotherapy drugs (producing testicular damage)
4. Digitalis (binds to estrogen receptors)
*5. Estrogen (esp. in prostate cancer treatment)
6. Methyldopa
7. Phenothiazines
8. Reserpine

PATHOLOGICAL

1. Bronchogenic carcinoma (secreting HCG)
2. Cirrhosis (increased conversion of androgens to estrogens)
3. Estrogen secreting tumor (eg, adrenal tumor; Leydig cell tumor)
4. Hyperthyroidism
*5. Hypogonadism (eg, castration; Klinefelter S. {XXY S.})
6. Hypopituitarism (incl. acromegaly)
7. Hypothyroidism, esp. infantile (cretinism)
8. Testicular feminization (androgen insensitivity)
9. Testicular tumor (eg, teratoma secreting HCG)

SYNDROMES

1. Cowden S. (multiple hamartoma S.)
2. Gorlin S. (nevoid basal cell carcinoma S.)
3. Paraneoplastic syndromes

*Common.

References

1. Bassett LW, Jackson VP, Jahan R, Fu YS, Gold RH: The Male Breast. In: Diagnosis of Diseases of the Breast. Philadelphia: WB Saunders, 1997, pp 501–518
2. Kopans DB: The male breast. In: Breast Imaging. New York: JB Lippincott Co., 1989, p 342
3. Kopans DB: Breast Imaging. (ed 2) Philadelphia: Lippincott-Raven, 1998, p. 378

Gamut I-13

ANECHOIC BREAST LESIONS ON ULTRASOUND

COMMON

1. Cyst (simple)
2. [Ultrasound equipment, malfunctioning or with very incorrect settings]

UNCOMMON

1. Fibroadenoma (rarely)
2. Lymphoma$_g$; leukemia

[ ] This condition does not actually cause the gamuted imaging finding, but can produce imaging changes that simulate it.

References

1. Friedrich M, Sickles EA: Radiologic Diagnosis of Breast Diseases. New York: Springer, 2000
2. Jackson VP: Management of solid breast nodules: what is the role of sonography? Radiology 1995;196:14–15
3. Kopans DB: Breast Imaging. (ed 2) Philadelphia: Lippincott-Raven, 1998
4. Powell DE, Stelling CB: The Diagnosis and Detection of Breast Disease. St. Louis: Mosby-Year Book, Inc., 1994, p 8
5. Smathers RL: Personal communication.
6. Stavros AT, Thickman D, Rapp CL, et al: Solid breast nodules: use of sonography to distinguish between benign and malignant lesions. Radiology 1995;196:123–124
7. Stavros A: Breast Ultrasound. Philadelphia: Lippincott-Williams & Wilkins, 2002

Gamut I-14

HYPOECHOIC BREAST LESIONS ON ULTRASOUND

COMMON

1. Abscess
2. Carcinoma
3. Cyst, complicated (proteinaceous; punctured by partial needle aspiration; inflammatory; infected; mildly hemorrhagic)
4. Fibroadenoma
5. Fibrocystic change
6. Intramammary lymph node
7. Papilloma
8. Sebaceous cyst

UNCOMMON

1. Keratinaceous cyst
2. Lactational adenoma
3. Lymphoma$_g$; leukemia
4. Phyllodes tumor (formerly cystosarcoma phyllodes; giant fibroadenoma)
5. Pseudoangiomatous stromal hyperplasia
6. Steatocystoma (simple or complex)
7. Superficial thrombophlebitis (Mondor's disease)
8. Tubular adenoma

References
1. Friedrich M, Sickles EA: Radiologic Diagnosis of Breast Diseases. New York: Springer, 2000
2. Jackson VP: Management of solid breast nodules: what is the role of sonography? Radiology 1995;196:14–15
3. Kopans DB: Breast Imaging. (ed 2) Philadelphia: Lippincott-Raven, 1998
4. Powell DE, Stelling CB: The Diagnosis and Detection of Breast Disease. St. Louis: Mosby-Year Book, Inc., 1994, p 8
5. Smathers RL: Personal communication.
6. Stavros AT, Thickman D, Rapp CL, et al: Solid breast nodules: use of sonography to distinguish between benign and malignant lesions. Radiology 1995;196:123–124
7. Stavros A: Breast Ultrasound. Philadelphia: Lippincott-Williams & Wilkins, 2002

Gamut I-15

HYPERECHOIC OR MIXED ECHOGENICITY BREAST LESIONS ON ULTRASOUND

COMMON

1. Carcinoma (calcified)
2. Fat necrosis (traumatic; postsurgical; postbiopsy scar; idiopathic)
3. Fibroadenoma (calcified)
4. [Metallic or other artifact; biopsy marker; foreign body]
5. "Milk of calcium" crystals in cyst fluid (dependent crystal layer in hyperechoic)
6. Scarring with or without scar calcification
7. Silicone extravasation (leakage or rupture)

UNCOMMON

1. Lipoma
2. Cyst, complex (inspissate, hemorrhagic)

[ ] This condition does not actually cause the gamuted imaging finding, but can produce imaging changes that simulate it.

References
1. Friedrich M, Sickles EA: Radiologic Diagnosis of Breast Diseases. New York: Springer, 2000
2. Jackson VP: Management of solid breast nodules: what is the role of sonography? Radiology 1995;196:14–15
3. Kopans DB: Breast Imaging. (ed 2) Philadelphia: Lippincott-Raven, 1998
4. Powell DE, Stelling CB: The Diagnosis and Detection of Breast Disease. St. Louis: Mosby-Year Book, Inc., 1994, p 8
5. Smathers RL: Personal communication.
6. Stavros AT, Thickman D, Rapp CL, et al: Solid breast nodules: use of sonography to distinguish between benign and malignant lesions. Radiology 1995;196:123–124
7. Stavros A: Breast Ultrasound. Philadelphia: Lippincott-Williams & Wilkins, 2002

Gamut I-16

AXILLARY LYMPHADENOPATHY SEEN ON MAMMOGRAPHY (USUALLY ON MLO VIEW)

COMMON
1. Dermatopathic (psoriasis; rheumatoid arthritis)
2. Lymphoma$_g$; leukemia
3. Metastatic disease from breast primary
4. Tuberculosis or fungus disease (may calcify)

UNCOMMON
1. Metastatic disease, other (eg, from melanoma; carcinoma of lung or ovary)

Reference
1. Smathers RL: Mammography Diagnosis and Intervention CD-ROM. Moraga, CA: Medical Interactive, 1995

Gamut I-17

ASYMMETRY OF PECTORALIS MUSCLE ON MAMMOGRAPH (USUALLY ON MLO VIEW)

1. Inadequate or improper positioning
2. Muscular dystrophy
3. Normal variant
4. Poland syndrome (pectoral muscle aplasia-syndactyly)
5. Poliomyelitis
6. Prior surgery injuring pectoralis with atrophy (eg, multiple difficult implant placements and removals with or without silicone extravasation)
7. Stroke
8. Trauma (esp. in childhood)

Reference
1. Smathers RL: Mammography Diagnosis and Intervention CD-ROM. Moraga, CA: Medical Interactive, 1995

Gamut I-18-S

MAMMOGRAPHY MISTAKES AND PITFALLS FOR RADIOLOGISTS AND PHYSICIANS

1. Reading mammograms under poor viewing conditions:
   a. With any room light reflected off films (overhead lights, lamps, hallway, other viewboxes)
   b. Without large, good quality magnifier
   c. With regular viewbox or dim light source (strong light source needed for mammogram reading)
2. Assuming a lesion is benign (especially a nodule) based on screening films only without proper workup (eg, magnification views or ultrasound).
3. Recommendation for biopsy of benign milk of calcium crystals due to failure to perform true lateral views or magnification views.
4. Mistaking a hypoechoic mass for an anechoic cyst on ultrasound. Many solid lesions including carcinomas can appear as hypoechoic masses with acoustic enhancement.
5. Failure to recommend biopsy for a carcinoma because it was thought to be a benign radial scar.
6. Incomplete or inaccurate assessment of a palpable lesion due to failure to correlate the palpable area with the imaging findings (esp. during ultrasound).
7. Failure to recognize microcalcification pattern of DCIS when there is no associated mass density.
8. Calling a patient back or recommending biopsy for the muscle shadow sometimes seen medially on the CC view (sternalis muscle or medial extension of the pectoralis muscle).
9. Correct assessment of the margins of a nodule or mass as poorly circumscribed, circumscribed, or well circumscribed. Also halo versus moat distinction.
10. Failure to do an axillary view for abnormal lymph nodes during diagnostic workup of a probable carcinoma in the breast.
11. Recommend unnecessary workup or biopsy due to failure to recognize benign axillary or intramammary lymph node characteristics.
12. Failure to make diagnosis of lymphadenopathy due to not looking in axillary region or not recognizing signs of lymph node abnormalities.
13. Failure to spot an early breast cancer developing when

multiple bilateral lesions are present (nodules, calcification clusters, or both).

14. Recommending unnecessary biopsy of post-traumatic or postbiopsy fat necrosis.
15. Attempting to biopsy dermal calcifications due to failure to obtain tangential views.
16. Leaving the tip of the localization wire short or proximal to the lesion due to bad positioning or use of a needle that is insufficiently long.
17. Calling a patient back or recommending biopsy of a lesion which appears to show an interval change on comparison to one prior mammogram when review of older mammograms show the lesion is actually unchanged for years.
18. Recommending biopsy of a complicated cyst because the gauge of the needle used for aspiration was too small and no fluid was drained. Some complicated cysts require an 18 gauge needle and a 10 cc syringe to aspirate thick or inspissated fluid, mucin, or grummous contents.
19. False ultrasound diagnosis of a hypoechoic lesion in the retroareolar region due to shadowing caused by the skin of the nipple and areola.
20. Absent, vague, or indecisive recommendation in written report leading to failure or delay of patient or physician to proceed to the next appropriate procedure. One common example is the ultrasound report which ends with just the impression "complicated cyst" without giving a specific recommendation such as biopsy or aspiration.
21. Failure to call a patient back or recommend biopsy of a lesion which appears to be stable on comparison to prior mammograms over a less than 3 year interval when it is actually an indolent carcinoma (esp. DCIS).
22. Calling a patient back or recommending biopsy for a false microcalcification cluster due to a fingerprint or scratch artifact.
23. Failure to notice unilateral diffuse increase in breast density due to widespread malignancy such as inflammatory carcinoma.
24. Interventional biopsy of the wrong lesion due to the presence of multiple lesions. This most often occurs when a partial field preliminary view is done which happens to make a second area look like the area of concern when actually the area of concern is outside the field of view.

Reference
1. Smathers RL: Mammography Diagnosis and Intervention CD-ROM. Moraga, CA: Medical Interactive, 1995

2. Smathers RL: Mammography for Technologists. CD-ROM. Moraga, CA: Medical Interactive, 2000

Gamut I-19-S

MAMMOGRAPHY MISTAKES AND PITFALLS FOR TECHNOLOGISTS

1. Films too light due to technique or poor compression.
2. Doing routine screening without carefully reviewing images before letting patient leave. This is especially true for mammography certified technologists (R.T.(M)) whose special training allows them to aid in the detection of breast cancer.
3. Failure to mark skin mote or other skin lesion leading to callback of the patient for workup of possible breast nodule.
4. Failure to mark the site of scars on the patient history sheet and/or on the skin leading to unnecessary patient recall.
5. Failure to obtain nipple profile view when nipple not profiled on either CC or MLO view.
6. Failure to do at least one magnification view for possible microcalcification cluster.
7. Poor or no visualization of the pectoralis muscle on the MLO view indicating failure to adequately show the upper outer quadrant and axillary region.
8. Exclusion of posterior breast tissue due to poor positioning (inadequate posterior nipple line distance).
9. Failure to do spot compression view for possible architectural distortion in dense tissue.
10. Failure to notice and correct artifacts on screens which can simulate microcalcification clusters.
11. Failure to show a lesion located near the skin (esp. within 1 cm of the skin) with ultrasound. Good imaging of nearfield lesions often needs special focusing, or the use of an offset pad or waterbath attachment.
12. Adding excessive fluid or failing to drain excessive fluid from breast biopsy specimens (esp. core biopsies) prior to specimen radiography.

Reference
1. Smathers RL: Mammography Diagnosis and Intervention CD-ROM. Moraga, CA: Medical Interactive, 1995
2. Smathers RL: Mammography for Technologists. CD-ROM. Moraga, CA: Medical Interactive, 2000

Multiple Systems: Miscellaneous

J

A LISTING OF DISEASES COMMON TO THE TROPICS AND DEVELOPING COUNTRIES BASED ON THE BODY SYSTEM AND ORGAN INVOLVED*

ABNORMALITIES OF THE ALIMENTARY TRACT

Esophagus
1. Chagas' disease (megaesophagus)
2. Fungus diseases (esp. candidiasis)
3. Malignant disease (esp. carcinoma)
4. Schistosomiasis (varices)
5. Tuberculosis
6. Other (eg, corrosive strictures; achalasia; hiatus hernia)

Stomach
1. Anisakiasis
2. Ascariasis
3. Fungus diseases (esp. candidiasis)
4. Malignant disease (incl. carcinoma; Burkitt's lymphoma; Kaposi sarcoma)
5. Schistosomiasis
6. Strongyloidiasis
7. Tuberculosis
8. Other (eg, peptic ulcer disease; gastric outlet obstruction; hiatus hernia)

Duodenum and Small Bowel
1. Amebiasis
2. Anisakiasis
3. Angiostrongyliasis costaricensis
4. Ascariasis
5. Chagas' disease
6. Fungus diseases (esp. candidiasis; histoplasmosis)
7. Giardiasis
8. Hookworm disease
9. Intestinal capillariasis
10. Kwashiorkor; malnutrition

11. Malignant disease (incl. carcinoma; lymphoma$_g$; Burkitt's lymphoma, Kaposi sarcoma)
12. *Salmonella* infections
13. Schistosomiasis
14. Strongyloidiasis
15. Taeniasis saginata (beef tapeworm)
16. Tropical sprue
17. Tuberculosis
18. Typhoid and paratyphoid fever
19. Other (eg, intestinal obstruction; intussusception; small bowel volvulus, hernia; obstructed hernia)

Colon
1. Amebiasis
2. Angiostrongyliasis costaricensis
3. Ascariasis
4. Bacillary dysentery (shigellosis)
5. Chagas' disease (megacolon)
6. Fungus diseases; actinomycosis
7. Helminthoma
8. Lymphogranuloma venereum
9. Malignant disease (esp. carcinoma)
10. *Salmonella* infections
11. Schistosomiasis
12. Strongyloidiasis
13. Trichuriasis
14. Tuberculosis
15. Other (eg, intestinal obstruction; intussusception; sigmoid volvulus; hernia; obstructed hernia; polyps)

Rectum and Anus
1. Amebiasis
2. Bacillary dysentery (shigellosis)
3. Chagas' disease
4. Lymphogranuloma venereum
5. Malignant disease (esp. carcinoma)
6. Schistosomiasis
7. Trichuriasis
8. Tuberculosis
9. Other (eg, hemorrhoids; fissures; strictures; recto-vaginal fistulae)

(continued)

Liver

1. Amebiasis
2. Ascariasis
3. Clonorchiasis; opisthorchiasis; fascioliasis
4. Fungus diseases (esp. histoplasmosis); actinomycosis
5. Hydatid disease
6. Kala-azar
7. Kwashiorkor
8. Malignant disease (esp. hepatoma; cholangio-carcinoma; Burkitt's lymphoma)
9. Pentastomiasis (*Armillifer* infection)
10. Schistosomiasis
11. Toxoplasmosis
12. Tuberculosis
13. Other (eg, cirrhosis; portal hypertension)

Gallbladder and Biliary Tract

1. Ascariasis
2. Biliary calculi (esp. in hemoglobinopathies)
3. Clonorchiasis; opisthorchiasis; fascioliasis
4. Oriental cholangiohepatitis

Jaundice

1. Ascariasis (esp. in children)
2. Calculi
3. Cirrhosis
4. Clonorchiasis; opisthorchiasis; fascioliasis
5. Hydatid disease
6. Oriental cholangiohepatitis

Spleen

1. Hemoglobinopathies (esp. sickle cell disease; thalassemia)
2. Hydatid disease
3. Kala-azar
4. Malaria
5. Malignant disease (esp. lymphoma$_g$)
6. Melioidosis
7. Pentastomiasis (*Armillifer* infection)
8. Schistosomiasis
9. Tropical splenic abscess

10. Tropical splenomegaly syndrome
11. Tuberculosis
12. Typhoid and paratyphoid fever

Pancreas

1. Carcinoma
2. Pancreatitis
3. Pancreatic lithiasis

RESPIRATORY TRACT

Nasopharynx, Mouth, Hypopharynx, and Trachea

1. Fungus diseases (esp. zygomycosis; {mucormycosis}; phycomycosis; rhinosporidiosis; rhinoentomophthoromycosis)
2. Malignant disease (eg, postnasal carcinoma; Burkitt's lymphoma)
3. Noma (cancrum oris)
4. Rhinoscleroma
5. Yaws; syphilis

Lungs

1. Amebiasis
2. Ascariasis
3. Capillariasis philippinensis
4. Fungus diseases
5. Gnathostomiasis
6. Hookworm disease
7. Hydatid disease
8. Malaria (pulmonary edema and shock lung)
9. Malignant disease, primary or metastatic carcinoma; Kaposi sarcoma
10. Melioidosis
11. Paragonimiasis
12. Plague
13. *Pneumocystis carinii* pneumonia, cytomegalovirus, and other opportunistic infections (esp. in AIDS)
14. Pentastomiasis (*Armillifer* infection)
15. Schistosomiasis
16. Strongyloidiasis
17. Tropical eosinophilia

18. Tuberculosis; atypical mycobacterial infections
19. Other (eg, bronchiectasis; unusual pneumonias—esp. measles; whooping cough; blackfat lipid pneumonia)

Mediastinum, Pleura, and Chest Wall

1. Amebiasis
2. Cysticercosis
3. Dracunculiasis (guinea worm infection)
4. Fungus diseases; actinomycosis; nocardiosis
5. Hydatid disease
6. Malignant disease (incl. Burkitt's lymphoma; metastatic disease)
7. Melioidosis
8. Paragonimiasis
9. Plague
10. Pentastomiasis (*Armillifer* infection)
11. Tuberculosis; atypical mycobacterial infections
12. Other (eg, rib and pleural lesions)

CARDIOVASCULAR SYSTEM

Heart

1. Amebiasis (pneumopericardium after abscess rupture)
2. Aneurysms (subvalvular or idiopathic aortic)
3. Aortitis, idiopathic
4. Burkitt's lymphoma
5. Cardiomegaly (idiopathic; puerperal)
6. Chagas' disease
7. Cysticercosis
8. Endomyocardial fibrosis (African myocardiopathy)
9. Hemoglobinopathies
10. Hydatid disease
11. Hypertension, systemic or pulmonary (eg, secondary to schistosomiasis)
12. Kwashiorkor; malnutrition
13. Tuberculosis

Pericardial Effusion

1. Amebiasis
2. Hemoglobinopathies
3. Hydatid disease
4. Kaposi sarcoma
5. Malignant disease

6. Rheumatic fever
7. Tuberculosis
8. Viral disease

Aorta, Pulmonary Arteries, Peripheral Arteries and Veins

1. Aneurysms
2. Idiopathic arteritis (Takayasu's disease)
3. Peripheral vascular disease; idiopathic gangrene; varicose veins
4. Pulmonary embolus and infarction
5. Pulmonary hypertension (secondary to schistosomiasis)

GENITOURINARY TRACT

Kidneys

1. Calculi
2. Filariasis (with chyluria)
3. Fungus diseases (esp. candidiasis)
4. Hemoglobinopathies (eg, sickle cell disease with papillary necrosis)
5. Hydatid disease
6. Idiopathic arteritis (Takayasu's disease)
7. Malaria
8. Malignant disease (incl. Burkitt's lymphoma)
9. Schistosomiasis
10. Tuberculosis

Ureters and Bladder

1. Calculi; calcification of ureteral or bladder wall (eg, schistosomiasis; tuberculosis)
2. Fungus diseases$_g$ (esp. candidiasis)
3. Hydatid disease
4. Malignant disease
5. Schistosomiasis
6. Tuberculosis

Urethra, Vagina, Penis, Seminal Vesicles, *and Prostate

1. Amebiasis
2. Filariasis; elephantiasis

(continued)

3. Lymphogranuloma venereum
4. Malignant disease
5. Rectovaginal and vesicovaginal fistulae
6. Schistosomiasis
7. Tuberculosis
8. Urethral strictures

CENTRAL NERVOUS SYSTEM

Brain and Meninges
1. African trypanosomiasis
2. Amebiasis
3. Angiostrongyliasis cantonensis
4. Cysticercosis
5. Fungus diseases (esp. cryptococcosis)
6. Hydatid disease
7. Malaria
8. Malignant disease
9. Neurotrichinosis
10. Paragonimiasis
11. Schistosomiasis
12. Sparganosis
13. Toxoplasmosis, cytomegalovirus, other opportunistic infections (esp. in AIDS)
14. Tuberculosis

Spine, Including Paraplegia
1. Brucellosis
2. Cysticercosis
3. Fungus diseases
4. Hemoglobinopathies
5. Hydatid disease
6. Malignant disease (incl. Burkitt's lymphoma)
7. Schistosomiasis
8. Spondylitis (eg, typhoid; pyogenic)
9. Syphilis
10. Tetanus
11. Tuberculosis

Peripheral Nerves
1. Leprosy

SOFT TISSUES

Soft Tissue Nodules Without Obvious Calcification
1. Dracunculiasis (guinea worm infection)
2. Filariasis (esp. onchocerciasis)
3. Fungus diseases; mycetoma
4. Gnathostomiasis
5. Hydatid disease
6. Kala-azar
7. Leprosy
8. Malignant disease (esp. Burkitt's lymphoma; Kaposi sarcoma)
9. Sparganosis
10. Tropical ulcer
11. Tuberculosis
12. Tumoral calcinosis
13. Yaws; syphilis

Calcifications in the Soft Tissue
1. Cysticercosis
2. Dracunculiasis (guinea worm infection)
3. Filariasis
4. Hydatid disease
5. Kikuyu bursa
6. Loiasis (*Loa loa*)
7. Medicinal injection sites
8. Onchocerciasis
9. Pentastomiasis (*Armillifer* infection)
10. Sarcocystis
11. Tuberculosis (lymph nodes)
12. Tumoral calcinosis

Other Soft Tissue Abnormalities (eg, Edema, Inflammation, Ulceration, Malignancy)
1. Ainhum
2. Amebiasis
3. Cysticercosis
4. Dracunculiasis (guinea worm infection)
5. Filariasis; elephantiasis
6. Fungus diseases; mycetoma
7. Gnathostomiasis
8. Hydatid disease

9. Leprosy
10. Loiasis (*Loa loa*)
11. Lymphogranuloma venereum
12. Malignant disease (eg, Kaposi sarcoma)
13. Melioidosis
14. Noma (cancrum oris)
15. Onchocerciasis
16. Rhinoscleroma
17. Trauma
18. Tropical pyomyositis
19. Tropical ulcer; Buruli ulcer
20. Tumoral calcinosis
21. Yaws; endemic syphilis

Lymphadenopathy (In addition to all the usual "nontropical" diseases, consider the following)

1. Brucellosis
2. Dracunculiasis (guinea worm infection)
3. Filariasis
4. Fungus diseases
5. Kala-azar
6. Leprosy
7. Lymphogranuloma venereum
8. Malignant disease (incl. Burkitt's lymphoma; Kaposi sarcoma)
9. Plague
10. Tuberculosis; atypical mycobacterial infection
11. Yaws

SKELETON

Skull, Facial Bones, and Spine

1. Brucellosis
2. Cysticercosis
3. Fluorosis
4. Fungus diseases; mycetoma
5. Hemoglobinopathies
6. Hydatid disease
7. Leprosy
8. Malignant disease (incl. Burkitt's lymphoma)
9. Noma (cancrum oris)
10. Rhinoscleroma
11. Spondylitis (eg, typhoid; pyogenic)

12. Tetanus
13. Tuberculosis
14. Yaws; endemic syphilis

Long Bones, Hands, and Feet

1. Ainhum
2. Brucellosis
3. Fungus diseases (esp. mycetoma)
4. Hemoglobinopathies
5. Hydatid disease
6. Leprosy
7. Malignant disease (incl. Burkitt's lymphoma; Kaposi sarcoma)
8. Melioidosis
9. Osteomyelitis (eg, salmonella; other pyogenic)
10. Smallpox (residual effects only)
11. Tropical ulcer
12. Tuberculosis
13. Yaws; endemic syphilis
14. Others (eg, anomalies; carpal fusions; congenital hip dislocation; tibia vara)

Arthritis and Other Joint Diseases (Acute, Chronic, Neuropathic)

1. Brucellosis
2. Dracunculiasis (guinea worm infection)
3. Filariasis
4. Fungus diseases
5. Hemoglobinopathies
6. Hydatid disease
7. Leprosy
8. Malignant disease (eg, synovial sarcoma)
9. Smallpox (residual effects only)
10. Tropical "arthritis"
11. Tuberculosis
12. Tumoral calcinosis
13. Yaws; syphilis

* When searching for the differential diagnosis of an abnormal finding on a radiograph of a patient or visitor from the tropics, it will be helpful to consult this list, which refers to the major parasitic, infectious, neoplastic, and other diseases that affect specific organs or systems. When used in conjunction with Gamut J-2, which details the geographic distribution of these diseases, a tentative diagnosis may often be suggested in such a patient.

(continued)

Reference

1. Palmer PES, Reeder MM: The Imaging of Tropical Diseases, with Epidemiological, Pathological and Clinical Correlation. (ed 2) Heidelberg: Springer-Verlag, 2001, pp XIX–XXIV

Gamut J-2-S

GEOGRAPHIC DISTRIBUTION OF TROPICAL INFECTIOUS AND PARASITIC DISEASES*

DISEASES FOUND WORLDWIDE THROUGHOUT THE TROPICS AND OCCASIONALLY IN TEMPERATE ZONES

1. AIDS
2. Amebiasis
3. Ascariasis
4. Bacillary dysentery (shigellosis)
5. Brucellosis
6. Cysticercosis
7. Filarial diseases
8. Fungus diseases
9. Giardiasis
10. Hookworm disease
11. Hydatid disease (more common in temperate zones)
12. Kala-azar
13. Kwashiorkor
14. Leprosy
15. Lymphogranuloma venereum
16. Malaria
17. Plague
18. Pyomyositis
19. Schistosomiasis (Bilharziasis)
20. Strongyloidiasis
21. Taeniasis saginata or solium (tapeworm infection)
22. Tetanus
23. Toxoplasmosis
24. Trichinosis (esp. neurotrichinosis)
25. Trichuriasis (whipworm infection)
26. Tropical myositis
27. Tuberculosis
28. Typhoid and paratyphoid fever
29. Yaws and syphilis

WEST INDIES AND CARIBBEAN
Diseases in Worldwide list, plus
1. Tropical sprue

CENTRAL AMERICA, MEXICO, AND PANAMA
Diseases in Worldwide list, plus
1. Angiostrongyloidiasis costaricensis
2. Chagas' disease
3. Paragonimiasis (rare)
4. Tropical ulcer

SOUTH AMERICA
Diseases in Worldwide list, plus
1. Chagas' disease
2. Melioidosis (rare)
3. Paragonimiasis (rare)
4. Sparganosis

EAST AFRICA, NORTH AFRICA, ARABIA, AND MIDDLE EAST
Diseases in Worldwide list, plus
1. Dracunculiasis (guinea worm infection)
2. Gnathostomiasis (Israel)
3. Helminthoma
4. Pentastomiasis (*Armillifer* infection)
5. Smallpox (residual effects only)
6. Sparganosis

WEST AFRICA
Diseases in Worldwide list, plus
1. Dracunculiasis (guinea worm infection)
2. Helminthoma
3. Loiasis
4. Paragonimiasis
5. Pentastomiasis (*Armillifer* infection)
6. Smallpox (residual effects only)

CENTRAL AND SOUTHERN AFRICA

Diseases in Worldwide list, plus
1. Dracunculiasis (guinea worm infection)
2. Helminthoma
3. Pentastomiasis (*Armillifer* infection)
4. Smallpox (residual effects only)

INDIA AND SRI LANKA

Diseases in Worldwide list, plus
1. Dracunculiasis (guinea worm infection)
2. Gnathostomiasis
3. Paragonimiasis
4. Pentastomiasissis (*Armillifer* infection)
5. Tropical sprue

ASIA (INCLUDING JAPAN AND THE PACIFIC ISLANDS)

Diseases in Worldwide list, plus
1. Angiostrongyloidiasis cantonensis
2. Anisakiasis (esp. Japan)
3. Clonorchiasis, opisthorchiasis, and other liver fluke diseases; Oriental cholangiohepatitis
4. Gnathostomiasis
5. Intestinal capillariasis
6. Melioidosis (esp. Southeast Asia)
7. Paragonimiasis
8. Pentastomiasis (*Armillifer* infection) (esp. Philippines)
9. Sparganosis

* This list is arranged alphabetically and the order does not in any way suggest the relative risks or frequencies of the various diseases. If used together with the list of differential diagnoses based on the organ or system involved (Gamut J-1), the possible cause of illness in a traveler or immigrant from the tropics may be suggested. Only infectious and parasitic diseases are listed.

Reference
1. Palmer PES, Reeder MM: The Imaging of Tropical Diseases, with Epidemiological, Pathological and Clinical Correlation. (ed 2) Heidelberg: Springer-Verlag, 2001, pp XIX–XXIV

Gamut J-3-S

DISORDERS ASSOCIATED WITH AMYLOIDOSIS

CHRONIC INFLAMMATORY DISEASES
1. Bronchiectasis
2. Cholecystitis
3. Crohn's disease
4. Leprosy
5. Osteomyelitis
6. Pyelonephritis
7. Reiter S.
8. Schistosomiasis
9. Syphilis
10. Tuberculosis
11. Ulcerative colitis
12. Whipple's disease

DERMATOSES
1. Dystrophic epidermolysis bullosa
2. Hidradenitis suppurativa
3. Psoriatic arthritis
4. Stasis ulcer

OTHER CHRONIC DISEASES
1. Collagen disease$_g$ (esp. scleroderma; dermatomyositis; lupus erythematosus)
2. Diabetes
3. Paraplegia
4. Rheumatoid arthritis
5. Senility

PLASMA CELL DYSCRASIAS AND NEOPLASIAS
1. Heavy chain disease (Franklin's disease)
2. Plasma cell myeloma
3. Waldenström's macroglobulinemia

NEOPLASMS
1. Calcifying odontogenic tumor of Pindborg
2. Hodgkin's disease

(continued)

3. Medullary carcinoma of thyroid
4. Renal cell carcinoma (hypernephroma)

HEREDOFAMILIAL DISEASES

1. Amyloid cardiopathy
2. Amyloid nephropathy
3. Amyloid polyneuropathy
4. Cutaneous amyloid
5. Mediterranean fever

References
1. Fraser RS, Müller NL, Coleman N, Paré PD (eds): Fraser & Paré: Diagnosis of Diseases of the Chest. (ed 4) Philadelphia: WB Saunders, 1999
2. Gross BH, Felson B, Birnberg FA: The respiratory tract in amyloidosis and the plasma cell dyscrasias. Semin Roentgenol 1986;21:113–127
3. Pear BL: Radiographic studies of amyloidosis. CRC Crit Rev Radiol Sci 1972;3:425–452

Gamut J-4-S

MUCOPOLYSACCHARIDOSES, MUCOLIPIDOSES, AND OTHER LYSOSOMAL STORAGE DISORDERS* (See D-1)

MUCOPOLYSACCHARIDOSES (MPS)

I-H   Hurler S.
I-S   Scheie S.
II   Hunter S.
III   Sanfilippo S.
IV   Morquio S.
VI   Maroteaux-Lamy S.
VII   Beta-glucuronidase deficiency S. (Sly S.)

MUCOLIPIDOSES (MLS)

I   Sialidosis (neuraminidase deficiency)
II   I-cell disease (Leroy)
III   Pseudopolydystrophy

GLYCOPROTEIN STORAGE DISEASES (OLIGOSACCHARIDOSES)

1. Aspartylglucosaminuria
2. Fucosidosis, types I and II
3. GM_1 gangliosidosis
4. Mannosidosis

* Producing dysostosis multiplex.

References
1. Ampola MG: Metabolic Diseases in Pediatric Practice. Boston: Little, Brown, 1982
2. Beighton P, et al: International nomenclature of constitutional diseases of bone: May 1983 revision. Ann Radiol 1984;27:275–280

Gamut J-5-S1

MULTIPLE ENDOCRINE NEOPLASIA (MEN) SYNDROMES

Men S. Type I (Wermer S.)

COMMON (PPP)

1. *P*ancreatic islet cell tumor or hyperplasia (See J-5-S-2)
2. *P*arathyroid neoplasm or hyperplasia
3. *P*ituitary adenoma (microadenoma)

UNCOMMON

1. Adrenal cortical hyperplasia or adenoma
2. Carcinoid tumor (gastrointestinal, bronchial, thymic)
3. Thyroid adenoma, hyperplasia, medullary carcinoma
4. Zollinger-Ellison S.

MEN S. TYPE IIA OR APUDOMA S. (Amine Precursor Uptake and Decarboxylation)

COMMON (PTA)

1. *P*arathyroid neoplasm or hyperplasia
2. *T*hyroid medullary carcinoma
3. *A*drenal pheochromocytoma

Men S. Type IIB (Sipple S.)

COMMON (TAG)
1. *T*hyroid medullary carcinoma
2. *A*drenal pheochromocytoma
3. *G*anglioneuromas, multiple (incl. gastrointestinal)

Men S., Mixed

References
1. Alberts WM, McMeekin JO, George JM: Mixed multiple endocrine neoplasia syndromes. JAMA 1980;244:1236–1237
2. Dodd GD: The radiologic features of multiple endocrine neoplasia Type IIA and IIB. Semin Roentgenol 1985;20:64–90
3. Doppman JL: Overview: Multiple endocrine syndromes—A nightmare for the endocrinologic radiologist. Semin Roentgenol 1985;20:7–16
4. Muhletahler CA: Radiology of the Zollinger-Ellison syndrome. Rev Interamer Radiol 1982;7:87–93

TYPES OF ISLET CELL TUMOR

1. Gastrinoma
2. Glucagonoma
3. Insulinoma
4. Mixed
5. Somatostatinoma
6. VIPoma (*V*asoactive *I*nhibitory *P*olypeptide)

References
1. Dodds WJ, Wilson SD, Thorsen MK, et al: MEN I syndrome and islet cell lesions of the pancreas. Semin Roentgenol 1985;20:17–63
2. Doppman JL: Overview: Multiple endocrine syndromes—A nightmare for the endocrinologic radiologist. Semin Roentgenol 1985;20:7–16
3. Muhletahler CA: Radiology of the Zollinger-Ellison syndrome. Rev Interamer Radiol 1982;7:87–93

MRI

INTRODUCTION

The organization of the MRI gamuts is heavily based on the appearance of lesions on T1- and T2-weighted images. For those readers less familiar with magnetic resonance imaging, let me add that a T1-weighted spin echo image is one with a short repetition time (TR) and a short echo delay time (TE) (which are both operator-selectable imaging parameters). ("Short" in the context of TR is less than 500 msec and "short" in the context of TE is ideally less than 20 msec—for a high-field system—or 30 msec for a low or mid field system.) T1-weighted gradient echo images are acquired with flip angles larger than 45 degrees and echo delay times generally less than 10 msec. If the repetition times are less than 200 msec, then either RF or gradient spoiling should be used. Such T1-weighted gradient echo techniques are known as FLASH (Siemens), SPGR (for spoiled GRASS, GE), or RF-Spoiled FAST (Picker).

T2-weighted spin echo images are those produced with a long TR and a long TE. "Long" in the context of TR is greater than 2000 msec for applications outside the brain at any field strength. For brain imaging, a long TR at 0.5 Tesla (or below) is 2000 msec while above 0.5 Tesla the TR should be in the 2500–3000 msec range for a T2-weighted image. "Long" in the context of TE is generally on the order of 80 msec or greater. While gradient echo images are never truly T2-weighted, there are certain parameter adjustments that can increase the T2 (or, more correctly, T2*) influence on image contrast. These in-clude a long TE (greater than 18 msec), a short TR (less than 100 msec *without* spoiling), and a low flip angle (less than 30°). (While the low flip angle actually results in proton density weighting, T2 and proton density tend to track together in disease.)

The organization of the MRI gamuts is slightly different than that of the preceding x-ray-based gamuts. The reader is therefore advised to become familiar with the main, organ-systems based organization as well as the suborganization for the brain in Section A prior to extensive use.

A project of this magnitude is rarely the result of one person's thinking; therefore, I would like to acknowledge a number of unwitting contributors. After an initial "free association" phase, I went through the textbook *Magnetic Resonance Imaging* (3rd edition) edited by David Stark and myself (Mosby, St. Louis, 1999) in some detail. Thus, I wish to acknowledge the authors of many of the clinical chapters in that textbook who inadvertently contributed to the gamuts that follow. I would like to thank my colleagues, Louis Teresi, MD; John Barrow, DO; and William Mullin, MD, for manuscript editing.

Finally, I owe a great deal of thanks to my personal assistant of 13 years, Kaye Finley, for the untold hours spent in formatting, reformatting, editing, and reorganizing this material. Without her help over many evenings and weekends, this project would not have been possible.

William G. Bradley, Jr., MD, PhD, FACR

M

BRAIN

PARENCHYMAL

	M-1	Isointense to Gray Matter on T1- and T2-Weighted Images, Nonspecific Parenchymal Location, Mass Effect
	M-2	Dark on T1-Weighted Image, Bright on T2-Weighted Image, Nonspecific Parenchymal Location, No Mass Effect, Nonenhancing
	M-3	Dark on T1-Weighted Image, Bright on T2-Weighted Image, Nonspecific Parenchymal Location, No Mass Effect, Enhancing
	M-4	Dark on T1-Weighted Image, Bright on T2-Weighted Image, Nonspecific Parenchymal Location, Mass Effect, Nonenhancing
	M-4-S1	Parenchymal Hemorrhage
	M-4-S2	Stages of Hemorrhage on MRI
	M-4-S3	Dural Sinus Thrombosis
	M-4-S4	Causes of Vasculitis
	M-5	Dark on T1-Weighted Image, Bright on T2-Weighted Image, Parenchymal, Posterior Paramedian Location, Nonenhancing
	M-6	Dark on T1-Weighted Image, Bright on T2-Weighted Image, Nonspecific Parenchymal Location, Mass Effect, Enhancing
	M-7	Dark on T1-Weighted Image, Bright on T2-Weighted Image, Subependymal, Nonenhancing
	M-8-1	Dark on T1-Weighted Image, Bright on T2-Weighted Image, Subependymal, Enhancing
	M-8-2	Subependymal Tumor Spread
	M-9	Dark on T1-Weighted Image, Bright on T2-Weighted Image, Periventricular, No Mass Effect, Nonenhancing
	M-10-1	Dark on T1-Weighted Image, Bright on T2-Weighted Image, Periventricular, No Mass Effect, Enhancing
	M-10-2	Periventricular Disease in AIDS
	M-10-S	Leukodystrophies with Macrocephaly (in Infants), and with Normocephaly
	M-11	Dark on T1-Weighted Image, Bright on T2-Weighted Image, Periventricular, Mass Effect, Nonenhancing
	M-12	Dark on T1-Weighted Image, Bright on T2-Weighted Image, Periventricular, Mass Effect, Enhancing
	M-13	Dark on T1-Weighted Image, Bright on T2- Weighted Image, Subcortical, No Mass Effect, Nonenhancing
	M-13-S	Causes of Cerebral Emboli
	M-14	Dark on T1-Weighted Image, Bright on T2-Weighted Image, Subcortical, No Mass Effect, Enhancing
	M-15	Dark on T1-Weighted Image, Bright on T2-Weighted Image, Subcortical, Mass Effect, Nonenhancing

M

M

M

M

M

M

KIDNEY	M-154-1	Renal Mass (Intermediate Signal Intensity on T2-Weighted Image)
	M-154-2	Renal Mass (Bright on T2-Weighted Image)
	M-154-3	Renal Mass (Dark on T2-Weighted Image)
	M-154-4	Renal Mass (Bright on T1-Weighted Image)
UTERUS	M-155-1	Endometrial Uterine Mass (Very Bright on T2-Weighted Image—Compared with Myometrium)
	M-155-2	Endometrial Uterine Mass (Intermediate Signal on T2-Weighted Image—Mildly Bright Compared with Myometrium)
	M-155-3	Endometrial Uterine Mass (Dark on T2-Weighted Image)
	M-155-4	Endometrial Uterine Mass (Bright on T1-Weighted Image)
	M-156-1	Myometrial Uterine Mass (Bright on T2-Weighted Image)
	M-156-2	Myometrial Uterine Mass (Intermediate on T2-Weighted Image—Increased Signal Compared with Myometrium)
	M-156-3	Myometrial Uterine Mass (Dark on T2-Weighted Image)
	M-156-4	Myometrial Uterine Mass (Bright on T1-Weighted Image)
ADNEXA	M-157-1	Adnexal Mass (Bright on T2-Weighted Image)
	M-157-2	Adnexal Mass (Dark on T2-Weighted Image)
	M-157-3	Adnexal Mass (Bright on T1-Weighted Image)
PROSTATE	M-158-1	Prostate Mass (Bright on T2-Weighted Image)
	M-158-2	Prostate Mass (Dark on T2-Weighted Image)
	M-158-3	Prostate Mass (Bright on T1-Weighted Image)

M

Gamut M-1

ISOINTENSE TO GRAY MATTER ON T1- AND T2-WEIGHTED IMAGES, NONSPECIFIC PARENCHYMAL LOCATION, MASS EFFECT

1. Hamartoma
2. Heterotopic gray matter
3. Meningioma
4. Tuberous sclerosis

References
1. Boyko OB: Chapter 54. Adult Brain Tumors. In: Stark DD, Bradley WG (eds): Magnetic Resonance Imaging. (ed 3) St. Louis: Mosby, 1999, pp 1231–1254
2. Zimmerman RA, Bilaniuk LT: Chapter 62. Pediatric Cerebral Anomalies. In: Stark DD, Bradley WG (eds): Magnetic Resonance Imaging. (ed 3) St. Louis: Mosby, 1999, pp 1403–1424

Gamut M-2

DARK ON T1-WEIGHTED IMAGE, BRIGHT ON T2-WEIGHTED IMAGE, NONSPECIFIC PARENCHYMAL LOCATION, NO MASS EFFECT, NONENHANCING

1. Glioma, low-grade, small
2. Gliomatosis cerebri
3. Gliosis (following trauma; infarction; infection)
4. Multiple sclerosis
5. Shearing injury, bland
6. Tuberous sclerosis

References
1. Boyko OB: Chapter 54. Adult Brain Tumors. In: Stark DD, Bradley WG (eds): Magnetic Resonance Imaging. (ed 3) St. Louis: Mosby, 1999, pp 1231–1254

2. Evans SJJ, Gean AD: Chapter 59. Craniocerebral Trauma. In: Stark DD, Bradley WG (eds): Magnetic Resonance Imaging. (ed 3) St. Louis: Mosby, 1999, pp 1347–1369
3. Lakhanpal SK, Maravilla KR: Chapter 61. Multiple Sclerosis. In: Stark DD, Bradley WG (eds): Magnetic Resonance Imaging. (ed 3) St. Louis: Mosby, 1999, pp 1379–1402

Gamut M-3

DARK ON T1-WEIGHTED IMAGE, BRIGHT ON T2-WEIGHTED IMAGE, NONSPECIFIC PARENCHYMAL LOCATION, NO MASS EFFECT, ENHANCING

1. [Flow artifact]
2. Glioma, small
3. Infection, indolent
4. Metastasis, small
5. Multiple sclerosis, acute
6. [Normal vein]
7. Scarring (eg, following surgery)
8. Sterile tissue (eg, tumor following radiation)
9. Vascular malformation, small

[ ] This condition does not actually cause the gamuted imaging finding, but can produce imaging changes that simulate it.

References
1. Bradley WG: Chapter 11. Flow Phenomena. In: Stark DD, Bradley WG (eds): Magnetic Resonance Imaging. (ed 3) St. Louis: Mosby, 1999, pp 231–256
2. Boyko OB: Chapter 54. Adult Brain Tumors. In: Stark DD, Bradley WG (eds): Magnetic Resonance Imaging. (ed 3) St. Louis: Mosby, 1999, pp 1231–1254
3. Litt AW, Maltin EP: Chapter 57. Cerebrovascular Abnormalities. In: Stark DD, Bradley WG (eds): Magnetic Resonance Imaging. (ed 3) St. Louis: Mosby, 1999, pp 1317–1328
4. Lakhanpal SK, Maravilla KR: Chapter 61. Multiple Sclerosis. In: Stark DD, Bradley WG (eds): Magnetic Resonance Imaging. (ed 3) St. Louis: Mosby, 1999, pp 1379–1402

DARK ON T1-WEIGHTED IMAGE, BRIGHT ON T2-WEIGHTED IMAGE, NONSPECIFIC PARENCHYMAL LOCATION, MASS EFFECT, NONENHANCING

1. Acute disseminated encephalomyelitis (ADEM) (postviral leukoencephalopathy)
2. Cerebritis, early
3. Contusion
4. Encephalitis, viral
5. Glioma, low-grade
6. Hemorrhage, hyperacute (dark border on T2-weighted image) (See A-99 and M-4-S-1)
7. Infarction, acute
8. Multiple sclerosis, tumefactive
9. Parasitic disease (*Cysticercus; Paragonimus; hydatid cyst*)

References
1. Boyko OB: Chapter 54. Adult Brain Tumors. In: Stark DD, Bradley WG (eds): Magnetic Resonance Imaging. (ed 3) St. Louis: Mosby, 1999, pp 1231–1254

2. Evans SJJ, Gean AD: Chapter 59. Craniocerebral Trauma. In: Stark DD, Bradley WG (eds): Magnetic Resonance Imaging. (ed 3) St. Louis: Mosby, 1999, pp 1347–1369
3. Sze GK: Chapter 60. Infection and Inflammation. In: Stark DD, Bradley WG (eds): Magnetic Resonance Imaging. (ed 3) St. Louis: Mosby, 1999, pp 1361–1378

PARENCHYMAL HEMORRHAGE (See A-99)

1. Amyloid angiopathy (peripheral location; elderly patients)
2. Aneurysm, ruptured
3. Angioma, cavernous
4. Arteriovenous malformation
5. Infarction, hemorrhagic (embolic; mass effect)
6. Infarction, subacute, hemorrhagic (petechial; no mass effect)
7. Infarction, venous (with dural sinus thrombosis) (See M-4-S3)
8. Postoperative
9. Shearing injury, hemorrhagic (diffuse axonal injury)
10. Trauma
11. Tumor (usually high grade)
12. Vasculitis (See M-4-S4)

STAGES OF HEMORRHAGE ON MRI

Stage	Time	Compartment	Hemoglobin	T1	T2
Hyperacute*	0–24 hours	intracellular	oxyhemoglobin	gray	bright
Acute	1–3 days	intracellular	deoxyhemoglobin	gray	dark
Early subacute	3–7 days	intracellular	methemoglobin	bright	dark
Late subacute	7–14 days	extracellular	methemoglobin	bright	bright
Chronic	14+ days	center	hemichromes	gray	bright
		rim	hemosiderin	gray	dark

* All hyperacute parenchymal hematomas have a deoxyhemoglobin border around them.

References
1. Atlas SW, Thulborn KR: MR detection of hyperacute parenchymal hemorrhage of the brain. Am J Neuroradiol 1998;19:1471–1477
2. Bradley WG: Chapter 58. Hemorrhage. In: Stark DD, Bradley WG (eds): Magnetic Resonance Imaging. (ed 3) St. Louis: Mosby, 1999, pp 1329–1346

Gamut M-4-S3

DURAL SINUS THROMBOSIS

1. Angioma
2. Arteriovenous malformation
3. Antithrombin III deficiency
4. Birth control pills
5. Heart failure
6. Dehydration
7. Disseminated intravascular coagulation (DIC)
8. Infection
9. Lupus anticoagulant
10. Malignant neoplasm invasion
11. Polycythemia vera
12. Pregnancy
13. Sickle cell disease
14. Thrombocytosis
15. Vasculitis, primary

Reference
1. Jensen MD, Brant-Zawadzki M, Jacobs BC: Chapter 55. Ischemia. In: Stark DD, Bradley WG (eds): Magnetic Resonance Imaging. (ed 3) St. Louis: Mosby, 1999, pp 1255–1276

Gamut M-4-S4

CAUSES OF VASCULITIS

PROBABLY IMMUNE COMPLEX DESPOSITION MECHANISM

1. Allergic angitis and granulomatosis
2. Connective tissue disease (collagen vascular disease)$_g$ with vasculitis (eg, lupus erythematosus; polyarteritis nodosa; mixed connective tissue disease {MCTD})
3. Henoch-Schönlein purpura
4. Hypersensitivity vasculitis
5. Hypocomplemenemic vasculitis
6. Malignancy with vasculitis
7. Mixed cryoglobulinemia
8. Necrotizing angiitis (eg, polyarteritis nodosa; rheumatic fever; hypersensitivity angiitis; giant cell arteritis; temporal arteritis)
9. Serum sickness (or serum sickness-like) vasculitis
10. Systemic necrotizing vasculitis

PROBABLY CELL-MEDIATED MECHANISM WITH ROUND CELL GRANULOMA FORMATION

1. Granulomatous angiitis
2. Lymphomatoid granulomatosis
3. Takayasu's arteritis
4. Wegner's granulomatosis

MISCELLANEOUS

1. Amphetamine/cocaine abuse
2. Arterial spasm (eg, subarachnoid or cerebral hemorrhage; migraine)
3. Arteriovenous malformation
4. Behçet S.
5. Bowel bypass dermatitis
6. Cerebral thrombosis (eg, sickle cell disease; oral contraceptives)
7. Cogan S.
8. Embolism (eg, subacute bacterial endocarditis; atrial myxoma)
9. Erythema nodosum
10. Idiopathic
11. [Increased intracranial pressure]
12. Infection (eg, herpes, tuberculosis, syphylis–rare)
13. Inflammatory disease of brain (eg, abscess; purulent or tuberculous meningitis)
14. Kawasaki S. (mucocutaneous lymph node S.)
15. Multiple progressive intracranial artery occlusions with telangiectasia (moyamoya)
16. Neurocutaneous syndromes (eg, neurofibromatosis; Sturge-Weber S.; tuberous sclerosis)
17. Radiation therapy
18. Sarcoidosis
19. Thromboangiitis obliterans (Buerger's disease)
20. Trauma

[ ] This condition does not actually cause the gamuted imaging finding, but can produce imaging changes that simulate it.

(continued)

References
1. Ferris EJ, Levine HL: Cerebral arteritis: Classification. Radiology 1973; 109:327–3412.
2. Grainger RG, Allison DJ (eds): Diagnostic Radiology: An Anglo-American Textbook of Imaging. (ed 2) Edinburgh: Churchill Livingstone, 1992, vol 3, pp 1993–1994
3. Hilal SK, Solomon GE, Gold AP, et al: Primary cerebral arterial occlusive disease in children. Radiology 1971;99:71–94
4. Jensen MD, Brant-Zawadzki M, Jacobs BC: Chapter 55. Ischemia. In: Stark DD, Bradley WG (eds): Magnetic Resonance Imaging. (ed 3) St. Louis: Mosby, 1999, pp 1255–1276
5. Leeds NE, Rosenblatt R: Arterial wall irregularities in intracranial neoplasms. Radiology 1972;103:121–124

Gamut M-5

DARK ON T1-WEIGHTED IMAGE, BRIGHT ON T2-WEIGHTED IMAGE, PARENCHYMAL, POSTERIOR PARAMEDIAN LOCATION, NONENHANCING

1. Cyclosporine toxicity (negative DWI—diffusion weighted imaging)
2. Hypertensive encephalopathy (eg, pre-eclampsia; negative DWI)
3. Infarction of posterior circulation (positive DWI)
4. Thrombosis of superior sagittal sinus (venous infarct)
5. Tuberous sclerosis

Reference
1. Cooney MJ, Bradley WG, Symko SC, Patel ST, Groncy PK: Hypertensive encephalopathy: complication in children treated for myeloproliferative disorders—report of three cases. Radiology 2000;214:711–716

Gamut M-6

DARK ON T1-WEIGHTED IMAGE, BRIGHT ON T2-WEIGHTED IMAGE, NONSPECIFIC PARENCHYMAL LOCATION, MASS EFFECT, ENHANCING

CENTRALLY ENHANCING

1. Cerebritis
2. Ganglion cell tumors (rare)
3. Glioma, high grade
4. Lymphoma$_g$ (primary or metastatic)
5. Metastasis
6. PNET (primitive neuroectodermal tumor)
7. Radiation necrosis

RIM ENHANCING

1. Abscess
2. ADEM (acute disseminated encephalomyelitis) (partial rim)
3. Cysticercosis
4. Lymphoma (occas.)
5. Metastasis (occas.)
6. Multiple sclerosis, tumefactive (partial rim)
7. Paragonimiasis

References
1. Boyko OB: Chapter 54. Adult Brain Tumors. In: Stark DD, Bradley WG (eds): Magnetic Resonance Imaging. (ed 3) St. Louis: Mosby, 1999, pp 1231–1254
2. Boyko OB: Chapter 65. Pediatric Brain Tumors. In: Stark DD, Bradley WG (eds): Magnetic Resonance Imaging. (ed 3) St. Louis: Mosby, 1999, pp 1467–1482
3. Lakhanpal SK, Maravilla KR: Chapter 61. Multiple Sclerosis. In: Stark DD, Bradley WG (eds): Magnetic Resonance Imaging. (ed 3) St. Louis: Mosby, 1999, pp 1379–1402

Gamut M-7

DARK ON T1-WEIGHTED IMAGE, BRIGHT ON T2-WEIGHTED IMAGE, SUBEPENDYMAL, NONENHANCING

SMOOTH
1. Edema, centrally tracking vasogenic
2. Interstitial edema
3. [Normal caudate body]
4. Small vessel ischemic change
5. Subependymal demyelination following interstitial edema

LUMPY
1. Hamartomas of tuberous sclerosis
2. Heterotopic gray matter

[ ] This condition does not actually cause the gamuted imaging finding, but can produce imaging changes that simulate it.

References
1. Jensen MD, Brant-Zawadzki M, Jacobs BC: Chapter 55. Ischemia. In: Stark DD, Bradley WG (eds): Magnetic Resonance Imaging. (ed 3) St. Louis: Mosby, 1999, pp 1255–1276
2. Bradley WG, Quencer RM: Chapter 66. Hydrocephalus and Cerebrospinal Fluid Flow. In: Stark DD, Bradley WG (eds): Magnetic Resonance Imaging. (ed 3) St. Louis: Mosby, 1999, pp 1483–1508

Gamut M-8-1

DARK ON T1-WEIGHTED IMAGE, BRIGHT ON T2-WEIGHTED IMAGE, SUBEPENDYMAL, ENHANCING

SMOOTH
1. Subependymal tumor spread, early (See M-8-2)
2. Ventriculitis/ependymitis (eg, cytomegalovirus infection)

LUMPY
1. Giant cell astrocytoma (tuberous sclerosis)
2. Subependymal hamartomas (tuberous sclerosis)
3. Subependymal tumor spread, late (See M-8-2)

Gamut M-8-2

SUBEPENDYMAL TUMOR SPREAD

1. Ependymoma
2. Glioblastoma
3. Lymphoma$_g$
4. Medulloblastoma
5. Metastatic disease (eg, carcinoma of breast or lung; melanoma)

Reference
1. Boyko OB: Chapter 54. Adult Brain Tumors. In: Stark DD, Bradley WG (eds): Magnetic Resonance Imaging. (ed 3) St. Louis: Mosby, 1999, pp 1231–1254

Gamut M-9

DARK ON T1-WEIGHTED IMAGE, BRIGHT ON T2-WEIGHTED IMAGE, PERIVENTRICULAR, NO MASS EFFECT, NONENHANCING

PATIENT UNDER 40

COMMON

1. ADEM (acute disseminated encephalomyelitis; postviral leukoencephalopathy)
2. AIDS (HIV) encephalitis (See M-10-2)
3. Lupus erythematosus
4. Migraine
5. Multiple sclerosis

UNCOMMON

1. Leukodystrophies (rare) (See M-10-S)
2. Lyme disease
3. Neurofibromatosis type I (spongiform change)
4. [Normal late myelinating fibers (thalamoparietal tracts)]
5. Periventricular leukomalacia
6. Sickle cell disease
7. Subacute sclerosing panencephalitis (SSPE) (rare)

PATIENT OVER 40

1. Marchiafava-Bignami disease (rare)
2. Multiple sclerosis
3. [Normal (ependymitis granularis)]
4. Radiation-induced white matter changes
5. Small vessel ischemic change in deep white matter

NONSPECIFIC WITH RESPECT TO AGE

1. Diffuse necrotizing leukoencephalopathy (DNL)
2. Hamartomas of tuberous sclerosis
3. Heterotopic gray matter
4. Neurofibromatosis
5. Shearing injury

[ ] This condition does not actually cause the gamuted imaging finding, but can produce imaging changes that simulate it.

References

1. Boyko OB: Chapter 54. Adult Brain Tumors. In: Stark DD, Bradley WG (eds): Magnetic Resonance Imaging. (ed 3) St. Louis: Mosby, 1999, pp 1231–1254
2. Dietrich RB: Chapter 63. Maturation, Myelination, and Dysmyelination. In: Stark DD, Bradley WG (eds): Magnetic Resonance Imaging. (ed 3) St. Louis: Mosby,1999, pp 1425–1448
3. Dietrich RB: Chapter 64. Pediatric Anoxic-Ischemic Injury. In: Stark DD, Bradley WG (eds): Magnetic Resonance Imaging. (ed 3) St. Louis: Mosby, pp 1449–1466, 1999.
4. Lakhanpal SK, Maravilla KR: Chapter 61. Multiple Sclerosis. In: Stark DD, Bradley WG (eds): Magnetic Resonance Imaging. (ed 3) St. Louis: Mosby, 1999, pp 1379–1402
5. Sze GK: Chapter 60. Infection and Inflammation. In: Stark DD, Bradley WG (eds): Magnetic Resonance Imaging. (ed 3) St. Louis: Mosby, 1999, pp 1361–1378
6. Zimmerman RA, Bilaniuk LT: Chapter 62. Pediatric Cerebral Anomalies. In: Stark DD, Bradley WG (eds): Magnetic Resonance Imaging. (ed 3) St. Louis: Mosby, 1999, pp 1403–1424

Gamut M-10-1

DARK ON T1-WEIGHTED IMAGE, BRIGHT ON T2-WEIGHTED IMAGE, PERIVENTRICULAR, NO MASS EFFECT, ENHANCING

1. AIDS (HIV) infection
2. Cytomegalovirus (CMV) infection
3. Infarct, subacute
4. Leukodystrophies (enhancing active border [rare])
5. Metastatic disease, early
6. Toxoplasmosis, early (See M-10-S1)

Gamut M-10-2

PERIVENTRICULAR DISEASE IN AIDS

1. Cytomegalovirus (CMV) infection
2. AIDS (HIV) encephalitis
3. Kaposi sarcoma
4. Lymphoma$_g$
5. Progressive multifocal leukoencephalopathy (PML)
6. Toxoplasmosis

Gamut M-10-S

LEUKODYSTROPHIES

WITH MACROCEPHALY (IN INFANTS)
1. Alexander's disease (anterior, sparing of internal capsule, enhances with gadolinium)
2. Canavan's disease (peripheral to central, early involvement of subcortical U-fibers)

WITH NORMOCEPHALY
1. Adrenoleukodystrophy (males, posterior, enhances with gadolinium)
2. Krabbe's disease (central to peripheral, nonenhancing)
3. Metachromatic leukodystrophy (central to peripheral, nonenhancing)
4. Pelizaeus-Merzbacher disease (males, central to peripheral, nonenhancing, brain stem atrophy)

Reference
1. Dietrich RB: Chapter 63. Maturation, Myelination, and Dysmyelination. In: Stark DD, Bradley WG (eds): Magnetic Resonance Imaging. (ed 3) St. Louis: Mosby,1999, pp 1425–1448

Gamut M-11

DARK ON T1-WEIGHTED IMAGE, BRIGHT ON T2-WEIGHTED IMAGE, PERIVENTRICULAR, MASS EFFECT, NONENHANCING

1. Acute disseminated encephalomyelitis (ADEM) (postviral leukoencephalopathy)
2. Glioma of visual pathway, low grade (neurofibromatosis)
3. Hamartoma (eg, in tuberous sclerosis)
4. Infarction (eg, from vasculitis; sickle cell disease)
5. Multiple sclerosis, tumefactive
6. Porencephalic cysts (porencephaly)

References
1. Boyko OB: Chapter 54. Adult Brain Tumors. In: Stark DD, Bradley WG (eds): Magnetic Resonance Imaging. (ed 3) St. Louis: Mosby, 1999, pp 1231–1254
2. Lakhanpal SK, Maravilla KR: Chapter 61. Multiple Sclerosis. In: Stark DD, Bradley WG (eds): Magnetic Resonance Imaging. (ed 3) St. Louis: Mosby, 1999, pp 1379–1402

Gamut M-12

DARK ON T1-WEIGHTED IMAGE, BRIGHT ON T2-WEIGHTED IMAGE, PERIVENTRICULAR, MASS EFFECT, ENHANCING

1. Abscess (eg, cytomegalovirus infection; toxoplasmosis); cryptococcosis
2. Astrocytoma, giant cell (tuberous sclerosis)
3. Glioma of visual pathway, degenerated (neurofibromatosis)
4. Lymphoma$_g$
5. Metastasis, parenchymal or intraventricular drop (eg, from glioblastoma)
6. Multiple sclerosis, tumefactive

(continued)

References
1. Boyko OB: Chapter 54. Adult Brain Tumors. In: Stark DD, Bradley WG (eds): Magnetic Resonance Imaging. (ed 3) St. Louis: Mosby, 1999, pp 1231–1254
2. Lakhanpal SK, Maravilla KR: Chapter 61. Multiple Sclerosis. In: Stark DD, Bradley WG (eds): Magnetic Resonance Imaging. (ed 3) St. Louis: Mosby, 1999, pp 1379–1402
3. Sze GK: Chapter 60. Infection and Inflammation. In: Stark DD, Bradley WG (eds): Magnetic Resonance Imaging. (ed 3) St. Louis: Mosby, 1999, pp 1361–1378

Gamut M-13

DARK ON T1-WEIGHTED IMAGE, BRIGHT ON T2-WEIGHTED IMAGE, SUBCORTICAL, NO MASS EFFECT, NONENHANCING

1. Infarction, embolic (See M-13-S)
2. Progressive multifocal leukoencephalopathy (PML)
3. Shearing injury (nonhemorrhagic)
4. Tuberous sclerosis

Gamut M-13-S

CAUSES OF CEREBRAL EMBOLI

SOURCE DISTAL TO LUNGS
1. Embolus (from cardiac mural thrombus; carotid dissection; open heart surgery; angiogram)
2. Infection (eg, infective endocarditis; subacute bacterial endocarditis)
3. Platelet embolus (from ulcerated carotid plaque)
4. Thrombus, cardiac mural
5. Tumor (atrial myxoma; choriocarcinoma; marantic endocarditis)

SOURCE PROXIMAL TO LUNGS—requires right to left shunt (rare)
1. Amniotic fluid embolism
2. Fat embolus (following trauma)

3. Thrombus (from inferior vena cava or thrombophlebitis)

Reference
1. Jensen MD, Brant-Zawadzki M, Jacobs BC: Chapter 55. Ischemia. In: Stark DD, Bradley WG (eds): Magnetic Resonance Imaging. (ed 3) St. Louis: Mosby, 1999, pp 1255–1276

Gamut M-14

DARK ON T1-WEIGHTED IMAGE, BRIGHT ON T2-WEIGHTED IMAGE, SUBCORTICAL, NO MASS EFFECT, ENHANCING

1. Carcinomatosis, leptomeningeal
2. Lymphoma$_g$
3. Meningitis
4. Sarcoidosis

References
1. Boyko OB: Chapter 54. Adult Brain Tumors. In: Stark DD, Bradley WG (eds): Magnetic Resonance Imaging. (ed 3) St. Louis: Mosby, 1999, pp 1231–1254
2. Sze GK: Chapter 60. Infection and Inflammation. In: Stark DD, Bradley WG (eds): Magnetic Resonance Imaging. (ed 3) St. Louis: Mosby, 1999, pp 1361–1378

Gamut M-15

DARK ON T1-WEIGHTED IMAGE, BRIGHT ON T2-WEIGHTED IMAGE, SUBCORTICAL, MASS EFFECT, NONENHANCING

1. Glioma, low grade
2. Heterotopic gray matter
3. Progressive multifocal leukoencephalopathy (PML)

References
1. Boyko OB: Chapter 54. Adult Brain Tumors. In: Stark DD, Bradley WG (eds): Magnetic Resonance Imaging. (ed 3) St. Louis: Mosby, 1999, pp 1231–1254

2. Sze GK: Chapter 60. Infection and Inflammation. In: Stark DD, Bradley WG (eds): Magnetic Resonance Imaging. (ed 3) St. Louis: Mosby, 1999, pp 1361–1378

Gamut M-16

DARK ON T1-WEIGHTED IMAGE, BRIGHT ON T2-WEIGHTED IMAGE, SUBCORTICAL, MASS EFFECT, ENHANCING

1. Abscess
2. Emboli (See M-13-S)
3. Metastasis
4. Multiple sclerosis, acute tumefactive
5. Sarcoidosis

References
1. Boyko OB: Chapter 54. Adult Brain Tumors. In: Stark DD, Bradley WG (eds): Magnetic Resonance Imaging. (ed 3) St. Louis: Mosby, 1999, pp 1231–1254
2. Sze GK: Chapter 60. Infection and Inflammation. In: Stark DD, Bradley WG (eds): Magnetic Resonance Imaging. (ed 3) St. Louis: Mosby, 1999, pp 1361–1378

Gamut M-17

DARK ON T1-WEIGHTED IMAGE, BRIGHT ON T2-WEIGHTED IMAGE, CORTICAL, NO MASS EFFECT, NONENHANCING

1. Gliosis, postbleed
2. Gliosis, postinfarct
3. Gliosis, postinfection
4. Gliosis, postoperative
5. Gliosis, posttraumatic

References
1. Bradley WG: Chapter 58. Hemorrhage. In: Stark DD, Bradley WG (eds): Magnetic Resonance Imaging. (ed 3) St. Louis: Mosby, 1999, pp 1329–1346
2. Evans AJJ, Gean AD: Chapter 59. Craniocerebral Trauma. In: Stark DD, Bradley WG (eds): Magnetic Resonance Imaging. (ed 3) St. Louis: Mosby, 1999, pp 1347–1360
3. Sze GK: Chapter 60. Infection and Inflammation. In: Stark DD, Bradley WG (eds): Magnetic Resonance Imaging. (ed 3) St. Louis: Mosby, 1999, pp 1361–1378

Gamut M-18

DARK ON T1-WEIGHTED IMAGE, BRIGHT ON T2-WEIGHTED IMAGE, CORTICAL, NO MASS EFFECT, ENHANCING

1. Angiomatosis, leptomeningeal (Sturge-Weber S.)
2. Carcinomatosis, leptomeningeal
3. Infarction, subacute
4. Lymphoma$_g$
5. Meningitis

References
1. Boyko OB: Chapter 54. Adult Brain Tumors. In: Stark DD, Bradley WG (eds): Magnetic Resonance Imaging. (ed 3) St. Louis: Mosby, 1999, pp 1231–1254

(continued)

2. Sze GK: Chapter 60. Infection and Inflammation. In: Stark DD, Bradley WG (eds): Magnetic Resonance Imaging. (ed 3) St. Louis: Mosby, 1999, pp 1361–1378
3. Zimmerman RA, Bilaniuk LT: Chapter 62. Pediatric Cerebral Anomalies. In: Stark DD, Bradley WG (eds): Magnetic Resonance Imaging. (ed 3) St. Louis: Mosby, 1999, pp 1403–1424

Gamut M-19

DARK ON T1-WEIGHTED IMAGE, BRIGHT ON T2-WEIGHTED IMAGE, CORTICAL, MASS EFFECT, NONENHANCING

COMMON

1. Cortical dysplasia
2. Glioma, low grade
3. Hamartoma (cortical tuber; tuberous sclerosis)
4. Infarction, acute
5. Vasculopathy, ischemic (eg, lupus erythematosus)

UNCOMMON

1. Dysembryoplastic neuroepithelial tumor (DNET)
2. Gangliocytoma
3. Pleomorphic xanthoastrocytoma

References
1. Boyko OB: Chapter 54. Adult Brain Tumors. In: Stark DD, Bradley WG (eds): Magnetic Resonance Imaging. (ed 3) St. Louis: Mosby, 1999, pp 1231–1254
2. Boyko OB: Chapter 65. Pediatric Brain Tumors. In: Stark DD, Bradley WG (eds): Magnetic Resonance Imaging. (ed 3) St. Louis: Mosby, 1999, pp 1467–1482
3. Jensen MD, Brant-Zawadzki M, Jacobs BC: Chapter 55. Ischemia. In: Stark DD, Bradley WG (eds): Magnetic Resonance Imaging. (ed 3) St. Louis: Mosby, 1999, pp 1255–1276
4. Zimmerman RA, Bilaniuk LT: Chapter 62. Pediatric Cerebral Anomalies. In: Stark DD, Bradley WG (eds): Magnetic Resonance Imaging. (ed 3) St. Louis: Mosby, 1999, pp 1403–1424

Gamut M-20

DARK ON T1-WEIGHTED IMAGE, BRIGHT ON T2-WEIGHTED IMAGE, CORTICAL, MASS EFFECT, ENHANCING

1. Carcinomatosis, leptomeningeal
2. Infarct, acute (vascular enhancement due to stasis, pial collaterals)
3. Infarct, subacute (gyral enhancement)
4. Meningitis, fungal

References
1. Boyko OB: Chapter 54. Adult Brain Tumors. In: Stark DD, Bradley WG (eds): Magnetic Resonance Imaging. (ed 3) St. Louis: Mosby, 1999, pp 1231–1254
2. Jensen MD, Brant-Zawadzki M, Jacobs BC: Chapter 55. Ischemia. In: Stark DD, Bradley WG (eds): Magnetic Resonance Imaging. (ed 3) St. Louis: Mosby, 1999, pp 1255–1276
3. Sze GK: Chapter 60. Infection and Inflammation. In: Stark DD, Bradley WG (eds): Magnetic Resonance Imaging. (ed 3) St. Louis: Mosby, 1999, pp 1361–1378

Gamut M-21

DARK ON T1-WEIGHTED IMAGE, BRIGHT ON T2-WEIGHTED IMAGE, BASAL GANGLIA

COMMON

1. Infarcts, lacunar
2. Ischemic-anoxic events (eg, near-drowning)
3. Multiple sclerosis
4. Neurofibromatosis type I (spongiform change)

UNCOMMON

1. Aminoacidemia
2. Behçet S.
3. Extrapontine myelinolysis

4. Jakob-Creutzfeld disease (nearly isointense on T1WI)
5. Leigh's disease (necrotizing encephalopathy)
6. MELAS
7. MERRF
8. Methanol intoxication
9. Oligopontocerebellar degeneration
10. Poisoning (eg, carbon monoxide; cyanide; ethylene glycol)
11. Wernicke encephalopathy (alcoholism)

References

1. Dietrich RB: Chapter 64. Pediatric Anoxic-Ischemic Injury. In: Stark DD, Bradley WG (eds): Magnetic Resonance Imaging. (ed 3) St. Louis: Mosby, pp 1449–1466, 1999.
2. DiPaolo DP, Zimmerman RA, Rorke LB, et al: Neurofibromatosis type 1: pathologic substrate of high-signal-intensity foci in the brain. Radiology 1995;195:721–724
3. Jensen MD, Brant-Zawadzki M, Jacobs BC: Chapter 55. Ischemia. In: Stark DD, Bradley WG (eds): Magnetic Resonance Imaging. (ed 3) St. Louis: Mosby, 1999, pp 1255–276
4. Lakhanpal SK, Maravilla KR: Chapter 61. Multiple Sclerosis. In: Stark DD, Bradley WG (eds): Magnetic Resonance Imaging. (ed 3) St. Louis: Mosby, 1999, pp 1379–1402
5. Pomeranz SJ, Smith PJ: Gamuts & Pearls in Neurologic MRI. Cincinnati: MRI-EFI Publ, 1998
6. Zimmerman RA, Bilaniuk LT: Chapter 62. Pediatric Cerebral Anomalies. In: Stark DD, Bradley WG (eds): Magnetic Resonance Imaging. (ed 3) St. Louis: Mosby, 1999, pp 1403–1424

6. Lupus erythematosus
7. Multiple sclerosis
8. Myelinolysis, central pontine
9. Progressive multifocal leukoencephalopathy (PML)
10. Shearing injury (posterolateral upper brain stem)
11. Wallerian degeneration (eg, secondary to stroke or adrenoleukodystrophy)

[ ] This condition does not actually cause the gamuted imaging finding, but can produce imaging changes that simulate it.

References

1. Boyko OB: Chapter 54. Adult Brain Tumors. In: Stark DD, Bradley WG (eds): Magnetic Resonance Imaging. (ed 3) St. Louis: Mosby, 1999, pp 1231–1254
2. Bradley WG: Chapter 51. Brainstem: Normal Anatomy and Pathology. In: Stark DD, Bradley WG (eds): Magnetic Resonance Imaging. (ed 3) St. Louis: Mosby, 1999, pp 1187–1208
3. Dietrich RB: Chapter 64. Pediatric Anoxic-Ischemic Injury. In: Stark DD, Bradley WG (eds): Magnetic Resonance Imaging. (ed 3) St. Louis: Mosby, pp 1449–1466, 1999.
4. Jensen MD, Brant-Zawadzki M, Jacobs BC: Chapter 55. Ischemia. In: Stark DD, Bradley WG (eds): Magnetic Resonance Imaging. (ed 3) St. Louis: Mosby, 1999, pp 1255–1276
5. Lakhanpal SK, Maravilla KR: Chapter 61. Multiple Sclerosis. In: Stark DD, Bradley WG (eds): Magnetic Resonance Imaging. (ed 3) St. Louis: Mosby, 1999, pp 1379–1402

Gamut M-22

DARK ON T1-WEIGHTED IMAGE, BRIGHT ON T2-WEIGHTED IMAGE, BRAIN STEM, NO MASS EFFECT, NONENHANCING

1. Amyotrophic lateral sclerosis
2. [CSF flow artifact (rare)]
3. Glioma, small, low-grade
4. Infarct
5. Ischemic change, small vessel (isointense on T1WI)

DARK ON T1-WEIGHTED IMAGE, BRIGHT ON T2-WEIGHTED IMAGE, BRAIN STEM, NO MASS EFFECT, ENHANCING

1. Capillary telanglectasia (may be isointense on T1- and T2-weighted images)
2. Multiple sclerosis, acute
3. Tumor, small (primary or metastasis)
4. Wernicke encephalopathy (alcoholism)

References

1. Lakhanpal SK, Maravilla KR: Chapter 61. Multiple Sclerosis. In: Stark DD, Bradley WG (eds): Magnetic Resonance Imaging. (ed 3) St. Louis: Mosby, 1999, pp 1379–1402
2. Litt AW, Maltin EP: Chapter 57. Cerebrovascular Abnormalities. In: Stark DD, Bradley WG (eds): Magnetic Resonance Imaging. (ed 3) St. Louis: Mosby, 1999, pp 1317–1328

Gamut M-24

DARK ON T1-WEIGHTED IMAGE, BRIGHT ON T2-WEIGHTED IMAGE, BRAIN STEM, MASS EFFECT, NONENHANCING

1. Encephalitis
2. Glioma, low-grade
3. Infarct
4. Ramsey Hunt S. (retrograde spread of varicella virus)

References

1. Boyko OB: Chapter 54. Adult Brain Tumors. In: Stark DD, Bradley WG (eds): Magnetic Resonance Imaging. (ed 3) St. Louis: Mosby, 1999, pp 1231–1254
2. Hirbawi IA, Hasso AN: Chapter 52. Cranial Nerves: Normal Anatomy and Pathology. In: Stark DD, Bradley WG (eds): Magnetic Resonance Imaging. (ed 3) St. Louis: Mosby, 1999, pp 1209–1224

3. Jensen MD, Brant-Zawadzki M, Jacobs BC: Chapter 55. Ischemia. In: Stark DD, Bradley WG (eds): Magnetic Resonance Imaging. (ed 3) St. Louis: Mosby, 1999, pp 1255–1276
4. Sze GK: Chapter 60. Infection and Inflammation. In: Stark DD, Bradley WG (eds): Magnetic Resonance Imaging. (ed 3) St. Louis: Mosby, 1999, pp 1361–1378

Gamut M-25

DARK ON T1-WEIGHTED IMAGE, BRIGHT ON T2-WEIGHTED IMAGE, BRAIN STEM, MASS EFFECT, ENHANCING

1. Abscess
2. Behçet S. with encephalitis
3. Encephalitis, brain stem
4. Ependymoblastoma (rare)
5. Ependymoma
6. Glioma of brain stem
7. Lymphoma$_g$
8. Metastasis
9. Multiple sclerosis, tumefactive
10. Myelinolysis, acute central pontine
11. Perineural spread of carcinoma (squamous cell and adenoid cystic)
12. Primitive neuroectodermal tumor (PNET)$_g$

References

1. Boyko OB: Chapter 54. Adult Brain Tumors. In: Stark DD, Bradley WG (eds): Magnetic Resonance Imaging. (ed 3) St. Louis: Mosby, 1999, pp 1231–1254
2. Hirbawi IA, Hasso AN: Chapter 52. Cranial Nerves: Normal Anatomy and Pathology. In: Stark DD, Bradley WG (eds): Magnetic Resonance Imaging. (ed 3) St. Louis: Mosby, 1999, pp 1209–1224
3. Jensen MD, Brant-Zawadzki M, Jacobs BC: Chapter 55. Ischemia. In: Stark DD, Bradley WG (eds): Magnetic Resonance Imaging. (ed 3) St. Louis: Mosby, 1999, pp 1255–1276
4. Sze GK: Chapter 60. Infection and Inflammation. In: Stark DD, Bradley WG (eds) Magnetic Resonance Imaging. (ed 3) St. Louis: Mosby, 1999, pp 1361–1378

Gamut M-26-1

CEREBELLAR MASS IN A CHILD

1. Astrocytoma, cystic or pilocytic
2. Lhermitte Duclos disease (rare)
3. Medulloblastoma (PNET)

Reference
1. Boyko OB: Chapter 65. Pediatric Brain Tumors. In: Stark DD, Bradley WG (eds): Magnetic Resonance Imaging. (ed 3) St. Louis: Mosby, 1999, pp 1467–1482

Gamut M-26-2

CEREBELLAR MASS IN AN ADULT

1. Astrocytoma
2. Hemangioblastoma
3. Metastasis
4. Multiple sclerosis, tumefactive

Reference
1. Boyko OB: Chapter 54. Adult Brain Tumors. In: Stark DD, Bradley WG (eds): Magnetic Resonance Imaging. (ed 3) St. Louis: Mosby, 1999, pp 1231–1254

Gamut M-27

DARK ON T1-WEIGHTED IMAGE, BRIGHT ON T2-WEIGHTED IMAGE, CRANIAL NERVE, ENHANCING

1. Carcinomatosis, leptomeningeal
2. Neuritis, viral (eg, Bell's palsy)
3. Perineural spread of carcinoma (eg, squamous cell and adenoid cystic)
4. Schwannoma (neurinoma)

Reference
1. Hirbawi IA, Hasso AN: Chapter 52. Cranial Nerves: Normal Anatomy and Pathology. In: Stark DD, Bradley WG (eds): Magnetic Resonance Imaging. (ed 3) St. Louis: Mosby, 1999, pp 1209–1224

Gamut M-28

DARK ON T1-WEIGHTED IMAGE, BRIGHT ON T2-WEIGHTED IMAGE, SELLA REGION LESION, SELLAR/PARASELLAR ORIGIN, ENHANCING

1. Carotid aneurysm (cavernous or suprasellar)
2. Chordoma
3. Craniopharyngioma
4. Germinoma (ectopic pinealoma; multiple midline tumor syndrome)
5. Glioma, high grade, of hypothalamus or visual pathway
6. Hypophysitis, lymphocytic
7. Meningioma
8. Metastasis to pituitary
9. Mucocele (sphenoid sinus)
10. Packing (fat or muscle) from previous transsphenoidal hypophysectomy
11. Pituitary macroadenoma
12. Rathke cleft cyst

Reference
1. Zhu M, Maeda M, Lee GJ, Yuh WTC: Chapter 53. Sellar Lesions. In: Stark DD, Bradley WG (eds): Magnetic Resonance Imaging. (ed 3) St. Louis: Mosby, 1999, pp 1225–1230

DARK ON T1-WEIGHTED IMAGE, BRIGHT ON T2-WEIGHTED IMAGE, SELLA REGION LESION, ENLARGED PITUITARY STALK, ENHANCING

1. Carcinomatosis, leptomeningeal (esp. from breast or lung)
2. Langerhans cell histiocytosis$_g$
3. Leukemia; lymphoma$_g$
4. Meningitis
5. Metastasis (rare)
6. Sarcoidosis

References
1. Boyko OB: Chapter 54. Adult Brain Tumors. In: Stark DD, Bradley WG (eds): Magnetic Resonance Imaging. (ed 3) St. Louis: Mosby, 1999, pp 1231–1254
2. Sze GK: Chapter 60. Infection and Inflammation. In: Stark DD, Bradley WG (eds): Magnetic Resonance Imaging. (ed 3) St. Louis: Mosby, 1999, pp 1361–1378

DARK ON T1-WEIGHTED IMAGE, BRIGHT ON T2-WEIGHTED IMAGE, SELLA REGION LESION, HYPOTHALAMIC ORIGIN, NONENHANCING

1. Glioma, low grade hypothalamic
2. Hamartoma of tuber cinereum (rare: usually isointense to brain)

Reference
1. Zhu M, Maeda M, Lee GJ, Yuh WTC: Chapter 53. Sellar Lesions. In: Stark DD, Bradley WG (eds): Magnetic Resonance Imaging. (ed 3) St. Louis: Mosby, 1999, pp 1225–1230

DARK ON T1-WEIGHTED IMAGE, BRIGHT ON T2-WEIGHTED IMAGE, SMALL PITUITARY LESION, NONENHANCING

1. Cyst of pars intermedia
2. Fibrosis
3. Hemorrhage, chronic
4. [Partial volume averaging cavernous carotid artery]
5. Pituitary microadenoma

[ ] This condition does not actually cause the gamuted imaging finding, but can produce imaging changes that simulate it.

Reference
1. Zhu M, Maeda M, Lee GJ, Yuh WTC: Chapter 53. Sellar Lesions. In: Stark DD, Bradley WG (eds): Magnetic Resonance Imaging. (ed 3) St. Louis: Mosby, 1999, pp 1225–1230

DARK ON T1-WEIGHTED IMAGE, BRIGHT ON T2-WEIGHTED IMAGE, PINEAL REGION TUMOR

PINEAL ORIGIN
1. [Benign cystic pineal gland]
2. Pineoblastoma
3. Pineocytoma

GERM CELL ORIGIN
1. Choriocarcinoma (rare)
2. Embryonal carcinoma (rare)
3. Germinoma (common; usually males)
4. Teratoma

[ ] This condition does not actually cause the gamuted imaging finding, but can produce imaging changes that simulate it.

Reference
1. Boyko OB: Chapter 65. Pediatric Brain Tumors. In: Stark DD, Bradley WG (eds): Magnetic Resonance Imaging. (ed 3) St. Louis: Mosby, 1999, pp 1467–1482

Gamut M-33

CSF INTENSITY LESION, PARENCHYMAL DISEASE, NO MASS EFFECT

1. Cryptococcal pseudocysts (early)
2. Cyst, developmental parenchymal
3. Encephalomalacia, macrocystic (following stroke, trauma, bleed, surgery)
4. Marchiafava-Bignami disease (corpus callosum)
5. Mucopolysaccharidosis
6. Myelinolysis, extrapontine
7. Neuroepithelial cyst (eg, choroid fissure)
8. [Perivascular ("Virchow-Robin") space]
9. Porencephalic cyst

[ ] This condition does not actually cause the gamuted imaging finding, but can produce imaging changes that simulate it.

Reference
1. Sze GK: Chapter 60. Infection and Inflammation. In: Stark DD, Bradley WG (eds): Magnetic Resonance Imaging. (ed 3) St. Louis: Mosby, 1999, pp 1361–1378

Gamut M-34

CSF INTENSITY LESION, PARENCHYMAL DISEASE, MASS EFFECT, NONENHANCING

1. Arachnoid cyst
2. Cryptococcal pseudocysts (late)
3. Cysticercus cyst (alive)

4. Hydatid cyst (alive)
5. Parenchymal cyst

Reference
1. Sze GK: Chapter 60. Infection and Inflammation. In: Stark DD, Bradley WG (eds): Magnetic Resonance Imaging. (ed 3) St. Louis: Mosby, 1999, pp 1361–1378

Gamut M-35

CSF INTENSITY LESION, PARENCHYMAL DISEASE, MASS EFFECT, ENHANCING RIM OR NODULE

1. Cysticercus cyst (dead)
2. Hydatid cyst (dead)
3. Metastasis, cystic (eg, from ovarian carcinoma)

Reference
1. Sze GK: Chapter 60. Infection and Inflammation. In: Stark DD, Bradley WG (eds): Magnetic Resonance Imaging. (ed 3) St. Louis: Mosby, 1999, pp 1361–1378

Gamut M-36

CSF INTENSITY LESION, BRAIN STEM

1. Infarct, old
2. Myelinolysis, central pontine
3. [Perivascular space]
4. Syringobulbia

[ ] This condition does not actually cause the gamuted imaging finding, but can produce imaging changes that simulate it.

Reference
1. Bradley WG: Chapter 51. Brainstem: Normal Anatomy and Pathology. In: Stark DD, Bradley WG (eds): Magnetic Resonance Imaging. (ed 3) St. Louis: Mosby, 1999, pp 1187–1208

Gamut M-37

CSF INTENSITY LESION, SELLAR/SUPRASELLAR REGION

1. Arachnoid cyst
2. Cephalocele, sphenoid
3. Empty sella

References

1. Zhu M, Maeda M, Lee GJ, Yuh WTC: Chapter 53. Sellar Lesions. In: Stark DD, Bradley WG (eds): Magnetic Resonance Imaging. (ed 3) St. Louis: Mosby, 1999, pp 1225–1230
2. Zimmerman RA, Bilaniuk LT: Chapter 62. Pediatric Cerebral Anomalies. In: Stark DD, Bradley WG (eds): Magnetic Resonance Imaging. (ed 3) St. Louis: Mosby, 1999, pp 1403–1424

Gamut M-38

CSF INTENSITY LESION, POSTERIOR FOSSA

1. Arachnoid cyst
2. Cysticercosis
3. Dandy-Walker cyst (or variant)
4. Epidermoid
5. Mega cisterna magna
6. Trapped fourth ventricle

References

1. Boyko OB: Chapter 54. Adult Brain Tumors. In: Stark DD, Bradley WG (eds): Magnetic Resonance Imaging. (ed 3) St. Louis: Mosby, 1999, pp 1231–1254
2. Zimmerman RA, Bilaniuk LT: Chapter 62. Pediatric Cerebral Anomalies. In: Stark DD, Bradley WG (eds): Magnetic Resonance Imaging. (ed 3) St. Louis: Mosby, 1999, pp 1403–1424

Gamut M-39

DARK ON T1- AND T2-WEIGHTED IMAGES, NONSPECIFIC LOCATION, NO MASS EFFECT

1. Calcification, esp. from old infection (eg, cysticercosis; tuberculosis; TORCH: toxoplasma, rubella, cytomegalovirus, herpes)
2. Cavernous or venous angioma (hemosiderin from chronic bleeding)
3. Contusion, old hemorrhagic
4. Shearing injury, hemorrhagic, acute (deoxyhemoglobin) or chronic (hemosiderin)

References

1. Evans SJJ, Gean AD: Chapter 59. Craniocerebral Trauma. In: Stark DD, Bradley WG (eds): Magnetic Resonance Imaging. (ed 3) St. Louis: Mosby, 1999, pp 1347–1369
2. Sze GK: Chapter 60. Infection and Inflammation. In: Stark DD, Bradley WG (eds): Magnetic Resonance Imaging. (ed 3) St. Louis: Mosby, 1999, pp 1361–1378

Gamut M-40

DARK ON T1- AND T2-WEIGHTED IMAGES, NONSPECIFIC LOCATION, MASS EFFECT

1. Aneurysm, acutely clotted
2. Cavernous angioma, old
3. Chloroma (leukemia)
4. Hemorrhage, acute (intracellular deoxyhemoglobin) (See A-99)
5. Leukoencephalopathy, hemorrhagic (autoimmune)
6. Lymphoma$_g$
7. Metastases, hemorrhagic (from carcinoma of breast, lung, kidney or thyroid; choriocarcinoma; melanoma)
8. Metastases, Short T2 (mucinous adenocarcinoma of colon; carcinoma of prostate; melanoma; osteosarcoma)

References
1. Boyko OB: Chapter 54. Adult Brain Tumors. In: Stark DD, Bradley WG (eds): Magnetic Resonance Imaging. (ed 3) St. Louis: Mosby, 1999, pp 1231–1254
2. Bradley WG: Chapter 58. Hemorrhage. In: Stark DD, Bradley WG (eds): Magnetic Resonance Imaging. (ed 3) St. Louis: Mosby, 1999, pp 1329–1346
3. Litt AW, Maltin EP: Chapter 57. Cerebrovascular Abnormalities. In: Stark DD, Bradley WG (eds): Magnetic Resonance Imaging. (ed 3) St. Louis: Mosby, 1999, pp 1317–1328

Gamut M-41

DARK ON T1- AND T2-WEIGHTED IMAGES, CORTICAL, NO MASS EFFECT, NONENHANCING

1. Infarct, old hemorrhagic (hemosiderin)
2. Siderosis, superficial (following surgery or subarachnoid hemorrhage)

Reference
1. Bradley WG: Chapter 58. Hemorrhage. In: Stark DD, Bradley WG (eds): Magnetic Resonance Imaging. (ed 3) St. Louis: Mosby, 1999, pp 1329–1346

Gamut M-42

DARK ON T1- AND T2-WEIGHTED IMAGES, CORTICAL, NO MASS EFFECT, ENHANCING

1. Infarction, hemorrhagic (subacute)
2. Metastases, leptomeningeal, hemorrhagic (Short T2)
3. [Vein]
4. Venous angioma

[ ] This condition does not actually cause the gamuted imaging finding, but can produce imaging changes that simulate it.

Reference
1. Bradley WG: Chapter 58. Hemorrhage. In: Stark DD, Bradley WG (eds): Magnetic Resonance Imaging. (ed 3) St. Louis: Mosby, 1999, pp 1329–1346

Gamut M-43

DARK ON T1- AND T2-WEIGHTED IMAGES, CORTICAL, MASS EFFECT

1. Contusion, acute hemorrhagic (deoxyhemoglobin)
2. Infarction, acute hemorrhagic

Reference
1. Bradley WG: Chapter 58. Hemorrhage. In: Stark DD, Bradley WG (eds): Magnetic Resonance Imaging. (ed 3) St. Louis: Mosby, 1999, pp 1329–1346

Gamut M-44

DARK ON T1- AND T2-WEIGHTED IMAGES, BASAL GANGLIA

1. Calcification, idiopathic
2. Carbon monoxide poisoning
3. Ferrocalcinosis (eg, hemorrhagic lacunar infarct)
4. Hallervorden-Spatz disease
5. Hemorrhage, acute (intracellular deoxyhemoglobin)
6. Iron deposition following ischemic-anoxic event in child (eg, near-drowning)
7. [Normal ferritin deposition (globus pallidus; putamen)]
8. Parkinson's plus (eg, Shy-Drager S.; progressive supranuclear palsy)

[ ] This condition does not actually cause the gamuted imaging finding, but can produce imaging changes that simulate it.

References
1. Bradley WG: Chapter 51. Brainstem: Normal Anatomy and Pathology. In: Stark DD, Bradley WG (eds): Magnetic Resonance Imaging. (ed 3) St. Louis: Mosby, 1999, pp 1187–1208
2. Bradley WG: Chapter 58. Hemorrhage. In: Stark DD, Bradley WG (eds): Magnetic Resonance Imaging. (ed 3) St. Louis: Mosby, 1999, pp 1329–1346

DARK ON T1-AND T2-WEIGHTED IMAGES, INTRAVASCULAR

1. Calcific atherosclerosis
2. [Normal flow void]
3. Thrombosis, acute (deoxyhemoglobin)

[ ] This condition does not actually cause the gamuted imaging finding, but can produce imaging changes that simulate it.

Reference

1. Bradley WG: Chapter 58. Hemorrhage. In: Stark DD, Bradley WG (eds): Magnetic Resonance Imaging. (ed 3) St. Louis: Mosby, 1999, pp 1329–1346

DARK ON T1- AND T2-WEIGHTED IMAGES, BRAIN STEM

NORMAL STRUCTURES

1. [Corticospinal tracts]
2. [Medial lemnisci]
3. [Medial longitudinal fasciculi]

ABNORMAL

1. Arteriovenous malformation (AVM)
2. Cavernous angioma (hemosiderin)
3. Hemorrhage, acute (eg, from hypertension) (intracellular deoxyhemoglobin)
4. Tortuous basilar or vertebral artery

[ ] This condition does not actually cause the gamuted imaging finding, but can produce imaging changes that simulate it.

References

1. Bradley WG: Chapter 51. Brainstem: Normal Anatomy and Pathology. In: Stark DD, Bradley WG (eds): Magnetic Resonance Imaging. (ed 3) St. Louis: Mosby, 1999, pp 1187–1208

2. Bradley WG: Chapter 58. Hemorrhage. In: Stark DD, Bradley WG (eds): Magnetic Resonance Imaging. (ed 3) St. Louis: Mosby, 1999, pp 1329–1346
3. Litt AW, Maltin EP: Chapter 57. Cerebrovascular Abnormalities. In: Stark DD, Bradley WG (eds): Magnetic Resonance Imaging. (ed 3) St. Louis: Mosby, 1999, pp 1317–1328

BRIGHT ON T1- AND T2-WEIGHTED IMAGES, NONSPECIFIC LOCATION

1. Aneurysm, late subacute thrombosis
2. Cavernous angioma (methemoglobin)
3. [Flow artifact]
4. Hemorrhage, late subacute (extracellular methemoglobin) (See A-99, M-4-S-2)

[ ] This condition does not actually cause the gamuted imaging finding, but can produce imaging changes that simulate it.

References

1. Bradley WG: Chapter 58. Hemorrhage. In: Stark DD, Bradley WG (eds): Magnetic Resonance Imaging. (ed 3) St. Louis: Mosby, 1999, pp 1329–1346
2. Litt AW, Maltin EP: Chapter 57. Cerebrovascular Abnormalities. In: Stark DD, Bradley WG (eds): Magnetic Resonance Imaging. (ed 3) St. Louis: Mosby, 1999, pp 1317–1328

BRIGHT ON T1- AND T2-WEIGHTED IMAGES, SELLA REGION

1. Aneurysm, thrombosed cavernous carotid (late subacute hemorrhage)
2. Colloid cyst
3. Craniopharyngioma (cystic)
4. Dermoid (cystic)
5. [Diamagnetic susceptibility artifact]

6. Pituitary hemorrhage, late subacute, esp. Sheehan S. (Simmonds disease) (postpartum pituitary necrosis or following bromocryptine therapy)
7. Rathke cleft cyst

[ ] This condition does not actually cause the gamuted imaging finding, but can produce imaging changes that simulate it.

References
1. Bradley WG: Chapter 58. Hemorrhage. In: Stark DD, Bradley WG (eds): Magnetic Resonance Imaging. (ed 3) St. Louis: Mosby, 1999, pp 1329–1346
2. Litt AW, Maltin EP: Chapter 57. Cerebrovascular Abnormalities. In: Stark DD, Bradley WG (eds): Magnetic Resonance Imaging. (ed 3) St. Louis: Mosby, 1999, pp 1317–1328
3. Zhu M, Maeda M, Lee GJ, Yuh WTC: Chapter 53. Sellar Lesions. In: Stark DD, Bradley WG (eds): Magnetic Resonance Imaging. (ed 3) St. Louis: Mosby, 1999, pp 1225–1230

Gamut M-49

BRIGHT ON T1-WEIGHTED IMAGE, DARK ON T2-WEIGHTED IMAGE, NONSPECIFIC LOCATION

1. Aneurysm, clotted (early subacute hemorrhage)
2. Calcification ("milk of calcium")
3. Dermoid
4. [Flow artifact]
5. Hemorrhage, early subacute (intracellular methemoglobin) (See M-4-S2)
6. Lipoma (on conventional spin echo only; bright on T2-weighted fast spin echo)
7. Shearing injury (early subacute)
8. "White" epidermoid (liquid triglyceride)

[ ] This condition does not actually cause the gamuted imaging finding, but can produce imaging changes that simulate it.

References
1. Bradley WG: Chapter 58. Hemorrhage. In: Stark DD, Bradley WG (eds): Magnetic Resonance Imaging. (ed 3) St. Louis: Mosby, 1999, pp 1329–1346

2. Evans SJJ, Gean AD: Chapter 59. Craniocerebral Trauma. In: Stark DD, Bradley WG (eds): Magnetic Resonance Imaging. (ed 3) St. Louis: Mosby, 1999, pp 1347–1369
3. Litt AW, Maltin EP: Chapter 57. Cerebrovascular Abnormalities. In: Stark DD, Bradley WG (eds): Magnetic Resonance Imaging. (ed 3) St. Louis: Mosby, 1999, pp 1317–1328

Gamut M-50

BRIGHT ON T1-WEIGHTED IMAGE, DARK ON T2-WEIGHTED IMAGE, PUTAMEN

1. Aluminum toxicity
2. Calcification, idiopathic
3. Hepatic encephalopathy
4. Hyperalimentation
5. Wilson's disease

Reference
1. Pomeranz SJ, Smith PJ: Gamuts & Pearls in Neurologic MRI. Cincinnati: MRI-EFI Publ, 1998

Gamut M-51

BRIGHT ON T1-WEIGHTED IMAGE, DARK ON T2-WEIGHTED IMAGE, SELLA REGION

1. Dermoid (fatty)
2. Ectopic posterior lobe of pituitary (following distal stalk transection)
3. Lipoma
4. [Normal posterior lobe of pituitary]
5. Pituitary hemorrhage, early subacute (intracellular methemoglobin)
6. "White" epidermoid (liquid triglyceride)

[ ] This condition does not actually cause the gamuted imaging finding, but can produce imaging changes that simulate it.

(continued)

References

1. Bradley WG: Chapter 58. Hemorrhage. In: Stark DD, Bradley WG (eds): Magnetic Resonance Imaging. (ed 3) St. Louis: Mosby, 1999, pp 1329–1346
2. Zhu M, Maeda M, Lee GJ, Yuh WTC: Chapter 53. Sellar Lesions. In: Stark DD, Bradley WG (eds): Magnetic Resonance Imaging. (ed 3) St. Louis: Mosby, 1999, pp 1225–1230

Gamut M-52

SIGNAL VOID, NONSPECIFIC LOCATION

1. Aneurysm
2. Arteriovenous malformation; venous angioma
3. Bone fragment (posttrauma)
4. Calcification, dense (See M-53-S)
5. Hemosiderin
6. Metallic artifact (eg, aneurysm clip)
7. [Normal vessel (artery; dural sinus)]
8. Pneumocephalus
9. Shunt tube
10. Medullary vein, enlarged
11. Collateral vessels (eg, in basal ganglia due to moya-moya)

[ ] This condition does not actually cause the gamuted imaging finding, but can produce imaging changes that simulate it.

References

1. Bradley WG: Chapter 11. Flow Phenomena. In: Stark DD, Bradley WG (eds): Magnetic Resonance Imaging. (ed 3) St. Louis: Mosby, 1999, pp 231–256
2. Bradley WG: Chapter 58. Hemorrhage. In: Stark DD, Bradley WG (eds): Magnetic Resonance Imaging. (ed 3) St. Louis: Mosby, 1999, pp 1329–1346
3. Jensen MD, Brant-Zawadzki M, Jacobs BC: Chapter 55. Ischemia. In: Stark DD, Bradley WG (eds): Magnetic Resonance Imaging. (ed 3) St. Louis: Mosby, 1999, pp 1255–1276
4. Litt AW, Maltin EP: Chapter 57. Cerebrovascular Abnormalities. In: Stark DD, Bradley WG (eds): Magnetic Resonance Imaging. (ed 3) St. Louis: Mosby, 1999, pp 1317–1328

Gamut M-53-S

DENSE INTRACRANIAL CALCIFICATION(S) (See A-46–50)

1. Congenital transplacental infection (eg, TORCH [toxoplasma, rubella, cytomegalovirus, herpes]; AIDS)
2. Hemorrhage, old (ferrocalcinosis)
3. Infection, old (eg, tuberculosis; cysticercosis; paragonimiasis; syphilis)
4. Tumor, benign (eg, oligodendroglioma)

Reference

1. Sze GK: Chapter 60. Infection and Inflammation. In: Stark DD, Bradley WG (eds): Magnetic Resonance Imaging. (ed 3) St. Louis: Mosby, 1999, pp 1361–1378

Gamut M-54

SIGNAL VOID, SUBEPENDYMAL

1. Arteriovenous malformation; venous angioma
2. Hamartoma, calcified (tuberous sclerosis)
3. Shunt tube

References

1. Bradley WG, Quencer RM: Chapter 66. Hydrocephalus and Cerebrospinal Fluid Flow. In: Stark DD, Bradley WG (eds): Magnetic Resonance Imaging. (ed 3) St. Louis: Mosby, 1999, pp 1483–1508
2. Litt AW, Maltin EP: Chapter 57. Cerebrovascular Abnormalities. In: Stark DD, Bradley WG (eds): Magnetic Resonance Imaging. (ed 3) St. Louis: Mosby, 1999, pp 1317–1328

Gamut M-55

SIGNAL VOID, SELLA REGION

1. Aneurysm (cavernous or supraclinoid carotid; basilar tip)
2. Carotid-cavernous fistula
3. "Kissing carotids"
4. Meningioma, densely calcified
5. [Metallic artifact (from clipped aneurysm)]
6. Pneumatized posterior clinoid

[ ] This condition does not actually cause the gamuted imaging finding, but can produce imaging changes that simulate it.

References
1. Boyko OB: Chapter 54. Adult Brain Tumors. In: Stark DD, Bradley WG (eds): Magnetic Resonance Imaging. (ed 3) St. Louis: Mosby, 1999, pp 1231–1254
2. Litt AW, Maltin EP: Chapter 57. Cerebrovascular Abnormalities. In: Stark DD, Bradley WG (eds): Magnetic Resonance Imaging. (ed 3) St. Louis: Mosby, 1999, pp 1317–1328

Gamut M-56

SMALL VENTRICLES, SMALL SULCI

1. Edema, diffuse brain
2. [Normal variant]
3. Pseudotumor cerebri

[ ] This condition does not actually cause the gamuted imaging finding, but can produce imaging changes that simulate it.

Reference
1. Jensen MD, Brant-Zawadzki M, Jacobs BC: Chapter 55. Ischemia. In: Stark DD, Bradley WG (eds): Magnetic Resonance Imaging. (ed 3) St. Louis: Mosby, 1999, pp 1255–1276

Gamut M-57

SYMETRICALLY ENLARGED VENTRICLES, SMALL SULCI

1. Central atrophy (eg, deep white matter ischemia; near-drowning or other ischemia-anoxia event; chronic multiple sclerosis)
2. Culpocephaly (dilated occipital horns only)
3. Hydrocephalus, communicating, chronic (See A-114, M-57-2)
4. Hydrocephalus, obstructive (See A-114, M-57-3)

References
1. Bradley WG, Quencer RM: Chapter 66. Hydrocephalus and Cerebrospinal Fluid Flow. In: Stark DD, Bradley WG (eds): Magnetic Resonance Imaging. (ed 3) St. Louis: Mosby, 1999, pp 1483–1508
2. Zimmerman RA, Bilaniuk LT: Chapter 62. Pediatric Cerebral Anomalies. In: Stark DD, Bradley WG (eds): Magnetic Resonance Imaging. (ed 3) St. Louis: Mosby, 1999, pp 1403–1424

Gamut M-58-1

ASYMMETRICALLY ENLARGED LATERAL VENTRICLES

1. Dyke-Davidoff-Masson S. (hemiatrophy)
2. Entrapment/obstruction at one foramen of Monro
3. Mesial temporal sclerosis (temporal horn only)
4. Normal variant
5. Paragonimiasis

Reference
1. Zimmerman RA, Bilaniuk LT: Chapter 62. Pediatric Cerebral Anomalies. In: Stark DD, Bradley WG (eds): Magnetic Resonance Imaging. (ed 3) St. Louis: Mosby, 1999, pp 1403–1424

Gamut M-58-2

ENLARGED TEMPORAL HORN (ISOLATED)

1. Entrapment (by atrial mass-unilateral)
2. Mesial temporal sclerosis (usually unilateral, leading to partial complex seizures)

Reference
1. Bradley WG, Quencer RM: Chapter 66. Hydrocephalus and Cerebrospinal Fluid Flow. In: Stark DD, Bradley WG (eds): Magnetic Resonance Imaging. (ed 3) St. Louis: Mosby, 1999, pp 1483–1508

Gamut M-59

ENLARGED VENTRICLES, LARGE SULCI

1. Alcoholism
2. Atrophy (due to AIDS; Alzheimer's disease; chronic multiple sclerosis; radiation therapy; chemotherapy; postinfectious; posttraumatic; global ischemia; dehydration)
3. Catabolic steroids
4. Cushing S.
5. Jakob-Creutzfeldt disease
6. Protein and/or calorie deprivation (eg, starvation; malnutrition; kwashiorkor; anorexia nervosa)

Reference
1. Bradley WG, Quencer RM: Chapter 66. Hydrocephalus and Cerebrospinal Fluid Flow. In: Stark DD, Bradley WG (eds): Magnetic Resonance Imaging. (ed 3) St. Louis: Mosby, 1999, pp 1483–1508

Gamut M-60

ABNORMAL VENTRICULAR CONFIGURATION

1. Agenesis of corpus callosum (high-riding third ventricle between lateral ventricles)
2. Asymmetry of lateral ventricles (See M-58-1)
3. Cavum of the velum interpositum (triangular CSF space separating posterior lateral ventricular bodies)
4. Cavum septum pellucidum and vergae (separation of lateral ventricles)
5. Hemimegalencephaly (single, enlarged, misshapen lateral ventricle with surrounding heterotopic gray matter)
6. Holoprosencephaly, alobar and semilobar (single ventricle)
7. Parasitic disease (esp. paragonimiasis; neurocysticercosis)
8. Periventricular leukomalacia (enlarged, irregular lateral ventricles)
9. Schizencephaly (lateral ventricular wall tethered laterally by gray matter-lined cleft)

Reference
1. Zimmerman RA, Bilaniuk LT: Chapter 62. Pediatric Cerebral Anomalies. In: Stark DD, Bradley WG (eds): Magnetic Resonance Imaging. (ed 3) St. Louis: Mosby, 1999, pp 1403–1424

Gamut M-61

INTRAVENTRICULAR MASS, CSF INTENSITY

1. Arachnoid cyst
2. "Black" epidermoid (solid cholesterol/cholesterin)
3. Cysticercosis
4. Dandy-Walker cyst or variant (enlarged fourth ventricle)

References

1. Bradley WG, Quencer RM: Chapter 66. Hydrocephalus and Cerebrospinal Fluid Flow. In: Stark DD, Bradley WG (eds): Magnetic Resonance Imaging. (ed 3) St. Louis: Mosby, 1999, pp 1483–1508
2. Zimmerman RA, Bilaniuk LT: Chapter 62. Pediatric Cerebral Anomalies. In: Stark DD, Bradley WG (eds): Magnetic Resonance Imaging. (ed 3) St. Louis: Mosby, 1999, pp 1403–1424

Gamut M-62

INTRAVENTRICULAR MASS, DARK ON T1-WEIGHTED IMAGE, BRIGHT ON T2-WEIGHTED IMAGE, NONENHANCING

1. "Black" epidermoid (solid cholesterol/cholesterin)
2. Colloid cyst (third ventricle)
2. Neuroepithelial cyst (choroid plexus)

Gamut M-63

INTRAVENTRICULAR MASS, DARK ON T1-WEIGHTED IMAGE, BRIGHT ON T2-WEIGHTED IMAGE, ENHANCING

1. Astrocytoma
2. Central neurocytoma (rare)
3. Choroid plexus papilloma or carcinoma
4. Colloid cyst
5. Ependymoma
6. Giant cell astrocytoma (in tuberous sclerosis—increases in size)
7. Hamartoma, subependymal (in tuberous sclerosis—does not increase in size)
8. Meningioma
9. Metastasis to choroid plexus (esp. from carcinoma of lung, colon, or breast; melanoma)
10. Metastasis, intraventricular (eg, spread of high-grade glioma)
11. Subependymoma (rare)

References

1. Boyko OB: Chapter 54. Adult Brain Tumors. In: Stark DD, Bradley WG (eds): Magnetic Resonance Imaging. (ed 3) St. Louis: Mosby, 1999, pp 1231–1254
2. Pomeranz SJ, Smith PJ: Gamuts & Pearls in Neurologic MRI. Cincinnati: MRI-EFI Publ, 1998

Gamut M-64

INTRAVENTRICULAR MASS, DARK ON T1- AND T2-WEIGHTED IMAGES

1. Glomus of choroid plexus, calcified
2. Hematoma, acute (deoxyhemoglobin)
3. Meningioma, densely calcified

References
1. Boyko OB: Chapter 54. Adult Brain Tumors. In: Stark DD, Bradley WG (eds): Magnetic Resonance Imaging. (ed 3) St. Louis: Mosby, 1999, pp 1231–1254
2. Bradley WG: Chapter 58. Hemorrhage. In: Stark DD, Bradley WG (eds): Magnetic Resonance Imaging. (ed 3) St. Louis: Mosby, 1999, pp 1329–1346

Gamut M-65

INTRAVENTRICULAR MASS, BRIGHT ON T1-WEIGHTED IMAGE, DARK ON T2-WEIGHTED CONVENTIONAL SPIN ECHO IMAGE

1. Dermoid
2. Hemorrhage, early subacute (intracellular methemoglobin)
3. Lipoma
4. Pantopaque
5. Xanthogranuloma of choroid plexus

References
1. Boyko OB: Chapter 54. Adult Brain Tumors. In: Stark DD, Bradley WG (eds): Magnetic Resonance Imaging. (ed 3) St. Louis: Mosby, 1999, pp 1231–1254
2. Bradley WG: Chapter 58. Hemorrhage. In: Stark DD, Bradley WG (eds): Magnetic Resonance Imaging. (ed 3) St. Louis: Mosby, 1999, pp 1329–1346

Gamut M-66

INTRAVENTRICULAR MASS, BRIGHT ON T1- AND T2-WEIGHTED IMAGES

1. Hemorrhage, late subacute (extracellular methemoglobin)
2. Lipoma (fast spin echo)

References
1. Bradley WG, Chen D-Y, Atkinson DJ, Edelman RR: Chapter 7. Fast Spin-Echo and Echo-Planar Imaging. In: Stark DD, Bradley WG (eds): Magnetic Resonance Imaging. (ed 3) St. Louis: Mosby, 1999, pp 150–158
2. Bradley WG: Chapter 58. Hemorrhage. In: Stark DD, Bradley WG (eds): Magnetic Resonance Imaging. (ed 3) St. Louis: Mosby, 1999, pp 1329–1346

Gamut M-67

INTRAVENTRICULAR SIGNAL VOID

1. Arteriovenous malformation (AVM)
2. Hyperdynamic CSF flow (communicating hydrocephalus; shunt-responsive normal pressure hydrocephalus)
3. Normal CSF flow (near aqueduct and foramen of Monro)
4. Pneumocephalus (postoperative; posttraumatic)
5. Vein of Galen "aneurysm" (posterior third ventricle)

References
1. Bradley WG, Quencer RM: Chapter 66. Hydrocephalus and Cerebrospinal Fluid Flow. In: Stark DD, Bradley WG (eds): Magnetic Resonance Imaging. (ed 3) St. Louis: Mosby, 1999, pp 1483–1508
2. Litt AW, Maltin EP: Chapter 57. Cerebrovascular Abnormalities. In: Stark DD, Bradley WG (eds): Magnetic Resonance Imaging. (ed 3) St. Louis: Mosby, 1999, pp 1317–1328

Gamut M-68

SUBARACHNOID SPACE LESION, HYPERINTENSE TO BRAIN ON FLAIR

1. [CSF flow related enhancement]
2. Hemorrhage, acute subarachnoid (protein effect)
3. Meningitis

[ ] This condition does not actually cause the gamuted imaging finding, but can produce imaging changes that simulate it.

References
1. Bradley WG: Chapter 11. Flow Phenomena. In: Stark DD, Bradley WG (eds): Magnetic Resonance Imaging. (ed 3) St. Louis: Mosby, 1999, pp 231–256
2. Bradley WG: Chapter 58. Hemorrhage. In: Stark DD, Bradley WG (eds): Magnetic Resonance Imaging. (ed 3) St. Louis: Mosby, 1999, pp 1329–1346
3. Bradley WG, Quencer RM: Chapter 66. Hydrocephalus and Cerebrospinal Fluid Flow. In: Stark DD, Bradley WG (eds): Magnetic Resonance Imaging. (ed 3) St. Louis: Mosby, 1999, pp 1483–1508
4. Sze GK: Chapter 60. Infection and Inflammation. In: Stark DD, Bradley WG (eds): Magnetic Resonance Imaging. (ed 3) St. Louis: Mosby, 1999, pp 1361–1378

Gamut M-69

SUBARACHNOID SPACE LESION, HYPERINTENSE TO BRAIN ON T1-WEIGHTED IMAGE

1. [CSF flow-related enhancement]
2. Dermoid
3. Hemorrhage, subacute subarachnoid (methemoglobin)
4. Lipoma (eg, cerebellopontine angle)
5. Pantopaque
6. "White" epidermoid (liquid triglyceride)

[ ] This condition does not actually cause the gamuted imaging finding, but can produce imaging changes that simulate it.

References
1. Bradley WG: Chapter 11. Flow Phenomena. In: Stark DD, Bradley WG (eds): Magnetic Resonance Imaging. (ed 3) St. Louis: Mosby, 1999, pp 231–256
2. Bradley WG, Quencer RM: Chapter 66. Hydrocephalus and Cerebrospinal Fluid Flow. In: Stark DD, Bradley WG (eds): Magnetic Resonance Imaging. (ed 3) St. Louis: Mosby, 1999, pp 1483–1508

Gamut M-70

SUBARACHNOID SPACE LESION, ISOINTENSE TO CSF

1. Arachnoid cyst
2. Cysticercosis (basilar racemose form)

Reference
1. Sze GK: Chapter 60. Infection and Inflammation. In: Stark DD, Bradley WG (eds): Magnetic Resonance Imaging. (ed 3) St. Louis: Mosby, 1999, pp 1361–1378

Gamut M-71

SUBARACHNOID SPACE, SIGNAL VOID

1. [Juxta-arterial CSF dephasing]
2. [Metallic (clip) artifact]
3. [Normal flow in artery]
4. [Normal CSF flow]
5. Third ventriculostomy

[ ] This condition does not actually cause the gamuted imaging finding, but can produce imaging changes that simulate it.

References
1. Bradley WG: Chapter 11. Flow Phenomena. In: Stark DD, Bradley WG (eds): Magnetic Resonance Imaging. (ed 3) St. Louis: Mosby, 1999, pp 231–256
2. Bradley WG, Quencer RM: Chapter 66. Hydrocephalus and Cerebrospinal Fluid Flow. In: Stark DD, Bradley WG (eds): Magnetic Resonance Imaging. (ed 3) St. Louis: Mosby, 1999, pp 1483–1508

Gamut M-72

MASS IN THE CEREBELLOPONTINE ANGLE CISTERN—ENHANCING

COMMON
1. Acoustic schwannoma
2. Meningioma
3. Trigeminal schwannoma (may have "dumbbell" shape with second mass in cavernous sinus)

UNCOMMON
1. Aneurysm of vertebral artery
2. Chordoma
3. Exophytic tumor (ependymoma or brain stem glioma)
4. Glomus tumor (jugulare, tympanicum, vagale)

References
1. Boyko OB: Chapter 54. Adult Brain Tumors. In: Stark DD, Bradley WG (eds): Magnetic Resonance Imaging. (ed 3) St. Louis: Mosby, 1999, pp 1231–1254
2. Litt AW, Maltin EP: Chapter 57. Cerebrovascular Abnormalities. In: Stark DD, Bradley WG (eds): Magnetic Resonance Imaging. (ed 3) St. Louis: Mosby, 1999, pp 1317–1328

Gamut M-73

MASS IN THE CEREBELLOPONTINE ANGLE CISTERN—NONENHANCING

1. Arachnoid cyst
2. Epidermoid
3. Lipoma

Reference
1. Boyko OB: Chapter 54. Adult Brain Tumors. In: Stark DD, Bradley WG (eds): Magnetic Resonance Imaging. (ed 3) St. Louis: Mosby, 1999, pp 1231–1254

Gamut M-74

FOCAL LEPTOMENINGEAL ENHANCEMENT

1. Carcinomatosis, leptomeningeal (eg, from carcinoma of breast or lung; melanoma)
2. Hyperemia, post-ictal
3. Infarction, subjacent acute (leptomeningeal collaterals) or subacute
4. Lymphoma$_g$
5. Meningitis, localized (eg, tuberculous)
6. Sarcoidosis
7. Scar, postoperative
8. Vasculitis

References
1. Boyko OB: Chapter 54. Adult Brain Tumors. In: Stark DD, Bradley WG (eds): Magnetic Resonance Imaging. (ed 3) St. Louis: Mosby, 1999, pp 1231–1254
2. Sze GK: Chapter 60. Infection and Inflammation. In: Stark DD, Bradley WG (eds): Magnetic Resonance Imaging. (ed 3) St. Louis: Mosby, 1999, pp 1361–1378

Gamut M-75

DIFFUSE LEPTOMENINGEAL ENHANCEMENT

1. Carcinomatosis, leptomeningeal (eg, from carcinoma of breast or lung; melanoma; or ependymoma)
2. Hemorrhage, post-subarachnoid
3. Hypotension, intracranial (after lumbar puncture or CSF leak)
4. Meningitis
5. Sarcoidosis
6. Postoperative (late finding)
7. Posttraumatic (late finding)

References
1. Bradley WG, Quencer RM: Chapter 66. Hydrocephalus and Cerebrospinal Fluid Flow. In: Stark DD, Bradley WG (eds): Magnetic Resonance Imaging. (ed 3) St. Louis: Mosby, 1999, pp 1483–1508
2. Sze GK: Chapter 60. Infection and Inflammation. In: Stark DD, Bradley WG (eds): Magnetic Resonance Imaging. (ed 3) St. Louis: Mosby, 1999, pp 1361–1378

Gamut M-76

PACHYMENINGEAL (DURAL) NONENHANCING LESION

1. Calcification, dense (black)
2. Meningioma, densely calcified
3. Ossification of falx (black rim, fatty center)

Reference
1. Sze GK: Chapter 60. Infection and Inflammation. In: Stark DD, Bradley WG (eds): Magnetic Resonance Imaging. (ed 3) St. Louis: Mosby, 1999, pp 1361–1378

Gamut M-77

PACHYMENINGEAL (DURAL) ENHANCEMENT

1. Fibrosis, benign meningeal (following shunt, subarachnoid hemorrhage, or surgery)
2. Hypotension, intracranial (after lumbar puncture or CSF leak)
3. Local tumor spread (eg, from glioblastoma)
4. Meningioma, dural tail
5. Meningitis (eg, tuberculous)
6. Metastasis, dural (eg, neuroblastoma)
7. [Normal (esp. at high field with high-dose gadolinium)]

[ ] This condition does not actually cause the gamuted imaging finding, but can produce imaging changes that simulate it.

Reference
1. Sze GK: Chapter 60. Infection and Inflammation. In: Stark DD, Bradley WG (eds): Magnetic Resonance Imaging. (ed 3) St. Louis: Mosby, 1999, pp 1361–1378

Gamut M-78

EXTRAAXIAL FLUID COLLECTION, CSF INTENSITY

1. Arachnoid cyst
2. Arachnoid rent, posttraumatic ("subdural hygroma")
3. Benign external hydrocephalus (immature arachnoidal granulations under age 1)
4. Benign subdural effusions (in neonatal meningitis)
5. Brain atrophy
6. Cysticercosis

References
1. Bradley WG, Quencer RM: Chapter 66. Hydrocephalus and Cerebrospinal Fluid Flow. In: Stark DD, Bradley WG (eds): Magnetic Resonance Imaging. (ed 3) St. Louis: Mosby, 1999, pp 1483–1508
2. Evans AJJ, Gean AD: Chapter 59. Craniocerebral Trauma. In: Stark DD, Bradley WG (eds): Magnetic Resonance Imaging. (ed 3) St. Louis: Mosby, 1999, pp 1347–1360

Gamut M-79

EXTRAAXIAL FLUID COLLECTION, DARK ON T1-WEIGHTED IMAGE, BRIGHT ON T2-WEIGHTED IMAGE

1. Empyema, subdural/epidural
2. Hematoma, chronic subdural/epidural

Reference
1. Bradley WG: Chapter 58. Hemorrhage. In: Stark DD, Bradley WG (eds): Magnetic Resonance Imaging. (ed 3) St. Louis: Mosby, 1999, pp 1329–1346

Gamut M-80

EXTRAAXIAL FLUID COLLECTION, DARK ON T1- AND T2-WEIGHTED IMAGES

1. Air, extraaxial (postoperative; posttraumatic)
2. Hematoma, acute subdural/epidural

Reference
1. Bradley WG: Chapter 58. Hemorrhage. In: Stark DD, Bradley WG (eds): Magnetic Resonance Imaging. (ed 3) St. Louis: Mosby, 1999, pp 1329–1346

Gamut M-81

EXTRAAXIAL FLUID COLLECTION, BRIGHT ON T1- AND T2-WEIGHTED IMAGES

1. Hematoma, late subacute epidural (extracellular methemoglobin)
2. Hematoma, late subacute subdural (extracellular methemoglobin)

Reference
1. Bradley WG: Chapter 58. Hemorrhage. In: Stark DD, Bradley WG (eds): Magnetic Resonance Imaging. (ed 3) St. Louis: Mosby, 1999, pp 1329–1346

Gamut M-82

EXTRAAXIAL FLUID COLLECTION, BRIGHT ON T1-WEIGHTED IMAGE, DARK ON T2-WEIGHTED IMAGE

1. Hematoma, early subacute epidural (intracellular methemoglobin)
2. Hematoma, early subacute subdural (intracellular methemoglobin)

Reference
1. Bradley WG: Chapter 58. Hemorrhage. In: Stark DD, Bradley WG (eds): Magnetic Resonance Imaging. (ed 3) St. Louis: Mosby, 1999, pp 1329–1346

Gamut M-83

EXTRAAXIAL MASS, NONENHANCING

1. Arachnoid cyst (dark on diffusion imaging)
2. Epidermoid (bright on diffusion imaging)

Reference
1. Moseley ME, Butts K: Chapter 68. Diffusion and Perfusion. In: Stark DD, Bradley WG (eds): Magnetic Resonance Imaging. (ed 3) St. Louis: Mosby, 1999, pp 1515–1538

Gamut M-84

EXTRAAXIAL MASS, ENHANCING

1. Hemangiopericytoma of meninges (angioblastic meningioma), rare
2. Meningioma
3. Metastasis to dura
4. Neurofibroma, upper cervical, extending through foramen magnum
5. Schwannoma of cranial nerve (eg, acoustic)

Reference
1. Boyko OB: Chapter 54. Adult Brain Tumors. In: Stark DD, Bradley WG (eds): Magnetic Resonance Imaging. (ed 3) St. Louis: Mosby, 1999, pp 1231–1254

Gamut M-85

EXTRACRANIAL MASS, CSF INTENSITY

1. Encephalocele
2. Meningocele
3. Pseudomeningocele (postoperative CSF leak)

Gamut M-86

EXTRACRANIAL MASS, DARK ON T1-WEIGHTED IMAGE

1. Cephalohematoma, acute (dark on T2-weighted image) (intracellular deoxyhemoglobin)
2. Cephalohematoma, chronic (bright on T2-weighted image)
3. Hemangioma
4. Lymphangioma
5. Sebaceous cyst

References
1. Boyko OB: Chapter 65. Pediatric Brain Tumors. In: Stark DD, Bradley WG (eds): Magnetic Resonance Imaging. (ed 3) St. Louis: Mosby, 1999, pp 1467–1482
2. Bradley WG: Chapter 58. Hemorrhage. In: Stark DD, Bradley WG (eds): Magnetic Resonance Imaging. (ed 3) St. Louis: Mosby, 1999, pp 1329–1346

Gamut M-87

EXTRACRANIAL MASS, BRIGHT ON T1-WEIGHTED IMAGE

1. Cephalohematoma, subacute (methemoglobin)
2. Lipoma

Reference
1. Bradley WG: Chapter 58. Hemorrhage. In: Stark DD, Bradley WG (eds): Magnetic Resonance Imaging. (ed 3) St. Louis: Mosby, 1999, pp 1329–1346

Gamut M-88

INTRAMEDULLARY LESION, CSF INTENSITY

1. Cysticercosis
2. Hydromyelia (See M-89-S)
3. Posttraumatic cystic myelomalacia
4. Syringomyelia (See M-89-S)
5. [Truncation artifact]

[ ] This condition does not actually cause the gamuted imaging finding, but can produce imaging changes that simulate it.

References
1. Haughton V, et al: Chapter 85. Cervical Spine. In: Stark DD, Bradley WG (eds): Magnetic Resonance Imaging. (ed 3) St. Louis: CV Mosby and Co., 1999
2. Najem ES, et al: Chapter 86. Thoracic Spine. In: Stark DD, Bradley WG (eds): Magnetic Resonance Imaging. (ed 3) St. Louis: CV Mosby and Co., 1999

Gamut M-89-S

CAUSES OF SYRINGOMYELIA AND HYDROMYELIA

1. Arachnoiditis
2. Chiari I malformation
3. Chiari II (Arnold Chiari malformation)
4. Communicating hydrocephalus
5. Herniation of cerebellar tonsils through foramen magnum due to posterior fossa mass
6. Postinfarction
7. Posttraumatic
8. Spinal stenosis
9. Spondylosis, severe
10. Tumor (rostral or caudal to cyst; intra- or extra-medullary)
11. Vascular impression

Reference
1. Houghton V, et al: Chapter 85. Cervical Spine. In: Stark DD, Bradley WG (eds): Magnetic Resonance Imaging. (ed 3) St. Louis: CV Mosby and Co., 1999

Gamut M-90

INTRAMEDULLARY LESION, DARK ON T1-WEIGHTED IMAGE, BRIGHT ON T2-WEIGHTED IMAGE, NO MASS EFFECT

1. Acute disseminated encephalomyelitis (ADEM) (postviral leukoencephalopathy)
2. Amyotrophic lateral sclerosis
3. Arteriovenous malformation (AVM)
4. [CSF flow artifact]
5. Cord edema (eg, due to herniated disk)
6. Devic's syndrome (demyelination of cord and optic neuritis)
7. Gliosis
8. HIV myelopathy

9. Lyme disease
10. Multiple sclerosis
11. Nitrous oxide
12. Small glioma
13. Small nonhemorrhagic contusion
14. Subacute combined degeneration (B_{12} deficiency)
15. Subacute infarct
16. [Truncation artifact]

[ ] This condition does not actually cause the gamuted imaging finding, but can produce imaging changes that simulate it.

Reference
1. Houghton V, et al: Chapter 85. In: Stark DD, Bradley WG (eds): Magnetic Resonance Imaging. (ed 3) St. Louis: CV Mosby and Co., 1999

Gamut M-91

INTRAMEDULLARY LESION, DARK ON T1-WEIGHTED IMAGE, BRIGHT ON T2-WEIGHTED IMAGE, MASS EFFECT

COMMON

1. Acute disseminated encephalomyelitis (ADEM) (postviral leukoencephalopathy)
2. Astrocytoma
3. Contusion, acute
4. Ependymoma
5. Hemangioblastoma
6. Leptomeningeal carcinomatosis (eg, breast)
7. Myelitis, viral
8. Tumefactive multiple sclerosis

UNCOMMON

1. Acute infarct (arterial or venous occlusion)
2. Drop metastasis to central canal (eg, medulloblastoma)
3. Gangliocytoma; ganglioglioma

4. Lymphoma_g
5. Meningitis, spinal
6. "Pre-syrinx"
7. Radiation necrosis

References

1. Houghton V, et al: Chapter 85. Cervical Spine. In: Stark DD, Bradley WG (eds): Magnetic Resonance Imaging. (ed 3) St. Louis: CV Mosby and Co., 1999
2. Fischbein NJ, Dillon WP, Cobbs C, Weinstein PR: The "presyrinx" state: a reversible myelopathic condition that may precede syringomyelia. AJNR 1999;20:7–20
3. Najem ES, et al: Chapter 86. Thoracic Spine. In: Stark DD, Bradley WG (eds): Magnetic Resonance Imaging. (ed 3) St. Louis: CV Mosby and Co., 1999

Gamut M-92

POTENTIALLY ENHANCING CORD LESIONS

1. Acute disseminated encephalomyelitis (ADEM) (postviral leukoencephalopathy)
2. Arteriovenous malformation (AVM)
3. Devic's syndrome (demyelination of cord and optic neuritis)
4. Glioma
5. Hemangioblastoma
6. Leptomeningeal carcinomatosis
7. Lyme disease
8. Lymphoma_g
9. Metastasis to central canal (eg, medulloblastoma)
10. Multiple sclerosis
11. Subacute infarct
12. Syphilis
13. Tuberculosis

Gamut M-93

DIFFUSELY SMALL CORD

1. AIDS myelopathy
2. Amyotrophic lateral sclerosis

3. Atrophy
4. Collapsed syrinx
5. Cord tethering
6. Cord transection
7. Diffuse multiple sclerosis
8. Juvenile amyotrophy
9. Kyphoscoliosis
10. Post-radiation therapy
11. Postsurgical
12. Primary lateral sclerosis
13. Subacute combined degeneration
14. Wallerian degeneration

References

1. Houghton V, et al: Chapter 85. Cervical Spine. In: Stark DD, Bradley WG (eds): Magnetic Resonance Imaging. (ed 3) St. Louis: CV Mosby and Co., 1999
2. Najem ES, et al: Chapter 86. Thoracic Spine. In: Stark DD, Bradley WG (eds): Magnetic Resonance Imaging. (ed 3) St. Louis: CV Mosby and Co., 1999
3. Pomeranz SJ: Gamuts and Pearls in Neurologic MRI. St. Louis: MRI-EFI Publications, Inc., 1998

Gamut M-94

FOCALLY SMALL CORD

1. Bony spinal stenosis
2. Collapsed syrinx
3. Compression due to herniated disk, epidural tumor, or extramedullary mass (eg, arachnoid cyst)
4. Multiple sclerosis
5. Myelomalacia
6. Post-infarct
7. Postsurgical
8. Posttraumatic

Gamut M-95

INTRAMEDULLARY LESION, DARK ON T1- AND T2-WEIGHTED IMAGES, NO MASS EFFECT

1. Focal calcification
2. Hemosiderin (eg, from cavernous angioma or AVM)
3. [Metallic artifact from previous surgery]
4. Osseous spur in diastematomyelia

[ ] This condition does not actually cause the gamuted imaging finding, but can produce imaging changes that simulate it.

Gamut M-96

INTRAMEDULLARY LESION, BRIGHT ON T1- AND T2-WEIGHTED IMAGES

1. Late subacute hematomyelia (extracellular methe-moglobin from tumor, AVM, trauma)
2. Tumor cyst

Gamut M-97

INTRAMEDULLARY LESION, BRIGHT ON T1-WEIGHTED IMAGE, DARK ON T2-WEIGHTED IMAGE

1. Early subacute hematomyelia (intracellular methe-moglobin from tumor, AVM, trauma)

Gamut M-98

EXTRAMEDULLARY, INTRADURAL LESION WITH CSF INTENSITY

1. Arachnoid cyst
2. Cysticercosis
3. Epidermoid (bright on diffusion imaging)
4. Multicystic arachnoiditis

Gamut M-99

EXTRAMEDULLARY, INTRADURAL LESION, DARK ON T1-WEIGHTED IMAGE, BRIGHT ON T2-WEIGHTED IMAGE, NO MASS EFFECT

1. Cytomegalovirus infection
2. Drop metastases, small
3. [Flow artifact]
4. Fungal meningitis
5. Postradiation (enlarged vessels)

[ ] This condition does not actually cause the gamuted imaging finding, but can produce imaging changes that simulate it.

References
1. Houghton V, et al: Chapter 85. Cervical Spine. In: Stark DD, Bradley WG (eds): Magnetic Resonance Imaging. (ed 3) St. Louis: CV Mosby and Co., 1999
2. Najem ES, et al: Chapter 86. Thoracic Spine. In: Stark DD, Bradley WG (eds): Magnetic Resonance Imaging. (ed 3) St. Louis: CV Mosby and Co., 1999
3. Tam JK, Bradley WG Jr., Goergen SK, et al: Patterns of contrast enhancement in the pediatric spine at MR imaging with single- and triple-dose gadolinium. Radiology 1996;198: 273–278

Gamut M-100

EXTRAMEDULLARY, INTRADURAL LESION, DARK ON T1-WEIGHTED IMAGE, BRIGHT ON T2-WEIGHTED IMAGE, MASS EFFECT

NONENHANCING

1. Arachnoiditis, chronic
2. "Black" epidermoid (solid cholesterol/cholesterin) (bright on diffusion imaging)
3. Dermoid (cystic)
4. Hemorrhage, hyperacute
5. Neurenteric cyst

ENHANCING

1. Arachnoiditis, acute
2. Drop metastasis, large
3. Exophytic glioma (apparent extramedullary)
4. Meningioma
5. Neurofibroma
6. Schwannoma

References

1. Houghton V, et al: Chapter 85. Cervical Spine. In: Stark DD, Bradley WG (eds): Magnetic Resonance Imaging. (ed 3) St. Louis: CV Mosby and Co., 1999
2. Najem ES, et al: Chapter 86. Thoracic Spine. In: Stark DD, Bradley WG (eds): Magnetic Resonance Imaging. (ed 3) St. Louis: CV Mosby and Co., 1999
3. Ross JE, et al: Chapter 87. Lumbar Spine. In: Stark DD, Bradley WG (eds): Magnetic Resonance Imaging. (ed 3) St. Louis: CV Mosby and Co., 1999

Gamut M-101-S

SOURCES OF DROP METASTASES TO SPINAL SUBARACHNOID SPACE

CNS SOURCES

COMMON

1. Astrocytoma
2. Ependymoma
3. Glioblastoma multiforme
4. Medulloblastoma

UNCOMMON

1. Choroid plexus carcinoma
2. Pineoblastoma
3. Pineocytoma
4. Teratoma

NON-CNS SOURCES

1. Metastatic carcinoma of breast
2. Metastatic carcinoma of lung
3. Metastatic lymphoma
4. Metastatic malignant melanoma

Reference

1. Najem ES, et al: Chapter 86. Thoracic Spine. In: Stark DD, Bradley WG (eds): Magnetic Resonance Imaging. (ed 3). St. Louis: CV Mosby and Co, 1999

Gamut M-102

EXTRAMEDULLARY, INTRADURAL LESION, BRIGHT ON T1-WEIGHTED IMAGE, DARK ON T2-WEIGHTED IMAGE*

1. Dermoid (fatty)
2. Fatty filum terminale
3. Lipoma
4. Pantopaque
5. "White" epidermoid (liquid triglyceride)

* Dark on T2-weighted conventional spin echo—bright on T2-weighted fast spin echo.

Reference
1. Najem ES, et al: Chapter 86. Thoracic Spine. In: Stark DD, Bradley WG (eds): Magnetic Resonance Imaging. (ed 3) St. Louis: CV Mosby and Co., 1999

Gamut M-103

EXTRAMEDULLARY, INTRADURAL SIGNAL VOID

1. Acute hemorrhage (deoxyhemoglobin)
2. Air (eg, post-lumbar puncture)
3. Arteriovenous malformation (AVM)
4. [CSF flow artifact]
5. [Metallic artifact]

[ ] This condition does not actually cause the gamuted imaging finding, but can produce imaging changes that simulate it.

Gamut M-104

NERVE ROOT ENHANCEMENT

1. Arachnoiditis
2. Compression (from disk herniation or spinal stenosis)
3. Cytomegalovirus infection (esp. in AIDS)
4. Fungal meningitis
5. Guillain-Barré S.
6. Leptomeningeal carcinomatosis ("zücherguss"— German: sugar coating)
7. Lymphomatous meningitis
8. [Normal]
9. Postradiation (enlarged vessels)
10. Postoperative
11. Sarcoidosis
12. Tuberculosis
13. Viral neuritis

[ ] This condition does not actually cause the gamuted imaging finding, but can produce imaging changes that simulate it.

Gamut M-105

ENLARGED NERVE ROOTS

1. Charcot-Marie-Tooth S.
2. Déjérine-Sottas S.
3. Guillain-Barré S.
4. Langerhans cell histiocytosis$_g$
5. Leptomeningeal carcinomatosis
6. Leukemia
7. Lymphoma$_g$
8. Neuritis
9. Neurofibromatosis
10. Sarcoidosis
11. Toxic neuropathy

Reference
1. Pomeranz SJ: Gamuts and Pearls in Neurologic MRI. St. Louis: MRI-EPI Publications, Inc., 1998

Gamut M-106

EXTRADURAL LESION WITH NORMAL ADJACENT BONE (See C-63)

AT LEVEL OF DISK ONLY

1. Disk bulge
2. Disk extrusion
3. Disk protrusion
4. Epidural scar (eg, after disk surgery)
5. Marginal osteophyte
6. [Normal epidural veins]
7. [Spondylolisthesis (axial image only)]

NOT NECESSARILY AT LEVEL OF DISK

1. Amyloidosis
2. Arachnoid cyst
3. Arachnoiditis
4. Conjoined root sleeve
5. Epidural abscess
6. Epidural granuloma (eg, tuberculosis; fungus disease; sarcoidosis)
7. Epidural hematoma
8. Epidural lipomatosis (eg, obesity; steroid therapy; Cushing S.)
9. Epidural metastases (eg, lymphoma$_g$)
10. Extramedullary hematopoiesis
11. Extruded or sequestered disk
12. [Iatrogenic (needle point defect; extradural injection of Pantopaque)]
13. Ligamentum flavum thickening; intraspinal ligament ossification (eg, DISH; primary—esp. in Japanese)
14. Lipoma (spinal dysraphism)
15. Lymphoma$_g$
16. Meningioma (with intradural component)
17. Neurogenic tumor (eg, neurofibroma)
18. Parasitic disease (eg, cysticercosis; schistosomiasis)
19. "Pseudomass" at dens due to C1-2 subluxation in rheumatoid arthritis, etc.
20. Retroperitoneal neoplasm extending through intervertebral foramen (eg, neuroblastoma; lymphoma$_g$)
21. Root sleeve avulsion (pseudomeningocele)
22. Root sleeve diverticulum
23. Root sleeve ectasia
24. Synovial cyst from facet joint
25. Tarlov (perineural) cyst
26. Teratoma; dermoid; epidermoid

[ ] This condition does not actually cause the gamuted imaging finding, but can produce imaging changes that simulate it.

References

1. Najem ES, et al: Chapter 86. Thoracic Spine. In: Stark DD, Bradley WG (eds): Magnetic Resonance Imaging. (ed 3) St. Louis: CV Mosby and Co., 1999
2. Stevens JM: The Spine and Spinal Cord. In: Sutton D, Young JWR (eds): A Short Textbook of Clinical Imaging. London: Springer-Verlag, 1990, pp 791–802

Gamut M-107

EXTRADURAL LESION WITH ABNORMAL ADJACENT BONE (See C-63)

1. Extramedullary hematopoiesis
2. Hydatid disease
3. Langerhans cell histiocytosis$_g$ (esp. eosinophilic granuloma)
4. Lymphoma$_g$
5. Neoplasm of spine, benign or malignant (eg, aneurysmal bone cyst; giant cell tumor; hemangioma; osteoblastoma; osteochondroma; bone sarcoma; multiple myeloma; chordoma) (See C-38-S)
6. Neurogenic tumor (eg, neurofibroma; ganglioneuroma; neuroblastoma)
7. Osseous metastasis with epidural soft tissue extension
8. Osteomyelitis with adjacent cellulitis; epidural abscess or granuloma (esp. tuberculosis; brucellosis; pyogenic)
9. Osteoporosis with fracture and granulation tissue
10. Paget's disease (uncalcified osteoid)

(continued)

11. Posttraumatic fracture fragment, dislocation, or hematoma
12. Spinal stenosis; spondylosis; spondylolisthesis; osteophyte

References
1. Houghton V, et al: Chapter 85. Cervical Spine. In: Stark DD, Bradley WG (eds): Magnetic Resonance Imaging (ed 3). St. Louis: CV Mosby and Co., 1999
2. Najem ES, et al: Chapter 86. Thoracic Spine. In: Stark DD, Bradley WG (eds): Magnetic Resonance Imaging. (ed 3) St. Louis: CV Mosby and Co., 1999
3. Stevens JM: The Spine and Spinal Cord. In: Sutton D, Young JWR (eds): A Short Textbook of Clinical Imaging. London: Springer-Verlag, 1990, pp 791–802

Gamut M-108

FOCAL VERTEBRAL BODY ABNORMALITY WITH LOW SIGNAL ON T1-WEIGHTED IMAGE, HIGH SIGNAL ON T2-WEIGHTED IMAGE

1. [Flow artifact from aorta or iliac arteries]
2. Fracture, acute
3. GCSF (granulocyte colony stimulating factor) therapy (eg, post bone marrow transplant)
4. Infection (from osteomyelitis or diskitis)
5. Marrow replacement
6. Osseous metastasis
7. Plasmacytoma; multiple myeloma
8. Primary bone tumor (eg, Ewing sarcoma; osteo-sarcoma; lymphoma)
9. Type I degenerative endplate changes

[ ] This condition does not actually cause the gamuted imaging finding, but can produce imaging changes that simulate it.

Reference
1. Najem ES, et al: Chapter 86. Thoracic Spine. In: Stark DD, Bradley WG (eds): Magnetic Resonance Imaging. (ed 3) St. Louis: CV Mosby and Co., 1999

Gamut M-109

FOCAL VERTEBRAL BODY ABNORMALITY WITH HIGH SIGNAL ON T1-WEIGHTED IMAGE, LOW SIGNAL ON T2-WEIGHTED IMAGE

1. Fat island
2. Fatty replacement following radiation
3. Type II degenerative endplate changes

References
1. Ross JS, et al: Chapter 87. Lumbar Spine. In: Stark DD, Bradley WG (eds): Magnetic Resonance Imaging. (ed 3) St. Louis: CV Mosby and Co., 1999
2. Najem ES, et al: Chapter 86. Thoracic Spine. In: Stark DD, Bradley WG (eds): Magnetic Resonance Imaging. (ed 2) St. Louis: CV Mosby and Co., 1999

Gamut M-110

FOCAL VERTEBRAL BODY ABNORMALITY WITH HIGH SIGNAL ON T1-WEIGHTED IMAGE, HIGH SIGNAL ON T2-WEIGHTED SPIN ECHO IMAGE

1. Fat island on fast/turbo spin echo images
2. Hemangioma

References
1. Ross JS, et al: Chapter 87. Lumbar Spine. In: Stark DD, Bradley WG (eds): Magnetic Resonance Imaging. (ed 3) St. Louis: CV Mosby and Co., 1999
2. Najem ES, et al: Chapter 86. Thoracic Spine. In: Stark DD, Bradley WG (eds): Magnetic Resonance Imaging. (ed 2) St. Louis: CV Mosby and Co., 1999

Gamut M-111

DIFFUSE VERTEBRAL BODY ABNORMALITIES, BRIGHT ON T1-WEIGHTED IMAGE

1. Aplastic anemia
2. Postradiation

Gamut M-112

DIFFUSE VERTEBRAL BODY ABNORMALITIES, INTERMEDIATE INTENSITY ON T1-WEIGHTED IMAGE

1. Anemia
2. Diffuse marrow replacement by tumor (multiple myeloma; diffuse metastatic disease)
3. [Menstruating woman]
4. Myelophthisic marrow replacement (eg, Gaucher disease)
5. [Normal elderly with osteoporosis]
6. Polycythemia vera

[ ] This condition does not actually cause the gamuted imaging finding, but can produce imaging changes that simulate it.

Gamut M-113

DIFFUSE VERTEBRAL BODY ABNORMALITIES, DARK ON T1-WEIGHTED IMAGE

1. Hemochromatosis
2. Hemosiderosis
3. Myelofibrosis; myelosclerosis
4. Osteoblastic metastases (eg, carcinoma of prostate or breast)

5. Osteopetrosis
6. Renal osteodystrophy (secondary hyperparathyroidism)

Reference
1. Pomeranz SJ: Gamuts and Pearls in MRI. Richmond: Wm Byrd Press, 1990

Gamut M-114

LESION OF THE GLOBE

BRIGHT ON T2-WEIGHTED IMAGE

COMMON
1. Choroidal metastasis (esp. from carcinoma of breast or lung)
2. Retinal detachment

UNCOMMON
1. Choroidal hemangioma
2. Retinal cyst

DARK ON T2-WEIGHTED IMAGE

COMMON
1. Melanoma (primary or metastatic)
2. Retinoblastoma (child)

UNCOMMON
1. Astrocytic hamartoma
2. Endophthalmitis
3. Glass prosthesis
4. Melanocytoma (benign)
5. Phthisis bulbi
6. Pseudotumor of orbit
7. Sarcoidosis

Reference
1. Stark DD, Bradley WG (eds): Magnetic Resonance Imaging. (ed 3) St. Louis: CV Mosby and Co., 1999

Gamut M-115

OPTIC NERVE/NERVE SHEATH LESION

INTERMEDIATE SIGNAL ON T2-WEIGHTED IMAGE

COMMON

1. Meningioma of optic nerve sheath
2. Optic glioma
3. Optic neuritis

HIGH SIGNAL ON T2-WEIGHTED IMAGE

UNCOMMON

1. Dural ectasia

Reference
1. Stark DD, Bradley WG (eds): Magnetic Resonance Imaging. (ed 3) St. Louis: CV Mosby and Co., 1999

Gamut M-116

RETROBULBAR MASS

ISOINTENSE TO FAT ON T2-WEIGHTED IMAGE

COMMON

1. Dermoid
2. Lacrimal gland tumor (See B-23)
3. Lymphoma$_g$
4. Meningioma of optic nerve sheath
5. Pseudotumor of orbit
6. Thyroid orbitopathy (Graves' disease)

UNCOMMON

1. Amyloidosis
2. Arteriovenous malformation (AVM)

3. Lipoma
4. Myeloma
5. Sarcoidosis

BRIGHTER THAN FAT ON T2-WEIGHTED IMAGE

COMMON

1. Cavernous hemangioma
2. Dermoid
3. Extraconal meningioma
4. Hematoma following trauma or surgery
5. Lacrimal gland tumor (See B-23)
6. Plexiform neurofibroma
7. Schwannoma

UNCOMMON

1. Bacterial infection
2. Brown tumor of hyperparathyroidism
3. Langerhans cell histiocytosis$_g$
4. Lymphangioma
5. Metastasis (children: neuroblastoma, leukemia, Ewing sarcoma; adults: carcinoma of breast or lung)

Reference
1. Stark DD, Bradley WG (eds): Magnetic Resonance Imaging. (ed 3) St. Louis: CV Mosby and Co., 1999

Gamut M-117

EXTRAOCULAR MUSCLE ENLARGEMENT

ISOINTENSE TO FAT ON T2-WEIGHTED IMAGE

1. Acromegaly
2. Infection
3. Pseudotumor of orbit
4. Sarcoidosis
5. Thyroid orbitopathy (bilateral)
6. Venous obstruction

BRIGHTER THAN FAT
ON T2-WEIGHTED IMAGE

1. Bacterial infection (from adjacent sinus infection)
2. Carotid—cavernous fistula (traumatic; dural AVM)
3. Hematoma
4. Leukemia
5. Lymphangioma
6. Lymphoma$_g$
7. Metastasis (esp. from carcinoma of breast or lung)
8. Rhabdomyosarcoma (child)
9. Trauma

Reference
1. Stark DD, Bradley WG (eds): Magnetic Resonance Imaging. (ed 3) St. Louis: CV Mosby and Co., 1999

LATERAL EXTRACONAL LESION

BRIGHT ON T2-WEIGHTED IMAGE

1. Inflammation of lacrimal gland (eg, sarcoidosis—generally bilateral)
2. Metastatic disease
3. Primary tumor of lacrimal gland (benign mixed tumor; adenoid cystic carcinoma; lymphoma$_g$ [usually bilateral])

DARK ON T2-WEIGHTED IMAGE

1. Extraconal meningioma
2. [Normal lacrimal gland]

[ ] This condition does not actually cause the gamuted imaging finding, but can produce imaging changes that simulate it.

Reference
1. Stark DD, Bradley WG (eds): Magnetic Resonance Imaging. (ed 3) St. Louis: CV Mosby and Co., 1999

ENLARGED SUPERIOR
OPHTHALMIC VEIN

1. Carotid—cavernous fistula (traumatic; dural AVM)
2. [Normal variant]
3. Orbital apex mass
4. Pseudotumor of orbit
5. Thyroid orbitopathy
6. Varix; varicocele; venous angioma

[ ] This condition does not actually cause the gamuted imaging finding, but can produce imaging changes that simulate it.

Reference
1. Stark DD, Bradley WG (eds): Magnetic Resonance Imaging. (ed 3) St. Louis: CV Mosby and Co., 1999

THROMBOSIS OF SUPERIOR
OPHTHALMIC VEIN

1. Adjacent orbital infection
2. Cavernous-sinus thrombosis (secondary to tumor, inflammation, trauma)
3. Dural arteriovenous malformation (AVM)
4. Varix

Reference
1. Stark DD, Bradley WG (eds): Magnetic Resonance Imaging. (ed 3) St. Louis: CV Mosby and Co., 1999

ORBITAL WALL LESION

HYPOINTENSE ON T2-WEIGHTED IMAGE

1. Chondrosarcoma
2. Fibrous dysplasia
3. Langerhans cell histiocytosis$_g$
4. Meningioma with hyperostosis
5. Osteoblastic osteosarcoma
6. Osteoma

HYPERINTENSE ON T2-WEIGHTED IMAGE

1. Chondrosarcoma (cystic)
2. Epidermoid
3. Ewing sarcoma
4. Frontonasal encephalocele
5. Giant cell granuloma
6. Giant cell tumor
7. Infection
8. Lymphangioma
9. Lymphoma$_g$
10. Metastatic disease
11. Mucocele
12. Neuroblastoma (child)

References

1. Pomeranz SJ: Gamuts and Pearls in MRI. Richmond: Wm Byrd Press, 1990
2. Stark DD, Bradley WG (eds): Magnetic Resonance Imaging. (ed 3) St. Louis: CV Mosby and Co., 1999

SINONASAL MASS WITHOUT BONE CHANGES

BRIGHT ON T2-WEIGHTED IMAGE

COMMON

1. Acute infection (sinusitis)
2. Mucous retention cyst
3. Polyp

UNCOMMON

1. Epidermoid
2. Lymphoma$_g$

DARK ON T2-WEIGHTED IMAGE

1. [Air]
2. Dentigerous (follicular) cyst
3. Dried secretions
4. Hemorrhage (acute)
5. Mycetoma (eg, aspergillosis)
6. Osteoma
7. Sinolith
8. Undescended maxillary tooth

[ ] This condition does not actually cause the gamuted imaging finding, but can produce imaging changes that simulate it.

Reference

1. Stark DD, Bradley WG (eds): Magnetic Resonance Imaging. (ed 3) St. Louis: CV Mosby and Co., 1999

Gamut M-123

SINONASAL MASS WITH BONY REMODELING WITHOUT EROSION

COMMON
1. Mucocele
2. Pyomucocele

UNCOMMON
1. Esthesioneuroblastoma
2. Histiocytic lymphoma
3. Inverting papilloma
4. Minor salivary gland tumor
5. Sarcoma
6. Schwannoma

Reference
1. Stark DD, Bradley WG (eds): Magnetic Resonance Imaging. (ed 3) St. Louis: CV Mosby and Co., 1999

Gamut M-124

SINONASAL MASS WITH BONY EROSION

COMMON
1. Adenoid cystic carcinoma (perineural extension)
2. Angiofibroma (boys)
3. Squamous cell carcinoma (adults)

UNCOMMON
1. Adenocarcinoma
2. Extracranial meningioma
3. Minor salivary gland carcinoma (high-grade)

Reference
1. Stark DD, Bradley WG (eds): Magnetic Resonance Imaging. (ed 3) St. Louis: CV Mosby and Co., 1999

Gamut M-125

VASCULAR SINONASAL MASS WITH FLOW VOIDS

COMMON
1. Juvenile angiofibroma (boys)
2. Metastatic disease (esp. from carcinoma of kidney or thyroid)

UNCOMMON
1. Hemangioma
2. Hemangiopericytoma

Reference
1. Stark DD, Bradley WG (eds): Magnetic Resonance Imaging. (ed 3) St. Louis: CV Mosby and Co., 1999

Gamut M-126

FIBRO-OSSEOUS OR OSTEOGENIC LESION OF A PARANASAL SINUS

DARK ON T2-WEIGHTED IMAGE
1. Fibrous dysplasia
2. Nonossifying fibroma
3. Ossifying fibroma
4. Osteoma

BRIGHT ON T2-WEIGHTED IMAGE
1. Osteoblastoma
2. Osteosarcoma

Reference
1. Stark DD, Bradley WG (eds): Magnetic Resonance Imaging. (ed 3) St. Louis: CV Mosby and Co., 1999

Gamut M-127

SKULL BASE LESION

BRIGHT ON T2-WEIGHTED IMAGE

COMMON
1. Chondroma; osteochondroma
2. Epidermoid
3. Ewing sarcoma
4. Hemangioma/vascular hamartoma of facial nerve
5. Osseous metastasis
6. Paraganglioma (glomus tympanicum)
7. Schwannoma of fifth and eighth cranial nerves
8. Squamous cell carcinoma extending through basal foramina

UNCOMMON
1. Aneurysmal bone cyst
2. Chordoma
3. Cholesterol granuloma
4. Fibrosarcoma (complicating Paget's disease; fibrous dysplasia; osteomyelitis; radiation therapy)
5. Giant cell tumor
6. Petrous apicitis
7. Pituitary macroadenoma
8. Plasmacytoma
9. Schwannoma of cranial nerves VII and IX–XII

DARK ON T2-WEIGHTED IMAGE
1. Langerhans cell histiocytosis$_g$ (child)
2. Meningioma

Reference
1. Stark DD, Bradley WG (eds): Magnetic Resonance Imaging. (ed 3) St. Louis: CV Mosby and Co., 1999

Gamut M-128

SALIVARY GLAND LESION

INTERMEDIATE ON T2-WEIGHTED IMAGE

COMMON
1. Benign mixed tumors (pleomorphic adenomas {most common in superficial lobe of parotid})
2. Epidemic parotitis (mumps)
3. Intraparotid lymphadenopathy (See M-129)
4. Lipoma
5. Mucoepidermoid carcinoma (low grade)
6. Sarcoidosis
7. Schwannoma/neurofibroma
8. Lymphoma$_g$ (systemic)

BRIGHT ON T2-WEIGHTED IMAGE

COMMON
1. Branchial cleft cyst
2. Cystic hygroma (lymphangioma)
3. Hemangioma
4. Parotid lymphoepithelial cysts (in AIDS)
5. Ranula

UNCOMMON
1. Actinomycosis
2. Acute suppurative sialadenitis
3. Carcinoma (eg, adenocarcinoma; adenoid cystic carcinoma; high-grade mucoepidermoid carcinoma {more often in deep lobe of parotid}; squamous cell carcinoma; undifferentiated carcinoma)
4. Chronic recurrent sialadenitis
5. Chronic sialectasis
6. Lymphoepithelial sialadenopathy
7. Lymphoma$_g$ (primary)
8. Metastatic disease (from cutaneous squamous cell carcinoma; melanoma; carcinoma of lung, breast, or kidney)
9. Sarcoma
10. Sialolithiasis

11. Syphilis
12. Tuberculosis

Reference
1. Stark DD, Bradley WG (eds): Magnetic Resonance Imaging. (ed 3) St. Louis: CV Mosby and Co., 1999

Gamut M-129

INTRAPAROTID LYMPHADENOPATHY

1. AIDS
2. Chronic autoimmune sialadenitis (Sjögren syndrome)
3. Lymphadenitis
4. Metastatic disease
5. Sarcoidosis
6. Toxoplasmosis
7. Tuberculosis

Reference
1. Stark DD, Bradley WG (eds): Magnetic Resonance Imaging. (ed 3) St. Louis: CV Mosby and Co., 1999

Gamut M-130

MASS IN THE NECK

INTERMEDIATE ON T2-WEIGHTED IMAGE

COMMON

1. Goiter
2. Jugular thrombophlebitis (acute; early subacute)
3. Lipoma
4. Lymphadenopathy (infectious; metastatic disease; lymphoma)
5. Thyroid adenoma
6. Thyroid carcinoma

UNCOMMON

1. Neuroblastoma (child)
2. Plexiform neurofibroma
3. Teratoma (fatty or solid)

BRIGHT ON T2-WEIGHTED IMAGE

COMMON

1. Abscess
2. Hemangioma
3. Jugular thrombophlebitis (late subacute; chronic)
4. Thyroglossal duct cyst (midline)

UNCOMMON

1. Colloid cyst of thyroid gland
2. Hygroma
3. Laryngocele
4. Lymphocele
5. Paraganglioma (glomus caroticum)
6. Schwannoma
7. Second branchial cleft cyst (lateral)
8. Teratoma (cystic)
9. Thymic cyst
10. Tracheoesophageal cyst

Reference
1. Stark DD, Bradley WG (eds): Magnetic Resonance Imaging. (ed 3) St. Louis: CV Mosby and Co., 1999

Gamut M-131

INCREASED SIGNAL IN SUPRASPINATUS TENDON ON PROTON DENSITY-WEIGHTED IMAGE

1. Contusion
2. [Magic angle effect (nonthickened tendon)]
3. [Normal (fat between tendinous insertions)]
4. Tear
5. Tendonitis (thickened tendon)
6. Tendinosis (degeneration)

[ ] This condition does not actually cause the gamuted imaging finding, but can produce imaging changes that simulate it.

Reference
1. Stark DD, Bradley WG (eds): Magnetic Resonance Imaging. (ed 3) St. Louis: CV Mosby and Co., 1999

Gamut M-132

INCREASED SIGNAL IN SUPRASPINATUS TENDON ON T2-WEIGHTED IMAGE

1. Partial tear or tendonitis (nondisplaced musculo-tendinous junction)
2. Posttraumatic contusion
3. Tear (displaced musculotendinous junction)

Reference
1. Stark DD, Bradley WG (eds): Magnetic Resonance Imaging. (ed 3) St. Louis: CV Mosby and Co., 1999

Gamut M-133

LINEAR SIGNAL IN KNEE MENISCUS

1. Degeneration
2. Frank tear
3. Intrasubstance tear
4. Postoperative repair (scar)
5. Pitfalls (See M-133-S)

Reference
1. Stark DD, Bradley WG (eds): Magnetic Resonance Imaging. (ed 3) St. Louis: CV Mosby and Co., 1999

Gamut M-133-S

PITFALLS INVOLVING POSTERIOR HORN OF LATERAL MENISCUS

1. Magic angle
2. Meniscofemoral ligament insertion
3. Popliteus tendon sheath
4. Posterior ligaments of Humphry and Wrisberg
5. Pulsation artifact from popliteal artery
6. Transverse ligaments
7. Truncation artifact

Gamut M-134

ABSENT BOW-TIE SIGN IN KNEE MENISCI*

1. Bucket handle tear
2. Medial flipped flap tear
3. Osteoarthritis
4. Postoperative
5. Radial tear

* On sagittal MR images of the knee two consecutive body segments of the meniscus should be seen.

Gamut M-135

BRIGHT INTRAMEDULLARY SIGNAL ON T2-WEIGHTED IMAGE OF KNEE WITH INTACT CORTEX

1. Bone bruise (contusion; trabecular fracture)
2. Leukemia
3. Lymphoma_g
4. Metastasis
5. Osteosarcoma
6. Regional migratory osteoporosis
7. Regrowth of hemopoietic marrow

Reference
1. Stark DD, Bradley WG (eds): Magnetic Resonance Imaging. (ed 3) St. Louis: CV Mosby and Co., 1999

Gamut M-136

HIGH INTRAMEDULLARY SIGNAL ON T2-WEIGHTED IMAGE OF KNEE WITH DISRUPTED CORTEX

1. Osteochondritis dessicans (chronic recurrent trauma)
2. Posttraumatic osteonecrosis
3. Spontaneous osteonecrosis
4. Type II bone contusion

Reference
1. Stark DD, Bradley WG (eds): Magnetic Resonance Imaging. (ed 3) St. Louis: CV Mosby and Co., 1999

Gamut M-137

MARKED LOW SIGNAL IN MARROW (DIFFUSE) ON T1- AND T2-WEIGHTED IMAGES

1. Granulocyte colony stimulating factor (GCSF) therapy
2. Hemochromatosis
3. Hemosiderosis
4. Myelofibrosis

Gamut M-138

INTRA-ARTICULAR MASS WITH LOW SIGNAL ON T2-WEIGHTED IMAGE

1. Amyloidosis
2. Gout
3. Pigmented villonodular synovitis

Gamut M-139

HOFFA'S FAT PAD MASS IN INFRAPATELLAR REGION

1. Chondroma
2. Ganglion
3. Pigmented villonodular synovitis
4. Synovial osteochondromatosis

Gamut M-140-S

CHRONIC LATERAL ANKLE PAIN

1. Anterolateral impingement
2. Lateral ligament tears
3. Longitudinal split tear of peroneus brevis
4. Loose body
5. Osteoarthritis
6. Sinus tarsi syndrome

Gamut M-141-1

FOCAL SIGNAL ABNORMALITY IN THE LIVER (BRIGHT ON T2-WEIGHTED IMAGE)

COMMON

1. Abscess (pyogenic, amebic, fungal, hydatid)
2. Biloma
3. Cholangiocarcinoma
4. Cyst
5. Dilated bile ducts
6. Fibrosis, confluent (usually wedge shaped)
7. [Flow artifact from aorta]
8. Focal nodular hyperplasia
9. Granuloma (eg, sarcoidosis or tuberculosis)
10. Hemangioma (incl. cavernous)
11. Hepatitis (post-radiation)
12. Hepatocellular adenoma
13. Hepatocellular carcinoma
14. Hematoma
15. Hydatid cyst
16. Infarct (usually wedge shaped)
17. Lymphoma$_g$
18. Metastasis
19. [Normal portal veins]
20. Peribiliary cyst (cirrhosis)
21. Portal vein thrombosis

UNCOMMON

1. Angiomyolipoma
2. Angiosarcoma
3. Biliary cystadenoma/cystadenocarcinoma
4. Biliary hamartoma
5. Caroli's disease (saccular biliary dilatation)
6. Ciliated hepatic foregut cyst
7. Extramedullary hematopoiesis
8. Fibrolamellar hepatocellular carcinoma
9. Hemangioendothelioma (children)
10. Hepatoblastoma (children)
11. Hepatic vein thrombosis (Budd-Chiari S.)
12. Inflammatory pseudotumor
13. Mesenchymal hamartoma (children)
14. Regenerative nodules (cirrhosis; Budd-Chiari S.)
15. Undifferentiated (embryonal) sarcoma of liver (children)

References

1. Krinsky GA, Lee VS, Thiese ND, et al: Hepatocellular carcinoma and dysplastic nodules in patients with cirrhosis: Prospective diagnosis with MR imaging and explantation correlation. Radiology 2001;219:445–454
2. Mitchell DG, Semelka RC: Chapter 22, In: Stark DD, Bradley WG (eds): Magnetic Resonance Imaging (ed 3). St. Louis: CV Mosby and Co., 1999
3. Mortele KJ, Ros PR: Cystic focal liver lesion in the adult: Differential CT and MR imaging features. RadioGraphics 2001; 21:895–910
4. Semelka RC (ed): MR imaging of the liver II: Diseases. Magnetic Resonance Imaging Clin North Am 10:1
5. Semelka RC, Braga K, Armao D, et al: Chapter 2, In: Semelka RC (ed): Abdominal-Pelvic MRI. New York: Wiley-Liss, Inc., 2002
6. Vilgrain V, Lewin M, Vons C, et al: Hepatic nodules in Budd-Chiari syndrome: Imaging features. Radiology 1999; 210:443–450

3. Mitchell DG, Semelka RC: Chapter 22, In: Stark DD, Bradley WG (eds): Magnetic Resonance Imaging (ed 3). St. Louis: CV Mosby and Co., 1999
4. Semelka RC (ed): MR imaging of the liver II: Diseases. Magnetic Resonance Imaging Clin North Am 10:1
5. Semelka RC, Braga K, Armao D, et al: Chapter 2, In: Semelka RC (ed): Abdominal-Pelvic MRI. New York: Wiley-Liss, Inc., 2002

Gamut M-141-2

FOCAL SIGNAL ABNORMALITY IN THE LIVER (BRIGHT ON T1-WEIGHTED IMAGE)

COMMON

1. Abscess
2. [Flow artifact from aorta]
3. Focal fatty infiltration
4. Hematoma, intratumoral (eg, in angiomyolipoma, hepatocellular adenoma, hepatocellular carcinoma, metastasis) or posttraumatic
5. Hepatic vein thrombosis
6. Hepatocellular adenoma
7. Hepatocellular carcinoma
8. Metastasis (esp. from mucin-producing carcinoma of colon, ovary, or pancreas; melanoma; multiple myeloma)
9. Nodule, dysplastic or regenerative
10. Portal vein thrombosis

UNCOMMON

1. Angiosarcoma
2. Angiomyolipoma
3. Biliary cystadenoma/cystadenocarcinoma
4. Cholangiocarcinoma
5. Ciliated hepatic foregut cyst
6. Cyst (hemorrhagic)
7. Hemangioma (>3 cm; heterogeneous)
8. Lipoma

[ ] This condition does not actually cause the gamuted imaging finding, but can produce imaging changes that simulate it.

References
1. Krinsky GA, Lee VS, Thiese ND, et al: Hepatocellular carcinoma and dysplastic nodules in patients with cirrhosis: Prospective diagnosis with MR imaging and explantation correlation. Radiology 2001; 219:445–454
2. Maetani Y, Itoh K, Watanabe C, et al: MR imaging of intrahepatic cholangiocarcinoma with pathologic correlation. AJR 2001;176:1499–1507

Gamut M-141-3

FOCAL SIGNAL ABNORMALITY IN THE LIVER (DARK ON T2-WEIGHTED IMAGE)

COMMON

1. Aneurysm of hepatic artery or portal vein
2. [Flow artifact from aorta]
3. Gas
4. Granuloma (eg, sarcoidosis or tuberculosis)
5. Hematoma, acute posttraumatic
6. Intratumoral hemorrhage, acute (in angiomyolipoma, hepatocellular adenoma, hepatocellular carcinoma, or metastasis)
7. Lymphoma_g
8. Metastasis (esp. treated or from melanoma)
9. Neoplasm (treated)
10. Nodule, siderotic (dysplastic or regenerative)
11. Vascular malformation

UNCOMMON

1. Hepatocellular carcinoma (low grade)
2. Iron deposition (focal)
3. Mesenchymal hamartoma

[ ] This condition does not actually cause the gamuted imaging finding, but can produce imaging changes that simulate it.

References
1. Krinsky GA, Lee VS, Thiese ND, et al: Hepatocellular carcinoma and dysplastic nodules in patients with cirrhosis: Prospective diagnosis with MR imaging and explantation correlation. Radiology 2001; 219:445–454

continued

2. Mitchell DG, Semelka RC: Chapter 22, In: Stark DD, Bradley WG (eds): Magnetic Resonance Imaging (ed 3). St. Louis: CV Mosby and Co., 1999
3. Semelka RC (ed): MR imaging of the liver II: Diseases. Magnetic Resonance Imaging Clin North Am 10:1
4. Semelka RC, Braga K, Armao D, et al: Chapter 2, In: Semelka RC (ed): Abdominal-Pelvic MRI. New York: Wiley-Liss, Inc., 2002

Gamut M-142-1

GADOLINIUM ENHANCEMENT CHARACTERISTICS OF FOCAL LIVER LESIONS WITH ABNORMAL SIGNAL— ARTERIAL HYPERENHANCEMENT

COMMON

1. Fibrolamellar hepatocellular carcinoma
2. [Flow artifact from aorta]
3. Focal nodular hyperplasia
4. Hemangioma (peripheral and nodular)
5. Hepatoblastoma (child)
6. Hepatocellular adenoma
7. Hepatocellular carcinoma
8. Metastasis (from carcinoma of breast, kidney, or thyroid; islet cell carcinoma; carcinoid; melanoma)
9. Nodule, dysplastic

UNCOMMON

1. Angiomyolipoma
2. Angiosarcoma
3. Biliary cystadenoma/cystadenocarcinoma
4. Extramedullary hematopoiesis
5. Hemangioendothelioma (child)
6. Inflammatory pseudotumor
7. Lymphoma$_g$
8. Nodule, regenerative (Budd-Chiari S.)

[ ] This condition does not actually cause the gamuted imaging finding, but can produce imaging changes that simulate it.

Gamut M-142-2

GADOLINIUM ENHANCEMENT CHARACTERISTICS OF FOCAL LIVER LESIONS WITH ABNORMAL SIGNAL— PORTAL VENOUS HYPERENHANCEMENT

COMMON

1. Abscess (pyogenic, amebic, fungal, hydatid) (rim enhancement)
2. Cholangiocarcinoma (may be seen best on equilibrium phase)
3. Granuloma (eg, sarcoidosis or tuberculosis)
4. Hemangioma (seen on arterial phase also)
5. Hepatocellular adenoma
6. Hepatocellular carcinoma
7. Lymphoma$_g$
8. Metastasis (from carcinoma of colon, lung, ovary, pancreas, prostate, or stomach; also transitional cell carcinoma)
9. [Normal portal veins]

UNCOMMON

1. Biliary hamartoma
2. Fibrosis, confluent (usually wedge-shaped)
3. Focal nodular hyperplasia
4. Mesenchymal hamartoma (child)
5. Nodules, dysplastic or regenerative
6. Undifferentiated embryonal sarcoma of liver (child)

[ ] This condition does not actually cause the gamuted imaging finding, but can produce imaging changes that simulate it.

Gamut M-142-3

GADOLINIUM ENHANCEMENT CHARACTERISTICS OF FOCAL LIVER LESIONS WITH ABNORMAL SIGNAL— NO ENHANCEMENT

COMMON

1. Biloma
2. Cyst, simple hepatic
3. Dilated bile ducts
4. [Flow artifact from aorta]
5. Hematoma
6. Hydatid cyst
7. Infarct
8. Metastasis (treated)
9. Peribiliary cyst
10. Portal vein thrombosis

UNCOMMON

1. Biliary cystadenoma
2. Caroli's disease (saccular biliary dilatation)
3. Ciliated hepatic foregut cyst
4. Hepatic vein thrombosis (Budd-Chiari S.)

[ ] This condition does not actually cause the gamuted imaging finding, but can produce imaging changes that simulate it.

References

1. Krinsky GA, Lee VS, Thiese ND, et al: Hepatocellular carcinoma and dysplastic nodules in patients with cirrhosis: Prospective diagnosis with MR imaging and explantation correlation. Radiology 2001;219:445–454
2. Maetani Y, Itoh K, Egawa H, et al: Benign hepatic nodules in Budd-Chiari syndrome. AJR 2002; 178:869–875
3. Mitchell DG, Semelka RC: Chapter 22, In: Stark DD, Bradley WG (eds): Magnetic Resonance Imaging (ed 3). St. Louis: CV Mosby and Co., 1999
4. Mortele KJ, Ros PR: Cystic focal liver lesion in the adult: Differential CT and MR imaging features. RadioGraphics 2001; 21:895–910
5. Semelka RC (ed): MR imaging of the liver II: Diseases. Magnetic Resonance Imaging Clin North Am 10:1
6. Semelka RC, Braga K, Armao D, et al: Chapter 2, In: Semelka RC (ed): Abdominal-Pelvic MRI. New York: Wiley-Liss, Inc., 2002

Gamut M-143

FOCAL ARTERIAL OR PORTAL VENOUS ENHANCEMENT IN ISOINTENSE (T1 AND T2) LIVER

Arterial Enhancement

COMMON

1. Focal nodular hyperplasia
2. Vascular shunting (adjacent hypervascular mass; cirrhosis; portal or hepatic venous compression or thrombosis; posttraumatic) (frequently wedge shaped)

UNCOMMON

1. Hepatocellular adenoma
2. Hepatocellular carcinoma

Portal Venous Enhancement

UNCOMMON

1. Lymphoma$_g$

References

1. Lane MJ, Jeffrey RB, Katz DS: Spontaneous intrahepatic vascular shunts. AJR 2000; 174:125–131
2. Semelka RC (ed): MR imaging of the liver II: Diseases. Magnetic Resonance Imaging Clin North Am 10:1
3. Semelka RC, Braga K, Armao D, et al: Chapter 2, In: Semelka RC (ed): Abdominal-Pelvic MRI. New York: Wiley-Liss, Inc., 2002
4. Yu JS, Kim KW, Jeong MG, et al: Non-tumorous hepatic arterial-portal venous shunts: MR imaging findings. Radiology 2000; 217:750–756

Gamut M-144

CENTRAL SCAR IN FOCAL LIVER LESION ON MRI

COMMON
1. Fibrolamellar hepatocellular carcinoma
2. Focal nodular hyperplasia (scar is bright on T2 and shows delayed enhancement)
3. Hemangioma (>3 cm)

UNCOMMON
1. Cholangiocarcinoma
2. Hepatocellular adenoma
3. Hepatocellular carcinoma
4. Metastasis
5. Nodule, regenerative (Budd-Chiari S.)

References
1. Maetani Y, Itoh K, Egawa H, et al: Benign hepatic nodules in Budd-Chiari syndrome. AJR 2002;178:869–875
2. Maetani Y, Itoh K, Watanabe C, et al: MR imaging of intrahepatic cholangiocarcinoma with pathologic correlation. AJR 2001;176:1499–1507
3. Semelka RC (ed): MR imaging of the liver II: Diseases. Magnetic Resonance Imaging Clin North Am 10:1
4. Semelka RC, Braga K, Armao D, et al: Chapter 2, In: Semelka RC (ed): Abdominal-Pelvic MRI. New York: Wiley-Liss, Inc., 2002

Gamut M-145-1

DIFFUSE SIGNAL ABNORMALITY IN THE LIVER (BRIGHT ON T1- AND DARK ON T2-WEIGHTED IMAGES)

COMMON
1. Fatty liver

UNCOMMON
1. Glycogen storage disease

Gamut M-145-2

DIFFUSE SIGNAL ABNORMALITY IN THE LIVER (DARK ON T1- AND BRIGHT ON T2-WEIGHTED IMAGES)

COMMON
1. Cirrhosis
2. Infectious hepatitis

UNCOMMON
1. Postradiation hepatitis

Gamut M-145-3

DIFFUSE SIGNAL ABNORMALITY IN THE LIVER (DARK ON T1- AND T2-WEIGHTED IMAGES)

COMMON

1. Hemochromatosis
2. Hemosiderosis (multiple transfusions; cirrhosis; anemia with hyperplastic marrow; intravascular hemolysis)

References

1. Mitchell DG, Semelka RC: Chapter 22, In: Stark DD, Bradley WG (eds): Magnetic Resonance Imaging (ed 3). St. Louis: CV Mosby and Co., 1999
2. Semelka RC (ed): MR imaging of the liver II: Diseases. Magnetic Resonance Imaging Clin North Am 10:1
3. Semelka RC, Braga K, Armao D, et al: Chapter 2, In: Semelka RC (ed): Abdominal-Pelvic MRI. New York: Wiley-Liss, Inc., 2002
4. Tani I, Kurihara Y, Kawaguchi A, et al: MR imaging of diffuse liver disease. AJR 2000; 174:965–971

Gamut M-146

PORTAL VEIN THROMBOSIS

COMMON

1. Cholangiocarcinoma
2. Cirrhosis with portal hypertension
3. Compression or obstruction of portal vein by lymphadenopathy or mass
4. Fibrolamellar hepatocellular carcinoma
5. Hepatocellular carcinoma
6. Hypercoagulable states
7. Inflammation secondary to pancreatitis, appendicitis, diverticulitis
8. Sclerosing cholangitis

UNCOMMON

1. Metastasis

References

1. Mitchell DG, Semelka RC: Chapter 22, In: Stark DD, Bradley WG (eds): Magnetic Resonance Imaging (ed 3). St. Louis: CV Mosby and Co., 1999
2. Semelka RC, Braga K, Armao D, et al: Chapter 2, In: Semelka RC (ed): Abdominal-Pelvic MRI. New York: Wiley-Liss, Inc., 2002

Gamut M-147

PERIPORTAL BRIGHT SIGNAL ON T2-WEIGHTED IMAGE

COMMON

1. Bile leak
2. Cholangitis (pyogenic, viral or AIDS)
3. Hemorrhage, posttraumatic
4. Hepatitis, acute or chronic
5. Liver transplant
6. Malignant infiltration (cholangiocarcinoma; leukemia; lymphoma$_g$; metastasis)
7. Metastases to porta hepatis (obstructs lymphatics)
8. Peribiliary cysts (cirrhosis)
9. Portal hypertension
10. Portal vein thrombus
11. Sclerosing cholangitis
12. Vascular resuscitation (posttrauma patients)

UNCOMMON

1. Budd-Chiari syndrome

References

1. Ly JN, Miller FH: Periportal contrast enhancement and abnormal signal intensity on state-of-the-art MR images. AJR 2001;176:891–897
2. Mitchell DG, Semelka RC: Chapter 22, In: Stark DD, Bradley WG (eds): Magnetic Resonance Imaging (ed 3). St. Louis: CV Mosby and Co., 1999
3. Semelka RC, Braga K, Armao D, et al: Chapter 2, In: Semelka RC (ed): Abdominal-Pelvic MRI. New York: Wiley-Liss, Inc., 2002

MASS IN THE PORTA HEPATIS

1. Adenocarcinoma of gallbladder
2. Carcinoma of pancreas with direct invasion
3. Cavernous transformation of portal vein
4. Cholangiocarcinoma
5. Choledochal cyst
6. Lymphadenopathy
7. Pancreatic pseudocyst
8. Peritoneal metastasis

References

1. Mitchell DG, Semelka RC: Chapter 22, In: Stark DD, Bradley WG (eds): Magnetic Resonance Imaging (ed 3). St. Louis: CV Mosby and Co., 1999
2. Semelka RC, Braga K, Armao D, et al: Chapter 2, In: Semelka RC (ed): Abdominal-Pelvic MRI. New York: Wiley-Liss, Inc., 2002

Gamut M-149

DILATATION OF BILIARY AND/OR PANCREATIC DUCTS ON MRCP

DILATED INTRAHEPATIC DUCTS

COMMON

1. Calculus, biliary
2. Cholangitis (pyogenic, viral or AIDS)
3. Compression of biliary ducts by lymphadenopathy or mass
4. Neoplasm of biliary ducts
5. Sclerosing cholangitis
6. Stricture of common bile duct (inflammatory; post-operative; posttraumatic)

UNCOMMON

1. Caroli's disease
2. Primary biliary cirrhosis
3. Recurrent pyogenic cholangitis

DILATED COMMON BILE DUCT AND INTRAHEPATIC DUCTS

COMMON

1. Ampullary stenosis
2. Calculus, biliary (present or recent passage)
3. Cholangitis (pyogenic, viral or AIDS)
4. Choledochal cyst
5. Compression of biliary ducts by lymphadenopathy or mass
6. Neoplasm of pancreas, common duct, or ampulla
7. Pancreatitis, chronic
8. Stricture of distal common bile duct (inflammatory; postoperative; posttraumatic)

UNCOMMON

1. Caroli's disease
2. Choledochocele
3. Recurrent pyogenic cholangitis
4. Sclerosing cholangitis

DILATED COMMON BILE DUCT, INTRAHEPATIC DUCTS AND PANCREATIC DUCT ("DOUBLE DUCT SIGN")

COMMON

1. Ampullary stenosis
2. Calculus, biliary (present or recent passage)
3. Intraductal papillary mucinous tumor
4. Neoplasm of pancreas, common duct, or ampulla
5. Pancreatitis, chronic
6. Stricture of distal common bile duct (inflammatory; postoperative; posttraumatic)

UNCOMMON

1. Choledochocele
2. Sclerosing cholangitis

ISOLATED PANCREATIC DUCT DILATATION

COMMON

1. Calculus in pancreatic duct
2. Carcinoma of pancreas

3. Intraductal papillary mucinous tumor
4. Pancreatitis, chronic
5. Stricture of pancreatic duct

UNCOMMON

1. Metastasis
2. Neuroendocrine tumor

References
1. Bader TR, Semelka RC, Reinhold C: Chapter 3, In: Semelka RC (ed): Abdominal-Pelvic MRI. New York: Wiley-Liss, Inc., 2002
2. Hahn PF: Chapter 23, In: Stark DD, Bradley WG (eds): Magnetic Resonance Imaging (ed 3). St. Louis: CV Mosby and Co., 1999
3. Levy AD, Murakata LA, Abbott RA, Rohrmann CA: Benign tumors and tumorlike lesions of the gallbladder and extrahepatic bile ducts: Radiologic-pathologic correlation. RadioGraphics 2002;22:387–413

Gamut M-150

FILLING DEFECT IN THE BILIARY TRACT ON MRCP

COMMON

1. [Air bubble]
2. [Arterial pulsation (band-like)]
3. Blood clot
4. Calculus, biliary
5. Cholangiocarcinoma
6. [Flow artifact, biliary]
7. Pseudocalculus (distal common bile duct)
8. Sludge
9. Stent
10. [Surgical clips; metallic susceptibility]

UNCOMMON

1. Neoplasm, benign (adenoma; cystadenoma; granular cell tumor; neurofibroma)
2. Parasites (*Ascaris; Clonorchis; Opisthorchis; Fasciola*); remnants of perforated amebic abscess or hydatid cyst

[ ] This condition does not actually cause the gamuted imaging finding, but can produce imaging changes that simulate it.

References
1. Bader TR, Semelka RC, Reinhold C: Chapter 3, In: Semelka RC (ed): Abdominal-Pelvic MRI. New York: Wiley-Liss, Inc., 2002
2. Hahn PF: Chapter 23, In: Stark DD, Bradley WG (eds): Magnetic Resonance Imaging (ed 3). St. Louis: CV Mosby and Co., 1999
3. Levy AD, Murakata LA, Abbott RA, Rohrmann CA: Benign tumors and tumorlike lesions of the gallbladder and extrahepatic bile ducts: Radiologic-pathologic correlation. RadioGraphics 2002;22:387–413

Gamut M-151-1

INTRALUMINAL GALLBLADDER SIGNAL ABNORMALITY (DARK ON T2-WEIGHTED IMAGE—COMPARED WITH LIVER SIGNAL)

COMMON

1. Gallstone
2. Gas
3. Hematoma, posttraumatic
4. Iodinated contrast media
5. Sludge, tumefactive

UNCOMMON

1. Cholecystitis, hemorrhagic

Gamut M-151-2

INTRALUMINAL GALLBLADDER SIGNAL ABNORMALITY (BRIGHT ON T2-WEIGHTED IMAGE—COMPARED WITH LIVER SIGNAL)

COMMON

1. Adenomyomatosis
2. Carcinoma of gallbladder
3. Hematoma, posttraumatic
4. Polyp, cholesterol or inflammatory

UNCOMMON

1. Cholecystitis, hemorrhagic
2. Metastasis
3. Neoplasm, benign (adenoma; carcinoid; granular cell tumor; neurofibroma)
4. Neoplasm, other malignant (carcinoid; lymphoma)
5. Xanthogranulomatous cholecystitis

Gamut M-151-3

INTRALUMINAL GALLBLADDER SIGNAL ABNORMALITY (BRIGHT ON T1-WEIGHTED IMAGE—COMPARED WITH LIVER SIGNAL)

COMMON

1. Hematoma, posttraumatic
2. Iodinated contrast media
3. Sludge

UNCOMMON

1. Cholecystitis, hemorrhagic
2. Gallstone

References

1. Bader TR, Semelka RC, Reinhold C: Chapter 3, In: Semelka RC (ed): Abdominal-Pelvic MRI. New York: Wiley-Liss, Inc., 2002
2. Hahn PF: Chapter 23, In: Stark DD, Bradley WG (eds): Magnetic Resonance Imaging (ed 3). St. Louis: CV Mosby and Co., 1999
3. Levy AD, Murakata LA, Abbott RA, Rohrmann CA: Benign tumors and tumorlike lesions of the gallbladder and extra-hepatic bile ducts: Radiologic-pathologic correlation. Radio-Graphics 2002;22:387–413
4. Semelka RC (ed): MR imaging of the liver II: Diseases. Magnetic Resonance Imaging Clin North Am 10:1

Gamut M-152

ABNORMAL SIGNAL IN THE INFERIOR VENA CAVA

COMMON

1. Blood clot
2. Carcinoma with direct invasion of IVC (eg, adrenal, hepatocellular, or renal cell carcinoma)
3. [Flow-related enhancement]
4. IVC filter (eg, for thromboembolism or schisto-somiasis)
5. Nephroblastoma with invasion of IVC (child)

UNCOMMON

1. Angiosarcoma
2. Leiomyosarcoma
3. Malignant fibrous histiocytoma

[ ] This condition does not actually cause the gamuted imaging finding, but can produce imaging changes that simulate it.

Reference

1. Kelekis NL, Semelka RC: Chapter 10, In: Semelka RC, Ascher SM, Reinhold C (eds): MRI of the Abdomen and Pelvis. New York: Wiley-Liss, Inc., 1997
2. Semelka RC, Pedro MS, Armao D, Ascher SM: Chapter 7, In: Semelka RC (ed): Abdominal-Pelvic MRI. New York: Wiley-Liss, Inc., 2002

Gamut M-153-1

ADRENAL MASS (BRIGHT ON T2-WEIGHTED IMAGE)

COMMON
1. Adrenocortical carcinoma
2. Cyst (posttraumatic or simple)
3. Hemorrhage (newborn or posttraumatic)
4. Metastasis (necrotic)
5. Neuroblastoma
6. Pheochromocytoma

UNCOMMON
1. Adenoma
2. Ganglioneuroma/ganglioneuroblastoma
3. Granuloma (esp. tuberculosis)
4. Hemangioma
5. Myelolipoma

Gamut M-153-2

ADRENAL MASS (INTERMEDIATE SIGNAL ON T2-WEIGHTED IMAGE)

COMMON
1. Adenoma
2. Adrenocortical carcinoma
3. Hyperplasia (due to ectopic ACTH production)
4. Metastasis
5. Myelolipoma
6. Neuroblastoma

UNCOMMON
1. Ganglioneuroblastoma/ganglioneuroma
2. Granuloma (esp. tuberculosis)
3. Lymphoma$_g$
4. Pheochromocytoma

Gamut M-153-3

ADRENAL MASS (BRIGHT ON T1-WEIGHTED IMAGE)

COMMON
1. Hematoma (newborn or posttraumatic)
2. Hemorrhage, intratumoral (in adrenocortical carcinoma; adenoma; metastasis; neuroblastoma; pheochromocytoma)
3. Myelolipoma

UNCOMMON
1. Adenoma (mild hyperintensity)

References
1. Burton SS, Ros PR: Chapter 24, In: Stark DD, Bradley WG (eds): Magnetic Resonance Imaging (ed 3). St. Louis: CV Mosby and Co., 1999
2. Nagase LL, Semelka RC, Armao D: In: Semelka RC (ed): Abdominal-Pelvic MRI. New York: Wiley-Liss, Inc., 2002

Gamut M-154-1

RENAL MASS (INTERMEDIATE SIGNAL INTENSITY ON T2-WEIGHTED IMAGE)

COMMON
1. Adenoma
2. Angiomyolipoma
3. Hematoma
4. Infarction
5. Lymphoma$_g$
6. Metastasis
7. Oncocytoma
8. Pyelonephritis
9. Renal cell carcinoma (hypernephroma)
10. Transitional cell carcinoma
11. Wilms' tumor (child)

UNCOMMON

1. Granulocytic sarcoma (chloroma)
2. Mesoblastic nephroma (child)
3. Nephroblastomatosis
4. Teratoma
5. Xanthogranulomatous pyelonephritis

Gamut M-154-2

RENAL MASS (BRIGHT ON T2-WEIGHTED IMAGE)

COMMON

1. Abscess (renal or perinephric)
*2. Acquired cystic disease of dialysis
3. Angiomyolipoma (esp. with tuberous sclerosis)
4. Adenoma
5. Calyceal diverticulum
*6. Cyst, simple
7. Hemorrhage (posttraumatic or intratumoral)
8. Hydronephrosis
9. Infarction
*10. Parapelvic cyst
11. Polycystic kidney disease
12. Pyelonephritis
13. Renal cell carcinoma (cystic, hemorrhagic or necrotic)
14. Renal vein thrombus
15. Urinoma

UNCOMMON

*1. Medullary cystic disease
2. Multilocular cystic nephroma

* No enhancement post-gadolinium injection.

Gamut M-154-3

RENAL MASS (DARK ON T2-WEIGHTED IMAGE)

1. Gas
2. Hemorrhage (posttraumatic; intratumoral; hemorrhagic cyst)
3. Leukemic infiltrate
4. Lymphoma$_g$

Gamut M-154-4

RENAL MASS (BRIGHT ON T1-WEIGHTED IMAGE)

1. Abscess
2. Angiomyolipoma (fat)
3. Cyst (hemorrhagic or proteinaceous)
4. Hematoma, posttraumatic
5. Hemorrhage, intratumoral (in angiomyolipoma; renal cell carcinoma; Wilms' tumor)
6. Lymphoma$_g$
7. Renal vein thrombus

References

1. Semelka RC, Braga L, Armao D, Cooper H: Chapter 9, In: Semelka RC (ed): Abdominal-Pelvic MRI. New York: Wiley-Liss, Inc., 2002
2. Torres GM, Ros PR: Chapter 25, In: Stark DD, Bradley WG (eds): Magnetic Resonance Imaging (ed 3). St. Louis: CV Mosby and Co., 1999

Gamut M-155-1

ENDOMETRIAL UTERINE MASS
(VERY BRIGHT ON T2-WEIGHTED IMAGE—COMPARED WITH MYOMETRIUM)

COMMON

1. Carcinoma of endometrium
2. Endometrial hyperplasia
3. Endometrial polyp
4. Endometritis
*5. Gestational trophoblastic disease
6. Hematometra
7. Intrauterine pregnancy
8. Obstructed endometrium or cervix with fluid/mucous
9. Pyometra
10. Retained products of conception
*11. Tamoxifen changes

UNCOMMON

*1. Leiomyoma (submucosal with degeneration or edema)

Gamut M-155-2

ENDOMETRIAL UTERINE MASS
(INTERMEDIATE SIGNAL ON T2-WEIGHTED IMAGE—MILDLY BRIGHT COMPARED WITH MYOMETRIUM)

COMMON

1. Carcinoma of cervix
2. Carcinoma of endometrium
3. Endometrial polyp
4. Hematometra

UNCOMMON

1. Sarcoma (usually mixed Müllerian tumor)
*2. Leiomyoma (submucosal with degeneration or edema)

Gamut M-155-3

ENDOMETRIAL UTERINE MASS
(DARK ON T2-WEIGHTED IMAGE)

COMMON

1. Hematometra, chronic (especially in imperforate hymen or cervical stenosis)
2. Intrauterine device (IUD)
3. Leiomyoma (submucosal)
4. Septate uterus

UNCOMMON

*1. Tamoxifen changes

Gamut M-155-4

ENDOMETRIAL UTERINE MASS
(BRIGHT ON T1-WEIGHTED IMAGE)

COMMON

1. Carcinoma of endometrium with hemorrhage
2. Endometritis
*3. Gestational trophoblastic disease with hemorrhage
4. Hematometra, secondary to obstructed endometrium or cervix (carcinoma; cervical stenosis; obstructed horn in uterine didelphys; imperforate hymen)
5. Retained products of conception with hemorrhage

UNCOMMON

*1. Leiomyoma (submucosal with hemorrhage)
*2. Sarcoma with hemorrhage (usually mixed Müllerian tumor)

* Usually heterogeneous.

References

1. Kubik-Huch RA, Reinhold C, Semelka RC, et al: Chapter 14, In: Semelka RC (ed): Abdominal-Pelvic MRI. New York: Wiley-Liss, Inc., 2002

(continued)

2. Sahdev A, Sohaib SA, Jacobs I, et al: MR imaging of uterine sarcomas. AJR 2001;177:1307–1311
3. Scoutt LM, McCarthy SM: Chapter 28, In: Stark DD, Bradley WG (eds): Magnetic Imaging. (ed 3) St. Louis: CV Mosby and Co., 1999

Gamut M-156-1

MYOMETRIAL UTERINE MASS
(BRIGHT ON T2-WEIGHTED IMAGE)

*1. Adenomyosis (ectopic endometrial rests or cystic changes)
2. Hematoma
*3. Leiomyoma (with degeneration or edema)
4. Myometritis
5. Postoperative changes
6. Vessels
*7. Sarcoma with necrosis (usually leiomyosarcoma)

Gamut M-156-2

MYOMETRIAL UTERINE MASS
(INTERMEDIATE ON T2-WEIGHTED IMAGE— INCREASED SIGNAL COMPARED WITH MYOMETRIUM)

COMMON
1. Carcinoma of cervix, invasive
2. Carcinoma of endometrium, invasive
*3. Leiomyoma (with degeneration)
4. Lymphoma$_g$
*5. Sarcoma with necrosis (usually leiomyosarcoma)

UNCOMMON
1. Metastasis

Gamut M-156-3

MYOMETRIAL UTERINE MASS
(DARK ON T2-WEIGHTED IMAGE)

COMMON
1. Adenomyosis (thickened junctional zone)
2. Contraction of uterus
3. Hematoma
4. Leiomyoma

UNCOMMON
1. Lymphoma$_g$
*2. Sarcoma (usually leiomyosarcoma)

Gamut M-156-4

MYOMETRIAL UTERINE MASS
(BRIGHT ON T1-WEIGHTED IMAGE)

COMMON
*1. Adenomyosis (ectopic hemorrhagic endometrial rests)
2. Hematoma
*3. Leiomyoma with hemorrhage

UNCOMMON
1. Lipoleiomyoma
*2. Sarcoma with hemorrhage (usually leiomyosarcoma)

* Usually heterogeneous.

References
1. Kubik-Huch RA, Reinhold C, Semelka RC, et al: Chapter 14, In: Semelka RC (ed): Abdominal-Pelvic MRI. New York: Wiley-Liss, Inc., 2002
2. Sahdev A, et al: MR imaging of uterine sarcomas. AJR 2001;177:1307–1311

3. Scoutt LM, McCarthy SM: Chapter 28, In: Stark DD, Bradley WG (eds): Magnetic Resonance Imaging. (ed 3) St. Louis: CV Mosby and Co., 1999
4. Siegelman ES, Outwater EK: Tissue characterization in the female pelvis by means of MR imaging. Radiology 1999; 212:5–18

Gamut M-157-1

ADNEXAL MASS
(BRIGHT ON T2-WEIGHTED IMAGE)

COMMON

1. Clear cell adenocarcinoma
2. Cystadenoma/cystadenocarcinoma (serous or mucinous)
3. Ectopic pregnancy
4. Endometrioid carcinoma
5. Hydrosalpinx
6. Leiomyoma (submucosal or broad ligament, with degeneration or edema)
7. Malignant germ cell tumors
8. Metastasis (from carcinoma of breast, gastrointestinal tract, pancreas, or uterus)
9. Ovarian cyst, simple (corpus luteum; paraovarian; polycystic ovary disease; theca lutein)
10. Ovarian torsion
11. Pyosalpinx
12. Sex cord stromal tumor (granular cell tumor)
*13. Teratoma (mature)
14. Tubo-ovarian abscess
15. Varices

UNCOMMON

*1. Brenner tumor (cystic degeneration)
2. Carcinoma of fallopian tube
*3. Endometrioma
*4. Fibrothecoma (cystic degeneration)
5. Hematosalpinx
6. Struma ovarii

* Usually heterogeneous.

Gamut M-157-2

ADNEXAL MASS
(DARK ON T2-WEIGHTED IMAGE)

COMMON

1. Arteriovenous malformation
2. Brenner tumor
3. Endometrioma
4. Leiomyoma (subserosal or broad ligament)
5. Fibrothecoma
*6. Metastasis, Krukenberg subtype (small foci or peripheral dark signal)
7. Ovarian cyst (hemorrhagic)
*8. Teratoma (mature with calcification)

UNCOMMON

1. Hematosalpinx
2. Struma ovarii

* Usually heterogeneous.

Gamut M-157-3

ADNEXAL MASS
(BRIGHT ON T1-WEIGHTED IMAGE)

COMMON

1. Cystadenoma/cystadenocarcinoma (mucinous)
2. Ectopic pregnancy with hemorrhage
3. Endometrioma
4. Metastasis (Krukenberg subtype)
5. Ovarian cyst (hemorrhagic)
*6. Ovarian torsion with hemorrhage
7. Pyosalpinx
*8. Teratoma (mature)
9. Tubo-ovarian abscess

(continued)

UNCOMMON

1. Hematosalpinx
2. Leiomyoma (subserosal or broad ligament, with hemorrhage)
*3. Struma ovarii

* Usually heterogeneous.

References

1. Baumgarten DA, Ascher SM, Semelka RC, et al: Chapter 15, In: Semelka RC (ed): Abdominal-Pelvic MRI. New York: Wiley-Liss, Inc., 2002
2. Scoutt LM, McCarthy SM: Chapter 28, In: Stark DD, Bradley WG (eds): Magnetic Resonance Imaging. (ed 3) St. Louis: CV Mosby and Co., 1999
3. Siegelman ES, Outwater EK: Tissue characterization in the female pelvis by means of MR imaging. Radiology 1999; 212:5–18

Gamut M-158-1

PROSTATE MASS
(BRIGHT ON T2-WEIGHTED IMAGE)

COMMON

1. Abscess
2. Benign prostatic hypertrophy
3. Hematoma (usually post-biopsy)
4. Müllerian duct cyst
5. Prostatitis, acute
6. Retention cyst
7. Utricle cyst

UNCOMMON

1. Adenocarcinoma (high mucin content)

Gamut M-158-2

PROSTATE MASS
(DARK ON T2-WEIGHTED IMAGE)

1. Adenocarcinoma
2. Benign prostatic hypertrophy
3. Calcification
4. Hematoma (usually post-biopsy)
5. Infarction
6. Intraglandular dysplasia
7. Prostatitis, chronic

Gamut M-158-3

PROSTATE MASS
(BRIGHT ON T1-WEIGHTED IMAGE)

COMMON

1. Hematoma (usually post-biopsy)

UNCOMMON

1. Adenocarcinoma (high mucin content)

References

1. Noone TC, Semelka RC, Kubik-Huch RA, Braga L: Chapter 12, In: Semelka RC (ed): Abdominal-Pelvic MRI. New York: Wiley-Liss, Inc., 2002
2. Schwartz CP, McCauley TR, Rifkin MD: Chapter 30, In: Stark DD, Bradley WG (eds): Magnetic Resonance Imaging. (ed 3) St. Louis: CV Mosby and Co., 1999

O

Obstetrical Ultrasound

O

O

COMMON INDICATIONS FOR OBSTETRICAL ULTRASOUND

1. Confirmation of intrauterine pregnancy and viability
2. Detection of fetal anomalies
3. Detection of placenta previa or abruptio
4. Diagnosis of ectopic pregnancy
5. Estimation of gestational age
6. Evaluation of complicated pregnancy (early)
7. Guidance for amniocentesis, chorionic villus sampling, cordocentesis

Reference

1. Fleischer AC, Boehm FK James AE Jr: Ultrasonography in obstetrics and gynaecology: obstetric radiology. In: Grainger RG, Allison DJ: Diagnostic Radiology. (ed 2) Edinburgh: Churchill Livingstone, 1992, pp 1809–1819

FETAL ANOMALIES DETECTABLE BY ULTRASOUND

CENTRAL NERVOUS SYSTEM

1. Agenesis of corpus callosum
2. Anencephaly
3. Arachnoid cyst
4. Choroid plexus cyst or papilloma
5. Dandy-Walker malformation
6. Encephalocele
7. Holoprosencephaly
8. Hydranencephaly
9. Hydrocephalus
10. Meningocele; meningomyelocele
11. Microcephaly
12. Porencephalic cyst (porencephaly)

FACE AND NECK

1. Cervical teratoma
2. Cleft lip or palate
3. Cyclops
4. Hypertelorism; hypotelorism
5. Lymphangioma (cystic hygroma)

CHEST

1. Cardiac arrhythmias
2. Congenital heart disease
3. Congenital diaphragmatic hernia
4. Mediastinal tumor
5. Pleural effusion

GASTROINTESTINAL TRACT AND ABDOMEN

1. Abdominal cyst (eg, mesenteric, choledochal, gut duplication, ovarian, urachal, or renal cyst; cystic teratoma)
2. Body stalk anomaly (absent umbilicus and cord)
3. Congenital diaphragmatic hernia
4. Esophageal atresia
5. Gastroschisis; omphalocele; Cantrell S.
6. Meconium peritonitis
7. Small bowel obstruction (eg, duodenal, jejunal or ileal atresia or stenosis; annular pancreas)

URINARY TRACT

1. Bladder dilatation (eg, posterior urethral valves)
2. Infantile polycystic kidney disease
3. Megaureter
4. Multicystic dysplastic kidney
5. Prune-belly S. (Eagle-Barrett S.)
6. Renal agenesis (bilateral)
7. Ureteropelvic junction obstruction

SPINE AND EXTREMITIES

1. Dwarfism; other skeletal dysplasias
2. Meningocele; meningomyelocele
3. Osteogenesis inperfecta
4. Sacral agenesis or deformity

(continued)

5. Sacrococcygeal teratoma
6. Vertebral defects; spina bifida

References

1. Eisenberg RL: Clinical Imaging: An Atlas of Differential Diagnosis. (ed 3) Philadelphia: Lippincott-Raven, 1997, pp 1196–1207
2. Fleischer AC, Boehm FK James AE Jr: Ultrasonography in obstetrics and gynaecology: obstetric radiology. In: Grainger RG, Allison DJ: Diagnostic Radiology. (ed 2) Edinburgh: Churchill Livingstone, 1992, p 1813

Gamut O-3

LARGE FOR DATES FETUS

COMMON

1. Inaccurate dating
2. Multiple gestation
3. Maternal obesity
4. Maternal diabetes

UNCOMMON

1. Beckwith-Wiedemann syndrome

Reference

1. Carlson DE: Chapter 18. Growth disturbances: Large-for-date and small-for-date fetuses. In: McGahan JP, Goldberg BB (eds): Diagnostic Ultrasound. Philadelphia: Lippincott-Raven, 1997

Gamut O-4

SMALL FOR DATES FETUS

FETAL FACTORS

1. Aneuploidy (trisomy; triploidy)
2. Skeletal dysplasias
3. Structural anomalies (syndromes)

MATERNAL FACTORS

COMMON

1. Hypertension
2. Medication (Warfarin; hydantoin {Dilantin}; cytotoxic drugs; isotretinoin)
3. Renal failure
4. Substance abuse

UNCOMMON

1. Collagen vascular disease$_g$
2. Cyanotic cardiopulmonary disease
3. Infection (syphilis; viral infections; malaria; Chagas disease; listeria)
4. Thyrotoxicosis

Reference

1. Carlson DE: Chapter 18. Growth disturbances: Large-for-date and small-for-date fetuses. In: McGahan JP, Goldberg BB (eds): Diagnostic Ultrasound. Philadelphia: Lippincott-Raven, 1997

Gamut O-5

INTRAUTERINE GROWTH RETARDATION

FETAL OR PLACENTAL FACTORS

1. Chorioangioma of placenta
2. Congenital infection (toxoplasmosis; rubella; cytomegalic inclusion disease; herpes; syphilis)
3. Congenital malformation or syndrome
4. Fetal chromosomal abnormality; trisomy
5. Multiple gestation
6. Placental vascular insufficiency or infarction
7. Twin-to-twin transfusion S.

MATERNAL FACTORS

1. Age below 17 years or over 35 years
2. Maternal illness (eg, cardiovascular disease; renal disease; malnutrition; anemia)
3. Substance abuse (drugs; alcohol; tobacco)

Reference
1. Powers GT: Gamut: Causes of intrauterine growth retardation (IUGR). Semin Roentgenol 1982–17:163

Gamut O-6

FAILURE OF FETAL HEAD TO ENGAGE DURING LABOR

FETAL FACTORS
1. Hydrops, hydrocephalus, or other fetal deformity
2. Low-lying placenta
3. Multiple gestation
4. Umbilical cord twist or shortening

MATERNAL FACTORS
1. Cephalopelvic disproportion
2. Distended bladder or rectum
3. Extrauterine pregnancy
4. Pelvic neoplasm or cyst
5. Spondylolisthesis; ischial spine prominence; other pelvic girdle deformity
6. Uterine malformation; persistent uterine contraction ring

Reference
1. Bishop PA: Radiologic Studies of the Gravid Lufterus. New York: Harper & Row, 1965, pp 39–84, 268–269

Gamut O-7

FETAL CRANIAL DEFORMITY

COMMON
1. Anencephaly
2. Cephalocele
3. Exencephaly
4. Fetal demise
5. Microcephaly
6. Open neural tube defect

UNCOMMON
1. Cloverleaf skull deformity (Kleeblatt-Schädel anomaly)
2. Craniosynostosis (See A-1)
3. Limb-body wall complex (body stalk anomaly)
4. Osteogenesis imperfecta

Reference
1. McGahan JP, Thurmond AS: Chapter 10. Fetal head and brain. In: McGahan JP, Goldberg BB (eds): Diagnostic Obstetrical Ultrasound. Philadelphia: Lippincott-Raven, 1997

Gamut O-8

FETAL BRAIN—MIDLINE CYSTIC MASS

COMMON
1. Agenesis of corpus callosum
2. Aneurysm of Vein of Galen
3. Dandy-Walker malformation
4. Holoprosencephaly

UNCOMMON
1. Arachnoid cyst
2. Cystic neoplasm

Reference
1. McGahan JP, Thurmond AS: Chapter 10. Fetal head and brain. In: McGahan JP, Goldberg BB (eds): Diagnostic Ultrasound. Philadelphia: Lippincott-Raven, 1997

Gamut O-9

FETAL BRAIN—LATERAL OR ASYMMETRICAL CYSTIC MASS

COMMON

1. Arachnoid cyst
2. Choroid plexus cyst
3. Porencephaly
4. Schizencephaly

UNCOMMON

1. Cystic neoplasm
2. Hydrocephalus (unilateral)
3. Intracranial hemorrhage

Reference

1. McGahan JP, Thurmond AS: Chapter 10. Fetal head and brain. In: McGahan JP, Goldberg BB (eds): Diagnostic Ultrasound. Philadelphia: Lippincott-Raven, 1997

3. Fragile X S.
4. Intracranial mass (brain neoplasm; arachnoid cyst)
5. Lissencephaly
6. Meckel-Gruber S.
7. Nasal-facial-digital S.
8. Osteogenesis imperfecta
9. Osteopetrosis (Albers Schönberg disease)
10. Posthemorrhagic
11. Postinflammatory
12. Roberts S.
13. Smith-Lemli-Opitz S.
14. Thanatophoric dysplasia
15. Trisomy 13 S.
16. Trisomy 18 S.
17. Vein of Galen aneurysm
18. Walker-Warburg S.

Reference

1. Nyberg DA, et al: Cerebral malformations. In: Nyberg DA, Mahoney BS, Pretorius DH (eds): Diagnostic Ultrasound of Fetal Anomalies: Text and Atlas. Chicago: Year Book, 1993

Gamut O-10

FETAL VENTRICULOMEGALY (HYDROCEPHALUS)

COMMON

1. Agenesis of corpus callosum
2. Aqueductal stenosis
3. Cephalocele
4. Dandy-Walker malformation
5. Holoprosencephaly
6. Hydranencephaly
7. Open neural tube defect (Arnold-Chiari II malformation)

UNCOMMON

1. Achondroplasia
2. Acrocephalosyndactyly (Apert type)

Gamut O-11

MASSIVE FETAL INTRACRANIAL FLUID COLLECTIONS

1. Alobar holoprosencephaly
2. Hydranencephaly
3. Massive hydrocephalus

Reference

1. McGahan JP, Thurmond AS: Chapter 10. Fetal head and brain. In: McGahan JP, Goldberg BB (eds): Diagnostic Ultrasound. Philadelphia: Lippincott-Raven, 1997

Gamut O-12

FETAL INTRACRANIAL CALCIFICATIONS

COMMON

1. Cytomegalovirus infection in utero
2. Herpes simplex type II infection in utero
3. Toxoplasmosis infection in utero

UNCOMMON

1. Brain tumor
2. Rubella infection in utero (congenital rubella S.)

Reference

1. McGahan, JP, Thurmond AS: Chapter 10. Fetal head and brain. In: McGahan JP, Goldberg BB (eds): Diagnostic Obstetrical Ultrasound. Philadelphia: Lippincott-Raven, 1997

Gamut O-13

STRAIGHT FETAL SPINE

COMMON

1. Abdominal pregnancy
2. Breech presentation
3. Hydramnios; anencephaly
4. Hydrops fetalis
5. Multiple gestation
6. Placental abnormality (enlarged or malpositioned)

UNCOMMON

1. Fetal abdominal mass (eg, Wilms' tumor; infantile polycystic kidneys; hydronephrosis; hepatic tumor)
2. Maternal pelvic mass (eg, uterine fibroids)
3. Meconium peritonitis

References

1. Barnett E, Naim A: A study of foetal attitude. Br J Radiol 1965;38:338–349
2. Daw E: Generalized deflexion of the foetal spine. Br J Radiol 1970;43:240–241

Gamut O-14

FETAL NECK MASS

COMMON

1. Hydrops fetalis
2. Lymphangioma (cystic hygroma)
3. Nonfused amnion (1st trimester)
4. Nuchal cord

UNCOMMON

1. Branchial cleft cyst
2. Cephalocele
3. Goiter
4. Hemangioendothelioma
5. Hemangioma
6. Iniencephaly
7. Meningomyelocele (cervical)
8. Neuroblastoma
9. Nuchal thickening (Down S.)
10. Teratomoa (cervical)
11. Twin sac of blighted ovum
12. Klippel-Tretaunay-Weber S.; Parkes Weber S.

References

1. McGahan JP, Coates TL, LeScale KB, et al: Chapter 12. Fetal neck and spine. In: McGahan JP, Goldberg BB (eds): Diagnostic Obstetrical Ultrasound. Philadelphia: Lippincott-Raven, 1997
2. Williamson MR: Chapter 8. Obstetrical ultrasound. In: Essentials of Ultrasound. Philadelphia: WB Saunders, 1996, p 180

Gamut O-15

FETAL CHEST MASS

COMMON

1. Bronchogenic cyst
2. Congenital diaphragmatic hernia
3. Cystic adenomatoid malformation

(continued)

4. Hydrothorax
5. Neurenteric cyst
6. Sequestration of lung

UNCOMMON

1. Bronchial atresia
2. Neuroblastoma
3. Rhabdomyoma
4. Teratoma

References

1. Goldstein RB: Chapter 13. Fetal thorax. In: McGahan JP, Goldberg BB (eds): Diagnostic Obstetrical Ultrasound. Philadelphia: Lippincott-Raven, 1997
2. Williamson MR: Chapter 8. Obstetrical ultrasound. In: Essentials of Ultrasound. Philadelphia: WB Saunders, 1996, p 181

Gamut O-16

FETAL CARDIAC MASS

UNCOMMON

1. Aneurysm of foramen ovale
2. Fibroma
3. Hemangioma
4. Myxoma
5. Rhabdomyoma
6. Teratoma
7. Thickening of chordae tendineae

Reference

1. Williamson MR: Chapter 8. Obstetrical ultrasound. In: Essentials of Ultrasound. Philadelphia: WB Saunders, 1996, p 183

Gamut O-17

NONVISUALIZATION OF FETAL STOMACH

COMMON

1. CNS disorder
2. Diaphragmatic hernia
3. Esophageal atresia
4. Normal (empty stomach)
5. Oligohydramnios

UNCOMMON

1. Facial clefts
2. [Situs inversus]

Reference

1. Porto M, Steiger RM: Chapter 15. Fetal abdomen and pelvis. In: McGahan JP, Goldberg BB (eds): Diagnostic Obstetrical Ultrasound. Philadelphia: Lippincott-Raven, 1997

Gamut O-18

ECHOGENIC FETAL BOWEL

COMMON

1. Artifact (excessive gain)
2. Normal variant (2nd trimester)
3. Trisomy 21 S. (Down S.)

UNCOMMON

1. Blood in amniotic fluid
2. Cytomegalovirus infection
3. Meconium ileus (cystic fibrosis)

Reference

1. Porto M, Steiger RM: Chapter 15. Fetal abdomen and pelvis. In: McGahan JP, Goldberg BB (eds): Diagnostic Obstetrical Ultrasound. Philadelphia: Lippincott-Raven, 1997

Gamut O-19

FETAL HEPATOSPLENOMEGALY

COMMON

1. Congenital transplacental infection (toxoplasmosis; rubella; cytomegalovirus; herpes; hepatitis)
2. Fetal anemia
3. Heart failure
4. Hydrops fetalis

UNCOMMON

1. Beckwith-Wiedemann S.
2. Leukemia
3. Metastatic neuroblastoma
4. Neoplasm of liver or spleen (eg, hepatoblastoma; hemangioendothelioma)

Reference

1. Porto M, McGahan JP: The fetal abdomen and pelvis. In: McGahan JP, Porto M (eds): Diagnostic Obstetrical Ultrasound. Philadelphia: JB Lippincott, 1994.

Gamut O-20-1

FETAL CYSTIC ABDOMINAL MASS

COMMON

1. Choledochal cyst
2. Cystic renal disease (eg, multicystic dysplastic kidney; infantile polycystic kidney disease)
3. Hepatic cyst
4. Hydronephrosis/hydroureter
5. Ovarian cyst

UNCOMMON

1. Anterior sacral meningocele
2. Hydrometrocolpos
3. Intestinal atresia
4. Meconium pseudocyst

5. Megacystic-microcolon-hypoperistalsis syndrome
6. Mesenteric or omental cyst
7. Sacrococcygeal teratoma
8. Splenic cyst
9. Umbilical vein varix
10. Urachal cyst
11. Ureterocele
12. Urinoma

Reference

1. Porto M, Steiger RM: Chapter 15. Fetal abdomen and pelvis. In: McGahan JP, Goldberg BB (eds): Diagnostic Obstetrical Ultrasound. Philadelphia: Lippincott-Raven, 1997

Gamut O-20-2

FETAL CYSTIC ABDOMINAL MASS—UPPER ABDOMEN

RIGHT UPPER QUADRANT

1. Choledochal cyst
2. Hepatic cyst

LEFT UPPER QUADRANT

1. Splenic cyst

Gamut O-20-3

FETAL CYSTIC ABDOMINAL MASS—MID ABDOMEN AND POSTERIOR (RENAL)

POSTERIOR RENAL

1. Hydronephrosis
2. Renal cyst
3. Urinoma

(continued)

MID-ABDOMEN

1. Meconium pseudocyst
2. Mesenteric cyst
3. Omental cyst
4. Umbilical vein varix

Gamut O-20-4

FETAL CYSTIC ABDOMINAL MASS—LOWER ABDOMEN AND PELVIS

LOWER ABDOMEN AND PELVIS

COMMON

1. Hydrometrocolpos
2. Ovarian cyst
3. Ureterocele
4. Urachal cyst

UNCOMMON

1. Anterior sacral meningocele
2. Sacrococcygeal teratoma

Reference
1. Porto M, McGahan JP: The fetal abdomen and pelvis. In: McGahan JP, Porto M (eds): Diagnostic Obstetrical Ultrasound. Philadelphia: JB Lippincott, 1994

Gamut O-21

FETAL INTRA-ABDOMINAL CALCIFICATIONS

COMMON

1. Meconium peritonitis

UNCOMMON

1. Cholelithiasis
2. Congenital viral infection (cytomegalovirus; varicella; rubella; toxoplasmosis)
3. Hepatic infarction
4. Tumor (hemangioma; hepatoblastoma; teratoma; neuroblastoma)

Reference
1. Porto M, Steiger RM: Chapter 15. Fetal abdomen and pelvis. In: McGahan JP, Goldberg BB (eds). Diagnostic Ultrasound. Lippincott-Raven, 1997

Gamut O-22

LARGE FETAL ABDOMEN DURING LAST TRIMESTER

COMMON

1. Ascites (incl. urine ascites) (See O-23)
2. Edema, generalized (eg, hemolytic disease; hydrops fetalis; maternal diabetes)
3. Hydronephrosis, massive
4. Polycystic kidneys

UNCOMMON

1. Gastrointestinal neoplasm or cyst
2. Hepatic neoplasm (eg, hepatoblastoma; hemangioendothelioma) or cyst (eg, polycystic liver disease)
3. Hydrometrocolpos
4. Neuroblastoma

5. Ovarian tumor or cyst (eg, teratoma)
6. Prune-belly S. (Eagle-Barrett S.)
7. Wilms' tumor

Reference
1. Moncado R, Wang JJ, Love L, et al: Neonatal ascites associated with urinary outlet obstruction (urine ascites). Radiology 1968;90:1165–1170

Gamut O-23

FETAL ASCITES

COMMON
1. Dead fetus
2. Heart failure, fetal (eg, atrioventricular shunt; arrhythmia; myocardial disorder; coarctation or interruption of aorta; placental tumor)
3. Hydrops fetalis (with pleural and/or pericardial effusions and skin edema)
4. Idiopathic
5. Posterior urethral valves with bladder outlet obstruction (urine ascites)
6. [Pseudoascites]
7. Rh isoimmunization

UNCOMMON
1. Biliary atresia
2. Intestinal obstruction with perforation (eg, atresia; stenosis; volvulus)
3. Turner S.
4. Twin to twin transfusion S.
5. Viral infection (eg, cytomegalovirus)

References
1. Eisenberg RL: Clinical Imaging: An Atlas of Differential Diagnosis (ed 3) Philadelphia: Lippincott-Raven, 1997, pp 1212–1213
2. Fleischer AC, James AE Jr: Diagnostic Sonography. Principles and Clinical Applications. Philadelphia: WB Saunders, 1989

3. Porto M, Steiger RM: Chapter 15. Fetal abdomen and pelvis. In: McGahan JP, Goldberg BB (eds): Diagnostic Obstetrical Ultrasound. Philadelphia: Lippincott-Raven, 1997

Gamut O-24

FETAL ANTERIOR ABDOMINAL WALL DEFECT

COMMON
1. Gastroschisis
2. Normal bowel herniation (8th–12th weeks)
3. Omphalocele; Cantrell S.

UNCOMMON
1. Allantoic cyst
2. Beckwith-Wiedemann S.
3. Ectopia cordis
4. Exstrophy of bladder
5. Exstrophy of cloaca
6. Limb-body wall complex (body stalk anomaly)
7. Omphalomesenteric cyst
8. Urachal cyst

References
1. Porto M, Steiger RM: Chapter 15. Fetal abdomen and pelvis. In: McGahan JP, Goldberg BB (eds): Diagnostic Obstetrical Ultrasound. Philadelphia: Lippincott-Raven, 1997
2. Williamson MR: Chapter 8. Obstetrical ultrasound. In: Essentials of Ultrasound. Philadelphia: WB Saunders, 1996 p 187

Gamut O-25

FETAL SKIN THICKENING (DIFFUSE HYPERTRICHOSIS)

COMMON
1. Hydrops fetalis
2. Lymphangiectasis (eg, Turner S.)

(continued)

UNCOMMON

1. Fetal akinesia deformation sequence (Pena-Shokeir S. type I)
2. Myotonic dystrophy
3. Thanatophoric dysplasia

Reference

1. Goldstein RB: Chapter 13. Fetal thorax. In: McGahan JP, Goldberg BB (eds): Diagnostic Obstetrical Ultrasound. Philadelphia: Lippincott-Raven, 1997.

Gamut O-26

OLIGOHYDRAMNIOS

COMMON

1. Fetal distress
2. Fetal malformations, other
3. Intrauterine growth retardation (IUGR) (See O-5)
4. Normal (reduction in amniotic fluid late in pregnancy; postmaturity)
5. Polycystic renal disease (infantile or adult)
6. Posterior urethral valves
7. Premature rupture of membranes
8. Prune-belly S. (Eagle-Barrett S.)
9. Renal agenesis (bilateral)
10. Renal or bladder obstruction

UNCOMMON

1. Caudal regression S.
2. Cytogenetic-triploidy S.
3. Idiopathic
4. Impending fetal death
5. Multicystic dysplastic kidneys (bilateral)
6. Trisomies
7. Urethral agenesis

References

1. Eisenberg RL: Clinical Imaging: An Atlas of Differential Diagnosis. (ed 3) Philadelphia: Lippincott-Raven, 1997, pp 1210–1211

2. Fleischer AC, James AE Jr: Diagnostic Sonography. Principles and Clinical Applications. Philadelphia: WB Saunders, 1989
3. Williamson MR: Chapter 8. Obstetrical ultrasound. In: Essentials of Ultrasound. Philadelphia: WB Saunders, 1996, p 195

Gamut O-27-1

FETAL ABNORMALITIES ASSOCIATED WITH POLYHYDRAMNIOS

CENTRAL NERVOUS SYSTEM

1. Anencephaly
2. Cebocephaly
3. Encephalocele; meningocele
4. Hydrocephalus; hydranencephaly
5. Porencephalic cyst (porencephaly)

GASTROINTESTINAL

1. Biliary atresia
2. Diaphragmatic hernia
3. Duodenal obstruction (atresia; annular pancreas)
4. Esophageal atresia
5. Gastroschisis
6. Omphalocele

CARDIOVASCULAR

1. Chorioangioma of placenta
2. Coarctation or interruption of fetal aorta
3. Fetal anemia
4. Fetal arteriovenous fistulas
5. Myocardial abnormalities; cardiac dysrhythmias
6. Twin-twin transfusion in monochorionic twins

MISCELLANEOUS

1. Chest or abdominal mass, other (eg, pancreatic cyst)
2. Congenital chylothorax
3. Fetal hydrops
4. Idiopathic

5. Mesonephric nephroma
6. Multicystic dysplastic kidneys
7. Pulmonary hypoplasia
8. Short limb dwarf syndromes (eg, thanatophoric dysplasia; asphyxiating thoracic dysplasia {Jeune S.})
9. Teratoma (sacrococcygeal or cervical)
10. Trisomy 18 S.

References
1. Eisenberg RL: Clinical Imaging: An Atlas of Differential Diagnosis. (ed 3) Philadelphia: Lippincott-Raven, 1997, pp 1208–1209
2. Fleischer AC, James AE Jr: Diagnostic Sonography. Principles and Clinical Applications. Philadelphia: WB Saunders, 1989

Gamut O-27-2

MATERNAL FACTORS ASSOCIATED WITH POLYHYDRAMNIOS

1. Diabetes mellitus
2. Heart failure
3. Idiopathic
4. Pre-eclampsia
5. Rh incompatibility
6. Syphilis

Gamut O-28

THIN PLACENTA

COMMON
1. Congenital fetal anomalies
2. Infection
3. Intrauterine growth retardation (IUGR)
4. Maternal factors
   a. Cardiovascular disease
   b. Diabetes mellitus
   c. Hypertension
   d. Renal disease
   e. Toxemia

Reference
1. Williamson MR: Chapter 8. Obstetrical ultrasound. In: Essentials of Ultrasound. Philadelphia, WB Saunders, 1996, p 166

Gamut O-29

THICKENED PLACENTA

COMMON
1. Hydrops (nonimmune)
2. Maternal diabetes mellitus
3. Maternal or fetal anemia
4. Normal variant
5. Rh isoimmunization

UNCOMMON
1. Beckwith-Wiedemann S.
2. Congenital fetal anomaly
3. Hydatidiform mole
4. Infection
5. Maternal heart failure
6. Neoplasm of uterus (chorioangioma)
7. Placental hemorrhage
8. Sacrococcygeal teratoma
9. Triploidy; other chromosomal abnormalities

Reference
1. Williamson MR: Chapter 8. Obstetrical ultrasound. In: Essentials of Ultrasound. Philadelphia: WB Saunders, 1996, p 166

Gamut O-30

SOLID PLACENTAL MASS

COMMON

1. Choriepithelioma (chorioangioma)

UNCOMMON

1. Teratoma

Gamut O-31

HYPOECHOIC PLACENTAL LESIONS

COMMON

1. Gestational trophoblastic disease (eg, hydatiform mole)
*2. Intervillous thrombosis
3. Maternal lake
4. Mature placenta
5. Normal subplacental complex
*6. Septal cyst
7. Subchorionic lake

UNCOMMON

1. Choriangioma
2. Circumvallate placenta
3. Hematoma
4. Infarct
5. Metastasis
*6. Perivillous or subchorionic fibrin deposition
7. Subchorionic thrombosis
8. Teratoma

* Anechoic or hypoechoic intraplacental collection, usually of no clinical significance.

References
1. Levine D: Chapter 28. Female pelvis. In: McGahan JP, Goldberg BB (eds): Diagnostic Ultrasound. Philadelphia: Lippincott-Raven, 1997

2. Spirit BA, Gordon LP: Chapter 8. Placenta and cervix. In: McGahan JP, Goldberg BB (eds): Diagnostic Ultrasound. Philadelphia: Lippincott-Raven, 1997
3. Williamson MR: Chapter 8. Obstetrical ultrasound. In: Essentials of Ultrasound. Philadelphia: WB Saunders, 1996, p 167

Gamut O-32

RETROPLACENTAL MASS

1. Abruptio placentae
2. Leiomyoma (fibroid) of uterus
3. Retroplacental hematoma
4. Submembranous hematoma

Reference
1. Spirit BA, Gordon LP: Chapter 8. Placenta and cervix. In: McGahan JP, Goldberg BB (eds): Diagnostic Ultrasound. Philadelphia: Lippincott-Raven, 1997

Gamut O-33

UMBILICAL CORD ENLARGEMENT OR MASS

COMMON

1. Hydrops (diffuse swelling)
2. Knotted umbilical cord
3. Localized deposition of Wharton's jelly
4. Thrombosis of umbilical vessels
5. Umbilical cord angioma
6. Umbilical cord cyst

UNCOMMON

1. Teratoma
2. Umbilical artery aneurysm
3. Umbilical vein varix

Reference
1. Finberg HJ: Chapter 9. Umbilical cord and amniotic membranes. In: McGahan JP, Goldberg BB (eds): Diagnostic Ultrasound. Philadelphia: Lippincott-Raven, 1997

Gamut O-34-S

RADIOLOGICAL SIGNS OF INTRAUTERINE PREGNANCY (FIRST TRIMESTER)

1. Double decidual sign
2. Fetal pole with uterine cavity
3. Gestational sac with yolk sac within endometrial cavity
4. Intradecidual sign

Gamut O-35

ENDOMETRIAL FLUID COLLECTION WITH POSITIVE BETA HCG

1. Decidual cyst (ectopic pregnancy)
2. Gestational sac (intrauterine pregnancy)
3. Missed abortion
4. Pseudogestational sac (ectopic pregnancy

Gamut O-36

OVARIAN MASS IN PREGNANCY

COMMON
1. Corpus luteum cyst (1st trimester)
2. Dermoid cyst of ovary
3. Endometrioma
4. Hemorrhagic corpus luteum cyst
5. Torsion of ovary

UNCOMMON
1. Malignant ovarian neoplasm

Abbreviations

ADEM	Acute disseminated encephalomyelitis	ie	That is
AIDS	Acquired immune deficiency syndrome	incl	Including
ANGIO	Angiography, arteriography	IUD	Intrauterine device
AP	Anteroposterior	IUGR	Intrauterine growth retardation
APVC	Anomalous pulmonary venous connection, total (T) or partial (P)	IVC	Inferior vena cava
		L	Left
ARDS	Adult respiratory distress syndrome	LA	Left atrium
ASD	Atrial septal defect	LLL	Left lower lobe
AV	Atrioventricular (communis or canal)	LUL	Left upper lobe
AVM	Arteriovenous malformation	LV	Left ventricle
CABG	Coronary artery bypass graft	MCTD	Mixed connective tissue disease
CHF	Congestive heart failure	MEN S.	Multiple endocrine neoplasia syndrome
CNS	Central nervous system	MRI	Magnetic resonance imaging
COPD	Chronic obstructive pulmonary disease	Occas	Occasionally
CPPD	Calcium pyrophosphate dihydrate crystal deposition disease	PA	Posteroanterior
		PDA	Patent ductus arteriosus
CREST S.	Calcinosis-Raynaud's-sclerodactyly-telangiectasia	PEEP	Positive end-expiratory pressure
		PIE	Pulmonary infiltrate with eosinophilia (a clinical entity almost exclusively of young women)
CSF	Cerebrospinal fluid		
CT	Computed tomography		
DIP	Distal interphalangeal (joint)	PIP	Proximal interphalangeal (joint)
DISH	Diffuse idiopathic skeletal hyperostosis	PML	Progressive multifocal leukoencephalopathy
eg	For example		
g	Consult Glossary	PNET	Primitive neuroectodermal tumor
GI	Gastrointestinal	PS	Pulmonary stenosis
GU	Genitourinary	pulm	Pulmonary
GYN	Gynecology	R	Right
HADD	Hydroxyapatite deposition disease	RA	Right atrium
HIV	Human immunodeficiency syndrome	RLL	Right lower lobe
IHSS	Idiopathic hypertrophic subaortic stenosis	RML	Right middle lobe

RUL	Right upper lobe	US	Ultrasound
RV	Right ventricle	VATER S.	Vertebral (or vascular) anomalies; anal anomalies (or auricular defects); tracheoesophageal fistula; esophageal atresia (or ring), renal anomalies (or radial defects, rib anomalies)
S	Syndrome		
SVC	Superior vena cava		
TORCH	Toxoplasmosis, rubella, cytomegalovirus, herpes simplex transplacental fetal infections		
		VSD	Ventricular septal defect

Glossary

ABSCESS, ABDOMINAL Abdominal wall, appendiceal, flank, greater or lesser sac, hepatic, pancreatic, psoas, renal, splenic, subhepatic, subphrenic, tuboovarian

ALVEOLAR PATTERN See CONSOLIDATION PATTERN

ANEMIA, PRIMARY Erythroblastosis, hemolytic anemia, pyruvate kinase deficiency, sickle cell disease and variants, spherocytosis, thalassemia and variants

ANEURYSM Arteriosclerotic, dissecting, false, mycotic, poststenotic, syphilitic, berry, fusiform, saccular

ANGIOMA Arteriovenous malformation, cirsoid aneurysm, hemangioma (incl. capillary and cavernous), lymphangioma, varices

ARDS Adult respiratory distress syndrome, shock lung, respirator lung, adult hyaline membrane disease, and many other synonyms: A confusing term, widely used and poorly defined, associated with widespread pulmonary involvement

ARTERIOSCLEROTIC HEART DISEASE Coronary artery disease

ARTERIOVENOUS MALFORMATION (AVM) See Angioma

BLEEDING OR CLOTTING DISORDER Anticoagulant effect, coagulopathy (eg, disseminated intravascular coagulation {DIC}), hemophilia, Christmas disease, leukemia, purpura (eg, Henoch-Schönlein), thrombocytopenia

BRONCHOGENIC OR BRONCHIAL CYST OF LUNG A cyst containing air and/or fluid, lined by respiratory mucosa. Unrelated to mediastinal bronchogenic cyst

CONNECTIVE TISSUE DISEASE (COLLAGEN VASCULAR DISEASE) Rheumatoid disease, lupus erythematosus, scleroderma, dermatomyositis, polyarteritis nodosa, mixed connective tissue disease (MCTD), CREST syndrome (calcinosis-Raynaud's-sclerodactyly-telangiectasia), Sjögren's syndrome

CONSOLIDATION PATTERN Alveolar pattern, air space pattern, peripheral airways pattern: identified by fluffy margins, early coalescence, air bronchogram or alveologram, and butterfly distribution

DUPLICATION (BRONCHOGENIC OR ENTERIC) CYST OF MEDIASTINUM Bronchogenic, enteric, or neurenteric cyst: a congenital cyst related to anomalous foregut development. Unrelated to bronchogenic cyst of lung (bronchial cyst)

EOSINOPHILIC LUNG DISEASE Acute eosinophilic pneumonia, idiopathic Löffler syndrome; chronic eosinophilic pneumonia; hypereosinophilic syndrome, PIE (pulmonary infiltrate with eosinophilia), drug-induced, parasite-induced (tropical pulmonary eosinophilia), fungus induced, eosinophilic lung disease with connective tissue disease and/or vasculitis

FAT EMBOLISM Incl. diffuse embolization of fatty bone marrow (after fracture), amniotic fluid, or oily contrast medium

FUNGUS DISEASE Aspergillosis, blastomycosis, coccidiomycosis, cryptococcosis (torulosis), moniliasis (candidiasis), histoplasmosis, paracoccidiomycosis (South American blastomycosis), sporotrichosis, zygomycosis (mucormycosis). Actinomycosis and nocardiosis have been reclassified as gram-positive bacteria, resembling fungi.

GASTROINTESTINAL STROMAL TUMOR   Fibroma, leiomyoma, neurofibroma, and their sarcomatous counterparts.

GLYCOGEN STORAGE DISEASE   von Gierke (Type I), Pompe (Type II), Cori (Type III), McArdle (Type V)

HAMARTOMA   A benign nodule composed of mature cells that normally occur in the affected part. In the lung it is usually a slow-growing chondroma, sometimes called a hamartochondroma.

HYDROCARBON ASPIRATION   Aspiration of furniture polish, gasoline, kerosene, lighter fluid, turpentine

HYPOPLASTIC LEFT HEART SYNDROME   Includes aortic stenosis or atresia, cor triatriatum, hypoplastic aorta, hypoplastic left ventricle, interrupted aortic arch, infantile coarctation, severe mitral stenosis or atresia

IATROGENIC   Instrumentation; catheterization; intubation; endoscopy; biopsy; instillation of fluid, blood, or drugs

IMMUNOLOGIC DISORDERS   AIDS, agammaglobulinemia (Bruton S.) or dysgammaglobulinemia, ataxia-telangiectasia S., Bloom S., Buckley S., combined deficiency S., DiGeorge S., chronic granulomatous disease of childhood, Job S.

INTERSTITIAL FIBROSIS   Synonyms: end-stage (honeycomb) lung, fibrosing alveolitis, Hamman-Rich syndrome, idiopathic interstitial fibrosis, muscular cirrhosis of the lung, usual interstitial pneumonitis (UIP)

LANGERHANS CELL HISTIOCYTOSIS   Eosinophilic granuloma, Hand-Schüller-Christian disease, Letterer Siwe's disease (nonlipid histiocytosis), formerly called histiocytosis X

LIPOID PNEUMONIA   Mineral oil granuloma, oil aspiration pneumonia, paraffinoma

LYMPHOMA   Includes Burkitt's lymphoma, Hodgkin's disease, non-Hodgkin's lymphoma, leukemia (all varieties, including chloroma), pseudolymphoma, Sezary syndrome, angioimmunoblastic lymphadenopathy

MASS   Tumor, neoplasm, cyst, abscess, hematoma, aneurysm, hernia

MEDIASTINITIS   Mediastinal abscess, cellulitis, edema, fibrosis, granuloma, phlegmon, acute mediastinitis, chronic sclerosing (fibrosing) mediastinitis

MUCOPOLYSACCHARIDOSES   Also mucolipidoses and other lysosomal storage diseases (See Gamut J-4)

MUSCULAR DISORDERS   Duchenne muscular dystrophy, myasthenia gravis, muscular dystrophy, myotonic dystrophy, myotonia congenita, oculopharyngeal myopathy, steroid or thyrotoxic myopathy, visceral myopathy, other myopathies, myotonias, and myositis (See also NEUROLOGIC AND NEUROMUSCULAR DISORDERS)

NEOPLASMS, BENIGN   Adenoma, chemodectoma, chondroma, endometrioma, hamartoma, hemangioma, hemangiopericytoma, lipoma, polyp, pseudotumor, teratoma (See also SPINDLE CELL TUMOR)

NEUROGENIC NEOPLASM   Ganglioneuroma and paraganglioneuroma, ganglioneuroblastoma, neurilemoma, neuroblastoma, neurofibroma, neurosarcoma, schwannoma (neurinoma)

NEUROLOGIC AND NEUROMUSCULAR DISORDERS   Alzheimer's disease, amyotonia congenita (Oppenheim disease), amyotrophic lateral sclerosis, brain damage, bulbar or pseudobulbar palsy, cerebral palsy, Duchenne syndrome, meningomyelocele, multiple sclerosis, parkinsonism, poliomyelitis, paraplegia, quadriplegia, stroke, syringomyelia, Werdnig-Hoffmann disease (infantile spinal muscular atrophy) (See also MUSCULAR DISORDERS)

PARALYTIC DISORDER   Bulbar paralysis, paraplegia, peripheral paralysis, poliomyelitis, quadriplegia

PARASITIC DISEASES WITH IMAGING CHANGES   Amebiasis, armillifer infestation, anisakiasis, ascariasis, capillariasis, Chagas' disease (trypanosomiasis), clonorchiasis, cysticercosis, dirofilariasis (heartworm), filariasis, giardiasis, guinea worm infestation, hookworm disease, hydatid disease (echinococcosis), loiasis, malaria, paragonimiasis, schistosomiasis, strongyloidiasis, taeniasis, toxoplasmosis, tropical pulmonary eosinophilia (microfilaria)

PNEUMOCONIOSIS WITH CONGLOMERATE MASS   Silicosis, coal-worker's pneumoconiosis, asbestosis

PNEUMONIA   Pneumonia, common bacterial (*Actinomyces, E. coli, H. influenzae, Klebsiella, Legionella, Mycoplasma,* plague, *Pseudomonas,* staphylococcal, streptococcal); actinomycosis; nocardiosis pneumonia; common viral (eg, chickenpox, Coxsackie, cytomegalovirus, ECHO virus, influenza, measles) pneumonia; common parasitic (*Pneumocystis carinii,* amebiasis, ascariasis, paragonimiasis, strongyloidiasis, toxoplasmosis, tropical pulmonary eosinophilia (microfilaria) pneumonia, chlamydial (eg, psittacosis) pneumonia; rickettsial (eg, Rocky Mountain spotted fever, Q fever)

PRIMITIVE NEUROECTODERMAL TUMOR (PNET) Cerebellar medulloblastoma, ependymoblastoma, meduloepithelioma, pigmented medulloblastoma, supratentorial PNET (cerebral neuroblastoma, pineoblastoma)

PSEUDOTUMOR (OF LUNG), INFLAMMATORY Synonyms: Organized pneumonia, fibroxanthoma, plasma cell granuloma, sclerosing hemangioma

POLYP Adenomatous, eosinophlic, hamartomatous, hyperplastic, inflammatory (fibrous, granulomatous), juvenile, papilloma, villous

SPINDLE CELL TUMOR Fibroma, leiomyoma, neurofibroma, rhabdomyoma, and their malignant counterparts

TETRALOGY OF FALLOT Includes also pentalogy of Fallot (tetralogy of Fallot plus ASD), pseudotruncus arteriosus, pulmonary atresia with VSD and systemic pulmonary collateral arteries, trilogy of Fallot (pulmonary stenosis with ASD)

THYROID MASS Adenoma, carcinoma, goiter, intrathoracic goiter (substernal, retrosternal), struma, thyroiditis, ectopic thyroid tissue

VASCULAR RING Aberrant right subclavian artery, double aortic arch, right aortic arch types I and II

WEGENER'S GRANULOMATOSIS Includes also bronchocentric granulomatosis, Churg and Strauss or other granulomatosis, hypersensitivity angiitis of Zeek, lymphomatoid granulomatosis, midline lethal granuloma

References

The following books and articles provided invaluable source material in the preparation of this book. Their excellent lists and tables formed a nucleus for many gamuts.

GENERAL REFERENCES

1. Burgener FA, Kormano M: Differential Diagnosis in Conventional Radiology. (ed 2) New York: Thieme, 1991

2. Burgener FA, Kormano M: Differential Diagnosis in Computed Tomography. New York: Thieme, 1996

3. Chapman S, Nakielny R: Aids to Radiological Differential Diagnosis. (ed 3) London: WB Saunders, 1995

4. Ebel K-D, Blickman H, Willich E, Richter E: Differential Diagnosis in Pediatric Radiology. Stuttgart: Thieme, 1999

5. Eisenberg RL: Clinical Imaging: An Atlas of Differential Diagnosis. (ed 3) Philadelphia: Lippincott-Raven, 1997

6. Grainger RG, Allison DJ (eds): Diagnostic Radiology: An Anglo-American Textbook of Imaging. (ed 2) Edinburgh: Churchill Livingstone, 1992

7. Keats TE: Atlas of Normal Roentgen Variants That May Simulate Disease. (ed 4) Chicago: Year Book, 1988

8. Kirks DR: Practical Pediatric Imaging. (ed 3) Philadelphia: Lippincott-Raven, 1998

9. Kreel L: Outline of Radiology. New York: Appleton-Century-Crofts, 1971

10. Oh KS, Ledesma-Medina, J, Bender TM: Practical Gamuts and Differential Diagnosis in Pediatric Radiology. Chicago: Year Book, 1982

11. Reeder MM: Reeder and Felson's Gamuts in Radiology. (ed 3) New York: Springer-Verlag, 1993

12. Silverman FN, Kuhn JP (eds): Caffey's Pediatric X-ray Diagnosis. (ed 9) St. Louis: Mosby, 1993

13. Slone RM, Fisher AJ: Pocket Guide to Body CT Differential Diagnosis. New York: McGraw-Hill, 1999

14. Sutton D (ed): Textbook of Radiology and Imaging. (ed 6) New York: Churchill Livingstone, 1998

15. Swischuk LE: Imaging of the Newborn, Infant, and Young Child. (ed 3) Baltimore: Williams & Wilkins, 1989

16. Swischuk LE, John SD: Differential Diagnosis in Pediatric Radiology. (ed 2) Baltimore: Williams & Wilkins, 1995

17. Eplick JG, Haskin ME: Roentgenologic Diagnosis, vol. 2. (ed 3) Philadelphia: WB Saunders, 1976

18. Weissleder R, Rieumont MJ, Wittenburg J: Primer of Diagnostic Imaging. (ed 2) St. Louis, Mosby-Year Book, 1997

19. Wilson JD, et al.: Harrison's Principles of Internal Medicine. (ed 12) New York: McGraw-Hill, 1991

CONGENITAL SYNDROMES AND BONE DYSPLASIAS

1. Beighton P, et al.: International nomenclature of constitutional diseases of bone. May 1983 revision. Ann Radiol 1984;27:275–280
2. Felson B (ed): Dwarfs and other little people. Semin Roentgenol 1973;8:133–263
3. Gorlin RJ, Cohen MM Jr, Levin LS: Syndromes of the Head and Neck. (ed 3) New York: Oxford University Press, 1990
4. Jones KL: Smith's Recognizable Patterns of Human Malformation. (ed 5) Philadelphia: WB Saunders, 1997
5. Kozlowski K, Beighton P: Gamut Index of Skeletal Dysplasias. Berlin: Springer-Verlag, 1984
6. Spranger JW, Langer LO Jr, Wiedemann H-R: Bone Dysplasias. Philadelphia: WB Saunders, 1974, pp 269–273
7. Taybi H, Lachman RS: Radiology of Syndromes, Metabolic Disorders, and Skeletal Dysplasias. (ed 4) St. Louis: Mosby-Year Book, 1996

SECTION A: SKULL AND BRAIN

1. Atlas SW: Magnetic Resonance Imaging of the Brain and Spine. New York: Raven Press, 1991
2. Barkovich AJ: Pediatric Neuroimaging. (ed 3) Philadelphia: Lippincott Williams & Wilkins, 2000
3. Djang WT: Basics of Cerebral Angiography. In: Ravin CE, Cooper C (eds): Review of Radiology. Philadelphia: WB Saunders, 1990, pp. 189–191
4. Doyle FH: Radiology of the pituitary fossa. In: Lodge T, Steiner RE (eds): Recent Advances in Radiology, vol. 6. New York: Churchill Livingstone, 1979
5. Dubois PJ: Neuro-otology. In: Rosenberg RN (ed): The Clinical Neurosciences, vol. 4. New York: Chuurchill Livingstone, 1984
6. DuBoulay GH: Principles of X-Ray Diagnosis of the Skull. (ed 2) London: Butterworths, 1980
7. Eisenberg RL: Skull and Spine Imaging. An Atlas of Differential Diagnosis. New York: Raven Press, 1994
8. Enzmann DR: Imaging of Infections and Inflammations of the CNS: CT, Ultrasound, and NMR. New York: Raven Press, 1984
9. Harwood-Nash DCF, Fitz CR: Neuroradiology in Infants and Children, vol. 2. St. Louis: Mosby, 1976
10. Hasso AN, Smith DS: The cerebellopontine angle. Semin Ultrasound CT MR. 1989;10:280–301.
11. Hatam A, Bergstrom M, Greitz T: Diagnosis of sellar and parasellar lesions by computed tomography. Neuroradiology 1979;18:249–258
12. Huckman MS (ed): ARRS Neuroradiology Categorical Course Syllabus. Reston: American Roentgen Ray Society, 1992
13. Lane BA, Moseley IF, Theron J: Intracranial tumors. In: Grainger RG, Allison DJ (eds): Diagnostic Radiology, vol. 3. Edinburgh: Churchill Livingstone, 1992
14. Lange S, Grumme T, Meese W: Computerized Tomography of the Brain. Berlin: Schering Medico-Scientific Book Series, 1980
15. Lee SH, Rao KC: Cranial Computed Tomography and MRI. (ed 2) New York: McGraw-Hill, 1987
16. Newton TH, Potts DG: Radiology of the Skull and Brain, vol. 1, book 1. St. Louis: Mosby, 1971
17. Newton TH, Hasso AN, Dillon WP (eds): Modern Neuroradiology, vol. 3. Computed Tomography of the Head and Neck. New York: Raven Press, 1988
18. Osborn AG: Handbook of Neuroradiology. St. Louis: Mosby-Year Book, 1991
19. Taveras JM, Wood EH: Diagnostic Neuroradiology, vol. 1. (ed 2) Baltimore: Williams & Wilkins, 1976
20. Walker M: Malignant brain tumors—a synopsis. CA-Cancer J Clinic 1975;25:114–120

SECTION B: HEAD AND NECK

1. Batsakis JG: Tumors of the Head and Neck. Clinical and Pathological Considerations. (ed 2) Baltimore: Williams & Wilkins, 1979
2. Blaschke DP, Osborn AG: The mandible and teeth. In: Bergeron RT, Osborn AG, Som PM (eds): Head and Neck Imaging Excluding the Brain. St. Louis: Mosby, 1984
3. Bryan RN, Craig JA: The eye: CT of the orbit. In: Bergeron RT, Osborn AG, Som PM (eds): Head and Neck Imaging Excluding the Brain. St. Louis: Mosby, 1984

4. DelBalso AM: Lesions of the jaws. Semin Ultrasound CT MR. 1995;16:487–512

5. Farman AG, Nortje CJ, Wood RE: Oral and Maxillofacial Diagnostic Imaging. St. Louis: Mosby-Year Book, 1993

6. Hall RE, DelBalso AM, Carter LC: Radiography of the sinonasal tract. In: DelBalso AM: Maxillofacial Imaging. Philadelphia: WB Saunders, 1990, pp. 139–207

7. Hasso AN: MRI Atlas of the Head and Neck. London: Martin Dunitz, 1993, pp. 58–59

8. Hayden CK Jr, Swischuk LE: Head and neck lesions in children. In: Bergeron RT, Osborn AG, Som PM: Head and Neck Imaging Excluding the Brain. St. Louis: Mosby, 1984, pp. 708–715

9. Langlais RP: Radiology of the jaws. In: DelBalso AM: Maxillofacial Imaging. Philadelphia: WB Saunders, 1990, pp. 313–373

10. Lufkin R, Borges A, Villablanca P: Teaching Atlas of Head and Neck Imaging. New York: Thieme, 2000

11. Peyster RG, Hoover E: Computed Tomography in Orbital Disease and Neuroophthalmology. Chicago: Year Book, 1984

12. Prein J, Remagen W, Spiessl B, et al.: Atlas of Tumors of the Facial Skeleton. Berlin: Springer-Verlag, 1986

13. Reede DL, Bergeron RT, Osborn AG: CT of the soft tissues of the neck. In: Bergeron RT, Osborn AG, Som PM: Head and Neck Imaging Excluding the Brain. St. Louis: Mosby, 1984, pp. 491–530

14. Seifert G, Miehlke A, Haubrich J, Chilla R: Diseases of the Salivary Glands. New York: Thieme, 1986, pp. 171–318

15. Silvers AR, Som PM: Salivary glands. Radiol Clin North Am 1998;36:941–966

16. Slone RM, Fisher AJ: Pocket Guide to Body CT Differential Diagnosis. New York: McGraw-Hill, 1999

17. Sobel DF, Salvolini U, Newton TH: Ocular and orbital pathology. In: Newton TH, Hasso AN, Dillon WP (eds): Modern Neuroradiology, vol. 3. Computed Tomography of the Head and Neck. New York: Raven Press, 1988

18. Som PM, Sanders DE: The salivary glands. In: Bergeron RJ, Osborn AG, Som PM: Head and Neck Imaging Excluding the Brain. St. Louis: Mosby, 1984, pp. 186–234

19. Som PM, Biller HF, Lawson W, et al.: Parapharyngeal space masses: an updated protocol based upon 104 cases. Radiology 1984;153:149–156

20. Som PM, Curtin HD: Head and Neck Imaging. (ed 3) St. Louis: Mosby-Year Book, 1996

21. Stafine EC, Gibilisco JA: Oral Roentgenographic Diagnosis. (ed 4) Philadelphia: WB Saunders, 1975

22. Teresi LM, Lufkin RB, Warthan DG, et al.: Parotid masses: MR imaging. Radiology 1987;163:405–409

23. Teresi LM, Lufkin RB, Hanafee WN: Magnetic resonance imaging of the larynx. Radiol Clin North Am 1989;27:393–406

24. Unger JM: Handbook of Head and Neck Imaging. New York: Churchill Livingstone, 1987

25. Valvassori GE, Buckingham RA, Carter BL, Hanafee WN, Mafee MF: Head and Neck Imaging. New York: Thieme, 1988

26. Vogl TJ: Chapter 38. In: Stark DD, Bradley WG (eds): Magnetic Resonance Imaging. (ed 2) St. Louis: Mosby, 1992

27. Vogl TJ, Balzer J, Mack M, Steger W: Differential Diagnosis in Head and Neck Imaging. New York: Thieme, 1999

28. Warpeha RL: Masses in the neck. In: Wood NK, Goaz PW: Differential Diagnosis of Oral Lesions. (ed 4) St. Louis: Mosby-Year Book, 1991, pp. 616–637

29. Weissman JL: Imaging of the salivary glands. Semin Ultrasound CT MR 1995;16:546–568

30. Wood NK, Goaz PW: Differential Diagnosis of Oral Lesions. (ed 4) St. Louis: Mosby-Year Book, 1991

SECTION C: SPINE AND ITS CONTENTS

1. Daffner D: Imaging of Vertebral Trauma. (ed 2) Philadelphia: Lippincott Williams & Wilkins, 1998

2. Du Boulay GH (ed): A Textbook of X-Ray Diagnosis by British Authors. Neuroradiology. London: Lewis, 1984

3. Epstein BS: Spinal canal mass lesions. Radiol Clin North Am 1966;4:185–202

4. Epstein BS: The Spine. Philadelphia: Lea & Febiger, 1976

5. Harris JH Jr, Mirvis SE: The Radiology of Acute Cervical Spine Trauma. (ed 3) Baltimore: Williams & Wilkins, 1996

6. Kattan KR: Trauma and No-trauma of the Cervical Spine. Springfield, IL: Charles C Thomas, 1975

7. Lewtas N: The Spine and Myelography. In: Sutton D (ed): Textbook of Radiology and Imaging. (ed 5) Edinburgh: Churchill Livingstone, 1987

8. Lombardi G, Passerini A: Spinal Cord Diseases: A Radiologic and Myelographic Analysis. Baltimore: Williams & Wilkins, 1964

9. Moseley IF: Myelography. In: du Boulay GH (ed): A Textbook of Radiological Diagnosis. (ed 5) London: Lewis, 1984

10. Murphey MD, Batnitsky S, Bramble JM: Diagnostic imaging of spinal trauma. Radiol Clin North Am 1989;27:855–872

11. Murphey MD, Andrews CL, Flemming DJ, et al.: Primary tumors of the spine: Radiologic-pathologic correlation. RadioGraphics 1996;16:1131–1158

12. Silverman FN (ed): Caffey's Pediatric X-ray Diagnosis. (ed 8) Chicago: Year Book, 1985

13. Resnick D: Diagnosis of Bone and Joint Disorders. (ed 3) Philadelphia: WB Saunders, 1995

14. Schmorl G, Junghanns H: The Human Spine in Health and Disease. (ed 2) New York: Grune & Stratton, 1971

15. Stevens JM: The spine and spinal cord. In: Sutton D, Young JWR (eds): A Short Textbook of Clinical Imaging. London: Springer-Verlag, 1990, pp. 806–811

16. Taveras JM, Wood EH: Diagnostic Neuroradiology. (ed 2) Baltimore: Williams & Wilkins, 1976

17. Wackensheim A: Roentgen Diagnosis of the Craniovertebral Region. Berlin: Springer-Verlag, 1974, pp. 363–366

SECTION D: BONE, JOINTS, AND SOFT TISSUES

1. Beighton P, Cremin BJ: Sclerosing Bone Dysplasia. Berlin: Springer-Verlag, 1980

2. Beighton P, et al.: International Classification of Osteochondrodysplasia, 1992 (modified)

3. Brower AC: Arthritis in Black and White. (ed 2) Philadelphia: WB Saunders, 1997

4. Edeiken J, Dalinka M, Krasnick D: Edeiken's Roentgen Diagnosis of Diseases of Bone. (ed 4) Baltimore: Williams & Wilkins, 1989

5. Enzinger FM, Weiss SW: Soft Tissue Tumors. (ed 3) St. Louis: Mosby, 1995

6. Forrester DM, Brown JC, Nesson JW: The Radiology of Joint Disease. (ed 3) Philadelphia: WB Saunders, 1987

7. Green M: Pediatric Diagnosis. (ed 6) Philadelphia: WB Saunders, 1998, p. 276

8. Greenfield GB: Radiology of Bone Diseases. (ed 5) Philadelphia: Lippincott, 1990

9. Jacobson HG, Siegelman SS: Some miscellaneous solitary bone lesions. Semin Roentgenol 1966;1: 314–335

10. Jensen P: Chondrocalcinosis and other calcifications. Radiol Clin North Am 1988;26:1315–1325

11. Jeung MY, Gangi A, Gasser B, et al.: Imaging of chest wall disorders. RadioGraphics 1999;19:617–637

12. Kohler A, Zimmer EA: Borderlands of the Normal and Early Pathologic in Skeletal Radiology. New York: Grune & Stratton, 1968

13. Kransdorf MJ, Murphey MD: Imaging of Soft Tissue Tumors. Philadelphia: WB Saunders, 1997

14. Kuisk H: Technique of Lymphography and Principles of Interpretation. St. Louis: Warren H Green, 1971

15. Lachman RS: International Nomenclature and Classification of the Osteochondrodysplasias (1997). Pediatr Radiol 1998;28:737–744

16. Madewell JE, Ragsdale BD, Sweet DE: Radiologic and pathologic analysis of solitary bone lesions. Radiol Clin North Am 1981;19:715–748

17. Murray RO, Jacobson HG, Stoker D: The Radiology of Skeletal Disorders. (ed 3) Edinburgh: Churchill Livingstone, 1990

18. Nelson SW: Some fundamentals in the radiologic differential diagnosis of solitary bone lesions. Semin Roentgenol 1966;1:244–267

19. Oh KS, Ledesma-Medina J, Bender TM: Practical Gamuts and Differential Diagnosis in Pediatric Radiology. Chicago: Year Book, 1982, p. 146

20. Ozonoff MB: Pediatric Orthopedic Radiology. Philadelphia: WB Saunders, 1992, pp. 234–276

21. Poznanski AK: Foot manifestations of the congenital malformation syndromes. Semin Roentgenol 1970; 5:354–366

22. Poznanski AK, Gam SM, Holt JF: The thumb in the congenital malformation syndromes. Radiology 1971; 100:115–129

23. Poznanski AK, Holt JF: The carpals in congenital malformation syndromes. Am J Radiol 1971;112: 443–459

24. Poznanski AK: The Hand in Radiologic Diagnosis. (ed 2) Philadelphia: WB Saunders, 1984

25. Ragsdale BD, Madewell JE, Sweet DE: Radiologic and pathologic analysis of solitary bone lesions. Part II: Periosteal reactions. Radiol Clin North Am 1981; 19:749–783

26. Resnick D, Niwayama G: Diagnosis of Bone and Joint Disorders. Philadelphia: WB Saunders, 1981

27. Resnick D: Diagnosis of Bone and Joint Disorders. (ed 3) Philadelphia: WB Saunders, 1995

28. Rimoin DL: International Nomenclature and Classification of the Osteochondrodysplasias (1997). Am J Med Genetics 1998;79:376–382

29. Seeger LL, Yao L, Eckardt JJ: Surface lesions of bone. Radiology 1998;206:17–33

30. Unni KK: Dahlin's Bone Tumors. General Aspects and Data on 11,087 Cases. (ed 5) Philadelphia: Lippincott-Raven, 1996

31. Weissman BN: Radiographic evaluation of total joint replacement. In: Kelly WN, Harris ED Jr, Ruddy S, Sledge CB (eds): Textbook of Rheumatology. Philadelphia: WB Saunders, 1994

32. Weissman BN: Imaging of total hip replacement. Radiology 1997;202:611–623

SECTION E: CARDIOVASCULAR

1. Chen JTT: Essentials of Cardiac Roentgenology. Boston: Little, Brown, 1987

2. Duncan W: Color Doppler in Clinical Cardiology. Philadelphia: WB Saunders, 1988

3. Edwards JE, Carey LS, Neufeld HN, et al.: Congenital Heart Disease. Philadelphia: WB Saunders, 1965

4. Elliott LP: Cardiac Imaging in Infants, Children, and Adults. Philadelphia: Lippincott, 1991

5. Feigenbaum H: Echocardiology. (ed 4) Philadelphia: Lea& Febiger, 1986

6. Felson B (ed): Congenital heart disease, part I. Semin Roentgenol 1985;20:110, 220

7. Felson B (ed): Congenital heart disease, part II. Semin Roentgenol 1985;20:200

8. Fowler NO: Cardiac Diagnosis and Treatment. (ed 3) Hagerstown, MD: Harper & Row, 1980

9. Gedgaudas E, Moller JH, Castaneda-Zuniga WR, et al.: Cardiovascular Radiology. Philadelphia: WB Saunders, 1985

10. Goldberg S: Doppler Echocardiography. (ed 2) Philadelphia: Lea & Febiger, 1988

11. Kisslo J: Doppler Color Flow Imaging. New York: Churchill Livingstone, 1988

12. Lester RG: Radiological concepts in the evolution of heart disease. Mod Concepts Cardiovasc Dis 1968; 37:113–118

13. Meszaros WT: Cardiac Roentgenology. Springfield, IL: Charles C Thomas, 1969

14. Moes CAF, Freedom RM, Burrows PE: Anomalous pulmonary venous connections. Semin Roentgenol 1985;20:134–150

15. Moss AJ, Adams FH, Emmanouilides GC: Heart Disease in Infants, Children, and Adolescents. (ed 2) Baltimore: Williams & Wilkins, 1977

16. O'Brien KM: Congenital Syndromes with Congenital Heart Disease. Semin Roentgenol 1985;20: 104–105

17. Palmer PES, Cockshott WP: Cardiac Diseases in the Tropics. In: Palmer PES, Reeder MM: The Imaging of Tropical Diseases, with Epidemiological, Pathological, and Clinical Correlation. (ed 2) Heidelberg: Springer-Verlag, 2001

18. Prichard RW: Tumors of the heart: Review of the subject and report of one hundred anf fifth cases. Arch Pathol 1951;51:98–128

19. Rowe RD, Mehrizi A. The Neonate with Congenital Heart Disease. Major Problems in Clinical Pediatrics, vol. 5. Philadelphia: WB Saunders, 1968

20. Seward J, Fajek A, Edwards W, et al.: Two Dimensional Echocardiographic Atlas. New York: Springer-Verlag, 1987

21. Spindola-Franco H, Fish BG (eds): Radiology of the

Heart: Cardiac Imaging in Infants and Children. New York: Springer-Verlag.

22. Swischuk LE: Plain Film Interpretation in Congenital Heart Disease. (ed 2) Baltimore: Williams & Wilkins, 1979

23. Tonkin ILD: The Infant with Respiratory Distress. In: Elliott LP (ed): Cardiac Imaging in Infants, Children, and Adults. Philadelphia: Lippincott, 1991, p. 777

24. Viamonte M Jr: Intrathoracic extracardiac shunts. Semin Roentgenol 1967;2:342–367

25. Wesenberg RL: The Newborn Chest. Hagerstown, MD: Harper & Row, 1973

26. Wilde P, Hartnell GG: Ischemic heart disease. In Sutton D, Young JWR (eds): A Short Textbook of Clinical Imaging. London: Springer-Verlag, 1990, pp. 161–163

SECTION F: CHEST

1. Felson B, Weinstein AW, Spitz HB: Principles of Chest Roentgenology: A Programmed Text. Philadelphia: WB Saunders, 1965, p. 197

2. Felson B: Disseminated interstitial diseases of the lung. Ann Radiol 1966;9:325–345

3. Felson B: Thoracic calcifications. Chest 1969;56: 330–343

4. Felson B: Chest Roentgenology. Philadelphia: WB Saunders, 1973

5. Felson B: Neoplasms of the trachea and main stem bronchus. Semin Roentgenol 1983;18:23–37

6. Fraser RG, Pare PD, Fraser RS: Differential Diagnosis of Diseases of the Chest. Philadelphia: WB Saunders, 1991, pp. 11–20, 25–30

7. Fraser RS, Muller NL, Coleman N, Pare PD (eds): Fraser and Pare: Diagnosis of Diseases of the Chest. (ed 4) Philadelphia: WB Saunders, 1999

8. Gaensler EA: Unilateral hyperlucent lung. In: Simon M, Potchen J, LeMay M: Frontiers of Pulmonary Radiology. New York: Grune & Stratton, 1969

9. Godwin JD, Webb WR, Savoca CJ, et al.: Multiple, thin-walled cystic lesions of the lung. Am J Roentgenol 1980;135:593–604

10. Hartman GE, Shochat SJ: Primary pulmonary neoplasms of childhood: A review. Ann Thorac Surg 1983;36:108–119

11. Heitzman ER: The Mediastinum: Radiologic Correlation with Anatomy and Pathology. St. Louis: Mosby, 1977

12. Heitzman ER: The Lung: Radiologic-Pathologic Correlations. (ed 2) St. Louis: Mosby, 1984, p. 182

13. Meyer JS, Nicotra JJ: Tumors of the pediatric chest. Semin Roentgenol 1998;33:187–198

14. Muller NL: Lecture at 16th Masters Diagnostic Radiology Conference, Kauai, Hawaii, 1999

15. Naidich DP, Zerhouni EA, Siegelman SS, Kuhn JP (eds): Computed Tomography and Magnetic Resonance of the Thorax. (ed 2) New York: Raven Press, 1991, pp. 60–136

16. Reed JC: Chest Radiology. Plain Film Patterns and Differential Diagnoses. (ed 4) St. Louis: Mosby-Year Book, 1997, pp. 211–225

17. Rigsby CM, Sostman HD, Matthay RA: Drug-induced lung disease. In: Flenley DC, Petty TL (eds): Recent Advances in Respiratory Medicine. New York: Churchill Livingstone, 1983, pp. 131–158

18. Rivero HJ, Bowen AD, Bender TM, et al.: Radiological evaluation of diaphragm and juxtadiaphragmatic lesions. Scientific exhibit, American Roentgen Ray Society Meeting, Boston, 1985

19. Rosenow EC III, Wilson WR, Cockerill FR III: Pulmonary disease in the immunocompromised host (Part I). Mayo Clin Proc 1985;60:473–487

20. Salzman E: Lung Calcifications in X-ray Diagnosis. Springfield, IL: Charles C Thomas, 1968

21. Siegel MJ, Sagel SS, Reed K: The value of computed tomography in the diagnosis and management of pediatric mediastinal abnormalities. Radiology 1986; 142:149–155

22. Spencer H: Pathology of the lung (Excluding Pulmonary Tuberculosis). (ed 3) New York: Pergamon Press, 1977

23. Strollo DC, Rosado de Christenson M, Rett JR: Primary mediastinal tumors. Part I. Tumors of the inferior mediastinum. Chest 1997;112:511–522

24. Strollo DC, Rosado de Christenson M, Rett JR: Primary mediastinal tumors. Part II. Tumors of the middle and posterior mediastinum. Chest 1997;112: 1344–1357

25. Trapnell DH: The differential diagnosis of linear

shadows in chest radiographs. Radiol Clin North Am 1973;11:77–92

26. Webb WR, Muller NL, Naidich DP: High Resolution CT of the Lung. (ed 3) Philadelphia: Lippincott, Williams & Wilkins, 2001

27. Wesenberg RL: The Newborn Chest. Hagerstown, MD: Harper & Row, 1973

28. World Health Organization histological typing of lung tumors. Am J Clin Pathol 1982;77:123–136

SECTION G: GASTROINTESTINAL TRACT AND ABDOMEN

1. Ayers AB: The spleen. In: Grainger RG, Allison DJ: Diagnostic Radiology. An Anglo-American Textbook of Imaging, vol. 3. (ed 2) Edinburgh: Churchill Livingstone, 1992, p. 2408

2. Baker SR, Cho KC: The Abdominal Plain Film with Correlative Imaging. Norwalk, CT: Appleton & Lange, 1998

3. Baron RL, Gore RM: Diffuse liver disease. In: Gore RM, Levine MS: Textbook of Gastrointestinal Radiology. (ed 2) Philadelphia: WB Saunders, 2000, pp. 1590–1638

4. Berk RN, Clemett AR: Radiology of the Gallbladder and Bile Ducts. Philadelphia: WB Saunders, 1977

5. Cheszmar JL: Pancreatic neoplasms. In: Gore RM, Levine MS (eds): Textbook of Gastrointestinal Radiology. (ed 2) Philadelphia: WB Saunders, 2000, pp. 1796–1811

6. Clouse RE, Diamant NE: Motor physiology and motor disorders of the esophagus. In: Feldman M, Scharschmidt BF, Sleisenger MH: Gastrointestinal and Liver Disease. (ed 6) Philadelphia: WB Saunders, 2000, pp. 61–91

7. Cohen SM, Kurtz AB: Biliary sonography. Radiol Clin North Am 1991;29:1171–1192

8. Cosgrove DO: Liver and biliary tree. In: Barnett E, Morley P (eds): Clinical Diagnostic Ultrasound. Oxford: Blackwell, 1985, pp. 365–386

9. Eisenberg RL: Gastrointestinal Radiology: A Pattern Approach. (ed 3) Philadelphia: Lippincott, 1996

10. Feldman M, Scharschmidt BF, Slesisinger MH: Gastrointestinal and Liver Disease. (ed 6) Philadelphia: WB Saunders, 2000

11. Fernbach SK: Neonatal gastrointestinal radiology. In: Gore RM, Levine MS (eds): Textbook of Gastrointestinal Radiology. (ed 2) Philadelphia: WB Saunders, 2000, pp. 2042–2073

12. Gelfand DW: Gastrointestinal Radiology. New York: Churchill Livingstone, 1984

13. Goldberg HI, Sheft DJ: Abnormalities in small intestine contour and caliber. Radiol Clin North Am 1976;14:461–475

14. Gore RM: Inflammatory disease. In: Margulis AR: Modern Imaging of the Alimentary Tube. New York: Springer-Verlag, 1998, pp. 185–216

15. Gore RM, Miller FH, Yaghmai V: Acquired immunodeficiency syndrome (AIDS) of the abdominal organs; imaging features. Semin US, CT, and MR 1998; 19:175–189

16. Gore RM, Levine MS: Textbook of Gastrointestinal Radiology. (ed 2) Philadelphia: WB Saunders, 2000

17. Gore RM: Gallbladder and biliary tract: Differential diagnosis. In: Gore RM, Levine MS: Textbook of Gastrointestinal Radiology. (ed 2) Philadelphia: WB Saunders, 2000, pp. 1408–1414

18. Gore RM: Spleen: Differential diagnosis. In: Gore RM, Levine MS: Textbook of Gastrointestinal Radiology. (ed 2) Philadelphia: WB Saunders, 2000, pp. 1925–1928

19. Gore RM: Pancreas: Differential diagnosis. In: Gore RM, Levine MS (eds): Textbook of Gastrointestinal Radiology, 2nd ed. Philadelphia: WB Saunders, 2000, pp. 1836–1843

20. Halpert RD, Feczko PJ: Gastrointestinal Radiology: The Requisites. (ed 2) St. Louis: Mosby-Year Book, 1999

21. Jeffrey RB, Jr: Gastrointestinal tract and peritoneal cavity. In: McGahan JP, Goldberg BB (eds): Diagnostic Ultrasound. Philadelphia: Lippincott-Raven, 1997

22. Jones B: Functional abnormalities of the pharynx. In Gore RM, Levine MS: Textbook of Gastrointestinal Radiology. (ed 2) Philadelphia: WB Saunders, 2000, pp. 316–328

23. Kelekis NL, Burdeny DA, Semelka RC: Spleen. In: Semelka RC, Ascher SM, Reinhold C (eds): MRI of

the Abdomen and Pelvis. New York: Wiley-Liss, 1997, pp. 239–256

24. Kirks DR, Merten DF, Grossman H, Bowie JD: Diagnostic imaging of pediatric abdominal masses: An overview. Radiol Clin North Am 1981;19: 527–545

25. Laing FC: The gallbladder and bile ducts. The liver. In: Rumack CM, Wilson SR, Charboneau JW (eds): Diagnostic Ultrasound. St. Louis: Mosby, 1998, pp. 175–223

26. Lefkowitch JH: Pathologic diagnosis of liver disease. In: Zakim D, Boyer TD: Hepatology. (ed 3) Philadelphia: WB Saunders, 1996, pp. 844–874

27. Levine MS: Esophagus: Differential diagnosis. In: Gore RM, Levine MS: Textbook of Gastrointestinal Radiology. (ed 2) Philadelphia: WB Saunders, 2000, pp. 509–513

28. Macari M, Balthazar EJ: CT of bowel wall thickening: Significance and pitfalls of interpretaion. Am J Roentgenol 200;176:1105–1116

29. Marshak RH, Lindner AE, Maklansky D: Radiology of the Colon. Philadelphia: WB Saunders, 1980

30. Mathieson JR, Cooperberg PL: The spleen. In: Rumack CM, Wilson SR, Charboneau JW (eds): Diagnostic Ultrasound. (ed 2) St. Louis: Mosby, 1998, pp. 155–174

31. Melicow MM, Uson AC: Palpable abdominal masses in infants and children: A report based on a review of 653 cases.

32. Mergo PJ, Ros PR: Benign lesions of the liver. Radiol Clin North Am 1998;36:319–322

33. Meyers MA: Dynamic Radiology of the Abdomen. (ed 5) New York: Springer-Verlag, 2000

34. Nemcek AA, Vogelzang RL: Angiography and interventional radiology of the alimentary tract. In: Gore RM, Levine MS (eds): Textbook of Gastrointestinal Radiology. (ed 2) Philadelphia: WB Saunders, 2000, pp. 509–511

35. Nicolas AI, Ros PR: Imaging of the mesentery and omentum. In: Grainger RG, Allison DJ: Grainger & Allison's Diagnostic Radiology. (ed 3) New York: Churchill Livingstone, 1997, pp. 1059–1079.

36. Ott DJ: Motility disorders of the esophagus. In: Gore RM, Levine MS: Textbook of Gastrointestinal Radi-

ology. (ed 2) Philadelphia: WB Saunders, 2000, pp. 316–328

37. Paley MR, Ros PR: Hepatic metastases. Radiol Clin North Am 1998;36:349–364

38. Parulekar SG: Gallbladder and bile ducts. In: McGahan JP, Goldberg BB (eds): Diagnostic Ultrasound. Philadelphia: Lippincott-Raven, 1997, chapter 22

39. Reeders JW, Joosten FB, Rosenbusch G: Radiology of the esophagus. Radiology 2000;40:479–493

40. Rice RP, Thompson WM, Gedgaudas RK: The diagnosis and significance of extraluminal gas in the abdomen. Radiol Clin North Am 1982;20:819–837

41. Riley SA, Marsh MN: Maldigestion and malabsorption. In: Feldman M, Scharschmidt BF, Sleisenger MH: Gastrointestinal and Liver Disease. (ed 6) Philadelphia: WB Saunders, 2000, pp. 1501–1522

42. Ros PR: Bubbles and marbles of the belly: Cystic and solid masses of the mesentery and omentum. In: Balfe DM, Levine MS: RSNA Categorical Course in Diagnostic Radiology: Gastrointestinal. 1997, pp. 59–66

43. Ros PR, Taylor HM: Benign and malignant tumors of the liver. In: Gore RM, Levine MS: Textbook of Gastrointestinal Radiology. (ed 2) Philadelphia: WB Saunders, 2000, pp. 1487–1568

44. Ros PR, Taylor HM, Barreda R, et al.: Focal hepatic infections. In: Gore RM, Levine MS: Textbook of Gastrointestinal Radiology. (ed 2) Philadelphia: WB Saunders, 2000, pp. 1569–1589

45. Rosenthal P: Biliary atresia and neonatal disorders of the bile ducts. In: Wyllie R, Hyams JS: Pediatric Gastrointestinal Disease. Philadelphia: WB Saunders, 1999, pp. 568–578

46. Rubesin SE: Pharynx. In: Levine MS, Rubesin SE, Laufer I: Double Contrast Gastrointestinal Radiology. (ed 3) Philadelphia: WB Saunders, 2000, pp. 61–91

47. Rummeny E, Weissleder R, Stark DD, et al.: Primary liver tumors: Diagnosis by MR imaging. Am J Roentgenol 1989;152:63–72

48. Sato M, Ishida H, Konno K, et al.: Liver tumors in children and young patients: Sonographic and color Doppler findings. Abdom Imaging 2000;25:596–601

49. Semelka RC, Kelekis NL: Liver. In: Semelka RC, Ascher SM, Reinhold C (eds): MRI of the Abdomen and

Pelvis: A Text-Atlas. New York: Wiley-Liss, 1997, pp. 19–136

50. Semelka RC (ed): Abdominal-Pelvi MRI. New York: Wiley-Liss, 2002

51. Shehadi WH: Radiologic examination of the biliary tract. Radiol Clin North Am 1966;4.

52. Siegel MJ: Pediatric Body CT. Philadelphia: Lippincott, Williams & Wilkins, 1999

53. Silverman PM, Cooper C: Mesenteric and omental lesions. In: Gore RM, Levine MS (eds): Textbook of Gastrointestinal Radiology. (ed 2) Philadelphia: WB Saunders, 2000, pp. 1980–1992

54. Skolnick ML: Guide to the Ultrasound Examination of the Abdomen. New York: Springer-Verlag, 1986

55. Stephens DH, Sheedy PF, Hattery RR, et al.: Computed tomography of the liver. Am J Roentgenol 1977;128:579–590

56. Taylor HM, Ros PR: Hepatic imaging: An overview. Radiol Clin North Am 1998;36:237–245

57. Urrutia M, Mergo PJ, Ros LH, Torres GM, Ros PR: Cystic masses of the spleen: radiologic-pathologic correlation. RadioGraphics 1996;16:107–129

58. Weill FS: Ultrasound Diagnosis of Digestive Diseases. (ed 3 revised) Berlin: Springer-Verlag, 1990, pp. 239–246

59. Williamson MR: Abdominal ultrasound. In: Essentials of Ultrasound. Philadelphia: WB Saunders, 1996, p. 86

60. Withers CW, Wilson SR: The liver. In: Rumack CM, Wilson SR, Charboneau JW (eds): Diagnostic Ultrasound. St. Louis: Mosby, 1998, pp. 87–154

SECTION H: GENITOURINARY TRACT, RETROPERITONEUM, AND GYNECOLOGICAL ULTRASOUND

1. Amis ES Jr, Hartman DS: Renal ultrasonography 1984: A practical overview. Radiol Clin North Am 1984;22:315–332

2. Bisset RAL, Khan AN: Differential Diagnosis in Abdominal Ultrasound. London: Bailliére Tindall, 1990

3. Bree RL, Silver TM: Sonography of bladder and perivesical abnormalities. Am J Roentgenol 1981;136:1101–1104

4. Cochlin DL: Urinary tract. In: McGahan JP, Goldberg BB (eds): Diagnostic Ultrasound. Philadelphia: Lippincott-Raven, 1997

5. Davidson AJ: A systematic approach to the radiologic diagnosis of renal parenchymal disease. In: Pollack HM (ed): Clinical Urography. Philadelphia: WB Saunders, 1990

6. Davidson AJ: Radiologic Diagnosis of Renal Parenchymal Disease. Philadelphia: WB Saunders, 1977

7. Davidson AJ, Hartman DS: Radiology of the Kidney and Urinary Tract. In: Angiography in Diseases of the Kidney. Philadelphia: WB Saunders, 1994

8. Dunnick NR, et al.: Textbook of Uroradiology. Baltimore: Williams & Wilkins, 1997

9. Elkin M: Renal cystic disease: An overview. Semin Roentgenol 1975;10:99–102

10. Elyaderani MK, Gabriele OF: Ultrasound of renal masses. Semin Ultrasound 1981;11:21–43

11. Felson B, Moskowitz M: Renal pseudotumors: The regenerated nodule and other lumps, bumps, and dromedary humps. Am J Roentgenol 1969;107:720–729

12. Felson B (ed): Renal cystic disease. Semin Roentgenol 1975;10:93

13. Fleischer AC, James AE: Introduction to Diagnostic Sonography. New York: John Wiley & Sons, 1980

14. Fleischer AC, Boehm FH, James AE Jr: Ultrasonography in Obstetrics and Gynaecology: Obstetric Radiology. In: Grainger RG, Allison DJ: Diagnostic Radiology. (ed 2) Edinburgh: Churchill Livingstone, 1992, pp. 1809–1819

15. Friedenberg RM, Dunbar JS: Excretory urography. In: Pollack HM (ed): Clinical Urography. Philadelphia: WB Saunders, 1990, pp. 101–255

16. Friedland GW, et al. (eds): Uroradiology: An Integrated Approach. London: Churchill Livingstone, 1983

17. Goldman SM, Gatewood OMB: Neoplasms of the renal collecting system, pelvis, and ureters. In: Pollack HM (ed): Clinical Urography. Philadelphia: WB Saunders, 1990

18. Hartman DS: Overview of renal cystic disease. In: Pollack HM, McClennan BL (eds): Clinical Urogra-

phy. (ed 2) Philadelphia: WB Saunders, 2000, pp. 1245–1250

19. Heiken JP: Tumors of the testis and testicular adnexa. World Health Organization Classification of Testicular Germ Cell Tumors. In: Pollack HM, McClennan BL (eds): Clinical Urography. (ed 2) Philadelphia: WB Saunders, 2000, pp. 1716–1741

20. Johnstrude IS, Jackson DC: A Practical Approach to Angiography. Boston: Little, Brown, 1979

21. Koop CE: Abdominal mass in the newborn infant. N Engl J Med 1973;289:569–571

22. Kuligowska E, Pomeroy OH: Prostate. In: McGahan JP, Goldberg BB (eds): Diagnostic Ultrasound. Philadelphia: Lippincott-Raven, 1997

23. Levine D: Female pelvis. In: McGahan JP, Goldberg BB (eds): Diagnostic Ultrasound. Philadelphia: Lippincott-Raven, 1997

24. Levine E, King BF Jr: Adult malignant renal parenchymal neoplasms. In: Pollack HM, McClennan BL (eds): Clinical Urography. (ed 2) Philadelphia: WB Saunders, 2000, pp. 1440–1559

25. Madewell JE, Hartman DS, Lichtenstein JE: Radiologic-pathologic correlations in cystic disease of the kidney. Radiol Clin North Am 1979;17:261–279

26. Malik RS: Calculus disease of the genitourinary tract. In: Witten DM, Myers GH Jr, Utz DC: Emmett's Clinical Urography. (ed 4) Philadelphia: WB Saunders, 1977, p. 1177

27. Margolin EG, Cohen LH: Genitourinary calcification: An overview. Semin Roentgenol 1982;17:95–100

28. Mellins HZ: Cystic dilatations of the upper urinary tract: A radiologist developmental model. Radiology 1985;153:291–301

29. Morillo G: The differential diagnosis of the unilateral small kidney. CRC Crit Rev Diagn Imaging 1979;11:261–296

30. Newhouse JH, Pfister RC: The nephrogram. Radiol Clin North Am 1979;17:213–225

31. Ney C, Friedenberg R: Radiographic Atlas of the Genitourinary System. Philadelphia: Lippincott, 1966

32. Paltiel HJ, Kirks DR: Pediatric urological neoplasms. In: Pollack HM, McClennan BL (eds): Clinical Urog-

raphy. (ed 2) Philadelphia: WB Saunders, 2000, pp. 1743–1765

33. Parker M: Diagnostic skills. In: Friedland GW, Filly R, Goris ML, et al.: Uroradiology: An Integrated Approach. New York: Churchill Livingstone, 1983, p. 1654

34. Pollack HM, McClennan BL (eds): Clinical Urography. (ed 2) Philadelphia: WB Saunders, 2000

35. Ralls PW, Halls J: Hydronephrosis, renal cystic disease, and renal parenchymal disease. Semin Ultrasound 1981;11:49–60

36. Scoutt LM, Burns P, Brown JL, et al.: Ultrasound evaluation of the urinary tract. In: Pollack HM, McClennan BL: Clinical Urography. (ed 2) Philadelphia: WB Saunders, 2000, pp. 459–469

37. Spirnak JP, Resnick MI, Banner MP: Calculous disease of the urinary tract: General considerations. In: Pollack HM (ed): Clinical Urography. Philadelphia: WB Saunders, 1990

38. Tank ES, Poznanski AK Holt JF: The radiologic discrimination of abdominal masses in infants. J Urol 1973;109:128–132

39. Thurston W, Wilson SR: The urinary tract. In: Rumack CM, Wilson SR, Charboneau JW (eds): Diagnostic Ultrasound. St. Louis: Mosby, 1998, pp. 382–384

40. Wedge JJ, Grosfeld JL, Smith JP: Abdominal masses in the newborn: 63 cases. J Urol 1971;106:770–775

41. Williamson B Jr, King BF Jr: Benign neoplasms of the renal parenchyma. In: Pollack HM, McClennan BL (eds): Clinical Urography. (ed 2) Philadelphia: WB Saunders, 2000, pp. 1414–1439

42. Williamson MR: Renal ultrasound. In: Essentials of Ultrasound. Philadelphia: WB Saunders, 1996

43. Witten DM, Myers GH Jr, Utz DC: Emmett's Clinical Urography. (ed 4) Philadelphia: WB Saunders, 1996

44. Zagoria RJ, Tung GA: Genitourinary Radiology: The Requisites. St. Louis: Mosby, 1997

SECTION I: MAMMOGRAPHY

1. Bassett LW: Mammographic analysis of calcifications. Radiol Clin North Am 1992;30:93–105

2. Bassett LW, Jackson VP, Jahan R, Fu YS, Gold RH: Diagnosis of Diseases of the Breast. Philadelphia: WB Saunders, 1997, pp. 461–500

3. Bassett LW, Jackson VP, Jahan R, Fu YS, Gold RH: The male breast. In: Diagnosis of Diseases of the Breast. Philadelphia: WB Saunders, 1997, pp. 501–518

4. Bland KI, Copeland EM: The unknown primary presenting with axillary adenopathy. In: The Breast: Comprehensive Management of Benign and Malignant Diseases, vol. 2 (ed 2) Philadelphia: WB Saunders, 1991, pp. 1447–1452

5. DeParedes ES: Atlas of Film Screen Mammography. (ed 2) Baltimore: Williams & Wilkins, 1992, p. 134

6. Dershaw DD (ed): Interventional Breast Procedures. Edinburgh: Churchill Livingstone, 1996

7. Feig SA: Breast masses: Mammographic and sonographic evaluation. Radiol Clin North Am 1992; 30:67–92

8. Friedrich M, Sickles EA: Radiologic Diagnosis of Breast Diseases. New York: Springer-Verlag, 2000

9. Hoeffken W, Lanyi M: Mammography. Transl. by Rigler LG, et al. Philadelphia: WB Saunders, 1977

10. Kopans DB: The male breast. In: Breast Imaging. (ed 2) Philadelphia: Lippincott-Raven, 1998

11. Kopans DB: Breast Imaging. (ed 2) Philadelphia: Lipincott-Raven, 1998

12. Lanyi M: Differential diagnosis of microcalcifications. In: Friedrich M, Sickles EA (eds): Radiological Diagnosis of Breast Diseases. New York: Springer, 2000

13. Powell DE, Stelling CB: The Diagnosis and Detection of Breast Disease. Stromal. Vascular, Hematolymphoid, and Metastatic Breast Lesions. St. Louis: Mosby-Year Book, 1994

14. Sickles EA: Breast calcification: Mammographic evaluation. Radiology 1986;160:289–293

15. Sickles EA: Periodic mammographic following of probably benign lesions: results in 3,184 consecutive cases. Radiology 1991;179:463–468

16. Sickles EA: Non-palpable, circumscribed non-calcified solid breast masses: likelihood of malignancy based on lesion size and age of patient. Radiology 1994;192:439–442

17. Smathers RL: Mammography Diagnosis and Intervention CD-ROM. Moraga, CA: Medical Interactive, 1995

18. Smathers RL: Mammography for Technicians CD-ROM. Moraga, CA: Medical Interactive, 2000

19. Stavros A: Breast Ultrasound. Philadelphia: Lippincott, Williams & Wilkins, 2002

20. Tabar L, Dean PB: Teaching Atlas of Mammography, (ed 3) New York: Thieme, 2001, pp. 18–91

21. Tavassoli FA: Pathology of the Breast. (ed 2) New York: McGraw-Hill, 1999

SECTION J: TROPICAL IMAGING AND MISCELLANEOUS

1. Doppman JL: Overview: Multiple endocrine syndromes—A nightmare for the endocrinologist radiologist. Semin Roentgenol 1985;20:7–16

2. Palmer PES, Reeder MM: The Imaging of Tropical Diseases, with Epidemiological, Pathological, and Clinical Correlation. (ed 2) Heidelberg: Springer-Verlag, 2001, pp. XIX–XXIV

3. Pear BL: Radiographic studies of amyloidosis. CRC Crit Rev Radiol Sci 1972;3:425–452

SECTION M: MRI

1. Boyko OB: Adult brain tumors. In: Stark DD, Bradley WG (eds): Magnetic Resonance Imaging. (ed 3) St. Louis: Mosby, 1999, pp. 1231–1254

2. Bradley WG: Hemorrhage. In: Stark DD, Bradley WG (eds): Magnetic Resonance Imaging. (ed 3) St. Louis: Mosby, 1999, pp. 1329–1346

3. Ferris EJ, Levine HL: Cerebral arteritis: Classification. Radiology 1973;109:327–341

4. Grainger RG, Allison DJ (eds): Diagnostic Radiology. An Anglo-American Textbook of Imaging, vol. 3 (ed 2) Edinburgh: Churchill Livingstone, 1992, pp. 1993–1994

5. Mortele KJ, Ros PR: Cystic focal liver lesion in th adult: Differential CT and MR imaging features. RadioGraphics 2001;21:895–910

6. Pomeranz SJ: Gamuts and Pearls in MRI. Cincinnati: MRI Education Foundation, Inc., 1990

7. Semelka RC (ed): MR imaging of the liver II. Diseases. Magnet Reson Imaging Clin North Am 10:1

8. Semelka RC (ed): Abdominal-Pelvic MRI. New York: Wiley-Liss, 2002

9. Siegelman ES, Outwater EK: Tissue characterization in the female pelvis by means of MR imaging. Radiology 1999;212:5–18

10. Stark DD, Bradley WG (eds): Magnetic Resonance Imaging. (ed 3) St. Louis: Mosby, 1999

11. Stevens JM: The Spine and spinal cord. In: Sutton D, Young JWR (eds): A Short Textbook of Clinical Imaging. London: Springer-Verlag, 1990, pp. 791–802

12. Zimmerman RA, Bilaniuk LT: Pediatric cerebral anomalies. In: Stark DD, Bradley WG (eds): Magnetic Resonance Imaging. (ed 3) St. Louis: Mosby, 1999, pp. 1403–1424

SECTION O: OBSTETRICAL ULTRASOUND

1. Carlson DE: Growth disturbances. Large-for-date and small-for-date fetuses. In: McGahan JP, Goldberg BB (eds): Diagnostic Ultrasound. Philadelphia: Lippincott-Raven, 1997

2. Fleischer AC, James AE Jr: Diagnostic Sonography. Principles and Clinical Applications. Philadelphia: WB Saunders, 1989

3. Fleischer AC, Boehm FH, James AE Jr: Ultrasonography in obstetrics and gynaecology: Obstetric radiology. In: Grainger RG, Allison DJ: Diagnostic Radiology. (ed 2) Edinburgh: Churchill Livingstone, 1992, pp. 1809–1819

4. Goldstein RB: Fetal thorax. In: McGahan JP, Goldberg BB (eds): Obstetrical Ultrasound. Philadelphia: Lippincott-Raven, 1997

5. McGahan JP, Thurmond AS: Fetal head and brain. In: McGahan JP, Goldberg BB (eds): Diagnostic Obstetrical Ultrasound. Philadelphia: Lippincott-Raven, 1997

6. Nyberg DA, et al.: Cerebral malformations. In: Nyberg DA, Mahoney BS, Pretorius DH (eds): Diagnostic Ultrasound of Fetal Anomalies. Text and Atlas. Chicago: Year Book, 1993

7. Porto M, McGahan JP: The fetal abdomen and pelvis. In: McGahan JP, Porto M (eds): Diagnostic Obstetrical Ultrasound. Philadelphia: Lippincott, 1994

8. Williamson MR: Obstetrical ultrasound. In: Essentials of Ultrasound. Philadelphia: WB Saunders, 1996, p. 180

GENERAL ULTRASOUND

1. Abbitt PL: Ultrasound: A Pattern Approach. New York: McGraw-Hill, 1995

2. McGahan JP, Goldberg BB (eds): Diagnostic Ultrasound. Philadelphia: Lippincott-Raven, 1997

3. Rumack CM, Nilson SR, Charboneau JW (eds): Diagnostic Ultrasound. (ed 2) St. Louis: Mosby, 1998

4. Siegel MJ: Pediatric Sonography. (ed 3) Philadelphia: Lippincott, Williams & Wilkins, 2002

5. Skolnick ML: Guide to the Ultrasound Examination of the Abdomen. New York: Springer-Verlag, 1986

6. Stavros A: Breast Ultrasound. Philadelphia: Lippincott, Williams & Wilkins, 2002

7. Weill FS: Ultrasound Diagnosis of Digestive Diseases. (ed 3 revised) Berlin: Springer-Verlag, 1990, pp. 239–246

8. Williamson MR: Abdominal ultrasound. In: Essentials of Ultrasound. Philadelphia: WB Saunders, 1996, p. 86

Index

Gamut numbers are in boldface, followed by page numbers in regular type.

in size of bone or limb (hemihypertrophy or hemiatrophy), localized or generalized, **D-13,** 254–255

in size of hand bones, **D-147-1 to D-147-3,** 358–359

Atelectasis

lobar or segmental, **F-5,** 500–501

small pleural effusion with subsegmental, **F-115,** 584

Atlanto-axial subluxation or instability, **C-7-1,** 194

congenital syndromes with, **C-7-2,** 194–195

Atrial level

right to left shunt at, **E-10,** 456

shunts, complicated, **E-10-S,** 456

Atrophy

bone, **D-42,** 277–278

spinal cord, **C-60,** 222

Sudeck's, **D-42,** 277–278

Auditory canal

tumor, external, **B-35,** 123–124

Auditory meatus, internal, erosion or widening of, **A-29,** 28–29

Avascular lesions, of liver on angiography, contrast-enhanced CT, or MRI, **G-171,** 703

Avascular necrosis, **D-48,** 284–285

sites of predilection and eponyms for, **D-48-S,** 285

Avascular renal mass, **H-61,** 786

Avascular zone near brain surface on cerebral angiography, **A-106,** 86–87

Avulsion injuries, sites of, **D-109-S,** 330

Azygoesophageal recess, abnormality of, especially on CT, **F-98,** 573

Azygos vein dilatation, **E-69,** 489

Baker's (popliteal) cyst, **D-237,** 416–417

Ballooned bones, **D-12,** 253

Barium

double tracking of, in distal colon, **G-90,** 661

residual intestinal, after gastrointestinal study, **G-75,** 652

retention of, in hypopharynx, **G-1,** 611

study, rectal disease on, **G-100,** 666–667

Basal ganglia

calcification, **A-49,** 40

disease, **M-21, M-44,** 880–881, 887

Basilar cisterns

increased density within, on nonenhanced CT scan, **A-90-1,** 76

intense enhancement of, on CT, **A-90-2,** 76

Basilar invagination, **A-12,** 16–17

with thickening of skull vault, **A-13,** 17

Battered child, clues to, **D-95-S,** 321

Beaked vertebrae in child, **C-21,** 202–203

Biconcave ("fish") vertebrae, **C-19,** 201–202

Bilary ducts, dilatation of, **G-130,** 681

Bile ducts

cystic and saccular lesions of, **G-133-1, G-133-2,** 682–683

filling defect or segmental lesion in, on cholangiography, **G-134,** 683

narrowing or obstruction, distal, **G-137,** 684–685

Biliary-enteric fistula, **G-139,** 686

Biliary tract, **G-129 to G-140,** 680–686

abnormal, congenital syndromes with, **G-129,** 680–681

diseases common to tropics and developing countries, **J-1-S,** 851–855

Biliary tree, gas in, **G-128,** 680

Biparietal bossing, **A-9,** 15

Bladder, **H-96 to H-110,** 801–807

calcification in wall or lumen, **H-105,** 805–806

diseases common to tropics and developing countries, **J-1-S,** 851–855

distended, **H-96,** 801

diverticula, **H-109,** 807

extrinsic pressure deformity of, **H-99,** 802–803

filling defect in wall or lumen, **H-104,** 804–805

fistula, **H-108,** 806–807

gas in, **H-107,** 806

neurogenic, **H-98,** 802

outlet obstruction, **H-110,** 807

pear-shaped, **H-99,** 802–803

small or contracted, **H-97,** 801

teardrop, **H-99,** 802–803

tumors, **H-103,** 804

urinary tract obstruction below, in child, **H-111,** 808

wall

filling defect(s) in, **H-105,** 805–806

thickening, **H-100 to H-101,** 803–804

Blind loop syndrome, **G-58,** 642–643

Blister lesion of bone, **D-68,** 301

Block vertebrae, **C-11, C-25,** 197–198, 204

Blood vessels, gas embolism in, **E-46,** 477

Blow-out lesion of bone, **D-69-1,** 302

Bone

age

decreased, **D-17-1,** 256–257

increased, **D-16,** 256

asymmetry in size of

in hand, **D-147-1 to D-147-3,** 358–359

localized or generalized, **D-13,** 254–255

ballooned, **D-12,** 253

benign tumor-like lesions of, **D-80,** 310

blister (solitary cyst-like lesion expanding bone eccentrically), **D-68,** 301

blow-out lesion of, **D-69-1,** 302

bowed, single or multiple, **D-8,** 250–251

changes

neurotrophic, **D-150,** 360–361

sinonasal mass without, **M-122,** 910

classification of sclerosing dysplasias of, **D-2-S,** 245

combined lung and, disorder, **F-67,** 543–544

cortical disorders, **D-89-S to D-106,** 317–326

cyst, precursor lesions of aneurysmal, **D-80-S3,** 311

osteolytic lesion of, solitary, **D-70,** 303

cystic lesions, **D-57-1 to D-76,** 292–306

defect in skull, solitary or multiple, **A-23-2,** 24–25

demineralization, **D-41 to D-47,** 276–284

density

or matrix, osteolytic lesion of bone containing, **D-72,** 303–304

scattered areas of decreased and increased, in skeleton, **D-47,** 283–284

destruction

common bone lesions and their typical patterns, **D-62-S,** 298

diagram of patterns of, **D-61-S,** 297

or erosion of external conical surface of, **D-105,** 325–326

Calcification (*continued*)

in kidney, focal or annular, **H-23,** 767

in liver, **G-142,** 688

lower quadrant, **H-138,** 819

in lymph nodes, **D-249,** 424

in muscles and subcutaneous tissues, **D-245-1, D-245-2,** 420–422

of one or more intervertebral disks, **C-55,** 219–220

pancreatic, **G-218, G-219,** 724–725

pelvic, **H-138,** 819

periarticular or intra-articular, **D-243,** 419–420

pericardial, **E-45,** 476

pleural, **F-124,** 598

in scrotum, **H-164,** 827

sellar or parasellar, **A-48,** 39–40

soft tissue nodules without obvious, diseases common to tropics and developing countries, **J-1-S,** 851–855

soft tissue tumor with associated, **D-250,** 424–425

in soft tissues, diseases common to tropics and developing countries, complications of, **J-1-S,** 851–855

splenic (see Splenic, calcification), **G-203, G-204,** 718–719

thoracic (see Thoracic, calcification), **F-140, F-141,** 598–599

ureteral, **H-85,** 796

in vas deferens, seminal vesicle, or fallopian tube, **H-149,** 823

vascular, **D-247,** 423

Calcified

loose body in joint, **D-241,** 418

pulmonary metastases, **F-142,** 600

Calcium

concentrations, causes of altered, **D-45-S,** 282–283

osteolytic lesion of bone containing, **D-72,** 303–304

Calcium stones of urinary tract, classification of, **H-25-S,** 768

Calculi, urinary tract (see Urinary tract, calculi) **H-106,** 806

Callus formation, excess, **D-96,** 321

Calvarium (see also Skull)

abnormal contour of, **A-4,** 13

diffuse or widespread increased density, sclerosis, or thickening of, **A-15-1,** 18–19

localized bulge of, **A-10,** 16

localized increased density, sclerosis, or thickening, **A-14,** 17–18

Camptodactyly, **D-136,** 349–350

Carcinoid tumors, **G-84-S,** 657

Carcinomas, rate of frequency of metastases to bone from various primary, **D-87-S1,** 316

Cardiac (see also Heart)

abnormalities, **E-27 to E-50-S,** 465–479

conditions, common, diagnosed by echocardiography, **E-50-S,** 479

displacement, **E-26,** 464–465

failure, in neonate, infant, or child, **E-4 to E-6,** 451–453

neoplasm or cyst, **E-43,** 475

pleural effusion with enlarged heart, **F-116,** 585

position, abnormal, **E-26,** 464–465

Cardiomegaly, **E-6,** 452–453

Cardiophrenic angle lesion, right anterior, **F-97,** 572–573

Cardiospasm, of esophagus, **G-3,** 612–613

Cardiovascular

anomalies, associated with complete atrioventricular canal, **E-12-S2,** 458

anomalies, associated with VSD, **E-12-S1,** 457–458

disease, hypertensive, **E-37,** 471

gamuts, **E-1 to E-73-S,** 447–491

Carpal, **D-156 to D-160-S,** 364–368

angle, congenital syndromes associated with abnormal, **D-159-1, D-159-2,** 367

anomalies seen in common congenital syndromes, **D-160-S,** 368

bones, fragmented, irregular, or, sclerotic, **D-157-1,** 364–365

fusion, **D-158,** 366

ossicles, congenital syndromes with accessory, **D-156,** 364

small, congenital syndromes with, **D-157-2,** 365

Cartilage, calcification in articular, **D-242,** 418–419

Catheterization, complications of central venous, **E-73-S,** 491

(subclavian, jugular) or pulmonary artery, **E-73-S,** 491

Cavitary lesions

multiple, of lung, **F-49,** 534

sharply defined, of lung, **F-43-1, F-43-2,** 529–531

Cavitation, extensive pulmonary infiltrate with, **F-50,** 534–353

Cecal lesion, **G-96,** 664

Cecum, conical or contracted, **G-97,** 665

Central nervous system

complications of HIV infection and AIDS, **A-119,** 94

Central vein groove (prominent anterior canal) of, vertebral body, **C-14,** 199

Cerebellopontine angle

cistern, **M-72, M-73,** 896

mass, **A-81,** 71

Cerebellum, multiple enhancing lesions in, on CT, **A-60,** 54

Cerebral angiography

avascular zone near brain surface on, **A-106,** 86–87

intracranial arteriovenous shunting and early venous filling on, **A-104,** 86

Cerebral arterial disease on angiography, **A-102, A-103,** 85

Cerebral emboli, causes of, **M-13-S,** 878

Cerebral infarction (stroke) on CT, MRI, or angiography, **A-98,** 81–82

Cerebral vessels, pattern analysis of, on angiography, **A-101,** 84

Cerebrospinal fluid

overproduction of, **A-114-2,** 91–92

rhinorrhea, **A-118,** 94

Cerebrum, multiple enhancing lesions in, on CT, **A-60,** 54

Cervical

esophagus, extrinsic impression on, **G-5,** 613

metastatic lymphadenopathy on CT or MRI, **B-101-S,** 169

Cervical spine, **C-6-S1 to C-10,** 192–197

fusion of, **C-10,** 197

injuries

mechanism of injury, **C-6-S1,** 192–193

stability and, **C-6-S2,** 193

Charcot joint, **D-223,** 410

Chemicals that can induce lung disease, **F-73-S,** 553–554

Chest

eggshell calcifications in, **F-143,** 600

gamuts, **F-1 to F-143,** 499–600

pleural effusion with radiographic evidence of other disease in, **F-114,** 583–584

wall

conditions, **F-126 to F-132,** 590–594

diseases common to tropics and developing countries, **J-1-S,** 851–855

lesion, **F-126,** 590–591

Cholangiography, filling defect or segmental lesion in bile ducts on, **G-134,** 683

Chondrocalcinosis, **D-242,** 418–419

Chondrosarcoma, types of, **D-81-S3,** 313
Chylothorax, **F-120,** 587
Chylous ascites, **G-235,** 732–733
Clavicle, **D-171 to D-175,** 374–378
    aplastic, hypoplastic, or thin, **D-172-1,** 375
    broad, thickened, or enlarged, **D-174-1,** 376–377
    erosion, destruction, penciling, or defect of outer end of, **D-175,** 377–378
    handlebar, **D-172-2,** 375–376
    lesion of, in infant or child, **D-171,** 374–375
    sclerosis and periosteal reaction involving, **D-174-2,** 377
Claw-hand, **D-145,** 358
Cleft vertebrae, **C-13,** 198
Clinodactyly, of fifth finger, **D-123,** 340–341
Clivus, mass in, **A-70,** 63–64
Clubbing
    or destruction of renal calyces, **H-19,** 765
    of fingers or toes, **D-133,** 348
Clubfoot, congenital conditions associated with, **D-154,** 363–364
Codman triangle, **D-90,** 318
Colitis, **G-88,** 659–660
Collapsed vertebra, solitary, **C-17,** 200
Collapsed vertebrae, multiple, **C-18,** 201
Colon, **G-83 to G-95-1,** 656–663
    annular lesion of, **G-85,** 657–658
    aphthoid ulcers in, **G-67,** 646–647
    diseases common to tropics and developing countries, **J-1-S,** 851–855
    distal, double tracking of barium in, **G-90,** 661
    innumerable tiny nodules in, **G-68,** 647
    multiple filling defects in, **G-87,** 658–659
    segmental narrowing of, **G-86,** 658
    smooth, **G-91,** 661
    solitary filling defect in, **G-83,** 656–657
    "thumbprinting" of, **G-103,** 668
Colonic
    distention without obstruction, **G-92,** 661–662
    tumors, classification of, **G-84-S,** 657
Common bile duct, calcification in, **G-114,** 673
Computed tomography (see CT)
Cone-shaped epiphyses, **D-27,** 266–267
Congenital abnormalities
    of great toe, **D-122-1,** 339
    of temporal bone, **B-24,** 117–118
    of thumb, **D-117-1 to D-117-6,** 334–336
Congenital anomalies
    associated with Wilms' tumor, **H-41,** 777
    and variations of appendix, **G-82-S,** 656
    vascular, **B-24,** 117–118
Congenital conditions
    associated with clubfoot or other foot deformity, **D-154,** 363–364
    with increased density or thickening of skull, **A-15-2,** 19–20
Congenital defects
    posterior neural arches, **C-45-1,** 213
Congenital diseases, of heart and great vessels, **E-1 to E-26-S,** 447–465
Congenital heart disease
    acyanotic
        with increased pulmonary vascularity, **E-16,** 460
        with normal pulmonary vascularity, **E-15,** 459

    associated with anterior right aortic arch, **E-21-S,** 462
    congenital syndromes with, **E-1,** 447
    cyanotic, with increased pulmonary vascularly, **E-17,** 460
    with decreased pulmonary arterial vascularly, **E-19,** 461
    differential features of major cyanotic, **E-8-S,** 455
    flat or concave pulmonary artery segment in, **E-20,** 461
    key findings in neonatal, **E-3,** 450
    left to right shunt in, **E-7,** 453
    onset of cyanosis in, **E-9,** 455–456
    pulmonary arterial vascularly in common, **E-14,** 458–459
    relative incidence of various types of, **E-2-S,** 449
    right to left shunt or admixture lesion in, **E-8,** 454
Congenital sternal abnormality, **D-209-1,** 401
Congenital syndromes
    with abdominal calcifications, **G-241,** 735–736
    with abnormal acetabular angle, **D-194-2,** 392
    with abnormal biliary tract, **G-129,** 680–681
    with abnormal pelvis, **D-192,** 389–390
    with abnormal scapula, **D-169,** 373–374
    with absent, hypoplastic, dysplastic, bipartite, or dislocated patella, **D-180,** 380
    with accessory carpal or tarsal ossicles, **D-156,** 364
    associated with abnormal carpal angle, **D-159-1, D-159-2,** 367
    associated with hydrocephalus, **A-114-2,** 91–92
    associated with intestinal malrotation, **G-66,** 646
    with atlanto-axial subluxation or instability, **C-7-2,** 194–195
    carpal anomalies seen in common, **D-160-S,** 368
    with congenital heart disease, **E-1,** 447–449
    with coxa vara, **D-187-2,** 384–385
    with delayed closure of fontanelles, **A-39,** 33–34
    with delayed or defective dentition, **B-62,** 142–144
    with delayed or defective pubic ossification, **D-195,** 392–393
    with elbow anomaly, **D-165,** 371–273
    with eleven pairs of ribs, **D-198-1,** 394
    with flat or decreased acetabular angle, **D-194-1, D-194-2,** 391, 392
    with generalized brachydactyly, **D-142,** 354–355
    with generalized or widespread osteosclerosis, **D-55-2,** 290–291
    with hypertelorism, **B-3-2,** 102–103
    with hypospadias or other ambiguous external genitalia, **H-166,** 828
    with irregularity, fragmentation, or stippling of multiple epiphyses, **D-19-2,** 259–260
    with joint dislocation or subluxation, **D-213,** 404–405
    with joint laxity or hypermobility, **D-212,** 403–404
    with kidney malformation or anomaly, **H-1,** 755
    with limited joint mobility, **D-211,** 402–403
    with macrocephaly, **A-3-2,** 12–13
    with maxillary or malar (zygomatic) hypoplasia, **B-60,** 140
    with multiple missing teeth, **B-64,** 144–145
    with myocardiopathy, **E-40-2,** 373
    with one or more short middle phalanges, **D-124,** 341
    with pectus carinatum, **F-129,** 592–593
    with pectus excavatum, **F-130,** 593
    with premature craniosynostosis, **A-1-2,** 10
    with prognathism, **B-57-1,** 137
    with renal insufficiency or nephropathy, **H-2,** 755–756
    with retarded skeletal maturation, **D-17-2,** 257–258
    with short hands and feet, **D-142,** 354–355
    with short limbs, **D-6,** 248–249
    with short, narrow thoracic cage, **F-131,** 593–594
    with short metacarpals or metatarsals, **D-143-1 to D-143-3,** 355–357

Congenital syndromes (*continued*)
  with short middle phalanx of fifth finger, **D-123,** 340–341
  with small carpals, **D-157-2,** 365
  with splaying, flaring, or widening of metaphyses, **D-34-2,** 271–272
  with splenomegaly, **G-198,** 716–717
  with thirteen pairs of ribs, **D-198-2,** 394
  with vertebral abnormality, **C-1,** 187–189
Conical cecum, **G-97,** 665
Consolidation (alveolar, air space) patterns, **F-1-S to F-16,** 499–509
  diffuse pulmonary disease with mixed, **F-16,** 508–509
  disseminated, acute or chronic, **F-8, F-9,** 502–503
  localized segmental or lobar, **F-2,** 499–500
  in patient with leukemia or lymphoma, **F-14,** 507
Constitutional diseases of bone, international, **D-1-S,** 239–244
  nomenclature of, **D-1-S,** 239–244
Constriction, localized, of esophagus, **G-12,** 617–618
Constrictive pericarditis, **E-48,** 478
Contour abnormality
  of calvarium, **A-4,** 13
  of occiput in an infant
    flat, **A-6,** 14
    prominent, **A-7,** 14
Contour irregularity of vessel walls, **A-101,** 84
Contracted
  bladder, **H-97,** 801
  cecum, **G-97,** 665
  hands, **D-145,** 358
Contracture, of digits, **D-135,** 349
Contrast-enhanced CT
  avascular lesions of liver on, **G-171,** 703
  vascular lesions of liver on, **G-171, G-172,** 703, 704
Contrast enhancement patterns, of intracranial masses, on CT,
    A-58-1 to A-58-4, 51–52
Convolutional markings
  decreased or absent, **A-42,** 36
  increased, **A-43,** 36
Cor pulmonale, **E-54,** 481–482
Coronal cleft vertebrae, **C-13,** 198
Coronary artery, aneurysm of, **E-65,** 487–488
Cortex of bone, "split" or double layer, **D-103,** 325
Cortical disease
  mass effect, **M-43,** 887
    enhancing, **M-20,** 880
    nonenhancing, **M-19,** 880
  no mass effect
    enhancing, **M-18, M-42,** 879–880, 887
    nonenhancing, **M-17, M-41,** 879, 887
Cortical disorders, bone, **D-89-S to D-106,** 317–326
Cortical hyperostosis involving shaft of bone, **D-99,** 323
Cortical margin, scalloping, erosion, or resorption of inner, **D-104,**
    325
Cortical surface of bone, destruction or erosion of external, **D-105,**
    325–326
Cortical thickening
  localized (one or few bones), **D-100,** 323
  widespread, **D-101,** 324
Cortical thinning
  widespread, **D-102,** 324
Coxa valga, **D-188,** 385
Coxa vara, **D-187-1,** 384

congenital syndromes with, **D-187-2,** 384–385
Cranial nerve, enhancement, **M-27,** 883
Cranial ossification, delayed or defective, **A-37,** 32–33
Craniostenosis, **A-1-1,** 9
Craniosynostosis, premature, **A-1-1,** 9
  classification of primary (idiopathic), **A-1-S,** 9
  congenital syndromes with, **A-1-2,** 10
Craniovertebral junction abnormality, **C-9-1, C-9-2,** 196
Cranium (see also Skull), **A-1-1 to A-45-2,** 9–37
  unilateral small, **A-5,** 14
Cricopharyngeal achalasia, **G-1,** 611
CSF intensity lesion
  brain stem, **M-36,** 885
  mass effect
    enhancing, **M-35,** 885
    nonenhancing, **M-34,** 885
  no mass effect, **M-33,** 885
  posterior fossa, **M-38,** 886
  sellar/suprasellar region, **M-37,** 886
CT
  abdominal, abscess mimics on, **G-244-S,** 737
  abnormality of azygoesophageal recess especially on, **F-98,** 573
  attenuation (density) of various intracranial lesions (relative to
      normal brain), **A-57-1 to A-57-3,** 49–51
  bone disorder associated with otosclerosis on tomography or, **B-25,**
      118
  cerebral infarction (stroke) on MRI or angiography, **A-98,** 81–82
  characteristics of orbital masses in children, **B-7-S,** 107
  contrast enhancement patterns of intracranial mass on, **A-58-1 to**
      A-58-4, 51–52
  cystic mesenteric lesion identified on, **G-228,** 728
  cystic or necrotic mass in posterior fossa as seen on MRI or
      ultrasound or, **A-83,** 72–73
  cystic retroperitoneal mass, **H-131,** 816
  deformity and dimensional changes in eyeballs on MRI or, **B-18,**
      113–114
  distinct optic nerve with perineural enhancement on, **B-15,** 111
  enhancing ventricular margins on, **A-89,** 75–76
  enlargement of rectus muscles of eyes on MRI or, **B-16,** 111–112
  extradural lesion on myelography or MRI or, **C-63,** 223–224
  extraglobal calcification on, **B-21,** 115–116
  fat density in abdomen on, **G-258,** 744
  fatty liver on, **G-144,** 689–690
  features useful in, identification of various types of neoplasm,
      A-59-S, 53
  focal hyperdense liver lesions on, **G-182, G-183,** 708–709
  focal hypodense liver lesions on, **G-180, G-181,** 707–708
  gas within bone on, **D-116,** 334
  globe calcification on, **B-20,** 114–115
  high density renal cyst on, **H-34,** 773
  high-resolution (HRCT) patterns, **F-26 to F-34-3,** 515–523
    chronic air space consolidation on, **F-28,** 518
    chronic interstitial lung disease, **F-26,** 515–516
    ground-glass opacities on, **F-27,** 516–517
    increased lung lucency (usually cystic pattern) on, **F-30,** 519
    lower lung disease on, **F-32,** 520
    peribronchovascular interstitial thickening on, **F-29,** 518–519
    small nodule distribution on, **F-34-1 to F-34-3,** 522–523
    small nodule opacities on, **F-33,** 521–522
    upper lung disease on, **F-31,** 520

Diametaphysis (*continued*)
    wide, localized or generalized, **D-11,** 252–253
Diaphragm, **F-133 to F-139,** 594–598
    bilateral elevated, **F-134,** 595
    flat or depressed, unilateral or bilateral, **F-133,** 594–595
    unilateral elevated, **F-135,** 595–596
Diaphragmatic moguls (bumps) or masses, **F-138,** 597
Diaphyseal lesion, solitary lytic, **D-60,** 296
Diaphysis, wide, **D-12,** 253
Digits (see also Fingers, Toes, and Thumbs)
    acquired acro-osteolysis confined to single, **D-127-2,** 344
    amputation or absence of, **D-129-1, D-129-2,** 345–346
    broad distal phalanx of thumb, **D-121-2,** 338
    broad phalanges of, **D-121-3 to D-121-4,** 339
    contracture of, **D-135,** 349
    "drumstick" distal phalanges, **D-121-1,** 338
    flexion deformity of one or more, **D-136,** 349–350
    fusion of phalanges in, **D-134,** 348
    localized accelerated maturation, elongation, or overgrowth of,
        D-14, 255
    self-mutilation of, **D-129-3,** 346
    short distal phalanx of the thumb, **D-119-1, D-119-2,** 337–338
    short proximal phalanx of the thumb and/or other digits, acquired or
        congenital, **D-120,** 338
    soft tissue or bony union between adjacent, **D-137,** 350–351
Dilatation, of stomach without obstruction, **G-31,** 628
Diseases
    common to tropics and developing countries, listing of, based on
        body system and organ involved, **J-1-S,** 851–855
    geographic distribution of tropical infectious and parasitic, **J-2-S,**
        856–857
Disk spaces
    narrow, **C-52,** 218–219
    wide, **C-53,** 219
Disks, intervertebral, **C-52 to C-56,** 218–220
    calcification of one or more, **C-55,** 219–220
    gas in, **C-56,** 220
Disks, vacuum, **C-56,** 220
Dissecting aneurysm of ascending aorta or arch, **E-64,** 487
Distended bladder, **H-96,** 801
Diverticulum
    of esophagus, **G-10-1 to G-10-4,** 616–617
    small bowel, **G-51-1,** 638
Double-barrel esophagus, **G-9,** 615
Double bubble sign, **G-43,** 634
Double-layer cortex, **D-103,** 325
Double tracking of barium in distal colon, **G-90,** 661
Drop metastases to spinal subarachnoid space,
    sources of, **M-101-S,** 903
Drugs that can induce lung disease, **F-73-S,** 553–555
"Drumstick" distal phalanges, **D-121-1,** 338
Dumbbell bones, **D-35,** 272–273
Duodenal
    dilatation, without obstruction, **G-45,** 635
    disease, combined gastric antral and, **G-29,** 627
    loop, widening of, **G-36,** 630–631
    mass, solitary intrinsic, **G-37,** 631
    narrowing or obstruction, **G-42,** 634
    obstruction, in infant, **G-43,** 634
    ulceration, postbulbar, **G-41,** 633

Duodenum, **G-35 to G-45,** 630–635
    band like constriction of transverse, **G-44,** 635
    diminished or absent fold pattern in, **G-39,** 632
    diseases common to tropics and developing countries, **J-1-S,** 851–855
    extrinsic indentation on, **G-35,** 630
    multiple or diffuse filling defects in, **G-38,** 631–632
    nodular or thickened folds in, **G-40,** 632–633
Dural sinus thrombosis, causes of, **M-4-S3,** 873
Dusts, inorganic, that cause pneumoconiosis, **F-70-S,** 545–546
Dwarfism
    late-onset, **D-4,** 246–247
    lethal forms of, **D-3,** 246
    major syndromes of short limb (rhizomelic, mesomelic, acromelic),
        D-5-1 to D-5-3, 247–248
Dysmyelinating diseases, **A-95-1,** 79
Dysphagia, roentgen counterpart of, **G-1,** 611
Dysplasias, sclerosing bone, classification of, **D-2, D-2-S,** 244–245
Dysplastic pedicle, **C-41,** 212
Dysplastic sella, **A-25-4,** 26

Ear, **B-30, B-31, B-32, B-36,** 120–122, 124
Ear cartilage (pinna), calcification in, **B-36,** 124
Echo-free renal mass on sonography, **H-64,** 787
Echocardiography, common cardiac conditions diagnosed by, **E-50-S,** 479
Echogenicity
    generalized or multifocal decreased or increased, of liver on
        ultrasound, **G-147, G-148,** 691–692
    of pancreatic masses on ultrasound, **G-213 to G-217,** 722–724
    splenomegaly with decreased, on ultrasound, **G-200,** 717
    splenomegaly with increased, on ultrasound, **G-201,** 717–718
Edema, pulmonary (see Pulmonary edema), **F-10-1, F-10-2,** 504–505
Eggshell calcifications in chest, **F-143,** 600
Elbow
    anomaly, congenital syndromes with, **D-165,** 371–372
    fat pad, displaced, **D-167,** 372
Elongated sella, **A-25-2,** 26
Elongation
    of fibula, **D-178,** 379
    generalized or widespread, of skeleton, **D-15,** 255
    localized accelerated, of bone, digit, or limb, **D-14,** 255
Emboli, **E-67,** 488
    cerebral, causes of, **M-13-S,** 878
Emphysema
    infantile lobar, **F-54,** 537
    interstitial, of stomach, **G-32,** 628–629
    soft tissue, **D-269,** 439
Empyema, subdural, on CT or MRI, **A-99,** 82–83
Endometrial fluid collection with positive beta HCG, **O-35,** 945
Enlarged
    brain stem, **A-85,** 73
    clavicle, **D-174-1,** 376–377
    heart, grossly, **E-41,** 474
    intervertebral foramen, **C-44,** 213
    liver, **G-141-1, G-141-2,** 686–688
    medial femoral condyle, **D-184,** 382
    papilla of Vater, **G-138,** 685–686
    pedicle, **C-40-2,** 211
    sella turcica, **A-26,** 26–27

unilateral elevated, **F-135,** 595–596
Hemihypertrophy or hemiatrophy (asymmetry in size of bone or limb), localized or generalized, **D-13,** 254–255
Hemithorax, opacification of one, **F-122,** 588
Hemorrhage
  intracerebral, on CT, MRI, or angiography, **A-99,** 82–83
  parenchymal, on MRI, **M-4-S1,** 872
  perinephric, **H-55-3,** 782–783
  pulmonary, **F-12,** 506
  stages of, on MRI, **M-4-S2,** 872
Hepatic (see also Liver)
  vein thromboembolism or obstruction on angiography, **G-189,** 711
Hernias, nondiaphragmatic, **G-64-S,** 645–646
High
  density renal cyst on CT, **H-34,** 773
  output heart disease, **E-39,** 472
Hilar
  displacement, unilateral or bilateral, **F-108,** 579
  enlargement, unilateral, **F-106,** 578–579
  lesions, **F-103 to F-106,** 576–579
  lymph node enlargement, **F-103,** 576–577
  lymphadenopathy, marked, **F-104,** 577
  shadow, unilateral small, **F-107,** 579
Hilum, mass-like pulmonary infiltrate or lesion radiating from, **F-40,** 528
Hip
  replacement, local complications of total, **D-222-S1,** 409
  secondary osteoarthritis of, **D-221,** 408
HIV infection, central nervous system complications of, **A-119,** 94
Hollow viscus, perforated, in infant, **G-238,** 734
Honeycomb lung, **F-22,** 512–513
Humeral head, grooved defect, erosion, or deformity of, **D-168,** 373
Humerus, erosion of medial aspect of proximal metaphyses of, **D-39,** 275
Hydrocephalus, **A-114-1, A-114-2, M-57, O-10,** 90–92, 891, 936
  atrophic, **A-114-1,** 90–91
  causes of communicating, **A-114-1, M-57,** 90–91, 891
  causes of obstructive, **A-114-1, M-57,** 90–91, 891
  congenital syndromes associated with, **A-114-2,** 91–92
  fetal ventriculomegaly, **O-10,** 936
  nonabsorptive, **A-114-1,** 90–91
  obstructive, **A-114-1, M-57,** 90–91, 891
Hydromyelia, causes of, **M-89-S,** 900
Hydronephrosis, **H-49,** 780
  obstruction of ureter with or without, **H-93,** 799–800
Hypercalcemia, **D-45-S,** 282–283
Hypercalcemic hypercalciuria, **H-25-S,** 768
Hypercalciuria, **D-45-S,** 282–283
Hyperdense liver lesions, focal, on CT, **G-182, G-183,** 708–709
Hyperechoic
  focus in gallbladder wall on ultrasound, **G-121,** 677
  liver lesions, focal, on ultrasound, **G-147,** 691
Hyperlucent segment, lobe, or lung, unilateral, **F-53,** 536–537
Hyperostosis, marked cortical, **D-99,** 323
Hyperparathyroidism, sites of subperiosteal resorption in primary, **D-41-S,** 277
Hyperphosphatemia, **D-45-S,** 282–283
Hypersensitivity pneumonitis, **F-69,** 544–545
Hypertelorism, **B-3-1,** 101–102

congenital syndromes with, **B-3-2,** 102–103
Hypertension, **E-37,** 471
  portal, **G-191,** 712–713
  pulmonary arterial, **E-54,** 481–482
  pulmonary venous, **E-59,** 484–485
  unilateral renal lesion that may cause, **H-59-1 to H-59-2,** 784–785
Hypertensive cardiovascular disease, **E-37,** 471
Hypertrophic osteoarthropathy, **D-98,** 322
Hypervascularity, **A-101,** 84
  generalized pulmonary arterial, **E-51,** 479–480
Hypocalcemia, **D-45-S,** 282–283
Hypocalciuria, **D-45-S,** 282–283
Hypodense
  liver lesions, focal, on CT, **G-180, G-181,** 707–708
  (low attenuation) lesion in brain stem on CT, **A-86,** 74
  mass, focal, in liver on nonenhanced CT scan, **G-180,** 707–708
Hypodontia, **B-64,** 144–145
Hypoechoic liver lesions, focal, on ultrasound, **G-174,** 705
Hypopharynx
  diseases common to tropics and developing countries, **J-1-S,** 851–855
  lesions of, **B-111,** 175–176
  retention of barium in, **G-1,** 611
Hypophosphatemia, **D-45-S,** 282–283
Hypoplasia
  of base of skull, **A-11,** 16
  of fibula, **D-179,** 379
  odontoid (dens), **C-8,** 195–196
  of radius or thumb, **D-161,** 368–369
Hypoplastic
  clavicle, **D-172-1,** 375
  pedicle, **C-40-1,** 211
  (spindle-shaped or stubby) terminal phalanges, **D-126,** 342–343
Hypospadias, congenital syndromes with, **H-166,** 828
Hypotelorism (decreased interorbital distance), **B-3-1,** 101–102
Hypovascularity
  generalized pulmonary arterial, **E-58,** 483–484
  pulmonary, **E-57,** 483

Ileocecal valve, enlargement of, **G-98,** 665
Iliac horns in infant or child, **D-193-4,** 391
Iliac veins, obstruction of inferior vena cava or, **E-71,** 490
ILO 1980 international classification of radiographs of pneumoconioses, **F-71-S,** 546–552
Immunocompromised patients, pulmonary disease in, **F-77,** 557
Indentation, extrinsic, on duodenum, **G-35,** 630
Indistinct
  epiphyses, **D-24,** 264–265
  metaphyses, **D-38,** 275
Infections of brain identifiable on CT or MRI, **A-93,** 78
Infectious
  lesion of bone, well-defined, often cyst-like, **D-66,** 300
  and parasitic diseases, tropical, geographic distribution of, **J-2-S,** 856–857
Inferior vena cava
  abnormal sign in, **M-152,** 924
  anomalies of, **E-72-S,** 491
  or iliac veins, obstruction of, **E-71,** 490

Neoplasm (*continued*)
  salivary gland, **B-91,** 163
Neoplasm-like lesions, **F-35-S,** 524
Neoplastic intracranial mass, **A-55-1,** 47
Nephrocalcinosis, **H-27,** 769–770
Nephrogram
  dense or prolonged, on IV urography, **H-14,** 762–763
  focal defect in, **H-13,** 762
Nephropathy, congenital syndromes with, **H-2,** 755–756
Nerve roots, on MRI, **M-104, M-105,** 904
Nerves, calcification in, **D-246-3,** 423
Neural arches
  abnormal, **C-43 to C-46-2,** 212–214
  posterior, defective or destroyed, **C-45-1, C-45-2,** 213–214
Neurogenic bladder, **H-98,** 802
Neurotrophic arthropathy, **D-223,** 410
Neurotrophic bone changes, **D-150,** 360–361
Nodular patterns in lungs, **F-21,** 511–512
Nonabsorptive hydrocephalus, **A-114-1,** 90–91
Nondiaphragmatic hernias, **G-64-S,** 645–646
Nonenhanced CT scan
  focal hypodense mass in liver on, **G-180,** 707–708
  increased density within basilar cisterns on, **A-90-1,** 76
Nonepithelial tumor, **G-84-S,** 657
Noneruption, of teeth, **B-61-1, B-61-2,** 141–142
Nonneoplastic intracranial mass, **A-55-2,** 47–48
Nonneoplastic (tumor-like) lesions of bone, **G-84-S,** 657
Nonodontogenic radiolucent lesions, **B-71,** 148–149
Nonspinal conditions, associated with vertebral anomalies, **C-2-S,** 189
Nonvisualization, of gallbladder, **G-108,** 670–671
Normal skull variants, **A-35-S1,** 31
  simulating a fracture, **A-35-S2,** 31–32
Notching on urinary tract, **H-90,** 798

Obstetrical ultrasound, common indications for, **O-1-S,** 933
Obstruction
  at fourth ventricle outlet, **A-84,** 73
  intestinal (see Intestinal obstruction), **G-66 to G-78,** 646–654
  gastric outlet, **G-30,** 627–628
  upper airway, in a child, acute or chronic, **B-123,** 181
Obstructive hydrocephalus, **A-114-1,** 90–91
Occiput
  flat, in infants, **A-6,** 14
  prominent, in infants, **A-7,** 14
Odontogenic radiolucent lesions of jaws, **B-71,** 148–149
Odontoid (dens) absence, hypoplasia, or fragmentation, **C-8,** 195–196
Oesophagus (see Esophagus)
Ogilvie syndrome, **G-79,** 654–655
Oligohydramnios on sonography, **O-26,** 941–942
Oligosaccharidoses, **J-4-S,** 858
Omega sella, **A-25-3,** 26
Opacification
  complete, of one hemithorax, **F-122,** 588
  early venous, renal angiography, **H-62,** 786
  of nasal cavity, **B-37,** 124–125
  of one or more paranasal sinuses, **B-51,** 133–134
Opportunistic
  organisms, **F-75-S,** 556

pulmonary infection, conditions that predispose to, **F-76-S,** 556–557
Optic canal
  enlargement, **B-13,** 109–110
  localized bony defect or erosion about, **B-12,** 109
  small, **B-4,** 103
Optic nerve
  distinct, with perineural enhancement on CT, **B-15,** 111
  enlargement on CT or MRI, **B-14,** 110–111
  lesions, **M-115,** 908
  sheath lesions, **M-115,** 908
  "tram-track" sign (distinct optic nerve with perineural enhancement on CT), **B-15,** 111
Orbital
  lesions, **B-6-1 to B-8, M-114 to M-121,** 104–108, 907–910
  masses in children, CT characteristics of, **B-7-S,** 107
  roof or walls, sclerosis and thickening of, **B-9,** 108
  (sphenoidal) fissure, **B-10, B-11,** 108, 109
    enlarged superior, **B-11,** 109
    narrowed superior, **B-10,** 108
  wall lesions, **M-121,** 910
Orbits, **B-1 to B-23,** 101–117
  bony defect, erosion, or radiolucent lesion of, **B-8,** 107–108
  large, **B-5,** 103–104
  lesions involving, **B-6-1 to B-6-6,** 104–106
  malformation of, **B-1,** 101
  small, **B-4,** 103
Organic dust disease, **F-69,** 544–545
Oropharynx, lesions of, **B-106,** 173–174
Osseous lesions, preferential site within bone of various, **D-57-1 to D-57-4,** 292–293
Ossification
  centers, epiphyseal (see Epiphyseal ossification centers) **D-19-1, D-19-2,** 259–260
  cranial, delayed or defective, **A-37,** 32–33
  incomplete, of sutures, **A-40,** 34–35
  pubic, congenital syndromes with delayed or defective, **D-195,** 392–393
  soft tissue, **D-244,** 420
  soft tissue tumor with associated, **D-261,** 432–433
Osteoarthritis
  of hip, secondary, **D-221,** 408
  premature, **D-220,** 407–408
Osteoarthropathy, hypertrophic, **D-98,** 322
Osteoblastic metastases, **D-85,** 315
Osteolysis, **D-76,** 306
  generalized, of jaws, **B-69,** 147–148
Osteolytic
  lesion, moth eaten or permeative, **D-71,** 303
  lesion, solitary skull, **A-23-1,** 23–24
  metastases, **D-86,** 315–316
Osteomalacia, **D-44, D-44-S,** 280–282
  bone and soft tissue neoplasms associated with, **D-44-S,** 282
Osteopenia, **B-69, C-36,** 147–148, 209
  generalized, of jaws, **B-69,** 147–148
  spinal (loss of density), **C-36,** 209
Osteoporosis, **D-42 to D-43-2, D-228, D-229,** 277–280, 413, 414
  arthritis with little or no, **D-229,** 414
  arthritis with some, **D-228,** 413
  generalized, **D-43-1 to D-43-2,** 278–280

ISBN 0-387-95588-7